OPERATIVE HAND SURGERY

SECOND EDITION

Volume 2

OPERATIVE HAND SURGERY

SECOND EDITION

Edited by

DAVID P. GREEN, M.D.

Clinical Professor
Department of Orthopaedics
Former Chief, Hand Surgery Service
University of Texas Health Science Center
    at San Antonio
San Antonio, Texas

CHURCHILL LIVINGSTONE
New York, Edinburgh, London, Melbourne   1988

Library of Congress Cataloging-in-Publication Data

Operative hand surgery.

  Includes bibliographies and index.
  1. Hand—Surgery. I. Green, David P.
[DNLM: 1. Hand—surgery. WE 830 O61]
RD559.O63 1988   617'.575059   87-22409
ISBN 0-443-08481-5 (v. 1)

Second Edition © Churchill Livingstone Inc. 1988
First Edition © Churchill Livingstone Inc. 1982

Distributed in the United Kingdom by Churchill Livingstone, Robert Stevenson House, 1-3 Baxter's Place, Leith Walk, Edinburgh EH1 3AF, and by associated companies, branches, and representatives throughout the world.

Accurate indications, adverse reactions, and dosage schedules for drugs are provided in this book, but it is possible that they may change. The reader is urged to review the package information data of the manufacturers of the medications mentioned.

Acquisitions Editor: *Toni M. Tracy*
Copy Editor: *Leslie Burgess*
Production Designers: *Rosalie Marcus and Charlie Lebeda*
Production Supervisor: *Sharon Tuder*

Printed in the United States of America

First published in 1988

Dedicated to my father,

J. Leighton Green, M.D.
(1899–1986)

A physician and surgeon worthy of emulation

Contributors

Jerome E. Adamson, M.D.
Professor of Plastic Surgery, Department of Surgery, Eastern Virginia Medical School; Chief, Hand Service, Eastern Virginia Medical School and Affiliated Hospitals, Norfolk, Virginia

Bernard S. Alpert, M.D.
Assistant Clinical Professor, Division of Plastic, Reconstructive, and Hand Surgery, Department of Surgery, University of California, San Francisco, School of Medicine, San Francisco, California

Alexander C. Angelides, M.D.
Attending Hand Surgeon, Department of Orthopedics, Palmetto Hospital and Hialeah Hospital, Hialeah, Florida

Loui G. Bayne, M.D.
Clinical Associate Professor of Orthopaedic Surgery, Department of Orthopaedics, Emory University School of Medicine; Director, Hand Clinic, Scottish Rite Children's Hospital, Atlanta, Georgia

Robert D. Beckenbaugh, M.D.
Associate Professor of Orthopedic Surgery, Department of Orthopedics, Mayo Medical School, Mayo Foundation; Consultant in Orthopedic Surgery and Surgery of the Hand, Mayo Clinic, Rochester, Minnesota

William H. Bowers, M.D., M.S.
Private Practice of Hand Surgery, Hand Center of Greensboro; Attending Surgeon, Hand Service, Moses H. Cone Hospital and Wesley Long Hospital, Greensboro, North Carolina

Richard M. Braun, M.D.
Associate Clinical Professor of Orthopedic Surgery, Department of Surgery, University of California, San Diego, School of Medicine, La Jolla, California; Instructor in Surgery (Orthopedics) and Consultant in Upper Limb Rehabilitation, Rancho Los Amigos–University of Southern California Medical Center, Downey, California; Director of Upper Extremity Rehabilitation, Donald N. Sharp Memorial Community Hospital Rehabilitation Center, San Diego, California

Paul W. Brown. M.D.
Clinical Professor of Orthopedic Surgery and Plastic and Reconstructive Surgery, Department of Surgery, Yale University School of Medicine, New Haven, Connecticut

Earl Z. Browne, Jr., M.D.
Chairman, Department of Plastic and Reconstructive Surgery, The Cleveland Clinic Foundation, Cleveland, Ohio

William E. Burkhalter, M.D.
Professor of Orthopaedics and Chief, Division of Hand Surgery, Department of Orthopaedics and Rehabilitation, University of Miami School of Medicine, Miami, Florida

Richard I. Burton, M.D.
Professor of Orthopaedics and Co-Director, Hand Service, Department of Orthopaedics, The University of Rochester Medical Center, Rochester, New York

Robert E. Carroll, M.D.
Professor Emeritus, Department of Orthopedic Surgery, Columbia University College of Physicians and Surgeons; Consultant in Orthopedic (Hand) Surgery, Columbia-Presbyterian Medical Center, New York, New York

Harold M. Dick, M.D.
Frank E. Stinchfield Professor and Chairman, Department of Orthopedic Surgery, Columbia University College of Physicians and Surgeons; Director of Orthopedic Surgery, Columbia-Presbyterian Medical Center, New York, New York

George Peter Dingeldein, M.D.
Private Practice of Plastic and Reconstructive Surgery, Texarkana, Texas

James H. Dobyns, M.D.
Professor of Orthopedic Surgery, Department of Orthopedics, Mayo Medical School, Mayo Foundation; Consultant in Orthopedics and Surgery of the Hand, Mayo Clinic, Rochester, Minnesota

James R. Doyle, M.D.
Associate Professor, Department of Surgery and Chairman, Division of Orthopedic Surgery, University of Hawaii John A. Burns School of Medicine, Honolulu, Hawaii

Gregory J. Dray, M.D.
Attending Hand Surgeon, Memorial Mission Hospital and St. Joseph's Hospital, Asheville, North Carolina

Richard G. Eaton, M.D.
Associate Professor, Department of Surgery, Columbia University College of Physicians and Surgeons, New York, New York

William W. Eversmann, Jr., M.D.
Private Practice of Hand Surgery, Iowa Musculoskeletal Center, Cedar Rapids, Iowa

Paul G. Feldon, M.D.
Assistant Clinical Professor, Department of Orthopedic Surgery, Tufts University School of Medicine; Chief, Hand Surgery Service, St. Elizabeth's Hospital, Boston, Massachusetts

Donald C. Ferlic, M.D.
Assistant Clinical Professor of Orthopedic Surgery, Department of Orthopedics, University of Colorado Health Sciences Center School of Medicine, Denver, Colorado

Michael O. Fidler, M.D.
Clinical Assistant Professor, Department of Orthopedic Surgery, West Virginia University School of Medicine; Practicing Surgeon, Department of Orthopedics, Charleston Area Medical Center, Charleston, West Virginia

Earl J. Fleegler, M.D.
Assistant Clinical Professor of Plastic Surgery, Department of Surgery, Case Western Reserve University School of Medicine; Head, Section of Hand Surgery, Department of Plastic and Reconstructive Surgery, The Cleveland Clinic Foundation, Cleveland, Ohio

Albert F. Fleury, Jr., M.D.
Clinical Instructor of Surgery, Division of Plastic and Reconstructive Surgery, Department of Surgery, Georgetown University School of Medicine, Washington, D.C.

Waldo E. Floyd III, M.D.
Assistant Professor (Orthopaedics), Department of Surgery, Mercer University School of Medicine; Director of Hand Clinic, Medical Center of Central Georgia, Macon, Georgia

Guy Foucher, M.D.
Head of Emergency Hand Unit, S.O.S. Main, Strasbourg, France

Avrum I. Froimson, M.D.
Clinical Professor of Orthopedic Surgery, Department of Orthopedics, Case Western Reserve University School of Medicine; Director, Department of Orthopedic Surgery, The Mount Sinai Hospital, Cleveland, Ohio

David P. Green, M.D.
Clinical Professor, Department of Orthopaedics and Former Chief, Hand Surgery Service, University of Texas Health Science Center at San Antonio, San Antonio, Texas

James H. Herndon, M.D.
Professor and Chairman, Department of Orthopaedics, Brown University Program in Medicine; Surgeon-in-Chief, Department of Orthopaedics and Rehabilitation, Rhode Island Hospital, Providence, Rhode Island

Norman A. Hill, M.D.
Professor of Clinical Orthopedic Surgery, Department of Orthopedic Surgery, New York Medical College, Valhalla, New York; Attending Orthopedic Surgeon, St. Luke's–Roosevelt Hospital Center, New York, New York

M. Mark Hoffer, M.D.
Professor and Chief, Division of Orthopedics, Department of Surgery, University of California, Irvine, California College of Medicine, UCI Medical Center, Orange, California; Chief, Department of Children's Orthopedics, Rancho Los Amigos Medical Center, Downey, California

James H. House, M.D.
Professor of Orthopaedic Surgery and Director of Hand Surgery, Department of Orthopaedic Surgery, University of Minnesota Health Sciences Center, Minneapolis, Minnesota

James M. Hunter, M.D.
Professor, Department of Orthopaedic Surgery, Jefferson Medical College of Thomas Jefferson University, Philadelphia, Pennsylvania

L. Lee Lankford, M.D.
Clinical Professor, Division of Orthopedic Surgery, Department of Surgery, University of Texas Health Science Center at Dallas Southwestern Medical School; Member, Teaching Staff, Department of Orthopedics, Baylor University Medical Center; Founding Director, Parkland Memorial Hospital Hand Service, Dallas, Texas

Joseph P. Leddy, M.D.
Clinical Associate Professor and Chief, Section of Hand Surgery, Division of Orthopedic Surgery, Department of Surgery, University of Medicine and Dentistry of New Jersey Robert Wood Johnson Medical School, New Brunswick, New Jersey

Robert D. Leffert, M.D.
Associate Professor, Department of Orthopedic Surgery, Harvard Medical School; Chief, Surgical Upper Extremity Rehabilitation Unit and Department of Rehabilitation Medicine, Massachusetts General Hospital, Boston, Massachusetts

Ronald L. Linscheid, M.D.
Professor of Orthopedic Surgery, Department of Orthopedics, Mayo Medical School, Mayo Foundation; Consultant in Orthopedic Surgery and Surgery of the Hand, Mayo Clinic, Rochester, Minnesota

Graham Lister, M.B., Ch.B.
Professor, Department of Surgery, University of Utah School of Medicine; Chief, Division of Plastic Surgery, University of Utah Medical Center, Salt Lake City, Utah

Dean S. Louis, M.D., B.S.
Professor, Department of Surgery and Chief of Hand Surgery, Section of Orthopedics, University of Michigan Medical School, Ann Arbor, Michigan

Ralph T. Manktelow, M.D., F.R.C.S.(C)
Associate Professor, Department of Surgery and Chairman, Division of Plastic Surgery, Department of Surgery, University of Toronto Faculty of Medicine; Head, Division of Plastic Surgery, Toronto General Hospital, Toronto, Ontario, Canada

Stephen J. Mathes, M.D.
Professor of Surgery and Head, Division of Plastic, Reconstructive, and Hand Surgery, Department of Surgery, University of California, San Francisco, School of Medicine, San Francisco, California

James W. May, Jr., M.D.
Associate Clinical Professor, Department of Surgery, Harvard Medical School; Chief of Hand Surgery, Division of Plastic and Reconstructive Surgery, Department of General Surgery, Massachusetts General Hospital, Boston, Massachusetts

Charles L. McDowell, M.D.
Clinical Professor, Division of Orthopedic Surgery, Department of Surgery, Medical College of Virginia, Virginia Commonwealth University School of Medicine; Chief, Division of Hand Surgery, Children's Medical Center; Chief, Upper Extremity Surgery, Spinal Cord Injury Unit, McGuire Veterans Administration Medical Center, Richmond, Virginia

Gordon B. McFarland, Jr., M.D.
Head, Hand Surgery Division, Oschner Clinic, New Orleans, Louisiana

Robert M. McFarlane, M.D., M.Sc., F.R.C.S.(C), F.A.C.S.
Professor, Department of Surgery, University of Western Ontario Faculty of Medicine; Chief, Division of Plastic Surgery, University of Western Ontario and Victoria Hospital, London, Ontario, Canada

Lewis H. Millender, M.D.
Clinical Professor, Department of Orthopedic Surgery, Tufts University School of Medicine; Assistant Chief of Hand Surgery Service, New England Baptist Hospital, Boston, Massachusetts

J. Russell Moore, M.D.
Associate Professor, Department of Orthopedic Surgery, Johns Hopkins University School of Medicine, Baltimore, Maryland

Edward A. Nalebuff, M.D.
Clinical Professor, Department of Orthopedic Surgery, Tufts University School of Medicine; Chief, Hand Surgery Service, New England Baptist Hospital, Boston, Massachusetts

Robert J. Neviaser, M.D.
Professor, Department of Orthopaedic Surgery, George Washington University School of Medicine and Health Sciences; Director, Hand and Upper Extremity Division, George Washington University Medical Center, Washington, D.C.

William L. Newmeyer, M.D.
Associate Clinical Professor, Department of Surgery, University of California, San Francisco, School of Medicine, San Francisco, California

Eugene T. O'Brien, M.D.
Clinical Professor of Surgery, Department of Orthopaedics, University of Texas Health Science Center at San Antonio, San Antonio, Texas

George E. Omer, Jr., M.D., M.S., F.A.C.S.
Professor of Orthopaedics and Chairman, Department of Orthopaedics and Rehabilitation; Professor of Surgery and Chief, Division of Hand Surgery, Department of Surgery; and Professor, Department of Anatomy, University of New Mexico School of Medicine Medical Center, Albuquerque, New Mexico

Andrew K. Palmer, M.D.
Professor, Department of Orthopedic Surgery, State University of New York Health Science Center at Syracuse College of Medicine, Syracuse, New York

Somayaji Ramamurthy, M.D.
Professor, Department of Anesthesiology, University of Texas Health Science Center at San Antonio, San Antonio, Texas

Rodney J. Rohrich, M.D.
Instructor, Department of Surgery, Harvard Medical School; Hand Micro-Fellow, Division of Plastic and Reconstructive Surgery, Department of General Surgery, Massachusetts General Hospital, Boston, Massachusetts

Spencer A. Rowland, M.D.
Clinical Professor of Surgery, Department of Orthopaedics, University of Texas Health Science Center at San Antonio, San Antonio, Texas

Roger E. Salisbury, M.D.
Professor of Surgery and Chief, Division of Plastic and Reconstructive Surgery, Department of Surgery, New York Medical College; Director, Burn Center, Westchester County Medical Center, Valhalla, New York

William E. Sanders, M.D.
Clinical Associate Professor, Department of Orthopaedics, University of Texas Health Science Center at San Antonio, San Antonio, Texas

Lawrence H. Schneider, M.D.
Clinical Professor, Department of Orthopaedic Surgery, Jefferson Medical College of Thomas Jefferson University, Philadelphia, Pennsylvania

Richard J. Smith, M.D.
Clinical Professor, Department of Orthopedic Surgery, Harvard Medical School; Chief of Hand Surgery, Department of Orthopedics, Massachusetts General Hospital, Boston, Massachusetts

James W. Strickland, M.D.
Associate Professor, Department of Orthopaedic Surgery and Chief, Hand Surgery Rotation, Indiana University School of Medicine; Chief, Hand Surgery Section, St. Vincent Hospital and Health Care Center, Indianapolis, Indiana

Julio Taleisnik, M.D.
Clinical Professor of Orthopaedic Surgery, Department of Surgery, University of California, Irvine, California College of Medicine, Irvine, California

Kenya Tsuge, M.D.
Emeritus Professor, Department of Orthopaedic Surgery, Hiroshima University School of Medicine; Director, Hiroshima Prefectural Rehabilitation Center, Higashi-Hiroshima, Japan

Steven H. Turkeltaub, M.D.
Assistant Professor, Division of Plastic Surgery, Department of Surgery, University of Massachusetts Medical Center, Worcester, Massachusetts

James R. Urbaniak, M.D.
Professor and Chief, Division of Orthopaedic Surgery, Department of Surgery, Duke University Medical Center, Durham, North Carolina

Michael I. Vender, M.D.
Attending Hand and Orthopaedic Surgeon, Edward Hospital, Naperville, Illinois; Good Samaritan Hospital, Downers Grove, Illinois; and Hinsdale Hospital, Hinsdale, Illinois

H. Kirk Watson, M.D.
Associate Clinical Professor of Orthopaedic Surgery, Department of Orthopaedics, University of Connecticut School of Medicine, Farmington, Connecticut; Associate Professor, Departments of Orthopedics and Surgery, University of Massachusetts Medical Center Worcester, Massachusetts; Assistant Clinical Professor, Division of Plastic Surgery, Department of Surgery and Department of Orthopedics and Rehabilitation, Yale University School of Medicine, Yale-New Haven Hospital, New Haven, Connecticut; Chief, Connecticut Combined Hand Service, Hartford, Connecticut; Chief, Hand Service, Newington Children's Hospital, Newington, Connecticut; Senior Staff, Department of Orthopaedics, Hartford Hospital, Hartford, Connecticut

Andrew J. Weiland, M.D.
Professor of Orthopedic Surgery; Professor of Plastic Surgery; and Professor of Emergency Medicine; Johns Hopkins University School of Medicine, Baltimore, Maryland

E. F. Shaw Wilgis, M.D.
Associate Professor of Orthopedic Surgery and Plastic Surgery, Department of Surgery, Johns Hopkins University School of Medicine; Chief, Division of Hand Surgery, Union Memorial Hospital, Baltimore, Maryland

Virchel E. Wood, M.D.
Professor, Department of Orthopedic Surgery, Loma Linda University School of Medicine; Chief, Hand Surgery Service, Loma Linda University Medical Center, Loma Linda, California

Elvin G. Zook, M.D.
Professor of Surgery and Chairman, Division of Plastic and Reconstructive Surgery, Department of Surgery, Southern Illinois University School of Medicine, Springfield, Illinois

Preface to the Second Edition

The enthusiastic response to the publication of *Operative Hand Surgery* in 1982 has indeed been gratifying. I have been particularly pleased with the widespread acceptance of this book not only in the United States, but also in many other countries throughout the world. However, no book is ever as good as it might be, and certainly there is always room for improvement. We have therefore worked very hard to try to make this a better book.

Eight entirely new chapters have been added, four of which pertain to the remarkable advances that have been made in microvascular surgery. Chapters dealing with fractures of the distal radius, intercarpal arthrodesis, the rheumatoid elbow, and a more comprehensive approach to the patient with a malignant lesion in the upper extremity have been added as well.

Many of the existing chapters were extensively revised to eliminate obsolete or outmoded operations and concepts and to add new procedures. Several hundred new illustrations have been added to supplement new text material.

Operative Hand Surgery now contains some 9,025 bibliographic citations. In a continuing effort to make the references readily accessible to the reader who wishes to pursue more comprehensive study, my wife Marge has in the preparation of these two editions painstakingly looked up the original sources to verify the accuracy of more than 6,000 of these references.

Editing the two editions of this book has been a great learning experience for me, and I hope that using it will be equally worthwhile for the reader.

David P. Green, M.D.

Preface to the First Edition

Considering the recent flood of new books that has inundated the medical world, one might justifiably ask, "Why yet *another* book on hand surgery?" It is true that there are already a number of books on hand surgery, many of them quite good. In my opinion, however, a comprehensive book dedicated primarily to operative techniques in hand surgery, combined with an extensive bibliography, is not available. The goal of this book has thus been to compile this type of single comprehensive reference work for the reader.

It is hoped that this book will prove useful to all serious students of hand surgery, ranging from residents to experienced practitioners. The breadth of hand surgery has expanded so widely during the past 35 years that few hand surgeons can hope to remain expert in all phases of what was once a relatively narrow surgical subspeciality. It is for this reason that this book was produced in a multi-author format. Prior to writing his chapter, each author had already established his credentials and expertise in the area about which he was selected to write.

The major emphasis in this book is on operative technique, but possessing the technical skill to perform an operation is obviously not an indication to do that operation. Surgical judgment cannot be learned entirely from a book, but an effort has been made here to put each operative procedure into proper perspective. There are often many different ways to manage a given clinical situation, and selecting the most appropriate method for a specific problem in an individual patient frequently poses a perplexing dilemma for the surgeon. For this reason, each author has been encouraged to describe a variety of well-accepted techniques, indicating which of these he prefers, and why.

The general format and organization of the book will be more apparent to the reader if he or she takes a few moments to scan the Contents page. In addition, the running heads at the top of each page contain the title, author, and number of each chapter to aid the reader in locating a specific topic.

Finally, we must all keep in mind that concepts, operations, and even our knowledge of anatomy change, and no written word should be considered inviolate. I am frequently reminded of an admonition that one of my former teachers, Harrison McLaughlin, inscribed in his classic book on trauma: "To the New York Orthopaedic residents: Don't believe everything you read."

David P. Green, M.D.

Acknowledgements

I would like to express my deep appreciation and gratitude to the many people responsible for the completion of the second edition of *Operative Hand Surgery*. Among these are:

First and foremost, the contributors, who have again invested enormous amounts of time and energy in this project. A special word of thanks and a fond remembrance is due Richard J. Smith, who unselfishly spent some of the last days of his life to leave with us his unique understanding of malignant tumors of the upper extremity.

My wife, Marge, who has again been of immeasurable assistance in the preparation of references, as noted in the Preface to the second edition. Far beyond that, though, her support of my writing habit has exceeded mere tolerance, and it has been her active encouragement of these time-consuming endeavors that has enabled me to do what I enjoy.

The very talented Elizabeth Roselius, known in the first edition as Betty Montgomery, who has prepared 131 new drawings with her usual precision and clarity. A highly intelligent mind, truly gifted artistic skills, and the patience and perseverance to "get it right" combine to make her the consummate medical illustrator.

Toni M. Tracy, the President of Churchill Livingstone, whose integrity and efficiency have made her a pleasure to work with.

Leslie Burgess, whose careful attention to detail as copy editor has been critical to the quality of the finished book.

All of my professional colleagues who took the time to write or call me about errors in the first edition and to offer constructive criticism. Morton Spinner and Jimmy Adams were particularly helpful in this regard.

Suzanne Taubert, my highly skilled medical transcriptionist, who not only prepares meticulously precise manuscripts, but who has also maintained the lines of communication among authors, publisher, and editor in the preparation of this book.

The orthopaedic residents and other students with whom I work, by whom I continue to be taught.

David P. Green, M.D.

Contents

Volume 1

Volume 3

Fractures of the Carpal Bones

19

Julio Taleisnik

FRACTURES OF THE SCAPHOID

Among all wrist injuries the incidence of fractures of the scaphoid is second only to fractures of the distal radius.[21–23,28,31,49,200–202] Fractures of the scaphoid most frequently occur in the young adult male and usually involve the waist of the scaphoid. It is a rare injury in children, in whom the most common fracture is that of the distal third.[69] The traumatic episode, usually a fall on the dorsiflexed wrist, may be minimal, and the injury initially dismissed as "just a sprain," except for the persistence of the symptoms, pain and swelling, in the anatomic snuffbox area.

Diagnosis

Although the diagnosis of a fracture of the scaphoid is suggested by the patient's age, the mechanism of injury, and the presenting sign and symptoms, it is confirmed only by radiographic examination. Furthermore, in the presence of tenderness over the anatomic snuffbox without deformity, a fracture of the scaphoid should always be presumed until radiographic examination proves negative beyond doubt.[239] As many as 16 views have been proposed for an exhaustive study of the injured wrist,[101] but only 4 must be included in the initial routine examination: one posteroanterior, one lateral, and two oblique projections. For the posteroanterior study, it is best to place the hand with the fingers flexed into a fist[45,173,186,192,209] (Fig. 19-1A and B). This produces slight dorsiflexion and ulnar deviation and places the longitudinal axis of the scaphoid in a plane more closely parallel with that of the film. The addition of ulnar deviation (Fig. 19-2) may improve visualization of the fracture.[109,148,192,202] The lateral projection is helpful for the evaluation of carpal alignment and the determination of a possible carpal instability problem (Figs. 19-3 and 19-4). If initial studies are negative, it has been recommended that the wrist be immobilized in a splint and repeat radiographs be taken in 2 to 3 weeks.[9,31,37,38,113,148,186,199,201,202,226] Resorption may assist identification by widening the fracture line, making its detection possible at that time. However, other diagnostic tests may make this initial immobilization unnecessary. Terry and Ramin[221] have called attention to a small radiolucent area normally present next to the scaphoid in anteroposterior radiographs, which they named the *navicular fat stripe*. A fracture on the radial side of the wrist can either displace or obliterate this line. A preserved fat stripe is a strong indication that a fracture has not occurred (Fig. 19-5). This

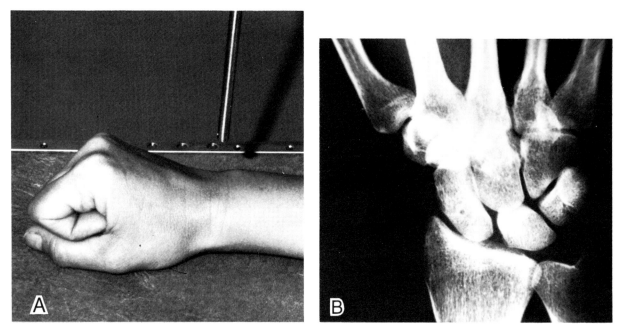

Fig. 19-1. (A) Positioning for a posteroanterior radiograph, obtained with the fingers flexed into a fist. (B) Slight dorsiflexion is produced, placing the longitudinal axis of the scaphoid in a plane more nearly parallel to that of the film.

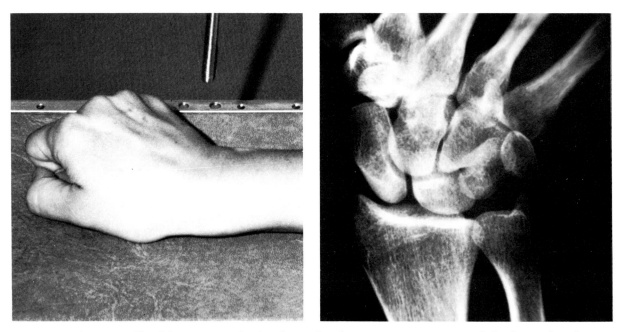

Fig. 19-2. A better profile of the entire scaphoid is obtained in the posteroanterior view with the fingers flexed into a fist and the wrist in ulnar deviation.

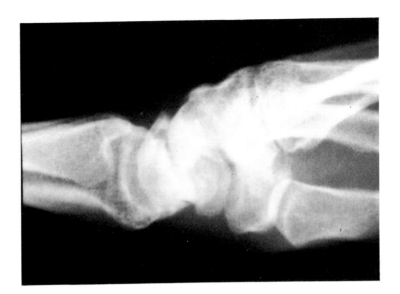

Fig. 19-3. Severe dorsal carpal instability (DISI) following a fracture of the scaphoid.

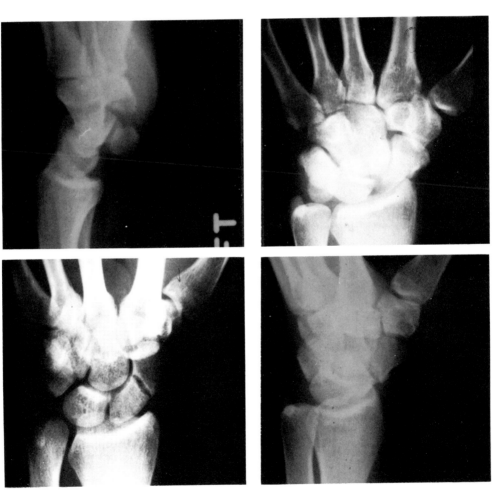

Fig. 19-4. Less frequent volar carpal instability (VISI) following a displaced fracture of the middle third of the scaphoid.

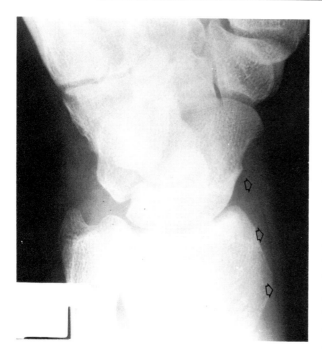

Fig. 19-5. Scaphoid ("navicular") fat stripe *(arrows),* seen in an oblique projection. (Taleisnik J: The Wrist. Churchill Livingstone, New York, 1985.)

sign is valuable only in fresh injuries, for the fat stripe may reappear as early as 5 days following a fracture. Carver and Barrington[43] suggested that soft-tissue swelling on the dorsum of the wrist would appear to be a more reliable radiologic sign than the displacement of the fat stripe. Other diagnostic techniques proposed for difficult to diagnose injuries include isotope scanning,[122] laminograms, and trispiral tomography[50] (Fig. 19-6). A negative isotope scan excludes the fracture. Increased focal activity soon after trauma, although not specific for fracture, suggests scaphoid injury, even if radiographs fail to demonstrate a fracture.[122,169,212] Therefore, when a strong clinical suspicion of fracture of the scaphoid exists with initial radiographs negative and the scaphoid fat stripe sign clearly positive, immobilization in a short arm thumb spica cast is justified, with repeat radiographs 2 to 3 weeks later. If the fat stripe sign is not conclusive, a negative isotope scanning obtained within 2 weeks of the injury should exclude a fracture. If the scan is positive, even with negative radiographs, an admittedly rare occurrence, a fracture must be strongly suspected, and the wrist immobilized for 2 to 3 weeks. Radiographs must then be repeated to confirm the diagnosis.[212]

Mechanism of Injury

Fractures of the scaphoid have been explained as bone failures caused by compressive or tension loads.[193] Todd[224] called the fracture a "snapped waist" fracture, similar to the response of a sugar lump subjected to a tension load. Cobey and White[48] suggested that the scaphoid actually breaks because of compression rather than tension loads; the compression is exerted against its concave surface by the head of the capitate. Radial or ulnar deviation was thought to determine whether the scaphoid would break at its waist, or proximal or distal to it.[61] Also, the degree of wrist dorsiflexion at impact was shown experimentally to be an important factor in localizing the fracture to the forearm, the distal radius, or the carpus. Frykman[87] subjected cadaver wrists to static loading and observed that greater dorsiflexion of the wrist resulted in more distal fractures, which required larger loads to develop. Thus, dorsiflexion of 35 degrees or less resulted in fractures of the forearm. With dorsiflexion of 90 degrees or more, injury occurred to the carpal bones. Fractures of the scaphoid were produced consistently after radial deviation was added. An additional factor is the point of application of the floor reaction force at impact.[60,217] This was confirmed by Weber and Chao on fresh cadaver specimens.[241] These authors demonstrated that for a fracture of the scaphoid to be consistently reproduced under experimental conditions, the load applied to the hand had to be concentrated on the radial half of the palm, with the wrist in 95 to 100 degrees dorsiflexion. While the proximal half of the scaphoid was stabilized between the radius, capitate, and volar capsular ligaments, bending loads were applied to the distal half, causing the fracture to occur between the supported and unsupported zones (Fig. 19-7). Torsion or rotation has also been considered important in producing this fracture.[81–83,93]

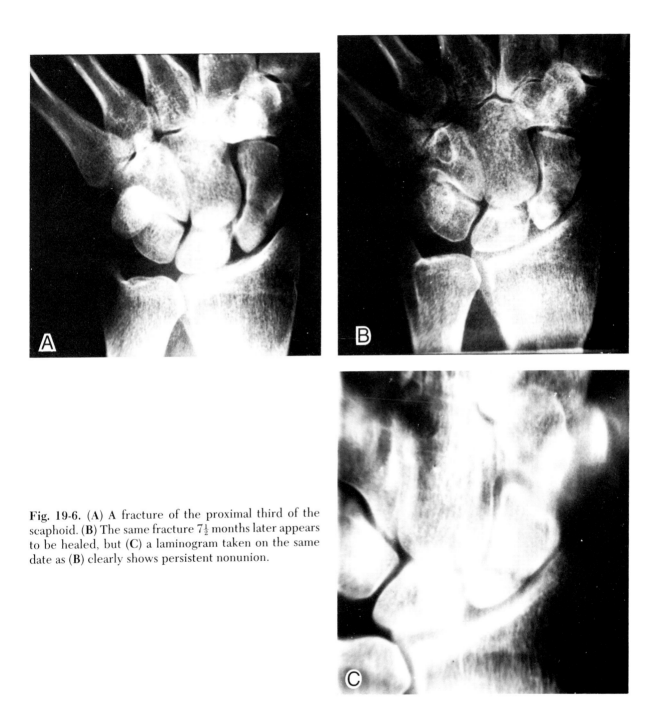

Fig. 19-6. (**A**) A fracture of the proximal third of the scaphoid. (**B**) The same fracture $7\frac{1}{2}$ months later appears to be healed, but (**C**) a laminogram taken on the same date as (**B**) clearly shows persistent nonunion.

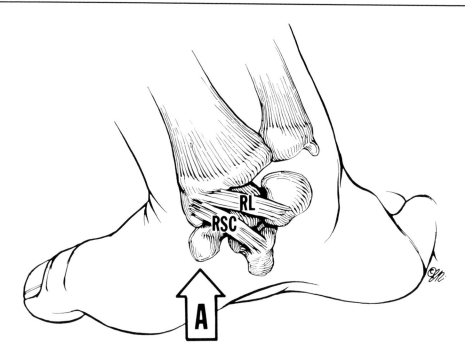

Fig. 19-7. Mechanism of fracture of the scaphoid according to Weber and Chao. Force applied to the radial half of the palm *(arrow A)* with the wrist in 95 to 100 degrees of dorsiflexion, produces bending loads to the unprotected distal half of the scaphoid. The proximal half is protected between the radius and the palmar radiocarpal ligaments (*RL*, radiolunate ligament; *RSC*, radioscaphocapitate ligament). (Taleisnik J: The Wrist. Churchill Livingstone, New York, 1985. © 1985, Elizabeth Roselius.)

Treatment

CONTROVERSIES REGARDING IMMOBILIZATION

Historically, there have been three main areas of disagreement in treating acute or fresh fractures of the scaphoid: (1) the position of the wrist in plaster, (2) the need to include joints other than the wrist in the cast, and (3) the duration of immobilization. A review of the literature regarding the first issue shows that there is enough lack of uniformity to suggest that immobilization itself is important, rather than the position in which the wrist is placed.[31] Actually, both the effectiveness of immobilization and the position of the wrist are meaningful. For treatment to be successful, immobilization must remain effective throughout its entire duration. If plaster immobilization is chosen, the cast must be changed frequently to remain effective. Otherwise, the newer, resined fiberglass materials are preferred, for these tend to remain snug longer.[9] It is important to allow the hand to function, for this seems to enhance the healing potential and reduce atrophy. The position of the wrist itself

should be such that radiographs taken after the cast is applied will show an anatomic coaptation of the fragments and a normal alignment of the carpus.

The second point of contention is the immobilization of joints other than the wrist. I always include the thumb, in a position of opposition, because the scaphoid is functionally related to the most radial of the digital rays. This effectively eliminates any potential disruptive action, particularly from the abductor pollicis longus[211] and brevis.[198,199] The inclusion of the elbow in the scaphoid cast was first suggested by Grace in 1929,[99] and again by Verdan in 1954.[232] Verdan placed great emphasis on eliminating the action of the volar radiocarpal ligament on the scaphoid during pronation and supination,[233] despite Stewart's report[211] (also in 1954) of 436 fractures treated in the US Army Medical Corps in a short arm thumb spica cast with a union rate approaching 95 percent. Against Stewart's experience is evidence presented by Broomé et al,[33] who reported that the results of comparable series treated with and without elbow immobilization showed a statistically significant reduction in the time needed for fracture healing when long arm plaster was utilized. King and co-authors[129] strongly support the use of a long arm plaster cast with the forearm in supination. Inclusion of the elbow in plaster has not been a problem in my experience, and removes an element of uncertainty from the treatment program. As the different types of fractures are discussed, it will be seen that in some the elbow may be left free, while others require above-elbow immobilization. In addition, when there is a strenuous objection from the patient, or a contraindication to elbow immobilization, an epicondylar bearing cast may be applied, thus restricting pronation-supination while allowing some flexion-extension of the elbow.[152] Immobilization of the fingers, either in a fist cast[179] or in the less objectionable three digit cast,[58] may be required for the potentially unstable scaphoid fractures in good alignment, and for the postoperative care of the unstable nonunion during the initial or vascular period of fracture healing. However, recent clinical and experimental data[129] based on Squire's concepts of carpal mechanics[204] support immobilization of even the "problem" fractures of the scaphoid (involving the proximal pole, displaced, or ununited) with the wrist in full ulnar deviation, some dorsiflexion, and the forearm supinated. I have no experience using this immobilization technique. Recovery of motion in all uninvolved joints is very prompt following removal of the cast, and even wrist motion can return to near normal in 1 to 5 weeks.[28,69,211]

The duration of immobilization was rather brief in early reports.[60,142] As experience accumulated, it became clear that longer periods of immobilization produced higher percentages of union. In 1960 Russe[186] stated that "since the period of immobilization may, in some cases, require many months, operative treatment by an experienced surgeon may be considered preferable." Therefore, the potential for economic hardship caused to young adults by prolonged immobilization and the availability of more consistently successful surgical techniques have been justification enough for many to recommend surgery not only for the older, ununited fractures, but also for delayed unions that have remained symptomatic after 3 to 4 months of adequate nonsurgical treatment.[31,37,48,49,57,64,70,113,151,227,229] More recently, electrical stimulation has become an alternative to surgery for the treatment of some of these patients.

FRACTURES OF THE MIDDLE THIRD OF THE SCAPHOID

This is the most common fracture of the scaphoid, and for years it has been notorious for a high percentage of slow or delayed unions or nonunions. These poor results have been explained by the frequent delay in initiating proper immobilization, either because of the patient's own failure to seek treatment following an injury often considered trivial, or because of a missed diagnosis.[15,149,233] Another reason may be the lack of recognition of associated carpal instability once the obvious fracture of the scaphoid is diagnosed.[81] The wrist is consequently treated as an isolated scaphoid injury, rather than as an injury with more extensive carpal involvement: the loss of scaphoid support renders the carpus unstable.[130] More frequently, the lunate becomes dorsiflexed; colinear alignment of radius, lunate, and capitate no longer exists. The carpus assumes a zigzag appearance, variously called "crumpling,"[93] "concertina,"[81] or DISI (dorsal intercalated segment instability)[136] deformity (Fig. 19-3). Less frequently, the lunate rotates into volarflexion and a VISI (volar intercalated segment instability) pattern exists (Fig. 19-4). Displacements and comminution of the fracture fragments and the direction of the fracture line can also indicate potential instability. (See Chapter 20 for further discussion of carpal instability.) Russe[186] classified scaphoid fractures into three types according to the relationship of the fracture line to the long axis of the scaphoid (Fig. 19-8). Horizontal oblique and transverse fractures are essentially stable and are expected to heal promptly, after a reasonably short period of immobilization of 6 to 12 weeks. Vertical oblique fractures have a high longitudinal shear component, are relatively unstable, and require long immobilization. Undisplaced fractures are stable and, for the most part, free of problem. When the fracture is angulated or displaced, regardless of the direction of the fracture line, some degree of carpal instability should be suspected.[240]

Nonoperative Treatment

Acute Fractures. There is now universal agreement that the vast majority of these fresh or acute scaphoid fractures will heal if immobilized

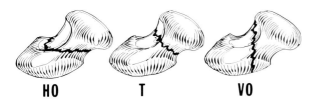

HO   **T**   **VO**

Fig. 19-8. Classification of fractures of the scaphoid (Russe). (*HO*, horizontal oblique; *T*, transverse; *VO*, vertical oblique.) (Taleisnik J: The Wrist. Churchill Livingstone, New York, 1985. © 1985, Elizabeth Roselius.)

properly and for a long enough period of time.[28,66,69,140,162,163,181,192,198,199,211] Based on a radiographic assessment of the stability of the fracture, Cooney et al[51] suggested a management program similar to that proposed by Herbert in 1974.[110] This program is, I believe, very reasonable and reliable. Stable fractures are those without displacement or angulation. They may be treated in below-elbow thumb spica plaster immobilization, with the wrist in some radial deviation and slight palmar flexion. In my opinion, this is satisfactory provided these fractures are less than 3 weeks old when first treated. When older than 3 weeks, I would favor initial immobilization in an above elbow cast. Unstable fractures are those showing either an offset greater than 1 mm between fragments, or angulation of fragments with an abnormal carpal alignment. Unstable fractures require above elbow immobilization, provided carpal and scaphoid alignments are acceptable or can be restored by manipulation or positioning. For instance, in a carpal collapse alignment, usually into DISI, lunate dorsiflexion may be corrected by full radial deviation of the wrist.[240] The absolute requisite is to accept nothing less than anatomic alignment. Otherwise, these unstable injuries should be treated by open reduction and internal fixation.

In summary, for the nonoperative treatment of recent fractures of the middle third of the scaphoid, it is my belief that short arm immobilization should be reserved for the stable, undisplaced, transverse-oblique fractures that are fresh. For fractures older than 3 weeks, and for all other undisplaced, but potentially unstable fractures, above elbow immobilization is recommended. For those patients with unsatisfactory displacement of the fracture fragments or with loss of normal carpal alignment, which cannot be restored by positioning or manipulation, open reduction and internal fixation must be considered.

Ununiting Fractures. In most instances, nonunions of the scaphoid are treated by surgical means. According to some reports, established nonunions, particularly if stable and without carpal collapse,[81] may not require any treatment, for they can remain essentially symptom-free.[31,61,139,148,149] Not infrequently, these injuries are surprising findings following minor trauma and respond well to a brief period of splinting, returning to their previous, nondisabling state.

Until recently, there was no clear-cut evidence to suggest that the incidence of post-traumatic osteoarthritis increased in these patients with the passage of time. This notion was challenged by Mack et al[143] and by Ruby and coauthors.[185] Both of these studies found a time-correlated increase in degenerative changes. The severity of osteoarthritis was greater for displaced fractures and for those with coexistent carpal instability. Actually, few of the nonunions remained stable or undisplaced, or free of arthritis, after 10 years. According to these authors, asymptomatic patients with stable undisplaced nonunions should be advised of the possibility of late degenerative changes. Mack et al[143] recommend that all displaced ununited scaphoid fractures be reduced and grafted, regardless of symptoms, before the onset of osteoarthritis. For the stable, undisplaced variety, although prolonged immobilization has been shown to produce a reversal of the nonunion process in a high percentage of patients,[28,211] this alone would seem to be a rather radical approach. For these nonunions, and for delayed unions, the use of electrical stimulation is, I believe, an excellent alternative to operation.

Electrical Stimulation

Although the mechanism of action is not fully understood, electrical stimulation has proven to be successful in treating nonunions. Electrical currents may be delivered directly to a fracture, either through surgical implantation of anode, cathode, and battery (the "invasive" method), or through percutaneous drilling of cathodes, the anode being

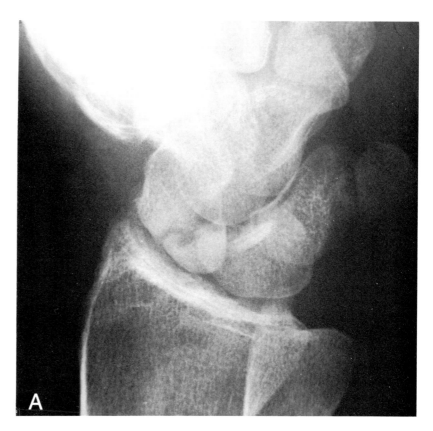

Fig. 19-9. Nonunion of a fracture of the scaphoid treated with immobilization and the application of pulsing electromagnetic field (PEMF) treatment. (A) Appearance after 6 months immobilization. (B) Localizer radiograph for the application of PEMF treatment. *(Figure continues.)*

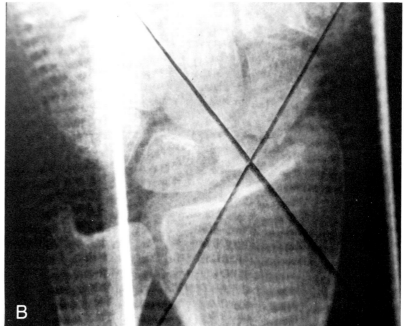

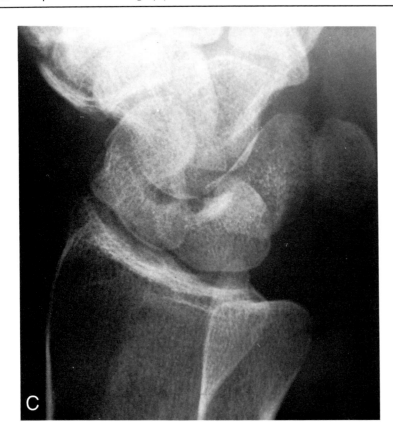

Fig. 19-9 *(Continued)*. (**C**) Four months later, the fracture is healed. (Taleisnik J: The Wrist. Churchill Livingstone, New York, 1985.)

attached to the skin surface (the "semi-invasive" method). By contrast, "noninvasive" methods create an electromagnetic field for the fracture through the incorporation of coils, centered at the fracture level, in the plaster immobilization. In 1974, Wilhelm, Feldmeier and Hauer[245] reported a limited experience in the treatment of 8 scaphoids using an electrical field created by a transformer connected to an AO screw. A variable success rate has been reported using the semi-invasive method.[11,29] More recently, Frykman, Taleisnik, Peters et al[88] presented their experience treating 44 nonunions, at least 6 months old, using noninvasive, pulsed electromagnetic field (PEMF) treatment. Thirty-five (80 percent) healed after a mean of 4.3 months of combined PEMF and plaster immobilization. Although these results are not as effective as those reported using the Russe bone-graft technique, they are satisfactory enough to merit incorporation of this modality into our armamentarium. I believe this in spite of experimental studies that doubt the efficacy of PEMF treat-

ment.[73] The clinical PEMF experience is particularly impressive in the treatment of the problem nonunions: those of the proximal third, and those accompanied by avascular necrosis (Fig. 19-9). In Frykman et al's series,[88] five of 8 fractures of the proximal third, and 8 of 9 with avascular necrosis went on to heal. The main problem in objectively evaluating the efficacy of PEMF treatment is the lack of a reliable double-blind study between like series of patients treated with immobilization alone, and those treated with immobilization and PEMF. Comparison of published series of nonunions of scaphoids treated by immobilization and this group treated with PEMF strongly suggest that PEMF is, indeed, effective and advantageous. This experience has been confirmed by others.[18] The technique is simple, low risk, and should be considered for nonunions that are undisplaced, without carpal instability, and less than 5 years old.[88] PEMF treatment is not inexpensive, although its cost compares favorably with the cost of surgical treatment and hospitalization.

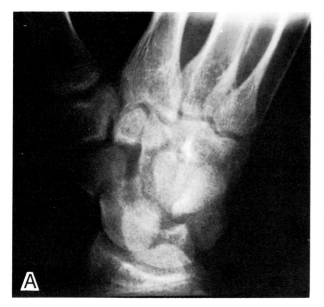

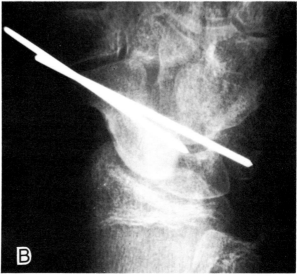

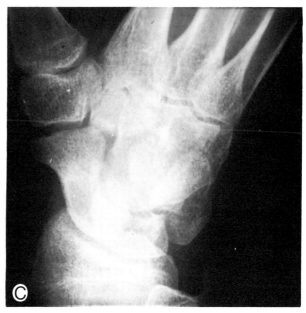

Fig. 19-10. (**A**) A displaced horizontal oblique fracture of the scaphoid. (**B**) The same fracture 6 weeks after open reduction and internal fixation with K-wires. (**C**) Follow-up radiograph at 3 months. The fracture is healed.

Operative Treatment

Fresh displaced or angulated fractures, or fresh fractures with loss of carpal alignment that cannot be satisfactorily corrected by manipulation or positioning of the wrist, or that can be corrected but not maintained by cast immobilization alone, should be treated by open reduction and internal fixation with K-wires (Fig. 19-10) or screws (Fig.

19-11).[80,82,110,136,147,151,233,240] The presence of displacement of the fracture fragments or of the carpus implies a more severe injury than just the scaphoid fracture itself, particularly suggesting that extensive ligamentous damage has occurred.[240] Unless comminution is present, bone grafts are not necessary for these recent injuries. Surgical treatment is also indicated for all painful delayed unions and nonunions that have failed to

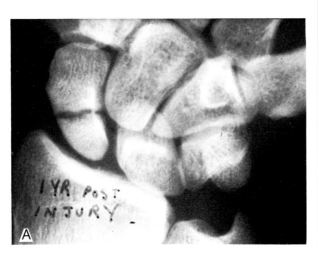 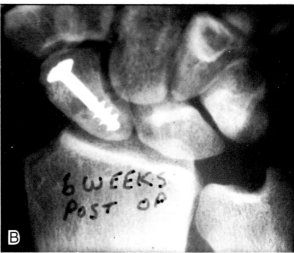

Fig. 19-11. (A) A transverse fracture of the scaphoid. (B) The same fracture 6 weeks following open reduction, minimal styloidectomy, and internal fixation with a screw. (Courtesy of Donald R. Huene, MD.)

heal and become asymptomatic after a reasonable trial of adequate nonoperative management, regardless of the presence of degenerative, avascular, or cystic changes. In their evaluation of treatment of nonunions of the scaphoid, the Pennsylvania Orthopaedic Society[172] concluded that "no one method of treatment can be used for types of disability caused by an ununited fracture of the carpal navicular." It was further stated that "a well stocked surgical armamentarium ready for any contingency does exist." The addition of new forms of treatment further supports this conclusion.

The choice of procedure will vary with the surgeon's preference and experience, the type of fracture, the patient's age, and the presence of periscaphoid arthrosis. The following is a discussion of frequently used surgical techniques for the operative treatment of scaphoid fractures. Partial fusions for the treatment of nonunions of the scaphoid are briefly reviewed (the techniques for these procedures are discussed in detail in Chapter 5). Implants, total fusions, and procedures considered unproven, obsolete, or uniformly unsuccessful, such as mutiple drilling and total or partial excision of major scaphoid fragments without implant, have been omitted. (Implant arthroplasty is discussed in Chapter 7; partial and total wrist arthrodeses in Chapters 5 and 6, respectively.)

Bone Graft. Bone grafts were first advocated by Adams in 1928.[1] In subsequent years, other authors, including Murray[162,163] and Burnett,[37,38] reported their experience with the use of tibial bone pegs introduced into holes drilled across the fracture site. In 1937 Matti[146] showed that fracture healing can also be achieved by cancellous bone chips packed into an excavated fracture site through a dorsal approach. This technique was modified by Russe[186] using a palmar approach to fill an egg-shaped cavity created within the scaphoid and across the fracture site with an oblong cancellous bone peg and additional cancellous bone chips. Most publications favor Russe's procedure.[64,66,69,151,161,227,229,233] In 1980, Russe reported a modification to his original technique[187] first presented in the English-language literature in 1985 by Green.[102] This most recent modification consists of using two corticocancellous grafts, inserted into the scaphoid excavation with their cancellous sides facing each other. The remainder of the cavity is filled with 2-mm-sized cancellous chips (Fig. 19-12). This procedure may be effective even in those ununited scaphoids with palmar angulation of the fragments, but will not adequately correct significant DISI deformity. Severe angulations are accompanied by carpal collapse, seen as a dorsiflexion of the lunate. Fisk[81] observed that in these cases, realignment of the fragments

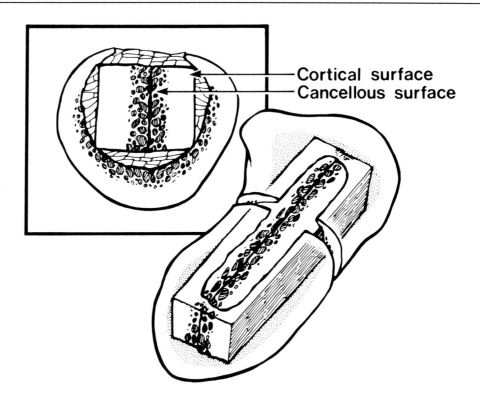

Cortical surface
Cancellous surface

Fig. 19-12. Modern Russe technique using two corticocancellous bone grafts. (Green DP: The effect of avascular necrosis on Russe bone grafting for scaphoid nonunion. J Hand Surg 10A:597–605, 1985.)

creates an anterior wedge-shaped defect, which requires an anterior, wedge-shaped bone graft (Fig. 19-13). Fisk showed that this procedure will correct the abnormal dorsiflexion of the lunate. Fisk proposed a lateral approach for this operation, with radial styloidectomy, using the radial styloid as the source of the wedge-graft, and relying on natural compressive forces for stabilization.[84,85] Recently, Fernandez[79] modified Fisk's technique by inserting a carefully measured iliac bone graft, through a palmar approach, and using internal fixation. I believe that both Russe's procedure and the Fernandez modification of Fisk's operation are excellent, and have clear-cut, well-defined indications. I have followed Russe's original precise guidelines and achieved a very satisfactory rate of success. This technique is indicated for all symptomatic, established nonunions and symptomatic delayed unions without osteoarthritis, with satisfactory carpal alignment, after immobilization or treatment using electrical stimulation have failed. The presence of cystic changes is not a contraindication,[161] but periscaphoid arthrosis is.[61] Although it may be successful in the presence of avascular

necrosis suggested by increased radiographic density of the proximal fragment, Green[102] pointed out that true avascular necrosis cannot always be accurately predicted by radiographic appearance. In his opinion, direct scrutiny for punctate bleeding points at the time of surgical excavation is the best method to determine scaphoid vascularity. His experience confirmed Russe's admonition that his operation is not likely to be successful if the proximal fragment is *totally* avascular. The success rate is also lower when vascularity is fair to poor. In the presence of a collapsed scaphoid nonunion with dorsal carpal instability, the anterior wedge-grafting operation is preferred.

Bone Graft Technique (Original Russe Method[186]). A 4- to 5-cm longitudinal incision is made along the radial border of the flexor carpi radialis tendon (Fig. 19-14A), centered at a level even with the tip of the radial styloid, which usually corresponds to the level of the fracture itself. The capsule is divided longitudinally (Fig. 19-14B), and the underlying deep volar radiocarpal ligaments are either divided partially and retracted, or completely severed and tagged for later repair (Fig.

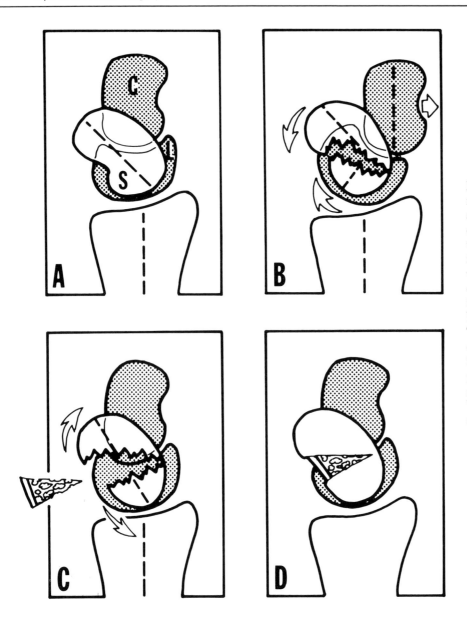

Fig. 19-13. **(A)** Schematic representation of normal alignment between scaphoid *(S)*, lunate *(L)*, and capitate *(C)*. **(B)** Nonunion of a fracture of the scaphoid with palmarflexion of the distal fragment, and a dorsal intercalated segment instability (DISI) pattern. **(C)** The scaphoid alignment is corrected. **(D)** It is maintained by the insertion of a palmar wedge-shaped bone graft. (Taleisnik J: The Wrist. Churchill Livingstone, New York, 1985. © 1985, Elizabeth Roselius.)

19-14C and D). An egg-shaped cavity is created well into both fracture fragments *without using power tools*. A cancellous bone graft is then obtained from the ipsilateral iliac crest and fashioned into an ovoid plug large enough to fit snugly into the scaphoid cavity (Fig. 19-14E). The graft is actually jammed into both fragments as these are forcibly distracted. Once the graft is in place, both fragments and the graft itself are impacted to produce a satisfactory degree of stability (Fig. 19-14F). Internal fixation is reserved for only those cases when

instability persists after the bone graft is in place. In such cases, I have preferred to use a couple of K-wires carefully inserted parallel to each other and to the longitudinal axis of the scaphoid. The radiocarpal ligaments are repaired, and the hand and wrist are immobilized in a compression-type dressing incorporated into a long arm cast. This is changed to a long arm thumb spica cast at 5 to 7 days and to a short arm thumb spica cast at 6 weeks postoperatively. In those cases in which the fracture is very unstable, or after reoperation, I prefer

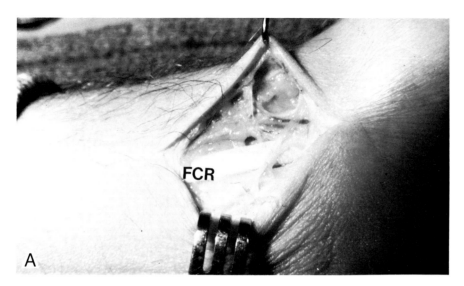

A

Fig. 19-14. Original Russe
bone graft technique. (A)
The incision. (FCR, Flexor
carpi radialis tendon.) (B)
The volar capsule (VC) is
divided longitudinally, exposing the deep volar radiocarpal ligaments (RC). (C)
The instrument is inserted
under the deep volar radiocarpal ligaments. (Figure
continues.)

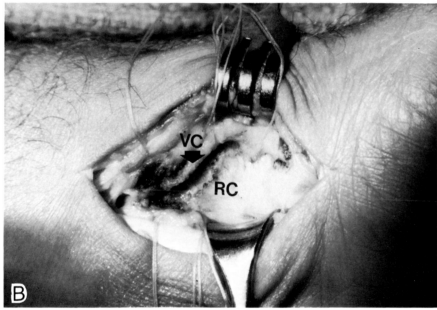

B

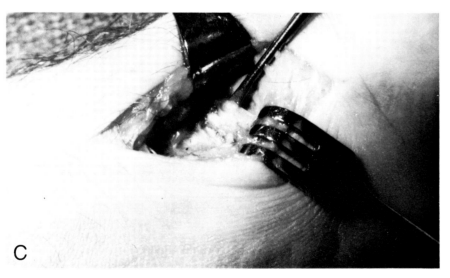

C

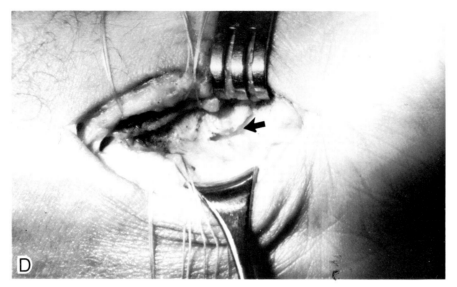

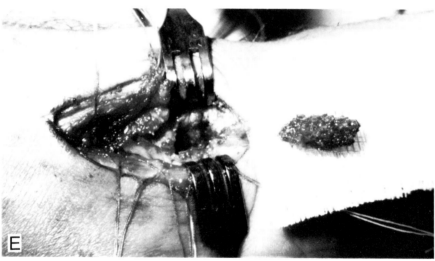

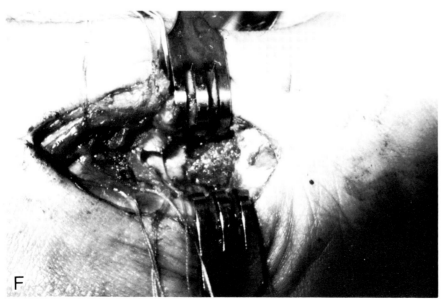

Fig. 19-14 *(Continued)*. **(D)** The radioscaphocapitate ligament and a portion of the radiolunate ligament have been divided *(arrow)*. **(E)** An egg-shaped cavity is created distal and proximal to the fracture line. A cancellous bone graft, usually obtained from the ipsilateral iliac crest, is fashioned to fit snuggly into this cavity. **(F)** The cancellous bone graft has been wedged into the cavity of the scaphoid. The stability of the graft and the fracture fragments should be satisfactory. If not, additional fixation with one or two K-wires is recommended.

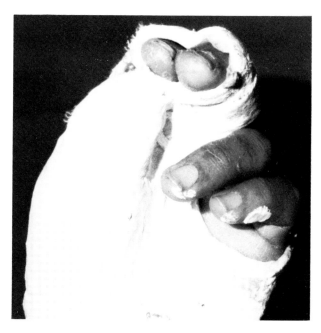

Fig. 19-15. For very unstable fractures, and after reoperations, I prefer a three-digit cast instead of the standard postoperative compression dressing-cast.

to use a three-digit cast (Fig. 19-15) for the initial 3 postoperative weeks, followed by the long arm thumb spica and short arm thumb spica casts in the same sequence described above. The total immobilization time for this procedure has averaged 12

to 14 weeks in my experience. Union in 90 percent or better of patients can be expected (Fig. 19-16).

Volar Wedge Bone Graft Technique (Fisk-Fernandez[79,84]). Tracings are obtained preoperatively of the injured and normal scaphoids. On these, the amount of resection and the size and shape of the bone graft are calculated (Fig. 19-17). The surgical approach is similar to that used for a Russe bone graft, extended distally to well expose the distal pole of the scaphoid, and medially to allow the dorsiflexed lunate to be seen. The resection is carried out using an oscillating saw. I like to "freshen up" the resulting surfaces using a rongeur. Fernandez advocates repeated drilling of the proximal fragment if it is sclerotic. A 0.035 K-wire may be used for this. A corticocancellous bone graft is obtained from the ipsilateral iliac crest. The scaphoid fragments are then distracted to correct flexion and length; at the same time an assistant tips the lunate into satisfactory alignment. A wedge-shaped, or trapezoidal graft is fashioned from the iliac bone, and is inserted with its cortical surface facing toward the palm. Protruding portions are trimmed flush. Two 0.045 K-wires are then introduced from the palmar aspect of the distal fragment, through the graft and into the dorsal aspect of the proximal fragment. Intraoperative radiographs or an image intensifier are used to insure satisfactory correction and placement of the internal fixation. Because of the considerable change in scaphoid dimensions,

Fig. 19-16. (A) Radiograph showing the preoperative appearance of the ununited scaphoid fracture depicted in Fig. 19-14. (B) Radiograph obtained 3 months after the Russe-type bone graft operation.

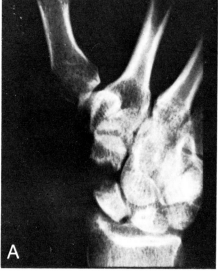
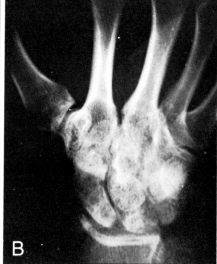

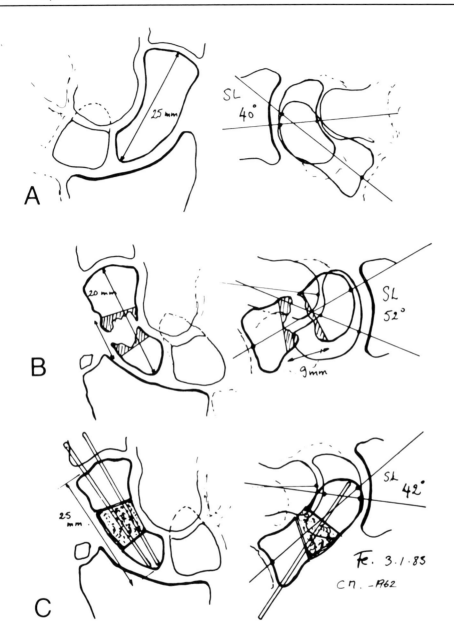

Fig. 19-17. Preoperative planning for the insertion of a wedge-shaped graft. (A) Tracing of the opposite uninjured wrist and measurement of scaphoid length and scapholunate angle. (B) Calculation of size and resection area and form of graft. (C) Definitive diagram of the operation. (Fernandez DL: A technique for anterior wedge-shaped grafts for scaphoid nonunions with carpal instability. J Hand Surg 9A:733–737, 1984.)

capsule closure may be difficult. In these cases, repair may be aided by using a portion of the flexor carpi radialis sheath, turned to cover the capsular defect.[123] Fernandez proposes postoperative immobilization in a below elbow cast for 8 weeks, followed by removable splinting until healing is proven with tomograms. The K-wires are removed at this point, which is on average 10 to 11 weeks after surgery.

Radial Styloidectomy. Radial styloidectomy is performed subperiosteally through the anatomic snuffbox. The radial styloid may also be used as a bone graft.[14] Styloidectomies alone have been unsatisfactory procedures,[148,172] but have proven successful when combined with bone grafts, either with or without internal fixation.[14,49,148,172] Although some authors consider styloidectomy to be an essential part of the treatment of nonunions,[202] the procedure does not seem to improve on the results of bone grafting alone, except in cases with localized scaphoid-styloid arthrosis. It may also be a factor of instability if performed carelessly (Fig. 19-18) and may preclude the subsequent use of a scaphoid implant, should this become indicated.

Bentzon's Procedure. This operation was initially used by Bentzon in 1939 and was first reported in 1941.[20] The concept is to convert a painful nonunion into a pain-free pseudarthrosis by the introduction of a soft tissue flap between the fracture fragments, based on the dorsoradial aspect of the wrist. In spite of its attractive simplicity, with very few exceptions[35,57] Bentzon's procedure has failed to become popular outside of Scandinavian countries.[3a,4,177] Results with this technique appear comparable to those obtained after bone grafting.[26] A recent long-term review by Boeckstyns and collaborators[27] showed persistent good results 22 to 39 years after Bentzon's operation. Carpal collapse, found in 15 of 25 patients, and osteoarthritis, present in 7, did not result in clinical disability.[27] These authors suggest that Bentzon's arthroplasty

may still be considered a satisfactory alternative when prolonged immobilization is contraindicated and after bone graft procedures have failed.

Osteosynthesis. Internal fixation of scaphoid fractures with K-wires or screws is always indicated following the treatment of trans-scaphoid perilunate fracture-dislocations, and for those fractures accompanied by more subtle forms of carpal instability.[81,89,147] K-wires, in my opinion, are easier to insert and remove, do not require a radial styloidectomy or extended approaches to facilitate exposure, and provide satisfactory stability. They can be used in the presence of avascular changes of the proximal fragment, when screws are formally contraindicated, and may actually be the only form of fixation possible in those comminuted fractures most in need of internal support. Bone grafts may be used in conjunction with internal fixation. Screw fixation was proposed by McLaughlin in 1954[150] and again more recently by several other authors.[33,34,81,107,110,147] The technique of screw osteosynthesis must be precise and meticulous to avoid unwanted complications, such as delayed union or nonunion perpetuated by poor screw insertion. Results can be disappointing[52,71,107]; however, Leyshon and co-authors[133] recently described their satisfactory experience treating acute and ununited fractures with an AO scaphoid lagscrew, inserted through an extended, lateral and volar bayonet-shaped incision. A radial styloidectomy was not required, and screw insertion could be accomplished under direct view. They advised against disturbing the fracture site, or using bone grafts in conjunction with the screw fixation. In 1982, Herbert[111] and in 1984, Herbert and Fisher,[112] published their experience with the use of a double-threaded bone-screw, with special instrumentation for its insertion, for the treatment of acute, unstable fractures, and for delayed and nonunions as well. This system was designed to overcome problems previously encountered with internal fixation. The screw is smaller in diameter, lacks a head, and presents threads that engage both fracture fragments. The thread on the leading edge of the screw has a greater pitch than that at the trailing end, to allow for compression as the screw is inserted (Fig. 19-19). It does not have to be removed, and may be used for smaller fragments and

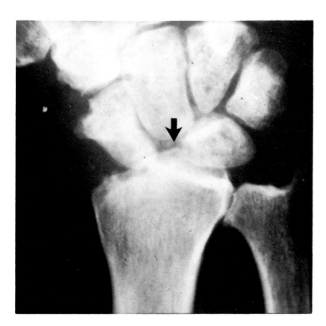

Fig. 19-18. An excessively generous radial styloidectomy may be a factor in carpal instability *(arrow)*, as shown here.

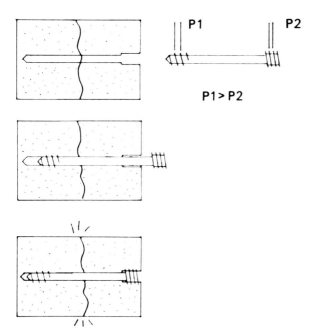

Fig. 19-19. Difference in pitch between the leading thread *(P1)* and the trailing thread *(P2)* of the Herbert screw governs the rate of "take-up" or drawing together of the two bone fragments, producing compression. (Herbert TJ, Fisher WE: Management of the fractured scaphoid using a new bone screw. J Bone Joint Surg 66B:114–123, 1984.)

with bone grafts. Because of the absent head, and the precision of its insertion, both ends of the screw remain buried under cartilage, without protruding into joints, and, consequently, do not interfere with attempts at early motion. A jig holds the fragments aligned and in apposition prior to inserting the screw, and provides guidance, both for the direction and for the depth of insertion. The Herbert screw is contraindicated for totally avascular small proximal fragments. Disadvantages of this technique are the technical demands of jig placement and the wide exposure required.[203]

Technique of Screw Osteosynthesis (Herbert and Fisher[112]). This is a difficult technique with a very narrow margin for error. Herbert's precise instructions should be studied carefully, and the operation practiced in a cadaver wrist before attempting it in a patient. The approach is similar to Russe's, extended distally into the base of the thenar eminence, in order to fully expose the distal

end of the scaphoid at the scaphotrapezial joint. Fresh fractures are reduced. Nonunions are aligned, and prepared for the insertion of a corticocancellous iliac bone graft and additional cancellous bone chips. The jig is positioned to insure correct screw placement, with the blade hooked around the proximal pole and the drill guide firmly clamped against its distal pole (Fig. 19-20). The length of the screw is read directly off the calibrated guide (Fig. 19-21). The screw is fully inserted and the jig is removed. When a graft is used, the screw traverses its center. Extra compression is provided by further turns of the screw. The graft is trimmed flush, and the incision is closed. Radiographs should be obtained in the operating room to confirm the satisfactory position of screw, fracture fragments, and bone graft. A compression dressing is applied. After sutures are removed, most patients are further protected with a removable splint. Active range of motion exercises are encouraged from the beginning following fixation of fresh fractures. When a bone graft is used, below elbow immobilization should be used for 4 to 6 weeks.

Proximal Row Carpectomy. Proximal row carpectomy has also been advocated for the treatment of ununited fractures of the scaphoid. Although Hill[113] finds the procedure indicated in older patients with a symptomatic nonunion who do not wish to accept a long period of immobilization, others[54,116,121] have used this treatment with very good functional and clinical results for younger, active workers who do heavy labor. Proximal row carpectomies may be preferable to fusions in some cases, except in the presence of radiocarpal arthrosis.

Technique of Proximal Row Carpectomy. For proximal row carpectomies done in traumatic cases, a transverse dorsal skin incision is preferred, along the radiocarpal joint projected immediately distal to Lister's tubercle (Fig. 19-22). A longitudinal incision, however, can be used when additional procedures are planned, for example, tendon transfers and synovectomy in the rheumatoid patient. The dorsal retinacular ligament is exposed, and the cutaneous branches of the ulnar and radial nerves are identified and retracted. The dorsal reti-

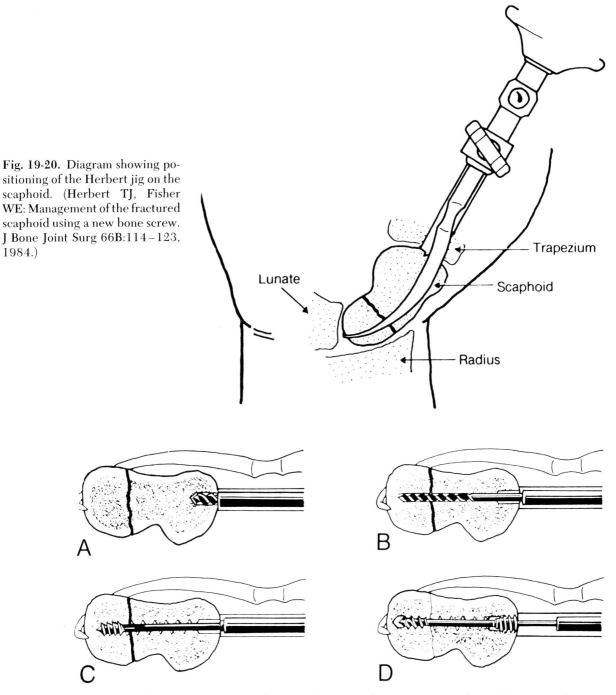

Fig. 19-20. Diagram showing positioning of the Herbert jig on the scaphoid. (Herbert TJ, Fisher WE: Management of the fractured scaphoid using a new bone screw. J Bone Joint Surg 66B:114–123, 1984.)

Trapezium

Scaphoid

Lunate

Radius

A

B

C

D

Fig. 19-21. Diagrams showing the stages of instrumentation for Herbert screw fixation. (**A**) The pilot drill (for trailing end of screw). (**B**) Long drill (for leading end of screw). (**C**) Tap (for leading thread). (**D**) The screw is inserted through the jig (the trailing thread is self-tapping). The jig is used to align all instruments and a built-in stop ensures drilling to the exact length required. (Herbert TJ, Fisher WE: Management of the fractured scaphoid using a new bone screw. J Bone Joint Surg 66B:114–123, 1984.)

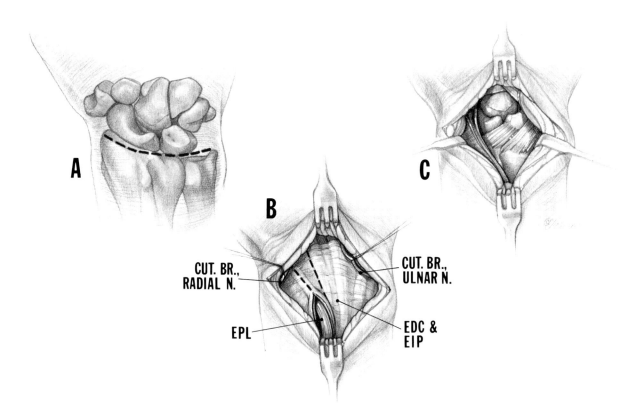

Fig. 19-22. Dorsal approach to the wrist using a transverse incision. (**A**) Incision. (**B**) The extensor pollicis longus tendon *(EPL)* is exposed. (*EDC*, extensor digitorum communis; *EIP*, extensor indicis proprius.) (**C**) Subcapsular and subperiosteal exposure of the joint through a longitudinal retinacular and capsular incision between the third and fourth dorsal extensor compartments. (Taleisnik J: The Wrist. Churchill Livingstone, New York, 1985. © 1985, Elizabeth Roselius.)

naculum is incised over the extensor pollicis longus tunnel. This tendon is unroofed, lifted, and retracted. The retinacular system separating this third dorsal wrist compartment from the extensor indicis propius and the extensor digitorum communis tendons is incised, and the entire dorsal retinaculum is reflected toward the ulna, together with the contents of the fourth dorsal extensor compartment. The entire lunate and triquetrum are removed, usually in that order. The scaphoid can be excised in its entirety, although I prefer to leave its distal one third attached to the trapezium and the trapezoid for additional support to the thumb ray. The proximal pole of the capitate is seated into the lunate concavity of the radius; if stability is questionable, a temporary K-wire is used for 3 to 4 weeks to maintain this position. I routinely divide

the posterior interosseous nerve, since entrapment of this nerve has been implicated as a possible cause of postoperative pain. The nerve can be found lying beneath the deep fascial layer, on the interosseous membrane, along the ulnar border of the radius. It is divided at least 2 to 3 cm proximal to the articular surface of the radius. The pisiform is not excised. Closure is in layers and includes the dorsal retinaculum. Immediate postoperative immobilization in a bulky compression dressing enclosed in plaster is used for 4 to 6 days and replaced then by a short arm cast for a total postoperative immobilization of 4 to 6 weeks. At the end of this period, gradual motion is allowed, while intermittent protection is provided by a removable splint, worn for 2 to 4 weeks, or until the patient is capable of free use of the wrist.

Partial Wrist Arthrodesis. In 1946, Sutro[213] and in 1952, Helfet[108] proposed to treat nonunions of the scaphoid by arthrodesing both fragments to the capitate when extensive sclerosis or resorption of the fragments exists, or when degenerative changes between scaphoid and capitate have occurred. When the radiocarpal joint is involved with osteoarthritis, and the scaphocapitate joint is satisfactory, a radioscapholunate fusion may be considered instead.[97] Other types of limited arthrodesis have been proposed.[100] In my opinion, the vast majority of nonunions of the scaphoid may be satisfactorily treated with techniques other than limited arthrodesis. Arthrodesis may be indicated, however, as a salvage procedure, particularly after repeated failures of bone grafts, and to prevent midcarpal collapse in unstable wrists when scaphoid implants are considered. The techniques of limited wrist arthrodesis are described in Chapter 5.

FRACTURES OF THE PROXIMAL THIRD OF THE SCAPHOID

Blood Supply Of The Scaphoid

In their study of vascular foramina in dried scaphoids, Obletz and Halbstein[166] found 13 percent without vascular perforations and 20 percent with only a single small foramen proximal to the waist. Therefore, in their opinion, 30 percent of middle third fractures could be expected to interfere with the blood supply to the proximal fragment and lead to avascular necrosis or nonunion. This potential is higher when the fracture is more proximal. Logroscino and DiMarchi[138] published a similar study. The scaphoid receives its blood supply through ligamentous attachments. The studies of Grettve,[104] Minne and co-authors,[157] and Taleisnik and Kelly[218] show three main arterial groups supplying the main body of the scaphoid. Because of their spatial relationship to the scaphoid, these groups were named laterovolar, dorsal, and distal[218] (Fig. 19-23). In support of this description, representative specimens in Obletz and Halbstein's study show major clusters of foramina just radial and proximal to the tubercle, corresponding to the point of entry of the laterovolar system. In a more recent investigation, Gelberman and

Menon[91] described two instead of three vascular systems: one dorsal, and the second a volar group limited to the tubercle, and therefore comparable to the distal vessels in Taleisnik and Kelly's description.[218] Furthermore, comparable specimens in both these papers show a strong resemblance between Gelberman and Menon's dorsal supply and Taleisnik and Kelly's laterovolar vessels. All of these studies demonstrate a strikingly poor blood supply to the proximal pole, particularly in comparison with the abundant supply to the distal two-thirds of the scaphoid. The proximal pole is an intraarticular structure completely covered with hyaline cartilage, with a single ligamentous attachment (the deep radioscapholunate ligament), and negligible or nonexistent independent blood supply. This entire anatomic arrangement is reminiscent of that of the head of the femur, and, just like the head of the femur, survival of the proximal pole of the scaphoid when isolated by a fracture is frequently compromised. There is, therefore, sufficient experimental data to explain the high incidence of nonunions and avascular necrosis of the proximal fragment among fractures of the proximal third of the scaphoid. Fractures in this location take an average of 6 to 11 weeks longer to heal than those in the middle third,[61,186,211] and have demonstrated an incidence of avascular necrosis of 14 to 39 percent in different series.[49,172,186]

Treatment

The treatment of proximal third fractures depends on the size and vascularity of the fragment and the age of the fracture. Fresh injuries may heal after prolonged, long-arm immobilization. Rehbein and Düben[180] report proximal third fractures healing with the use of their fist-cast. For those that fail to unite after 6 months, particularly for the fragments that are smaller than 30 percent of the scaphoid, pulsing electromagnetic field stimulation (PEMF) has added a viable alternative to surgical treatment. In a recent report,[88] 67 percent of established nonunions of the proximal third went on to heal in an average of 4.3 months after starting electrical stimulation. **PEMF** is a pain-free method that requires a very strict compliance from the patient for its success. It is noninvasive, may be used in the presence of infection, and is preferable, in

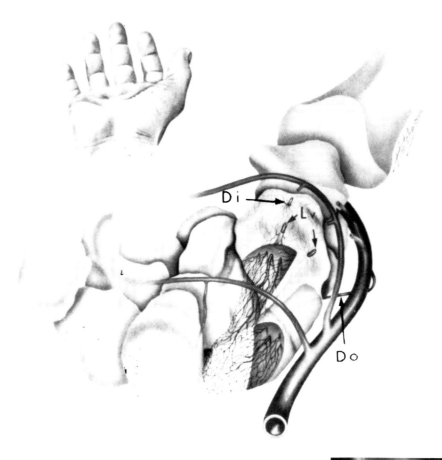

Fig. 19-23. Schematic representation of the blood supply of the scaphoid. (*Lv,* laterovolar vessels; *Do,* dorsal vessels; *Di,* distal vessels.) (Taleisnik J, Kelly PJ: The extraosseous and intraosseous blood supply of the scaphoid bone. J Bone Joint Surg 48A:1125–1137, 1966.)

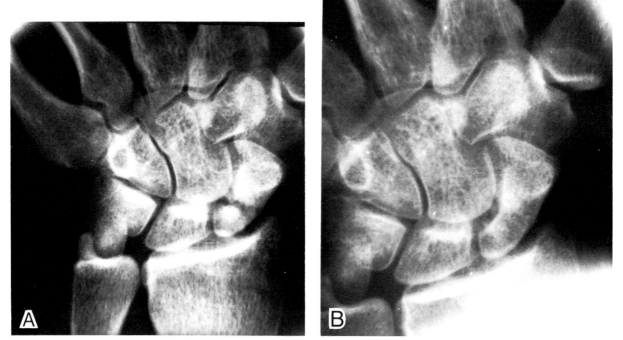

Fig. 19-24. (A) Preoperative radiograph of a fracture of the proximal third of the scaphoid. (B) Postoperative appearance 5 months after a volar bone graft procedure (Russe).

my opinion, to electrical stimulation with transcutaneous insertion of electrodes.[219]

The choice of operative treatment depends on the size and appearance of the proximal fragment. When this is a full one-third of the scaphoid, a bone graft using Russe's technique may be successful (Fig. 19-24). For smaller, viable fragments, Matti's original technique,[146,227] in which cancellous bone chips are packed tightly into the fracture from a dorsal approach, may be preferable. In either case, fixation *across* the proximal fragment, from the distal scaphoid into the lunate, with staples[235] or K-wires may considerably help to enhance healing through increased stability. After the union is solid, the K-wires or staples should be removed. If union fails to take place, or if the fragment is too small or avascular to justify reconstruction, and in the absence of carpal instability (Fig. 19-25), the fragment may be excised[14,21,22,31,113,145,199,211] and a silicone spacer used in its place. This may be carved from a silicone block[247] or cut out of a silicone scaphoid implant (Fig. 19-26). Michon in 1972[154] and Jones in 1982[119] proposed to excise the small

proximal fragment and to replace it with a silicone sphere. Irisarri et al[117] use instead a portion of silicone scaphoid implant, cut to match the space left by the excision of the fragment. This partial implant is carved to include a distal, central, rectangular stem, which is introduced into a similar opening drilled into the distal fragment (Fig. 19-27).

FRACTURES OF THE DISTAL THIRD OF THE SCAPHOID

Fractures in this location are infrequent.[61,113,172] They may be limited to just the tuberosity or may involve the entire distal third of the bone. Fractures of the *tuberosity* are extraarticular, usually stable, and have a generous blood supply.[75,138,166,218] They tend to heal promptly and are best treated in a short thumb spica cast worn for 3 to 6 weeks. In Russe's classification,[186] fractures of the *distal third* are commonly of the transverse, stable type, and in his experience united rapidly, usually after 4 to 8 weeks in a short arm thumb spica cast. Vertical fractures into the scaphotrape-

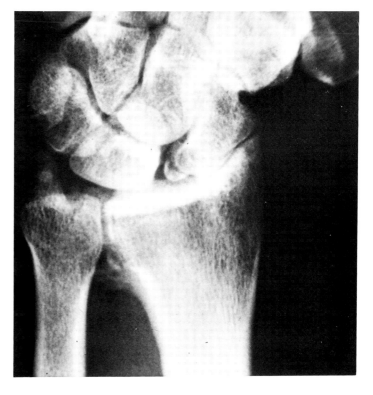

Fig. 19-25. An old ununited fracture with a very small proximal pole. Moderate scaphoid subluxation and early narrowing of the radioscaphoid joint space have occurred.

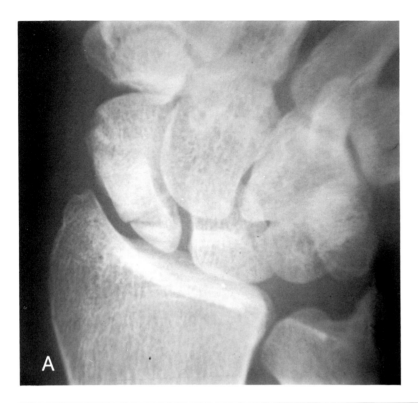

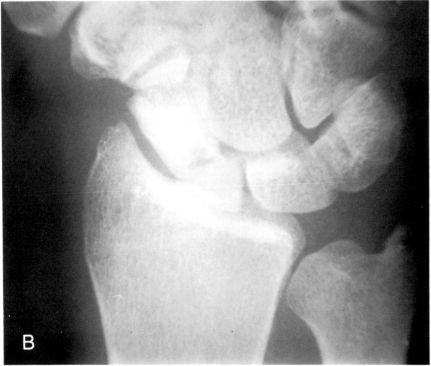

Fig. 19-26. Ununited fracture of the proximal pole of scaphoid treated by excision of fracture fragment and insertion of silicone spacer. (A) Preoperative radiograph. (B) Postoperative appearance. (Taleisnik J: The Wrist. Churchill Livingstone, New York, 1985.)

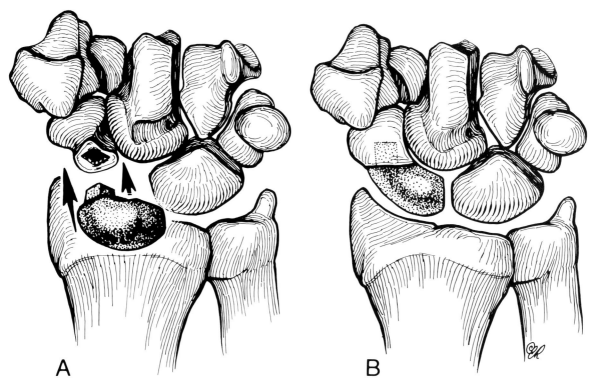

Fig. 19-27. Insertion of a partial, proximal scaphoid silicone implant with a carved rectangular stem into the distal fracture fragment.

zium-trapezoid joint have been described.[50] They may be difficult to detect, requiring special diagnostic views and techniques, such as trispiral tomography. Plaster immobilization is usually successful (Fig. 19-28). Just as for other intraarticular injuries, open reduction and internal fixation should be considered when the fracture fragments are unacceptably displaced or offset.

Author's Preferred Methods for Scaphoid Fractures

MIDDLE THIRD FRACTURES

1. *Fresh stable, undisplaced.* Short arm thumb spica cast.
2. *Fresh undisplaced but potentially unstable (vertical oblique or reduced trans-scaphoid dislocations) and stable fractures more than 3 weeks old.* Long arm thumb spica cast.

3. *Fresh displaced or angulated.* Open reduction and internal fixation (K-wires or Herbert screw).
4. *Nonunions, asymptomatic, stable.* Advise patient of strong likelihood of late osteoarthritis. Recommend PEMF treatment if fracture is less than 5 years old or Russe's bone graft. Otherwise, suggest yearly follow up with x-rays.
5. *Established symptomatic nonunions, without osteoarthritis, definitive avascular necrosis, or carpal collapse.* PEMF treatment may be used for stable, undisplaced nonunions less than 5 years old. Russe's bone graft for displaced fractures, or with bone resorption, and nonunions that are more than 5 years old.
6. *Nonunions with carpal collapse (DISI) without osteoarthritis or definitive avascular necrosis.* Anterior wedge bone graft with internal fixation (K-wires or Herbert screw).
7. *Nonunions with radioscaphoid osteoarthritis,*

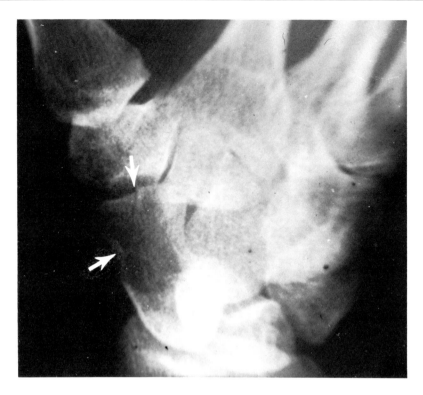

Fig. 19-28. A vertical fracture of the distal pole of the scaphoid *(arrows)*.

without avascular necrosis. Bone graft and limited styloidectomy.

8. *Nonunions with definitive avascular necrosis.* Replacement of proximal fragment with partial scaphoid implant.[117]

9. *Nonunions with osteoarthritis.* Partial or total arthrodesis, with or without concomitant use of a scaphoid implant.

PROXIMAL THIRD FRACTURES

1. *Fresh, full-third fractures.* 3-finger, long arm cast followed by short arm thumb spica cast.

2. *Delayed or nonunion, full-third fragment.* PEMF treatment in long arm thumb spica cast, followed by short arm thumb spica cast.

3. *Persistent nonunion, full-third, no avascular necrosis.* Matti or Russe bone graft, internal fixation across the proximal fragment into the lunate.

4. *Nonunion, after failed treatment, or with avascular fragment, and for very small proximal pole fractures.* Excise fragment and insert silicone partial implant.

DISTAL THIRD FRACTURES

1. *Fractures of the tuberosity.* Short arm thumb spica cast.

2. *Fractures of the distal third.* Short arm thumb spica cast.

3. *Intraarticular displaced.* Open reduction and internal fixation.

4. *Nonunions.* Very rare; may be amenable to Russe Bone graft.

ISOLATED FRACTURES OF OTHER CARPAL BONES

Fractures of the Triquetrum

Fractures of the triquetrum are more commonly associated with other carpal injuries (Fig. 19-29). Isolated fractures are much less frequent, although

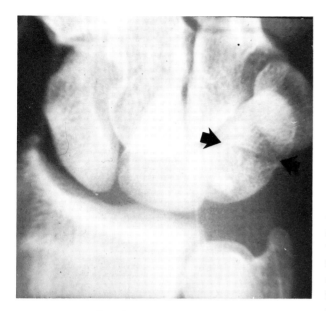

Fig. 19-29. A dorsal perilunate transtriquetral dislocation. Arrows point to a fracture in the body of the triquetrum.

they are reported to represent the second[16,28,192] or third[36,246] most common group of carpal bone fractures. The mechanism of injury may be a rotation or twisting motion, particularly if resisted[16,191]; a shear force applied by impingement of the hamate on the posteroradial projection of the triquetrum,[36] which occurs during falls with the wrist in dorsiflexion and ulnar deviation[36,60,62,192]; or a direct blow to the dorsum of the carpus.[16] There are two main types of triquetral fractures. The dorsal cortical fractures (Fig. 19-30A) are produced by either avulsion[16,191,192,234] or shear forces.[36] They are better seen in oblique and lateral radiographs and respond well to casting or splinting for 6 weeks. In my experience, these fractures become asymptomatic even in those cases with dorsal cortical fragments that remain ununited. The second type of fracture involves the main body of the triquetrum[16] (Fig. 19-30B). This type occurs less frequently than the dorsal cortical fracture, is usually

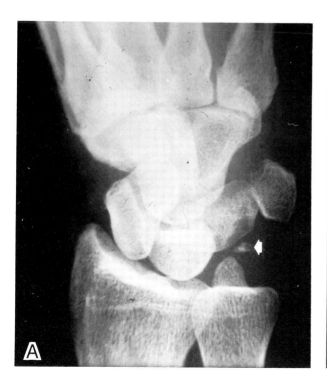

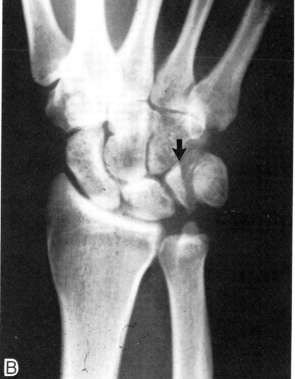

Fig. 19-30. Fractures of the triquetrum. **(A)** A dorsal cortical fracture *(arrow)*. **(B)** A fracture of the body of the triquetrum *(arrow)*.

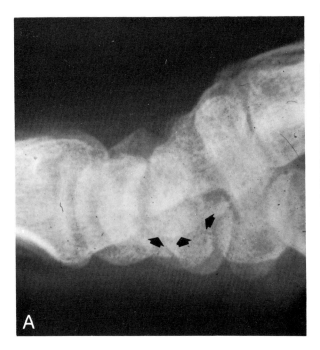

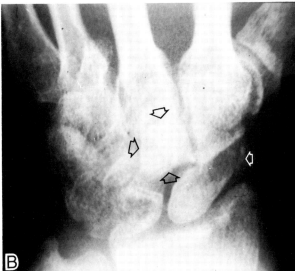

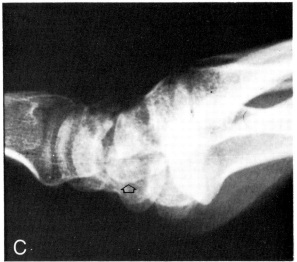

Fig. 19-31. Scaphocapitate fracture syndrome. (A) Initial lateral radiograph. The head of the capitate is rotated 90 degrees and lies volar to the body *(arrows)*. (B) Initial posteroanterior radiograph. Arrows point to fractures in the head of capitate and scaphoid. (C) Two year follow-up. The scaphoid fracture is healed. The head of the capitate remains displaced and ununited *(arrow)*. The patient is symptom-free. Wrist motion and strength are nearly normal.

undisplaced, and can be treated successfully by cast immobilization for 4 to 6 weeks. Nonunion can occur[68] but is exceedingly rare. Avascular necrosis has not been reported. Dislocation of the triquetrum is very rare, and should be reduced by closed or open means, as necessary.[219]

Fractures of the Capitate

Fractures of the capitate may be found in combination with other major carpal fractures or as isolated injuries to the body and neck of the capitate. A longitudinal fracture of the body was described by Guermonprez (quoted by Destot).[60] Bizarro[23] included six "incomplete" fractures of the os magnum in his series of carpal injuries, of which at least five were located within the body of this bone. In Böhler's review of 826 carpal injuries from 1926 to 1936,[28] only seven fractures of the capitate were found, a frequency of 0.8 percent. However, in 1962 Adler and Shaftan[2] reviewed 79 cases found in the literature and added 12 of their own. Forty-eight of these cases were isolated body fractures, 11 the so-called scaphocapitate syndrome, and 32 accompanied other carpal injuries.

The scaphocapitate syndrome consists of a fracture of the neck of the capitate with rotation of the proximal fragment, associated with a fracture of the waist of the scaphoid (naviculocapitate fracture syndrome)[153] (Fig. 19-31). The mechanism of injury may involve a direct blow to the dorsum of the wrist in volar flexion[36,78,230] or, more frequently, a fall on the outstretched hand with the wrist in dorsiflexion.[210] Fenton[77] postulated that dorsiflexion was accompanied by radial deviation, causing the waist of the scaphoid to be struck by the radial styloid. According to Fenton, the scaphoid fracture occurs first; when the injury force is not fully dissipated on the scaphoid, fracture of the neck of the capitate takes place; the malrotation of the proximal fragment was thought to take place consequent to a continuaton of the initial thrust. Stein and Seifel[210] demonstrated in cadaver specimens that the fracture of the capitate could be produced in forced dorsiflexion by the dorsal lip of the radius striking the capitate, while the scaphoid fractured in tension, created at the midcarpal joint level by the forced dorsiflexion. This mechanism of capitate

fracture had already been suggested by Destot.[60] With the loss of stability across the midcarpus secondary to this double fracture, an abnormal range of angulation in dorsiflexion becomes possible. The head of the capitate rotates together with the proximal fragment of the scaphoid. Upon cessation of injury, several radiographic patterns may be found,[230] most commonly a scaphocapitate fracture syndrome without dislocation (Fig. 19-31), or less frequently, accompanying a dorsal perilunate dislocation (Fig. 19-32). The diagnosis is entirely based on careful radiographic evaluation and can easily be missed. The injury may be labeled an isolated fracture of the scaphoid or a typical transscaphoid perilunate fracture-dislocation, and the lesion to the capitate overlooked.

In these cases, although carpal alignment may be restored promptly, either spontaneously or by manipulation, persistent displacement of the head of the capitate remains. Despite this, the fracture of the scaphoid can progress to union, and the patient may regain a pain-free wrist with minimal loss of function[2,230] (Fig. 19-31). Excision of the head fragment has been advised as the treatment for this condition.[77,78,141] Other authors[230] favor an anatomic surgical reduction of the head of the capitate, an opinion with which I concur. The reduction should be done if the injury is fresh or any time within the initial 3 to 4 weeks following injury. After this golden period, the handling of this injury becomes a matter of judgement, and nonoperative management may then be the treatment of choice, provided the fracture of the scaphoid goes on to heal and the patient remains relatively symptom-free. This can, of course, progress after several years to a painful midcarpal arthrosis, which may then be treated by a midcarpal fusion. When the injury is seen and surgically treated within the initial 3 to 4 weeks, internal fixation may be used for one or both of the carpal fractures (Fig. 19-32D), particularly if the reduction appears unstable. This should be followed by cast immobilization until union is apparent in both bones. Initial bone grafting procedures may be required for those fractures with severe comminution[242] and secondary bone grafts for delayed unions and nonunions. If the head of the capitate has become entirely avascular, as proven by direct observation in surgery, or is surrounded by poor articular surfaces, it may need

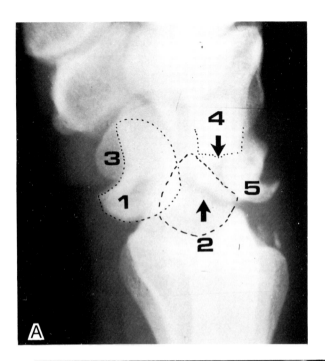

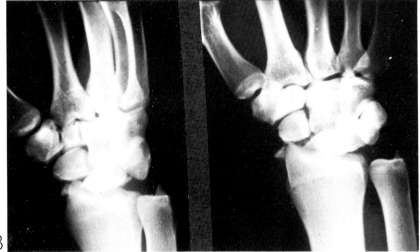

Fig. 19-32. A complex, comminuted transcaphoid, transcapitate dorsal perilunate fracture-dislocation. (**A**) Lateral radiograph. (*1*, Lunate; *2*, proximal scaphoid fragment; *3*, distal scaphoid fragment; *4*, neck of capitate; *5*, head of capitate.) (**B**) Posteroanterior radiographs. *(Figure continues.)*

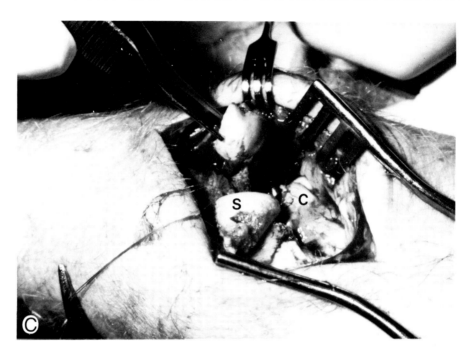

Fig. 19-32 *(Continued).* **(C)** Appearance at operation. Dorsal approach. The head of the capitate is held by forceps. (*S,* Scaphoid fragment; *C,* body of capitate.) **(D)** Radiographic appearance after open reduction and internal fixation. **(E)** Six months postoperatively.

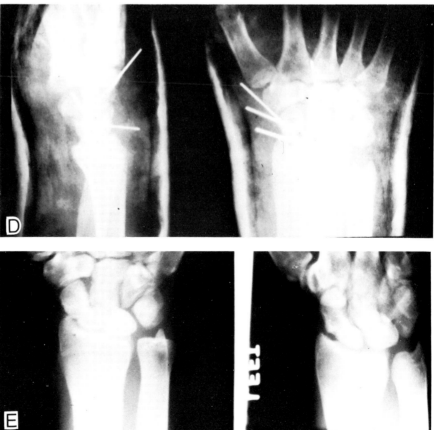

to be excised and treated by a fusion between capitate, scaphoid, and lunate. Kimmel and O'Brien[126] reported excision of an avascular head of the capitate and its replacement with an anchovy-type fascial graft.

Fractures of the Hamate

There are two main varieties of hamate fractures: those involving the body and those localized to the hamular process (hook).[155] From the clinical standpoint, these fractures may be remarkably similar. There is pain on the ulnar half of the wrist, localizing swelling, and tenderness, usually over the dorso-ulnar projection of the body of the hamate, even for those fractures of the hamulus without involvement of the body itself.[40,207]

FRACTURES OF THE BODY OF THE HAMATE

Detection of these fractures requires careful radiographic examination, often including several oblique projections until the plane of the fracture

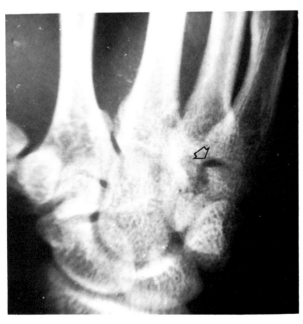

Fig. 19-33. A fracture of the body of the hamate *(arrow)*.

can be clearly seen (Fig. 19-33). The fracture line is usually oblique, either ulnar or, more frequently, radial to the radiographic projection of the hook.[155] Tomography or computerized tomography may also be of help in detection. Not infrequently, this type of fracture is accompanied by fractures at the base of the ulnar metacarpals. These are generally stable injuries and become asymptomatic after a period of immobilization of 4 to 6 weeks, even if fibrous union is present. This may be because the fracture line remains entirely extraarticular, or if it enters the carpometacarpal joint, it does so between the facets for the articulation of the fourth and fifth metacarpals. If the fracture fragments are displaced, an open reduction and internal fixation with K-wires should be done.[30,167]

FRACTURES OF THE HAMULAR PROCESS (HOOK OF THE HAMATE)

Fractures of the hook of the hamate may be easily missed. This injury should be strongly suspected when a deep, ill-defined pain is referred to the ulnar half of the wrist, particularly in golfers,[40,165,207,225] but also in tennis, baseball, and squash players.[40,207] Symptoms are aggravated when attempting to swing a golf club, tennis racquet, or baseball bat. Tenderness may be elicited by deep palpation over the tip of the hook of the hamate in the palm and by pressure on the dorsal ulnar aspect of this bone.[40,207] Lateral movements of the little finger against resistance increase the discomfort. Ulnar nerve involvement has been reported[114,194] and attributed to hemorrhage within the "loge de Guyon." [114,165,194] Flexor tendon ruptures may also occur by attrition against the rough irregularity of the fracture.[47,55,156,168,220] The fracture of the hamulus is most likely secondary to a direct blow produced by the butt end of a golf club, baseball bat, or tennis racquet, or following a fall, striking the base of the hypothenar area.[39,40,165,207,225] The diagnosis is confirmed by radiographic demonstration of the fracture. The carpal tunnel profile view described by Hart and Gaynor[105] is particularly helpful (Fig. 19-34). An oblique projection obtained with the hand in 45 degrees supination and the wrist in radial deviation[7] and dorsiflexion is also useful[165] (Fig. 19-35).

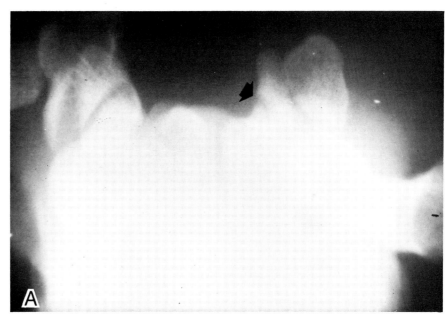

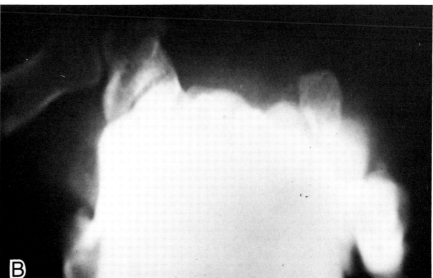

Fig. 19-34. (A) A fracture at the base of the hook of the hamate *(arrow)* in a carpal tunnel projection. (B) Post-operative appearance. The hook of the hamate has been excised.

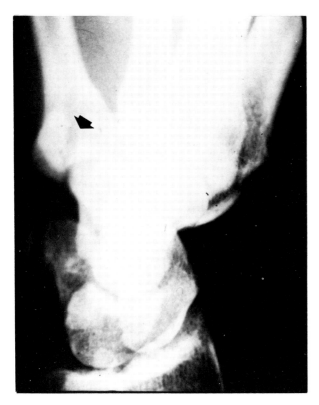

Fig. 19-35. A fracture of the hook of the hamate is seen in an oblique radiograph *(arrow)*, obtained in 45 degrees supination, slight radial deviation, and dorsiflexion.

In both these projections, demonstration of the hamulus may require several radiographs in slightly different degrees of rotation, until a satisfactory profile of the hook is obtained. Computerized tomography of the carpal tunnel is an excellent technique for allowing the hamulus to be seen.[176] With few exceptions,[155,225] the recommended treatment has been excision of the hook of the hamate fragment (Fig. 19-34B), even in fractures through the very base of the hamulus.

Technique of Excision of the Hook of Hamate

Aso, in 1984 (reported by Mizuseki et al[158]), and Mizuseki et al, in 1986,[158] proposed a medial approach, centered at the fifth carpometacarpal joint, and dorsal to the abductor digiti minimi. I have no experience with this approach. I have routinely excised the tip of the hamulus through a short palmar incision overlying the projection of the hook. Care should be taken to preserve the integrity of the motor branch of the ulnar nerve, which is in close proximity to the hamular process. In some patients there may be some difficulty localizing the fracture site, but subperiosteal dissection and gentle manipulation of the tip of the hamulus should lead to the site of nonunion. The fracture fragment is excised, smoothness to the base of the hook of the hamate is restored if possible, and this is covered by careful repair of the overlying periosteal layer. Postoperative cast immobilization is required only until acute tenderness subsides, after which a gradual return to full activities is allowed.

Fractures of the Trapezium

Isolated injuries of the trapezium are infrequent. Fractures are usually associated with fractures of other bones, usually the first metacarpal and the radius, while dislocations are extremely rare.[53,188] The mechanism of injury is not clear. Fractures may be secondary to direct injury, or may occur indirectly by longitudinal impact from the first metacarpal, rigidly fixed by thumb abduction.[103,127] Others[6,118] believe that the body of the trapezium may fracture as a result of thumb hyperextension, with the trapezium caught against the scaphoid[6] or the tip of the radial styloid.[118]

There are three main types of fractures: of the body, avulsion injuries, and fractures of the palmar ridge. The diagnosis may be suspected by the presence of localized tenderness and swelling following injury. Fractures of the ridge are tender immediately distal to the palpable distal tuberosity of the scaphoid. The tenderness in fractures of the body of the trapezium is more easily elicited anterior or dorsal to the tendon of the abductor pollicis longus, approximately 1 cm distal to the tip of the radial styloid. Thumb motions may be pain-free, but pinch between thumb and fingers is weak. Occasionally, fractures of the palmar ridge may result in symptoms of median nerve compression. The diagnosis is proven only by adequate radiographic examination. This should include the Bett's view,[219] obtained with the elbow raised from the cassette, the thumb extended and abducted, the hand somewhat pronated, and the hypothenar eminence rest-

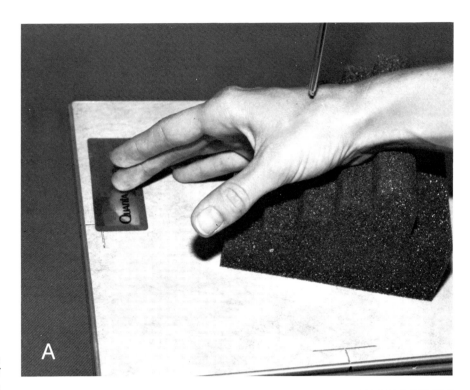

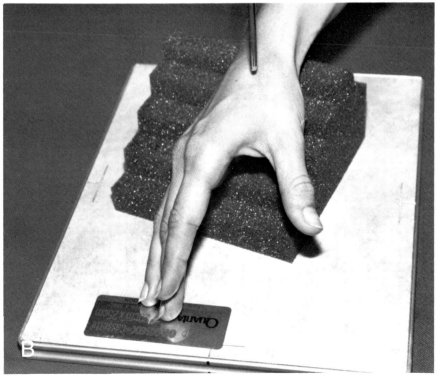

Fig. 19-36. Trapezium views (see text). **(A,B)** Position of the hand and wrist (Bett's view). (Taleisnik J: The Wrist. Churchill Livingstone, New York, 1985.)

ing on the plate. The center beam is directed to the scaphotrapezium-trapezoid joint (Fig. 19-36). A carpal tunnel view is mandatory when a fracture of the palmar ridge of the trapezium is suspected.

Undisplaced and avulsion fractures can usually be treated with plaster immobilization in a thumb spica cast for 4 weeks, followed by intermittent protective splinting and gradual mobilization. Displaced fractures are usually intraarticular into the trapeziometacarpal joint. The fracture line runs from this articulation to the dorsal and lateral surfaces of the trapezium, usually sparing the scaphotrapezium joint.[120] This creates a major fragment that, together with the first metacarpal, displaces dorsally and proximally.[120] These fractures must be exposed surgically, reduced accurately, and internally fixed with screws or, as I prefer, with K-wires.[53] Fractures of the ridge of the trapezium that remain symptomatic after a period of splinting are treated by surgical excision of the ununited fragment through a palmar approach.

For acute dislocations of the trapezium a closed reduction should be attempted. When this is unsuccessful, open reduction and temporary fixation for 3 to 4 weeks with K-wires is the procedure of choice. For neglected unreduced dislocations, when an open reduction fails, or with concomitant comminution, an excisional arthroplasty will produce a satisfactory result.[95,175] Aching pain, and weakness, may continue after intraarticular fractures have healed, usually due to progressive degenerative changes of the trapeziometacarpal joint. When these symptoms are disabling, treatment may be successfully provided by either a trapeziometacarpal arthrodesis, or an excisional arthroplasty of the trapezium with insertion of a soft tissue "anchovy."

KIENBÖCK'S DISEASE

Since 1910, when Kienböck[125] published his classic description of lunatomalacia, neither the etiology nor a reliable treatment for this condition has been established with certainty. Although Kienböck's own theory of the etiology of lunato-

malacia, attributing the collapse of the lunate to avascular changes, has been universally accepted, the actual cause leading to this vascular impairment has remained elusive.

Etiology

The loss of blood supply to the lunate has been attributed to primary circulatory problems,[13,132] to traumatic interference with circulation or ligament injury with subsequent degeneration and collapse,[65,125,144] or, more frequently, to single or multiple fracture resulting in secondary vascular impairment.[24,44,62,96,124,160,164,174,205,223] Although fracture-dislocations or dislocations of the carpus may frequently result in increased radiodensity of the lunate, this is a transient phenomenon that should not be confused with Kienböck's disease.[243] Whether fractures or fissures precede the avascular changes, or occur secondarily in the already weakened bone, has not been satisfactorily established.[219] There are actual simple fractures, following well-defined trauma, that do not develop into typical Kienböck's disease, and may heal without surgery. These fractures align along the frontal plane, and produce two large fragments of roughly equal size (Fig. 19-37).

In 1928, Hultén[115] published a study of the distal radioulnar relationship in normal wrists and in patients with Kienböck's disease. In 51 percent of the normal individuals, the distal articular surfaces of radius and ulnar were found to be at the same level; this was referred to as the *zero variant.* The ulna was proximal to the radius, the *ulna minus variant,* in only 23 percent. In contrast with this normal proportion, the majority of patients with Kienböck's disease (18 out of 23) showed an ulna minus stance (Fig. 19-38); only five cases showed a zero variant (Fig. 19-39). The ulna plus relationship was not present in any patient in this group of Kienböck's disease patients. Although no simple etiologic factor could be verified for this disease in Axelsson's extensive review,[12] enough objective data was found to support Hultén's minus variant theory. Gelberman and co-authors[90] also found a statistically significant relation between the ulna minus variant and Kienböck's disease, although it was not considered a *primary* etiologic association.

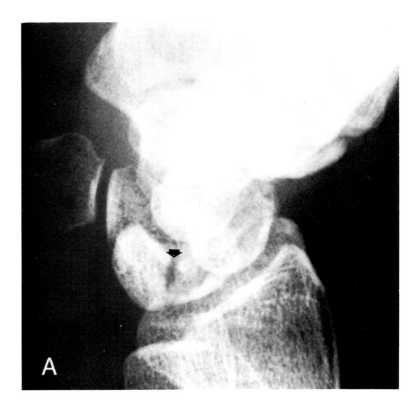

Fig. 19-37. (A) Lunate fracture *(arrow)* following a fall on the hand with the wrist in dorsiflexion, successfully treated by immobilization and the application of pulsing electromagnetic field treatment. (B) Appearance after 5 months of treatment. (Taleisnik J: The Wrist. Churchill Livingstone, New York, 1985.)

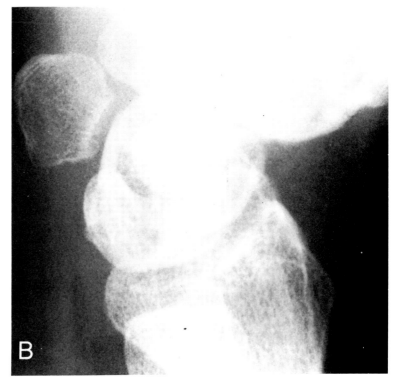

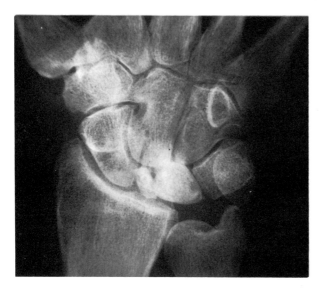

Fig. 19-38. A fragmented, avascular lunate. Note the ulna minus variant.

Stahl and Reis[206] observed the development of typical Kienböck's disease in the ipsilateral wrist of a patient with a pre-existent unilateral post-tramatic ulna minus deformity. They believed this to be additional evidence in favor of the etiologic relationship between lunatomalacia and ulna minus variants.

In 1966, Antuña Zapico[8] observed a relationship between the shape of the lunate and the length of the ulna (Fig. 19-40). He described a Type I lunate, seen in ulna minus wrists, presenting a proximal apex or crest (Fig. 19-40A). Types II and III were more rectangular or square, and coexisted with zero and plus variants (Fig. 19-40B and C). In Antuña Zapico's opinion, the trabecular pattern in Type I was the weakest (Fig. 19-40D), with a greater potential for bone fatigue and stress fracture under loads. Fragmentation was more frequent in ulna minus variants with Type I lunates. Razemon[178] pointed out that, in addition, ulna minus wrists provided poor coverage to the lunate; in these cases, there is a large portion of the lunate that is not covered by the radius, creating uneven stress under loads, with the radial half being the most susceptible to compression. A study of load stresses on the lunate[124] supports Hultén's theory, showing a concentration of forces on the lunate during dorsiflexion and ulnar deviation, and tensile forces on the distal surface of the lunate predisposing it to fracture. Armistead and co-authors[10] suggest that in extreme dorsiflexion, volar radiolunate

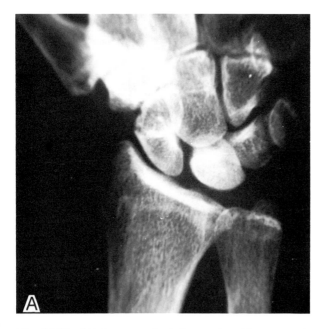

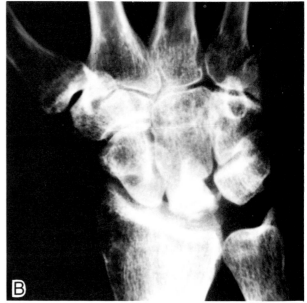

Fig. 19-39. (A) Lunatomalacia in a wrist with zero variant of radioulnar relationship. (B) Late lunate collapse and fragmentation in the same patient.

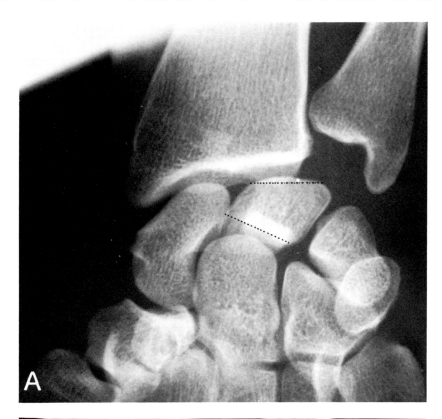

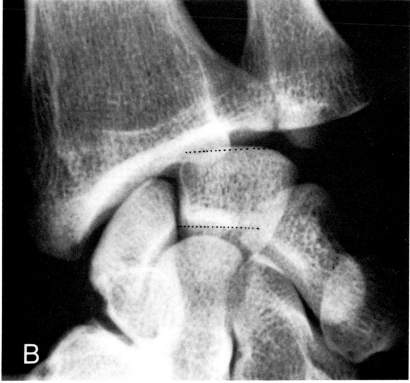

Fig. 19-40. Types of lunate and relationship with ulnar variance according to Antuña-Zapico. **(A)** Type I lunate coexists with ulna minus variant. *(Figure continues.)*

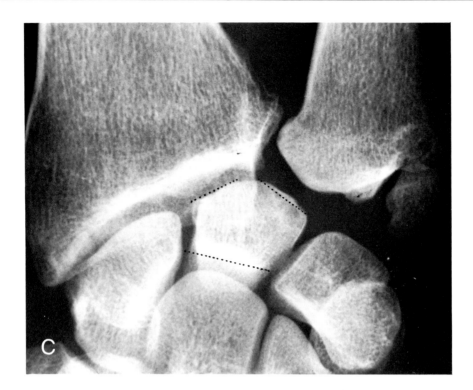

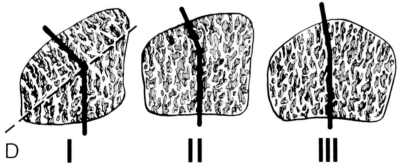

Fig. 19-40 *(Continued).*
(B), **(C)** Types II and III lunates coexist with zero and
ulna plus variants. **(D)** Trabecular patterns for Types I,
II and III lunates. (Taleisnik
J: The Wrist. Churchill Livingstone, New York,
1985.)

and lunotriquetral ligaments become tense. This is transmitted to the volar pole of the lunate. The triquetrum is able to shift proximally on the more compliant ulnocarpal complex, but the lunate is subjected to tension and "nutcracker" effect between the capitate and the radius (Fig. 19-41), resulting in failure, most frequently between the anterior and middle thirds of the lunate.

It is obvious that no single factor may be blamed for the development of Kienböck's disease. In all likelihood, lunatomalacia results from repeated compression strains and, more rarely, from a single severe compression force, possibly associated with tension loads on the concave distal surface of the lunate, producing a disruption of the intraosseous anatomy in patients with a vascular[92,131] or mechanical predisposition.[8] Synovitis, intraarticular effusion,[164] and the unavoidable continuous stress of normal function on this "carpal keystone"[144] interfere with any attempts at healing. This insidious combination of factors may render the lunate susceptible to a "nutcracker" effect between a

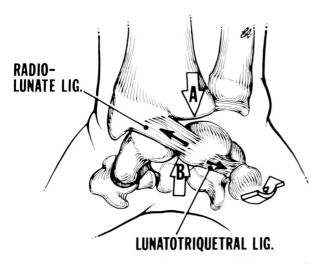

RADIO-LUNATE LIG.

LUNATOTRIQUETRAL LIG.

Fig. 19-41. In extreme dorsiflexion, the radiolunate and lunotriquetral ligaments become tense, producing equal forces of opposite directions acting on the lunate *(black arrows)*. The triquetrum is more likely to shift dorsally and proximally on the more compliant ulnocarpal cartilaginous complex *(right arrow)*. Added compression from the radius *(A)* and capitate *(B)* results in lunate failure. (See Ref. 10.) (Taleisnik J: The Wrist. Churchill Livingstone, New York, 1985. © 1985, Elizabeth Roselius.)

prominent radius and the head of the capitate, setting up a self-perpetuating mechanism of progressive lunate collapse.

Diagnosis

The diagnosis is made strictly upon radiographic examination. The condition may be suspected, particularly in young adults who present with pain and stiffness of the wrist and some swelling and tenderness localized dorsal to the lunate. A specific, severe traumatic event predating the onset of symptoms is frequently absent, although some form of injury is described by a significant number of patients. There is limitation of motion and a striking weakness of grip for the relative paucity of clinical findings. Symptoms of carpal tunnel syndrome have been reported,[17] stressing the importance of radiographic examination of patients with complaints of median nerve entrapment at the wrist, without symptoms suggestive of lunatomalacia.[219]

Radiographs may be negative initially, except for the ulna minus variant and a Type I lunate. If strongly suspected, early Kienböck's disease may sometimes be proven by trispiral tomography. Bone scintigraphy may show an abnormally high uptake by the lunate.[19] During the ensuing weeks, the typical radiographic findings, such as sclerosis of the lunate, progressive loss of lunate height, and eventually fragmentation, help to establish the diagnosis (Fig. 19-39). Later on, fragmentation of the lunate results in actual dissociation within the proximal carpal row, allowing the scaphoid and triquetrum to rotate in opposite directions: the scaphoid into palmar flexion (foreshortening), and the triquetrum into dorsiflexion (migrating distally on the hamate) (Fig. 19-42). The net effect is one of progressive loss of carpal height.[219] Eventually, degenerative joint changes develop (Fig. 19-43).

Treatment

The search for a universally acceptable treatment plan continues to this date, some 70 years after Kienböck's description. Although several authors have reported good results following simple excision of the lunate,[25,44,65,94,144,183] others have called this procedure a "crippling" or "mutilating" operation[205] and a useless procedure.[24] Ståhl[205] concluded that prolonged immobilization was the treatment of choice. This concept has never gained acceptance. Recently, however, evidence has been presented suggesting that patients not subjected to operative treatment rarely changed their occupations, while various surgical procedures resulted in inability to resume occupations in close to one half of cases.[190] Tajima surveyed 80 patients with Kienböck's disease seen during a 42-year period, without appreciable difference in the end results of nonoperative versus surgical treatment.[216] Evans and co-authors[74] also found satisfactory wrist function in long term follow-up of patients treated nonsurgically. A review of the literature, however, shows that a great number of different surgical procedures have been proposed for the correction of the multiple factors leading to lunate collapse or for the treatment of the collapsed lunate itself.[3,46,54,65,100,115,128,132,137,164,174,214] Attempts to revascularize the lunate[86] or to replace it with via-

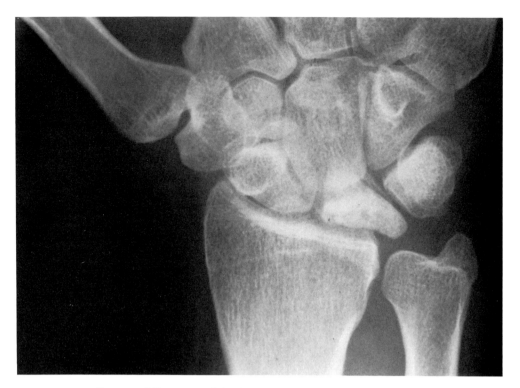

Fig. 19-42. Collapse and flattening of the lunate with radiographic evidence of opposite rotations of scaphoid (palmarflexed), and triquetrum (dorsiflexed). (Taleisnik J: The Wrist. Churchill Livingstone, New York, 1985.)

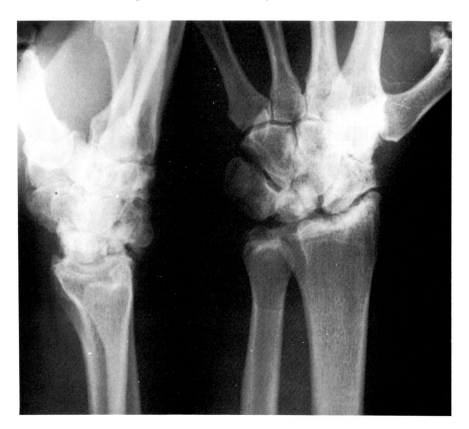

Fig. 19-43. Carpal collapse and degenerative changes 27 years following the onset of Kienböck's disease.

ble bone grafts[32,63,189] have produced inconclusive results. The following discussion is a review of those treatment modalities that have enjoyed more universal acceptance.

Lunate Implant Resection Arthroplasty

In an effort to prevent the shift of the remaining carpal bones after excision of the lunate, Vitallium,[137] acrylic,[3,56] and Silastic implants[214] have been proposed. Vitallium and acrylic prostheses have had only limited clinical trials, without widespread acceptance. Swanson's Silastic implant has been used extensively. Earlier problems with fitting and easy subluxation or dislocation of the implant (Fig. 19-44) have been solved to a considerable degree by changing its design to a deep-cupped shape, by careful reconstruction of the volar capsule or preservation of the volar cortex of the lunate,[17,214] and by the use of simultaneous limited intercarpal arthrodeses, when carpal instability and collapse are present (Fig. 19-45). Lichtman et al[134] correlated the results of lunate silicone replacement arthroplasty with four clinical and radiographic stages. In Stage I there is a linear or compression fracture, but otherwise normal architecture and density. In Stage II, density is abnormal, without lunate or carpal collapse. Lunate collapse indicates the onset of Stage III. In Stage IV extensive osteoarthritic changes are present. In Lichtman and co-author's experience,[135] and in that of Stark et al,[208] lunate replacement arthroplasties worked best for Stage III Kienböck's disease. Following this procedure, grip strength and motion improve, although never reaching preoperative values. In Stark and co-author's study[208] carpal collapse beyond that present preoperatively occurred in the majority of their patients after insertion of a hand-carved spacer. Hastings and co-workers[106] also found statistically significant collapse at an early postoperative date. Additional later collapse was not significant. Based on this experience, these authors advised against early use of implant arthroplasties of the lunate, recommending that they be deferred until after significant collapse of the lunate is present. In discussing this paper, Carroll[42] pointed out that symptomatic improvement is more important than maintenance of

carpal height, and suggested a longer follow-up before arriving at definitive conclusions.

Reports on the development of silicone particle synovitis[41,98,171,182,196,244] have resulted in increasing concern over the use of carpal implants (Fig. 19-46). The lunate implants, in particular, showed the greatest deformity, change in color, and opacification.[196] Smith and co-authors theorized that reducing compression loads on the implants by intercarpal arthrodesis might reduce deformity, fibrillation, and synovitis. They also suggested that, after intercarpal arthrodesis, the implant may serve little purpose. Therefore, there may be no need to remove or replace the lunate in these patients, an opinion also advanced by Watson et al.[238] My experience with lunate implants has been very satisfactory, perhaps because of the use of intercarpal arthrodesis whenever carpal collapse was actually or potentially present. However, it would seem reasonable to include yearly reexaminations in the postoperative protocol of these patients. Replacement of the implant, synovectomy and bone-grafting of reactive bone cysts, and the addition of intercarpal arthrodesis, when not previously done, may provide a satisfactory answer to these problems, if they are identified before major damage has occurred.

Technique of Lunate Implant Resection Arthroplasty. The following technique is based on Swanson's description, with minimal modifications. The wrist is approached through a longitudinal dorsal incision in line with the axis of the third metacarpal. Dorsal superficial sensory nerves are identified and preserved. It is convenient to unroof the extensor pollicis longus tendon and retract it laterally. The tendons in the fourth dorsal wrist compartment (extensor indicis propius and extensor digitorum communis) are left undisturbed within their retinacular synovial envelope and retracted medially, thus exposing the dorsal wrist capsule. This is carefully incised transversely, leaving attached to the dorsal lip of the radius a proximal capsular apron several millimeters long for capsular repair at the completion of the procedure. The lunate is best excised piecemeal, leaving, if possible, a very thin cortical wafer of bone still attached to the volar capsule. It is imperative that the volar capsule not be damaged. If a rent is created during excision of the lunate, it must be repaired. Traction and

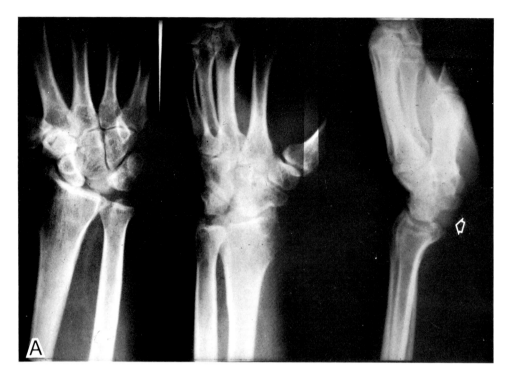

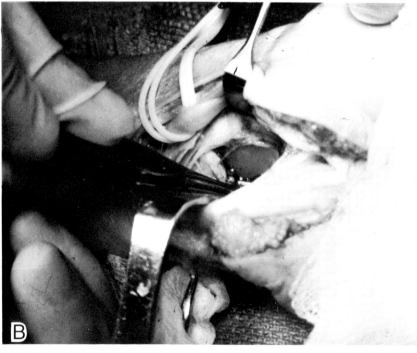

Fig. 19-44. Volar dislocation of a Silastic lunate implant. (**A**) The lunate dislocation is best seen in the lateral projection *(arrow).* (**B**) Volar dislocation of the lunate implant through the floor of the carpal canal. The causes of this complication are failure to repair a rent in the volar capsule and failure to support an unstable carpus through a simultaneous scaphotrapezium-trapezoid arthrodesis.

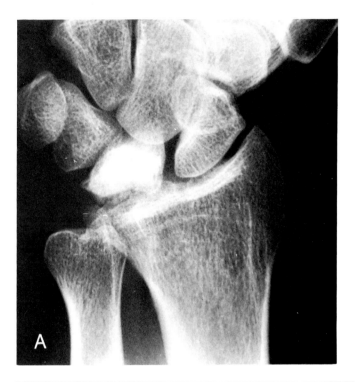

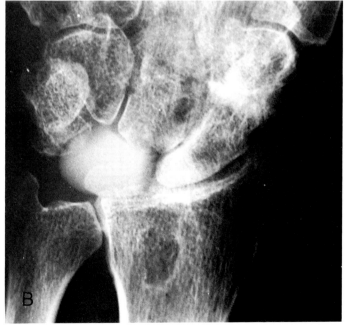

Fig. 19-45. Combined lunate implant arthroplasty and scaphotrapezium-trapezoid fusion for the treatment of Kienböck's disease. **(A)** Preoperative radiograph. **(B)** Radiographic appearance two years after scaphotrapezium-trapezoid fusion, and lunate implant arthroplasty. Carpal height and alignment are satisfactory and the patient is asymptomatic. (Taleisnik J: The Wrist. Churchill Livingstone, New York, 1985.)

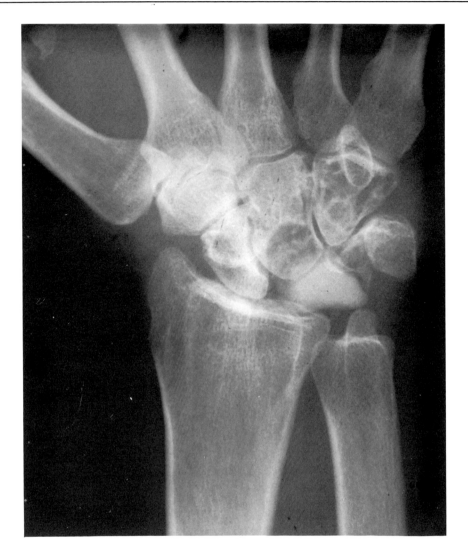

Fig. 19-46. Silicone particle synovitis after lunate implant arthroplasty for Kienböck's disease. Note carpal collapse, including ulnar translocation in this late (2½ year) follow-up radiograph. (Courtesy of David P. Green, MD.)

compression across the wrist at this point should provide information as to the potential carpal instability.[215] If this is present, a scaphotrapezium-trapezoid fusion should be considered (see Chapter 5). A proper size implant is selected, usually large enough to provide a snug fit with good stability as the wrist is taken through full passive motion; it should never be oversized. The stem in the implant is placed into a hole created in the triquetrum by impacting, rather than by removing bone. The implant may be sutured to the scaphoid using nonabsorbable material, secured through 1 mm drill-holes through the scaphoid (Fig. 19-47). A fine K-wire can also be used for additional fixation to

the scaphoid if necessary; it is left in situ 4 to 6 weeks. The newer high-performance elastomer allows placement of sutures and K-wires through the implant with reduced possibility of tear.[135] Although this penetration of the implant may theoretically increase the likelihood of particulate synovitis, this has not been my experience thus far. The capsule is repaired using nonasborbable sutures to the proximal capsular apron if strong enough, or to holes drilled through the distal radius for secure fixation. If the capsular layer is not sufficiently strong, it may be reinforced with a strip of extensor carpi radialis brevis tendon, woven through the capsule and the radius, dorsal to the

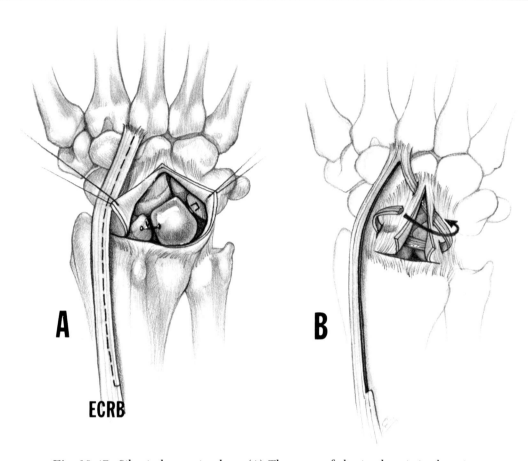

Fig. 19-47. Silastic lunate implant. (**A**) The stem of the implant is in the triquetrum; further fixation is secured by suture of the implant to the scaphoid with 2-0 nylon on an FS needle. (**B**) The ulnar third of the extensor carpi radialis brevis tendon is used to reinforce the dorsal capsular repair. The tendon slip should not be tenodesed to the radius to prevent loss of wrist flexion. (Taleisnik J: The Wrist. Churchill Livingstone, New York, 1985. © 1985, Elizabeth Roselius. Redrawn from Swanson AB: Stabilization Techniques for Carpal Bone Implants (Scaphoid, Lunate, Trapezium). Orthopaedic and Reconstructive Surgeons of Grand Rapids, Grand Rapids, Michigan, 1979.)

lunate (Fig. 19-47). Closure is completed and immobilization provided in a compression-type dressing for 5 to 7 days, followed by a short arm cast that is worn for a total postoperative immobilization of 6 weeks.

Intercarpal Arthrodesis

Partial carpal fusions have also been proposed for the treatment of Kienböck's disease.[67,76,100]

Capitate-Hamate Arthrodesis. Chuinard and Zeman[46] suggested that the capitate be fused to the hamate to prevent the proximal migration of the capitate–third metacarpal axis into the defect created by the gradual collapse of the lunate. According to these authors, this procedure should remove the distal pressure of the capitate on the lunate and allow revascularization (Fig. 19-48A). The carpal height is measured preoperatively, between the articular surface of the radius and the top of the head of the capitate, and is compared to that of the uninvolved side. When the difference in carpal height is 2 mm or less, only the capitate-hamate fusion is performed (Fig. 19-48B). When the difference is

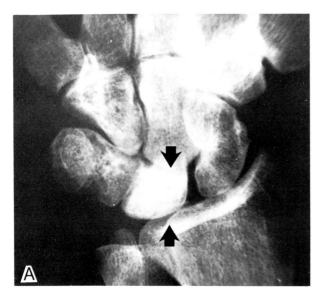

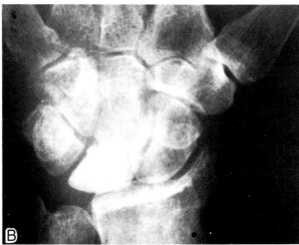

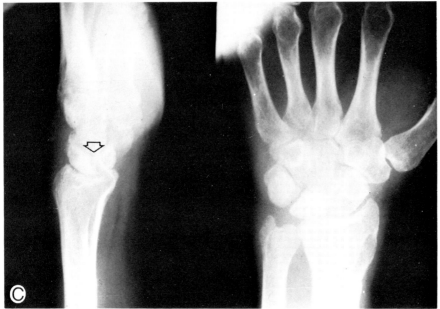

Fig. 19-48. (A) Lunatomalacia without loss of carpal height. Arrows represent the "nutcracker" effect of radius and capitate on the lunate. (B) Early postoperative appearance following capitate-hamate fusion. (C) Radiographic appearance 1 year after capitate-hamate fusion. Increased lunate density and a vertical fracture line *(arrow)* are still visible.

greater than 2 mm, Chuinard and Zeman recommend that, in addition to the fusion, the lunate be excised (Fig. 19-49). A replacement arthroplasty may be used in these cases. In my experience, this procedure has failed to maintain carpal height. In most patients the lunate has continued to show unchanged features of avascular necrosis or ununited fracture lines (Fig. 19-48C). In the normal wrist the capitate and hamate are already firmly bound by short, stout ligaments, and motion between them is virtually nil. Collapse of the lunate, and its fragmentation, allow collapse of the *entire* proximal carpal row, through foreshortening of the scaphoid and distal migration of the triquetrum on the hamate.[219] The lack of effectiveness of capitohamate fusions in reducing loads on the lunate has been shown experimentally.[228]

Scaphotrapezium-trapezoid Arthrodesis. Only a fusion designed to stabilize the midcarpal joint,

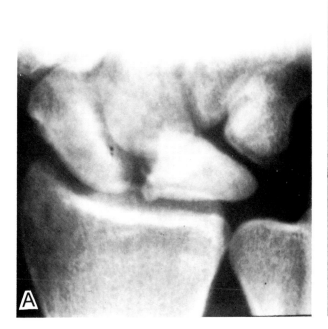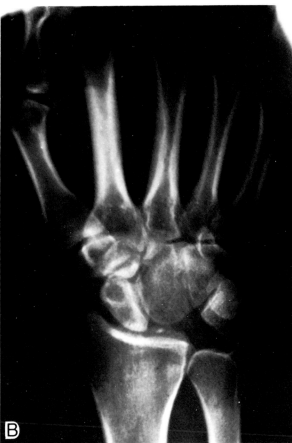

Fig. 19-49. (A) Lunatomalacia with carpal shortening greater than 2 mm. (B) Radiographic appearance 7 months after excision of the lunate and capitate-hamate fusion. Further proximal migration of the capitate is apparent. This wrist was eventually arthrodesed.

such as one between scaphoid, trapezium, and trapezoid,[236-238] can succeed in preventing carpal shortening (Fig. 19-45). The technique of scapho-trapezium-trapezoid arthrodesis is discussed in Chapter 5.

Ulnar Lengthening and Radial Shortening

The joint-leveling operations[12] (ulnar lengthening[10,59,74,174,197,223,231] and radial shortening[5,72,159,170,178,195]) have not, until recently, enjoyed much popularity in this country, in spite of the excellent late results reported. Their success is explained on the basis of postoperative changes in the radiolunate relationship. Of the two proce-

dures, shortening of the radius may be easier to perform, with less potential for postoperative pseudarthrosis and a more direct approach to decompressing the lunate from the corner of the radius. Ulnar lengthening works on the carpus by advancing the ulnocarpal complex "pad" ahead of the lengthened ulna. Disruption of distal radioulnar joint function has not been a problem. Although partial denervation of the wrist following this type of surgery may occur, this alone does not fully explain the long-lasting benefit obtained. Armistead and co-authors[10] have shown increased radiolunate distance following ulnar lengthening in intraoperative arthrograms obtained before and after ulnar lengthening. Trumble et al[228] have monitored lunate strain with electronic strain gauges, and found that bone leveling procedures were as effective as scaphotrapezium-trapezoid fusions in relieving lunate loading through a functional range of wrist and forearm motion. Their study revealed that a shortening of the radius or lengthening of the ulna of only 2 mm was required to maximize lunate decompression. This, of course, would greatly reduce the danger of postoperative radioulnar disruption, and eliminate the need to exactly make up the radioulnar length discrepancy.

The main attraction of "leveling" techniques is that the carpus is left undisturbed. They are indicated in patients with ulna minus variant, fair maintenance of lunate architecture,[184] preservation of the lunocapitate joint,[10] and absent degenerative changes. Joint "leveling" requires standardized radiographic techniques, to allow for exact measurements of radioulnar discrepancy (see Chapter 21 for a description of "zero rotation" radiographs).

Technique of Ulnar Lengthening[10] (Fig. 19-50). The distal third of the ulna is exposed subperios-

teally using a longitudinal incision along its subcutaneous border and between the extensor carpi ulnaris and the flexor carpi ulnaris. A partial osteotomy is performed through the medial three-fourths of the ulna. A plate with four or more slotted holes is placed, centered on the osteotomy. All screws are inserted closest to the osteotomy within each slot. The osteotomy is completed. A laminar spreader is used to distract the fragments to a width 1- to 2-mm greater than the ulna variant. A bicortical graft obtained from the iliac crest is inserted into the gap. Fixation is completed and the graft is trimmed as needed. Postoperatively, a long arm cast is used for 2 weeks, followed by a short arm cast for an additional 4 to 6 weeks.

Technique of Radial Shortening. Almquist and Burns[5] recommend a longitudinal radial-palmar approach to the distal radius. Dissection proceeds medial to the radial artery. The pronator quadratus and the origin of the flexor pollicis longus are exposed, the periosteum is incised along this inser-

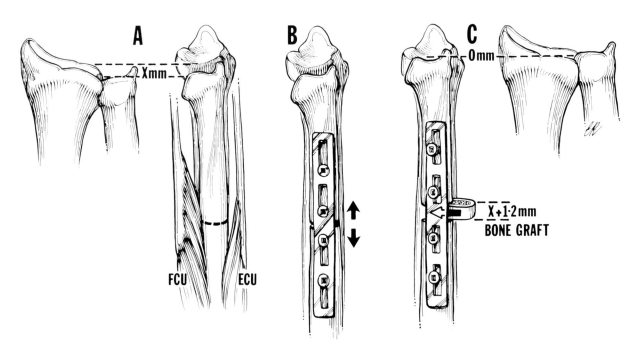

Fig. 19-50. Technique for lengthening the ulna. **(A)** Initial ulna minus variant. **(B)** Ulnar osteotomy and stabilization with a slotted plate. Distraction is applied *(arrows)*. **(C)** A bone graft is inserted, 1 to 2 mm wider than the ulnar variance. (Taleisnik J: The Wrist. Churchill Livingstone, New York, 1985. © 1985, Elizabeth Roselius. Redrawn from Armistead RB, Linscheid RL, Dobyns JH, Beckenbaugh RD: Ulnar lengthening in the treatment of Kienböck's disease. J Bone Joint Surg 64A:170, 1982.)

tion, and the radius is exposed subperiosteally. An osteotomy is performed and a wafer of radius as thick as the radioulnar discrepancy is removed. Fixation is provided using a T-shaped compression plate (Fig. 19-51). Closure is performed in layers. Immediate postoperative immobilization with a compression-type dressing incorporated into a long arm cast is changed 5 to 7 days later for a regular long arm cast. At 4 weeks, a short arm cast is used. The total postoperative immobilization is usually 8 to 12 weeks.

Wrist Arthrodesis

Radiocarpal fusion is indicated for those patients with Kienböck's disease who present degenerative joint changes at multiple levels or who show evidence of severe carpal instability, and for those cases that fail to improve following other surgical procedures (see Chapter 6).

Proximal Row Carpectomy

The indications for proximal row carpectomy[54,116,121] are similar to those of radiocarpal fusion, although its use for Kienböck's disease has been rather infrequent (see page 832 for the technique of this procedure).

Author's Preferred Method

Lichtman[134] suggested that treatment of Kienböck's disease must be correlated with the radiographic stage of the disease. In my opinion,[219] there are four variables to consider (Fig. 19-52): (1) the structural weakness of the lunate (common to all stages); (2) lunate collapse; (3) carpal collapse or instability; and (4) perilunate osteoarthritis. With this in mind, four stages may be considered. In Stage I, only the first factor is present. Treatment must be directed at "unloading" the lunate to prevent further damage. This may be accomplished by a scaphotrapezium-trapezoid arthrodesis or by a joint-leveling procedure. In Stage II, additional lunate collapse and fragmentation exists. Excision and replacement of the lunate, particularly if the lunocapitate joint is involved, is an excellent procedure. Silicone particle synovitis has not been a problem following lunate silicone arthroplasties in my experience. If fragmentation and joint disrup-

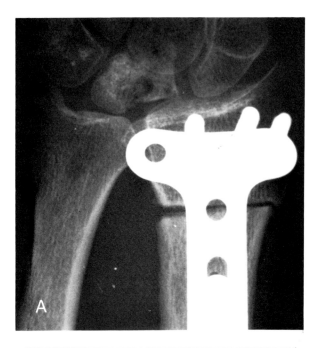

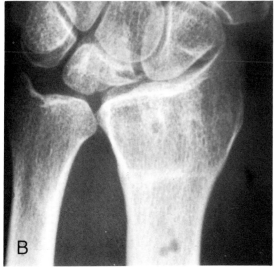

Fig. 19-51. Radial shortening for the treatment of Kienböck's disease. (**A**) Initial postoperative radiograph. (**B**) Late (2-year) postoperative radiograph. The patient is free of symptoms. The appearance of the lunate is improved. (Taleisnik J: The Wrist. Churchill Livingstone, New York, 1985. Courtesy of James R. Doyle, MD.)

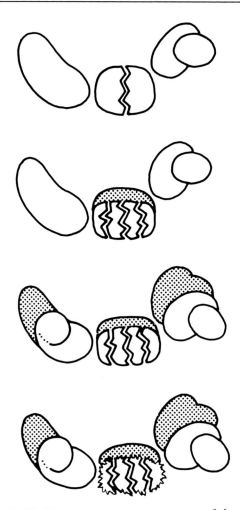

Fig. 19-52. Diagrammatic representation of the stages of progression of lunatomalacia (from top to bottom). (**1**) The lunate is not collapsed. Carpal alignment is normal. There is no osteoarthritis. (**2**) Lunate fragmentation and initial lunate collapse. Carpal height is normal. There is no osteoarthritis. (**3**) Lunate fragmentation and collapse, with carpal shortening and instability. There is no evidence of osteoarthritis. (**4**) The last stage, when perilunate osteoarthritic changes are present. (Taleisnik J: The Wrist. Churchill Livingstone, New York, 1985.)

tion are absent or minimal, an "unloading" technique may be used instead. When carpal instability appears (Stage III), my operation of choice has been excision of the lunate, replacement with a silicone implant, and correction of carpal collapse and restoration of loadbearing through a scapho-

trapezium-trapezoid arthrodesis. For Stage IV, more extensive arthrodesis, or a complete wrist fusion, should be considered.

REFERENCES

1. Adams JD: Fracture of the carpal scaphoid. A new method of treatment with a report of one case. New Engl J Med 198:401–404, 1928
2. Adler JB, Shaftan GW: Fractures of the capitate. J Bone Joint Surg 44A:1537, 1962
3. Agerholm JC, Goodfellow GW: Avascular necrosis of the lunate bone treated by excision and prosthetic replacement. J Bone Joint Surg 45B:110, 1963
3a. Agner O: Treatment of ununited fractures of the carpal scaphoid by Bentzon's operation. Acta Orthop Scand 33:57–65, 1963
4. Agner O, Rasmussen KB: Treatment of ununited fractures of the carpal scaphoid by Bentzon's operation. p. 131. In Stack HG, Bolton H (eds): Proceedings of the Second Hand Club, 1956–67. British Society for Surgery of the Hand, London, 1975
5. Almquist EE, Burns JF: Radial shortening for the treatment of Kienböck's disease. A 5 to 10 year followup. J Hand Surg 7:348–352, 1982
6. Anderson RL, Katz T: Function of the greater multangular bone (Report of two cases). West Virginia Med J 44:55, 1948
7. Andress MR, Peckar VG: Fracture of the hook of the hamate. Br J Radiol 43:141, 1970
8. Antuña Zapico JM: Malacia del semilunar. Tesis doctoral. Universidad de Valladolid. Industrias y Editorial Sever Cuesta, Valladolid, España, 1966
9. Archambault JL: Resined fiberglass cast for carpal navicular fractures. The Physician and Sports Medicine 8:83, 1980
10. Armistead RB, Linscheid RL, Dobyns JH, Beckenbaugh RD: Ulnar lengthening in the treatment of Kienböck's disease. J Bone Joint Surg 64A:170–178, 1982
11. Aversa JM: The electrical treatment of scaphoid nonunions. J Hand Surg 8:216, 1983
12. Axelsson R: Behandling av lunatomalaci. Elanders Boktrycker: Aktiebolag, Göteborg, Sweden, 1971
13. Axhausen G: Nickt malacie sondern nekrose des os lunatum carpi. Arch Klin Chir 129:26, 1924
14. Barnard L, Stubbins SG: Styloidectomy of the

radius in the surgical treatment of nonunion of the carpal navicular. J Bone Joint Surg 30A:98–102, 1948

15. Barr JS, Elliston WA, Musnick H, Delorme TL, Hanelin J, Thibodeau AA: Fracture of the carpal navicular (scaphoid) bone. An end-result study in military personnel. J Bone Joint Surg 35A:609, 1953

16. Bartone NF, Grieco RV: Fractures of the triquetrum. J Bone Joint Surg 38A:353–356, 1956

17. Beckenbaugh RD, Shives TC, Dobyns JH, Linscheid RL: Kienböck's disease: The natural history of Kienböck's disease and considerations of lunate fractures. Clin Orthop 149:98, 1980

18. Beckenbaugh RD: Noninvasive pulsed electromagnetic stimulation in the treatment of scaphoid nonunion. Orthop Trans 9:444, 1985

19. Bellinghausen HW, Weeks PM, Young LV, et al: Röentgen Rounds #62. Orthop Rev 11:73, 1982

20. Bentzon PGK: Redegorelse for virksomheden paa samfundet og hjemmet for vanfores orthopaediske hospital i Aarhus i 4-aarsperioden September 1936-September 1940. Nort Med 11:2366, 1941

21. Bentzon PGK, Madsen AR: Surgical therapy of pseudarthrosis following fractures of carpal scaphoid bone. Nord Med 21:524, 1944

22. Bentzon PGK, Madsen AR: On fracture of the carpal scaphoid: Method of operative treatment of inveterate fractures. Acta Orthop Scand 16:30, 1945

23. Bizarro AH: Traumatology of the carpus. Surg Gynecol Obstet 34:574–588, 1922

24. Blaine ES: Lunate osteomalacia. JAMA 96:492, 1931

25. Blanco RH: Excision of the lunate in Kienböck's disease: Long term results. J Hand Surg 10A:1008–1013, 1985

26. Boeckstyns MEH, Busch P: Surgical treatment of scaphoid pseudarthrosis: Evaluation of the results after soft tissue arthroplasty and inlay bone grafting. J Hand Surg 9A:378–382, 1984

27. Boeckstyns MEH, Kjäer L, Busch P, Holst-Nielson F: Soft tissue interposition arthroplasty for scaphoid nonunion. J Hand Surg 10A:109–114, 1985

28. Böhler L: Técnica del tratamiento de las fracturas. 3rd Ed. (Translated from German, Vol. 1, 7th Ed., by Schneider G, Jimeno Vidal F.) Editorial Labor SA, Barcelona, 1954

29. Bora FW, Ostermanm AL, Woodbury DF, Brighton CT: Treatment of nonunion of the scaphoid by direct current. Orthop Clin North Am 15:107–112, 1984

30. Bowen TL: Injuries of the hamate bone. Hand 5:235–238, 1973

31. Boyes JH: Bunnell's Surgery of the Hand. 5th Ed. JB Lippincott, Philadelphia, 1970

32. Braun RM: Pronator pedicle bone grafting in the forearm and proximal carpal row. Presented at the 38th Annual Meeting, American Society for Surgery of the Hand, Anaheim, March, 1983

33. Broomé A, Cedell CA, Colléen S: High plaster immobilization for fracture of the carpal scaphoid bone. Acta Chir Scand 128:42, 1964

34. Broström L-Å, Lindvall N, Stark A, et al: Compression screw fixation of nonunion of the carpal scaphoid: Long term results. Acta Orthop Scand 54:666, 1983

35. Brueckman FR: The Bentzon procedure for nonunion of the carpal navicular. Presented at the 1st meeting, Surg-Hands, Indianapolis, 1975

36. Bryan RS, Dobyns JH: Fractures of the carpal bones other than lunate or navicular. Clin Orthop 149:107–111, 1980

37. Burnett JH: Fracture of the (navicular) carpal scaphoid. N Engl J Med 211:56–60, 1934

38. Burnett JH: Further observations on treatment of fracture of the carpal scaphoid (navicular). J Bone Joint Surg 19:1099–1109, 1937

39. Cameron HU, Hastings DE, Fournasier VL: Fracture of the hook of the hamate: A case report. J Bone Joint Surg 57A:276–278, 1975

40. Carter PR, Eaton RG, Littler JW: Ununited fracture of the hook of the hamate. J Bone Joint Surg 59B:583–588, 1977

41. Carter PR, Benton LJ: Late osseous complications of carpal silastic implants. Presented at the 40th Annual Meeting, American Society for Surgery of the Hand, Las Vegas, January, 1985

42. Carroll RE: Discussion of carpal collapse deformity after lunate resection for Kienböck's disease. J Hand Surg 8:612, 1983

43. Carver RA, Barrington NA: Soft-tissue changes accompanying recent scaphoid injuries. Clin Radiol 36:423–425, 1985

44. Cave EF: Kienböck's disease of the lunate. J Bone Joint Surg 21:858–866, 1939

45. Cave EF: Injuries to the carpal bones. p. 376. In Cave EF (ed): Fractures and Other Injuries. Year Book Medical Publishers, Chicago, 1958

46. Chuinard RG, Zeman SC: Kienböck's disease: An analysis and rationale for treatment by capitate-hamate fusion. Orthop Trans 4:18, 1980

47. Clayton ML: Rupture of the flexor tendons in carpal tunnel (non-rheumatoid) with specific reference to fracture of the hook of the hamate. J Bone Joint Surg 51A:798, 1969

48. Cobey MC, White RK: An operation for nonunion

of fractures of the carpal navicular. J Bone Joint Surg 28:757–764, 1946

49. Cooney WP, Dobyns JH, Linscheid RL: Nonunion of the scaphoid. Analysis of the results from bone grafting. J Hand Surg 8:343–354, 1980

50. Cooney WP, Ripperger RR, Linscheid RL: Distal pole scaphoid fractures. Orthop Trans 4:18, 1980

51. Cooney WP, Dobyns JH, Linscheid RL: Fractures of the scaphoid: A rational approach to management. Clin Orthop 149:90–97, 1980

52. Cooney WP: Nonunion of the scaphoid. Orthop Trans 6:130, 1982

53. Cordrey LJ, Ferrer-Torells M: Management of fractures of the greater multangular. Report of five cases. J Bone Joint Surg 42A:1111–1118, 1960

54. Crabbe WA: Excision of the proximal row of the carpus. J Bone Joint Surg 46B:708–711, 1964

55. Crosby EB, Linscheid RL: Rupture of the flexor profundus tendon of the ring finger secondary to ancient fracture of the hook of the hamate. Review of the literature and report of two cases. J Bone Joint Surg 56A:1076–1078, 1974

56. Danis A: Osteomalacie du semi-lunaire traitée par exerese et prothese acrylique; résultat aprés trois ans. Acta Chir Belg 50:120, 1951

57. Dawkins AL: The fractured scaphoid: A modern view. Med J Aust 1:332, 1967

58. Dehne E, Deffer PA, Feighney RE: Pathomechanics of the fracture of the carpal navicular. J Trauma 4:96–114, 1964

59. Desenfens G: A propos de la maladie du semi-lunaire. Opération de Persson. Acta Chir Belg 1:58, 1953

60. Destot E: Injuries of the wrist: A radiological study. (Translated by Atkinson FRB) Ernest Benn, London, 1925

61. Dickinson JC, Shannon JG: Fractures of the carpal scaphoid in the Canadian Army. Surg Gynecol Obstet 79:225–239, 1944

62. Dobyns JH, Linscheid RL: Fractures and dislocations of the wrist. p. 345. In Rockwood CA Jr, Green DP (eds): Fractures. JB Lippincott, Philadelphia, 1975

63. Domoter E: Lunatum necrosis kezelese pisiform beuletessel. Magy Traumatol Orthop 17:192, 1974

64. Dooley BJ: Inlay bone grafting for non-union of the scaphoid bone by the anterior approach. J Bone Joint Surg 50B:102–109, 1968

65. Dornan A: The results of treatment in Kienböck's disease. J Bone Joint Surg 31B:518–520, 1949

66. Dunn AW: Fractures and dislocations of the carpus. Surg Clin North Am 52:1513–1538, 1972

67. Duparc J, Christel P: Traitement chirurgical des nécroses du semi-lunaire par arthrodése inter-carpienne. Ann Chir 32:565–569, 1978

68. Durbin FC: Non-union of the triquetrum. J Bone Joint Surg 32B:388, 1950

69. Eddeland A, Eiken O, Hellgren E, Ohlsson NM: Fractures of the scaphoid. Scand J Plast Reconstr Surg 9:234–239, 1975

70. Edelstein JM: Treatment of ununited fractures of the carpal navicular. J Bone Joint Surg 21:902–908, 1939

71. Edmunds JO Jr, Miller G, Stokes H, Haddad RJ, Riordan DS: Surgical management of carpal scaphoid non-union. Orthop Trans 6:360, 1982

72. Eiken O, Niechajev I: Radius shortening in malacia of the lunate. Scand J Plast Reconstr Surg 14:191, 1980

73. Enzler MA, Sumner-Smith G, Waelchli-Suter C, Perrin SM: Treatment of nonuniting osteotomies with pulsating electromagnetic fields. A controlled animal experiment. Clin Orthop 187:272–276, 1984

74. Evans G, Burke FD, Barton NJ: A comparison of conservative treatment and silicone replacement arthroplasty in Kienböck's disease. J Hand Surg 11B:98–102, 1986

75. Fajardo JC: Irrigacion del hueso escafoides de la mano. Rev Med Rosario 51:3, 1961

76. Fenollosa J, Valverde C: Résultats des arthrodeses intracarpiennes dans le traitement des necroses du semi-lunaire. Rev de Chir Orthop 56:745–754, 1970

77. Fenton RL: The naviculo-capitate fracture syndrome. J Bone Joint Surg 38A:681–684, 1956

78. Fenton RL, Rosen H: Fracture of the capitate bone: Report of two cases. Bull Hosp Joint Dis 11:134, 1950

79. Fernandez DL: A technique for anterior wedge-shaped grafts for scaphoid nonunions with carpal instability. J Hand Surg 9A:733–737, 1984

80. Fisk G: Carpal injuries. p. 101. In Pulvertaft RG (ed): Clinical Surgery: The Hand. Butterworths, Washington DC, 1966

81. Fisk G: Carpal instability and the fractured scaphoid. Ann R Coll Surg Engl 46:63, 1970

82. Fisk G: Unusual fractures of the carpal scaphoid. p. 129. In Stack HG, Bolton H (eds): Proceedings of the Second Hand Club, 1956–67. British Society for Surgery of the Hand, London, 1975

83. Fisk G: Treatment of fractures and joint injuries of the hand. p. 274. In Stack HG, Bolton H (eds): Proceedings of the Second Hand Club, 1956–67. British Society for Surgery of the Hand, London, 1975

84. Fisk G: Operative surgery, part II. p. 540. In Bent-

ley G (ed): Orthopaedics. Butterworths, Kent, England, 1979

85. Fisk G: Non-union of the carpal scaphoid treated by wedge grafting. J Bone Joint Surg 66B:277, 1984

86. Foucher G, Saffar Ph: Revascularization of the necrosed lunate, stages I and II, with a dorsal intermetacarpal arteriovenous pedicle. J Chir Main 1:259, 1982

87. Frykman G: Fractures of the distal radius including sequelae—Shoulder-hand-finger syndrome, disturbances in the distal radio-ulnar joint and impairment of nerve function. A clinical and experimental study. Acta Orthop Scand Suppl 108, 1967

88. Frykman GK, Taleisnik J, Peters G, Kaufman R, Helal B, Wood VE, Unsell RS: Treatment of nonunited scaphoid fractures by pulsed electromagnetic field and cast. J Hand Surg 11A:344–349, 1986

89. Gasser H: Delayed union and pseudoarthrosis of the carpal navicular: Treatment by compression-screw osteosynthesis. A preliminary report on 20 fractures. J Bone Joint Surg 47A:249–265, 1965

90. Gelberman RH, Salamon PB, Jurist JM, Posch JL: Ulnar variance in Kienböck's disease. J Bone Joint Surg 57A:674–676, 1975

91. Gelberman RH, Menon J: The vascularity of the scaphoid bone. J Hand Surg 5:508–513, 1980

92. Gelberman RH, Bauman TD, Menon J, Akeson WH: The vascularity of the lunate bone and Kienböck's disease. J Hand Surg 5:272, 1980

93. Gilford WW, Bolton RH, Lambrinudi C: The mechanism of the wrist joint, with special reference to fractures of the scaphoid. Guy's Hosp Rep 92:52, 1943

94. Gillespie HS: Excision of the lunate bone in Kienböck's disease. J Bone Joint Surg 43B:245–249, 1961

95. Goldberg I, Amit S, Bahar A, Seelenfreund M: Complete dislocation of the trapezium (multangulum majus). J Hand Surg 6:193–195, 1981

96. Goldsmith R: Kienböck's disease of the semilunar bone. Ann Surg 81:857–862, 1925

97. Gordon LH, King D: Partial wrist arthrodesis for old ununited fractures of the carpal navicular. Am J Surg 102:460–464, 1961

98. Gordon M, Bullough PG: Synovial and osseous inflammation in failed silicone-rubber prostheses. A report of six cases. J Bone Joint Surg 64A:574–580, 1982

99. Grace RV: Fracture of the carpal scaphoid. Ann Surg 89:752–761, 1929

100. Graner O, Lopes EI, Costa Carvalho B, Atlas S: Arthrodesis of the carpal bones in the treatment of Kienböck's disease, painful ununited fractures of the navicular and lunate bones with avascular necrosis, and old fracture-dislocations of carpal bones. J Bone Joint Surg 48A:767–774, 1966

101. Graziani A: L'esame radiologico del carpo. Radiol Med 27:382, 1940

102. Green DP: The effect of avascular necrosis on Russe bone grafting for scaphoid nonunion. J Hand Surg 10A:597–605, 1985

103. Green EI, Miller LF: Isolated fractures of the os magnum trapezium. J Bone Joint Surg 15:775, 1933

104. Grettve S: Arterial anatomy of the carpal bones. Acta Anat 25:331, 1955

105. Hart VL, Gaynor V: Roentgenographic study of the carpal canal. J Bone Joint Surg 23:382, 1941

106. Hastings H, Thornberry RL, Kleinman WB, Strickland JW, Steichen JB: Carpal collapse deformity after lunate resection for Kienböck's disease. J Hand Surg 8:612, 1983

107. Heim U, Pfeiffer KM: Small Fragment Set Manual. Technique recommended by the ASIF Group. p. 87. Spring-Verlag, New York, 1974

108. Helfet AJ: A new operation for ununited fracture of the scaphoid. J Bone Joint Surg 34B:329, 1952

109. Henry MG: Fractures of the carpal scaphoid bone in industry and in the military service. Arch Surg 48:278–283, 1944

110. Herbert TJ: Scaphoid fractures and carpal instability. Proc R Soc Med 678:1080, 1974

111. Herbert TJ: Management of the fractured scaphoid bone using a new surgical technique. Orthop Trans 6:464–465, 1982

112. Herbert TJ, Fisher WE: Management of the fractured scaphoid using a new bone screw. J Bone Joint Surg 66B:114–123, 1984

113. Hill NA: Fractures and dislocations of the carpus. Orthop Clin North Am 1:275, 1970

114. Howard FM: Ulnar nerve palsy in wrist fractures. J Bone Joint Surg 43A:1197–1201, 1961

115. Hultén O: Über anatomische Variationen der Handgelenkknochen. Acta Radiol Scand 9:155–168, 1928

116. Inglis AE, Jones EC: Proximal-row carpectomy for diseases of the proximal row. J Bone Joint Surg 59A:460–463, 1977

117. Irisarri C, Alcocer L, Galvan F, Perez-España M: Fracturas antiguas del escafoides carpiano. In Irisarri C (ed): Lesiones Traumaticas de la Muñeca y Mano. ENE Ediciones SA, Madrid, 1985

118. Jeanne LA, Mouchet A: Les lésions traumatiques fermées du poignet. 28th Congres Français de Chirurgie, 1919

119. Jones KG: Replacement of the proximal portion of

the scaphoid with a spherical implant for post-traumatic carporadial arthritis. Orthop Trans 6:474, 1982

120. Jones WA, Ghorbal MS: Fractures of the trapezium. A report of three cases. J Hand Surg 10B:227–230, 1985

121. Jorgensen EC: Proximal-row carpectomy: An end result study of 22 cases. J Bone Joint Surg 51A:1104–1111, 1969

122. Jorgensen TM, Andresen JH, Thommesen P, Hansen HH: Scanning and radiology of the carpal scaphoid bone. Acta Orthop Scand 50:663–665, 1979

123. Karev A: Utilization of a flexor carpi radialis tendon sheath flap for better closure of the capsule in the volar approach to the carpal navicular. J Orthop Surg Techniques 1:45–51, 1985

124. Kashiwagi D, Fujiwara A, Inoue T, Liang FH, Iwamoto Y: An experimental and clinical study on lunatomalacia. Orthop Trans 1:7, 1977

125. Kienböck R: Über traumatische Malazie des Mondbeins und Kompression Fracturen. Fortschr Roentgenstrahlen, 16:77–103, 1910–1911

126. Kimmel RB, O'Brien ET: Surgical treatment of avascular necrosis of the proximal pole of the capitate. Case report. J Hand Surg 7:284–286, 1982

127. Kindl J: Isolierte Handwurtzelknochenverletzungen. Beitr z Klin Chir 68:549, 1910

128. King AB: Kienböck's disease (Abstract). J Bone Joint Surg 46B:570, 1964

129. King RJ, Mackenney RP, Elnur S: Suggested method for closed treatment of fractures of the carpal scaphoid: Hypothesis supported by dissection and clinical practice. J Royal Soc Med 75:860–867, 1982

130. Landsmeer JM: Studies in the anatomy of articulation. I. The equilibrium of the "intercalated" bone. Acta Morphol Neerl Scand 3:287, 1961

131. Lee MLH: The intra-osseous arterial pattern of the carpal lunate bone and its relation to avascular necrosis. Acta Orthop Scand 33:43–55, 1963

132. Leriche R, Fontaine R: Contribution a l'etude de la maladie de Kienböck; son traitement par la sympathectomie perihumerale. Strassbourg Med 89:581, 1929

133. Leyshon A, Ireland J, Trichey EL: The treatment of delayed union and non-union of the carpal scaphoid by screw fixation. J Bone Joint Surg 66B: 124–127, 1984

134. Lichtman DM, Mack GR, MacDonald RI, Gunther SF, Wilson JN: Kienböck's disease: The role of silicone replacement arthroplasty. J Bone Joint Surg 59A:899–908, 1977

135. Lichtman DM, Alexander AH, Mack GR, Gunther SF: Kienböck's disease—Update on silicone replacement arthroplasty. J Hand Surg 7:343–347, 1982

136. Linscheid RL, Dobyns JH, Beabout JW, Bryan RS: Traumatic instability of the wrist: Diagnosis, classification, and pathomechanics. J Bone Joint Surg 54A:1612–1632, 1972

137. Lippman EM, McDermott LJ: Vitallium replacement of lunate in Kienböck's disease. Milit Surg 105:482–484, 1949

138. Logroscino D, DeMarchi E: Vascolarizzazione e trofo-patie delle ossa del carpo. Chir Organi Mov 23:499, 1938

139. London PS: The broken scaphoid bone. The case against pessimism. J Bone Joint Surg 43B:237–244, 1961

140. London PS: Ununited fracture of the scaphoid bone. p. 131. In Stack HG, Bolton H (eds): Proceedings of the Second Hand Club, 1956–67. British Society for Surgery of the Hand, London, 1975

141. Lucero B: Fractura del carpo en un niño. Bol y Trab Soc Arg de Cirujanos 10:260, 1943

142. Lutzeler H: Die Enstehungsursache der Pseudarthrose nach Bruch des Kahnbeins der Hand. Dtsch Z Chir 235:450, 1932

143. Mack GR, Bosse MJ, Gelberman RH, Yu E: The natural history of scaphoid non-union. J Bone Joint Surg 66A:504–509, 1984

144. Marek FM: Avascular necrosis of the carpal lunate. Clin Orthop 10:96–107, 1957

145. Margo MK, Seely JA: A statistical review of 100 cases of fracture of the carpal navicular bone. Clin Orthop 31:102–105, 1963

146. Matti H: Uber die Behandlung der Navicularefracture und der Refractura Patellae durch Plombierung mit Spongiosa. Zentralbl Chir 64:2353, 1937

147. Maudsley RH, Chen SC: Screw fixation in the management of the fractured scaphoid. J Bone Joint Surg 54B:432–441, 1972

148. Mazet R, Hohl M: Conservative treatment of old fractures of the carpal scaphoid. J Trauma 1:115–127, 1961

149. Mazet R, Hohl M: Fractures of the carpal navicular: Analysis of 91 cases and review of the literature. J Bone Joint Surg 45A:82–112, 1963

150. McLaughlin HL: Fracture of the carpal navicular (scaphoid) bone: Some observations based in treatment by open reduction and internal fixation. J Bone Joint Surg 36A:765–774, 1954

151. McLaughlin HL, Parkes JC: Fracture of the carpal navicular (scaphoid) bone: Gradations in therapy

based upon pathology. J Trauma 9:311–319, 1969

152. Melone CP Jr: Scaphoid fractures: Concepts of management. Clin Plast Surg 8:83, 1981

153. Meyers MH, Wells R, Harvey JP: Naviculo-capitate fracture syndrome: Review of the literature and case report. J Bone Joint Surg 53A:1383–1386, 1971

154. Michon J: Fractures et pseudarthroses du scaphoide carpien. Rev Chir Orthop 58:723–724, 1972

155. Milch H: Fracture of the hamate bone. J Bone Joint Surg 16:459–462, 1934

156. Minami A, Ogino T, Usui M, Ishii S: Finger tendon rupture secondary to fracture of the hamate. A case report. Acta Orthop Scand 56:96–97, 1985

157. Minne J, Depreux R, Mestdagh H, et al: Les pédicules artérieles du massif carpien. Lille Med 18:1174, 1973

158. Mizuseki T, Ikuta Y, Murakami T, Watari S: Lateral approach to the hook of hamate for its fracture. J Hand Surg 11B:109–111, 1986

159. Möberg E: Treatment of Kienböck's disease by shortening of the radius. Presented at the joint meeting of Japanese and American Hand Surgeons, Hiroshima, 1974

160. Mouat TB, Wilkie J, Harding HE: Isolated fracture of the carpal semilunar and Kienböck's disease. Br J Surg 19:577–592, 1931

161. Mulder JD: Pseudoarthrosis of the scaphoid bone (Abstract). J Bone Joint Surg 45B:621, 1963

162. Murray G: Bone graft for nonunion of the carpal scaphoid. Br J Surg 22:63–68, 1934

163. Murray G: End results of bone grafting for nonunion of the carpal navicular. J Bone Joint Surg 28:749–756, 1946

164. Nahigian SH, Li CS, Richey DG, Shaw DT: The dorsal flap arthroplasty in the treatment of Kienböck's disease. J Bone Joint Surg 52A:245–252, 1970

165. Nisenfield FG, Neviaser RJ: Fracture of the hook of the hamate: A diagnosis easily missed. J Trauma 14:612–616, 1974

166. Obletz BE, Halbstein BM: Non-union of fractures of the carpal navicular. J Bone Joint Surg 20:424–428, 1938

167. Ogunro O: Fracture of the body of the hamate bone. J Hand Surg 8:353–355, 1983

168. Okuhara T, Matsui T, Sugimoto Y: Spontaneous rupture of flexor tendon of a little finger due to projection of the hook of the hamate (case report). Hand 14:71–74, 1982

169. Olsen N, Schousen P, Dirksen H, Christofferson JK: Regional scintimetry in scaphoid fractures. Acta Orthop Scand 54:380–382, 1983

170. Ovesen J: Shortening of the radius in the treatment of lunatomalacia. J Bone Joint Surg 63B:231–232, 1981

171. Peimer CA, Medige J, Eckert BS, Wright JR, Howard CS: Invasive silicone synovitis of the wrist. Orthop Trans 9:193–194, 1985

172. Pennsylvania Orthopedic Society, Scientific Research Committee: Evaluation of treatment for non-union of the carpal navicular. J Bone Joint Surg 44A:169–174, 1962

173. Perschl L: Sur rontgenologischen Diagnostik der frischen Kahnbeinbruche der Hand. Rontgenpraxis 10:11, 1938

174. Persson M: Causal treatment of lunatomalacia. Further experiences of operative ulna lengthening. Acta Chir Scand 100:531–544, 1950

175. Peterson CL: Dislocation of the multangulum majus of trapezium and its treatment in two cases with extirpation. Arch Chir Neerl 2:369, 1950

176. Polivy KD, Millender LH, Newberg A, Phillips CA: Fractures of the hook of the hamate — A failure of clinical diagnosis. J Hand Surg 10A:101–104, 1985

177. Rasmussen KB: Bentzon's operation for pseudarthrosis of the scaphoid bone (Abstract). J Bone Joint Surg 45B:621, 1963

178. Razemon JP: Etude pathogénique de la maladie de Kienböck. Ann Chir Main 1:240, 1982

179. Rehbein F: Zur konservativen Behandlung der veralteten Kahnbeinbrüches und der Kahnbeinpseudarthrose der Hand. Arch Klin Chir 260:356, 1948

180. Rehbein F, Düben W: Zur konservativen behandlung des veralteten kahnbeinbruches und der kahnbeinpseudarthrose. Arch Orthop Unfall Chir 45:67, 1952

181. Robertson JM, Wilkins RD: Fracture of the carpal scaphoid. Br Med J 1:685, 1944

182. Rosenthal DI, Rosenberg AE, Schiller AL, Smith RJ: Destructive arthritis due to silicone: A foreign-body reaction. Radiology 149:69–72, 1983

183. Roth FB: Aseptic necrosis of the lunate bone: A case report with a study of the pathological changes. J Bone Joint Surg 25:683–687, 1943

184. Roullet J, Walch G: Technique d'allongement de l'ulna dans la maladie de Kienböck. Résultats au-delà de dix ans. Ann Chir Main 1:268, 1982

185. Ruby LK, Stinson J, Belsky MR: The natural history of scaphoid non-union. A review of fifty-five cases. J Bone Joint Surg 67A:428–432, 1985

186. Russe O: Fracture of the carpal navicular. Diag-

nosis, non-operative treatment, and operative treatment. J Bone Joint Surg 42A:759–768, 1960

187. Russe O: Die kahnbeinpseudarthrose, behandlung und ergebnisse. Hefte Unfallheikd 148:129–134, 1980

188. Russell TB: Inter-carpal dislocations and fracture-dislocations: A review of fifty-nine cases. J Bone Joint Surg 31B:524–531, 1949

189. Saffar Ph: Remplacement du semi-lunaire par le pisiforme. Description d'une nouvelle technique pour le traitement de la maladie de Kienböck. Ann Chir Main 1:276, 1982

190. Saffar Ph, Gentaz R: Comparaison entre le traitement medical et chirurgical de la maladie de Kienböck. Ann Chir Main 1:250, 1982

191. Scaramuzza RGJ: El movimiento de rotacion en el carpo y su relacion con la fisiopatologia de sus lesiones traumaticas. Bol y Trabajos de la Sociedad Argentina de Orthopedia y Traumatologia 34:337, 1969

192. Sgrosso JA: Traumatismos del carpo: Tratamiento. p. 1–140. Decimosexto Congreso Argentino de Cirugia, Buenos Aires, 1944

193. Sgrosso JA, Ananos V: Sobre el mecanismo de las fracturas del escafoides carpiano. Rev Ortop Traumatol 18:183, 1948

194. Shea JD, McClain EJ: Ulnar nerve compression syndromes at and below the wrist. J Bone Joint Surg 51A:1095–1103, 1969

195. Simmons EH, Dommissee IG: An investigation into the pathogenesis and treatment of Kienböck's disease. Presented at the 35th Annual Meeting, American Society for Surgery of the Hand, Atlanta, 1980

196. Smith RJ, Atkinson RE, Jupiter JB: Silicone synovitis of the wrist. J Hand Surg 10A:47–60, 1985

197. Sommelet J, Hahn P, Schmitt D, et al: L'allongement du cubitus dans le traitement de la maladie de Kienböck. Rev Chir Orthop 56:731, 1970

198. Soto-Hall R, Haldeman KO: Treatment of fractures of the carpal scaphoid. J Bone Joint Surg 16:822–828, 1934

199. Soto-Hall R, Haldeman KO: The conservative and operative treatment of fractures of the carpal scaphoid (navicular). J Bone Joint Surg 23:841–850, 1941

200. Speed K: Injuries of the carpal bones. Surg Clin North Am 25:1–13, 1945

201. Speed K: Fractures and dislocations of the carpus. Calif Med 72:93, 1950

202. Sprague B, Justis EJ: Nonunion of the carpal navicular: Modes of treatment. Arch Surg 108:692–697, 1974

203. Sprague HH, Koniuch MP, Osterman AL, Carter P, Burandt D, DuShuttle RP, Bora FW, Benton L: Use of the Herbert screw for scaphoid fractures. Orthop Trans 9:176, 1985

204. Squire M: Carpal mechanics and trauma. J Bone Joint Surg 41B:210, 1959

205. Ståhl F: On lunatomalacia (Kienböck's disease): Clinical and roentgenological study, especially on its pathogenesis and late results of immobilization treatment. Acta Chir Scand (suppl) 126:1–133, 1947

206. Stahl S, Reis D: Traumatic ulnar variance in Kienböck's disease. J Hand Surg 11A:95–97, 1986

207. Stark HH, Jobe FW, Boyes JH, Ashworth CR: Fracture of the hook of the hamate in athletes. J Bone Joint Surg 59A:575–582, 1977

208. Stark HH, Zemel NP, Ashworth CR: Use of a hand-carved silicone-rubber spacer for advanced Kienböck's disease. J Bone Joint Surg 63A:1359–1370, 1981

209. Stecher WR: Roentgenography of the carpal navicular bone. Am J Roentgenol 37:704–705, 1937

210. Stein F, Siegel MW: Naviculocapitate fracture syndrome. A case report: New thoughts on the mechanism of injury. J Bone Joint Surg 51A:391, 1969

211. Stewart MJ: Fractures of the carpal navicular (scaphoid): A report of 436 cases. J Bone Joint Surg 36A:998–1006, 1954

212. Stordahl A, Schjöth A, Woxholt G, Fjermeros H: Bone scanning of fractures of the scaphoid. J Hand Surg 9B:189–190, 1984

213. Sutro CJ: Treatment of nonunion of the carpal navicular bone. Surgery 20:536, 1946

214. Swanson AB: Silicone rubber implants for the replacement of the carpal scaphoid and lunate bones. Orthop Clin North Am 1:299–309, 1970

215. Swanson AB, Maupin BK, Swanson G de Groot, Ganzhorn RW, Moss SH: Lunate implant resection arthroplasty: Long term results. J Hand Surg 10A:1013–1024, 1985

216. Tajima T: An investigation of the treatment of Kienböck's disease. J Bone Joint Surg 48A:1649, 1966

217. Taleisnik J: Wrist: Anatomy, function and injury. p. 61. AAOS Instructional Course Lectures, Vol. 27. CV Mosby, St Louis, 1978

218. Taleisnik J, Kelly PJ: The extraosseous and intraosseous blood supply of the scaphoid bone. J Bone Joint Surg 48A:1125–1137, 1966

219. Taleisnik J: The Wrist. Churchill Livingstone, New York, 1985

220. Teissier J, Escare P, Asencio G, et al: Rupture of the flexor tendons of the little finger in fractures of

the hook of the hamate bone. Report of two cases. Ann Chir Main 2:319–327, 1983

221. Terry DW, Ramin JE: The navicular fat strip: A useful roentgen feature for evaluating wrist trauma. Am J Roentgenol 124:25–28, 1975

222. Therkelsen F, Andersen K: Lunatomalacia. Acta Chir Scand 97:503–526, 1949

223. Tillberg B: Kienböck's disease treated with osteotomy to lengthen ulna. Acta Orthop Scand 39:359–368, 1968

224. Todd AH: Fractures of the carpal scaphoid. Br J Surg 9:7–26, 1921

225. Torisu T: Fracture of the hook of the hamate by a golfswing. Clin Orthop 83:91–94, 1972

226. Torngren S, Sandqvist S: Pseudoarthrosis in the scaphoid bone treated by grafting with autogenous bone peg: A follow up study. Acta Orthop Scand 45:82–88, 1974

227. Trojan E: Grafting of ununited fractures of the scaphoid. Proc R Soc Med 67:1078, 1974

228. Trumble T, Glisson RR, Seaber AV, Urbaniak JR: A biomechanical comparison of the methods for treating Kienböck's disease. J Hand Surg 11A:88–93, 1986

229. Unger HS, Stryker WC: Nonunion of the carpal navicular: Analysis of 42 cases treated by the Russe procedure. South Med J 62:620–622, 1969

230. Vance RM, Gelberman RH, Evans EF: Scaphocapitate fractures: Patterns of dislocation, mechanism of injury, and preliminary results of treatment. J Bone Joint Surg 62A:271–276, 1980

231. Verbrugge J, Verjans H: L'allongement du cubitus comme traitement de choix de la maladie de Kienböck. Rev Chir Orthop 49:563, 1963

232. Verdan C: Le role du ligament anterieur radiocarpien dans les fractures du scaphoide: Deductions therapeutiques. Z Unfallmed Berufskr 54:299, 1954

233. Verdan C, Narakas A: Fractures and pseudoarthrosis of the scaphoid. Surg Clin North Am 48A:1083–1095, 1968

234. Wagner CJ: Fracture-dislocations of the wrist. Clin Orthop 15:181–196, 1959

235. Warner WC, Freeland AE, McAndrew JC: The scaphoid staple for stabilization of selected fractures and nonunions. Presented at the 35th Annual Meeting, American Society for Surgery of the Hand, Atlanta, 1980

236. Watson HK: Limited wrist arthrodesis. Clin Orthop 149:126–136, 1980

237. Watson HK, Hempton RF: Limited wrist arthrodesis. I. The triscaphoid joint. J Hand Surg 5:320–327, 1980

238. Watson HK, Ryu J, DiBella A: An approach to Kienböck's disease: Triscaphe arthrodesis. J Hand Surg 10A:179–187, 1985

239. Watson-Jones R: Fractures and Joint Injuries, Vol. 2, 4th Ed. Williams & Wilkins, Baltimore, 1960

240. Weber ER: Biomechanical implications of scaphoid waist fractures. Clin Orthop 149:83–89, 1980

241. Weber ER, Chao EY: An experimental approach to the mechanism of scaphoid waist fractures. J Hand Surg 3:142–153, 1978

242. Weseley MS, Barenfield PA: Trans-scaphoid, transcapitate, transtriquetral perilunate fracture dislocation of the wrist: A case report. J Bone Joint Surg 54A:1073–1078, 1972

243. White RE, Omer GE: Transient vascular compromise of the lunate after fracture-dislocation or dislocation of the carpus. J Hand Surg 9A:181–184, 1984

244. Wickham MG, Rudolph R, Abraham JL: Silicone identification in prosthesis-associated fibrous capsule. Science 199:437–439, 1978

245. Wilhelm K, Feldmeier C, Hauer G: Die behandlung von navikulare-frakturen und navikulare-pseudarthrosen mit elektrischen und magnetischen potentialen. Munch Med zzwschr 116:2191–2194, 1974

246. Wiot JF, Dorst JP: Less common fractures and dislocations of the wrist. Radiol Clin North Am 4:261, 1966

247. Zemel NP, Stark HH, Ashworth CR, Rickard TA, Anderson DR: Treatment of selected patients with an ununited fracture of the proximal part of the scaphoid by excision of the fragment and insertion of a carved silicone-rubber spacer. J Bone Joint Surg 66A:510–517, 1984

Carpal Dislocations and Instabilities

20

David P. Green

The past decade has seen a tremendous resurgence of interest in carpal bone injuries. Meticulous anatomic dissections, sophisticated biomechanical investigations, and many excellent clinical research studies have enhanced our knowledge of carpal anatomy, function, and derangement, but many questions remain unanswered and a number of clinical problems await a definitive, highly predictable method of treatment. In the short span of five years since this chapter was written for the first edition, there has been a veritable flood of papers related to this topic, and information from 141 new references has been incorporated into this revision. Again, an attempt has been made to summarize the current state of our knowledge, realizing that a truly comprehensive understanding of carpal bone injuries has not yet been achieved.

ANATOMY AND FUNCTION

Osseous Anatomy

Traditional Concept

The seven major carpal bones (excluding the pisiform, which is a sesamoid) are arranged into two transverse rows, proximal and distal, with the scaphoid bridging the two rows and in fact being part of each (Fig. 20-1A). The distal row consists of the hamate, capitate, trapezoid, trapezium, and distal pole of scaphoid; the proximal row consists of the triquetrum, lunate, and proximal pole of the scaphoid. Thus, the so-called wrist joint is actually two separate articulations, the radiocarpal and midcarpal joints. In 1943, Lambrinudi and his associates[77] pointed out that because of this arrangement, the wrist is a "link joint," which would be inherently unstable to compression forces were it not for the scaphoid, which acts as a bridge across the link to stabilize it (Fig. 20-2). Fisk[67] later expanded this concept by noting that if it is accepted that the scaphoid braces the midcarpal joint, it must be equally true that the intact midcarpal joint must support the scaphoid.

Columnar Carpus Concept

Taleisnik[222] reintroduced the concept of a vertical or columnar carpus that was originally proposed by Navarro in 1919 (Fig. 20-1B). As originally described, this theory suggested that the carpus is composed of three vertical columns: (1) the *central* flexion-extension) column, formed by the lunate, capitate, and hamate; (2) the *lateral* (mobile) column, composed of the scaphoid, trapezium, and trapezoid; and (3) the *medial* (rotation) column, consisting of the triquetrum and pisiform. The

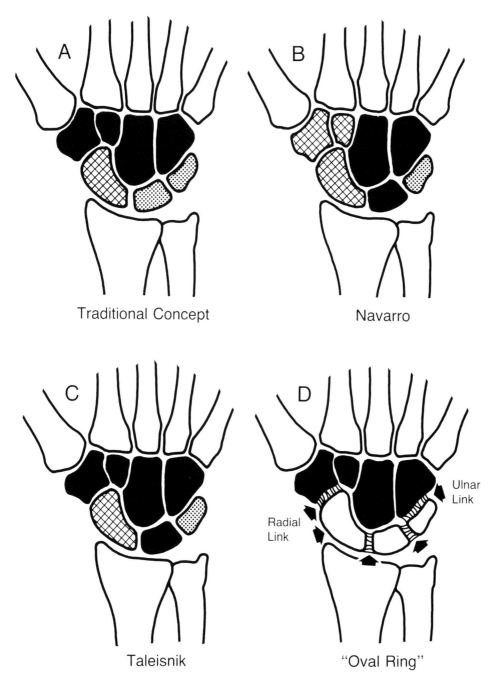

Fig. 20-1. Several theories have been postulated to describe the arrangement of the carpal bones with respect to function. (**A**) The traditional concept of two transverse rows with the scaphoid bridging the two; (**B**) Navarro's columnar carpus concept; (**C**) Taleisnik's modification of Navarro's theory; and (**D**) Lichtman's oval ring concept. (See text for descriptions of each). (**B,C,** and **D** redrawn from Lichtman DM, Schneider JR, Swafford AR, Mack GR: Ulnar midcarpal instability—Clinical and laboratory analysis. J Hand Surg 6:522, 1981.)

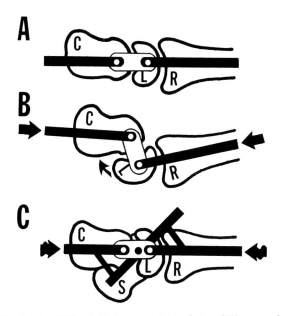

Fig. 20-2. Gilford, Bolton, and Lambrinudi[77] were the first to suggest the analogy between the wrist and a link joint, noting that it is inherently unstable in compression because of the intercalated segment (the proximal row, represented here by the lunate, *L*). The scaphoid *(S)* acts as a bridge across the link and stabilizes it against compression forces during normal flexion and extension of the wrist. (Modified from Gilford WW, Bolton RH, Lambrinudi C: The mechanism of the wrist joint with special reference to fractures of the scaphoid. Guy's Hosp Rep 92:52–59, 1943.)

major point of difference in this concept from the traditional concept is that the triquetrum is given recognition as an important part of the complex carpal anatomy. Taleisnik has proposed two modifications to this theory: (1) eliminate the pisiform, since it does not actually participate in carpal motion; and (2) include the trapezium and trapezoid as part of the central column, since they are integral parts of the distal carpal row (Fig. 20-1C). Thus, the central column is the main flexion-extension link along the axis of the radius, lunate, and capitate (with the entire distal row acting in concert with the capitate). The scaphoid maintains its previously well-recognized role as the stabilizing or connecting link for the midcarpal joint, and the triquetrum is introduced as the pivot point around which carpal and hand rotation takes place.

Oval Ring Concept

Lichtman[6,133] believes that the lunate should not be considered a part of the rigid central column because there is considerable mobility between the capitate and lunate, both in flexion and extension and in radial and ulnar deviation. He has therefore proposed the "oval ring" concept, which considers the carpus to be a ring with two physiological mobile links to permit reciprocal motion between the proximal and distal rows during radial and ulnar deviation. These links are the mobile scaphotrapezial joint and the rotatory triquetrohamate joint, but a break in the ring at *any* point (see arrows in Fig. 20-1D) will produce abnormal motion or carpal instability. That break can be a ligamentous disruption or a fracture.

Longitudinal Columns Concept

Weber's biomechanical studies[249] have led him to visualize the carpal bones from yet another, somewhat different, approach (Fig. 20-3). He divides the carpus into two longitudinal columns, as follows.

1. *Force-bearing column.* The bones on the radial side of the carpus transmit forces generated by the hand to the forearm unit. The force-bearing column thus consists of the distal radial articular surface, lunate, proximal two-thirds of the scaphoid, capitate, trapezoid, and bases of the second and third metacarpals.
2. *Control column.* Weber emphasizes the important role of the inclined slope of the triquetrohamate joint that serves to position the lunate relative to the stable capitate. Thus the control column consists of the distal ulna, triangular fibrocartilage, triquetrum, hamate, and bases of the fourth and fifth metacarpals. The helicoid configuration of the triquetrohamate joint causes compressive forces transmitted by the hamate to displace the triquetrum ulnarly.

The apparent contradictions among these various concepts of carpal function may tend to confuse rather than clarify, but it seems to me that each offers important principles necessary in trying to comprehend the complex nature of the wrist. The

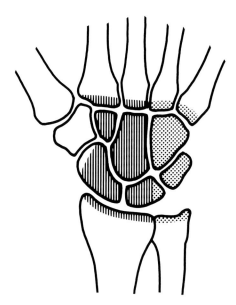

Fig. 20-3. Weber's view of the carpus is that of two longitudinal columns. The control column (stippled) occupies the ulnar portion of the wrist, emphasizing the importance of the helicoid configuration of the triquetrohamate joint. The force-bearing column (striped) is on the radial side. (Redrawn from Weber ER: Concepts governing the rotational shift of the intercalated segment of the carpus. Orthop Clin North Amer 15:196, 1984. Reprinted with permission from WB Saunders, Philadelphia.)

serious student of carpal bone injuries is encouraged to read the references cited for a more thorough understanding of carpal anatomy and function.

Ligamentous Anatomy

In 1976, Taleisnik[221] and Mayfield, Johnson, and Kilcoyne[149] published independent studies that have enhanced our knowledge of the intricate ligamentous anatomy of the wrist. Although there are minor differences in their interpretations of this difficult area of anatomy, the discrepancies are not contradictory, and in fact these two studies tend to support each other's findings. Table 20-1 lists the major ligamentous structures that they have identified in the wrist, attempting to reconcile their minor differences. More important than the discrepancies, however, are the major points of agreement found in both studies.

1. The major ligaments of the wrist are intracapsular, as originally emphasized by Lewis, Hamshere, and Bucknill.[131] This is the primary reason why they are difficult for the surgeon to see at operation, since they are covered by the joint capsule.
2. The volar ligaments (Fig. 20-4) are much more substantial (and thus apparently more important) than the dorsal ligaments.
3. The general configuration of the volar ligaments is a double V-shaped structure, with an area of potential weakness between them, called the space of Poirier. This weak area lies directly over the capitolunate articulation.

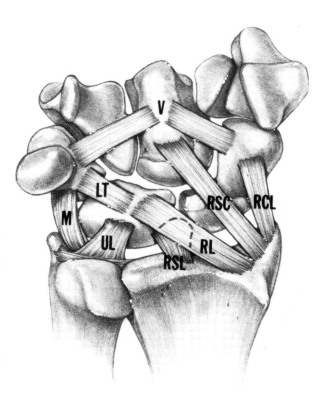

Fig. 20-4. The volar ligaments of the wrist as described by Taleisnik. The most important stabilizer of the proximal pole of the scaphoid is thought to be the radioscapholunate *(RSL)* ligament. (*RCL*, radial collateral ligament; *RSC*, radioscaphocapitate ligament; *RL*, radiolunate ligament; *RSL*, radioscapholunate ligament; *UL*, ulnolunate ligament; *M*, ulnocarpal meniscus homologue; *LT*, lunotriquetral ligament; *V*, V or deltoid ligament.) (Taleisnik J: The Wrist. p. 14. Churchill Livingstone, New York, 1985.)

Table 20-1. Ligamentous Anatomy of the Wrist

Taleisnik[221]	Mayfield, Johnson, and Kilcoyne[149]
Volar	
Deep volar radiocarpal ligament	Palmar radiocarpal ligament
1. Radioscaphocapitate	1. Radiocapitate
2. Radiolunate	2. Radio-(lunate)triquetral[a]
3. Radioscapholunate	3. Radioscaphoid (lunate)
Volar ulnocarpal ligament	Palmar ulnocarpal ligament
1. Ulnolunate	1. Ulnolunate
	2. Ulnotriquetrum[b]
Intrinsic (intercarpal) ligaments	Intercarpal ligament
A. Long	1. Capitotriquetral[c]
1. Volar intercarpal (V, deltoid, arcuate)	
B. Intermediate	
1. Lunate-triquetral	
2. Scapholunate	
3. Scaphotrapezium	
C. Short (bind the four bones of the distal row together)	
Dorsal	
1. Dorsal radiocarpal (radiolunate-triquetrum)	1. Dorsal radiocarpal (radiolunate-triquetrum)
Collateral	
1. Radial collateral ligament	1. Radial collateral ligament
2. Ulnar collateral ligament	2. Ulnar collateral ligament

Discrepancies:

[a] Mayfield and associates show the radiolunate ligament continuing on to the triquetrum; Taleisnik has it terminating on the lunate, but he identifies an intrinsic lunate-triquetral ligament.

[b] Mayfield and associates show the ulnocarpal ligament as dividing into separate ligaments, inserting onto the lunate and triquetrum, respectively; Taleisnik shows it inserting only into the lunate. However, both demonstrate that the origin of the ulnocarpal ligament is from the meniscus, not the head or styloid of the ulna.

[c] Mayfield and associates imply the presence of other specific intercarpal ligaments (e.g., scapholunate), but they do not list or label them.

4. The prime stabilizer of the proximal pole of the scaphoid is the volar radioscapholunate ligament, and rotary subluxation of the scaphoid cannot occur unless this ligament is torn. Although the scapholunate ligaments must also be torn for subluxation to take place, rupture of the scapholunate ligaments alone will not create instability of the proximal pole.[15]

5. The collateral ligaments probably do not exist as static collateral stabilizers of the wrist joint. In their classic article on the anatomy of the wrist joint in 1970, Lewis et al[131] concluded that "there is little to justify the concept of a definite ulnar collateral ligament arising from the tip of the ulnar styloid process." Taleisnik[221] agreed with this, describing the ulnar collateral liga-

ment as "little more than a thickening of the joint capsule." Kauer's[118] later studies further endorsed this concept, for he observed that the sheaths of the dorsal (extensor) tendons merge in part with the joint capsules, and at the radial and ulnar sides of the wrist joint these mergers can be interpreted erroneously as collateral ligaments.

From a practical point of view, these individual ligaments are, in my experience, difficult to identify at operation in a patient with a carpal dislocation, and consequently, virtually impossible to repair as individual structures. However, it is my opinion that attempts should be made to repair the ligamentous complexes, and this is technically feasible, as described later in this chapter. For this reason, even though one probably cannot repair the individual ligaments, a thorough appreciation of the ligaments is imperative for the surgeon who is confronted with a carpal dislocation and must make some attempt at ligamentous repair.

Kinematics

Dorsiflexion and palmar flexion of the wrist take place in both the radiocarpal and midcarpal joints,[24] although the relative contributions of each have been inconsistently reported in the literature (Table 20-2). The wide variances and absolute contradictions noted by various authors are yet another testimonial to the complexity of the kinematics of the wrist. Rather than attempt to assign a specific number of degrees or a percentage of motion to each of the two joints, it is perhaps better to accept the conclusions of Youm et al[260,261] that both the radiocarpal and midcarpal joints contribute to all phases of flexion and extension motion of the wrist.

Talesinik has noted that the position of the scaphoid determines the degree of participation of these two joints in the total range of wrist motion. As the wrist moves toward ulnar deviation or dorsiflexion, the scaphoid itself dorsiflexes, i.e., it becomes less vertical to the long axis of the radius, and it "locks" the midcarpal joint. As more ulnar deviation or dorsiflexion occurs, all subsequent motion takes place in the radiocarpal joint. Conversely, the midcarpal joint becomes "unlocked" as the wrist is

radially deviated or palmarflexed, allowing motion to occur in the midcarpal joint.

The axis of rotation in the wrist has been determined biomechanically to lie within the head of the capitate.[260] In ulnar deviation, the proximal row slides toward the radius, and the distal row rotates in reciprocal fashion in a clockwise direction (looking at the right wrist from a dorsal view). In radial deviation, the proximal row moves toward the ulna, and the distal row rotates counterclockwise. Although the proximal row appears to be moving as a unit, there are subtle changes taking place *within* the proximal row as the wrist moves from radial to ulnar deviation. Some understanding of these changes is very helpful in trying to sort out the various types of dislocations and instabilities that are described later in this chapter. When interpreting x-ray films in a clinical setting, the lunate is frequently used as a focal point, and therefore I have found it useful to try to understand the factors influencing the position of the lunate, which may be summarized as follows.

1. *Contact pressure exerted by the head of the capitate.* In ulnar deviation, the capitate is palmarflexed, and this tends to push the lunate into dorsiflexion (Fig. 20-5A). In radial deviation, the capitate dorsiflexes and pushes the lunate into palmarflexion (Fig. 20-5B).
2. *Wedge shape of the lunate.* The lunate has a shorter dorsal height and a longer volar lip, and thus has an inherent tendency to dorsiflex.[117,228]
3. *Attachments to the scaphoid.* In ulnar deviation the scaphoid dorsiflexes (i.e., becomes more co-

Table 20-2. Relative Contributions of the Radiocarpal and Midcarpal Joints to Flexion and Extension of the Wrist

Authors	Dorsiflexion		Volar Flexion	
	Radiocarpal	Midcarpal	Radiocarpal	Midcarpal
Horwitz (1940)[101]	42%	58%	21%	79%
Bunnell (1948)[30]	56%	44%	50%	50%
Wagner (1956, 1959)[240,241]	Slight	Primarily	Most	Less
Fisk (1970)[67]	First ⅔	Last ⅔	Last ½	First ½
Mayfield, Johnson and Kilcoyne (1976)[149]	Slight	Primarily	Primarily	Less
Sarrafian, Melamed, and Goshgarian (1977)[200]	66%	34%	40%	60%

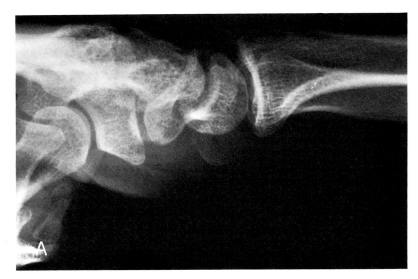

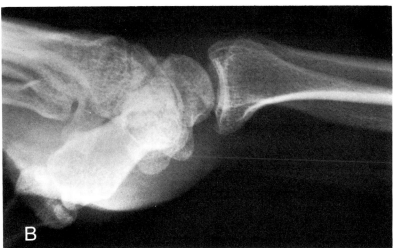

Fig. 20-5. Lateral radiographs of the wrist in (**A**) ulnar deviation and (**B**) radial deviation. Note that in ulnar deviation the lunate is in dorsiflexion and in radial deviation it tends to be palmarflexed.

linear with the long axis of the radius), which means that its proximal pole rotates into a more volar position. As it does so, it pulls the lunate along with it, forcing the lunate into dorsiflexion. In radial deviation, the scaphoid palmar flexes and its proximal pole shifts more dorsally, pulling the lunate along and forcing it into palmarflexion.

4. *Triquetrohamate "helicoid" joint.* The inclined plane of the triquetrohamate joint serves to position the lunate relative to the stable capitate.[248,249] In ulnar deviation (Fig. 20-6A), the triquetrum is in the "low" position, i.e., it lies more distal on the hamate articulation and closer to the base of the fifth metacarpal, but

also in a dorsiflexed attitude because of the slope of the triquetrohamate joint. Because of its attachments to the lunate, the triquetrum thus tends to force the lunate into dorsiflexion in ulnar deviation. In radial deviation (Fig. 20-6B), the triquetrum rides up the slope of the hamate to its "high" position (i.e., more proximal on the hamate and actually articulating with the capitate, but also in a palmarflexed attitude), thereby pulling the lunate into palmarflexion as well.

The result of all these forces is that in ulnar deviation the lunate is pushed into dorsiflexion and in radial deviation the lunate tends to be palmar-

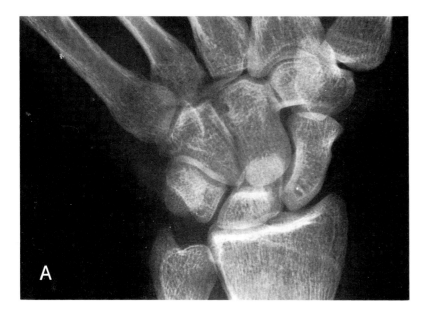

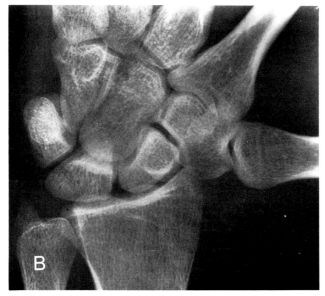

Fig. 20-6. PA radiographs of the wrist in (A) ulnar deviation and (B) radial deviation. In ulnar deviation, the triquetrum is in the "low" position, i.e., it lies more distal on the hamate articulation and closer to the base of the fifth metacarpal. Because of the slope of the helicoid triquetrohamate joint, it is also in a dorsiflexed attitude. In radial deviation, the triquetrum rides up the slope of the hamate to its "high" position, i.e., more proximal and palmarflexed.

flexed. Being aware of these normal reciprocal relationships among the carpal bones allows one to more carefully analyze x-ray films of patients with carpal instabilities. For a more thorough understanding of these important kinematic concepts, the reader is referred to the excellent articles by Taleisnik[228] and Weber.[248,249]

Another concept that may be useful as an adjunct in evaluating patterns of carpal instability is that of carpal height ratio, as proposed by Youm and colleagues.[158,260] *Carpal height* is a term used to designate the distance between the base of the third metacarpal and the distal articular surface of the radius measured along the proximal projection of the longitudinal axis of the third metacarpal (Fig. 20-7). When compared with the length of the third metacarpal, a constant ratio for carpal height was found to be 0.54 ± 0.03 in normal wrists.

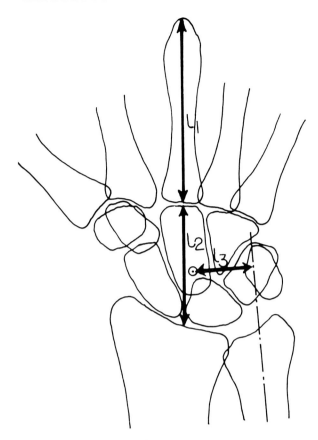

Fig. 20-7. The carpal height ratio is calculated by dividing the carpal height *(L2)* by the length of the third metacarpal *(L1)*. The normal is 0.54 ± 0.03. (Youm Y, McMurtry RY, Flatt AE, Gillespie TE: Kinematics of the wrist. I. An experimental study of radioulnar deviation and flexion-extension. J Bone Joint Surg 60A:423–431, 1978.)

MECHANISMS OF INJURY

Most major carpal dislocations are the result of extreme hyperextension (dorsiflexion) injuries, often due to violent trauma such as that sustained in falls from heights or in motorcycle accidents. In such cases, the most obvious dislocation occurs at the midcarpal joint, where the capitate is usually displaced dorsal to the lunate. Much attention in the past has been directed to the unique anatomic position of the scaphoid, which bridges the two carpal rows.[67,77,134,145,203] It is thus apparent that in

order for the capitate to dislocate dorsal to the lunate, the scaphoid must either fracture or tear its ligamentous attachments to the lunate[36,53,240,241] (Fig. 20-8). Applying Lichtman's oval ring concept,[6,133] another way to visualize this is to recognize that if the break in the ring occurs through the waist of the scaphoid, the result is a trans-scaphoid perilunate dislocation. If, on the other hand, the break in the ring is between the scaphoid and lunate, the result is a perilunate dislocation with scapholunate dissociation.

As with all ligamentous injuries, carpal dislocations and instabilities encompass a broad spectrum of injury ranging from minor sprains to frank disruptions such as the major dislocations noted above. In an effort to quantitate the degree of ligamentous damage and offer some logical sequence of injury, Mayfield, Johnson, and Kilcoyne[150–153] described what they termed "progressive perilunar instability" (PLI). The four stages of PLI, as illustrated in Fig. 20-9, describe the progressive disruption of ligamentous attachments and anatomic relations to the lunate, as follows:

Stage I. *Scapholunate instability.* Tearing of the scapholunate interosseous and volar ra-

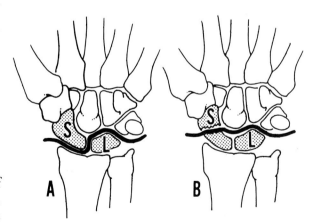

Fig. 20-8. The scaphoid occupies a unique anatomic position, bridging the proximal and distal carpal rows. When a midcarpal dislocation occurs (i.e., between the two rows), the scaphoid must either rotate or fracture. This results in the two major patterns of carpal dislocations: **(A)** perilunate dislocation or **(B)** trans-scaphoid perilunate dislocation.

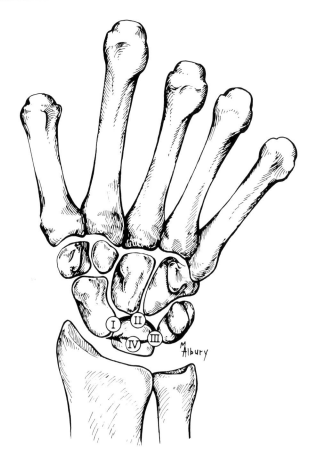

Fig. 20-9. In an effort to offer some logical sequence of injury pattern in carpal disruptions, Mayfield described what he termed "progressive perilunar instability" (PLI). See text for description. (Mayfield JK: Mechanism of carpal injuries. Clin Orthop 149:50, 1980.)

dioscaphoid ligaments results in scapholunate dissociation.

Stage II. *Capitate dislocation.* Dislocation of the capitate-lunate (midcarpal) joint through the space of Poirier.

Stage III. *Triquetral dislocation.* Separation of the triquetrum from the lunate due to tearing of the radiotriquetral ligament.

Stage IV. *Lunate dislocation.* Disruption of the dorsal radiocarpal ligament allows the lunate to rotate freely into the carpal tunnel on its intact palmar ligamentous hinge.

Thus, Mayfield and his colleagues have shown from their experimental studies what was suggested as early as 1925 by Destot[53]: volar dislocation of the lunate is the end stage of a dorsal perilunate dislocation. They have also demonstrated that scapholunate dissociation can exist as an isolated injury in the absence of midcarpal disruption, a clinical entity that has been recognized with increasing frequency in recent years.

The concept of PLI offers a rational explanation for dislocations and instabilities on the radial side of the carpus, but it does not offer much help in explaining the ulnar carpal instabilities. In fact, Mayfield et al did not see any ulnar perilunar instability without a radial component in their experimental studies. Perhaps, then, triquetrolunate injury may represent a "forme fruste" of stage III PLI as suggested by Lichtman et al,[132] in which triquetrolunate instability persists after the radial components have healed. There may be, however, other mechanisms of injury that have yet to be clearly defined.[70] Mayfield et al's experimental studies were done on cadaver wrists, and probably did not reflect all of the loading forces found in the usual clinical conditions. Taleisnik[103] believes that the position of the hand at the moment of impact influences the type of injury caused, and that carpal hyperpronation may be responsible for isolated ulnar instabilities.

Many types of subtle ligamentous injuries in the carpus are just being recognized, and our knowledge of the mechanisms of injury causing these problems is as elementary and incomplete as our understanding of their treatment.

Nevertheless, the concept that carpal ligamentous injuries represent a spectrum of injuries is important in the clinical setting. In the past, there has been a tendency to consider perilunate and lunate dislocations as separate and distinct entities. There may, however, be considerable diagnostic overlap between these two injuries. When a patient is first seen, the original lateral radiograph may show a "pure" dorsal perilunate dislocation or volar lunate dislocation, or it may depict a configuration of the carpal bones that lies somewhere in between these two extremes, i.e., with the lunate being displaced slightly volarly from its normal position, and the capitate partially articulating with the distal radius (Fig. 20-10). Moreover, the position of the bones when the patient is seen in the emergency room does not necessarily reflect the degree of instability or the full extent of the ligamentous damage. For example, a volar lunate dislocation may

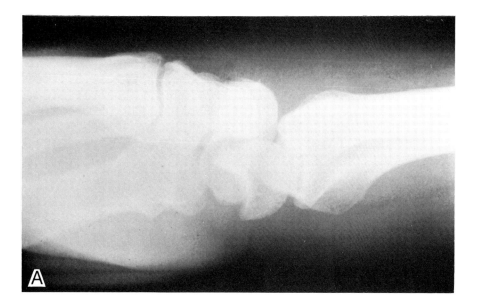

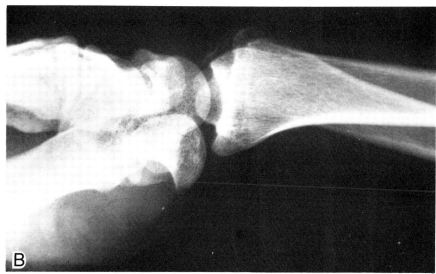

Fig. 20-10. Carpal dislocations comprise a spectrum of injury, and the initial lateral radiograph in a patient with a carpal dislocation may depict a configuration at any point in that spectrum. (A) A "pure" dorsal perilunate dislocation. (B) An intermediate stage. (C) A "pure" volar lunate dislocation.

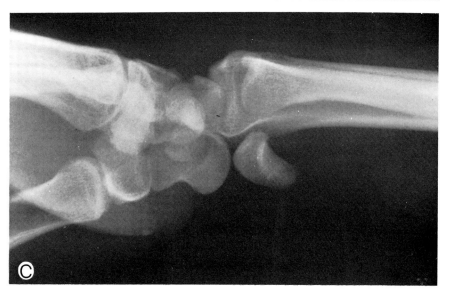

partially reduce and present as a dorsal perilunate dislocation. For these reasons, it has been my practice to consider perilunate and lunate dislocations as progressive stages of the same basic injury. The sections on management that follow are based on this concept.

CLASSIFICATION

Carpal dislocations and instabilities are difficult to classify partly because of the many subtle variations encountered clinically and the confusing and often conflicting terminology used throughout the literature, but perhaps more so because these complex injuries are not yet fully understood. In a previous publication, however, Green and O'Brien[88] attempted to offer a classification that would permit some sort of reasonably systematic approach to management. A modification of that classification, based upon newer concepts and a somewhat better understanding of these injuries, is shown in Table 20-3. It must be emphasized, however, that the entities listed in that classification are arbitrary designations, when in fact significant overlap exists among the various types. The classification is therefore used only as a frame of reference and as an outline to be followed in the subsequent sections on treatment.

DIAGNOSIS

Clinical Diagnosis

As previously noted, the various derangements of the carpal bones discussed in this chapter encompass a wide spectrum of injury. From the standpoint of clinical evaluation, there are really two separate types of situations with which the examiner must deal. At one end of the spectrum is the patient who presents following violent trauma, such as a fall from a height or a motorcycle acci-

Table 20-3. Classification of Carpal Dislocations & Instabilities

"Major" carpal dislocations
  Dorsal perilunate/volar lunate dislocation[a]
  Dorsal trans-scaphoid perilunate dislocation[a]
  Variants
    Transradial styloid perilunate dislocation
    Scaphocapitate syndrome
    Transtriquetral perilunate dislocation
  Volar perilunate/dorsal lunate dislocation
  Complete dislocation of the scaphoid
  Capitate-hamate diastasis

Carpal instability, dissociative (CID)
  Radial carpal instabilities
    Scapholunate dissociation[a]
    Dorsiflexion instability (DISI)[a]
  Ulnar carpal instabilities
    Triquetrohamate instability
    Triquetrolunate instability
    Volar flexion instability (VISI)
  Central carpal instability

Carpal instability, nondissociative (CIND)
  Nondissociative instability of the proximal carpal row
    Midcarpal joint
    Radiocarpal joint

[a] The most common patterns of injury

dent, who is likely to have a "major" dislocation. At the other end of the spectrum is the patient with a painful wrist who may not even recall a specific traumatic event, yet may have a significant carpal instability. In the former patient, the diagnosis of a major carpal dislocation may be fairly obvious, and in the latter, identification of a precise carpal instability pattern may be exceedingly difficult. The physical examination of patients with late carpal instabilities will be discussed separately under each specific heading; below is what one encounters in the patient with an acute injury.

ACUTE INJURIES

Except in the case of open dislocations, the physical findings in the patient with a "major" dislocation are frequently not particularly dramatic. Swelling is generally mild-to-moderate if the patient is seen early, although it may increase significantly if there has been a delay of a few days. Because of the extensive ligamentous and bony damage, tenderness can usually be elicited in a rather diffuse pattern about the wrist. Nonetheless, palpation for maximum areas of tenderness should be done over the scaphoid, scapholunate joint, lunate, triquetrum, hamate, carpal tunnel region, and radial styloid. Range of motion of the wrist is usually significantly limited by pain. If skin marks (abrasions, contusions) are present on the hypothenar or thenar eminences they may be helpful in ascertaining the mechanism of injury.

Careful assessment of the neurovascular status is imperative, with particular attention to the median nerve, which is frequently involved either by direct contusion at the moment of impact or later by subsequent swelling of the wrist.

Concomitant injuries known to result from the same mechanism of injury (carpometacarpal dislocation, radioulnar joint dislocation, radial head fracture, and elbow dislocation) should be specifically looked for as well.

Radiographic Diagnosis

TERMINOLOGY

Some confusion exists over the various terms used to describe the radiographic appearances of the sequelae of carpal dislocations. The two most widely recognized patterns of carpal instability are dorsiflexion and palmarflexion instability (Fig. 20-11). Of the two, dorsiflexion instability is by far the most common pattern resulting from trauma and is thus given the most attention in this chapter. As early as 1943, Lambrinudi and his associates[77] showed an illustration of this dorsiflexion instability pattern, commenting that they believed it to be "the most common derangement of the wrist but has been overlooked." Landsmeer[129] later referred to this as the "zigzag" configuration, noting that the angles of the two joints (radiocarpal and midcarpal) change in opposite directions, and Fisk[67] called it a "concertina" deformity. The acronym **DISI** *(dorsiflexed intercalated segment instability)*, coined by Dobyns and Linscheid[54,134,179,203] to describe the appearance of the proximal row when the unstable link system "collapses," is probably the most commonly used expression of dorsiflexion instability. The opposite situation, **VISI** or **PISI** *(volar* or *palmar flexed intercalated segment instability)*, has become more frequently recognized as a component of the ulnar carpal instabilities (see page 928).

Scapholunate dissociation and *rotary subluxation of the scaphoid*, described in more detail on page 912, are in my opinion synonymous terms. Scapholunate dissociation may be seen in conjunction with dorsiflexion instability or it may exist as an isolated entity without any evidence of dorsal tilting of the proximal row. In the latter situation, it represents stage I of Mayfield et al's[153] PLI (Progressive Perilunar Instability) (see page 883).

ROUTINE VIEWS

The initial routine radiographic examination in the patient with a suspected carpal dislocation should include three views of the wrist: anteroposterior, lateral, and oblique. The lateral view must be a true lateral, preferably with the wrist in neutral, to demonstrate displacement of the capitate and/or lunate or rotation of the lunate, the so-called spilled teacup sign (Fig. 20-12). The anteroposterior view should be taken with the forearm in supination (palm up) to best demonstrate scapholunate dissociation. If a fractured scaphoid is suspected, a PA (palm down) view with the wrist in ulnar deviation is likely to show that more clearly.

Gilula[79,196] has noted that in the PA view, three fairly smooth radiographic arcs can be drawn to define normal carpal relationships (Fig. 20-13). A break in the continuity of any of these arcs strongly suggests an abnormality at the site of the broken arc. He also pointed out that articulating bones normally have parallel apposing surfaces, and thus overlapping of two or more carpal bones is also suggestive of carpal instability.

The normal configuration of the lunate is trapezoidal, and it has long been taught that a triangular or wedge-shaped lunate is diagnostic of lunate dislocation (Fig. 20-14A). Gilula[79] has shown that whenever the lunate tilts in either direction (dorsiflexion or palmar flexion), it projects a more triangular shape in the PA view. Therefore, a triangular lunate does not necessarily mean dislocation, but it does imply an instability pattern of the lunate. Thus, a more subtle sign of lunate instability is elongation of the volar lip of the lunate in the **PA** view (Fig. 20-14B).

Curtis et al[51] have emphasized the importance of soft tissue changes in the evaluation of carpal bone injuries, noting that identification of swelling

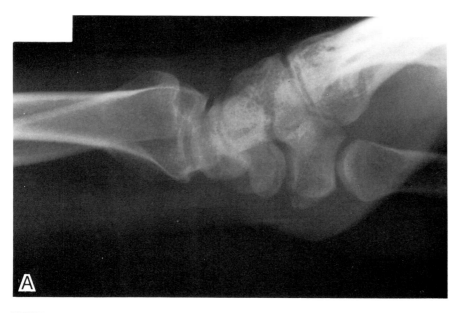

Fig. 20-11. The two major patterns of post-traumatic instability of the wrist are dorsiflexion (DISI) (A) and palmar flexion (VISI) (B) instability. Of the two, dorsiflexion instability is by far the more common pattern resulting from trauma.

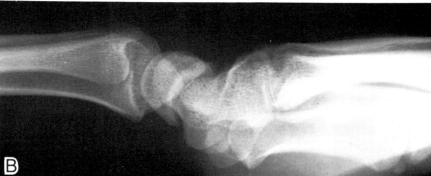

Fig. 20-12. The typical configuration of the lunate in the lateral radiograph of a volar lunate dislocation has been called the spilled teacup sign because the distal concavity of the bone is rotated nearly 90 degrees, pointing volarward instead of distally.

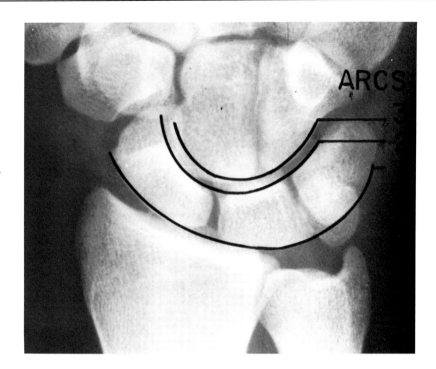

Fig. 20-13. Gilula and his colleagues have pointed out that three fairly smooth radiographic arcs can be drawn in the PA view to define normal carpal relationships. A break in the continuity of any of these arcs strongly suggests an abnormality at the site of the broken arc. (Bellinghausen HW, Gilula LA, Young LV, Weeks PM: Post-traumatic palmar carpal subluxation. Report of two cases. J Bone Joint Surg 65A:999, 1983.)

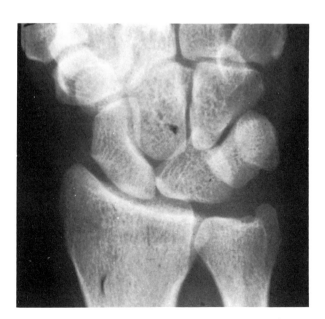

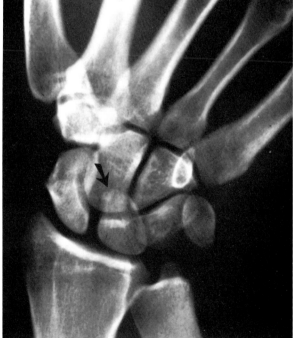

Fig. 20-14. It has long been taught that a triangular or wedge-shaped lunate (**A**) is diagnostic of lunate dislocation, but Gilula[79] has shown that tilting of the lunate in either direction (dorsiflexion or palmarflexion) results in a more triangular shape of the lunate as compared with its normal trapezoidal configuration. A more subtle sign of lunate instability is elongation of the volar lip of the lunate in the PA view (**B**).

should direct one's attention to possible occult areas of bone or joint injury. Obliteration and bulging of the navicular fat stripe[38,50,51,80.232] is suggestive of an injury to the scaphoid.

Concomitant radial styloid fractures are sufficiently common with carpal dislocations that in any patient with a radial styloid fracture, rotary subluxation of the scaphoid and/or intercalated segment instability should be specifically looked for with the radiographic views discussed below.

ADDITIONAL VIEWS

In patients with acute perilunate or lunate dislocations (with or without scaphoid fracture), the three routine views noted above are sufficient to establish the diagnosis before commencing treatment. These initial views, however, are often difficult to interpret because of overlap and displacement of the carpal bones. I have found it particularly advantageous to obtain anteroposterior and lateral radiographs with the hand suspended in finger-traps; these distraction views usually demonstrate the extent of bony damage much more clearly.

The radiographic evaluation of patients with more subtle carpal instabilities generally requires additional views. My routine "scaphoid series" of radiographs in the office consists of the following.

1. True lateral view with the wrist in neutral for evaluation of the overall alignment and measurement of the carpal bone angles.
2. PA (palm down) view in maximum ulnar deviation, the view most likely to show a scaphoid fracture.
3. AP (palm up) view with fist compression. Dobyns and his colleagues[54] have suggested that compression of the carpus by having the patient make a fist or by applying a longitudinal compression force on the wrist may accenuate scapholunate dissociation (Fig. 20-15).
4. Oblique view midway between neutral and full pronation to better visualize the ulnar side of the carpus in profile.

These four views are a good starting point, but specific areas of tenderness in the clinical examination or subtle changes seen in the four routine views may suggest the need for additional views. Several

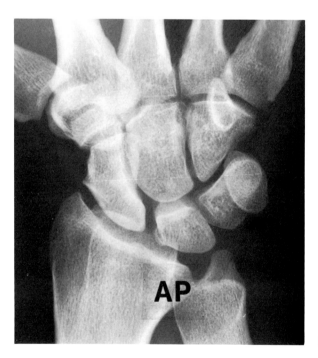
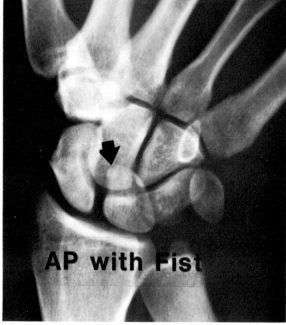

Fig. 20-15. Dobyns and his colleagues[54] have suggested that compression of the carpus by having the patient make a fist may accenuate scapholunate dissociation, as illustrated in these radiographs.

authors have suggested a routine "motion" series for any patient in whom there is a suggestion of carpal instability. Gilula[80] refers to this as his "instability series," which includes the following views:

1. PA in radial deviation, neutral, and ulnar deviation;
2. AP with fist compression;
3. Lateral in dorsiflexion, neutral, and volar flexion;
4. Oblique; and
5. Pisotriquetral view (lateral in 30 degrees supination).

Since Gilula recommends that x-ray films be taken of both wrists for comparison, his series includes 18 views. In my own practice, I prefer cineradiographs for those patients in whom I suspect subtle carpal instabilities, but in the absence of facilities to perform cines, static films comprising a "motion series" are an excellent substitute. Ironically, I have found that having studied many cineradiographs has enabled me to better interpret the static films.

For evaluating dynamic instabilities, the most useful plain films may be three lateral views obtained with the wrist in neutral, radial deviation, and ulnar deviation, with the forearm pronated and the x-ray beam directed horizontally against a vertical cassette. In evaluating these films, however, one must keep in mind the changes seen in the normal wrist as illustrated in Figures 20-5 and 20-6.

MEASUREMENT OF CARPAL BONE ANGLES

Calculation of the capitolunate, scapholunate, and radiolunate angles (Fig. 20-16) may also be helpful in diagnosing the more subtle variations of carpal dislocations. Clear distinction should be made between these different angles to avoid confusion. Although "normal" values are difficult to establish from the literature,[78,134,179,200,203] there are ranges of normal that are helpful to keep in mind when interpreting the radiographs. True lateral radiographs with the wrist in neutral (no dorsiflexion or volar flexion) are essential for proper interpretation of these angles.

SCAPHOLUNATE

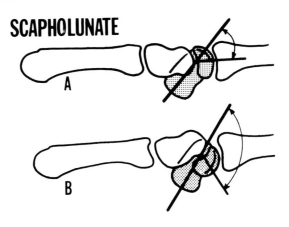

CAPITOLUNATE

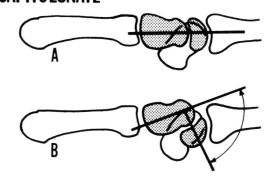

RADIOLUNATE

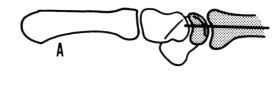

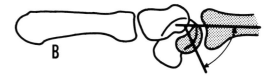

Fig. 20-16. The carpal bone angles are of considerable aid in identifying carpal instability patterns. In each illustration the normal is shown (**A**) in comparison with the abnormal angle seen in dorsiflexion instability (**B**). The *capitolunate* angle should theoretically be 0 degrees with the wrist in neutral, but the range of normal probably extends to as much as 15 degrees. The *scapholunate* angle is the most helpful, in my experience, and an angle greater than 80 degrees is definite evidence of dorsiflexion instability. The *radiolunate* angle is abnormal if it exceeds 15 degrees (see text).

Capitolunate Angle

The capitolunate angle is determined by measuring the longitudinal axes of the lunate and capitate. Although classically it has been stated that the long axes of the radius, lunate, capitate, and third metacarpal are co-linear, Sarrafian, Melamed, and Goshgarian[200] concluded that this is true in only a small percentage (11 percent) of normal subjects. As Gilula and Weeks[78] have demonstrated, however, precise localizations of these axes on the lateral radiograph are difficult to identify and subject to considerable error. The standard method of defining the lunate axis is to draw a line perpendicular to a line connecting the volar and dorsal tips of the lunate. Because of the frequent asymmetry of the lunate (the volar pole is often longer than the dorsal pole), this method may not be entirely accurate, and usually it is better to simply estimate a line through the midportion of the lunate. The capitate axis is identified by connecting a point in the center of the convexity of the head with a point at the center of its distal articular surface with the third metacarpal. Theoretically, the normal capitolunate axis should be 0 degrees with the wrist in neutral, but the range of normal probably extends to approximately 10 to 15 degrees.[100,138]

Scapholunate Angle

To determine the scaphoid axis, a line is drawn connecting the proximal (dorsal) and distal (volar) convexities of the bone. In my experience, this line is particularly difficult to define with precise accuracy and reproducibility, but I believe that the scapholunate angle is the most helpful of the carpal bone angles in identifying dorsiflexion instability (collapse deformity) of the carpus. As defined by Linscheid and colleagues,[134] normal values range from 30 to 60 degrees, with an average of 47 degrees. Angles greater than 80 degrees should be considered a definite indication of scapholunate dissociation.

Radiolunate Angle

The radiolunate angle provides further diagnostic information, giving objective evidence of the dorsal tilt of the lunate seen in dorsiflexion instability if the angle is greater than 15 degrees.[100]

CINERADIOGRAPHS

Although cineradiography is not necessary in the routine management of patients with carpal dislocations, it is a source of considerable information regarding the pathomechanics and various patterns of injury. It is also of value in evaluating the patient who has a painful snapping, clicking, popping, or "clunking" wrist, in whom routine and special views do not demonstrate the site of pathology.[8,110,174,189] I have seen several patients in whom cineradiographs clearly demonstrated scapholunate dissociation, despite normal plain films (including fist compression views).

Active motion may be studied by the use of fluoroscopy, videotape, or cines. Fluoroscopy provides no permanent record and thus does not allow deliberate study of the carpal kinematics. Cineradiographs provide much better detail than videotape, and for this reason cines are my preference. Most hospitals have 35-mm cineradiograph facilities that are used extensively by the cardiologists, and our cardiac cath lab technicians have been very cooperative in producing wrist cines for us when the facilities are not in use for cardiac catheterizations.

Our routine cineradiograph series includes active movement from radial to ulnar deviation in both AP and PA views; dorsiflexion and volar flexion in the lateral view; and radial and ulnar deviation in the lateral view. If the patient has a painful pop or clunk, it is important for that to be reproduced during the cine examination.

TOMOGRAPHY

Tomograms are not particularly helpful in the evaluation and treatment of carpal dislocations, but they may aid in localizing more subtle areas of injury, such as osteochondral fractures of the carpal bones. Routine tomograms (laminagrams) are of limited value in such cases because their 5-mm slices are likely to miss smaller areas of abnormality. If tomographic evaluation is indicated, it should be done with polytomes (trispiral tomography), which allow intervals as close together as 1.5 to 2.0 mm. As with any radiographic examination, two views at right angles to each other (AP and lateral) should be obtained.

BONE SCANS

Radioisotope bone scans are of no particular value in carpal dislocations, but I have found them to be especially useful in localization of the cause of obscure wrist pain. The bone scan is a nonspecific test, i.e., it does not tell us *what* is wrong, but it can be very useful in pinpointing *where* the problem is. Using the techniques recommended by Stein and his colleagues,[213] I have found bone scans to be very helpful in localizing obscure causes of wrist pain, such as chondral fractures of the carpal bones.

THREE-DIMENSIONAL IMAGING

In my experience, three-dimensional imaging[250] has not yet been developed into a useful clinical tool, but with the incredibly rapid advances being made in imaging systems and computer graphics, I would anticipate that this modality will soon begin to add to our knowledge of carpal kinematics and in some way enhance our ability to treat carpal instabilities.

ARTHROGRAPHY

Moneim and Omer[164] have reported that arthrographic findings have correlated well with the pathologic findings at surgery in patients with acute carpal injuries, but in my opinion insufficient additional information is yielded by wrist arthrography to warrant its routine use in acute injuries. It is of more value in delineating pathologic changes in chronic injuries, especially those involving the radioulnar joint.[121,127,160,179] Arthrography has also been used increasingly in the evaluation of patients with more subtle carpal instability problems such as scapholunate dissociation, ulnar (medial) carpal instabilities, and osteochondral fractures.[231] Experimental studies with arthrotomography[16,19] have shown that some of the volar ligaments of the wrist can be identified with this technique.

In the normal wrist, there is no communication between the radiocarpal and midcarpal joints, and thus wrist arthrography has been used to identify tears in the scapholunate and triquetrolunate ligaments. Several authors[80,180] have stressed that the most critical aspect of wrist arthrography is the *flow* of dye, which indicates the location of inter-

carpal ligament tears. A single film that shows dye in both the radiocarpal and midcarpal joints is of limited value; it is imperative to watch both the pattern and speed of the dye-flow in order to evaluate ligament tears. The problem, however, comes in trying to interpret the arthrographic findings. With our current imperfect and incomplete knowledge of carpal kinematics and injuries, it is difficult to truly understand the significance of tiny ligament tears and even more difficult to know how (and even whether or not) to treat them.

DORSAL PERILUNATE/VOLAR LUNATE DISLOCATION

For the reasons stated on page 884, I consider dorsal perilunate and volar lunate dislocations to be progressive stages of the same basic injury pattern, and the management of these is identical.

Anesthesia

Complete muscle relaxation is essential for an atraumatic reduction of a carpal dislocation. General anesthesia, brachial block, and intravenous regional anesthesia (Bier block) are all satisfactory; local infiltration anesthesia is not. If cineradiography or image intensification is planned, the tourniquet necessary for an intravenous regional block may be somewhat cumbersome in manipulating the hand. The specific details of these various techniques are described in Chapter 2.

Traction

An initial period of 5 to 10 minutes of uninterrupted traction is also very helpful prior to reduction. I prefer to use wire finger-traps, but the Weinberger apparatus is used by some (Fig. 20-17). Ten to fifteen pounds of counterweight should be applied across the upper arm, with the elbow flexed to 90 degrees.

Böhler[21,22] was the first to emphasize the necessity of continuous traction, but he used longitu-

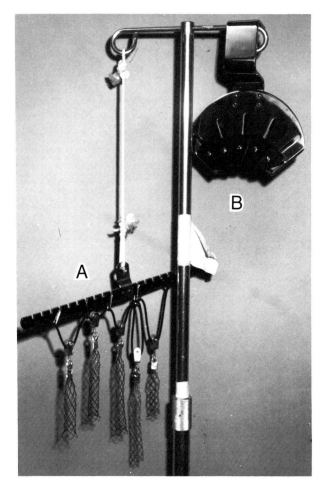

Fig. 20-17. Traction is essential prior to closed reduction of a carpal dislocation. I prefer to use the wire finger-traps (**A**), but the Weinberger apparatus (**B**) is used by some. Ten to 15 pounds of counterweight are applied across the upper arm, with the elbow flexed 90 degrees.

dinal traction as the sole means of reducing the dislocation, i.e., without manipulation. Stevenson[217] reemphasized the importance of sustained traction, extending its use with a skeletal distraction device continuously for up to 3 days in long-standing cases in which the 10-minute manual traction was unsuccessful.

I use traction only as an important preliminary to closed manipulation, not as a method of reduction in itself. During the period of traction, however, an excellent opportunity is provided to obtain AP and lateral radiographs with the carpus distracted (Fig.

20-18), and this should be done routinely. These films are of great value in delineating the full extent of damage to the carpal bones, and often more detail is visible than can be seen in the initial films taken before traction is applied.

Closed Reduction

During the 1920s when case reports of lunate dislocations began to appear, a variety of methods was suggested for closed reduction.[41,47,62,83,92,124, 130,146,176,215] Although no reference to the original source is given, Davis[52] in 1923 discussed "Gunn's law," an axiom that has filtered down through the orthopaedic literature for many years as an established principle. This rule states that the correct method of closed reduction places the dislocated member in the position it was in at the time of injury, and then reverses the force. Davis favored this technique in the treatment of lunate dislocations, and he added a broomstick, which he used as a fulcrum on the volar surface of the wrist to push the lunate back up into position while simultaneous traction was applied to increase the space between the radius and capitate and make enough room for the lunate. Conwell[44] advocated the broomstick technique, but added that "the use of the fluoroscope is indispensable in this type of case and should always be used." Adams[1] advised against the use of a hard surface, which he thought might damage the flexor tendons, suggesting that only the surgeon's fingers should be used as a fulcrum.

As noted above, Böhler[21,22] emphasized the concept of *sustained* traction for at least 10 minutes as the preferred method of reduction. He believed that levering movements in hyperextension of the wrist often resulted in damage to the median nerve.

MacConaill[145] advocated a slightly different method of reduction, employing a palmar flexion maneuver to lock the capitate into the distal concavity of the lunate, then reducing the capitate and lunate together as a unit by dorsiflexion movement.

Based on his studies in freshly amputated arms, Tanz[229] presented what he believed to be the importance of pronation and supination forces (of the hand on the radius, not forearm rotation) in the mechanism of carpal dislocation. He therefore advocated that closed reduction of a dislocated lunate

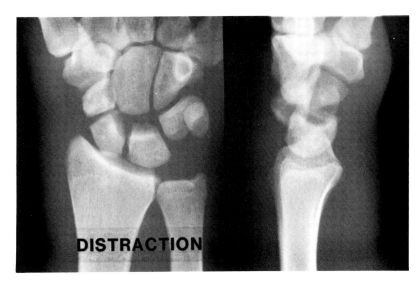

Fig. 20-18. AP and lateral radiographs taken with the fingers suspended in finger traps to show the carpus distracted often provide additional information not well visualized in the initial injury films, such as the osteochondral fragments seen in this patient in the capitate-lunate joint.

should include supination of the hand in addition to traction, and that pronation should be a part of the maneuver for reduction of a perilunate dislocation.

Technique

For dorsal perilunate/volar lunate dislocations, I routinely use the technique described by Tavernier[230] and popularized by Watson-Jones.[246,247] After 5 to 10 minutes of continuous traction, the finger-traps are removed, and the longitudinal traction force is maintained manually by the surgeon. With one hand, the patient's hand is dorsiflexed (maintaining longitudinal traction), while the thumb of the other hand stabilizes the lunate on the volar aspect of the wrist.[40] Gradual palmar flexion of the hand then allows the capitate to snap back into the concavity of the lunate. Our studies of this technique under cineradiography show that the reduction of the capitolunate articulation occurs very rapidly as the capitate is brought over into palmar flexion, and that the lunate is not actually pushed back into place by the operator's thumb; rather, the thumb simply stabilizes the lunate to prevent its being displaced forward by the capitate.

If performed within a few days of injury, closed reduction is usually quite easily accomplished, and the capitolunate joint is generally reasonably stable in neutral or palmar flexion, but unstable in dorsiflexion.

Postreduction Management

The recommended position of immobilization advocated in the literature ranges from full palmar flexion[246] to "just short of dorsiflexion."[145] Most authors have favored palmar flexion,[35,44,99,146,198] some neutral[115,116] and several dorsiflexion.[1,4,145,146] Russell[198] and Watson-Jones[246] suggested only 1 week in palmar flexion, followed by 2 weeks in neutral position.

For initial immobilization I prefer a dorsal short arm thumb spica plaster splint with the wrist in neutral or slight palmar flexion.

Postreduction radiographs are then taken in plaster to ascertain the adequacy of reduction. It is imperative to take enough different views to assess *very critically* the following specific points: (1) the relationship of the capitate and lunate (i.e., is there any intercalated segment instability?) and (2) the position of the scaphoid, i.e., is there any residual rotary subluxation of the scaphoid (scapholunate dissociation)? The minimum views required are a true lateral of the wrist and an anteroposterior (palm up) view, which is most likely to show scapholunate dissociation.

Rawlings[192] has emphasized the importance of assessing the scapholunate angle in the postreduction lateral view, pointing out that this is more likely to give a true reading of midcarpal instability than is the radioscaphoid angle, especially if the wrist is in some palmar flexion. He noted that in his series a scapholunate angle of greater than 80 degrees usually led to an unsatisfactory result, and that such a finding was an indication for repeat closed reduction, and if not improved, then for open reduction.

Period of Immobilization

If all of the above prerequisites for an acceptable reduction are satisfied (which is unusual), the patient is admitted to the hospital at least overnight for elevation of the hand and observation of the neurovascular status.

The period of plaster immobilization has also been a subject of considerable controversy in the literature. Several authors have favored early mobilization: Adams[1] at 48 hours, Conwell[44] at 5 days, and Cave[36,37] at 1 week. Most[92,115,198,246] have advocated 3 weeks of immobilization, although MacAusland[144] and Kaplan[116] recommended 6 weeks.

If the closed reduction is accepted and the wrist is immobilized with plaster only, *it is imperative to reassess the reduction radiographically weekly for at least the first 3 weeks.* At the end of 3 weeks, out-of-plaster films offer an opportunity to better evaluate the critical relationships of the scaphoid, lunate, and capitate. If the reduction has not been lost, I would continue immobilization in a short arm thumb spica cast for a total of 12 weeks (from day of reduction) in dorsal perilunate/volar lunate dislocations.

Closed Reduction and Percutaneous Pin Fixation

Because of the inherent instability of the scaphoid following closed reduction of perilunate/lunate dislocations and the likely recurrence of scapholunate dissociation, I favor internal fixation rather than relying on plaster immobilization to hold the reduction. This can occasionally be accomplished by closed reduction and percutaneous pin fixation. This is done *only* if *anatomic* reduction of the scaphoid, lunate, and capitate can be achieved by closed manipulation.

Technique

The image intensifier is essential in this technique, as our cineradiographic studies have demonstrated that there is no predictable position that will consistently reduce the bones in all cases. Ordinarily, the scaphoid subluxation can be reduced by slight radial deviation and dorsiflexion of the wrist, but this often results in redisplacement of the capitate dorsally. Therefore, I prefer to do percutaneous pin fixation under the image intensifier, first manipulating the wrist into a variety of positions to find the most acceptable position of reduction. It is preferable to do these manipulations before prepping the hand. If the image intensifier reveals that a satisfactory reduction can be achieved, the optimal position of reduction is noted, and the upper extremity is given a standard surgical prep.

A knowledgeable assistant is necessary, as the reduction must be held while the pins are inserted. Using a power drill, two smooth 0.045-inch K-wires are inserted from the anatomic snuffbox through the scaphoid into the capitate and lunate, respectively. Care must be taken to avoid the radial artery and the superficial branch of radial nerve. Occasionally, a third K-wire across the radial styloid, scaphoid, and capitate will provide additional stability. Although the placement of the pins is done under the image intensifier, adequacy of reduction and pin position should be checked by permanent radiographs. The K-wires are left protruding through the skin and are bent at right angles to facilitate later removal. Manipulation of the wrist after placement of the pins should be done very carefully, as this may result in bending of the K-wires (Fig. 20-19).

Postreduction Management

A well-padded thumb spica splint is applied immediately after the final radiographs have been obtained. This is converted to a thumb spica cast at 7 to 10 days after swelling has subsided and the pin tracts are seen to be free of infection. The protruding pins must be well padded to prevent local irritation beneath the plaster. Radiographs are taken in the new cast to ensure proper maintenance of reduction. The cast and pins are removed at 8 weeks and immobilization in plaster is continued for an

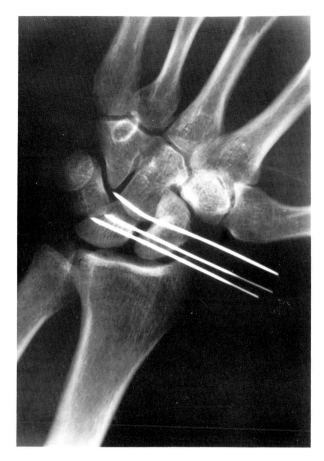

Fig. 20-19. Following percutaneous pin fixation of a perilunate dislocation, movement of the wrist should be done very carefully to avoid bending of the K-wires, as occurred in this patient.

additional 4 weeks, for a total of 12 weeks following reduction.

Open Reduction

If anatomic reduction and adequate stability of the scaphoid, lunate, and capitate cannot be accomplished by closed reduction (with or without percutaneous pinning), open reduction is indicated.

Much of the early literature regarding open reduction of these injuries focused only on the lunate dislocation, and most of these authors favored a dorsal approach,[36,37,119,146,154,246] fearing further vascular damage to the lunate from the volar side. In 1923 Davis[52] devised a "semilunate skid" that was designed to facilitate repositioning of the displaced lunate from the dorsal approach. Subsequent authors[21,22,34,99,146] have preferred the volar approach. Böhler's volar approach was used in conjunction with skeletal traction to open up the space between the capitate and radius. Eggers[59] thought that a direct volar approach was likely to cause adhesions in the flexor tendons, and he therefore devised a medial (ulnar) exposure beneath the flexor tendons.

In the first of their excellent articles, Campbell and colleagues[33] reported on open reduction using a dorsal approach in nine patients and a volar approach in four. They noted no avascular necrosis following surgery in any of the four patients in whom a volar approach had been used, a possible complication mentioned by earlier authors as a reason for not using this exposure. In their later article,[34] Campbell and colleagues favored the dorsal approach for two reasons: (1) it is usually necessary to clean out the space between the capitate and lunate, and this cannot be done adequately from the volar approach, and (2) the lunate dislocation may have been initially a perilunate dislocation, and it is therefore important to correct the scaphoid subluxation, which is more easily done dorsally. They were, moreover, perhaps the first to note that a volar incision was indicated (in addition to the dorsal incision) if the lunate was greatly displaced or if decompression of the median nerve was necessary.

Dobyns[55] has subsequently advocated combined dorsal and volar approaches to allow the surgeon to assess and repair the ligamentous and bony structures about both surfaces of the wrist.

Taleisnik[222] has recommended that these injuries always be exposed from the volar approach, as this is the site of major ligamentous change.

Adkinson and Chapman[3] recommended a dorsal approach only, offering their satisfactory results with this technique as evidence that maintenance of anatomic alignment with multiple K-wire fixation alone is sufficient to restore perilunate ligamentous integrity without the need for individual ligament repair or augmentation procedures.

Author's Preferred Method

In my experience, it is extremely difficult and highly unreliable to depend on closed reduction alone to maintain anatomic alignment of a dorsal perilunate/volar lunate dislocation. Prevention of late residual midcarpal instability or scapholunate dissociation with cast immobilization alone is unlikely, and my experience with closed reduction and percutaneous pinning of these injuries has not been particularly rewarding either. I would therefore agree with Adkinson and Chapman[3] that open reduction and internal fixation is the preferred treatment, although contrary to their recommendations, I do make an attempt to repair the ligaments at the same time.

As is true of all ligamentous injuries, early treatment is advised, and the sooner the open reduction is done, the easier it will be to adequately reduce the bones and repair the ligaments. Except in open injuries, however, these are rarely absolute emergencies, and satisfactory reduction and repair can be carried out anytime in the first few days. After about 7 to 10 days, however, the operation becomes more difficult and the result less predictable.

If the patient is seen on the day of injury and for some reason open reduction cannot be done immediately, I believe that a closed reduction of the midcarpal dislocation with the technique described on page 895 should be done at that time. The wrist is then splinted, the hand elevated, and the operation done as soon as feasible following the closed reduction.

Based on the assumption that dorsal perilunate and volar lunate dislocations are different stages of the same basic injury pattern, the operative treatment for these two injuries is identical. I routinely employ both dorsal and volar approaches, agreeing with Dobyns[55] that this gives the most comprehensive view of the pathology and a better opportunity to repair the extensive bony and ligamentous damage that is always present in these injuries.

Both exposures are made before proceeding with insertion of K-wires or repair of ligaments. Through a gentle lazy-S incision, and taking great care to identify and protect the superficial branch of radial nerve, the dorsal aspect of the carpus is exposed (Fig. 20-20A). After retracting the extensor tendons, the carpus comes immediately into view, as the entire ligamentous complex has usually been stripped completely off the bones.

The proximal pole of the scaphoid, having rotated dorsalward and radialward, protrudes vertically into the wound (Fig. 20-20B). Retracting this to the radial side exposes the bald base of the capitate, which is frequently dislocated dorsal to the lunate. On the volar side, a routine carpal tunnel incision is extended proximally across the wrist, with careful planning of the incision to avoid damage to the palmar cutaneous branch of median nerve (Fig. 20-21A). The flexor tendons and median nerve are retracted radially, revealing a consistent transverse rent in the volar capsule and ligaments (Fig. 20-21B). This tear has been present in all patients with both dorsal perilunate and volar lunate dislocations on whom I have operated, whether or not the lunate was displaced into the carpal tunnel on the preoperative radiographs.

After exposing both dorsal and volar sides, the lunate is easily reduced under direct vision from the volar approach by manually pushing it back in between the capitate and radius while an assistant applies gentle longitudinal traction on the hand (Fig. 20-21C). Although it is virtually impossible to identify and repair the individual intracapsular ligaments, it is relatively easy to repair the rent in the capsular-ligamentous complex with interrupted nonabsorbable sutures (Fig. 20-21D).

Returning to the dorsal exposure, the proximal pole of the capitate is reduced into the distal concavity of the lunate under direct vision. The proximal pole of the scaphoid, which has been displaced dorsally and radially by the injury, is rotated back down into its normal anatomic position (Fig. 20-20C). Using a power drill, two or three smooth 0.045-inch K-wires are inserted to stabilize the three key elements—the scaphoid, lunate, and capitate. The first two pins are inserted from the snuffbox across the scaphoid into the capitate and lunate, respectively (Fig. 20-20D). A third pin, inserted from the radial styloid through the scaphoid into the capitate, can be used to provide additional stability, if necessary. Anteroposterior, posteroanterior, and lateral radiographs are then taken to critically assess the reduction, with particular emphasis to ensure that: (1) the three key elements—scaphoid, lunate, and capitate—are anatomically

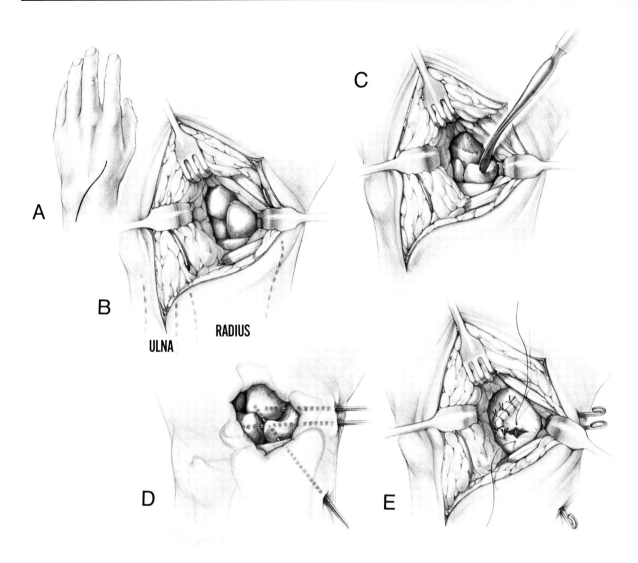

Fig. 20-20. Open reduction of dorsal perilunate/volar lunate dislocation (dorsal approach). The carpus is exposed through a gentle lazy-S incision (**A**), bringing the carpal bones into view (**B**). The scaphoid is reduced into its normal anatomic position and held in place (**C**) while K-wires are inserted to stabilize the scaphoid to the lunate and capitate (**D**), adding a third pin across the radial styloid to provide additional stability. Repair of the relatively weak (and frequently severely damaged) dorsal ligaments is then carried out (**E**). The dorsal approach is combined with the volar exposure shown in Figure 20-21. (See text for details and sequence of operation.)

reduced, and (2) the K-wires have solid purchase on each of the three bones. The pins are then bent at right angles outside of the skin to facilitate later removal.

Damage to the weak dorsal ligaments is often so extensive that repair is usually difficult and somewhat unsatisfying. In many instances it is possible only to tack the ligamentous complex back into po-

sition in rather gross fashion (Fig. 20-21E); rarely is there a clean tear on the dorsal side similar to that found on the volar aspect, and in my experience, never is there truly substantial ligamentous tissue to suture. Although I have not used tendon reconstruction to reinforce ligaments in any acute cases, the paucity of solid ligamentous tissue available for repair and the tendency for rotary subluxation of

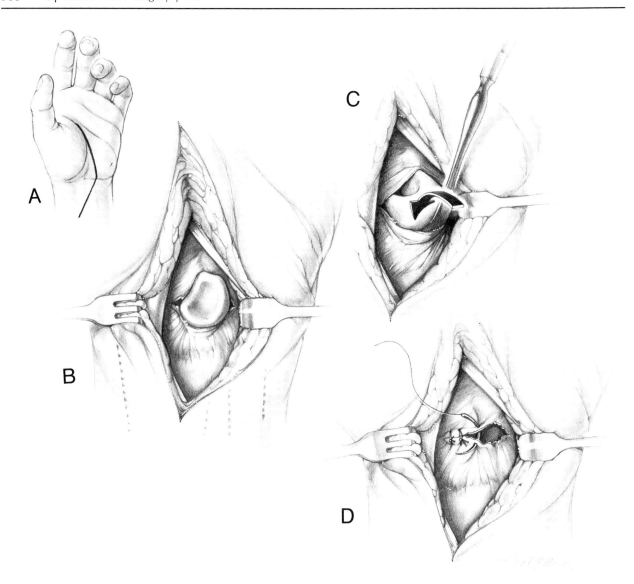

Fig. 20-21. Open reduction of dorsal perilunate/volar lunate dislocation (volar approach). A carpal tunnel incision is extended proximally across the wrist, taking care to avoid the palmar cutaneous branch of median nerve (**A**). A transverse rent in the volar capsule and ligaments is consistently found, whether the lunate is displaced into the carpal tunnel or not (**B**). While an assistant applies longitudinal traction to the hand, the lunate is reduced (**C**) and the transverse rent repaired with nonabsorbable sutures (**D**). The volar approach is used in combination with the dorsal approach shown in Figure 20-20. (See text for details and sequence of operation.)

the scaphoid to recur after removal of the K-wires suggest that some type of reinforcement may be desirable at the time of this initial operation. However, as noted on page 922, the unpredictable and inconsistent results of these ligamentous reconstructions in late cases have cautioned me against their use in acute injuries. Moreover, Palmer, Dobyns, and Linscheid[179] reported that although the intercarpal relationships were more consistently maintained when ligamentous reconstruction was used in their patients with acute injuries, there was no significant difference in symptoms or function from those in whom no reinforcement was done.

Osteochondral fractures of the carpal bones, especially of the capitate and lunate, are frequent concomitant injuries,[87] and probably contribute significantly to the postoperative stiffness seen in most of these patients. Often the damage to articular surfaces is rather extensive, and attempts should be made to remove small fragments and reattach larger ones if possible (occasionally they are avulsed by intercarpal ligaments).

Many of these patients have accompanying radial styloid fractures. If the styloid is a single, large fragment, it should be reduced anatomically and held with additional smooth K-wires. In some patients, the styloid is so severely comminuted that the most expeditious treatment may appear to be excision of the fragments. However, since this creates a potentially unstable situation by removing important bony, ligamentous, and possibly vascular support of the scaphoid, it is probably preferable to mold the fragments back into place as anatomically as possible.

Postoperative Management

A compression dressing incorporating a thumb spica plaster splint is applied in the operating room. Sutures are removed after 10 to 14 days, and a short arm thumb spica cast is applied. Radiographs are taken at this time to confirm maintenance of reduction and position of the wires. Manipulation of the wrist during cast changes should be avoided, as the K-wires traverse the radiocarpal and midcarpal joints.

The K-wires are left in place for at least 8 weeks. Initially they were removed earlier, but I have seen recurrence of the scaphoid subluxation following removal of the wires at 6 weeks. Plaster immobilization of the wrist is continued for an additional 4 weeks after pin removal, for a total of 12 weeks postoperatively.

Virtually all these patients will have some permanent limitation of motion, and several months of rehabilitation are required to regain range of motion and grip strength. In my experience, the average final range of motion in the wrist has been approximately 50 percent of normal, and in patients with more extensive articular damage, it is even

less. Return to heavy labor is rarely possible before 6 months, and more commonly requires up to 12 months.

TRANS-SCAPHOID PERILUNATE DISLOCATION

The initial management of trans-scaphoid perilunate dislocation, including the necessity of adequate anesthesia and preliminary traction, is identical to that described for dorsal perilunate dislocation on page 893. Radiographs taken with the hand suspended in finger-traps are particularly helpful in properly assessing the extent of damage to the carpal bones and should be obtained routinely before proceeding with closed reduction.

Closed Reduction

As noted on pages 884 and 898, the technique for closed reduction is the same regardless of whether the initial films show a typical dorsal trans-scaphoid perilunate dislocation or the less common situation in which the lunate and attached proximal pole of the scaphoid are dislocated volarly.

I use the technique described by Tavernier[230] and popularized by Watson-Jones.[246,247] After 5 to 10 minutes of continuous traction, during which time anteroposterior and lateral radiographs are obtained, the finger-traps are removed and the longitudinal traction force is maintained manually by the surgeon. With one hand, the patient's hand is dorsiflexed (maintaining longitudinal traction), while the thumb of the other hand stabilizes the lunate on the volar aspect of the wrist. Gradual palmar flexion of the hand then allows the capitate to snap back into the concavity of the lunate. The wrist is held in approximately 30 degrees volar flexion, and a dorsal plaster thumb spica splint is applied.

Postreduction radiographs are taken in plaster to ascertain the adequacy of reduction. It may be difficult to visualize the scaphoid fracture with the wrist in this position, but it is imperative to take enough different views to assess *very critically* the scaphoid fracture reduction. Usually, if the scaphoid is properly reduced, the midcarpal joint (capitate-lunate relationship) will be adequately reduced as well, but it is also important to look specifically for intercalated segment instability. The surgeon must not accept the reduction unless he is confident that the scaphoid fracture is reduced anatomically and that there is no intercalated segment instability.

Postreduction Management

If all of the above prerequisites for an acceptable reduction are satisfied, the patient is admitted to the hospital at least overnight for elevation of the hand and observation of the neurovascular status.

I generally leave the initial splint intact for 3 weeks, but *it is imperative to reassess the reduction radiographically weekly for at least the first 3 weeks.* At the end of 3 weeks, out-of-plaster films offer an opportunity to better evaluate the adequacy of the scaphoid fracture reduction and also detect the presence of intercalated segment instability. If the rigid criteria of reduction are still met, the wrist is brought from volar flexion to neutral, and immobilization of the wrist is continued in a short arm thumb spica cast until the scaphoid fracture is healed. The cast is removed for out-of-plaster radiographs at 6- to 8-week intervals. Gradual loss of reduction of the scaphoid fracture can occur, with resulting nonunion of the fracture and late dorsiflexion instability (Fig. 20-22). If a tendency toward this instability pattern is detected (this may be a gradual progression, and it is imperative to view each new set of radiographs in comparison with all previous films), open reduction and bone grafting of the scaphoid are indicated. In this situation, not only must the scaphoid be grafted, but an attempt must be made to restore proper alignment of the carpal bones, a goal that becomes more difficult to achieve the longer the interval since injury.

In those cases in which bone grafting is required several months after the initial injury, it is important to carefully evaluate the midcarpal joint. In many cases, especially those in which the scaphoid was not stabilized with open reduction primarily, there will be significant dorsiflexion instability (DISI). This is due to collapse and shortening of the volar cortex of the scaphoid, resulting in what Linscheid and Dobyns[136] have called the "humpback deformity." As several authors[12,68,69,89,96,136] have pointed out, an attempt must be made to correct the dorsiflexion deformity of the carpus by reestab-

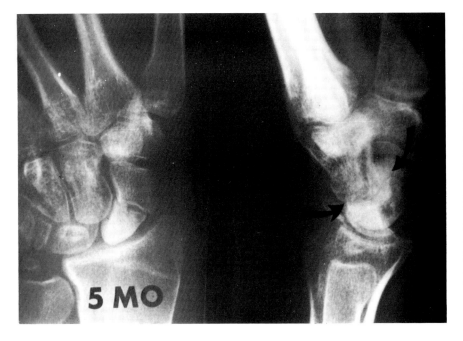

Fig. 20-22. This patient with a trans-scaphoid perilunate dislocation was treated by closed reduction and cast immobilization for 5 months. Not only does he now have a nonunion of the scaphoid and probably avascular necrosis of the proximal pole, but loss of the stabilizing effect of the scaphoid has allowed the wrist to develop a classic dorsiflexion instability pattern. This case demonstrates the importance of careful serial assessment of reduction in a patient treated with closed reduction. If anatomic reduction is not maintained, open reduction and internal fixation are indicated.

lishing the normal length of scaphoid. This is technically difficult to do and frequently results in incomplete correction with the standard Russe bone graft.[66,89] Fisk[67] first suggested that this type of scaphoid deformity should be corrected with a volar wedge-shaped bone graft, and Fernandez[66] has subsequently described a precise technique for doing this. Herbert[95] has advocated a similar procedure that combines a trapezoid-shaped corticocancellous graft with screw fixation. This late dorsiflexion instability problem due to the humpback scaphoid deformity is avoided by anatomic union of the scaphoid and is best prevented by primary stabilization of the scaphoid at the time of injury as described in the next section.

Open Reduction

It has long been recognized that failure to reduce the scaphoid fracture anatomically yields a poor result, but how to handle the unreduced scaphoid fracture has been a subject of considerable controversy. Earlier authors[144,145] recommended excision of the proximal fragment or proximal row carpectomy. Wagner[240,241] reported such uniformly poor results with open reduction that he advised primary arthrodesis of the wrist in all cases of transscaphoid perilunate dislocation in which anatomic reduction of the scaphoid could not be achieved by closed reduction. Few authors have shared that extreme degree of pessimism, and since Campbell and colleagues'[34] excellent article in 1965, several authors[10,34,87,99,258] have recommended open reduction and internal fixation if anatomic reduction of the scaphoid fracture cannot be achieved and maintained in plaster. Cave[36] actually advocated this principle in 1941. Several pertinent points, however, remain disputed: (1) the timing of operative intervention, (2) the operative approach, (3) the type of fixation, (4) whether or not bone grafting is indicated at the time of open reduction, and (5) the incidence of avascular necrosis of the proximal fragment.

Timing of Operative Intervention

Specific details concerning operative treatment of the displaced scaphoid fracture are skimpy in the many articles written about carpal dislocations.

What little mention there is about the timing of open reduction of the scaphoid is at wide variance. Cave[36] said that reduction must be done "within a few days," believing that later it may be impossible to satisfactorily realign the fragments. Worland and Dick[258] also favored immediate operative intervention, but Hill[99] preferred to defer open reduction until after 3 to 4 weeks of immobilization, to allow the intercarpal ligaments to heal. Theoretically, early stabilization of the fracture fragments should enhance the potential for healing and revascularization of the proximal pole.

Operative Approach

Cave's approach[36,37] was a curved radial incision exposing the scaphoid just volar to the tendons of the first dorsal compartment. Worland and Dick[258] advocated a dorsal approach for primary open reduction, as this necessitates no further dissection of the soft tissue structures because they are usually completely stripped off as a result of the perilunate dislocation. They reserved the volar (Russe type[197]) approach for later bone grafting, if indicated.

Moneim, Hoffmann, and Omer[163] also preferred the dorsal approach because it allowed good visualization not only of the scaphoid fracture fragments but also the area of the lunate and capitate to assure adequate reduction of the midcarpal joint.

Type of Fixation

The type of internal fixation favored by most authors has been K-wires,[33,87,94,165,258] although Cave[36] reported the successful use of dowel grafts taken from the tibia. McLaughlin[156] designed a lag screw for scaphoid fixation that was subsequently adopted by the AO group,[168] and later Huene[105,106] devised an alignment device to facilitate its insertion. An unstable scaphoid fracture in an acute trans-scaphoid perilunate dislocation is probably an ideal indication for the Herbert screw,[96] although I would recommend that it be used in this situation only if the surgeon is quite familiar with the instrumentation. Excellent rigid fixation can be achieved with the Herbert screw, but the technique is exacting and placement of the screw must be precise.

Use of Bone Graft

The need for bone graft at the time of open reduction has seldom been mentioned. Cave[11,36,37] used bone graft as the sole means of internal fixation, and Hill[99] reported that bone graft should be used in conjunction with internal fixation. As noted above, Worland and Dick[258] preferred to delay bone grafting for 6 weeks, using it only if there were signs of avascular necrosis or early nonunion. Although we have used supplemental bone graft in some of our open reductions, it is probably not necessary if the open reduction is done within 2 to 3 weeks of injury. I have frequently achieved successful union using only internal fixation without bone graft.[87]

Incidence of Avascular Necrosis

Broad disagreement exists as to the incidence of avascular necrosis of the proximal pole following trans-scaphoid perilunate dislocation. Campbell, Lance, and Yeoh[33] said that it is not common, but they did not report any figures about its incidence in their large series. Morawa, Ross, and Schock[165] had only two cases of avascular necrosis among their 21 patients. On the other hand, Wagner[240] said that the incidence was 50 percent with accurate reduction of the scaphoid and 100 percent without anatomic reduction, although he did not support this statement with clinical data. Hawkins and Torkelson[94] reported 100 percent avascular necrosis in their 16 patients, although all of the eight patients treated with open reduction had union of the fracture. Avascular necrosis of the proximal pole developed in eight of Worland and Dick's[258] nine cases, and in 13 of Russell's[198] 27 patients.

Perhaps the major reason for this disagreement over the incidence of avascular necrosis lies in the definition of avascular necrosis. It is my firm opinion that increased radiographic density of the proximal pole of the scaphoid does not *necessarily* establish the diagnosis of avascular necrosis, as shown in a recent study on Russe bone grafting.[89]

This same type of relative increased density can be seen in the lunate following fracture-dislocation or dislocation of the carpus.[182,255] The literature reflects that true avascular necrosis of the lunate is surprisingly uncommon even after complete lunate dislocation. White and Omer[255] reported three cases of increased radiographic density in the lunate, but none of these progressed to classic avascular necrosis, and these authors emphasized that this "transient vascular compromise" should not be confused with Kienböck's disease.

Author's Preferred Method

Based on the concept that the primary objective of open reduction in the patient with a trans-scaphoid perilunate dislocation is to stabilize the scaphoid and prevent subsequent midcarpal collapse deformity, I generally expose the scaphoid through a limited Russe-type approach, preferably within 2 weeks of injury. A 3-cm longitudinal incision is made just radial to the flexor carpi radialis tendon, curving outward over the base of the thenar eminence at the volar wrist crease for an additional 2 cm (Fig. 20-23A). The radial artery is identified and retracted radialward, the flexor carpi radialis tendon sheath opened, and the tendon retracted ulnarward. The wrist joint capsule is then opened longitudinally, exposing the fracture site (Fig. 20-23B). If the operation is done within the first 2 weeks following injury, anatomic reduction of the fracture is fairly easy to accomplish under direct vision. Beyond that time, accurate reduction becomes increasingly difficult, in my experience. Temporary placement of threaded 0.045-inch K-wires into each of the two fragments to use as "handles" often facilitates manipulation and reduction (Fig. 20-23C). Precise placement of the *smooth* 0.045-inch K-wires to stabilize the fracture is sometimes deceptively difficult. Usually, they can be inserted from the distal pole in retrograde fashion if the wrist is ulnarly deviated by an assistant, who must also hold the fracture reduced to prevent distraction of the scaphoid during insertion of the fixation wires (Fig. 20-23D). The K-wire "handles" mentioned earlier are particularly helpful in this regard, and a power-operated drill greatly facilitates accurate placement of the pins.

Following pin insertion, radiographic assessment of the adequacy of reduction and location of the K-wires is imperative. No distraction or displacement of the fracture should be accepted and the pins should not penetrate the proximal pole of the scaphoid into the radius.

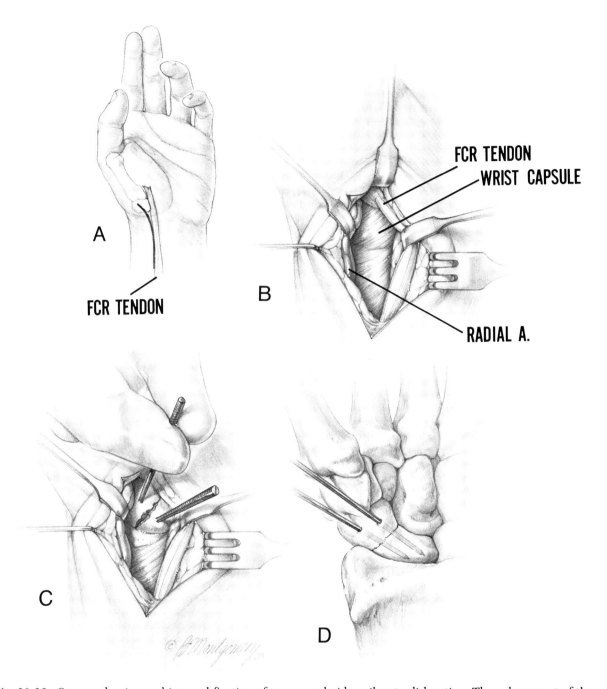

Fig. 20-23. Open reduction and internal fixation of trans-scaphoid perilunate dislocation. The volar aspect of the wrist is exposed through a Russe-type incision (**A**). Retracting the radial artery radialward and the flexor carpi radialis tendon ulnarward, the joint capsule is opened to expose the fracture site (**B**). Temporary placement of threaded K-wires into each of the two fragments to use as "handles" facilitates manipulation and reduction (**C**). While an assistant maintains the fracture reduction with the "handles" and ulnarly deviates the wrist, the surgeon inserts smooth K-wires from the distal pole of the scaphoid proximally (**D**). (See text for details.)

It is also extremely important at this stage to assess critically the reduction of the lunate as well. If fixation of the scaphoid adequately stabilizes the midcarpal joint, no further fixation is required. Since it is difficult to visualize the capitate-lunate joint directly through the limited Russe-type incision, it is imperative to look specifically for lunate (intercalated segment) instability in the postreduction films taken in the operating room. If there is the slightest tendency for volar subluxation or rotary instability of the lunate, additional operative exposure will generally be necessary to visualize and reduce the lunate and/or capitate. This requires extension of the volar incision and occasionally a dorsal approach as well. In such cases, additional K-wires should be introduced to stabilize the capitate-lunate joint in anatomic position. Failure to do this may result in late dorsiflexion instability.

As noted above, if the operation is done within 2 to 3 weeks of injury, bone graft is not used. If open reduction has been delayed for more than 3 weeks following injury, however, I may add bone graft at the time of internal fixation.

The tourniquet is released prior to closure to be sure that the radial artery has not been damaged during the operation. A secure capsular closure is then performed, and the skin is closed with subcuticular suture. A thumb spica splint is applied with the wrist in neutral.

Postoperative Management

Sutures are removed 10 to 14 days postoperatively, and a short arm thumb spica cast is applied with the wrist in neutral, leaving the distal joint of the thumb free. Radiographs are taken in the new cast to check the maintenance of the capitolunate reduction, especially if no K-wires were used for stabilization of these bones at operation.

The K-wires are usually removed in the office at 8 weeks, and a new thumb spica cast is applied. From this point on, management is identical to that for a routine acute scaphoid fracture. Progression of healing of the scaphoid fracture is monitored radiographically at 6- to 8-week intervals; these must be out-of-plaster films to adequately assess healing. The patient is usually seen every 3 to 4 weeks to check the condition of the plaster, as these patients are frequently aggressive, young males who are hard on casts.

The mere presence of increased radiographic density of the proximal pole is, in itself, not an indication for bone grafting.[87] I have seen several patients with transient radiographic changes suggestive of this, who nonetheless went on to successful healing of the fracture. If the fracture appears to be healing, I will continue immobilization for 6 months until radiographic union is present. If serial radiographs show no progression toward healing, I consider bone grafting as early as 4 months after injury. If grafting is necessary, I use the volar approach and the technique described by Russe[197] (see Chapter 19), although the volar wedge graft technique may be necessary if a "humpback" scaphoid and DISI deformity are present (see page 902).

Following removal of the cast, a period of rehabilitation is necessary, emphasizing wrist range of motion and grip-strengthening exercises. These

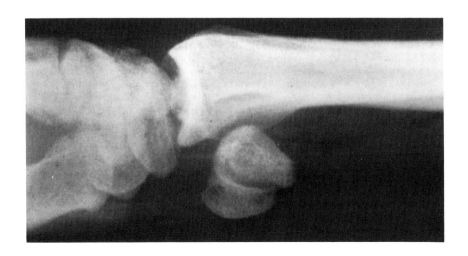

Fig. 20-24. In this patient with a trans-scaphoid perilunate dislocation, the proximal pole of the scaphoid remains attached to the lunate, and both have been dislocated volarly.

are severe injuries, and return to heavy use of the hand is generally not likely before 6 to 12 months. In my experience, the best results have been in younger patients and in patients in whom we were able to stabilize the entire carpus by fixation of the scaphoid alone through the limited Russe-type approach described earlier.

My worst results with carpal dislocations have been in those patients with trans-scaphoid perilunate dislocations in whom the lunate and proximal pole of the scaphoid have been dislocated volarly into the carpal tunnel[87] (Fig. 20-24). Although relatively uncommon, these tend to be open injuries with severe concomitant soft tissue damage, and in my hands the results have been poor despite early open reduction. Stern[215] reported two patients

with this injury who were asymptomatic following open reduction, although one had a scaphoid nonunion and early radioscaphoid arthrosis.

VOLAR PERILUNATE/DORSAL LUNATE DISLOCATION

Only a few isolated cases have been reported of this rare injury,[5,65,143,187,201,257] in which the capitate is displaced volar to the palmarflexed lunate. Like its more common dorsal counterpart, volar perilunate dislocation requires either a concomi-

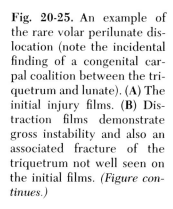

Fig. 20-25. An example of the rare volar perilunate dislocation (note the incidental finding of a congenital carpal coalition between the triquetrum and lunate). (A) The initial injury films. (B) Distraction films demonstrate gross instability and also an associated fracture of the triquetrum not well seen on the initial films. *(Figure continues.)*

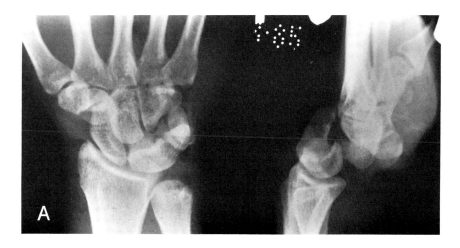

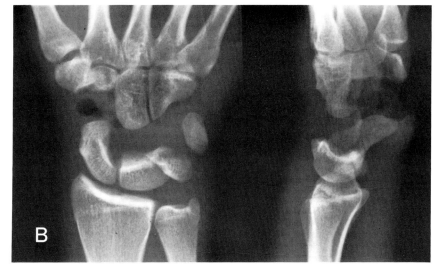

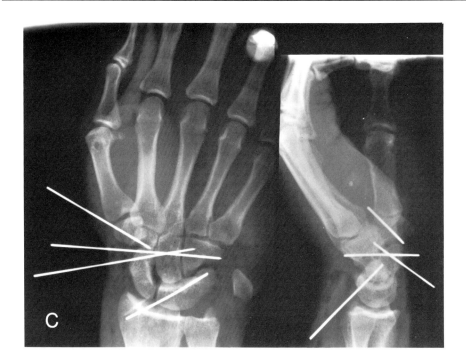

Fig. 20-25 *(Continued).* **(C)** Films taken in the operating room following open reduction and internal fixation.

tant fracture of the scaphoid or scapholunate dissociation.

Forced hyperflexion from a fall on the back of the hand has been proposed as the mechanism of injury by Aitken and Nalebuff.[5] O'Brien[88] reported a patient who died of other injuries two weeks after a volar perilunate dislocation. Manipulation of the dissected hand postmortem in this patient showed that the midcarpal displacement could be recreated by supination of the proximal segment on the extended distal segment, rotation occurring around the triquetrum. A fall on the hyperextended wrist with supination of the forearm and proximal row on the fixed hand and distal row may thus be the possible mechanism for this injury.

In acute injuries, closed reduction using finger trap traction should be the initial step in management. Although successful treatment has been reported with closed reduction alone,[65] careful assessment must be made after the closed manipulation to ascertain the anatomic alignment of the carpal bones. My very limited experience with this rare injury suggests to me that it is exceedingly unstable (Fig. 20-25), and open reduction is probably indicated in most cases to realign and stabilize the bones.

TRANSRADIAL STYLOID PERILUNATE DISLOCATION

This is not a truly separate entity, and is mentioned simply to emphasize the frequent concomitance of radial styloid fractures with carpal dislocations.[87,198,258] In my experience, radial styloid fractures are more commonly seen with dorsal perilunate dislocations, but they can also occur with trans-scaphoid perilunate dislocations.

The entire management of these injuries, from initial reduction to open reduction, if necessary, is identical to that described previously for the basic carpal dislocation pattern without the accompanying radial styloid fracture. What to do about the styloid fracture at the time of open reduction can occasionally be a cause for some concern. If it is a single, large fragment, it should be reduced anatomically and held with additional smooth K-wires. In some patients, the styloid is so severely comminuted that the most expeditious treatment may appear to be excision of the fragments. However, since this creates a potentially unstable situation by removing important bony, ligamentous, and possibly vascular support of the scaphoid, it is probably preferable to mold the fragments back into place as anatomically as possible.

SCAPHOCAPITATE SYNDROME

The scaphocapitate syndrome is a relatively uncommon variation of midcarpal dislocation in which the capitate is fractured, with the proximal pole rotating 90 or 180 degrees.[25,60] The first reported case in the English-language literature was by Nicholson[173] in 1940. Fenton[63,64] coined the term naviculocapitate syndrome, postulating that the fracture resulted from a force transmitted from the radial styloid through the waist of the scaphoid. Stein and Seigel[214] presented what appears to be the most logical mechanism of injury, i.e., direct compression of the capitate by the dorsal lip of the radius with the wrist in acute hyperextension, a theory also supported by Monahan and Galasko.[161]

As radiographic interpretation of this injury may be confusing,[194] films with the hand suspended in finger-trap traction should be obtained routinely. The squared-off end of the proximal capitate is easily seen in this view (Fig. 20-26).

Fenton and Rosen[64] advocated excision of the proximal pole as primary treatment because they believed avascular necrosis and nonunion were inevitable. Although Jones[113] and Adler and Shaftan[4] have described cases in which the fragment healed in its malrotated position, Marsh and Lampros[148] subsequently demonstrated that the fragment may undergo necrosis if left unreduced. Meyers, Wells, and Harvey[159] described a case in which union was accomplished by open reduction and internal fixation with K-wires. Weseley and Warenfeld[254] achieved successful healing in their single case with primary bone grafting after open reduction of the capitate. Adler and Shaftan[4] in their comprehensive article on capitate fractures, suggested that treatment of the displaced capitate fracture should be determined on the basis of other associated carpal injuries.

Vance, Gelberman, and Evans[238] made the important observation that the first step in operative treatment should be reduction and fixation of the

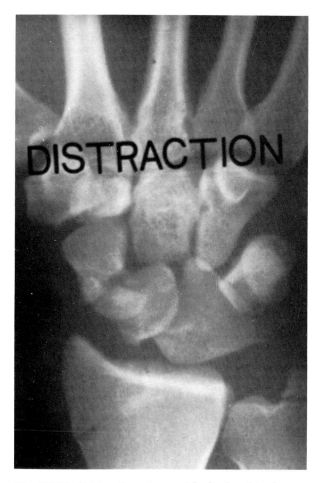

Fig. 20-26. Distraction views with the hand in finger-trap traction are useful in delineating the full extent of damage in carpal dislocations. These views are particularly helpful in depicting the squared-off end of the proximal pole of capitate in a scaphocapitate syndrome. (Green DP, O'Brien ET: Classification and management of carpal dislocations. Clin Orthop 149:68, 1980.)

capitate fracture (Fig. 20-27). If this is not done, the scaphoid tends to migrate medially (ulnarly) into the defect left by the carpal dislocation, making reduction of the scaphoid fracture difficult if not impossible without preliminary fixation of the capitate.

Author's Preferred Method

I believe that persistent displacement of a capitate fracture after closed reduction is an indication for open reduction. If performed within the first 2

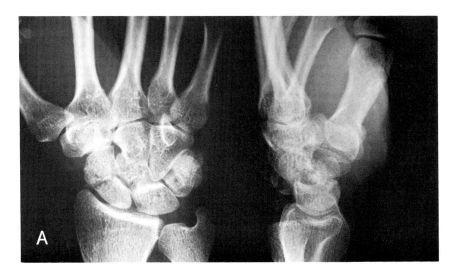

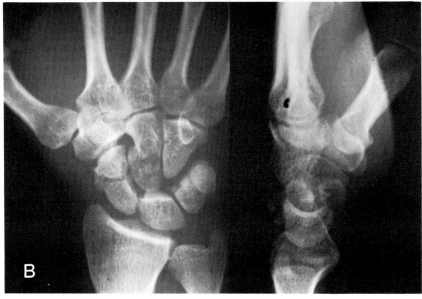

Fig. 20-27. Scaphocapitate syndrome. In the initial injury films (A), the fracture of the capitate is not well delineated, but distraction views (B) clearly show the transverse fracture in the capitate. *(Figure continues.)*

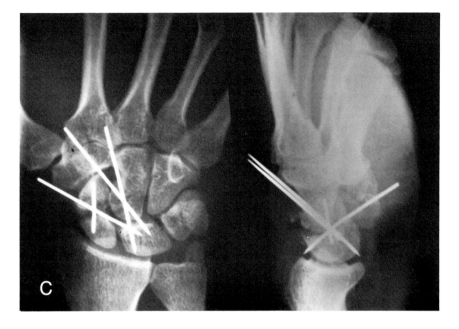

Fig. 20-27 *(Continued).* As pointed out by Vance et al,[238] it is important to fix the capitate fracture before attempting to stabilize the scaphoid **(C).** (Films courtesy of James W Adams, MD, Ogden, Utah).

weeks after injury, anatomic reduction of the capitate fracture can usually be accomplished under direct vision through a dorsal approach. Since the capitate fracture is only part of the carpal dislocation, it is equally important to achieve anatomic reduction and stabilization of the scaphoid and lunate using the techniques previously described for perilunate and trans-scaphoid perilunate dislocations (pages 897 and 904.).

Transient avascular changes in the proximal pole of the capitate are common, but healing usually occurs.

TRANSTRIQUETRAL PERILUNATE FRACTURE-DISLOCATION

In some carpal dislocations, the line of cleavage separating the midcarpal joint may extend through the triquetrum, leaving its proximal pole attached to the lunate and allowing the distal fragment to displace with the capitate. This can occur with the standard type of perilunate dislocation,[88] or, as in the case reported by Weseley and Warenfeld,[254] be a part of trans-scaphoid, transcapitate perilunate

dislocation (scaphocapitate syndrome). I have encountered this variant in several patients, noting that occasionally the triquetral fracture may be severely comminuted. I have directed no special attention to this particular aspect of the injury, except for removing nonviable free fragments of bone from the triquetrum. Generally, the triquetral fracture is restored into an acceptable position with reduction of the midcarpal joint.

COMPLETE DISLOCATION OF THE SCAPHOID

Isolated complete dislocation of the scaphoid without associated injuries to other carpal bones is an exceedingly rare injury. This entity is entirely different from rotary subluxation of the scaphoid, in which the proximal pole rotates dorsally, hinged upon the intact distal attachments.[56] As the name implies, complete dislocation of the scaphoid is a situation in which *all* the ligamentous attachments of the scaphoid are torn and the bone is totally displaced volarly from the remaining carpus.

Very few cases have been reported in the English-language literature since 1930.[7,27,31,39,43,98,128,147,169,202,233,242] On the basis of these articles, several pertinent points warrant mentioning. Most of the reported injuries appear to have resulted from force applied to the radial aspect of the hand with the wrist in dorsiflexion and ulnar deviation. In at least two of the cases,[31,43] there was an apparent separation between the bases of the third and fourth metacarpals, with proximal displacement of the entire radial side of the hand (capitate, trapezoid, trapezium, and first three metacarpals). Kuth's[128] case had an associated fracture of the trapezium, further suggesting some type of longitudinal force directed along the axis of the thumb.

In most cases, the diagnosis was easily made immediately after injury because of the presence of an abnormal bony prominence at the base of the thumb, adjacent to the radial styloid. This is in sharp contrast to isolated rotary subluxation of the scaphoid, in which the diagnosis is frequently delayed.

In six of the 10 cases, closed reduction was easily accomplished by traction on the fingers and direct manual pressure on the bony prominence. Results were uniformly good in these patients treated with closed reduction and plaster immobilization for periods ranging from 4 to 8 weeks.

Open reduction was necessary in only four of the reported cases. In two of these, the diagnosis had been delayed 2 and 6 weeks, respectively, and in one, closed manipulation failed to reduce the dislocation because of interposition of a flap of capsule discovered at the time of open reduction. In this latter case, reported by Murakami,[169] open reduction without K-wire fixation resulted in early loss of reduction and persistent rotary subluxation of the scaphoid.

Surprisingly, avascular necrosis did not occur in any case, even in the patient reported by Walker[242] in whom the scaphoid was removed, bathed in saline, and replaced at the time of open reduction (although transient increased radiographic density did appear in this case).

Author's Preferred Method

Having had no personal experience with this rare injury, I can offer nothing more than that which has been summarized above from the available literature. It would appear that an attempt at closed reduction is warranted, and consideration might be given to percutaneous pin fixation if anatomic reduction can be achieved by closed manipulation.

CAPITATE-HAMATE DIASTASIS

In 1985, Garcia-Elias et al[74] described a series of cases resulting from severe crush injuries of the carpus that showed remarkable similarities, the most notable feature being disruption of the carpal arch through the capitate-hamate articulation, with slight variations in the line of cleavage (Fig. 20-28). Primiano and Reef[188] had previously reported four cases with essentially identical patterns, and a careful retrospective review of other articles on carpal bone injuries[170] has revealed similar findings. For example, the case reports by Buzby[31] and Connell and Dyson[43] of dislocation of the scaphoid both showed capitate-hamate diastasis as concomitant radiographic abnormalities. Most of these patients have had extensive lacerations of the thenar eminence and massive swelling, suggestive of a bursting-type response to a severe crush injury. Although several of the cases reported were treated by closed reduction, Primiano and Reef[188] performed carpal tunnel releases in all of their four patients, and stabilization of the capitate-hamate diastasis by open reduction and internal fixation would appear to be a reasonable method of treatment.

SCAPHOLUNATE DISSOCIATION

Scapholunate dissociation (rotary subluxation of the scaphoid) is now recognized with much greater frequency than it was even a few years ago, and I share Taleisnik's[224] view that this is probably the most common form of carpal instability. It may be the late residual from a perilunate/lunate dislocation (see page 897), or it may exist as an isolated entity, representing stage I of Mayfield et al's PLI (see page 883). It is my impression that scapholu-

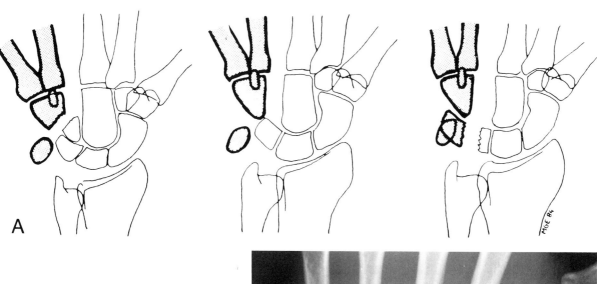

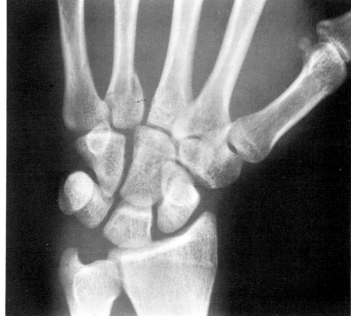

Fig. 20-28. (A) Three patterns of capitate-hamate diastasis as described by Garcia-Elias et al,[74] showing the main line of separation between the capitate and hamate, extending out between the third and fourth metacarpals. (B) This line of cleavage may be subtle and easy to overlook in the patient with a crush injury of the hand. (A from Garcia-Elias M, Abanco J, Salvador E, Sanchez R: Crush injury of the carpus. J Bone Joint Surg 67B:288, 1985.)

nate dissociation can exist with or without the midcarpal changes seen in dorsiflexion instability (DISI).

Diagnosis

CLINICAL DIAGNOSIS

Despite pleas in the literature emphasizing the importance of early diagnosis and treatment, scapholunate dissociation unfortunately rarely seems to be recognized early, especially those cases not associated with or residual from a perilunate/lunate dislocation. In those patients who recall a mechanism of injury, it is usually a fall on the outstretched hand with the wrist in dorsiflexion, but often there is no history of a specific traumatic episode, either recent or remote. Other less common causes have been reported,[48,166] and there is some suggestion that inherent ligamentous laxity may be a predisposing factor.[97,185,237] In some cases, therefore, radiographic examination of the opposite wrist may be indicated.

An important part of the physical examination is precise localization of maximum tenderness. Usually this will be on the dorsum of the wrist directly over the scapholunate joint, although most of these patients also have tenderness in the anatomic snuffbox as well. Wrist motion may be severely limited by pain, or there may be surprisingly little pain except at the extremes of motion.

Watson[90] has described a test for scapholunate dissociation that is useful, but somewhat difficult to perform. Experience with this test in many normal wrists is necessary before it can be evaluated with confidence. The examiner's four fingers of the same hand as that to be examined are placed behind the radius. The thumb is placed on the tuberosity (distal pole) of the scaphoid. The other hand is used to move the wrist passively from ulnar to radial deviation. In ulnar deviation, the scaphoid assumes a position in line with the forearm. In radial deviation, the scaphoid lies more perpendicular to the axis of the forearm than it does in ulnar deviation. Pressure on the tuberosity while the wrist is moved from ulnar deviation to radial deviation prevents the scaphoid from assuming the more transverse position, and the proximal pole will displace dorsally out of the elliptical fossa of the radius if there is sufficient ligamentous laxity. Comparison of the two sides is important. Watson's test is illustrated and described in Chapter 5.

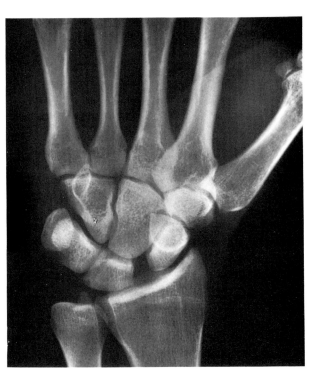

Fig. 20-29. The key radiographic features of rotary subluxation of the scaphoid (scapholunate dissociation) are seen on this anteroposterior view of the wrist: (1) widening of the space between the scaphoid and lunate; (2) a foreshortened appearance of the scaphoid; and (3) the cortical "ring" shadow, which represents an axial projection of the abnormally oriented scaphoid.

RADIOGRAPHIC DIAGNOSIS

The key radiographic features of scapholunate dissociation have been clearly established and repeatedly described in the literature. They are summarized here.

1. Widening of the space between the scaphoid and lunate in the anteroposterior projection (Fig. 20-29). This is usually seen better with the hand in full supination (AP rather than PA view),[234] or with the wrist in radial deviation.[85] Dobyns and his colleagues[54] have suggested that the scapholunate gap may be accentuated by compressing the carpus either by having the patient make a fist or by applying a longitudinal force to the hand. In my routine scaphoid series, I therefore include a view that incorporates those positions most likely to demonstrate scapholunate dissociation, namely an AP view combined with fist compression. If the patient has excessive pain that prevents adequate fist compression, an alternative view is that suggested by Moneim,[162] i.e., a PA view with the ulnar border of the hand elevated 20 degrees off the table (Fig. 20-30). This view directs the beam so that it is parallel to the adjacent surfaces of the scaphoid and lunate. A scapholunate gap greater than 3 mm is said to be diagnostic of scapholunate dissociation,[135] although in patients with a gap of 2 to 3 mm, I generally obtain comparison views of the opposite side. In such patients, the significance of this slightly increased gap may be difficult to interpret, and it must be considered in light of the history and

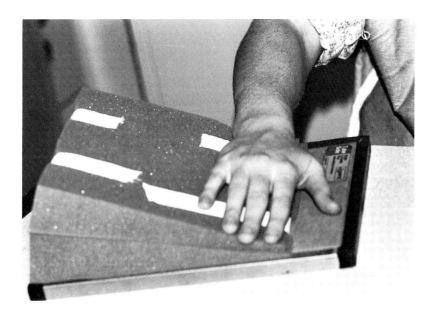

Fig. 20-30. Moneim has described an x-ray view in which the beam is directed parallel to the adjacent surfaces of the scaphoid and lunate, thereby giving a perhaps more precise reading of the gap between the two bones. The ulnar border of the hand is elevated 20 degrees off the table. (Moneim MS: The tangential posteroanterior radiograph to demonstrate scapholunate dissociation. J Bone Joint Surg 63A:1324, 1981.)

other radiographic and clinical findings. This scapholunate widening has also been called the "Terry Thomas" sign[72] after the famous English film comedian's dental diastema.

2. A foreshortened appearance of the scaphoid in the AP view.[18,233,239]
3. A cortical "ring" shadow seen in the AP view, which represents an axial projection of the abnormally oriented scaphoid.[18,49,109]
4. In the lateral view (Fig. 20-31), the scaphoid is palmarflexed, i.e., its long axis lies more perpendicular to the long axis of the radius rather than at its usual angle of 45 to 60 degrees.[134,239] The scapholunate angle is also increased (see page 891), with higher angles being seen when there is accompanying DISI.
5. Taleisnik's "V" sign.[222] In the normal wrist, lines drawn along the volar margins of the scaphoid and radius form a wide C-shaped pattern. When the scaphoid is subluxated, the volar outline of the scaphoid intersects the volar margin of the radius at an acute angle, forming a sharper, V-shaped pattern (Fig. 20-31).
6. The most subtle sign of scapholunate dissociation in my experience is lack of parallelism between the apposing articular surfaces of the scaphoid and lunate in the AP view (Fig. 20-32).[45] This finding in a patient with appropriate supporting findings on the clinical examination is in my opinion an indication for cineradiographs or a "motion series."

The diagnosis of scapholunate dissociation can usually be made on standard x-rays, and I routinely obtain a "scaphoid series" (see page 890) in any patient suspected of having this condition. There are, however, patients with what I call dynamic scapholunate dissociation, in whom the plain films may be normal except for the subtle sign noted above showing lack of parallelism between the scaphoid and lunate in the AP view. In such patients, cineradiographs[110,174,189] will frequently show abnormal movement between the scaphoid and lunate, especially as the wrist is moved actively in radial and ulnar deviation.

Arthrography has not been particularly useful to me in the diagnosis of scapholunate dissociation, although it may show abnormal leakage of dye from the radiocarpal joint into the midcarpal joint via the scapholunate interval, especially after the patient actively moves the wrist through a full range of motion. In patients with obscure wrist pain in which it is difficult to pinpoint the cause, arthrography may demonstrate more subtle and unusual findings such as a partial tear of the scapholunate ligament reported by Weeks et al[251] or the radiocarpal septum described by Wehbe and Karasick.[252]

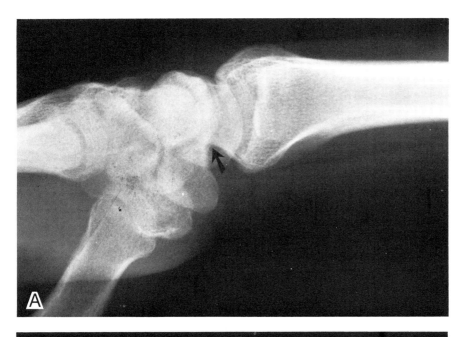

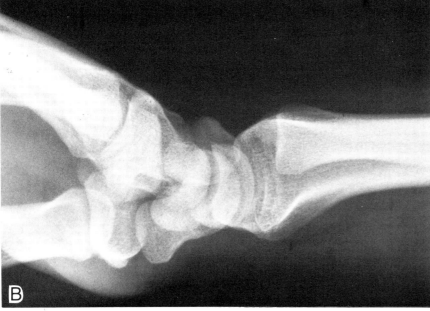

Fig. 20-31. Rotary subluxation of the scaphoid can also be seen in the lateral radiograph. Note the vertical orientation of the scaphoid lying at 90 degrees to the long axis of the radius. Taleisnik's V sign is also apparent; the volar margin of the scaphoid intersects the volar margin of the radius at an acute angle *(arrow)*. In the normal wrist (**B**), these lines form a wide C-shaped pattern.

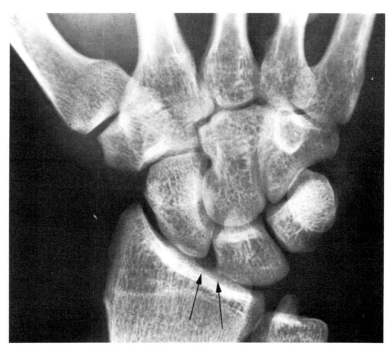

Fig. 20-32. A subtle sign of scapholunate dissociation may be lack of parallelism between the apposing articular surfaces of the scaphoid and lunate *(arrows)*. In the author's opinion, this finding in a patient with appropriate supporting findings on clinical examination is an indication for cineradiographs or a "motion series" of plain radiographs.

Methods of Treatment

Treatment of scapholunate dissociation is difficult and, given our present imperfect understanding of the carpus, not always predictable. Even Linscheid and Dobyns, clearly two of the most knowledgeable wrist authorities in the world, have recently stated that "treatment of this condition is seldom entirely satisfactory." [137] With this in mind, the following sections are intended to review the various alternatives for treatment that have been described for this difficult problem.

ACUTE SCAPHOLUNATE DISSOCIATION

As mentioned previously, scapholunate dissociation is diagnosed early rather infrequently. Even the definition of what constitutes an "acute" injury is debatable; Taleisnik[224] says within 3 weeks, Linscheid[135] suggests 3 months. Nonetheless, if we accept scapholunate dissociation as a ligamentous injury and apply the principles of ligamentous injuries in other joints, we would have to believe that primary treatment should be instituted within 2 to 3 weeks of injury in order to be effective.

Closed Reduction and Cast Immobilization

Despite occasional reports in the literature[2,13,123] suggesting that scapholunate dissociation can be successfully treated with cast immobilization alone, I share the opinion of most authors that it is virtually impossible to consistently maintain a satisfactory reduction in a cast alone. King[123] has recommended immobilization of the wrist in the "wine waiter's position" of full supination, middorsiflexion, and ulnar deviation, but our cineradiographic studies have demonstrated that there is no single position that will consistently reduce all cases of scapholunate dissociation.

Closed Reduction and Percutaneous Pin Fixation

Several authors[48,137,177,224] have recommended percutaneous pin fixation of acute scapholunate dissociation if satisfactory alignment can be achieved by closed manipulation. The procedure should be done under image intensification to insure anatomic alignment of the scaphoid and the lunate. O'Brien[177] recommends fixation with two pins through the scaphoid into the capitate and lunate, respectively. Linscheid and Dobyns[137] suggest one pin through the radial styloid into the lunate (after it has been positioned 60 percent in the lunate fossa), a second pin from the radial styloid into the scaphoid, and occasionally a third pin transfixing the scaphoid to the lunate. They note that introduction of the pins may displace the bones, and it is important for the surgeon to stabilize the carpus with his own hand as the pins are being inserted.

Taleisnik[224] has emphasized Mayfield et al's "paradox" of closed reduction of scapholunate dissociation. Believing that the volar ligaments (especially the radioscapholunate ligament) are the critical elements providing stability for the scaphoid, Taleisnik notes that theoretically the ends of these ligaments would be more closely approximated with the wrist in volar flexion, but this places the proximal pole of the scaphoid in an undesirable, unstable position. Conversely, if the scaphoid is reduced by dorsiflexing the wrist, the torn ends of the volar ligaments will be distracted. As a possible solution to this paradox, Crawford and Taleisnik[48] have suggested that the scaphoid first be reduced in dorsiflexion and, under cineradiographic control, stabilized with K-wires to the other carpal bones, specifically the lunate. The wrist is then volar flexed to approximate the torn ends of the ligament. If this is done, however, the wrist must be moved with great care under image intensification to prevent bending of the K-wires (see Fig. 20-19).

These authors recommend that the wires be left in for 8 weeks[177] to 10 weeks,[224] with protection in a removable splint for an additional 4 weeks[177] after motion is begun.

Open Reduction and Internal Fixation

Open reduction of acute scapholunate dissociation is controversial,[137] but it does offer the same advantages as primary operative repair of ligamentous injuries in other joints; e.g., assurance that the subluxation is reduced, visualization and treatment of associated damage, such as osteochondral fragments, and direct repair of torn ligaments. O'Brien[177] suggests a dorsal approach between the third and fourth extensor compartments, which allows direct visualization and repair of the dorsal scapholunate interosseous ligament. There is sometimes sufficient ligamentous tissue to permit a reasonable repair, and occasionally the scapholunate ligament has been avulsed with a small osteochondral fragment that can be very neatly tacked back down into its bed. Not infrequently, however, even in acute cases, the ligament is so badly damaged that satisfactory repair is impossible. In such cases, the surgeon may try to use some local capsule to reinforce the repair, although often this is tenous at best. The dorsal approach obviously does not allow visualization and repair of the important volar ligaments, but I am not aware of any series that has been reported with a volar approach for primary operative treatment of scapholunate dissociation, although Fisk[71] has mentioned this.

Re-creation of the Scapholunate Linkage

Linscheid[135] believes that if scapholunate dissociation is recognized early, an attempt should be made to "re-create the scapholunate linkage." Basically, what he describes is an augmentation procedure to use at the time of open reduction when inadequate tissue for repair of the dorsal scapholunate ligaments is encountered. Drill holes are made obliquely from the dorsal rim of the lunate to the denuded area from which the interosseous ligaments have been avulsed (Fig. 20-33A), allowing the ligament to be reapproximated with minimal intraarticular exposure. In some cases, further reinforcement is added by Linscheid with a strip of flexor carpi radialis tendon that is passed through a 3- to 4-mm drill hole in the scaphoid and sutured to the dorsal rim of the radius near Lister's tubercle (Fig. 20-33B).

Author's Preferred Method

I do not believe that scapholunate dissociation can be treated adequately with cast immobilization alone, and I have been a bit disappointed with closed reduction and percutaneous pin fixation. Therefore, in those rare patients that I see with acute scapholunate dissociation following a specific wrist injury, my preference is open reduction through a dorsal approach, repair of the dorsal scapholunate interosseous ligaments, and stabilization of the scaphoid to the lunate and capitate with two or more Kirschner wires.

Theoretically, the volar ligaments are the most

Fig. 20-33. In some cases of scapholunate dissociation, Linscheid uses small drill holes in the dorsal rim of the lunate (**A**) through which the scapholunate ligaments can be reattached. If further reinforcement is needed, he may also use a strip of flexor carpi radialis tendon passed through a 3- to 4-mm drill hole in the lunate (**B**). (Linscheid RL: Scapho-lunate ligamentous instabilities (dissociations, subdislocations, dislocations). Ann Chir Main 3:328, 1984.)

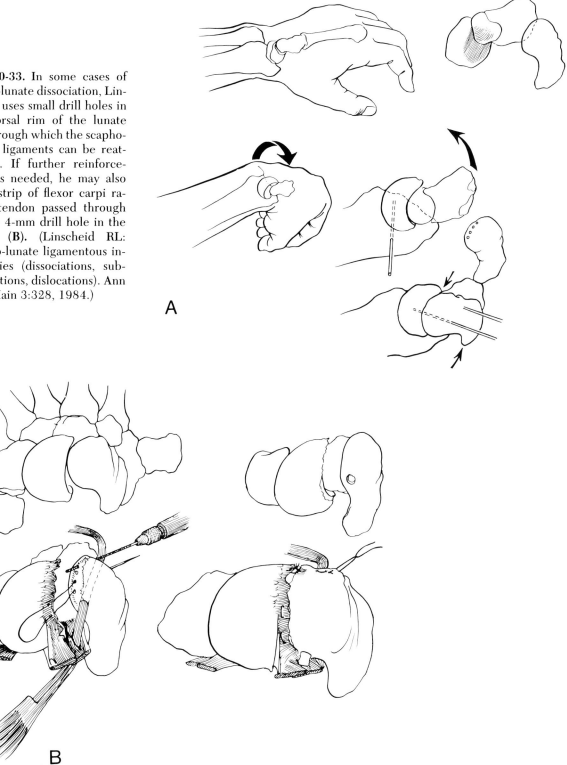

important stabilizers of the proximal pole of the scaphoid, but I prefer the dorsal approach mainly because it provides better visualization of the anatomic relationships of the scaphoid and lunate. If the scaphoid is reduced anatomically and stabilized with K-wires, it is hoped that the important volar radioscapholunate ligament should heal, especially if the wrist is immobilized in slight palmar flexion (see discussion of Mayfield's "paradox" of reduction on page 918).

In light of the inconsistent results with all forms of treatment for scapholunate dissociation, it is my opinion that open reduction and direct repair should offer the best chance of correcting the problem early. There is one caveat, however. Even the patient who has a typical dorsiflexion wrist injury with both clinical and radiographic findings diagnostic of acute scapholunate dissociation may in fact have a fresh wrist injury superimposed on pre-existing scapholunate instability. In such patients, the surgeon may be surprised at operation to find chronic changes with a paucity of local ligamentous tissue to repair, and he or she must thus be prepared to alter the operative game plan and employ one of the procedures described below for treatment of late carpal instability.

CHRONIC SCAPHOLUNATE DISSOCIATION

Although chronic scapholunate dissociation can theoretically exist alone without concomitant midcarpal instability, in most cases there will also be an element of DISI as well. Therefore, the discussion of chronic scapholunate dissociation has been included in the section that follows on late post-traumatic carpal instability, since it is very difficult to separate the various elements in the spectrum of deformity seen in the chronic state.

LATE POST-TRAUMATIC CARPAL INSTABILITY

Throughout this chapter, emphasis has been on early recognition and treatment of carpal dislocations, as delay in diagnosis is likely to lessen the chance of a successful result. Unfortunately, the surgeon is still more often confronted with patients in whom the diagnosis is made weeks, months, and even years after the acute injury. It is these patients with late post-traumatic carpal instability that present the greatest challenge in management, since the accumulated experience in the literature is insufficient to provide the surgeon with consistently reliable and predictable reconstructive procedures. Dobyns and Linscheid have been the major pioneers in this field, and their intensive studies of these difficult problems have been the foundation to which others have added important bits of knowledge. Taleisnik and Watson in particular have made major contributions to our management of these difficult problems.

Methods of Treatment

DIRECT LIGAMENT RECONSTRUCTION

The difference between acute and chronic injuries does not have a clear and distinct dividing line, and thus the first option for treatment of chronic carpal instability is identical to the last method described previously under acute injuries, re-creation of the scapholunate linkage. It was mentioned in that section that Linscheid[135] attempts to reapproximate the dorsal scapholunate interosseous ligament, but if that is not possible, he will use a strip of flexor carpi radialis tendon as reinforcement. Goldner's[84] preference for chronic scapholunate instability is quite similar, i.e., "pin fixation, complemented by dorsal capsular repair with nonabsorbable sutures passed through small drill holes in subchondral bone and existing capsular and ligamentous material. If an inadequate collagen covering is present, additional material such as a small free tendon graft is attached to the surfaces of the carpal bones by sutures. If the patient has hypermobile collagen in all joints, then palmar capsular plication may also be necessary."

DORSAL CAPSULODESIS

Blatt[20] has described a soft tissue technique for stabilization of chronic rotary subluxation of the scaphoid that he refers to as dorsal capsulo-ligamentosis. The concept of this operation is that a check-rein is created to prevent volar rotation of the distal pole of scaphoid. He believes that this procedure offers better postoperative range of motion with less surgical morbidity than intercarpal arthrodesis.

Technique

The radioscaphoid joint is exposed through a longitudinal dorsoradial incision. A 1.0-cm wide flap of dorsal capsulo-ligamentous tissue is raised, leaving its proximal edge securely attached to the dorso-ulnar aspect of the distal radius (Fig. 20-34A). The subluxated scaphoid is reduced by manipulation of the wrist, confirming reduction by restoring the anatomic appearance of the scapho-trapezial-trapezoidal joint. The reduced position is maintained with a single 0.045-inch K-wire passed obliquely from the distal pole of the scaphoid into the capitate. At a point well *distal* to the midaxis of rotation of the scaphoid, a notch is created down to fresh cancellous bone. The dorsal flap is then inserted into this notch and held in place with a pull-out suture tied over a button on the volar aspect of the wrist (Fig. 20-34B).

Postoperatively the patient wears a thumb spica cast for 2 months, at which time active range of motion exercises are begun. Blatt leaves the K-wire in for an additional month, removing this and al-

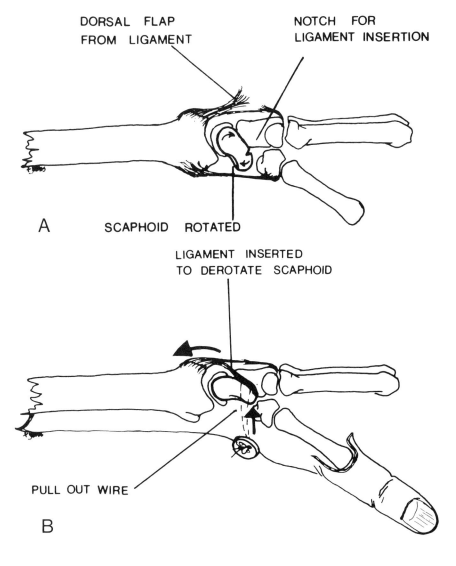

Fig. 20-34. Blatt's technique of dorsal capsulodesis for chronic rotary subluxation of the scaphoid. (A) A 1.0-cm wide strip of dorsal capsule is raised, leaving it attached to the dorsal rim of the distal radius. A notch is created in the distal pole of the scaphoid well distal to its axis of rotation. (B) After reducing the scaphoid anatomically and fixing it with a single K-wire to the capitate, the dorsal flap is inserted into the notch and tied over a button on the volar aspect of the wrist.

lowing intercarpal motion to begin 3 months post-operatively.

LIGAMENT RECONSTRUCTION USING TENDON GRAFTS

As Dobyns and Linscheid have noted[54,179] exact anatomic repair and reconstruction of the carpal ligaments are impossible at the present stage of our surgical art. The scapholunate and radioscapholunate ligaments are short, stout structures serving precise anatomic functions. A tendon running through drill holes in the carpal bones obviously does not lie in the same plane nor perform the same function as the original ligament, and thus far all attempts to reconstruct these ligaments have been rather crude compromises of actual anatomic structures. Even if the operation is performed with precise skill and technique, it is well known that all tenodeses have a tendency to attenuate and lose their effectiveness with time. Moreover, the extensive dissection and relatively large drill holes required for the operation introduce further undesirable eventualities: (1) the holes may produce a weakened area in the bone, which becomes the site of a potential fracture; (2) the blood supply of the bones may be compromised; and (3) postoperative scarring adds further injury and stiffness to a wrist that is already significantly damaged.

The reconstructive procedures described by Dobyns and Linscheid have dealt primarily with attempts to correct scapholunate dissociation (rotary subluxation of the scaphoid or dorsiflexion instability). In general, two types of reconstruction have received the most attention: reconstruction of the interosseous scapholunate ligaments and reconstruction of the radioscapholunate ligament. Several points need emphasis before considering the use of these procedures: (1) they are contraindicated in patients with established post-traumatic arthrosis; (2) some patients with chronic scapholunate dissociation or dorsiflexion instability are relatively asymptomatic and do not warrant operative treatment; (3) these procedures are technically demanding, requiring a thorough knowledge of the anatomy of the wrist and meticulous attention to detail in the operative techniques; and (4) the results of these operations are still somewhat unpredictable.[82]

Scapholunate Ligament Reconstruction (Fig. 20-35) (Technique of Dobyns and Linscheid[54,179])

Combined volar and dorsal approaches are recommended, as described for treatment of acute carpal dislocations (page 898). Anatomic reduction of the three key elements (scaphoid, lunate, and capitate) is the first priority, although this may be somewhat difficult in long-standing cases. The gap between the scaphoid and lunate is often filled with fibrous tissue, and rather extensive soft tissue dissection may be required to free up the scaphoid adequately to permit complete correction of the scaphoid subluxation. Obviously, this dissection should be limited to that required to achieve reduction, as excessive soft tissue stripping from the scaphoid may create further instability and also result in some devascularization of the scaphoid. Two or three K-wires are essential to hold the reduction of the three bones. Preparations for ligamentous reconstruction must be made before reduction and fixation are completed, since the necessary exposure is not available after reduction.

From the dorsal incision, a 10-cm strip of half of one of the radial wrist extensors (ECRL or ERCB) is prepared, leaving the distal end attached at the normal tendon insertion. A hole is carefully drilled (avoiding damage to the radial articular surface) from the dorsal portion of the proximal pole of the scaphoid, emerging on the scapholunate interarticular surface at a point below or palmar to the center of the scapholunate joint surface. A similar hole is drilled from the dorsal aspect to the lunate, emerging opposite the scaphoid tunnel. The final diameter of this tunnel should be large enough to accept a 5-mm Hunter tendon implant, which is used as the tendon passer. Curved ligature carriers can also be used to thread the tendon graft through the holes.

The graft is then passed from scaphoid to lunate, prior to actual reduction and fixation of the bones. After the bones have been reduced and stabilized with K-wires, the graft is pulled through the tunnel snugly and placed under slight tension. The graft, which emerges from the dorsal opening in the lunate, is then brought back across the scapholunate interval, sutured to itself, and further reinforced by

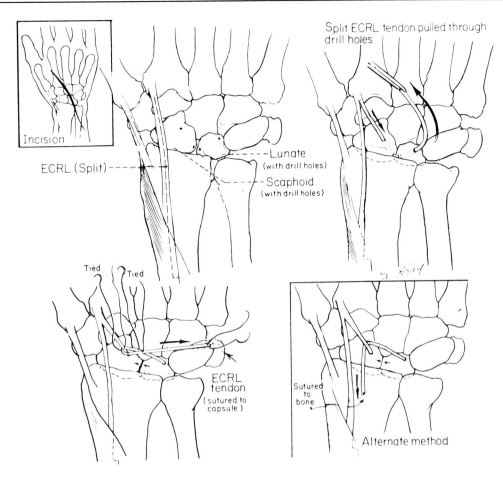

Fig. 20-35. Technique for reconstruction of the (dorsal) scapholunate ligaments (Dobyns and Linscheid). The extensor carpi radialis longus tendon is split longitudinally and a 10- to 15-cm segment is left attached distally at its insertion. This graft is passed through a tunnel from the dorsal aspect of the scaphoid across the scapholunate joint, emerging on the dorsum of the lunate. K-wires (not shown) are then used to stabilize the bones and the graft sutured to itself after being made snug. If sufficient graft remains, it is passed across the carpus and sutured into the capsule overlying the triquetrum. An alternate method of insertion into the dorsal periosteum of the radius is shown. (See text for details.) (Reproduced with permission from Dobyns JH, Linscheid RL, Chao EYS, Weber ER, Swanson GE: Traumatic instability of the wrist. p. 193. AAOS Instructional Course Lectures, Vol. 24. CV Mosby, St Louis, 1975.)

tacking it to the strong dorsal capsular fibers over the triquetrum or, alternatively, into the dorsal periosteum of the distal radius. All possible repairs of available ligamentous tissue are then carried out to further reinforce the dorsal capsule.

The authors have noted several critical points in technique: (1) careful drilling of the bone tunnels to avoid fracture of the roof of the tunnel; (2) passage of good quality tendon graft; (3) overreduc-tion of both the radiolunate-capitate and scaphoid alignment, preferably using three K-wires to hold the reduction; and (4) prolonged postoperative immobilization.

Postoperative Management. Dobyns and Linscheid recommend a bulky dressing extending above the elbow, incorporating a short arm plaster splint, until swelling has subsided, at which time a well-fitted short arm thumb spica cast is applied. The K-wires are removed at 6 to 8 weeks postoperatively, and part-time splinting is continued for an additional 6 weeks. Rehabilitation until maximum improvement is achieved will require a minimum of 6 months, extending to 12 months in severely damaged wrists.

Radioscapholunate Ligament Reconstruction (Fig. 20-36) (Technique of Taleisnik[222])

Combined volar and dorsal approaches are required. A strip of flexor carpi radialis tendon is prepared, leaving its distal insertion attached. The free

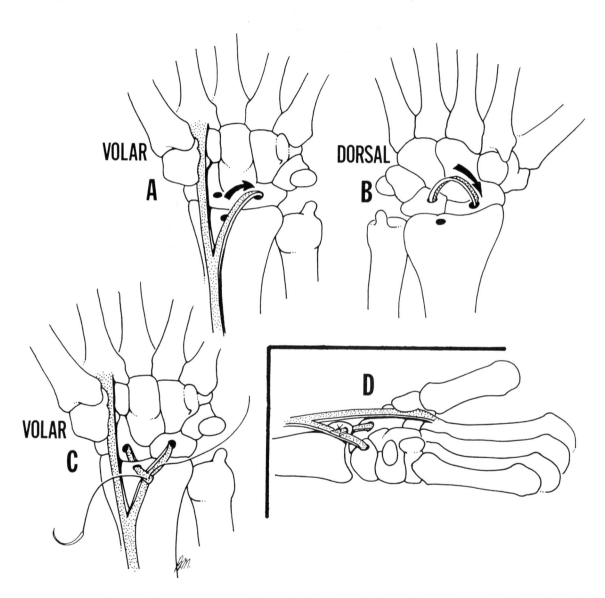

Fig. 20-36. Technique for reconstruction of the (volar) radioscapholunate ligament (Taleisnik). Combined volar and dorsal approaches are required. A strip of flexor carpi radialis tendon is prepared, leaving its distal insertion attached. The free end of the graft is passed dorsally through the lunate (**A**), across the scapholunate joint dorsally (**B**), back down through the scaphoid from dorsal to volar (**C**), and finally through the volar lip of the radius (from intraarticular to extraarticular) (**D**). (See text for details.)

end of the graft is passed vertically from volar to dorsal through the lunate, across the scapholunate joint dorsally, back down through the scaphoid from dorsal to volar, and finally through the volar lip of the radius (from intraarticular to extraarticular), suturing the end of the graft to the periosteum of the volar aspect to the radius. Dobyns and colleagues use K-wires to stabilize the bones in an overcorrected position, again passing the graft through the drill holes before finally reducing and pinning the bones. Taleisnik has used synthetic materials threaded together with the tendon graft instead of K-wires for stability.

Postoperative immobilization is continuous for a minimum of 6 to 8 weeks, followed by intermittent protective splinting and graduated mobilization for an additional 4 to 6 weeks.

It should be emphasized that Taleisnik himself notes that this technique is complex and not consistently reliable. He, too, is searching for simpler and more reliable methods of reconstruction.

INTERCARPAL ARTHRODESIS

Various types of intercarpal arthrodeses[17,32,86,93,114,126,186,226,236,244,245] have been described for the treatment of late post-traumatic carpal instability. Watson has been the prime advocate of what he refers to as "limited wrist arthrodesis," and a more detailed discussion of intercarpal arthrodesis is found in Chapter 5. However, some comments will be made here regarding the various types of intercarpal arthrodeses as they apply specifically to late post-traumatic carpal instability.

Scaphoid-Trapezium-Trapezoid (Triscaphoid) Arthrodesis

Triscaphoid arthrodesis (or triscaphe arthrodesis as Watson prefers to call it) has become a very popular method of treatment for chronic scapholunate dissociation over the past several years. The operation is technically difficult, and careful study of Watson's descriptions of the procedure in Chapter 5 and in his articles[243,244] is essential before attempting to perform this operation. Several particularly pertinent points bear emphasis here. It is important to maintain the normal anatomic align-

ment of the three bones to be fused, i.e., the external dimensions of the completed fusion unit must be the same as the external dimensions of the bones in the normal wrist. This means that after the articular cartilage and subchondral bone are removed, the gaps remaining between the bones must be filled in with cancellous bone graft, and the bones must not be pressed together. Watson recommends a very sharp, small dental ronguer for decorticating the bones, which allows the surgeon to contour the denuded surfaces more precisely than with an osteotome or saw. I have found Watson's technique of pin placement (Fig. 20-37) to create some difficulty not only at the time of insertion, but also at the time of removal, and K-wire removal occasionally has to be done in the operating room. Kleinman et al[126] modified the pin placement by fixing the scaphoid to the capitate and lunate with two K-wires in a manner similar to that described for percutaneous pin fixation of acute scapholunate dissociation (see page 917).

Perhaps the most difficult aspect of this operation is achieving correct anatomic alignment of the scaphoid. Even under direct visualization of the scapholunate joint and believing that I had reduced the bones anatomically, I have occasionally found that I either over- or underreduced the scaphoid. The latter fails to close the scapholunate gap correctly, and the former may result in more severely limited wrist motion postoperatively. Given the choice, *underreduction* is probably preferable, for it may provide relief of symptoms despite a persistent radiographic scapholunate gap, while *overreduction* leads to loss of radial deviation and severe limitation of palmar flexion.

Scapholunate Arthrodesis

Scapholunate arthrodesis would appear to be a logical method of treating late scapholunate dissociation since the surgical correction is carried out directly on the involved joint. However, several authors,[244] including Linscheid,[135] have commented that it is a difficult joint in which to achieve bony union. Eaton (personal communication) has apparently used this procedure for years, and while he acknowledges that bony union frequently does not occur, he has found that the resulting fibrous union between scaphoid and lunate is often strong

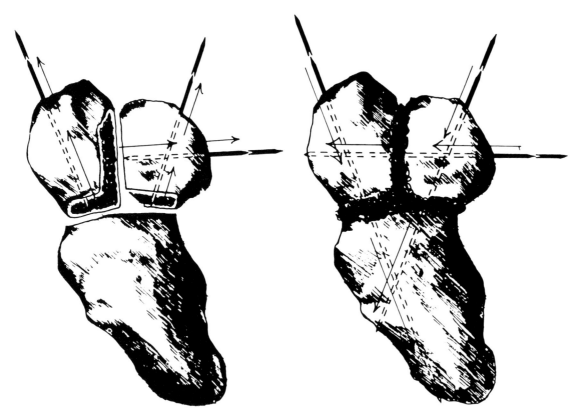

Fig. 20-37. Watson's triscaphoid (scaphoid-trapezium-trapezoid) arthrodesis has become a standard method of treating scapholunate dissociation. Careful attention to detail is essential in performing this operation (see text). (Watson HK, Hempton RF: Limited wrist arthrodesis. I. The triscaphoid joint. J Hand Surg 5:321, 1980.)

enough to significantly decrease the patient's symptoms.

Scapholunate-Capitate Arthrodesis

For patients who have late scapholunate dissociation with associated dorsiflexion instability, intercarpal arthrodesis of the scaphoid, lunate, and capitate offers an alternative method of treatment. Since this procedure eliminates motion in the midcarpal joint, postoperative wrist motion will be reduced by at least 50 percent of normal, but it may be a reasonable choice of operation in a patient with severe fixed dorsiflexion instability who does not yet have degenerative changes on the proximal pole of scaphoid and apposing articular surface of the radius.

AUTHOR'S PREFERRED METHOD

Chronic scapholunate dissociation is one of the most difficult problems in hand surgery, and I share the opinion of others[12,137,224] that a consistently successful solution to this problem has not yet been realized. In my experience, no single operation has been universally successful in treating late scapholunate dissociation with or without dorsiflexion instability, and I have had both good and poor results with several of the operations described in the preceding section. In general, my first choice is to try to do a late open reduction and reconstruction using local tissue. The wrist is approached through a dorsal lazy-S incision and the carpal bones are exposed between the third and fourth dorsal compartments, i.e., between the extensor pollicis longus and the extensor digitorum communis. I try to anatomically reduce the scaphoid, lunate, and capitate, utilizing as many K-wires as are necessary to stabilize these three bones. In some cases even several months after injury, one is fortunate enough to find sufficient local tissue to reconstruct the dorsal scapholunate ligaments by intraosseous sutures using the techniques advocated by Goldner and Linscheid described on page 920. In those patients with insufficient local tissue, my results with ligament reconstruction using tendon grafts have not been particularly rewarding, and I prefer to reinforce the ligaments with dorsal capsular tissue similar to the technique described by Blatt (page 920). If there is insufficient dorsal tissue with which to do an adequate local reconstruction, then I will do a triscaphoid arthrodesis, even though I am not convinced that this operation is *the* answer to late scapholunate dissociation. Properly performed, this operation succeeds in bringing the proximal pole of scaphoid under the dome of the radius and theoretically improves force transmission across the wrist, but it does not correct the scapholunate dissociation. Most if not all of these patients will show persistence of scapholunate instability on x-ray examination.

If I find at operation that the patient has loss of articular cartilage and definite post-traumatic arthritis in the radioscaphoid joint, then I will do one of the operations described in the next section.

Late Post-traumatic Carpal Instability with Established Arthrosis

Clearly, in patients with established post-traumatic arthrosis secondary to long-standing dorsiflexion instability, attempts at restoring the anatomy of the carpal bones and reconstructing the ligaments are not likely to significantly relieve pain. In such patients, the alternatives for operative treatment are numerous, although each has its relative disadvantages. Details of these procedures are described elsewhere in this book as noted, but the following discussion mentions some of the important points to be considered when deciding which choice of treatment to use in these difficult problems.

Styloidectomy

Although styloidectomy (see Chapter 19) is possibly indicated in patients with arthrosis specifically isolated to the radioscaphoid joint, it is at best a temporizing procedure and at worst may lead to further instability. Because styloidectomy may compromise later reconstructive procedures, it is, in my opinion, not a good choice for this particular problem, and I tend to use it only on very rare occasions.

Proximal Row Carpectomy

Proximal row carpectomy is a controversial operation, but all of the reasonably large series in the literature[46,91,107,157,171,209–211] have reported generally good results. Each author who has studied this procedure, however, has noted that it must be done before degenerative changes are present. Specifically, this means that a prerequisite for the operation is good articular cartilage on the proximal pole of capitate and in the lunate fossa of the radius. Although the operation would appear to be totally unphysiologic, the concept is to convert a complex link system into a simple hinge joint,[210] and in most cases this has proven to be surprisingly effective. The major advantage of proximal row carpectomy is that it can preserve reasonably good wrist motion while at the same time affording good relief of pain, although most of these patients will have some subjective weakness in grip strength. It has the added advantage of being convertible to a wrist arthrodesis or arthroplasty at a later date if it fails to relieve the patient's pain. The technique of proximal row carpectomy is described in Chapters 7 and 19.

Silastic Scaphoid Replacement Arthroplasty

Although reports of "silicone synovitis"[184, 205,219] have dampened somewhat the enthusiasm for replacement of the scaphoid with a Silastic implant, this procedure has been used rather widely for treatment of scaphoid nonunion with post-traumatic arthrosis. However, it is probably *not* a good choice for the patient with late post-traumatic instability for several reasons: (1) it is difficult if not impossible to properly seat the implant in a wrist with dorsiflexion instability; (2) replacing the scaphoid with an implant probably further enhances the midcarpal instability; and (3) it is not likely to retard further progression of post-traumatic arthrosis in the radiocarpal and midcarpal joints. The scaphoid implant may, however, have a place if used conjointly with midcarpal arthrodesis as suggested by Watson[245] for his SLAC wrist operation (see Chapter 5).

Total Wrist Arthroplasty

Recent advances in total joint replacement of the wrist (see Chapter 7) have made it a reasonably predictable operation with good likelihood of at least short-term relief of pain, with maintenance of some wrist motion. However, long-term follow-up in some of these patients has identified new problems that contraindicate its use in young patients or in patients who place heavy demands on the wrist. Unfortunately, most of the patients with late post-traumatic instability from carpal dislocations are young men who engage in heavy labor, and therefore in my opinion this procedure is not an acceptable choice in these patients.

Wrist Arthrodesis

In this age of total joint replacement, arthrodesis of any joint is anathema to many surgeons. However, in the heavy laborer with post-traumatic arthrosis of the wrist, arthrodesis may still be the procedure of choice and the one most likely to return him to his former occupation (see Chapter 6).

MEDIAL (ULNAR) CARPAL INSTABILITIES

Of all the sections in this chapter, probably the most significant advances in our understanding of carpal pathomechanics during the past several years has been in the area of medial carpal instability. Much more importance has been ascribed to the role of the helicoid triquetrohamate joint in controlling carpal movements, especially in radial and ulnar deviation (see Kinematics, page 881).

Lichtman[6,132] has drawn particular attention to the two forms of medial carpal instability, triquetrohamate and triquetrolunate dissociation, and Taleisnik[223,225] has also offered some insights into these fascinating problems.

Triquetrohamate Dissociation

Lichtman[6] has suggested that the main ligamentous structure stabilizing the midcarpal joint is the capitotriquetral fasicle of the arcuate (V) ligament. When this ligament is divided in a cadaver specimen, the triquetrum no longer moves smoothly on the hamate, but "jumps" from the low to the high position with a sudden, abrupt movement (see page 881). In the patient with triquetrohamate dissociation, movement from radial to ulnar deviation is frequently accompanied by a palpable, audible, and frequently painful "clunk." Since the triquetrolunate ligaments are intact, the lunate and triquetrum still move in concert, and when the triquetrum snaps into its low position on the hamate in ulnar deviation, the lunate is forced into dorsiflexion. Thus, these patients usually exhibit a dorsiflexion instability (DISI) pattern, although some may show a palmar flexion (VISI) deformity.[218] The critical feature that distinguishes this from the more common form of DISI that occurs with rotary subluxation of the scaphoid is that in medial carpal instability, there is no scapholunate dissociation, and the scaphoid and lunate move as a unit.[225]

The clinical clue to triquetrohamate instability is the characteristic audible and palpable clunk that the patient can reproduce with active motion of the wrist and that can often also be elicited by the examiner with passive radial and ulnar deviation. The diagnosis is best confirmed by cineradiography,[6] although the snap occurs so rapidly that careful frame-by-frame study of the cine is often necessary to clearly see the pathomechanics.

Treatment

Temporary relief as well as additional confirmation of the diagnosis can often be accomplished with steroid injection of the triquetrohamate joint, and some of these patients are not sufficiently symptomatic to warrant surgical treatment. However, if pain persists, stabilization of the triquetro-

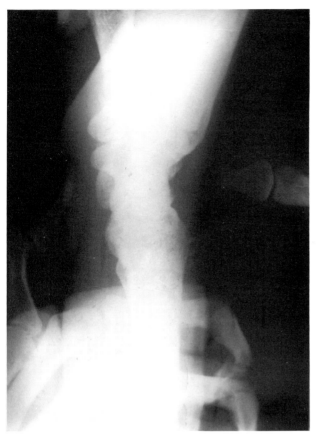

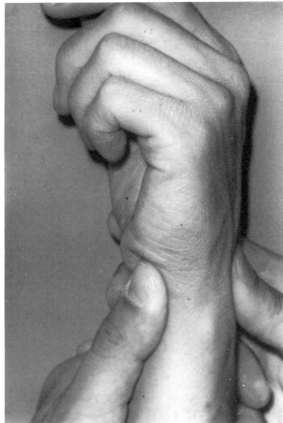

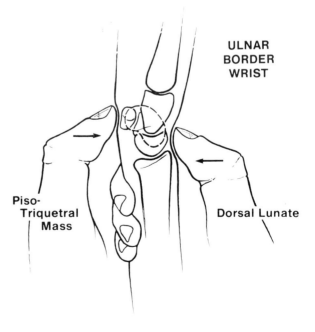

Fig. 20-38. The "shear" test as described by Kleinman is similar to the ballottment test described by Reagan et al.[193] This test is painful for the patient with a sprain or instability in the triquetrolunate joint. See text for details. (Illustrations courtesy of William B. Kleinman, MD, Indianapolis, Indiana.)

hamate joint would appear to be the treatment of choice.[133] If the "clunk" can only be reproduced in the preoperative examination by active motion but not by passive motion, then I prefer to explore the wrist under Neurolept anesthesia (see Chapter 2), which affords the opportunity to have the patient reproduce the instability under direct vision at the table. Intercarpal arthrodesis of the triquetrohamate joint is carried out as described in Chapter 5, taking care to preserve the normal spatial relationships of the bones. Recently, I have combined triquetrohamate arthrodesis with capitate-lunate fusion for two reasons: (1) the larger fusion mass seems to enhance the chances for successful union;[186] and (2) these two joints form the midcarpal joint, and fusing one effectively eliminates motion in the other joint anyway.

Triquetrolunate Dissociation

The other type of medial carpal instability pattern occurs between the triquetrum and lunate, and triquetrolunate injuries are also being diag-nosed with increasing frequency.[193] Most of these patients relate a specific injury of the wrist, usually dorsiflexion, and the major complaint is pain on the ulnar aspect of the wrist. Some patients will describe a painful click.

The most important physical finding is point tenderness directly over the triquetrolunate joint, and another helpful finding is a positive ballottement test as described by Reagan et al.[193] The lunate is firmly stabilized with the thumb and index finger of one hand while the triquetrum and pisiform are displaced dorsally and palmarly with the other hand. A positive result elicits pain, crepitus, and excessive laxity.

A modification of this test is the "shear" test described by Kleinman[125] (Fig. 20-38). With the patient's elbow resting on the table and the forearm in neutral rotation, the examiner's contralateral thumb is placed over the dorsal aspect of the lunate, just at the medial edge of the distal radius. With the lunate thus stabilized, the examiner's other thumb directly loads the pisotriquetral joint in a dorsal-volar plane, creating a shear force at the

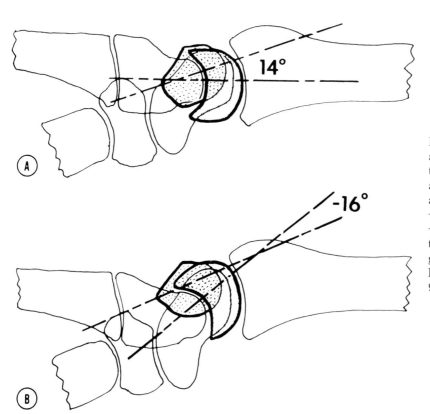

Fig. 20-39. The lunatotriquetral angle may be difficult to measure in the lateral radiograph, but the angle has been shown by Reagan et al to be decreased from its normal of +14 degrees (**A**) to an average of −16 degrees (**B**) in the patient with triquetrolunate dissociation. (Reagan DS, Linscheid RL, Dobyns JH: Lunotriquetral sprains. J Hand Surg 9A:506, 1984.)

triquetrolunate joint and causing pain in the patient with a sprain of this joint.

As with all ligamentous injuries, triquetrolunate sprains are thought to encompass a spectrum from partial tears to actual dissociation between the two bones. At the milder end of the spectrum, routine radiographs are usually normal, but arthrography may demonstrate a tear of the interosseous ligament by allowing abnormal communication of dye between the radiocarpal and midcarpal joints via the triquetrolunate interval.[6,26] In the more severe cases with actual dissociation, a palmar flexion instability (VISI) is seen because of the disruption between the triquetrum and lunate. Measurement of the LT (lunatotriquetral) angle on the lateral x-ray film has been shown by Reagan et al[193] to be decreased from its normal average of $+14$ degrees to -16 degrees (Fig. 20-39), but I have found this angle difficult to measure because of overlap of the carpal bones.

Treatment

Milder sprains can be adequately treated with immobilization, anti-inflammatory medications, and injections, but more severe dissociations may require operative treatment. The only reasonably large series of patients reported in the literature is that from the Mayo Clinic,[193] and their surgical procedures included ligament repair, ligament reconstruction, and intercarpal arthrodesis. Unfortunately, even their numbers are too few from which to glean solid guidelines regarding the optimal treatment for any given patient. Lichtman[6] has suggested that triquetrolunate arthrodesis is the preferred treatment since very little motion occurs normally at this articulation.

NONDISSOCIATIVE INSTABILITY OF THE PROXIMAL CARPAL ROW

Dobyns (personal communication, 1986) has recently introduced an entirely new concept that may aid in our understanding of the patient with a "clunking" wrist. Nondissociative instability of the

proximal row is yet another pattern of carpal instability that has the following features.

1. Lax ligamentous habitus, with the carpus easily translatable on the radius, i.e., capable of being shifted volarly by downward stress on the hand while the forearm is stabilized.
2. Sudden shift of the proximal row as a unit into either VISI or DISI with active radial and ulnar deviation movement as seen on cineradiographs. VISI is apparently more commonly seen.
3. Painful "clunking" of the wrist as this shift takes place.
4. Absence of scapholunate or triquetrolunate dissociation on x-ray, arthrograms, or surgical exploration.

The key feature of this type of instability is that there is destabilization between the distal and proximal carpal rows (i.e., scaphotrapezial-trapezoid, capitolunate, and triquetrohamate), in the absence of dissociation *within* the proximal carpal row. Similar destabilization may occur between the distal forearm (radius or ulna) and the proximal carpal row with similar radiologic and clinical features.

Since this entity has only recently been described, it is difficult to offer firm recommendations about treatment. Midcarpal (capitolunate and triquetrohamate) arthrodesis will obviously solve the problem, but that may be more than is needed, and Dobyns and Linscheid have preferred to treat most of their patients with some type of ligament reconstruction.

CENTRAL CARPAL INSTABILITY ("CLIP" WRIST)

Louis and his colleagues[140,256] have described what they consider to be a separate and distinct type of instability pattern in which the distal carpal row (represented by the capitate) can be manually displaced dorsally on the proximal carpal row (represented by the lunate), in the absence of any detectable angular (DISI or VISI) instability. Their eleven patients had pain and clicking in the region of the midcarpal joint and, at times, frank snapping, usually when lifting heavy objects. These authors have subsequently shown that this type of dynamic instability can be present in asymptomatic adults, and only one of their patients underwent operative treatment. The remaining ten patients reduced their symptoms by simply modifying their activities.

It is difficult to know exactly how to classify this instability pattern and how it fits into the spectrum of ligamentous injuries of the carpus, but it is my opinion that the so-called CLIP wrist is probably related to the medial (ulnar) carpal instabilities, about which our understanding is just beginning to emerge.

REFERENCES

1. Adams JD: Displacement of the semilunar carpal bone. J Bone Joint Surg 7:665–681, 1925
2. Adelaar RS: Traumatic wrist instabilities. Contemp Orthop 4:309–324, 1982
3. Adkison JW, Chapman MW: Treatment of acute lunate and perilunate dislocations. Clin Orthop 164:199–207, 1982
4. Adler JB, Shaftan GW: Fractures of the capitate. J Bone Joint Surg 44A:1537–1547, 1962
5. Aitken AP, Nalebuff EA: Volar transnavicular perilunar dislocation of the carpus. J Bone Joint Surg 42A:1051–1057, 1960
6. Alexander CE, Lichtman DM: Ulnar carpal instabilities. Orthop Clin North Am 15:307–320, 1984
7. Andrews FT: A dislocation of the carpal bones— The scaphoid and semilunar: Report of a case. J Mich State Med Soc 31:269, 1932.
8. Arkless R: Cineradiography in normal and abnormal wrists. Am J Roentgenol Radium Ther Nucl Med 96:837–844, 1966
9. Armstrong GWD: Rotational subluxation of the scaphoid. Can J Surg 11:306–314, 1968
10. Aufranc OE, Jones WN, Harris WH: Transnavicular retrolunar dislocation of the wrist. JAMA 181:131–133, 1962
11. Aufranc OE, Jones WN, Turner RN: Transnavicular perilunar carpal dislocation. JAMA 196:130–133, 1966
12. Beckenbaugh RD: Accurate evaluation and management of the painful wrist following injury. An approach to carpal instability. Orthop Clin North Am 15:289–306, 1984
13. Bell MJ: Perilunar dislocation of the carpus and an associated Colles' fracture. Hand 15:262–266, 1983
14. Bellinghausen HW, Gilula LA, Young LV, Weeks PM: Post-traumatic palmar carpal subluxation. Report of two cases. J Bone Joint Surg 65A:998–1006, 1983
15. Berger RA, Blair WF, Crowninshield RD, Flatt AE: The scapholunate ligament. J Hand Surg 7:87–91, 1982
16. Berger RA, Blair WF, El-Khoury GY: Arthrotomography of the wrist. Clin Orthop 186:224–229, 1984
17. Bertheussen K: Partial carpal arthrodesis as treatment of local degenerative changes in the wrist joints. Acta Orthop Scand 52:629–631, 1981
18. Bjelland JC, Bush JC: Secondary rotational subluxation of the carpal navicular. Ariz Med 34:267–268, 1977
19. Blair WF, Berger RA, El-Khoury GY: Arthrotomography of the wrist: An experimental and preliminary clinical study. J Hand Surg 10A:350–359, 1985
20. Blatt G: Capsulodesis in reconstructive hand surgery: Dorsal capsulodesis for the unstable scaphoid and volar capsulodesis following excision of the distal ulna. Hand Clinics 3:81–102, 1987
21. Böhler L: The Treatment of Fractures. 4th English Ed., pp. 235–247. William Wood, Baltimore, 1935
22. Böhler L: The Treatment of Fractures. 5th English Ed., pp. 826–854. Grune & Stratton, New York, London, 1956
23. Boyes JG: Subluxation of the carpal navicular bone. South Med J 69:141–144, 1976
24. Bradley KC, Sunderland S: The range of movement at the wrist joint. Anat Rec 116:139–145, 1953
25. Brekkan A, Karlsson J, Thorsteinsson T: Case Report 252. Skeletal Radiol 10:291–293, 1983
26. Brown DE, Lichtman DM: The evaluation of chronic wrist pain. Orthop Clin North Am 15:183–192, 1984
27. Brown RHL, Muddu BN: Scaphoid and lunate dislocation. A report on a case. Hand 13:303–307, 1981
28. Brumfield RH, Champoux JA: A biomechanical study of normal functional wrist motion. Clin Orthop 187:23–25, 1984
29. Brumfield RH, Nickel VL, Nickel E: Joint motion

in wrist flexion and extension. South Med J 59:909–910, 1966

30. Bunnell S: Surgery of the Hand. 2nd Ed., JB Lippincott, Philadelphia, 1948

31. Buzby BF: Isolated radial dislocation of carpal scaphoid. Ann Surg 100:553–555, 1934

32. Campbell CJ, Keokarn T: Total and subtotal arthrodesis of the wrist. Inlay technique. J Bone Joint Surg 46A:1520–1533, 1964

33. Campbell RD, Jr, Lance EM, Yeoh CB: Lunate and perilunar dislocations. J Bone Joint Surg 46B:55–72, 1964

34. Campbell RD, Jr, Thompson TC, Lance EM, Adler JB: Indications for open reduction of lunate and perilunate dislocations of the carpal bones. J Bone Joint Surg 47A:915–937, 1965

35. Cave EF: Fractures and dislocations of the carpal bones. pp. 39–54. In Wilson PD (ed): Management of Fractures and Dislocations. JB Lippincott, Philadelphia, 1938

36. Cave EF: Retrolunar dislocation of the capitate with fracture or subluxation of the navicular bone. J Bone Joint Surg 23:830–840, 1941

37. Cave EF: Injuries to the wrist joint. pp. 9–24. AAOS Instructional Course Lectures. Vol. 10. CV Mosby, St Louis, 1953

38. Chernin MM, Pitt MJ: Radiographic disease patterns at the carpus. Clin Orthop 187:72–80, 1984

39. Cleak DK: Dislocation of the scaphoid and lunate bones without fracture: A case report. Injury 14:278–281, 1982

40. Codman EA, Chase HM: The diagnosis and treatment of fracture of the carpal scaphoid and dislocation of the semilunar bone. Report of 30 cases. Ann Surg 41:863–885, 1905

41. Cohn I: Dislocations of the semilunar carpal bone. Ann Surg 73:621–628, 1921

42. Cone RO, Szabo R, Resnick D, Gelberman R, Taleisnik J, Gilula LA: Computed tomography of the normal soft tissues of the wrist. Invest Radiol 18:546–551, 1983

43. Connell MC, Dyson RP: Dislocation of the carpal scaphoid. J Bone Joint Surg 37B:252–253, 1955

44. Conwell HE: Closed reduction of acute dislocations of the semilunar carpal bone. Ann Surg 82:289–292, 1925

45. Cope JR: Rotatory subluxation of the scaphoid. Clin Radiol 35:495–501, 1984

46. Crabbe WD: Excision of the proximal row of the carpus. J Bone Joint Surg 46B:708–711, 1964

47. Cranmer RR, Foss AR: A report of three cases of dislocated semilunar bone. Minn Med 5:484–486, 1922

48. Crawford GP, Taleisnik J: Rotatory subluxation of the scaphoid after excision of dorsal carpal ganglion and wrist manipulation—A case report. J Hand Surg 8:921–925, 1983

49. Crittenden JJ, Jones DM, Santarelli AG: Bilateral rotational dislocation of the carpal navicular. Radiology 94:629–630, 1970

50. Curtis DJ: Injuries of the wrist: An approach to diagnosis. Radiol Clin North Am 19:625–644, 1981

51. Curtis DJ, Downey EF, Jr, Brower AC, Cruess DF, Herrington WT, Ghaed N: Importance of soft-tissue evaluation in hand and wrist trauma: Statistical evaluation. AJR 142:781–788, 1984

52. Davis GG: Treatment of dislocated semilunar carpal bones. Surg Gynecol Obstet 37:225–229, 1923

53. Destot E: Injuries of the Wrist: A Radiological Study. Translated by Atkinson FRB, Ernest Benn, London, 1925

54. Dobyns JH, Linscheid RL, Chao EYS, Weber ER, Swanson GE: Traumatic instability of the wrist. pp. 182–199. AAOS Instructional Course Lectures. Vol. 24. CV Mosby, St Louis, 1975

55. Dobyns JH, Swanson GE: Fracture conference: A 19-year-old with multiple fractures. Minn Med 56:143–149, 1973

56. Drewniany JJ, Palmer AK: Correspondence. J Bone Joint Surg 65A:871–872, 1983

57. Drewniany JJ, Palmer AK, Flatt AE: The scaphotrapezial ligament complex: An anatomic and biomechanical study. J Hand Surg 10A:492–498, 1985

58. Dunn AW: Fractures and dislocations of the carpus. Surg Clin North Am 52:1513–1538, 1972

59. Eggers GWN: Anterior dislocation of os lunatum. J Bone Joint Surg 15:394–400, 1933

60. El-Khoury GY, Usta HY, Blair WF: Naviculocapitate fracture–dislocation. AJR 139:385–386, 1982

61. England JPS: Subluxation of the carpal scaphoid. Proc R Soc Med 63:581–582, 1970

62. Farr CE: Dislocation of the carpal semilunar bone. Ann Surg 84:112–115, 1926

63. Fenton RL: The naviculo-capitate fracture syndrome. J Bone Joint Surg 38A:681–684, 1956

64. Fenton RL, Rosen H: Fracture of the capitate bone: Report of two cases. Bull Hosp Joint Dis 11:134–139, 1950

65. Fernandes HJA, Koberle G, Ferreira GHS, Camargo JN, Jr: Volar transscaphoid perilunar dislocation. Hand 15:276–280, 1983

66. Fernandez DL: A technique for anterior wedge-

shaped grafts for scaphoid non-unions with carpal instability. J Hand Surg 9A:733–737, 1984

67. Fisk GR: Carpal stability and the fractured scaphoid. Ann R Col Surg Engl 46:63–76, 1970

68. Fisk GR: An overview of injuries of the wrist. Clin Orthop 149:137–144, 1980

69. Fisk GR: Editorial. Hand 15:239–241, 1983

70. Fisk GR: The wrist. J Bone Joint Surg 66B:396–407, 1984

71. Fisk GR: Malalignment of the scaphoid after lunate dislocation. Ann Chir Main 3:353–356, 1984

72. Frankel VH: The Terry-Thomas sign. Clin Orthop 129:321–322, 1977

73. Ganel A, Engel J, Ditzian R, Farin I, Militeanu J: Arthrography as a method of diagnosing soft-tissue injuries of the wrist. J Trauma 19:376–380, 1979

74. Garcia-Elias M, Abanco J, Salvador E, Sanchez R: Crush injury of the carpus. J Bone Joint Surg 67B:286–289, 1985

75. Gerard FM: Post-traumatic carpal instability in a young child. A case report. J Bone Joint Surg 62A:131–133, 1980

76. Gibson PH: Scaphoid-trapezium-trapezoid dislocation. Hand 15:267–269, 1983

77. Gilford WW, Bolton RH, Lambrinudi C: The mechanism of the wrist joint with special reference to fractures of the scaphoid. Guy's Hosp Rep 92:52–59, 1943

78. Gilula LA, Weeks PM: Post-traumatic ligamentous instability of the wrist. Radiology 129:641–651, 1978

79. Gilula LA: Carpal injuries: Analytic approach and case exercises. AJR 133:503–517, 1979

80. Gilula LA, Destouet JM, Weeks PM, Young LV, Wray RC: Roentgenographic diagnosis of the painful wrist. Clin Orthop 187:52–64, 1984

81. Gilula LA, Totty WG, Weeks PM: Wrist arthrography. Radiology 146:555–556, 1983

82. Glickel SZ, Millender LH: Ligamentous reconstruction for chronic intercarpal instability. J Hand Surg 9A:514–527, 1984

83. Golden WW: Dislocations of the semilunar bone: Report of a case in which reduction was successful. JAMA 76:466, 1921

84. Goldner JL: Treatment of carpal instability without joint fusion—Current assessment (Guest editorial). J Hand Surg 7:325–326, 1982

85. Gordon SL: Scaphoid and lunate dislocation: Report of a case in a patient with peripheral neuropathy. J Bone Joint Surg 54A:1769–1772, 1972

86. Graner O, Lopes EI, Carvalho BC, Atlas S: Arthrodesis of the carpal bones in the treatment of Kienbock's disease, painful ununited fractures of the navicular and lunate bones with avascular necrosis, and old fracture-dislocations of carpal bones. J Bone Joint Surg 48A:767–774, 1966

87. Green DP, O'Brien ET: Open reduction of carpal dislocations: Indications and operative techniques. J Hand Surg 3:250–265, 1978

88. Green DP, O'Brien ET: Classification and management of carpal dislocations. Clin Orthop 149:55–72, 1980

89. Green DP: The effect of avascular necrosis on Russe bone grafting for scaphoid nonunion. J Hand Surg 10A:597–605, 1985

90. Green DP: The sore wrist without a fracture. pp. 300–313. AAOS Instructional Course Lectures. Vol. 34. CV Mosby, St Louis, 1985

91. Green DP: Proximal row carpectomy. Hand Clinics 3:163–168, 1987

92. Hamill RC: Forward dislocation of semilunar bone; undiagnosed. Int Clin 3:124–127, 1920

93. Hastings DE, Silver RL: Intercarpal arthrodesis in the management of chronic carpal instability after trauma. J Hand Surg 9A:834–840, 1984

94. Hawkins L, Torkelson R: Transnavicular perilunar fracture-dislocations of the wrist. (Abstract) J Bone Joint Surg 56A:1087, 1974

95. Herbert TJ: Herbert Screw Bone System. Surgical Technique. Zimmer Corp, 1982

96. Herbert TJ, Fisher WE: Management of the fractured scaphoid using a new bone screw. J Bone Joint Surg 66B:114–123, 1984

97. Hergenroeder PT, Penix AR: Bilateral scapholunate dissociation with degenerative arthritis. J Hand Surg 6:620–622, 1981

98. Higgs SL: Two cases of dislocation of carpal scaphoid. Proc R Soc Med 23:61–64, 1930

99. Hill NA: Fractures and dislocations of the carpus. Orthop Clin North Am 1:275–284, 1970

100. Hockley BJ: Carpal instability and carpal injuries. Aust Radiol 23:158–169, 1979

101. Horwitz T: An anatomical and roentgenologic study of the wrist joint. Surgery 7:773–783, 1940

102. Howard FM, Fahey T, Wojcik E: Rotatory subluxation of the navicular. Clin Orthop 104:134–139, 1974

103. Howard FM (Moderator): Carpal instability (Panel Discussion). Contemp Orthop 4:107–144, 1982

104. Hudson TM, Caragol WJ, Kaye JJ: Isolated rotatory subluxation of the carpal navicular. Am J Roentgenol 126:601–611, 1976

105. Huene DR: An alignment instrument for pin fixation of small bone fractures. Orthop Rev 6:93–95, 1977

106. Huene DR: Primary internal fixation of carpal na-

vicular fractures in the athlete. Am J Sports Med 7:175–177, 1979

107. Inglis AE, Jones EC: Proximal row carpectomy for diseases of the proximal row. J Bone Joint Surg 59A:460–463, 1977

108. Israeli A, Engel J, Ganel A: Recurrent volar carpal perilunate subluxation. Arch Orthop Traumat Surg 99:285–286, 1982

109. Israeli A, Ganel A, Engel J: Post-traumatic ligamentous instability of the wrist. Brit J Sports Med 15:17–19, 1981

110. Jackson WT, Protas JM: Snapping scapholunate subluxation. J Hand Surg 6:590–594, 1981

111. Johnson RP: The acutely injured wrist and its residuals. Clin Orthop 149:33–44, 1980

112. Johnston HM: Extension, ulnar and radial flexion. J Anat Physiology 41:109–122, 1907

113. Jones GB: An unusual fracture-dislocation of the carpus. J Bone Joint Surg 37B:146–147, 1955

114. Jonsson K, Sigfusson BF: Arthrosis of the lunate-capitate joint. Acta Radiologica Diagnosis 24:415–418, 1983

115. Jorgensen EC: Proximal row carpectomy: An end result study of twenty-two cases. J Bone Joint Surg 51A:1104–1111, 1969

116. Kaplan L: Treatment of fractures and dislocations of the hand and fingers. Surg Clin North Am 20:1695–1720, 1940

117. Kauer JMG: The interdependence of carpal articulation chains. Acta Anat 88:481–501, 1974

118. Kauer JMG: Functional anatomy of the wrist. Clin Orthop 149:9–20, 1980

119. Keenan CB, Wilkie AL: Dislocation of the semilunar bone of the wrist. Can Med Assoc J 20:639–641, 1929

120. Kellum HIJ, McGoey PF: Review of fractures and dislocations of the carpus. Can Med Assoc J 53:332–335, 1945

121. Kessler I, Silberman Z: An experimental study of the radiocarpal joint by arthrography. Surg Gynecol Obstet 112:33–40, 1961

122. Key JA, Conwell HE: The Management of Fractures, Dislocations and Sprains. 3rd Ed., p. 781. CV Mosby, St Louis, 1942

123. King RJ: Scapholunate diastasis associated with a Barton fracture treated by manipulation, or Terry-Thomas and the wine waiter. JR Soc Med 76:421–423, 1983

124. Kleinberg S: Dislocation of the carpal scaphoid and semilunar bones. JAMA 74:312–313, 1920

125. Kleinman WB: The "shear" test. Am Soc Surg Hand Corr Newsl 1985–51, 1985

126. Kleinman WB, Steichen JB, Strickland JW: Management of chronic rotary subluxation of the scaphoid by scapho-trapezio-trapezoid arthrodesis. J Hand Surg 7:125–136, 1982

127. Kricun ME: Wrist arthrography. Clin Orthop 187:65–71, 1984

128. Kuth JR: Isolated dislocation of the carpal navicular. J Bone Joint Surg 21:479–483, 1939

129. Landsmeer JMF: Studies in the anatomy of articulation. I. The equilibrium of the "intercalated" bone. Acta Morphol Neerl Scand 3:287–303, 1961

130. Lediard HA: Dislocation of the semilunar bone. Edinburgh Med J 30:244–245, 1923

131. Lewis OJ, Hamshere RJ, Bucknill TM: The anatomy of the wrist joint. J Anat 106:539–552, 1970

132. Lichtman DM, Noble WH, Alexander CE: Dynamic triquetrolunate instability: Case report. J Hand Surg 9A:185–188, 1984

133. Lichtman DM, Schneider JR, Swafford AR, Mack GR: Ulnar midcarpal instability—Clinical and laboratory analysis. J Hand Surg 6:515–523, 1981

134. Linscheid RL, Dobyns JH, Beabout JW, Bryan RS: Traumatic instability of the wrist: Diagnosis, classification and pathomechanics. J Bone Joint Surg 54A:1612–1632, 1972

135. Linscheid RL: Scapholunate ligamentous instabilities (dissociations, subdislocations, dislocations). Ann Chir Main 3:323–330, 1984

136. Linscheid RL, Dobyns JH: The unified concept of carpal injuries. Ann Chir Main 3:35–42, 1984

137. Linscheid RL, Dobyns JH: Athletic injuries of the wrist. Clin Orthop 198:141–151, 1985

138. Linscheid RL, Dobyns JH, Beckenbaugh RD, Cooney WP, Wood MB: Instability patterns of the wrist. J Hand Surg 8:682–686, 1983

139. Loeb TM, Urbaniak JR, Goldner JL: Traumatic carpal instability: Putting the pieces together. Orthop Trans 1:163, 1977

140. Louis DS, Hankin FM, Greene TL, Braunstein EM, White SJ: Central carpal instability—capitate lunate instability pattern. Diagnosis by dynamic placement. Orthop 7:1693–1696, 1984

141. Lourie JA: An unusual dislocation of the lunate and the wrist. J Trauma 22:966–967, 1982

142. Lowdon IMR, Simpson AHRW, Burge P: Recurrent dorsal trans-scaphoid perilunate dislocation. J Hand Surg 9B:307–310, 1984

143. Lowrey DG, Moss SH, Wolff TW: Volar dislocation of the capitate. Report of a case. J Bone Joint Surg 66A:611–613, 1984

144. MacAusland WR: Perilunar dislocation of the carpal bones and dislocation of the lunate bone. Surg Gynecol Obstet 79:256–266, 1944

145. MacConaill MA: The mechanical anatomy of the carpus and its bearings on some surgical problems. J Anat 75:166–175, 1941

146. Mahorner HR, Meade WH: Operation for dislocated semilunar bone of the wrist. Surgery 5:249–259, 1939

147. Maki NJ, Chuinard RG, D'Ambrosia R: Isolated, complete radial dislocation of the scaphoid. A case report and review of the literature. J Bone Joint Surg 64A:615–616, 1982

148. Marsh AP, Lampros PJ: The naviculocapitate fracture syndrome. Am J Roentgenol 82:255–256, 1959

149. Mayfield JK, Johnson RP, Kilcoyne RF: The ligaments of the human wrist and their functional significance. Anat Rec 186:417–428, 1976

150. Mayfield JK: Mechanism of carpal injuries. Clin Orthop 149:45–54, 1980

151. Mayfield JK: Patterns of injury to carpal ligaments. A spectrum. Clin Orthop 187:36–42, 1984

152. Mayfield JK: Wrist ligamentous anatomy and pathogenesis of carpal instability. Orthop Clin North Am 15:209–216, 1984

153. Mayfield JK, Johnson RP, Kilcoyne RK: Carpal dislocations: Pathomechanics and progressive perilunar instability. J Hand Surg 5:226–241, 1980

154. McBride ED: An operation for late reduction of the semilunar bone. South Med J 26:672–676, 1933

155. McGoey PF: Fracture-dislocation of a fused triangular and lunate (congenital): Report of a case. J Bone Joint Surg 25:928–929, 1943

156. McLaughlin HL: Fracture of the carpal navicular (scaphoid) bone. Some observations based on treatment by open reduction and internal fixation. J Bone Joint Surg 36A:765–774, 1954

157. McLaughlin HL, Baab OD: Carpectomy. Surg Clin North Am 31:451–461, 1951

158. McMurtry RY, Youm Y, Flatt AE, Gillespie TE: Kinematics of the wrist. II. Clinical applications. J Bone Joint Surg 60A:955–961, 1978

159. Meyers MH, Wells R, Harvey JP, Jr: Naviculo-capitate fracture syndrome: Review of the literature and a case report. J Bone Joint Surg 53A:1383–1386, 1971

160. Mikic ZDJ: Arthrography of the wrist joint. An experimental study. J Bone Joint Surg 66A:371–378, 1984

161. Monahan PRW, Galasko CSB: The scapho-capitate fracture syndrome: A mechanism of injury. J Bone Joint Surg 54B:122–124, 1972

162. Moneim MS: The tangential posteroanterior radiograph to demonstrate scapholunate dissociation. J Bone Joint Surg 63A:1324–1326, 1981

163. Moneim MS, Hoffmann KE, III, Omer GE: Trans-scaphoid perilunate fracture-dislocation. Result of open reduction and pin fixation. Clin Orthop 190:227–235, 1984

164. Moneim MS, Omer GE: Wrist arthrography in acute carpal injuries. Orthopedics 6:299–306, 1983

165. Morawa LG, Ross PM, Schock CC: Fractures and dislocations involving the navicular-lunate axis. Clin Orthop 118:48–53, 1976

166. Morgan W, Groves RJ: Scapholunate dissociation from a fall on the elbow. J Hand Surg 9A:845–847, 1984

167. Mueller JJ: Avascular necrosis and collapse of the lunate following a volar perilunate dislocation. A case report and review of this complication in dislocations of the wrist. Orthopedics 7:1009–1014, 1984

168. Muller ME, Allgower M, Willenegger H: Technique of Internal Fixation of Fractures. pp. 179–184. New York, Springer-Verlag, 1965

169. Murakami Y: Dislocation of the carpal scaphoid. Hand 9:79–81, 1977

170. Murphy JB: Dislocations of the left unciform bone. Surgical Clinics of Murphy 4:423–427, 1915

171. Neviaser RJ: Proximal row carpectomy for post-traumatic disorders of the carpus. J Hand Surg 8:301–305, 1983

172. Newman JH, Watt I: Avascular necrosis of the capitate and dorsal dorsi-flexion instability. Hand 12:176–178, 1980

173. Nicholson CB: Fracture-dislocation of the os magnum. JR Nav Med Serv 26:289–291, 1940

174. Nielsen PT, Hedeboe J: Posttraumatic scapholunate dissociation detected by wrist cineradiography. J Hand Surg 9A:135–138, 1984

175. Noble J, Lamb DW: Translunate scaphoradial fracture: A case report. Hand 11:47–49, 1979

176. Noon C: Dislocation of the semilunar bone: With notes of a case. Lancet 208:432–433, 1925

177. O'Brien ET: Acute fractures and dislocations of the carpus. Orthop Clin North Am 15:237–258, 1984

178. O'Carroll PF, Gallagher JE: Brief report. Irreducible transscaphoid perilunate dislocation. Int J Med Science 152:424–426, 1983

179. Palmer AK, Dobyns JH, Linscheid RL: Management of posttraumatic instability of the wrist secondary to ligament rupture. J Hand Surg 3:507–532, 1978

180. Palmer AK, Levinsohn EM, Kuzma GR: Arthrography of the wrist. J Hand Surg 8:15–23, 1983

181. Palmer AK, Wener FW, Eng MM, Murphy D, Glisson R: Functional wrist motion: A biomechanical study. J Hand Surg 10A:39–46, 1985

182. Panting AL, Lamb DW, Noble J, Haw CS: Disloca-

tions of the lunate with and without fracture of the scaphoid. J Bone Joint Surg 66B:391–395, 1984

183. Parkes JC, Stovell PB: Dislocation of the carpal scaphoid: A report of two cases. J Trauma 13:384–388, 1974

184. Peimer CA, Medige J, Eckert BS, Wright JR, Howard CS: Invasive silicone synovitis of the wrist. Orthop Trans 9:193–194, 1985

185. Pennes DR, Braunstein EM, Shirazi KK: Carpal ligamentous laxity with bilateral perilunate dislocation in Marfan Syndrome. Skeletal Radiol 13:62–64, 1985

186. Peterson HA, Lipscomb PR: Intercarpal arthrodesis. Arch Surg 95:127–134, 1967

187. Pournaras J, Kappas A: Volar perilunar dislocation: A case report. J Bone Joint Surg 61A:625–626, 1979

188. Primiano GA, Reef TC: Disruption of the proximal carpal arch of the hand. J Bone Joint Surg 56A:328–332, 1974

189. Protas JM, Jackson WT: Evaluating carpal instability with fluoroscopy. AJR 135:137–140, 1980

190. Rand JA, Linscheid RL, Dobyns JH: Capitate fractures. A long term follow-up. Clin Orthop 165:209–216, 1982

191. Rask MR: Carponavicular subluxation: Report of a case treated with percutaneous pins. Orthopedics 2:134–135, 1979

192. Rawlings ID: The management of dislocations of the carpal lunate. Injury 12:319–330, 1981

193. Reagan DS, Linscheid RL, Dobyns JH: Lunotriquetral sprains. J Hand Surg 9A:502–514, 1984

194. Resnik CS, Gelberman RH, Resnick D: Transscaphoid, transcapitate, perilunate fracture dislocation (scaphocapitate syndrome). Skeletal Radiol 9:192–194, 1983

195. Resnick D: Arthrography in the evaluation of arthritic disorders of the wrist. Diagnostic Radiology, 113:331–340, 1974

196. Rockwell WB, Destouet JM, Gilula LA, Young LV, Weeks PM: Radiographic approach to the painful wrist. Orthopaedic Review 14:43–52, 1985

197. Russe O: Fracture of the carpal navicular. J Bone Joint Surg 42A:759–768, 1960

198. Russell TB: Inter-carpal dislocations and fracture-dislocations: A review of fifty-nine cases. J Bone Joint Surg 31B:524–531, 1949

199. Sabato S, Porat S: Radial trans-scaphoid perilunate dislocation. J Trauma 21:330–331, 1981

200. Sarrafian SK, Melamed JL, Goshgarian GM: Study of wrist motion in flexion and extension. Clin Orthop 126:153–159, 1977

201. Saunier J, Chamay A: Volar perilunar dislocation of the wrist. Clin Orthop 157:139–142, 1981

202. Schlossbach T: Dislocation of the carpal navicular bone not associated with fracture. J Med Soc NJ 51:533–534, 1954

203. Sebald JR, Dobyns JH, Linscheid RL: The natural history of collapse deformities of the wrist. Clin Orthop 104:140–148, 1974

204. Simmons BP, McKenzie WD: Symptomatic carpal coalition. J Hand Surg 10A:190–193, 1985

205. Smith RJ, Atkinson RE, Jupiter JB: Silicone synovitis of the wrist. J Hand Surg 10A:47–60, 1985

206. Spar I: Bilateral perilunate dislocations. Case report with review of literature and anatomic study. J Trauma 18:64–65, 1978

207. Speed K: Fractures and dislocations of the carpus. Calif Med 72:93–98, 1950

208. Squire M: Carpal mechanics and trauma. J Bone Joint Surg 41B:210, 1959

209. Stack JK: End results of excision of carpal bones. Arch Surg 57:245–252, 1948

210. Stamm TT: Excision of the proximal row of the carpus. Proc R Soc Med 38:74, 1944

211. Stamm TT: Excision of the proximal row of the carpus. Guy's Hosp Rep 112:6–8, 1963

212. Stark WA: Recurrent perilunar subluxation. Clin Orthop 73–152, 1970

213. Stein F, Miale A, Stein A: Enhanced diagnosis of hand and wrist disorders by triple phase radionuclide imaging. Bull Hosp J Dis 44:477–484, 1984

214. Stein F, Seigel MW: Naviculocapitate fracture syndrome: A case report. J Bone Joint Surg 51A:391–395, 1969

215. Stern PJ: Transscaphoid-lunate dislocation: A report of two cases. J Hand Surg 9A:370–373, 1984

216. Stern WC: Dislocations of the carpal semilunar bone. JAMA 75:1389–1391, 1920

217. Stevenson DL: Dislocations of the carpal lunate. Br Med J 1:126, 1940

218. Sutro CJ: Bilateral recurrent intercarpal subluxation. Am J Surg 72:110–113, 1946

219. Swanson AB: Long-term bone response around carpal bone implants. Orthop Trans 9:194, 1985

220. Tachakra SS: A case of trapezio-scaphoid subluxation. Br J Clin Pract 31:162, 1977

221. Taleisnik J: The ligaments of the wrist. J Hand Surg 1:110–118, 1976

222. Taleisnik J: Wrist: Anatomy, function and injury. pp. 61–87. AAOS Instructional Course Lectures. Vol. 27. CV Mosby, St Louis, 1978

223. Taleisnik J: Post-traumatic carpal instability. Clin Orthop 149:73–82, 1980

224. Taleisnik J: Scapholunate dissociation. Ch. 39. In Strickland JW, Steichen JB (eds.): Difficult Problems in Hand Surgery, CV Mosby, St Louis, 1982

225. Taleisnik J: Triquetrohamate and triquetrolunate

instabilities (medial carpal instability). Ann Chir Main, 3:331–343, 1984

226. Taleisnik J: Subtotal arthrodeses of the wrist joint. Clin Orthop 187:81–88, 1984

227. Taleisnik J: The Wrist. Churchill Livingstone, New York, 1985

228. Taleisnik J, Malerich M, Prietto M: Palmar carpal instability secondary to dislocation of scaphoid and lunate: Report of case and review of the literature. J Hand Surg 7:606–612, 1982

229. Tanz SS: Rotation effect in lunar and perilunar dislocations. Clin Orthop 57:147–152, 1968

230. Tavernier L: Les deplacements traumatiques du semilunaire. pp. 138–139. These, Lyon, 1906

231. Tehranzadeh J, Labosky DA: Detection of intraarticular loose osteochondral fragments by double-contrast wrist arthrography. A case report of a basketball injury. Am J Sports Med 12:77–79, 1984

232. Terry DW, Ramin JE: The navicular fat stripe. A useful roentgen feature for evaluating wrist trauma. Am J Roentgen 124:25–28, 1975

233. Thomas HO: Isolated dislocation of the carpal scaphoid. Acta Orthop Scand 48:369–372, 1977

234. Thompson TC, Campbell RD, Jr, Arnold WD: Primary and secondary dislocation of the scaphoid bone. J Bone Joint Surg 46B:73–82, 1964

235. Tullos HS, Erwin WD, Fain RH: Isolated subluxation of the carpal scaphoid associated with secondary displacement of the capitate. South Med J 66:568–574, 1973

236. Uematsu A: Intercarpal fusion for treatment of carpal instability: A preliminary report. Clin Orthop 144:159–165, 1979

237. Vance RM, Gelberman RH, Braun RM: Chronic bilateral scapholunate dissociation without symptoms. J Hand Surg 4:178–180, 1979

238. Vance RM, Gelberman RH, Evans EF: Scaphocapitate fractures. Patterns of dislocation, mechanisms of injury, and primary results of treatment. J Bone Joint Surg 62A:271–276, 1980

239. Vaughan-Jackson OJ: A case of recurrent subluxation of the carpal scaphoid. J Bone Joint Surg 31B:532–533, 1949

240. Wagner CJ: Perilunar dislocations. J Bone Joint Surg 38A:1198–1230, 1956

241. Wagner CJ: Fracture-dislocations of the wrist. Clin Orthop 15:181–196, 1959

242. Walker GBW: Dislocation of the carpal scaphoid reduced by open operation. Br J Surg 30:380–381, 1943

243. Watson HK, Hempton RF: Limited wrist arthrodesis. I. The triscaphoid joint. J Hand Surg 5:320–327, 1980

244. Watson HK: Limited wrist arthrodesis. Clin Orthop 149:126–136, 1980

245. Watson HK, Ballet FL: The SLAC wrist: Scapholunate advanced collapse pattern of degenerative arthritis. J Hand Surg 9A:358–365, 1984

246. Watson-Jones R: Carpal semilunar dislocations and other wrist dislocations with associated nerve lesions. Proc R Soc Med 22:1071–1086, 1929

247. Watson-Jones R: Fractures and Joint Injuries. 3rd Ed. pp. 568–577. E & S Livingstone, Edinburgh, 1943

248. Weber ER: Biomechanical implications of scaphoid waist fractures. Clin Orthop 149:83–90, 1980

249. Weber ER: Concepts governing the rotational shift of the intercalated segment of the carpus. Orthop Clin North Am 15:193–207, 1984

250. Weeks PM, Vannier MW, Stevens WG, Gayou D, Gilula LA: Three-dimensional imaging of the wrist. J Hand Surg 10A:32–39, 1985

251. Weeks PM, Young VL, Gilula LA: A cause of painful clicking wrist: A case report. J Hand Surg 4:522–525, 1979

252. Wehbe MA, Karasick D: Radiocarpal septum after trauma. J Hand Surg 10A:498–502, 1985

253. Weiss C, Laskin RS, Spinner M: Irreducible transscaphoid perilunate dislocation: A case report. J Bone Joint Surg 52A:565–568, 1970

254. Weseley MS, Barenfeld PA: Trans-scaphoid, trans-capitate, transtriquetral, perilunar fracture-dislocation of the wrist: A case report. J Bone Joint Surg 54A:1073–1078, 1972

255. White RE, Omer GE: Transient vascular compromise of the lunate after fracture-dislocation or dislocation of the carpus. J Hand Surg 9A:181–184, 1984

256. White SJ, Louis DS, Braunstein EM, Hankin FM, Greene TL: Capitate-lunate instability: Recognition by manipulation under fluoroscopy. AJR 143:361–364, 1984

257. Woodward AH, Neviaser RJ, Nisenfeld F: Radial and volar perilunate trans-scaphoid fracture-dislocation: A case report. South Med J 68:926–928, 1975

258. Worland RL, Dick HM: Transnavicular perilunate dislocations. J Trauma 15:407–412, 1975

259. Wright RD: A detailed study of movement of the wrist joint. J Anat 70:137–143, 1936

260. Youm Y, McMurtry RY, Flatt AE, Gillespie TE: Kinematics of the wrist. I. An experimental study of radial-ulnar deviation and flexion-extension. J Bone Joint Surg 60A:423–431, 1978

261. Youm Y, Flatt AE: Kinematics of the wrist. Clin Orthop 149:21–32, 1980

The Distal Radioulnar Joint 21

William H. Bowers

The information contained in this chapter in the first edition was derived from the literature and my experience prior to 1979. Since that time there has been an explosion of interest in disorders of the ulnar side of the wrist and the distal radioulnar joint. This chapter has been extensively revised. The new material presented can be classified as follows: (1) a description of the pathologic disorders; (2) diagnostic methods; and (3) operative techniques.

Painful derangements of this complex area are now more commonly recognized and treated. Diagnosis remains difficult and often delayed, however, because of associated injuries of the radius and carpus and because significant derangements may occur with minimal radiographic evidence. A systematic approach to diagnosis is most important. The supervising physician must possess a thorough understanding of the anatomy and function of this area in order to evaluate the data gathered. A careful history is the first step and should be followed by a thorough physical examination. Diagnosis may then proceed using standard radiographic projections of the wrist, plus provocative positional and grip loading of various ligamentous structures, fluoroscopy with provocative stressing, arthrography (videotaped for exhaustive perusal), and arthroscopy. Any of these may be combined with selective anesthetic blocks. Bone scanning is helpful in localizing obscure pathology. The newer techniques of digital reconstruction from CT scans can provide three-dimensional images of carpal architecture. Surgical exploration remains an excellent diagnostic maneuver, but only if the physician is equipped with the requisite knowledge of pathology and reconstructive techniques to allow a sound treatment decision to be made on the spot.

Congenital and developmental disorders of this joint area do occur. Their diagnosis and treatment are covered in other chapters. Likewise, for disorders of the distal radioulnar joint occurring in the rheumatoid diseases, the reader is referred to Chapters 7 and 44. The disorders discussed in this chapter are those resulting from acquired or iatrogenic affectations.

A classification of conditions is presented in Table 21-1, which also defines the scope and organization of this chapter. The classification overlaps in one specific area. Acute problems when untreated or undiagnosed become chronic problems. At times the management for the chronic problem is no different from the acute, except for the degree of operative difficulty and extended period of postoperative rehabilitation. In other instances, a reconstructive approach is more direct and effective at some sacrifice to anatomy. Here judgment and

Table 21-1. Derangements of the Distal Radioulnar Joint

I. *Acute Fractures*

    A. FRACTURES INVOLVING THE SIGMOID NOTCH OF THE RADIUS. Colles', Barton's, distal radial metaphyseal fractures with comminution (Frykman's[44] Classification V-VIII), distal radial epiphyseal fractures or separations

    B. ULNAR ARTICULAR SURFACE FRACTURES INCLUDING CHONDRAL FRACTURES.[44,128]

    C. ULNAR STYLOID FRACTURES.[52] Isolated or associated with fractures of the radius (see II-B below)

II. *Acute Joint Disruption*

    A. TFCC DISRUPTION WITH DISLOCATION OR INSTABILITY ASSOCIATED WITH FRACTURES OR OTHER DISLOCATIONS (see I-C above).
       1. Fracture separation of radial epiphysis
       2. Moore's fracture[93] (Colles' fracture with disruption of distal radioulnar joint)
       3. Radial shaft or metaphysis fracture (Darrach,[24] Galleazi-Hughston,[58] Milch,[91] Smith[120])
       4. Radial head fractures (Essex-Lopresti)[42,84]
       5. Isolated ulnar fractures[133]
       6. Combined fractures of the radius and ulna[133]
       7. Proximal radioulnar joint dislocations—traumatic or infantile[133]
       8. Radiocarpal joint dislocations[133]
       9. Monteggia's injury[133] (fracture of the ulna with proximal radioulnar dislocation)

    B. ISOLATED TFCC DISRUPTION WITH INSTABILITY (see I-C, III-B)[2,8,11,12,22,23,33,45,47,52,53,55,57,113,120,133]

    C. ISOLATED TFC DISRUPTION WITHOUT INSTABILITY (see III-A)[19,32,60,74,85,95,97,100,128,134]

III. *Chronic Or Late-appearing Joint Disruption—without Radiographic Arthritis*

    A. TFC INJURY, ISOLATED WITHOUT INSTABILITY (See II-C)

    B. TFCC DISRUPTION WITH RECURRENT DISLOCATION OR INSTABILITY
       1. Isolated (see I-C, II-B)
       2. Associated with Shaft Deformity (see II-A)

IV. *Joint Disorders*

    A. THE ULNOCARPAL IMPINGEMENT SYNDROME[11-13,32,77,87,90,100,101,126]—A LENGTH DISCREPANCY WITH THE ULNA LONG RELATIVE TO THE RADIUS
       1. Premature closure of radial epiphysis secondary to trauma (acquired Madelung's deformity[82,91] or premature wrist fusion[133])
       2. Excision or "settling" of radial head (or shaft) secondary to trauma, tumor, infection[42,54,84]
       3. Occupational overload of a "normal variant" long ulna[11-13]
       4. Reconstruction of radial or ulnar shaft for trauma, tumor, or infection

    B. ARTHRITIS[1,11-13,18,24,31,35,44,68,81,91,117,133] INCLUDING OSTEOARTHRITIS, ARTHRITIS FOLLOWING TRAUMA, AND ARTICULAR CHONDROMALACIA—WITH OR WITHOUT INSTABILITY

V. *Other Disorders*

    A. SNAPPING OR DISLOCATING EXTENSOR CARPI ULNARIS[16,36,107,121]

    B. FIXED ROTATIONAL DEFORMITY[5,11,12]

experience become paramount. The overlap is therefore necessary for a thorough consideration of the injury spectrum.

Table 21-2 is a summary of the author's recommendations for management of disorders of the distal radioulnar joint; Table 21-3 is a classification of TFCC abnormalities as devised by Palmer (Palmer AK: Personal communication). Although in this chapter I have presented a discussion of abnormalities focusing on the TFCC, I believe that the classification is sufficiently important to include here. As one reads the description of TFCC injuries as I have presented them, frequent referral to Table 21-3 will help to provide what I feel is a

Table 21-2. Disorders of the Distal Radioulnar Joint: Management Recommendations

Disorder	Surgical Management[a]
I. *Fractures*	
A. Sigmoid Notch	
Fragment (large)	Open reduction and internal fixation (ORIF)
Comminuted	External fixation
B. Ulnar Articular Surface	
Small fragment	Excise (open or with arthroscope)
Large fragment	ORIF
Comminution	Hemi-resection interposition arthroplasty (HIT)[13]
Chrondral	Debride or HIT[13]
C. Ulnar Styloid	ORIF[11,12,52] if closed reduction not satisfactory
II. *Joint Disruption — Acute*	
A. TFCC Disruption in Association with Fractures or Other Dislocations	Repair TFCC (or ORIF styloid fracture) plus management of other injury
B. TFCC Disruption — Isolated	Closed reduction and immobilization — ORIF if unsatisfactory
C. TFC Tears — No Instability	
1. Positive variant with or without chondromalacia	Limited debridement of tear with ulnar recession[11,12,32]
2. Neutral variant with chondromalacia	Same as above
3. Minus variant	Limited debridement of tear[60,85,97,100] (open or with arthroscope)
III. *Joint Disruption — Chronic or Late-Appearing — No Evidence of Arthritis*	
A. TFC Tears — No Instability	As in II-C[1-3]
B. TFCC Disruption — Recurrent Dislocation or Instability	
1. Isolated	Repair by styloid or TFCC reattachment if possible.[11,12,52] If not possible, TFCC reconstruction (Hui[57] or similar procedure); consider pronator advancement[61]
2. Associated with shaft deformity	
(a) Translational	As above PLUS radial angular osteotomy with graft
(b) Rotational	As above PLUS rotational osteotomy; alternatives: Darrach modification (Tsai[130]); HIT (Bowers[13]); Sauve-Kapandji
IV. *Joint Disorders*	
A. Ulnocarpal Impingement Syndrome	
1. Premature closure radial epiphysis in children	Ulnar epiphyseal arrest
2. Other ulna long conditions	
(a) Without radioulnar arthrosis	Ulnar recession[10,32,90]
(b) With radioulnar arthrosis	HIT with ulnar recession (Bowers[13]); Sauve-Kapandji[117,127]; Darrach modified (Tsai[130])
B. Arthritis[b]	HIT[13] (with or without shortening of ulna); Sauve-Kapandji[117,127]; Darrach modified (Tsai[130]); arthrodesis[17]
V. *Other Disorders*	
A. Snapping or Dislocating ECU	Stabilization — Bowers modification[11-13] of Spinner[121]
B. Fixed Rotational Deformity	
1. No motor control of rotation	Radioulnar arthrodesis[17]
2. Acceptable motor control of rotation	Soft tissue release of contracture; HIT[13]; Sauve-Kapandji[117,127]; Baldwin[5]

[a] In most cases nonsurgical management is either not indicated or is assumed to have been tried without success.
[b] For rheumatoid arthritis, see Chapters 7 and 44.

Table 21-3. TFCC Abnormalities[a]

CLASS I — Traumatic
  A. Central Perforation
  B. Medial Avulsion (ulnar attachment)
       with distal ulnar fracture
       without distal ulnar fracture
  C. Distal Avulsion (carpal attachment)
  D. Lateral Avulsion (radial attachment)
       with sigmoid notch fracture
       without sigmoid notch fracture

CLASS II — Degenerative (Ulnocarpal impingement
           syndrome)
Stage 1. TFCC wear
Stage 2. TFCC wear
       + lunate and/or ulnar chondromalacia
Stage 3. TFCC perforation
       + lunate and/or ulnar chondromalacia
Stage 4. TFCC perforation
       + lunate and/or ulnar chondromalacia
       + L-T ligament perforation
Stage 5. TFCC perforation
       + lunate and/or ulnar chondromalacia
       + L-T ligament perforation
       + ulnocarpal arthritis

[a] A classification of traumatic and degenerative conditions of the TFCC devised by Andrew K. Palmer, MD (personal communication). The Class I lesion emphasizes that injuries can occur to the three major attachment areas of the TFCC (IB, C, D), as well as to the central portion of the TFC (IA, II).

valuable viewpoint of this central structure. The table classifies both degenerative and traumatic lesions in a unique way.

ANATOMY, BIOMECHANICS, AND KINETICS

The anatomy of the distal radioulnar joint is complex. Accurate anatomic concepts are necessary for communication, diagnosis, surgical techniques, and new developments. This section may therefore be the most valuable portion of the chapter. The distal radioulnar joint, its stabilizing ligaments, its overlying fascia and retinacula, and the musculotendinous units in the area will be reviewed. The description offered is based largely on the author's dissection of fresh, unembalmed specimens, ranging in age from 15 to 50, and on a number of operative cases. The study was guided by the works of Lewis, Hamshere and Bucknill,[72] Kauer,[65] Kaplan,[64] and Spinner.[121] Recent contributions of great value are those of Palmer and Werner,[102] Taleisnik,[125] and Ekenstam.[38,39]

The distal radioulnar joint articulation is trochoid, as is the proximal radioulnar joint. The semi-cylindrical, concave sigmoid articular notch is variable in its depth (Fig. 21-1). Its dimensions are on average 1.5 cm dorsovolar and 1 cm proximaldistal. There are three distinct margins to the notch: dorsal, distal, and volar. The dorsal margin is acutely angular in cross-section, the volar less so. The carpal (distal) margin is the junction between the notch and the distally facing lunate facet. The two are separated by the attachment of the triangular fibrocartilage to the radius. The prominent volar beak of the distal radius seen on the lateral radiograph represents these two adjacent articular surfaces. Thus, fractures of the lunate facet are also fractures of the distal radioulnar joint and viceversa. The head of the ulna, or articular "seat" on which the radius rotates, is semi-cylindrical as well. The cylindrical articular surface is inclined 15 degrees toward the ulna and has 130 degrees in its dorsovolar arc. The articulation of the ulnar head with the sigmoid notch is not congruous as the radius of the shallow arc of the sigmoid notch is greater than that of the ulnar convexity.[20,38] For this reason the forearm movements of pronation and supination must include a sliding as well as a rotational component. In addition, even in the presence of "normal" ligamentous support, the dysharmonic radii of the two surfaces dictate that there is significant dorsovolar translation, particularly in the zero position of rotation. In this midrange the sigmoid notch accepts 60 to 80 degrees of the 130 degrees articular convexity, but in the extremes of rotation less than 10 percent of this surface may be in contact with the dorsal (in pronation) or volar (in supination) margins of the notch. Implicit in this anatomic observation is the importance of ligamentous stability in the rotational extremes of the joint (see Fig. 21-6). The semi-cylindrical ulnar head is flattened distally as it faces the underside of the triangular fibrocartilage. The periphery of this flattened dome is articular cartilage. An eccentric concavity of the dome lies at the base of the styloid and is the attachment area for the ulnar apex of the triangular fibrocartilage (TFC)

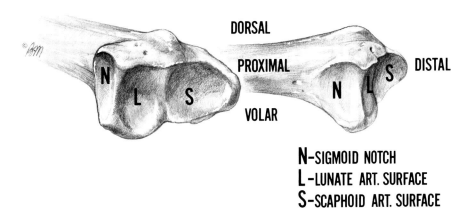

Fig. 21-1. On the left, the distal radius is viewed from the ulnar aspect of the carpus, and on the right from directly ulnar. Note the confluence of the lunate facet and the sigmoid notch (ulnar facet).

DORSAL

PROXIMAL   DISTAL

VOLAR

N-SIGMOID NOTCH
L-LUNATE ART. SURFACE
S-SCAPHOID ART. SURFACE

and ulnocarpal ligaments (UCL). The area is replete with vascular foramina, allowing communicating vessels to supply the ligament complex, ulnar metaphysis, and distal radioulnar joint synovium. The concavity flows dorsally onto the shaft-head junction, forming a sulcus for the extensor carpi ulnaris sheath (Figs. 21-2 and 21-3). The ulnar styloid is a continuation of the prominent subcutaneous ridge of the shaft of the ulna. It projects distally toward the triquetrum for a variable distance (2–6 mm), providing an increased area of attachment for the ligament complex. The structure attaching the radius to the ulna is variously known as the triangular fibrocartilage, carpal articular disc, discus articularis, triangular ligament, triangular cartilage, triangular disc, and, most unfortunately, meniscus. The latter designation is confusing, as it should be reserved for a nearby anatomic structure related to the triangular fibrocartilage but distinct from it (see the Meniscus sec-

tion). The triangular fibrocartilage is but part of an extensive fibrous system that arises from the carpal margin of the sigmoid notch of the radius, cups the lunate and triquetral bones, and reaches the volar base of the fifth metacarpal (Fig. 21-4). The center of this complex (triangular fibrocartilage and ulnocarpal ligaments) has been termed the ulnocarpal complex (UCC) by Taleisnik,[125] the triangular fibrocartilage complex (TFCC) by Palmer and Werner,[101] and the ulnocarpal ligament complex (UCLC) by me.[11] None of the terms is particularly accurate or satisfying, although all of us agree that we are referring to the same structure. The terms may be used interchangeably. I will use the designation triangular fibrocartilage complex (TFCC) for this structure in deference to the historically well-known triangular fibrocartilage (TFC). The triangular fibrocartilage complex supplies the demands of articulation by (1) providing a continuous gliding surface across the entire distal face of the

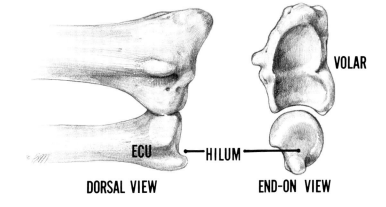

Fig. 21-2. The radioulnar articulation in neutral or zero rotation as viewed from the dorsum and from end on. Note that the arc of the notch circumscribes a circle of greater diameter than that of the ulnar head.

VOLAR

ECU   ───HILUM───

DORSAL VIEW   END-ON VIEW

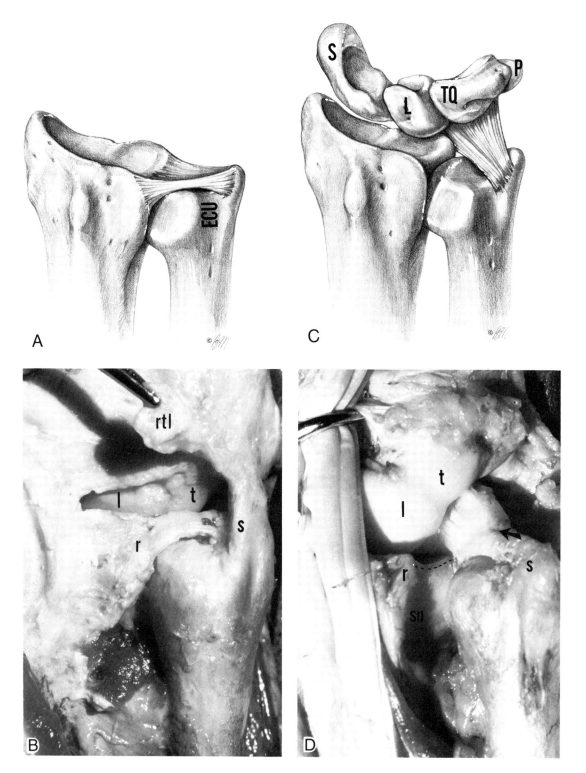

Fig. 21-3. **(A)** A diagrammatic representation of the TFC as an isolated structure (*ECU*, groove for the extensor carpi ulnaris). **(B)** The TFC, as seen in a dissected specimen, viewed from the dorsum. The radioulnar articulation is in neutral or zero rotation. (*rtl*, radiotriquetral ligament; *l*, lunate; *t*, triquetrum; *r*, radius; *s*, styloid.) **(C)** The ulnocarpal or V ligament shown diagrammatically as an isolated structure. This V ligament is also part of the ulnocarpal complex. **(D)** The ulnocarpal V ligament *(arrow)* as seen in a dissected specimen. The TFC has been removed, and the dotted line represents its radial attachment (*sn*, sigmoid notch). *(Figure continues.)*

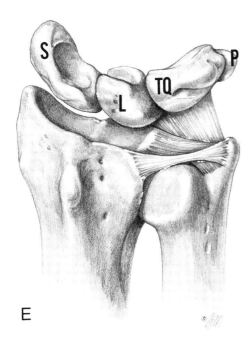

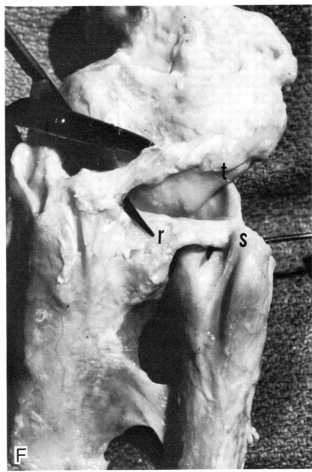

Fig. 21-3 *(Continued).* **(E)** The combined TFC and ulnocarpal V ligament shown diagrammatically. Geometrically, these represent two equilateral triangles perpendicular to one another. **(F)** A dissected specimen showing the combined TFC and ulnocarpal V ligament. The scissors are under the distal radiotriquetral ligament. Note the marked groove in the ulnar styloid, which represents the floor of the extensor carpi ulnaris tendon sheath. The combined TFC-UCLC cups the ulnar side of the carpus, yet provides a stable rotational attachment for the distal ulna. **(G)** The same specimen with the radioulnar joint distracted, emphasizing the so-called ligamentum subcruentum *(arrow).* This is actually part of the origin of the V ligament shown in Figure 21-3C and D (*vc*, volar capsule).

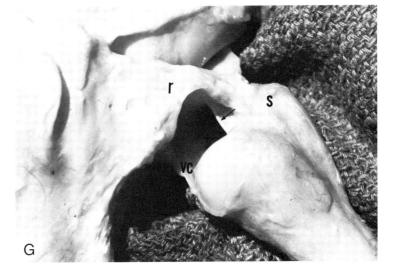

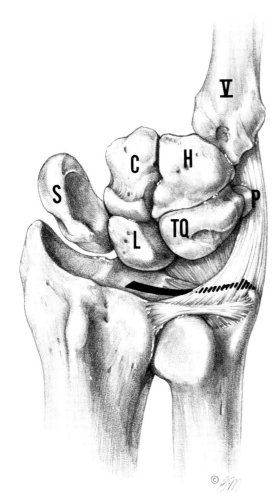

Fig. 21-4. A diagrammatic drawing of the meniscal reflection and the prestyloid recess. The meniscal reflection runs from the dorsoulnar radius to the ulnovolar carpus. The arrow denotes access under the reflection to the tip of the styloid—the so-called prestyloid recess. Its relationship to the ulnocarpal complex can be appreciated when compared to Figure 21-3.

two forearm bones for carpal flexion and extension and translational movements; (2) providing a flexible mechanism for stable rotational movements of the radiocarpal unit around the ulnar axis; (3) suspending the ulnar carpus from the dorsal ulnar face of the radius; (4) cushioning the forces transmitted through the ulnocarpal axis; and (5) solidly connecting the ulnar axis to the volar carpus. As we further discuss the elements of the triangular fibrocartilage complex, I will try to relate them to these functional demands.

The Triangular Fibrocartilage

The portion of the TFCC called the triangular fibrocartilage (TFC) is triangular in shape, and 1 to 2 mm thick at its base, the distal margin of the sigmoid notch. The biconcave body (Fig. 21-3A and B) of the structure stretches across the ulnar-articular dome, and its apex is attached to the eccentric concavity of the head and projecting styloid, where it may be as much as 5 mm thick. Viewed from within the radioulnar joint, the styloid attachment appears folded. Between the folds, vessels enter the TFCC from the hilar foramina previously mentioned. This intraarticular fold and its vascular hilum have been termed the ligamentum subcruentum (Fig. 21-3E–G). The folded appearance is actually the confluence of the TFC and V-shaped ligament that proceeds from the styloid hilar area (its apex) to twin insertions on the volar surface of the lunate and triquetral bones (Fig. 21-3C and D). The peripheral margins of the triangular cartilage are thick lamellar collagen, structurally adapted to bear tensile loading. These are often referred to as the dorsal and volar radioulnar ligamentous margins. The thin central portion, occasionally referred to as the articular disk, is chondroid fibrocartilage morphologically seen in structures that bear compressive loads. This central area is occasionally absent (congenital perforations) and often so thin as to be translucent. The load-bearing function of the triangular fibrocartilage is a subject of much discussion and little concrete information.[39,102] Compressive force across the carpalulnar articulation is partially transmitted through the center of the triangular fibrocartilage to the ulnar dome. This same force tends to separate the radius and ulna (particularly in a neutral or negative variant wrist). The triangular fibrocartilage resists this tendency, thus converting some of the compressive loading to tensile loading within the lamellar collagen of the periphery of the triangular fibrocartilage. The triangular fibrocartilage is assisted in meeting this functional demand (demand No. 4) by the muscular action of the pronator quadratus and the interosseous membrane. The portion of the compressive load not converted to tensile loading is accepted by the stable and fixed ulnar dome. This is the case in static power grip. The picture becomes more complicated when grip forces are applied as the forearm is rotated. Loaded rotational grip requires that the forces be accepted by a triangular fibrocartilage that is being twisted at its apex and an ulnar dome that is moving beneath it. More of the load may be borne by the periphery of the triangular fibrocartilage and redistributed as tension in this mode. The distribution of the load is greatly influenced by the length of the ulna relative to the radius (ulnar variance). In an ulnar-positive variant (ulna longer than radius), the compressive load through the center of the triangular fibrocartilage to the underlying ulnar dome may be greatly increased. Palmer et al[102] have shown experimentally that in the neutral variant, 80 percent of the static axial load is borne by the radius, while 20 percent is borne by the ulna (Fig. 21-5). If relative ulnar length is varied from −2 mm to +2.5 mm, the load borne by the ulna increases from 5 to 40 percent. The full significance of the negative variant is unknown, but more of the force is probably converted to tension.

Ulnocarpal Ligaments

The second major element of the triangular fibrocartilage complex is the combined volar ulnolunate and ulnotriquetral ligament (Fig. 21-3C and D). This ligament duo begins at the base of the styloid coextensive with the triangular fibrocartilage apical attachment, spreads distally passing the triangular fibrocartilage at its volar margin, and proceeds to insert volarly on the lunate and triquetrum. The general shape of the two ligaments together is triangular with the apex at the ulnar styloid and the base across the lunate and triquetrum. As this combined ligament passes the volar margin of the triangular fibrocartilage, it is so intimately blended with the triangular fibrocartilage that, viewed from within the radiocarpal joint, the triangular fibrocartilage and ulnocarpal ligaments (UCL) appear to be a singular structure (hence the term triangular fibrocartilage complex; Fig. 21-3F) beginning at the radius and cupping the ulnar carpus with intermediate attachment to the ulnar styloid. This anatomic combination supplies the functional demand of suspending the volar-ulnar carpus from the dorso-ulnar margin of the radius (demand No. 3). It resists the volar-ulnar displacement forces generated on the carpus by the flexors in power grip, a displacement well seen in rheumatoid arthritis when progressive destruction of this ligament occurs. The styloid attachment of the complex provides a mechanism for a stable, flexible attachment of the radiocarpal unit to the ulnar axis (functional demand No. 2). These two structures (TFC and UCL) are morphologically distinct and have individual roles even though the complex functions as a unit. The individual role of the combined ulnocarpal ligaments is to provide a stable connection between the ulna and the volar-ulnar carpus. This ligament resists dorsal displacement of the distal ulna relative to the carpus and radiocarpal unit. It is taut in supination and less so in pronation, a position in which the styloid and volar carpus are more nearly approximated. Destruction of this ligament by attenuation (rheumatoid arthritis) will allow volar displacement of the carpus in relation to the distal ulna, a condition even more obvious in pronation (the "supinated" carpal unit of rheumatoid arthritis).

The individual role of the TFC on the other hand, along with the ulnar articular surface, provides radioulnar stability, particularly in the rotational ex-

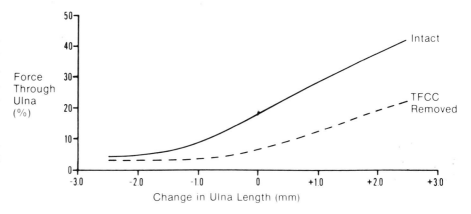

Fig. 21-5. Axial load transmission through the ulnar column. This shows the percentage of total forearm load as the ulna is lengthened by a 2.5-mm distance. (Palmer AK, Werner FW: Biomechanics of the distal radioulnar joint. Clin Orthop 187:26–34, 1984.)

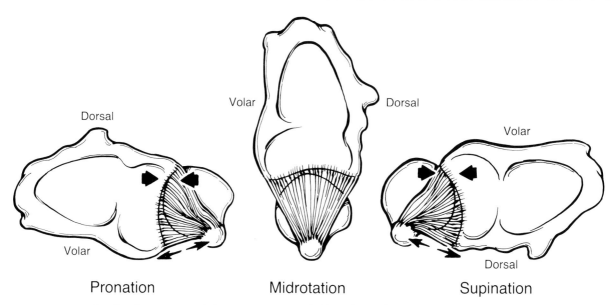

Pronation   Midrotation   Supination

Fig. 21-6. Distal radioulnar joint stability in pronation (left) is dependent on (1) tension developed in the volar margin of the TFC plus (2) compression between the contact areas of the radius and ulna (volar surface of ulnar articular head and dorsal margin of sigmoid notch). A tear of the volar TFC would therefore allow dorsal displacement of the ulna in pronation. The reverse is true in supination where a tear of the dorsal margin of the TFC would allow volar displacement of the ulna relative to the radius as this rotational extreme is reached.

tremes (Fig. 21-6).[38] The volar margin of the TFC is taut in pronation, developing this tension as the dorsal margin of the radius and the volar portion of the ulnar articular surface are compressed. Should the volar margin of the TFC become attenuated or torn, dorsal subluxation of the distal ulna would occur in pronation as the ulnocarpal ligaments are relaxed somewhat in this position. Similarly, the dorsal margin of the TFC becomes taut in supination while the volar margin of the sigmoid notch and dorsal portion of the ulnar articular surface are compressed. Should the dorsal margin of the TFC become attenuated or torn, volar or anterior subluxation might occur. The integrity of the osseous shape of the convexity of the ulnar articular surface and the margins of the sigmoid notch obviously play corresponding roles in this rotational stability.

Other Stabilizing Factors

The triangular fibrocartilage and ulnocarpal ligaments provide the heart of the triangular fibrocartilage complex. Stability of the radioulnar carpal unit is additionally influenced by the conformation of the sigmoid notch, the interosseous membrane, the extensor retinaculum, and the dynamic forces of the extensor carpi ulnaris and the pronator quadratus, as well as by the dorsal carpal ligament complex. The latter can be visualized as a "star" centered over and blending with the dorsal peripheral margin of the triangular fibrocartilage complex (Fig. 21-7). The proximal and distal legs are the extensor carpi ulnaris sheath extending from the extensor carpi ulnaris groove to the dorsal base of the fifth metacarpal. The radial legs are the proximal and distal radiotriquetral ligaments and the dorsal transverse carpal ligament. The ulnar leg is a wide ligament band proceeding from the center of the star around the ulnar aspect of the triquetrum distal to the styloid attaching to the pisotriquetral joint capsule.

I attach no functional or anatomic significance to the oft-described ulnar collateral ligaments and dorsal and volar radioulnar ligaments, except as these terms may be used to describe the dorsal and volar margins of the TFC (see Fig. 21-19). These ligament designations are probably figments of imaginations that supposed that they should exist and, if continued, serve only to confuse the understanding of the area. The distal radioulnar joint capsule is uniformly thin and cannot be construed to offer stability in the usual sense. Dorsally, the capsule is minimally reinforced by the obliquely passing radiotriquetral capsular ligament. It offers no coverage to the ulnar head. Spinner[121] has called attention to the importance of the extensor carpi ulnaris musculotendinous unit in stabilizing the joint. The emphasis is warranted but should be shared by both the rather strong sheath system through which it runs and the strong volar ligament complex. Johnson and Shrewsbury[62] have demonstrated that the dual structure of the pronator quadratus stabilizes the distal radioulnar joint by ac-

tively maintaining coaptation of the ulnar head in the notch in pronation and passively by viscoelastic forces in supination.

Meniscus

The last element to be covered is the meniscus (Fig. 21-4). This element of the ulnar wrist is often confused with the triangular fibrocartilage. It is found in a minority of wrists explored; when present, it lies within the ulnocarpal joint. It has a concave, free margin (resembling the meniscus of the knee) and, when fully developed, overlies the triangular fibrocartilage – ulnocarpal ligament-styloid, extending from dorsal triangular fibrocartilage to the volar ulnar aspect of the triquetrum. It may exclude the presentation of the styloid tip from the ulnocarpal joint. If one passes a probe or arthrographic dye beneath the meniscus, one enters the prestyloid recess. The meniscus may lie fused (or scarred) to the triangular fibrocartilage in which case neither probe nor dye will reach the prestyloid recess. In the usual case, in which the meniscus is underdeveloped, an arthrogram will show a sharp indentation just distal to the styloid. In this case the styloid may present within the joint clothed in articular cartilage, and dye enters the prestyloid recess freely. When the meniscus is more developed it may contain an ossicle (os lanula, 4 percent) which can be misinterpreted as a styloid fracture. The meniscus, lanula, and prestyloid recess, as well as variations in the length of the styloid, are variations in the presentation of normal ulnar phylogeny. With the exception of ulnar variance it is unclear what role, if any, they play in the pathology of this area.

ULNAR VARIANCE

There is a final comment to make concerning ulnar variance. According to several studies,[46,59,92] the relative lengths of the radius and ulna may differ. This is usually referred to as Hulten's variance[59] (Fig. 21-8): ulna zero (both the same length), ulna plus (ulna 1 – 5 mm longer), and ulna minus (1 – 6 mm shorter). This is apparently an expression of the normal regression of the ulna from its embryonic carpal articulation.[65,72]

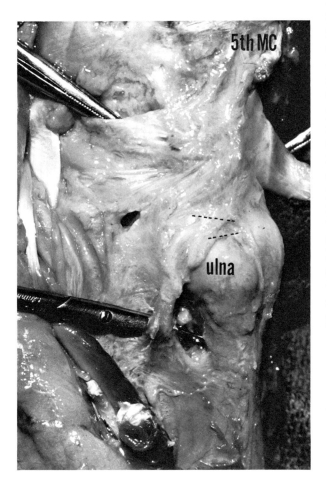

Fig. 21-7. The dorsal ulnar wrist ligament complex. This complex overlies and blends with the TFC (shown in dotted lines).

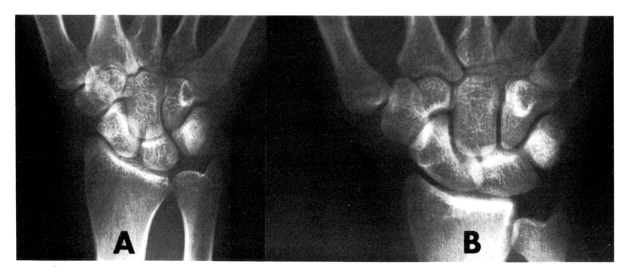

Fig. 21-8. Radiographs demonstrating positive (**A**) and negative (**B**) ulnar variance.

Ulnar variance is usually estimated by looking at a wrist x-ray. Studies have correlated negative variance with Kienböck's disease[46,59,92] and, on an empiric basis, the procedure of ulnar lengthening has gained favor as a surgical alternative to treat this disorder. This relationship must be tempered by Taleisnik's[126] observation that Kienböck's has not been reported following excision of the distal ulna. Recent work by Palmer and Werner[101] has demonstrated a correlation between triangular fibrocartilage perforation and ulnolunate chondromalacia with the positive variant. This correlation is substantiated by the studies of Mikic,[87] who observed triangular fibrocartilage perforation and ulnolunate chrondromalacic changes with aging. Data on ulnar column loading related to variance is available only from Palmer[102] and Ekenstam.[39] Epner et al[41] have demonstrated that the measurement of variance is influenced by forearm rotation, wrist positioning, and roentgenographic technique. They have recommended a method for standardizing a technique of wrist x-rays that eliminates these variables as sources of error in measurement (see below).

FOREARM ROTATION

The rotational freedom within the upper extremity of man may be developmentally related to the period of the great apes when arboreal brachiation became important as a means of movement. The hinges of rotation are the proximal and distal radioulnar joints. There are several opinions as to where the axis of rotation lies. Perhaps the best discussion is provided by Kapandji,[63] who concludes that there are several rotational axes, depending on which of the upper extremity bones is fixed. The most common axis, used with the tridigital grip, passes through the lower radius near the sigmoid notch. The radius rotates about this axis while the ulna translates without rotation. Understanding of rotational mechanics is elusive yet essential to the restoration of this capacity.

TECHNIQUES IN DIAGNOSIS

In an area where pathoanatomic processes are only gradually becoming well-defined clinical presentations, one must methodically gather data until a correlation becomes very clear. Only then is treatment rational.

HISTORY

The selection of treatment options is often based on the occupational demands of the patient, and therefore a careful work history is essential prior to any sequence of diagnostic maneuvers. It is critical to obtain a thorough understanding of the wrist motion, repetitions, and load to which a surgical procedure will be subjected. After this is first obtained, history-taking should include age, dominance, symptom characteristics, and provocative questions designed to firmly fix in the examiner's mind the mechanism of injury or symptom production. Identical mechanisms may produce different injuries; nevertheless, there are some typical patterns. Carpal hypersupination with ulnar deviation is often recalled in patients who have developed extensor carpi ulnaris instability. Hyperpronation and dorsiflexion is a common mechanism for producing lunate-triquetral ligament injuries. Repeated pronation and supination may produce chondromalacia of the ulnar head, and, if associated with a long ulna, the "ulnocarpal impingement syndrome." Sudden onset of pain accompanied by redness and swelling points to an inflammatory process, frequently calcific tendonitis.

CLINICAL EXAMINATION

Specific palpation is most important because of the intimate location of these joints and their supporting structures. Palpation should be methodical and is often assisted by pressure with the eraser end of a pencil. Each joint is then — to the extent possible — individually stressed and manipulated in order to detect crepitation, pain, or snaps. These are meaningful only if they reproduce the patient's pain. The patient then should be asked to duplicate the motion or attitude that causes the symptoms, and this should be confirmed by the examiner's directed maneuvers. The usual tendency is for the examiner to examine the dorsum of the wrist with the forearm pronated and the volar aspect with the forearm supinated. The subluxating or dislocating extensor carpi ulnaris may be obvious only by examining the dorsum of the wrist with the forearm supinated.

Screening x-rays are then obtained, and if not contributory, selective injection of a suspected joint or structure with a local anesthetic may be helpful. Other joints should be evaluated on other days with this technique.

RADIOGRAPHIC EVALUATION

Standard Films

A joint that both rotates and moves in space demands a standardized technique for accuracy and comparison follow-up studies. This is increasingly important because radioulnar joint and carpal pathologies are defined in terms of measurements (variance, carpal height, scapholunate angle, intercarpal distance, etc.), and these measurements are then used for surgical decision-making.

Evans[43] in 1945 published a method for estimating forearm rotation by comparing sequential x-ray projections of the bicipital tuberosity of the radius in progressive degrees of rotation. This was recommended as an aid in aligning fractures. A similar concept can be applied distally to the ulna.[11,41] In this technique we can ascertain forearm rotation by comparing the x-ray projection of the ulnar styloid to that of the shaft of the ulna and to the radius. We can also determine carpal deviation by comparing the position of the lunate to the radius.

In the normal configuration of the ulna, the ulnar styloid is posterior (dorsal) just as the olecranon is posterior. The two are in constant relationship, connected by the subcutaneous ridge of the ulna. The central radian of the articular convexity of the ulnar head is anterior and remains in a fixed relationship to the coronoid process of the ulna. Thus, with the radius in zero or midposition of forearm rotation, a lateral wrist film will show the ulnar styloid exactly in the center of the ulna and the radius superimposed upon it (Fig. 21-9A). An AP or PA film of this wrist position will show the radial and ulnar styloids farthest apart, at the extreme medial and lateral edges, respectively, of each bone (Fig. 21-9A). Thus, an AP or PA wrist x-ray showing the ulnar styloid directly opposite to the radius defines a wrist in the mid- or zero position of rotation. In full pronation the ulnar styloid will be in the center of the ulnar head on the PA or AP view, but volar in relation to the radius on the lateral view (Fig. 21-9C). Similarly, in full supination the ulnar styloid will again be in the center of the ulnar head on the AP or PA view, but dorsal in relation to the radius on the lateral view (Fig. 21-9B). Additionally, if the shafts of the radius and the ulna are noted to converge proximally on a PA

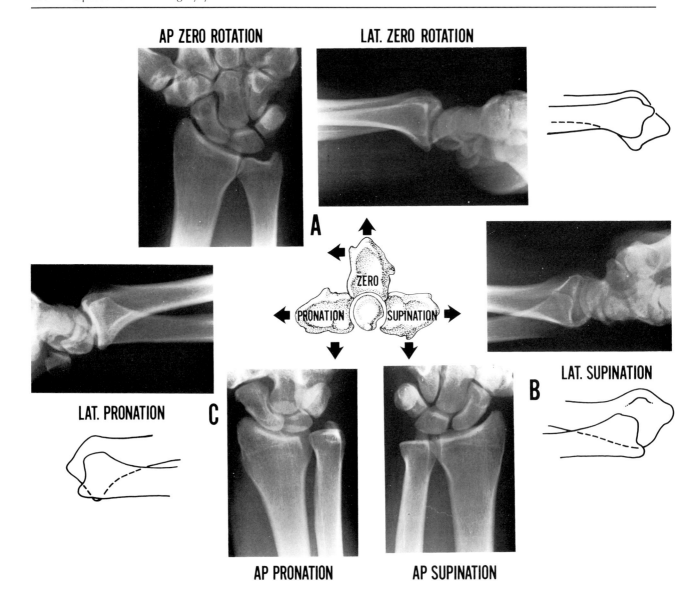

Fig. 21-9. The determination of forearm rotation using the ulnar styloid as a reference point. (**A**) Anteroposterior and lateral in zero rotation, the preferred standard position. (**B**) Anteroposterior and lateral in full pronation. (**C**) Anteroposterior and lateral in full supination.

or AP wrist film this further suggests the forearm bones are crossed or pronated (Fig. 21-9C). When they appear parallel or divergent, the position is either zero rotation or supination (Fig. 21-9B and C).

Wrist deviation can be estimated using the lunate as a landmark. It is a recognized anatomic fact that in neutral or radial deviation the osseous shadow of the lunate on a PA or AP x-ray film is half on and half off the ulnar border of the radius at the distal radioulnar joint, and it is completely over the radius (lying in the lunate facet of the distal radiocarpal articulation) if the wrist is in full ulnar deviation (Fig. 21-10). Thus a full ulnar deviation PA or AP view can be easily recognized as such if the lunate is fully over the radius. We have selected from these views as a standard position the zero rotation–ulnar deviation PA and the zero rota-

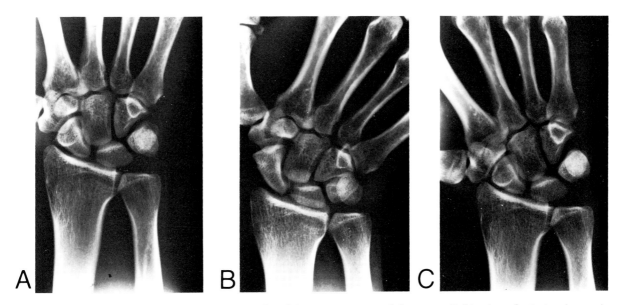

Fig. 21-10. Standard zero rotation PA radiographs of the wrist in neutral deviation (left), ulnar deviation (center), and radial deviation (right). Note that only in full ulnar deviation is the lunate completely over the radius.

tion – neutral deviation lateral.[11,41] These films can be instantly recognized as such by using the internal reference standards of ulnar styloid and lunate as noted above. They are neutral with regard to the changes in ulnar variance and are useful in

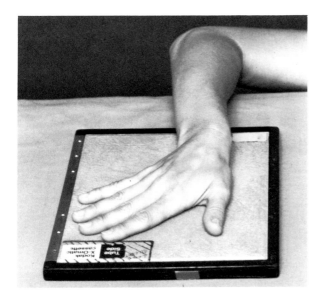

Fig. 21-11. Positioning for the standard zero rotation – ulnar deviation PA radiograph.

recognizing common maladies, such as scaphoid fractures, scapholunate injuries, and so forth. The PA view is an excellent screening view for rheumatoid arthritis (the lack of movement of the lunate radially on attempted ulnar deviation of the wrist is recognized as an early predictive abnormality in the progression of radiocarpal arthritis[4]).

To obtain the standard zero rotation – ulnar deviation PA, the patient is positioned with shoulder abducted 90 degrees, elbow flexed 90 degrees, forearm in a zero position of rotation, and the wrist in ulnar deviation (Fig. 21-11). To obtain the standard zero rotation – neutral deviation lateral, the arm is brought to the side (zero degrees shoulder abduction) while the forearm is maintained in zero rotation. Placing the wrist on the cassette brings the wrist into neutral deviation (Fig. 21-12). The tube-to-cassette distance should be constant, the elbow flexed 90 degrees, and the beam direction should as nearly as possible be at a right angle to the wrist. Variations are known to influence the measurement of ulnar variance.[41]

This unique, standard radiograph can be identified by noting the position of the ulnar styloid with reference to the ulna itself and to the radial styloid. Wrist deviation can be appreciated by using the lunate as an internal reference point. When used as

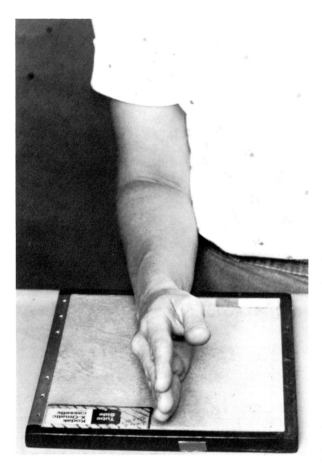

Fig. 21-12. Positioning for the standard zero rotation – neutral deviation lateral radiograph.

a standard wrist film technique, variations from zero rotation and ulnar deviation can be "read" as such and discarded as inappropriate to use for accurate measurements. Any film, other than the standard, can, of course, be used for measurement, but only if the most careful attention is given to obtaining subsequent films in this nonstandard position. This rigid control assures valid comparisons throughout the patient's management, whatever the diagnosis may be.

Semi-Pronated View

The ulnar border of the hand is against the cassette, the forearm and hand pronated 45 degrees. This view helps visualize dorso-ulnar structures.

Semi-Supinated View

This view is also sometimes called a "reversed oblique" or "ballcatcher" view. It is obtained as above, with the forearm and hand supinated 30 to 45 degrees. This is useful in evaluation of the volar ulnar quadrant of the wrist, especially the pisotriquetral joint and hook of the hamate.

Dynamic, Provocative, or Loaded Views

Application of compressive forces across the wrist joint loads the radial and ulnar columns and tends to displace the unstable distal radioulnar joint. The patient is asked to make a firm fist; more reliably to squeeze an object such as the standard wrist dynamometer. When compared to the opposite side and nonloaded views, instability may be recognized. Loaded PA radial and ulnar deviation views show the proximal row as it moves in relation to the TFC and radius. Loss of normal lunate movement may support the diagnosis of lunate chondromalacia, especially in a patient with a positive variant ulna. It is also a valuable sign in early radiocarpal involvement in patients with rheumatoid arthritis (see above). Taleisnik[125,126] has suggested that lateral views of the pronated wrist, with deviation designed to provoke the patient's symptoms, may reveal abnormal midcarpal motion.

SPECIAL DIAGNOSTIC TECHNIQUES

Tomography

Two-plane trispiral tomography[78,104] may be very helpful in detecting small avulsion type fractures—indicative of a ligament disruption. It is also useful in detecting fractures of the hook of the hamate.

Computerized Tomography and Digital Reconstruction

The computerized tomographic scan has proved its usefulness in evaluating distal radioulnar joint subluxation or dislocation[20,85,118] (Fig. 21-13). Its advantages are that it does not require precise positioning and it can be done through plaster casts, although films of the normal side are recom-

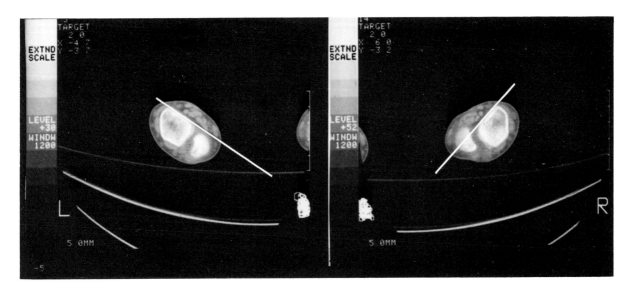

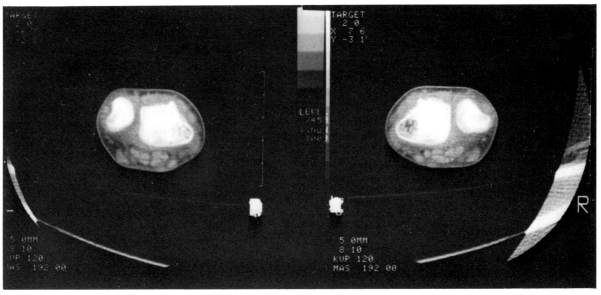

Fig. 21-13. Comparison CT scans of both wrists in (top) full pronation and (bottom) full supination. The clinical problem was volar dislocation of the right ulna relative to the radius occurring in supination. The patient had a rotational malunion of the radius and ulna subsequent to a double-bone forearm fracture, as well as a disruption of the TFCC from the ulnar styloid. A comparison of the two ulnas (in pronation) shows an approximate 30 degree pronation deformity of the right ulna relative to the left ulna. Compare this scan carefully with Figure 21-6. The patient was effectively treated by supination osteotomy of the ulna and reattachment of the TFCC to the styloid.

mended. Digital reconstruction[112] is a new technique that takes computerized tomographic data and constructs a picture in any desired plane, not just in a cross-section. The construction is limited only by the interpolation required for the area be-

tween scan cuts. Recently developed computerized tomographic programs allow the construction of data such that a three-dimensional facsimile of the wrist is obtained. The image may then be exploded or manipulated so that all surface areas and contours may be evaluated. Although not widely available, the technique holds tremendous promise.

Bone Scintigraphy

Radioisotope scans may be very useful to evaluate obscure pain syndromes.[6] Focal uptake may make subsequent films or arthrography more valuable as attention can be directed to these specific areas. Scans should be obtained prior to using invasive diagnostic techniques, such as arthrography or arthroscopy, as these may result in artificially increased uptake.

Arthroscopy

This technique is in its infancy for the wrist joint. It offers little at the present time except for the possible visualization of lunate-triquetral or triangular fibrocartilage ligament tears. This exciting technique has been made possible by borrowing from the field of knee arthroscopy. The techniques are still new and relatively untried, but the field holds tremendous promise for intraarticular diagnosis and perhaps treatment. A major advantage of arthroscopy is that it is a relatively noninvasive diagnostic method that allows better visualization of the structures in the volar and ulnar wrist compartments than can be obtained even with an extensive open procedure. Entry into the midcarpal and distal radioulnar joints is more difficult, but equally rewarding from a diagnostic standpoint. The newer, small, angled telescopes and chip cameras make this technique one that should not be ignored.

Arthrography

The distal radioulnar joint and ulnocarpal joints and the interposed triangular fibrocartilage complex (TFCC) are best evaluated with the following arthrographic technique. The patient is seated next to the fluoroscopic table with his arm resting upon it. The hand is placed palm down with the wrist flexed over a triangular radiolucent sponge. The forearm is positioned to make the normal volar tilt of the distal radial articular surface parallel to the vertical fluoroscopic x-ray beam. Under x-ray control a lead "zero" is positioned over the radiocarpal joint just lateral to the scapholunate ligament to avoid an inadvertent puncture of the midcarpal joint. After skin preparation a small amount of local anesthetic prepares the way for a 22-gauge, 1.5-inch, short bevel needle puncture into the radiocarpal joint. Joint fluid should be aspirated for culture and to avoid dilution prior to dye injection. Following this, 2 to 3 cc of the positive contrast dye material are injected and the needle and foam pillow removed. It is my recommendation that the physician who has pursued the diagnosis to this point actually do the injection and subsequent manipulation, suggesting to the radiologist appropriate spot films of record. If this is not possible, the responsible physician should at least be present to observe and direct the study. The entire procedure, from preinjection manipulation to postinjection manipulation, should be recorded on videotape, especially the first few seconds of injection and initial dye distribution. These few seconds, studied under stop frame projection, may show the exact location of tears that are obscured by further addition of contrast and the final dye distribution. (A newer technique of digital arthrography,[111] with or without subtraction films, holds promise for similar detection of subtle abnormalities in the wrist's ligaments. This technique has not been used extensively at the date of this writing.) The wrist is then briefly manipulated to distribute the contrast material and filming is begun. Several standard and oblique films are obtained. It is my practice to arrange with the radiologist ahead of time to obtain anteroposterior tomograms of the contrast study. These arthrotomograms are exceptionally valuable to precisely localize triangular fibrocartilage tears and to detect lunate or ulnar chondromalacia.[9] As the dye begins to fade from the radiocarpal injection, a second injection is made to define the distal radioulnar joint if it remains unfilled by the initial injection.

Normal findings in the arthrogram include the prestyloid recess and communication with the pisotriquetral joint (Fig. 21-14A and B). Abnormal findings are penetration of the dye from the radiocarpal joint to either the distal radioulnar joint (Fig. 21-14B) or vice-versa; to the intercarpal joints, or to tendon sheaths, especially the extensor carpi ulnaris or flexor carpi ulnaris. Reports of arthrographic studies and pathoanatomic dissections have clearly shown that asymptomatic age-related attritional ruptures or perforations occur in the scapholunate ligament (36 percent), lunate triquetral ligament (40 percent), and TFC (50–60 percent).[65,68,72,74,89,98,103,106,110,134] Since significant age-related changes begin as early as the third decade and increase rapidly by age 50, virtually all wrists will have significant degeneration of ligamentous structures, and 50 percent or more will have arthrographically demonstrable lesions. Some authors report congenital central TFC fenestrae[68,110,134] as well. This technique thus adds more precise detail to the diagnostic data collection, but positive findings do not prove causal relationships to the trauma or condition in question. Some reports suggest that peripheral, as opposed to central, tears or leaks are more commonly related to trauma.[19,95,134]

ACUTE FRACTURES INVOLVING THE DISTAL RADIOULNAR JOINT

Fractures Involving the Sigmoid Notch of the Radius

Nonunion or malunion of these fractures is frequently associated with pain, instability or weakness, and loss of motion.[44] Recognition and accurate diagnosis are essential for management. Initial films are seldom sufficient for complete diagnosis. Both collapse and rotational deformity may obscure major articular displacements. A two-plane zero rotation study with the patient relaxed and in finger-trap traction will often yield the necessary information concerning number, size, and location of fragments. It should not be assumed that the distal radioulnar joint derangement will "do well" if attention is devoted only to the length and volar articular tilt of the radius, although this is sometimes the case. Some contend that the carpus or radius will "do well" if attention is instead focused on the distal radioulnar joint.[44,58,73,128] For an acceptable reduction, intraarticular radioulnar fractures must be anatomically aligned, and joint congruity must exist. The ulnar articular surface must

not be translated proximally, distally, dorsally, or volarly on the sigmoid notch.

I prefer to manage this problem using external fixation similar to that reported by Green[51] or Cooney, Linscheid, and Dobyns.[21,44] If it can be ascertained that the lunate facet and its tangent portion of the sigmoid notch are significantly displaced as a single, large fragment, open reduction with appropriate internal fixation is indicated. In my opinion, severe comminution of the distal radius involving the distal radioulnar joint is best managed by closed techniques.[21,44,51]

Ulnar Articular Surface Fractures, Including Chondral Fractures

These fractures should be opened and fixed with small K-wires or small compression screws if anatomic closed reduction is not obtained. Comminuted fractures of the head are best treated with primary resection of the head, preserving the shaft-styloid axis if possible (see the sections on Operative Exposure and Hemi-resection Interposition Arthroplasty[13]) or Darrach's resection (modified as below) if this axis cannot be preserved. Chondral fractures are difficult to diagnose, and their frequency of occurrence is unknown. Persistent ulnar-sided wrist pain and limitation of motion following injury should prompt an early arthrogram, which may show the chondral fragment. Arthrotomography is very helpful in delineating these injuries.[7,9] Excision is warranted if a fragment can be seen on the arthrogram.

Ulnar Styloid Fractures — Isolated or in Association with Fractures of the Radius

Ulnar styloid fractures may occur independent of other wrist fractures and should be recognized for what they are — an avulsion fracture of the major stabilizing ligaments of the distal ulna.[11,12,52,108,128] In cases where the styloid is avulsed at its base, a serious potential derangement of the joint has occurred (Fig. 21-14B). Nonunion may result in painful limited rotation and grip weakness. Minimal displacement may be ade-

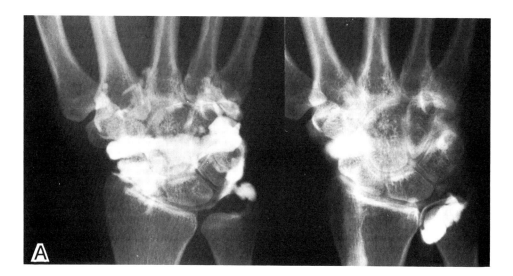

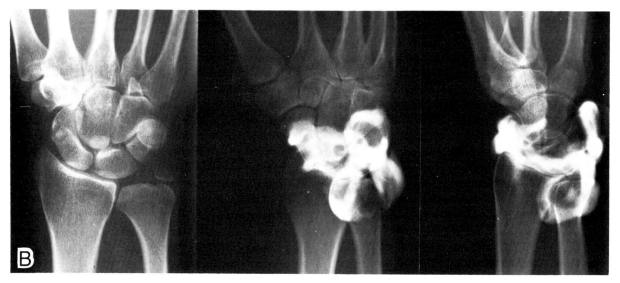

Fig. 21-14. (A) Arthrogram showing the radiocarpal and the radioulnar joints in sequential injections. No perforation of the TFC exists, but dye penetration into the intercarpal joints is seen via a surgically demonstrated triquetral lunate disruption. The prestyloid recess is well seen, as well as dye penetration from the midcarpal joints into the flexor carpi radialis tendon sheath. (B) These radiographs were taken following a single radiocarpal injection in a different patient. They show communication of dye into the distal radioulnar joint through a chronic perforation. The dye collection in the prestyloid area may indicate a chronic detachment of the TFC via an avulsion of the styloid rather than a TFC perforation (see Fig. 21-20). Dye also communicates with the pisotriquetral joint (see far right), but not the midcarpal joints.

quately treated by immobilization in a well-fitted below-elbow cast using the technique of interosseous molding to prevent more than midrange forearm rotation. The wrist should be in neutral rotation and slight ulnar deviation as the cast is applied.

It is particularly important to avoid extreme forced positioning, either in pronation, supination, flexion, or ulnar deviation, as subluxation may be easily provoked. The moderately or severely displaced styloid requires accurate closed reduction, or the joint should be opened and the TFCC and styloid anatomically replaced. Fixation by intraosseous compression wire techniques (24-gauge wire or larger) (see Fig. 21-17) and a long arm cast for 4 weeks is necessary to assure a good result. Late excision of the mobile, painful styloid fragment has been advocated.[108] Motion may be demonstrated by fluoroscopy or standard films with wrist deviation, rotation, or applied traction. The pain should be isolated to the styloid by appropriate relief of pain following specific injection of this area, and a simple shelling out of the styloid should be performed without interfering with the surrounding ulnocarpal complex. I advocate this only if the distal radioulnar joint is stable.

OPERATIVE EXPOSURE OF THE DISTAL RADIOULNAR JOINT AND TFC

The keys to exposure are the extensor carpi ulnaris and extensor digiti minimi tendons (Fig. 21-15A and B). As it enters the retinacular compartment, the extensor carpi ulnaris lies on top of the ulnar styloid in any of the positions of forearm rotation. The extensor digiti minimi changes from muscle to tendon as it enters its retinacular compartment. The first centimeter or so of this tendon lies on the radial attachment of the TFC in any position of forearm rotation. The ulnar head invariably can be made to present between these two tendons if the arm is pronated (Figs. 21-15B and 21-16B). For exposure of the major portion of the ulnar articular surface, the procedure is begun in full pronation. The incision is begun laterally three finger-breadths proximal to the styloid along the ulnar shaft and curved gently around the distal side of the head to end dorsally at midcarpus. For further distal exposure, the incision can be curved back ulnarly. The incision lies just dorsal to the dorsal ulnar sensory branch, which must be found and protected from vigorous retraction or pressure during the entire procedure (Fig. 21-16A). As the skin flaps are developed, dorsal veins are retracted rather than cut if possible, and dissection is carried to the obliquely lying extensor retinacular fibers. At the proximal border of the retinaculum the capsule of the ulnar head presents between the extensor digiti minimi and extensor carpi ulnaris (Fig. 21-15B and 21-16B). A V-shaped portion of ulnar

shaft disappears proximally between the deep-lying extensor indicis proprius muscle belly (Fig. 21-15B, arrow, and 16-B). The proximal and ulnar half of the extensor retinaculum is reflected radially, uncovering the extensor carpi ulnaris tendon and extensor digiti minimi tendons (Fig. 21-16C). The base of this flap is the septum between the extensor digiti minimi and the extensor digitorum communis compartment. Care is taken not to enter the extensor digitorum communis compartment unnecessarily. The extensor digiti minimi is retracted, revealing the dorsal margin of the sigmoid notch of the radius and the TFC (Fig. 21-16D). The capsule is sharply detached from the radius, leaving a 1-mm cuff for later repair. The capsule is then reflected toward the ulna, exposing the ulnar head for approximately 100 degrees of its total convexity. A small lamina spreader may be used to view the sigmoid notch. For better exposure of the underside of the TFC, the forearm should be brought to midrotation and a nerve hook or small right angle retractor used to expose this area. Magnification is helful in observing the pathologic changes in the TFC. To further expose the TFC, both the extensor digiti minimi and extensor carpi ulnaris must be released from their retinacular compartments (Fig. 21-16E). This can be accomplished by reflecting the distal half of the extensor retinaculum toward the ulna opposite to the first flap. The retinaculum is divided along the extensor digiti minimi septum; the base of the flap is the attachment of the extensor carpi ulnaris compartment nearest to the ulna. The extensor carpi ulnaris, where its groove is most pronounced, lies 1 to 2 mm ulnar to the attachment of the TFC (Fig. 21-3B and D). The ECU should be fully released only if it is pathologically involved. The unviolated sixth compartment may be subperiosteally dissected from the ulnar shaft for exposure without disturbing its stabilizing function.

When the extensor digiti minimi and extensor carpi ulnaris are reflected to either side, one observes the transverse-lying fibers of the dorsal radiotriquetral ligament (Figs. 21-7 and 21-16E). This ligament may be incised along its course for a good look at the lunate and triquetral surfaces of the TFC. For excellent exposure of the styloid, the forearm is carried to full supination, using the groove of the extensor carpi ulnaris to mark its dor-

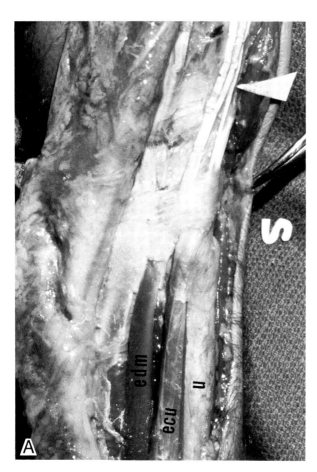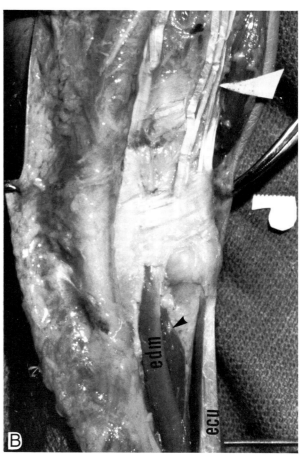

Fig. 21-15. (A) Exposure of the dorsum of the distal radioulnar joint as seen with the forearm in full supination. Note that the extensor carpi ulnaris *(ecu)* and extensor digiti minimi *(edm)* are adjacent *(u,* ulnar shaft). The paper arrow represents an aberrant slip of the extensor carpi ulnaris going to the extensor hood of the little finger. (B) The same specimen fully pronated. The ulnar head presents between the extensor carpi ulnaris and extensor digiti minimi. Note the position of the extensor indicis proprius muscle belly *(arrow).* (See Fig. 21-16B for comparison.)

sal base. The reflected capsule may be used as an interpositional arthroplasty flap if fracture comminution or arthritis dictates ulnar head extirpation, as described below (Fig. 21-16F). The extensor carpi ulnaris should be returned to its styloid groove, and the first retinacular flap can be used to stabilize this location of the tendon if necessary. Alternative retinacular flaps have been described by others.[76,121]

The intact distal radioulnar joint surfaces and ulnocarpal joint structures cannot be fully explored by any single approach because of the intimacy of contact between the radius and ulna and the trian-

gular fibrocartilage. The dorsal approach, as above, allows visualization of the dorsal 60 percent of the ulnar head and the carpal face of the triangular fibrocartilage, the lunate-triquetral ligament, the triquetrum, the meniscus, the prestyloid recess, and most of the distal radioulnar joint synovial cavity. If carefully dissected and replaced, none of this exposure should alter joint mechanics or stability. A volar approach is possible that allows the remainder of the articular surface to be seen. This approach is appropriate for release of soft tissue pronation contracture involving the volar capsular structures. The flexor carpi ulnaris and ulnar nerve

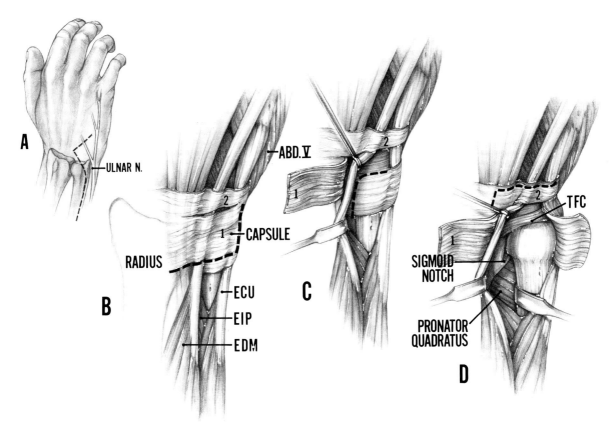

Fig. 21-16. Operative exposure of the distal radioulnar joint (see text for details). (**A**) The incision, emphasizing the location of the ulnar sensory nerve. (**B**) The exposed capsule in pronation (see Fig. 21-15B). (**C**) The proximal retinacular flap *(1)* and capsular incision *(dotted line)*. (**D**) The capsular flap reflected with exposure of the sigmoid notch using retractors or a baby lamina spreader. *(Figure continues.)*

and artery are retracted ulnarly, and the flexor group is retracted radially. A corner of the pronator quadratus is reflected. In a supinated wrist the synovial cavity is easily opened for a look. There may be significant scar tissue here in the post-traumatic wrist. When joint stability is unimpaired, release of this scar may be all that is required for a resistant pronation contracture.

OPEN REDUCTION AND INTERNAL FIXATION

The surgical exposure just described (exploration) is adequate for open reduction and internal fixation of the sigmoid notch and lunate facet in comminuted fractures of this portion of the distal radius, for styloid fractures, and for intraarticular fractures of the articular surface of the distal ulna. For distal shaft fractures of the ulna, exposure of the triangular fibrocartilage complex and ulnocarpal joint is unnecessary. The exposure can be extended proximally to allow the shaft to be seen. It is important to see the articular surface of the distal radioulnar joint to ensure that internal fixation of the distal shaft does not compromise motion of the joint itself. The technique of open reduction and internal fixation of the styloid fracture is not difficult. A compression screw or intraosseous wiring technique is recommended.[52] I prefer the latter. The fracture is opened, and, under direct view, two drill holes, using K-wires for drill points, are made proximally from the fracture to exit facing the

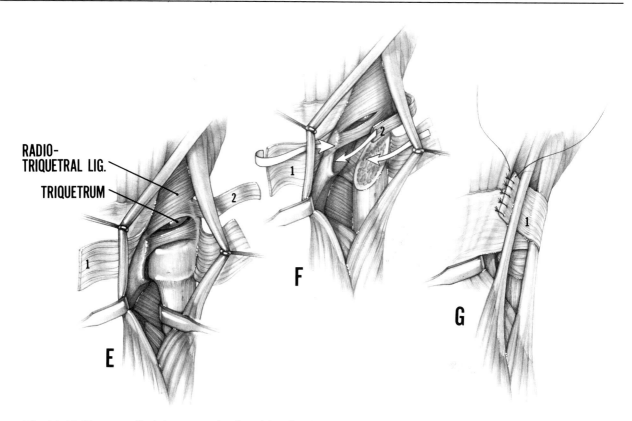

RADIO-
TRIQUETRAL LIG.

TRIQUETRUM

E

F

G

Fig. 21-16 *(Continued).* (**E**) Retinacular flap *(2)* is developed and reflected to expose the radiotriquetral ligaments and the TFC and its carpal face (see Fig. 21-3B). (**F**) The ulnar head has been resected and the capsular flap covers the cancellous resection area. The capsule is attached volarly. Retinacular flap *(2)* is used to cover the radioulnar articulation by suturing it to the previous capsular attachment on the radius. (**G**) The first retinacular flap *(1)* is used to stablize the extensor carpi ulnaris tendon.

radius at the axilla of the ulnar shaft and its articular surface. An appropriately sized wire (24-gauge or larger) is then passed either around or through the styloid using similar drill holes, and the two free ends of the wire are then passed proximally through the fracture site into the previously prepared drill holes in the proximal shaft (Fig. 21-17). The wire is then twisted, compressing the styloid to the shaft. Tightening of the wire is done with the forearm in neutral position. The forearm is then immobilized in neutral position in a long arm cast with the wrist in slight ulnar deviation for a period of 4 weeks. At that time limited motion is allowed using an ulnar gutter splint for an additional 2 weeks. Unrestricted motion is then permitted. This procedure is indicated when the styloid fracture is imperfectly reduced and the distal radioulnar joint

is unstable following acute injuries. The intraosseous wiring technique is also useful for stabilizing repairs of the triangular fibrocartilage complex (TFCC) when this complex has been avulsed from the styloid at its attachment, either in acute or recurrent instabilities. It is also my method of choice when shortening of the ulna is done coincident with hemi-resection interposition arthroplasty (see Fig. 21-31).

EXTERNAL FIXATION

External fixation is of value when comminuted fractures of the sigmoid notch may not be handled best by open reduction and internal fixation. The fixation should be from radius to metacarpals allowing forearm rotational motion to mold the frac-

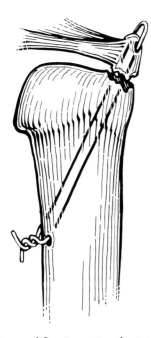

Fig. 21-17. Internal fixation using the intraosseous wire technique. The same method may be employed to repair a destabilizing tear of the TFCC when no fracture is present or where ulnar shortening is done in conjunction with a hemi-resection arthroplasty. The wire should be at least 24-gauge.

tured surface of the sigmoid notch. This technique alone is contraindicated when fractures of the sigmoid notch are associated with instability of the distal radioulnar joint itself. In that case external fixation may be employed only after the triangular fibrocartilage complex has been explored and repaired or the ulnar styloid fracture has been internally fixed (see the foregoing section).

ACUTE JOINT DISRUPTION

This group includes all disruptions of the static ligament system stabilizing the distal radioulnar joint. Whether these ligaments are the TFCC — as the author believes — or the dorsal and volar radioulnar ligaments and the ulnar collateral ligaments — as other authors have stated[53,79,89] — the disruption allows abnormal joint positioning (static joint subluxation or dislocation) and potentially allows abnormal transmission of force (dynamic joint subluxation or dislocation). Recognition of the injury is the key element in preventing disability (Fig. 21-18).[95] (See also Table 21-3.)

Fig. 21-18. Two radiographs showing a radial fracture with a locked volar dislocation of the distal ulna. The excellent anteroposterior view of the radiocarpal relationship makes the overlapping ulna hard to miss. The true lateral of the radius and carpus makes the volar position of the ulna obvious. Not all cases of distal radioulnar dislocation are so clearly demonstrated radiographically. Those who are wary will not interpret these films as oblique views, but the temptation is great to do so.

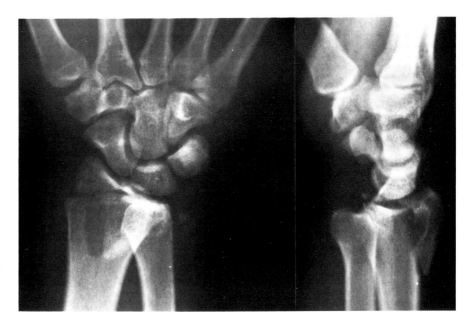

TFCC DISRUPTION WITH DISTAL RADIOULNAR JOINT DISLOCATION OR INSTABILITY IN ASSOCIATION WITH FRACTURES OR OTHER DISLOCATIONS

When the ligament disruption is associated with radial or ulnar fractures or other dislocations, accurate closed reduction of the dislocation, as well as of the fracture, followed by appropriate cast immobilization, will often suffice. The best position for management of distal radioulnar joint disruption associated with fractures is midrotation, with slight ulnar deviation and volar flexion and support of the volar ulnar side of the wrist. Extreme rotation and forced wrist positioning (e.g., Cotton-Loder position for Colles' fracture) will often produce an unsatisfactory wrist, as the ulnar fulcrum is unstable.[38,82,93] Compromised positioning may be necessary due to the nature of the fracture. However, optimal position for the joint must be recognized and distal radioulnar joint instability dealt with rather than ignored. In some cases alternative fracture management should be considered rather than accepting abnormal joint positioning. When the fracture or other dislocation must be open and distal radioulnar joint disruption is evident, ligament repair should not be left undone.

Fractures of the radial head may be associated acutely or chronically with distal radioulnar joint ligament derangement (Essex-Lopresti fracture).[42,54,84,94,105,124] Some authors have proposed that a radial head prosthesis be employed as a method of stabilizing the proximal and distal radioulnar joints following radial head excision.[42,124] I favor the approach that deals with the derangement later, if it becomes symptomatic.[54,94,105]

ISOLATED TFCC DISRUPTION WITH DISLOCATION OR INSTABILITY

It has been pointed out that it would be more appropriate to call this injury a periulnar dislocation of the radiocarpal mass, since the ulna remains in its normal relationship at the elbow.[53,91] Although this is anatomically correct, the lesion has been universally described as a dislocation of the distal end of the ulna. This is the way it appears clinically and on radiographs, and therefore the description has the merit of simplicity and probably will endure. Isolated dislocations will respond to cast immobilization of 6 weeks if an accurate closed reduction can be obtained. Dislocation with the ulna volar is reduced by pronation, and with the ulna dorsal by supination.[53] Reduction may require regional anesthesia. The criterion of acceptability should be joint congruity as assessed by 90-degree two-plane zero position radiographs. It has been recommended that a long arm cast be employed, with the forearm in full supination for ulnar dorsal and full pronation for ulnar volar. I favor positioning in neutral rotation and slight ulnar deviation for both injuries after reduction.

If the dislocation is locked or the reduction is incongruous, the joint should be opened and reduced and the TFCC repaired.

TFCC REPAIR

An operative exposure such as that shown in Figure 21-19 should be carried out. The TFCC is usually disrupted from an unfractured styloid as marked by the heavy lines in this illustration. The disruption may extend along the two ulnocarpal ligaments (ulnolunate and ulnotriquetral ligament) and be associated with a lunate-triquetral ligament tear as in an ulnar perilunate dislocation pattern. Direct repair should be accomplished using the intraosseous wire technique (Fig. 21-17) with 24-gauge or larger wire. Because of the torque and stress placed on this structural relationship, the repair should be tight and supported by cast immobilization for 6 to 8 weeks. The cast immobilization should be long-arm with the elbow flexed, the forearm in zero position, and wrist neutral. Closed and/or open reduction should be attempted as long as 2 to 3 months after injury. After this time a reconstructive approach might be considered (see the section on Chronic Joint Derangements).

ISOLATED TEARS OF THE TFC WITHOUT INSTABILITY

Complete excision has been proposed as a treatment alternative for presumed isolated traumatic lesions of the TFC.[19,96] The authors who have championed this treatment have presented a combined series of 26 patients seen after a period of

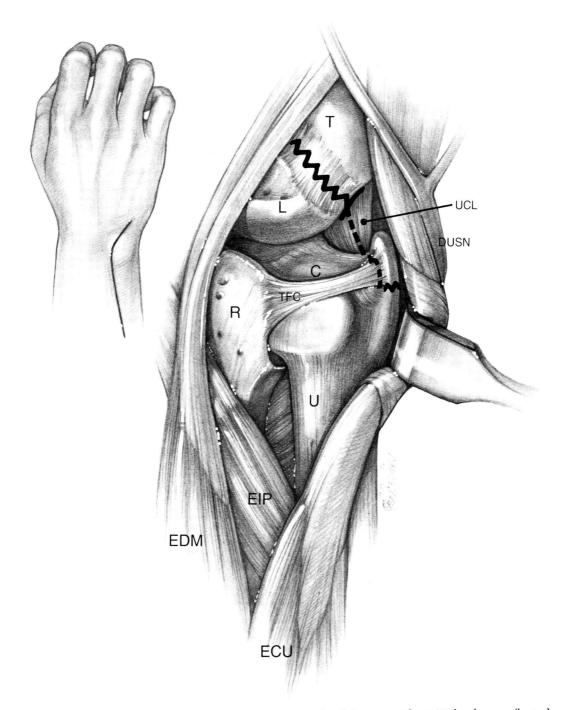

Fig. 21-19. Author's concept of an extensive exposure of the ulnar side of the wrist. The ECU has been reflected subperiosteally in its compartment and the dorsal ulnocarpal ligaments (see Fig. 21-7) have been conceptually removed. The dark lines at the styloid, which extend distally between the ulnotriquetral ligament and the ulnolunate ligament and then as a zigzag line between lunate and triquetrum, represent one of the more common patterns of a destabilizing TFCC injury. The pattern represents the ulnar half of a perilunate ligament disruption and probably accounts for the high percentage of lunate-triquetral ligament tears seen on post-traumatic arthrograms. The same injury pattern may be accompanied by a styloid fracture. (*C*, central TFC; *ECU*, extensor carpi ulnaris; *EDM*, extensor digiti minimi; *EIP*, extensor indicis proprius; *DUSN*, dorsal ulnar sensory nerve; *L*, lunate; *R*, radius; *T*, triquetrum, *U*, ulna; *UCL*, ulnocarpal ligament.)

between 2 and 12 months of symptoms. Fifteen patients were rated as having good results. Those who did well were noted at surgery to have peripheral or attachment tears of the TFC. While I do not doubt the results, I remain convinced that complete excision of the TFC in peripheral or attachment tears is contraindicated based on anatomic considerations presented herein. In my opinion, repair rather than excision should be attempted in these lesions.

The diagnosis is suggested by a history of a blow to the ulnar palm producing dorsiflexion and pronation. Persistent tenderness and pain localized to the dorsum of the distal radioulnar joint, increased local symptoms with sudden or forceful resisted rotation, or occasional "clicking" associated with localized pain or tenderness are associated findings. Only occasionally is mild radioulnar instability noted. Arthrograms have been said to be helpful, but no specifics were given.[19,96] The stable, isolated injury is certainly a rare lesion. If the treating physician can make a presumptive diagnosis with some assurance, exploration of the TFC is indicated using the approach previously described (Figs. 21-16 and 21-19). The major portion of the two surfaces of the TFC can be seen. The surface facing the ulnar head in its volar half cannot be seen well, if at all, even with a needle arthroscope. If a significant structural tear cannot be seen, empiric TFC excision is unwise. Rather, a search for other local pathology should be made. Some other possible causes of symptoms or clicking in the area are lunate-triquetral ligament disruption, pisotriquetral arthritis, a snapping extensor carpi ulnaris, or subluxation of the distal radioulnar joint because of a shallow notch or chronic ligamentous laxity. If a significant tear is seen and it is felt that the interposition or enfolding of the torn margins is interfering with wrist or distal radioulnar joint function, subtotal or partial excision of the torn elements of the TFC is indicated.[12,60,85,97,100,103] This tear most often will be in the central portion of the TFC (C in Fig. 21-19). Excision of this limited area will not affect the function of the TFCC. Care must be taken not to disturb the critical TFC margins and the ulnocarpal ligaments. If the tear is associated with a positive variant ulna, I would recommend an ulnar recession (shortening) to accompany the

treatment of the tear itself.[11,12,31] If a zero variant is present and articular changes of the carpus or ulna are also present, I would also do the ulnar recession. If an ulna minus is present, no treatment other than debridement of the tear is indicated.

LATE-APPEARING OR CHRONIC JOINT DISRUPTION (LONGER THAN 2 MONTHS) WITHOUT RADIOGRAPHIC ARTHRITIS

This section presents the management choices for the symptomatic distal radioulnar joint after preventive options have expired. The major clinical effort in this group is to causally relate the pathology and presenting symptoms. Physical findings include point tenderness over the articulation, restricted or painful motion, and instability. In addition, assessment should include grip strength and documentation of instability. Documentation should begin with 90-degree two-plane zero rotation radiographs and proceed to grip-loaded two-plane films. Subluxation may be provoked by full pronation, full supination, or ulnar deviation or grip loading in these positions. Fluoroscopic examination is helpful. The evaluation may be extended by computerized tomographic studies and arthrotomography.

Isolated Triangular Fibrocartilage Tears Without Instability

Management is identical to that for acute triangular fibrocartilage tears without instability as discussed in the previous section. It is again emphasized that if exploration is undertaken, all other sources of ulnar wrist pain should be carefully considered before debridement, with or without ulnar recession, is accepted as the sole surgical maneuver to be employed.

Triangular Fibrocartilage Complex Disruption With Recurrent Dislocation or Instability

WITHOUT RADIAL OR ULNAR SHAFT DEFORMITY

Before considering TFCC disruption with recurrent instability and without radial or ulnar shaft deformity,[2,8,22,23,33,45,47,53,55,113,132] the anatomy should be carefully reviewed, in particular the sections on the stabilizing functions of the osseous anatomy and the changes in stability with rotation. The diagnosis of instability is difficult — particularly when considering that some dorsovolar translation is permitted by the normal joint. The history of injury is usually remote and may not be well documented. Obvious subluxation or dislocation with the ulna dorsal are associated with a prominent ulnar head dorsally and a limitation of supination. With the ulna subluxating or dislocating volarly, pronation is limited, and the ulnar displacement is provoked by supination. Clinically, there is a dimple or depression replacing the normal contour of the ulna when the wrist is examined in supination (Fig. 21-20). Diagnosis can be made by zero-rotation lateral or comparison right- and left-wrist computerized tomographic scans in the position that provokes the instability (Fig. 21-13). Pain and limitation of function should dictate treatment, as some patients tolerate the instability with few complaints.

WITH RADIAL OR ULNAR SHAFT DEFORMITY

TFCC disruption with recurrent instability and radial or ulnar shaft deformity[24,42,58,84,91,93,119,132] usually occurs in association with a fracture. If the TFCC disruption is missed but the fracture is perfectly reduced and stabilized, the disruption may heal unaided; normal osseous anatomy protects this complex from other than normal stresses, making a good outcome possible. If the fracture union is imperfect, stresses on the disrupted TFCC may stretch the newly formed scar tissue and, if so, distal radioulnar joint derangement is probable. When malunion results in a longitudinal discrepancy of the radius and ulna (such as with most injuries listed in Table 21-1), derangement may be expressed mainly as a variant of the "ulnocarpal

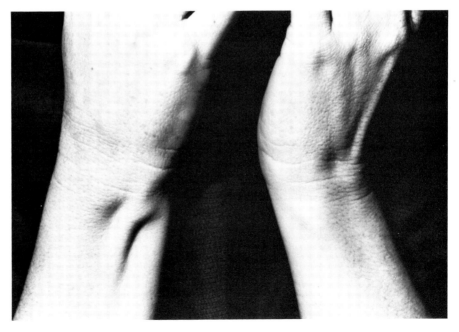

Fig. 21-20. The clinical appearance of a volar dislocation of the patient's right distal ulna as provoked by supination.

impingement syndrome" (see that section under Joint Disorders). If the malunion is expressed as a rotational or dorsovolar translational malalignment of the forearm bones, then the derangement will be expressed as a subluxation or dislocation of the distal radioulnar joint. Although it is possible that rotational or translational malunions could stress an uninjured TFCC to such a degree that instability would eventuate, it is unlikely. The expected expression of this circumstance would be limitation of forearm rotation without instability.

The fractures most often resulting in rotational malunions are isolated fractures of the radial or ulnar shafts and, particularly, double-bone forearm fractures in children. The fractures most often associated with translational malunions are isolated distal radius fractures in adults and children. Early diagnosis is based on an awareness of the potential for TFCC disruption to accompany shaft fractures. Later, when a dislocation presents as the primary problem, we must again recall this association and persistently seek a history of forearm fractures. Establishing the presence of a rotational or translational malunion is best accomplished by exact comparison full-length zero-rotation PA and lateral films of the entire forearm. Landmarks to use are the bicipital tuberosities of the radius as compared to the distal metaphysis, the ulnar styloid in relation to the coronoid process of the ulna, and, of course, the radius to the ulna. The use of comparison computerized tomographic scans at two levels is also an excellent method. The scan should be done with the right and left arm compared at the levels of the distal radioulnar joint (styloid of ulna) and the bicipital tuberosity. Each level should be done in maximum pronation, maximum supination, and zero rotation. Management of the distal radioulnar joint instability must include correction of the rotational or translational malunion, or the soft tissue repair or reconstruction is certain to fail.

Management of Chronic Joint Instability

Repair of the TFCC as suggested (Fig. 21-17) is recommended if the TFCC is detached by a styloid fracture. If the TFCC is detached without a fracture, then repair as suggested in Figure 21-19 is recommended. Even after 2 to 3 months this ideal should be sought with the admonition that rotational or translational deformity must be corrected at the same time as the repair of the TFCC. Although this approach should be considered first, problems such as contracture, painful rotation, or loss of tissue may demand a reconstructive approach. There are no excellent procedures available, but the following have received some support. All are, I believe, contraindicated if rotational or translational malunions, length discrepancies, or arthritic changes are present and cannot be simultaneously corrected.

TFCC RECONSTRUCTION AND/OR SUBSTITUTION

Reconstruction

I believe, mainly on theoretical grounds, that for successful soft tissue reconstruction, the essential elements of the TFCC (see Fig. 21-3) — (1) a smooth carpal articulation; (2) a flexible rotational tether, radius to ulna; (3) suspension of the ulnar carpus to the radius; (4) an ulnocarpal cushion; and (5) ulnar shaft and ulnar carpal connection — must be duplicated in an effective fashion. The Bunnell-Boyes[15] procedure as a working approach is good, but does not attempt to provide elements 1, 3, and 4 (Fig. 21-21). This technique is, however, innovative and carefully anatomic insofar as reconstruction of distal radioulnar joint instability and capacity for rotation are concerned. Reconstruction of the volar ulnocarpal ligaments as diagrammed in Figure 21-21D was first conceptualized in a case reported by Hill[55] (see Fig. 21-25H). Recent reports by Hui[57] (Fig. 21-22) and Tsai[130] (Fig. 21-23) use this feature of the Bunnell-Boyes reconstruction to advantage in operations for dorsal distal radioulnar joint instability. Both employ distally based portions of the flexor carpi ulnaris (FCU) harvested proximally and stripped distally to the pisiform attachment. The new ligament is stabilized distally by weaving it through the remaining volar capsule. This relieves possible torque stress on the pisotriquetral joint. This "new" ligament is then passed through a drill hole in the styloid area to exit in the axilla of the ulnar articular surface. The repair is completed with imbrication of the

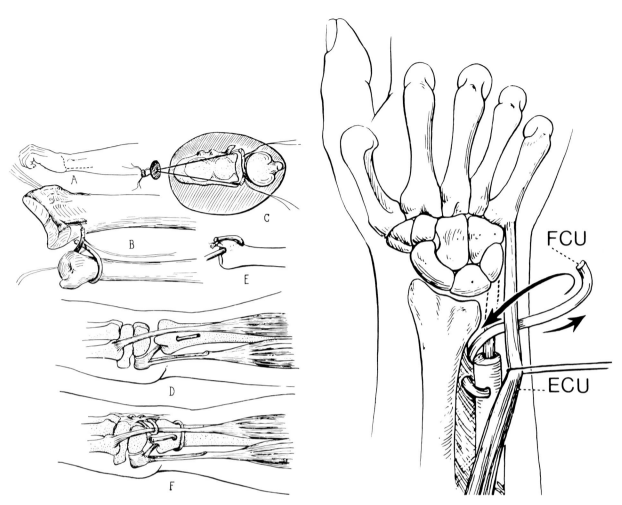

Fig. 21-21. The Boyes/Bunnell reconstruction of the distal radioulnar articulation. (Boyes JH: Bunnell's Surgery of the Hand, 5th Ed. pp. 229–302. JB Lippincott, Philadelphia, 1970.)

Fig. 21-23. Stabilization of the ulnar stump using the flexor carpi ulnaris—a modification of the Darrach procedure. (Tsai T, Stillwell JH: Repair of chronic subluxation of the distal radioulnar joint (ulna dorsal) using flexor carpi ulnaris tendon. J Hand Surg 9B:289–293, 1984.)

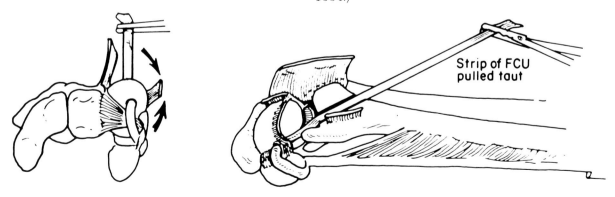

Fig. 21-22. Stabilization of the distal radioulnar joint by substitution of the volar ulnocarpal ligament. Compare carefully to Figure 21-21D and F. (Hui FC, Linscheid RL: Ulnotriquetral augmentation tenodesis. J Hand Surg 7:230, 1982.)

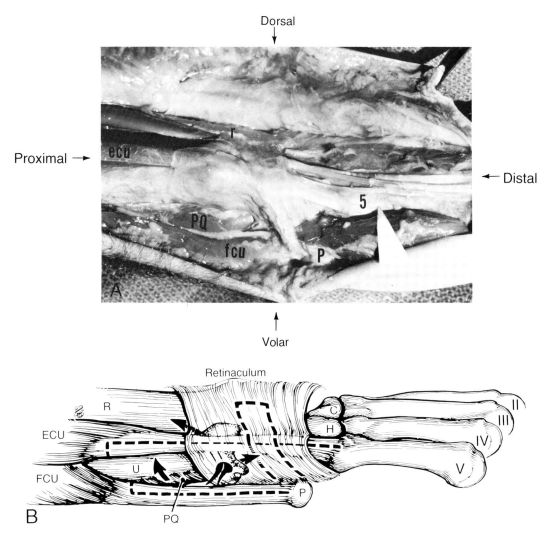

Fig. 21-24. (**A,B**) Strips of retinaculum, extensor carpi ulnaris *(ECU)*, or flexor carpi ulnaris *(FCU)* may be dissected to their distal attachments and used in the reconstruction of ulnar-sided ligaments. The drill hole from distal to proximal through the ulna would allow the use of any of these strips to stabilize the ulna-to-volar structures. In order to accomplish this, the ECU must first be taken volarly, attached to the wrist capsule on its volar aspect, and then brought through the drill hole, whereas the retinaculum and FCU and their normal attachment to the pisiform may be used without re-routing. It is, however, essential that they be woven through the volar capsule. This would avoid abnormal stresses on (and possibly pain from) the pisotriquetral joint. The horizontally placed drill hole through the ulnar styloid suggests an alternate route for any of these tissues, providing a firm attachment to the styloid area if tissue is necessary for reconstruction of the TFC itself. The author has used this technique only in isolated instances and does not necessarily recommend its use. It represents an idea that may be expanded upon in the future. In addition, the direction of pronator advancement[61,62] is shown (*black arrow* in **B**). (*PQ*, pronator quadratus; *P*, pisiform; *U*, ulna; *5*, *V*, fifth metacarpal; *R*, radius; *white arrow* (in **A**), base of fifth metacarpal.)

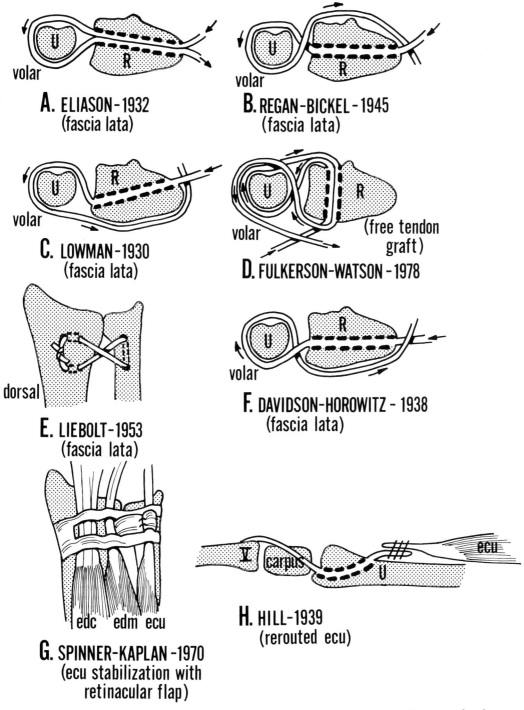

A. ELIASON-1932
(fascia lata)

B. REGAN-BICKEL-1945
(fascia lata)

C. LOWMAN-1930
(fascia lata)

D. FULKERSON-WATSON-1978
(free tendon graft)

E. LIEBOLT-1953
(fascia lata)

F. DAVIDSON-HOROWITZ - 1938
(fascia lata)

G. SPINNER-KAPLAN-1970
(ecu stabilization with
retinacular flap)

H. HILL-1939
(rerouted ecu)

Fig. 21-25. A sampling of soft tissue reconstructions suggested in the literature for the unstable distal radioulnar joint. (G is redrawn from Spinner M, Kaplan EB: Extensor carpi ulnaris—Its relationship to stability of the distal radio-ulnar joint. Clin Orthop 68:124–129, 1970.)

dorsal capsule. The techniques are said to be contraindicated in volar dislocations. If the technique faithfully recreates a portion of the normal TFCC, I find it not "contraindicated," just incomplete. The method of Tsai[130] may be employed as a modification to the Darrach procedure. This aspect of TFCC reconstruction has met with some success. Suspension of the ulnar carpus from the radius (element 3) and reconstruction of the radius-to-ulnar tether (element 2) and a cushion (element 4) have been elusive if the ulnar articular dome is left intact. If some elements are intact, the missing elements may be selectively augmented by using locally available tissue (Fig. 21-24).

Substitution

The radioulnar tether procedures are the historical approach to substitution.[15,22,45,75,86,89,109,129] These procedures attempt to supply one function of the triangular fibrocartilage complex—the radioulnar connection. As a group they approach the problem at a level proximal to the radioulnar articulation and attempt, by weaving a tendon graft around or through the bones, to pull them together. Each series reports success in a limited number of patients. Follow-up has been insufficient to allow meaningful statements to be made. Criticism generally reflects that the procedures are ineffective in preventing instability or that rotation is restricted if anteroposterior stability is achieved. A review of these procedures is shown in Figure 21-25.

Some support can be given to the rationale of Johnson,[61] who has proposed advancing the pronator quadratus from its normal insertion on the ulna to a more lateral and dorsal insertion. He postulates that this might increase radioulnar joint stability, particularly in dorsal instability situations. It could additionally be used to augment repair of the triangular fibrocartilage, although he has not proposed it for this purpose. His method may be visualized by a review of Figure 21-24 and 21-26.

Osteotomy

Osteotomy is an integral part of several procedural approaches to disorders of the distal radioulnar joint. The types of osteotomy vary, but the uses are to correct abnormal angulation, rotation, or

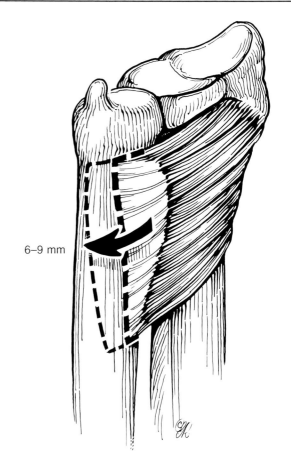

6–9 mm

Fig. 21-26. The pronator advancement as described by Johnson.[61] The perspective is volar.

length discrepancies between the two forearm bones.

Osteotomy of the Distal Radius. This technique is to be considered when correction of malunion or deformity of the distal radius is desired. The desired results are often to reestablish length, volar tilt, and ulnar inclination of the radius. The technique usually requires a strong plate and the addition of a uni- or bicortical bone graft. Some excellent results have been reported using a wide radial approach and a strong volar plate with a trapezoidal bone graft.[69] If the original injury or insult involved the sigmoid notch, then one must presume that this surface of the distal radioulnar joint is abnormal. An osteotomy done proximal to this level might not correct the sigmoid irregularity, but instead simply change its angular relationship to the distal ulnar articular surface, therefore solving the abnormal radiocarpal relationships and perhaps unloading the ulnocarpal impingement, though perhaps not addressing radioulnar incongruity. An osteotomy done through the notch would be more direct, but also more difficult. If the deformity is the result of an injury not involving the notch, one might expect a well-done osteotomy to be highly beneficial if radial length, tilt, and inclination are well corrected. A detailed description of the technique for osteotomy of the distal radius in presented in Chapter 22.

Rotational Osteotomy of the Ulna. For an explanation of this topic, refer to the discussion of ulnar recession osteotomy that follows.

JOINT DISORDERS

Length Discrepancy Exhibiting a Long Ulna Relative to the Radius (Ulnocarpal "Loading" or "Impingement Syndrome")

This section will be best understood if the reader reviews the anatomy section of this chapter dealing with the TFC portion of the TFCC and its load-bearing characteristics (see also Fig. 21-5), as well as the comments on ulnar variance. Milch[90] described in 1941 a loss of radial length associated with severe Colles' fractures. He stated that "the ulnar head impinges against the carpus, with resultant limitation of rotation and subsequent relaxation of the ligamentous fixation of the wrist." He devised a "cuff resection" of the ulna (resection of a variable amount of the distal ulnar diaphysis, followed by a wire suture to hold the osteotomy in position for healing) which was a more formal version of one described earlier by Darrach.[26] His procedure is known today as the "Milch procedure," "shortening osteotomy," or "ulnar recession osteotomy." It is a useful procedure in dealing with symptomatic "ulna long" forearm bone-length discrepancies. These disorders are collected

currently as the "ulnocarpal loading" or "impingement syndrome."[11,12,32,78,87,90,101] They are generally characterized by ulnar wrist pain, particularly with rotational or ulnar deviation loading; clicks or crepitus localized to the TFCC area; and radiographic findings of a long ulna relative to the radius (Fig. 21-27). Additionally, sclerotic or cystic changes may be seen in the lunate or ulnar head, arthrograms may show TFC perforations, and arthrotomography may show narrowing and/or chondromalacia in the cartilage of the lunate or ulna or both. Lunate-triquetral ligament tears are a frequent associated finding. The syndrome may occur over a wide age range (adolescence to geriatric) and in either sex. The presumption for understanding this syndrome is that the ulnocarpal axis is primarily structured for rotational movements and handles loading poorly when it is in excess of its usual 18 to 20 percent of the force across the wrist. The further presumption is that a long ulna increases this load transmission greatly and that the loaded structures degenerate, tear, or "hurt." The theory is supported by research data, pathoanatomic studies, and clinical treatment results. It has become one of the more well-defined ulnar wrist disorders. A number of conditions may predispose the patient to this syndrome: a premature closure of the radial epiphysis secondary to trauma[82] (acquired Madelung's deformity, Fig. 21-27), or premature wrist fusion,[132] excision of the radial head or shaft (for trauma, tumor, or infection), fracture malunions with shortening of the radius (Colles'-type shaft or head), or a "normal variant long ulna with occupational overload" (common in occupations or sports where rotational or ulnar deviation loading is required).

Treatment is chosen to fit the patient. In the lightly used wrist the derangement may not be a functional disability. If the condition is functionally disabling and cannot be managed by occupational alteration, then surgical management may be considered. In children the relative discrepancy may be corrected by an ulnar epiphyseal arrest.[91] In addition, the condition is well managed by the Milch shortening osteotomy or one of its modern variations (Figs. 21-28 and 21-29). Management of the ulnocarpal impingement syndrome by this technique alone is contraindicated if the TFCC is not functionally adequate or if the new portion of

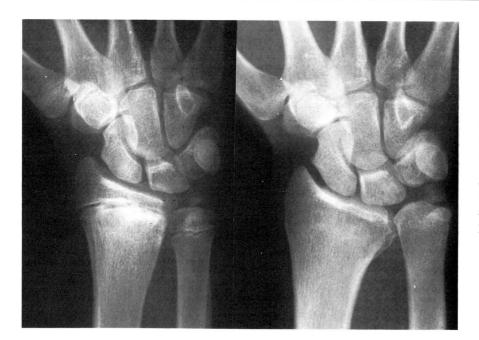

Fig. 21-27. Longitudinal radioulnar discrepancy secondary to early closure of radial epiphyseal injury (acquired Madelung's deformity). This is an example of an adolescent ulnocarpal inpingement syndrome.

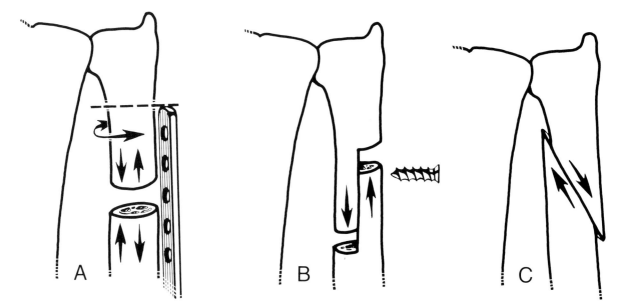

Fig. 21-28. Techniques for ulnar osteotomy. The transverse osteotomy (**A**) may be used for shortening, lengthening (with bone graft), or rotational corrections. The osteotomy should be planned so that the distal end of the plate does not impinge as the forearm rotates. Step-cut (**B**) and oblique (**C**) osteotomy techniques are most applicable for shortening. Compression screw or plate fixation may be used.

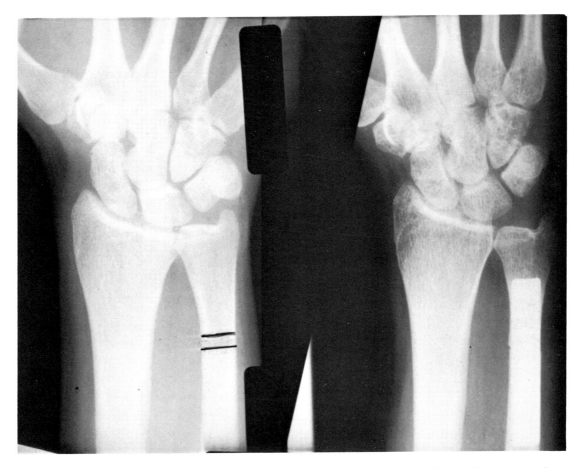

Fig. 21-29. Milch's shortening osteotomy for wrist pain in a young professional tennis player. The positive ulnar variance was changed to a slightly negative variance by removal of a 3-mm section of ulna. Early degenerative changes were noted on the ulnar dome and the underside of the TFC. The lines on the left mark only the amount of bone removed, not the osteotomy site.

the ulnar articular surface relative to the sigmoid notch will be predictably incongruous. Thus, prior to ulnar shortening the TFCC should be examined arthrotomographically and by direct visual inspection at operation. Attritional perforation or non-destabilizing tears are not a contraindication — in fact, they are an indication. If the TFCC is destabilized it must be repaired along with the shortening. Problems with distal radioulnar joint incongruity produced by ulnar shortening may be predicted in some cases of old, acquired Madelung's (Fig. 21-27) or Colles' malunions. For these instances, a variety of procedures have been proposed: ulnar head excision (Darrach[25] and modifications); ulnar

recession and fusion of the ulnar head to the radius, with restoration of forearm motion by creation of a proximal pseudarthrosis[117,127] (Sauve-Kapandji procedure); or hemi-resection interposition arthroplasty with shortening (Bowers)[13]. Moderate-to-severe chondromalacia of the distal radioulnar joint found at surgery may be a relative contraindication to the recession procedure alone, calling instead for one of the other alternatives. Darrow[32] and his co-authors at the Mayo Clinic believe that if the obvious chondromalacia is surgically debrided, the recession will increase stability and alter distal radioulnar joint contact areas sufficiently to be an effective form of treatment.

ULNAR OSTEOTOMY FOR SHORTENING, ROTATION, OR ANGULATION

Chevron, stepcut, transverse, and oblique osteotomies have been stabilized by wiring, compression screws, or plates. The operation was popularized by Darrach[26] who credits Dr. Kirby Dwight. Milch[90,91] developed the concept and provided the best description of this procedure, which is outlined in the first edition of this book. Since then, precision techniques of osteotomy and internal fixation have provided a more predictable outcome for this important procedure. A recent report by Darrow et al[32] provides the first good evidence of its efficacy.

Author's Preferred Method

I prefer the following surgical technique for ulnar shortening. The distal ulna is exposed as shown in Figure 21-16. Following exposure, all maneuvers are performed with the forearm in zero rotation to ensure accurate measurements, osteotomy positioning, and plate application. The planned site is 3 to 4 cm proximal to the proximal extent of the sigmoid notch. A four-hole compression plate is placed over the chosen site and clamped to the ulna. (The use of a four-hole compression plate is not universally recommended. I have had no problems with delayed union using this plate, but others have recommended the use of longer plates.) The forearm is carried to full supination. If impingement of the plate and radius occurs, the site is adjusted proximally. The site is marked on the bone. The osteotomy is transverse. All of the bone removed is proximal to the marked site so that the distal margin of the plate does not change its relative position to the sigmoid notch. The amount to be removed is predetermined by radiographic measurements. When the desired shortening is accomplished, the osteotomy is stabilized by application of the plate (Fig. 21-29). A long arm cast with the forearm in zero rotation is used for 4 weeks, after which range of motion exercises are begun. An orthoplast forearm brace with the wrist and elbow free is used to protect the arm between exercise periods until the osteotomy is healed. Healing time varies from 1.5 to 7 months, with the usual time being less than 3 months. If rotation or angular correction is needed, the procedure is a little different. Angular changes are achieved with a wedge cut and a small bend in the plate. Rotational changes are best predetermined from a computerized tomographic scan and can be estimated at surgery using wires drilled into the shaft perpendicular to its long axis. I have noticed, though, that when ulnar rotational changes are needed, the distal ulnar fragment will automatically derotate to assume the correct position relative to the radius upon completion of the osteotomy. This is probably a result of the energy stored in an abnormally tensioned TFCC.

ARTHRITIS

The conditions of post-traumatic and degenerative osteoarthritis are etiologically different but present a similar problem. They are characterized by painful rotation produced by inadequate joint surfaces. Marginal osteophytes, articular incongruity, and cartilage-wear debris make reconstructive approaches necessary if limiting use of the wrist is impractical. Surgical alternatives are (1) excision of the distal end of the ulna, using the classic technique as popularized by Darrach[24,25,26,27,30,31]; (2) one of the many modifications of this technique[10,35,48,67,115,130]; (3) hemi-resection interposition arthroplasty[13]; (4) resection and replacement arthroplasty (Swanson)[123,124];(5) arthrodesis and creation of a proximal ulnar pseudarthrosis to restore rotation[117,127] (Sauve-Kapandji); or (6) arthrodesis.[17] A review of these operations follows.

Resection of the Distal End of the Ulna (The Darrach Procedure)

In 1912 William Darrach[24] presented to the New York Surgical Society a patient with an unreduced palmar dislocation of the distal ulna treated by subperiosteal resection of its "lower inch." He credited Dr. Kirby Dwight with the idea, although the procedure was first mentioned by Desault[34] and later by Moore,[93] von Lesser,[71] Lauenstein,[70] Van Lennep,[131] and Angus.[3] In further publications, Darrach specified the indications and technical principles for this procedure. The procedure now carries his name and has weathered the test of time and critical review.[1,8,35,56,67,81] It is a worthy member of the surgical armamentarium for management of post-traumatic arthritis and rheumatiod arthritis. As recommended by Darrach, an incision is extended proximally from the ulnar styloid process. The bone is approached by separating the extensor carpi ulnaris and flexor carpi ulnaris tendons, avoiding the dorsal cutaneous branch of the ulnar nerve. The periosteum is incised and reflected from the distal 3 cm of the ulna. An osteotomy is made about 3 cm proximal to the styloid or at the level of the proximal extent of the sigmoid notch. The osteotomy is best done by predrilling the cortex, then completing the cut with small, sharp osteotomes or a bone biter. The distal fragment is then dissected free, and the ulnar styloid process is osteotomized at its base and left in situ. The periosteal sleeve is closed to provide a firm attachment for the styloid process and its ulnar collateral ligament, which will prevent abduction laxity. The wound is closed in layers. As instructed by Darrach, no splint is applied, and active motion is encouraged in 24 hours.

The general indication for Darrach's resection is any condition that causes derangement of the surfaces of the distal radioulnar joint, interfering with the action of the joint and resulting in limited and/or painful motion. This resection may be used for any of the disorders in this classification with expectation of good results, particularly in malunited Colles' fractures or in the late sequelae of intraarticular fractures. Dingman[35] has reviewed the procedure with regard to the technical points of extra- or subperiosteal resection, the obliquity of the cut, whether or not to remove the styloid, and the amount of bone to be resected (Fig. 21-30). His study suggested that none of these factors other than the amount of bone resection was a critical determinant of a good result. He considered the amount of bone resected to be the major factor influencing outcome of the procedure, and suggested that only the ulna adjacent to the sigmoid notch of the radius be removed. His preference was that the styloid process be left in situ and the resection be subperiosteal, because those patients in whom regeneration had occurred appeared to have had better results. The shorter the period of immobilization after operation, the sooner the return to work. I agree with these findings, particularly the amount of ulna resected and, in fact, have employed in many cases resection of the articular prominence of the ulnar head only, leaving the shaft-styloid axis along with the TFCC intact (see the Hemi-resection Arthroplasty section).

The Darrach procedure is not without its difficulties; however, two unsubstantiated criticisms are (1) increased ulnocarpal translocation and (2) decreased grip strength. I know of no reports of a

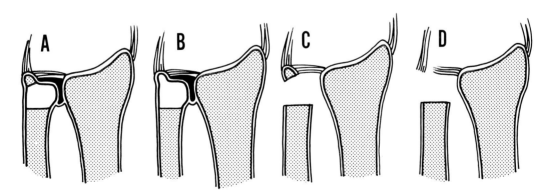

Fig. 21-30. The Darrach procedure and its modifications as presented by Dingman (see text). (Redrawn from Dingman PVC: Resection of the distal end of the ulna (Darrach operation). J Bone Joint Surg 34A:893–900, 1952.)

post-Darrach ulnar carpal slide in patients who have not also had their radiocarpal ligaments disrupted by trauma or rheumatoid arthritis. Thus, the "slide" is probably not a valid criticism of the Darrach procedure itself but of its application in rheumatoid arthritis. There are no reports documenting decreased grip strength. I have noticed increased grip strength in patients in whom the procedure has been appropriately used. The Darrach procedure does, however, destroy the bony support for the triangular fibrocartilage complex. In addition to creating ulnocarpal instability, it creates "unstable" rotation of the radiocarpal unit around the ulnar axis. With muscular action, the ulnar stump may abut the radius or fray the overlying tissues. This may present as painful snapping, or cause rupture of tendons, or both.[10,48,67,83,98,99,11] If this occurs, the temptation to remove more of the ulna must be resisted, as a poor result may easily be converted into a disaster. There are no excellent salvage procedures for the painful instability of the "too short" Darrach resection. Some options may be found in the next section. I have found some success by instituting long-term usage of a forearm brace (elbow and wrist free, with pronounced molding of the interosseous space), a concept borrowed from Sarmiento.[116] For these reasons, the use of the Darrach procedure today should be very selective. It may be useful in the ulnocarpal impingement or loading syndrome when the distal radioulnar joint surfaces will not permit a successful Milch shortening osteotomy, and also in the advanced rheumatoid group where it should be combined with a radiolunate fusion or other radiocarpal stabilization procedures.

Technical Modifications to Improve the Darrach Procedure

In order to mitigate the instability created by the Darrach excision, a variety of modifications have been proposed. Swanson has capped the distal ulna with a silicone implant, which provides a soft end for the stump, maintains its length, and provides a focus about which ligament reconstruction may take place.[123,124] Although it has theoretical application in traumatic and attritional disorders, its greatest proven application is in the rheumatoid

distal radioulnar joint. Disruption and dislocation of the implant are problems. The reader is referred to Chapter 7 for technical details of this procedure. Blatt and Ashworth[10] have sutured a flap of the volar capsule to the dorsal ulnar stump to hold it down. Ruby[115] has suggested tethering the distal ulnar stump with a distally based strip of extensor carpi ulnaris. The intact portion of the extensor ulnaris is stabilized in permanent dorsal position as Spinner and Kaplan[121] have suggested. Kessler and Hecht[67] suggest a dynamic stabilization of the ulnar stump by looping a strip of tendon around the distal ulnar stump and the ECU and tying the two together. Goldner and Hayes[48] have formalized these recommendations by passing a strip of the extensor carpi ulnaris (detached distally) through a drill hole in the ulnar stump with the forearm in supination. Tsai and Stillwell[130] have employed a distally based portion of the flexor carpi ulnaris tendon to stabilize the ulnar stump and then looped this tendon to stabilize the extensor carpi ulnaris over the ulnar stump as well (Fig. 21-23). They reported its usefulness in three patients. I have used this procedure with some success in failed Darrach procedures. A further adjunct in the management of the unstable distal ulnar stump may be the pronator advancement of Johnson[61] (Fig. 21-26).

The Hemi-resection Interposition Technique of Arthroplasty (HIT)

This procedure is an outgrowth of what Dingman[35] describes as the "best" Darrach procedures, i.e., those in which minimal resection was followed by regeneration of the ulnar shaft within the retained periosteal sleeve. The technique involves resection of the ulnar articular head only, leaving the shaft/styloid relationship intact. An interposition "anchovy" of tendon or muscle or capsule is placed in the vacant distal radioulnar joint synovial cavity to limit contact of the radial and ulnar shafts which tend to approach one another after this procedure. The procedure presupposes an intact or reconstructible TFCC. Figure 21-31 illustrates the use of the procedure and its modifications. It should not be employed in situations where ulnar variance is positive unless the ulna is shortened as

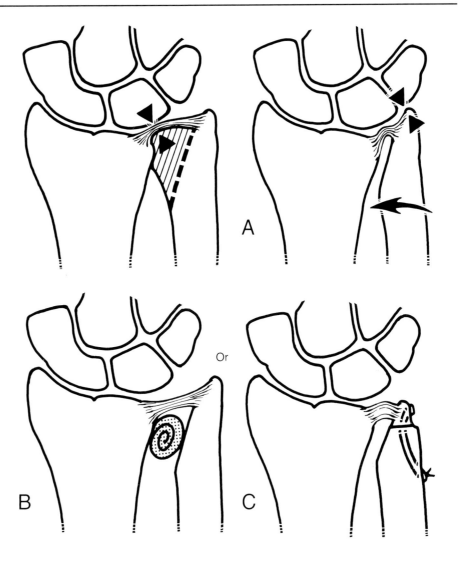

Fig. 21-31. The hemi-resection technique of arthroplasty employed in the ulnocarpal impingement syndrome. In (**A**) the still-too-long ulna produces stylocarpal impingement, a condition caused by the approximation of the radius and ulna allowed when the articular dome is removed. To obviate this, the alternatives of (**B**) interposition or (**C**) shortening are necessary. In every instance where this method is employed, intraoperative consideration of this possible complication is mandatory.

part of the procedure. Figures 21-32 and 21-33 illustrate a patient with distal radioulnar joint arthrosis following a failed "tether" attempt. The HIT is safely employed without shortening, because with grip loading (Fig. 21-31B) the styloid is not an impingement problem even though it nears the radius as a result of muscular action of the pronator quadratus once the arthritic surface is removed. Figure 21-34A and B illustrates the need for shortening. With the HIT alone in this patient, the styloid would surely produce the same impingement that the ulnar articular surface did preoperatively (Fig. 21-31A).

Author's Technique of Hemi-resection Interposition Arthroplasty

The initial exposure is as illustrated in Figure 21-16 and described on page 959. There is no need to enter the radiocarpal joint or expose the carpal surface of the TFC unless pathology is suspected therein. The retinacular flaps are developed for exposure and to conserve tissue for dorsal stabilization of the ECU (first or proximal flap) or augmentation of a deficient TFCC (second or distal flap). If not needed for these purposes the flaps may be reattached, used for deep cover of the

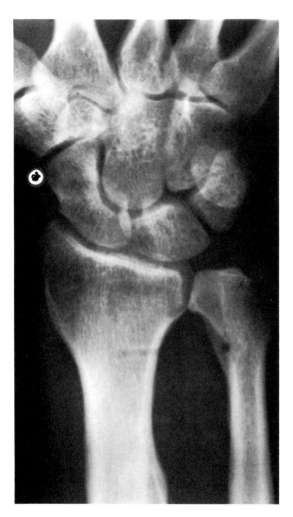

Fig. 21-32. Distal radioulnar arthrosis after an unsuccessful "tether" procedure for instability.

passed around the ECU, the distal end is sewn to the fourth compartment wall distal to its takeoff. This ensures a sling rather than a noose (Fig. 21-16G). After development of the retinacular flaps the capsule of the distal radioulnar joint is detached distally, radially, and proximally, and turned ulnarly to expose the articular surface. A synovectomy is done and the ulnar articular surface and subchondral bone is removed with small osteotomes and rongeurs. Inadequate bone removal is the likely technical error at this point. Large osteophytes around the sigmoid notch and all of the bone of the ulnar head under the articular surfaces must be removed. The remaining shaft and styloid axis should be round in cross-section and resemble a tapering 1-cm diameter dowel. A volar portion of the head is particularly easy to miss in this resection. The now vacant distal radioulnar joint cavity is cleaned of remaining synovium, and the TFC is carefully inspected. Lesions of the TFC will be readily apparent. If centrally located, these perforations or tears are now functionally inconsequential, since resection of the ulnar head has accomplished full decompression. Repair of central perforations is unnecessary. The lesions may be cleaned up with minor debridement. A decision about shortening, begun preoperatively with the radiographic impressions about possible stylocarpal impingement, should be completed at this point. The radial and ulnar shaft should be compressed and rotated with the wrist ulnarly deviated. If there is any question about impingement, the ulna should be shortened. Shortening may be done through the metaphyseal base at the site of the previous ulnar head, or by more proximal osteotomy with plating (Fig. 21-28A). If the former site is chosen, fixation is accomplished with a compression intraosseous wire loop (Fig. 21-31C). If the preoperative assessment is equivocal (zero variant +/− 1 mm) and the intraoperative assessment is equivocal, then the radioulnar space may be maintained by placing a carefully made ball of tendon or muscle about the size of the resected dome into the vacant distal radioulnar joint cavity (Fig. 21-31C) and stabilizing it to dorsal and volar capsules with a few sturdy sutures. The material may be obtained from the palmaris longus (preferred), ECU, or FCU. This added interposition bulk seems to adequately counter radioulnar shaft approximation

arthroplasty site, or excised. The ECU need not be removed from its retinacular compartment if it is stable. Subperiosteal lateral reflection of the ECU compartment is possible and allows excellent exposure of the distal ulnar area with the potential that when returned to its position it will reassume its stabilizing function. ECU stabilization is done only if it is displaced palmarly or if it is unstable in its compartment. In these instances the ECU is freed to its insertion on the fifth metacarpal. The first (proximal) flap is then used to create a sling. The technique is similar to that recommended by Spinner and Kaplan[121] but varies in that, after the flap is

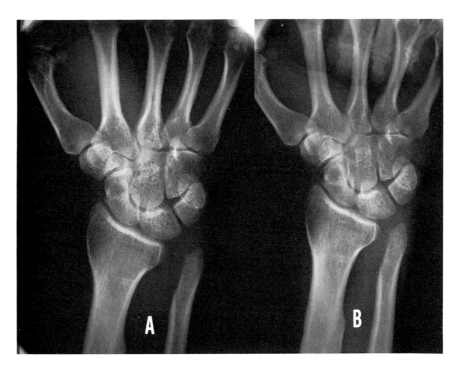

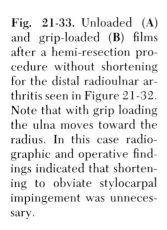

Fig. 21-33. Unloaded (**A**) and grip-loaded (**B**) films after a hemi-resection procedure without shortening for the distal radioulnar arthritis seen in Figure 21-32. Note that with grip loading the ulna moves toward the radius. In this case radiographic and operative findings indicated that shortening to obviate stylocarpal impingement was unnecessary.

and therefore obviates stylocarpal impingement in the borderline cases (zero variant +/− 1 mm).

Closure is accomplished as discussed in the approach to the joint on page 959. The extensor carpi ulnaris compartment is replaced in its original position or stabilized using the sling. If no shortening is done, the postoperative dressing is a short arm bulky dressing with dorsopalmar plaster reinforcement. Finger motion is encouraged while forearm rotation is neither encouraged nor discouraged. At 2 weeks, suture removal is accomplished, and a wrist splint is applied for 2 more weeks allowing unrestricted rotation. If ulnar shortening is done in association with the HIT, the initial plaster reinforcement splint goes above the elbow and, by supracondylar molding, limits forearm rotation to a few degrees. The operative dressing is converted to a short arm cast with interosseous space molding at 2 weeks. This allows slightly more rotation and is removed 2 weeks later (4 weeks postoperatively). A wrist splint is then used for the transition to full use over the next several weeks. The osteotomy, if done at the site of the ulnar head resection, will usually heal in 6 weeks. If the recession is done at shaft level, the osteosynthesis should be protected until full healing (8–12 weeks).

Indications for This Procedure. The indications include (1) unreconstructible fractures of the ulnar head or displaced fractures entirely within the articular area which will likely eventuate in radioulnar joint incongruity; (2) ulnocarpal impingement syndrome with distal radioulnar joint surface incongruity or arthrosis; (3) the early stages of rheumatoid arthritis unresponsive to medical management, with impending instability or tendon rupture; (4) arthritis after trauma and ostearthritis of the distal radioulnar joint; or (5) chronic TFC attritional or traumatic lesions associated with severe radioulnar chondromalacia or arthrosis, such that ulnar recession alone (Fig. 21-28) is a questionable first choice.

Contraindications. The basis for the procedure is a functionally adequate or reconstructible TFCC (see page 968 for the section entitled TFCC Reconstruction or Substitution). Without this, no advantage over the Darrach or its modifications is realized. The large majority of cases in which the TFCC will be unreconstructible are those with advanced rheumatoid arthritis. Here a modified Darrach procedure coupled with a radiolunate arthrodesis is a good choice.[18] Another alternative is

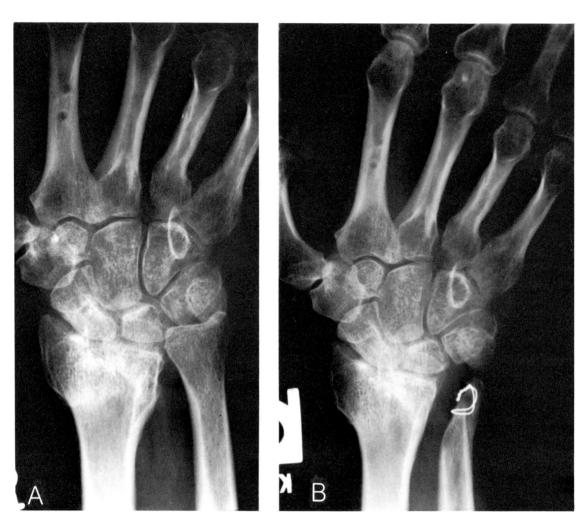

Fig. 21-34. (**A**) An "ulnocarpal impingment" resulting from shortening of a distal radius fracture. If only the articular dome were removed (standard **HIT**), the styloid would then become the source of impingement. Shortening is required (**B**) to allow a stable rotational axis to persist without impingement.

the Sauve-Kapandji procedure discussed next. An additional contraindication is preoperative evidence of ulnar carpal translation (post-traumatic or arthritic).

Distal Radioulnar Fusion with Surgical Pseudarthrosis of the Ulna (The Sauve-Kapandji Procedure)

In 1936, Sauve and Kapandji[117] proposed an operation consisting of a radioulnar joint fusion and creation of a pseudarthrosis proximal to the fusion (Fig. 21-35). This procedure was advanced as an alternative in the management of distal radioulnar joint disorders previously treated by excision of the ulnar head. Steindler[122] and Goncalves[49] have apparently erroneously attributed this procedure to Lauenstein, a mistake perpetuated by me in the first edition of this book. To date, there is little evidence in the literature to validate the efficacy of this procedure. Vergoz and Choussat,[133] Bunnell,[15] and Goncalves[49] have indicated their use of the procedure. Goncalves reported that in 22 patients results were "consistently better" than the Darrach procedure. Taleisnik[127] has reported his sur-

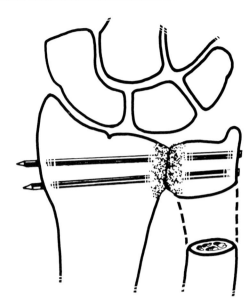

Fig. 21-35. The Sauve-Kapandji procedure as described by Taleisnik.[127]

gical technique (below) and results in 24 patients with greater than one-year follow-up. Elimination of pain, restoration of satisfactory forearm rotation, and few complications have led him to express general satisfaction with the procedure. The theoretically predictable complications of an unstable proximal ulnar stump were observed in only three of the 24 patients. Indications are similar to those for the Darrach procedure when dealing with a younger, more vigorous population. These indications include: (1) osteoarthritis or severe chondromalacia of the distal radioulnar joint, (2) post-traumatic ulnocarpal impingement associated with distal radioulnar joint arthrosis, (3) younger rheumatoid arthritic patients with ulnar translocation in addition to distal radioulnar joint disease, and (4) rheumatoid arthritis patients who may need a stable radioulnar surface for support of an arthroplasty or implant.

Taleisnik's Technique for Radioulnar Joint Arthrodesis and Proximal Pseudarthrosis (Sauve-Kapandji Procedure)

A longitudinal incision is preferred, placed along the space between the extensor and flexor carpi ulnaris tendons from 2 to 3 cm proximal to the prominence of the ulnar head to just distal to it. In this fashion, the dorsal branch of the ulnar nerve will remain distal to the operative field as it traverses in a dorsal and distal direction bisecting the space between the ulnar styloid and the pisiform. The pretendinous retinaculum is exposed and incised. Since the pretendinous retinaculum is not adherent to the underlying capsule, it can be lifted with ease. The neck of the ulna is exposed subperiosteally, and the periosteum along the intended pseudarthrosis site is completely excised. The ulnar head is grasped with a large towel clip. This will serve to manipulate it. An osteotomy is performed transversely, tangential to the proximal margin of the flare of the ulnar head, no more than 1 to 2 mm proximal to the border of its articular cartilage (Fig. 21-35). When radioulnar length discrepancy is present and needs correction, usually because of the ulna being too long, the ulnar head must be recessed proximally until it faces the sigmoid cavity of the radius. In all cases, after this radioulnar relationship is restored, a segment of ulna is excised measuring 12 to 15 mm. The head of the ulna is then hinged away from the radius, thus exposing both opposing radioulnar articular surfaces. These are decorticated down to cancellous bone. The ulnar head is then brought against the radius and is pinned to it using two crisscross 0.0625-inch or 0.045-inch K-wires. The wires are driven through the radius until their tips are palpable under the skin on the radial aspect of the wrist. On the medial side they are flush with the cortex of the head of the ulna. Bone grafts obtained from the portion of the ulna that was excised may be inserted into the fusion site to enhance healing. Periosteum within the ulnar pseudarthrosis must be entirely excised. The pronator quadratus is next brought into the pseudarthrosis gap and is sutured to the sheath of the extensor carpi ulnaris, as described by Sauve and Kapandji. If the ulnar stump still appears unstable, particulary with the forearm in pronation, then a palmar capsular flap can be brought over the dorsum of the cut end of the ulna in a manner similar to that descibed by Blatt and Ashworth.[10] Postoperative mobilization is provided in a short arm splint. Gentle motion is allowed a few days after operation, and progression of motion continues depending on the level of pain. The distal radioulnar fusion is protected for a period of 4 to 6 weeks. Usually 3 to 4 weeks postoperatively one of the two Kirschner wires is removed. The second wire is removed after the fusion appears radiographically solid (6–8 weeks following surgery).

Radioulnar Arthrodesis

If a stable forearm is paramount and rotation can be sacrificed, the technique of Carroll and Imbriglia[17] is trustworthy (success in 60 of 65 patients). This procedure may be a good choice in the paralytic instability of an otherwise unreconstructible brachial plexus injury or in spastic rotational contractures. The technique of arthrodesis is graphically demonstrated in Figure 21-36.

The Carroll and Imbriglia Technique of Radioulnar Fusion

A dorsal curvilinear incision is made over the distal radioulnar joint. The exposure continues as described on page 959. The periosteum is stripped from the ulna just proximal to the articular surface. The dorsal radioulnar ligaments are stripped sharply, and if the distal ulna is still remaining, the articular cartilage is removed with osteotomes. If the distal ulna has been removed or part of the distal ulna is missing, the remaining portion of the distal ulna is decorticated. The radius is then prepared using a drill and small osteotomes. A notch is made in the ulnar aspect of the distal radius where the distal ulna can be slotted. The level of the decorticated notch in the radius depends on the length of the ulna. The ulna is manually compressed into the notch, holding the forearm in 10 to 15 degrees of pronation. When the surgeon is satisfied with the position, a K-wire is driven from the ulna into the radius and two 4-mm compression (lag) screws are driven from the outer aspect of the ulna through both cortices of the radius. The compression aspect of the technique is very important because the ulna tends to distract laterally. Simple K-wire fixation is not recommended, nor does single screw fixation seem to provide enough strength. Once the forearm has been stabilized, the extensor retinaculum is reconstructed and the skin closed. A long arm cast is applied and immobilization is continued for 8 weeks.

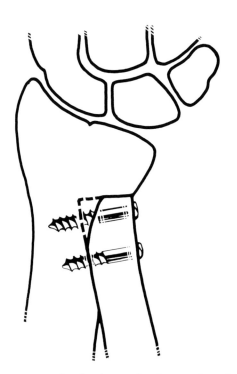

Fig. 21-36. Distal radioulnar arthrodesis as described by Carroll and Imbriglia.[17]

OTHER DISORDERS

Snapping or Dislocating Extensor Carpi Ulnaris[16,36,107]

The arrangement of the fibrous septa about the extensor carpi ulnaris creates an angular approach of the tendon to its insertion in the position of full supination. This angle results in an ulnar translation stress on the tendon sheath during ECU contraction, particularly with the forearm in supination and the wrist ulnarly deviated (Fig. 21-20). This is the position most often recalled by patients suffering traumatic dislocation of the tendon. The patient complains of a painful, soft snap. For acute injuries, the initial treatment is a cast with the forearm in pronation and the wrist dorsiflexed with slight radial deviation. Chronic subluxations require surgical reconstruction of a tunnel as described by Spinner and Kaplan.[121]

Operative Technique of Spinner and Kaplan for Extensor Carpi Ulnaris Stabilization

The operative exposure is the same as that described on page 959. A flap of extensor retinaculum beginning at Lister's tubercle is developed with the base on the ulnar side of the sheath of the extensor digiti minimi. The flap is $\frac{3}{8}$-inch wide at its radial side and $\frac{1}{2}$-inch wide at its base adjacent to the tendon of the extensor digiti minimi. The flap is mobilized. The intramuscular septum of the extensor retinaculum to the ulnar side of the common extensor compartment is released, as well as the radial septum for the compartment of the extensor digiti minimi. The flap is passed under the extensor carpi ulnaris from the radial side of the tendon so that the synovial side passes around and over the extensor carpi ulnaris tendon. The free end of the flap is sutured to itself and to the adjacent soft tissue of the radial side of the compartment for the extensor carpi ulnaris (Fig. 21-25G). Separate sutures are necessary to stabilize the flap on the ulnar side to the periosteum and adjacent soft tissue in line with the ulnar styloid. The fibroosseous tunnel for the extensor carpi ulnaris is thus reconstructed, and the tendon is recentralized on the dorsum of the distal ulna.

Three weeks of immobilization in a short arm cast is followed by the use of a simple wrist splint for two weeks; at that time, unrestricted use of the wrist may resume.

Fixed Pronation or Supination Deformity

These deformities may be the result of trauma or spasticity. Stable positioning may be attained by radioulnar arthrodesis. Various resections of the ulnar head (Darrach) or shaft (Baldwin or Sauve-Kapandji) may restore the rotation if suitable motor control is available. The Baldwin[5,49] procedure accepts the ankylosed distal radioulnar joint and creates a proximal pseudarthrosis similar to the Sauve-Kapandji procedure. I have had some success with soft tissue pronation contractures by a volar approach to the distal radioulnar joint and release of scar in the volar radioulnar joint capsule (see Operative Exposure of the Distal Radioulnar Joint and TFC section).

REFERENCES

1. Albert SM, Wohl MA, Rechtman AM: Treatment of the disrupted radio-ulnar joint. J Bone Joint Surg 45A:1373–1381, 1963
2. Alexander AH: Bilateral traumatic dislocation of the distal radioulnar joint, ulna dorsal: Case report and review of the literature. Clin Orthop 129:238–244, 1977
3. Angus: Dislocation of head of the ulna caused by a "backfire" in starting a motor car. North Humberland and Durham Med J 18;23, 1908–1909
4. Arkless R: Rheumatoid wrists: Cineradiography. Radiology 88:543–549, 1967
5. Baldwin WI: Orthopedic surgery of injuries. p. 251. In Jones, Sir Robert (ed): Pub. Joint Com. of Henry Frowde, Vol. 1. Hodder and Stroughton, London, 1921
6. Bastillas J, Vasilas A, Pizzi WF: Bone scanning in the detection of occult fractures. J Trauma, 21:564–569, 1981
7. Berger RA, Blair WF, El-Khoury GY: Arthrotomography of the wrist: The triangular fibrocartilage complex. Clin Orthop 172:257–264, 1983
8. Birch-Jensen A: Luxation of the distal radio-ulnar joint. Acta Chir Scand 101:312–317, 1951
9. Blair WF, Berger RA, El-Khoury GY: Arthrotomography of the wrist: An experimental and preliminary clinical study. J Hand Surg 10A:350–359, 1985
10. Blatt G, Ashworth CR: Volar capsule transfer for stabilization following resection of the distal end of the ulna. Orthop Trans 3:13–14, 1979
11. Bowers WH: The distal radioulnar joint. p. 743. In: Green DP (ed.): Operative Hand Surgery, Vol. 1. Churchill-Livingstone, New York, 1982
12. Bowers WH: Problems of the distal radioulnar joint. Adv Orthop Surg 7:289–303, 1984
13. Bowers WH: Distal radioulnar joint arthroplasty: The hemiresection-interposition technique. J Hand Surg 10A:169, 1985
14. Boyd HB, Stone MM: Resection of the distal end of the ulna. J Bone Joint Surg 26:313–321, 1944

15. Boyes JH: Bunnell's Surgery of the Hand. 5th Ed. pp. 299–303. JB Lippincott, Philadelphia, 1970

16. Burkhart SS, Wood MB, Linscheid, RL: Post-traumatic recurrent subluxation of the extensor carpi ulnaris tendon. J Hand Surg 7:1, 1982

17. Carroll RE, Imbriglia JE: Distal radioulnar arthrodesis. Orthop Trans 3:269, 1979

18. Chamay A, Santa DD, Vilaseca A: Radiolunate arthrodesis—Factor of stability for the rheumatoid wrist. Ann Chir Main 2:5–17, 1983

19. Coleman HM: Injuries of the articular disc at the wrist. J Bone Joint Surg, 42B:522–529, 1960

20. Cone RO, Szabo R, Resnick D, et al: Computed tomography of the normal radioulnar joints. Invest Radiol 18:541–545, 1983

21. Cooney WP, Linschied RL, Dobyns JH: External pin fixation for unstable Colles' fracture. J Bone Joint Surg 61A:840–845, 1979

22. Cox FJ: Anterior dislocation of the distal extremity of the ulna. Surgery 12:41–45, 1942

23. Dameron TB: Traumatic dislocation of the distal radiounlar joint. Clin Orthop 83:55–63, 1972

24. Darrach W: Forward dislocation at the inferior radio-ulnar joint, with fracture of the lower third of the shaft of the radius. Ann Surg 56:801, 1912

25. Darrach W: Anterior dislocation of the head of the ulna. Ann Surg 56:802–803, 1912

26. Darrach W: Partial excision of lower shaft of ulna for deformity following Colles' fracture. Ann Surg 57:764–765, 1913

27. Darrach W: Habitual forward dislocation of the head of the ulna. Ann Surg 57: 928–930, 1913

28. Darrach W: Fractures of the lower extremity of the radius. Diagnosis and treatment. J Am Med Assoc 89:1683, 1927

29. Darrach W: Discussion following Eliason EL: An operation for recurrent inferior radioulnar dislocation. Ann Surg 96:27–35, 1932

30. Darrach W: Colles' fracture. N Engl J Med 226:594–596, 1942

31. Darrach W, Dwight K: Derangements of the inferior radio-ulnar articulation. Med Red 87:708, 1915

32. Darrow JC, Linscheid RL, Dobyns JH, Mann JM, Wood MB, Beckenbaugh RD: Distal ulnar recession for disorders of the distal radioulnar joint. J Hand Surg 10A:482–491, 1985

33. Davidson, AJ, Horwitz MT: Recurrent or habitual dislocation of the inferior radio-ulnar articulation. Am J Surg 41:115–117, 1938

34. Desault M: Extrait d'un memoire de M. Desault sur la luxation de l'extremite inferieure du radius. J Chir I: 78, 1791

35. Dingman PVC: Resection of the distal end of the ulna (Darrach operation). An end result study of twenty-four cases. J Bone Joint Surg 34A:893–900, 1952

36. Eckhardt WA, Palmer AK: Recurrent dislocation of the extensor carpi ulnaris tendon. J Hand Surg 6:629–631, 1981

37. Ekenstam F, Engvist O, Wadin K: Results from resection of the distal end of the ulna after fractures of the lower end of the radius. Scan J Plast Reconstr Surg 16(2):177–181, 1982

38. Ekenstam F: The distal radioulnar joint—An anatomical, experimental, and clinical study. Acta Univ. Abstr Uppsala, Dissertion from the Faculty of Medicine, 505:1–55, Uppsala ISBN 91-554-161H-7, 1984

39. Ekenstam F, Palmer AK, Glisson RR: The load on the radius and ulna in different position of the wrist and forearm. Acta Ortho Scand 55:363–365, 1984

40. Eliason EL: An operation for recurrent inferior radioulnar dislocation. Ann Surg 96:27–35, 1932

41. Epner RA, Bowers WH, Guilford WB: Ulna variance: The effect of wrist positioning and roentgen filming technique. J Hand Surg 7:298–305, 1982

42. Essex-Lopresti P: Fractures of the radial head with distal radioulnar dislocation: Report of two cases. J Bone Joint Surg 33B:244–247, 1951

43. Evans EM: Rotational deformity in the treatment of fractures of both bones of the forearm. J Bone Surg 27:373–379, 1945

44. Frykman G: Fracture of the distal radius including sequelae-shoulder-hand-finger syndrome, disturbance in the distal radioulnar joint and impairment of nerve function. Acta Orthop Scand (suppl.) 108:27, 1967

45. Fulkerson JP, Watson HK: Congenital anterior sublaxation of the distal ulna. A case report. Clin Orthop. 131:179–182, 1978

46. Gelberman RH, Salamon PB, Jurist JM, Posch JL: Ulnar variance in Kienböck's disease. J Bone Joint Surg 57A:674–676, 1975

47. Gibson A: Uncomplicated dislocation of the inferior radio-ulnar joint. J Bone Joint Surg 7:180–189, 1925

48. Goldner JL, Hayes MD: Stabilization of the remaining ulna using one-half of the extensor carpi ulnaris tendon after resection of the distal ulna. Orthop Trans 3:330–331, 1979

49. Goncalves D: Correction of disorders of the distal radio-ulnar joint by artificial pseudarthrosis of the ulna. J Bone Joint Surg 56B:462–463, 1974

50. Gould JS, Nicholson B: Prosthetic replacement of

the distal ulna. 2d Congress — Intl Fed Soc Surg Hand, Abstract 47, p. 22, Boston, 1983

51. Green DP: Pins and plaster treatment of comminuted fractures of the distal end of the radius. J Bone Joint Surg 57A:304 – 310, 1975

52. Hagart CG: Functional aspects of the distal radioulnar joint. (Abstract) J Hand Surg 4:585, 1979

53. Heiple KG, Freehafer AA, Van't Hof A: Isolated traumatic dislocation of the distal end of the ulna or distal radio-ulnar joint. J Bone Surg 44A:1387 – 1394, 1962

54. Hergenroeder PT, Gelberman RH: Distal radioulnar joint subluxation secondary to excision of the radial head. Orthopedics 3:649 – 650, 1980

55. Hill RB: Habitual dislocation of the distal end of the ulna. J Bone Joint Surg 21:780, 1939

56. Hucherson DC: The Darrach operation for lower radioulnar derangement. Am J Surg 53:237 – 241, 1941

57. Hui FC, Linscheid RL: Ulnotriquetral augmentation tenodesis. A reconstructive procedure for dorsal subluxation of the distal radioulnar joint. J Hand Surg 7:230 – 236, 1982

58. Hughston JC: Fracture of the distal radial shaft: Mistakes in management. J Bone Joint Surg 39A:249 – 264, 1957

59. Hulten O: Uber anatomische Variationen der Hand — Gelenk – knochen. Acta Radiol 9:155 – 169, 1928

60. Imbriglia JE, Boland DS: Tears of the articular disc of the triangular fibrocartilage complex and Results of excision of the articular disc. (Absract) J Hand Surg, 8:620, 1983

61. Johnson RK: Muscle-tendon transfer for stabilization of the distal radioulnar joint. J Hand Surg 10A:437, 1985

62. Johnson RK, Shrewsbury MM: The pronator quadratus in motions and in stabilization of the radius and ulna at the distal radioulnar joint. J Hand Surg 1:205 209, 1976

63. Kapandji IA: The inferior radioulnar joint and pronosupination. pp. 121 – 129. In: Tubiana R (ed): The Hand, Vol. 1. WB Saunders, Philadelphia, 1981

64. Kaplan EB: Functional and Surgical Anatomy of the Hand. 2nd Ed. pp. 114-140. JB Lippincott, Philadelphia, 1965

65. Kauer JMG: The articular disc of the hand. Acta Anat 93:590 – 605, 1975

66. Kauer JMG: Functional anatomy of the wrist. Clin Orthop 149:9 – 20, 1980

67. Kessler I, Hecht O: Present application of the Darrach procedure. Clin Orthop 72:254 – 260, 1970

68. Kessler I, Silberman Z: An experimental study of the radiocarpal joint by arthrography. Surg Gynecol Obstet 112:33 – 40, 1961

69. Lanz U, Kron W: Nueve Technik zur Korrektur in Fehlstllung verheilter distaler Radiusfrakturen. Handchirurgie 8:203 – 206, 1976

70. Lauenstein C: Zur behandlung der nach karpaler vorderarm-fraktur zuruckbleibenden storoung der-und supinations — bewegung. Centralblatt fur Chirurgie 23:433, 1887

71. Lesser L von: Zur behandlung fehlerhaft geheilter bruch den karpalen radiusepiphyse. Centralblatt fur Chirurgie 15:265 – 270, 1887

72. Lewis OJ, Hamshere RJ, Bucknill TM: The anatomy of the wrist joint. J Anat 106:539 – 552, 1970

73. Lidstrom A: Fractures of the distal end of the radius — A clinical and statistical study of end results. Acta Orthop Scand (suppl.) 41, 1959

74. Liebolt FL: Surgical fusion of the wrist joint. Surg Gynecol Obstet 66:1008 – 1023, 1938

75. Liebolt FL: A new procedure for treatment of luxation of the distal end of the ulna. J Bone Joint Surg 35A:261 – 262, 1953

75. Linscheid RL, Dobyns JH: Rheumatoid arthritis of the wrist. Orthop Clin North Am 2:662, 1971

77. Linscheid RL, Dobyns JH, Younge DK: Trispiral tomography in the evaluation of wrist injuries. Bull Hosp Joint Dis 44:297 – 308, 1984

78. Linscheid RL: Symposium on distal radioulnar joint. Contemp Orthop 7:81, 1983

79. Lippmann, RK: Laxity of the radioulnar joint following Colles' fracture Arch Surg 35: 772 – 786, 1937

80. Lowman CL: The use of fascia lata in the repair of disability at the wrist. J Bone Joint Surg 12:400 – 402, 1930

81. Lugnegard H: Resection of the head of the ulna in post-traumatic dysfunction of the distal radioulnar joint. Scand J Plast Reconstr Surg 3:65 – 69, 1969

82. Matev I, Karagancheva S: The Madelung deformity. Hand 7:152 – 158, 1975

83. Mauer I: Reconstruction following posttraumatic derangement of the distal radioulnar joint. Bull Hosp Joint Dis 22:95 – 104, 1961

84. McDougall A, White J: Sublaxation of the inferior radio-ulnar joint complicating fracture of the radial head. J Bone Joint Surg 39B:278 – 287, 1957

85. Menon J, Wood VE, Shoene HR, Frykman GK, Hohl JC, Bestard EA: Isolated tears of the triangular fibrocartilage of the wrist: Results of partial excision. J Hand Surg 9A:527 – 530, 1984

86. Mino DE, Palmer AK, Levinsohn EM: The role of radiography and computerized tomography in the

diagnosis of subluxation and dislocation of the distal radioulnar joint. J Hand Surg 8:23–31, 1983

87. Mikic ZD: Age changes in the triangular fibrocartilage of the wrist joint. J Anat 126:367–384, 1978

88. Mikic ZD: Arthrograpy of the wrist joint. An experimental study. J Bone Joint Surg 66A:371–378, 1984

89. Milch, H: Dislocation of the end of the ulna—suggestion for a new operative procedure. Am J Surg 1:141–146, 1926

90. Milch H: Cuff resection of the ulna for malunited Colles' fracture. J Bone Joint Surg 23:311–313, 1941

91. Milch H: So-called dislocation of the lower end of the ulna. Ann Surg 116:282–292, 1942

92. Moberg E: Discussion of the dorsal flap arthroplasty in the treatment of Kienböck's disease by Nahigian SH, Li CS, Richey DG, and Shaw DT. J Bone Joint Surg 52A:251–252, 1970

93. Moore EM: Three cases illustrating luxation of the ulna in connection with Colles' fracture. Med Rec NY 17:305–308, 1880

94. Morrey BF, Chao EY, Hui FC: Biomechanical study of the elbow following excision of the radial head. J Bone Joint Surg 61A:63–68, 1979

95. Morrissy RT, Nalebuff EA: Dislocation of the distal radioulnar joint: Anatomy and clues to prompt diagnosis. Clin Orthop 144:154–158, 1979

96. Mossing N: Isolated lesions of the radio-ulnar disk treated with excision. Scand J Plast Reconstr Surg 9:231–233, 1975

97. Neviaser RJ, Palmer AK: Traumatic perforation of the articular disc of the triangular fibrocartilage complex of the wrist. Bull Hosp Joint Dis 44:376, 1984

98. Newmeyer WL, Green DP: Rupture of extensor tendons following resection of the distal ulna. J Bone Joint Surg 64A:178–182, 1982

99. Noble J, Arafa M: Stabilization of the distal ulna after excessive Darrach procedure. Hand 15:70–76, 1983

100. Palmer AK: Symposium on distal ulnar injuries. Contemp Orthop 7:81, 1983

101. Palmer AK, Werner FW: The triangular fibrocartilage complex of the wrist: Anatomy and function. J Hand Surg 6:153–161, 1981

102. Palmer AK, Werner FW: Biomechanics of the distal radioulnar joint. Clin Orthop 187:26–34, 1984

103. Palmer AK, Levinsohn EM, Kuzma GR: Arthrography of the wrist. J Hand Surg 8:15–23, 1983

104. Posner MA, Greenspan A: Trispiral tomography in the diagnosis of wrist problems. J Hand Surg 9A:602, 1984

105. Radin EL, Riseborough EJ: Fractures of the radial head. A review of 88 cases and analysis of the indications for excision of the radial head and non-operative treatment. J Bone Joint Surg 48A:1055–1064, 1966

106. Ranawat CS, Freiberger RH, Jordan LR, Straub LR: Arthrography in the rheumatoid wrist joint: A preliminary report. J Bone Joint Surg 51A:1269–1280, 1969

107. Rayan GM: Recurrent dislocation of the extensor carpi ulnaris in athletes. Amer J Sports Med 11:183–184, 1983

108. Reeves B: Excision of the ulnar styloid fragment after Colles' fracture. Int Surg 45:46–52, 1966

109. Regan JM, Bickel WH: Fascial sling operation for instability of the lower radioulnar joint. Mayo Clin Proc 20:202–208, 1945

110. Resnik O: Rheumatoid arthritis of the wrist. Med Radiogr Photogr 52:50–87, 1976

111. Resnik D, Andre M, Kerr R, Pineda C, Guerra J, Atkinson D: Digital arthrography of the wrist: A radio-graphic-pathological investigation. Amer J Radiol 142:1187–1190, 1984

112. Roberts D, Ram C, Udupa J, Herman G, Manders EK, Graham WP III: Computerized 3-D image reconstruction from computerized tomographic scans. p. 16. Abstract 136, 2nd Congress. Intl Fed Soc Surg Hand, Boston, 1983

113. Rose-Innes AP: Anterior dislocation of the ulna at the inferior radio-ulnar joint. J Bone Joint Surg 42B:515–521, 1960

114. Rowland SA: Stabilization of the ulnar side of the rheumatoid wrist following radiocarpal arthroplasty and resection of the distal ulna. Orthop Trans 6:474, 1982

115. Ruby LK: Correspondence letter, 1983-70. Amer Soc Surg Hand, 1983

116. Sarmiento A, Kinman PB, Murphy RB: The treatment of ulnar fractures by functional bracing. J Bone Joint Surg 58A:1104–1107, 1976

117. Sauve-Kapandji: Nouvelle technique traitement chirurical des luxations recidivantes isolees de l'extremite inferieure du cubitus. J de Chirurgie 47:589–594, 1936

118. Sclafani SJA: Dislocation of the distal radioulnar joint. J Comput Assist Tomogr 5:450, 1981

119. Smith JA, Homans J: Fracture of the lower end of the radius associated with fracture or dislocation of the lower end of ulna. Boston Med Surg J 187:401–407, 1922

120. Snook GA, Chrisman OD, Wilson TC, Wietsma RD: Subluxation of the distal radioulnar joint by hyperpronation. J Bone Joint Surg 51A:1315–1323, 1969

121. Spinner M, Kaplan EB: Extensor Carpi ulnaris. Its relationship to stability of the distal radio-ulnar joint. Clin Orthop 68:124–129, 1970

122. Steindler A: Orthopedic Operations. Indications, Techniques and Results. First printing, Charles C Thomas, Springfield, IL 1946

123. Swanson AB: Flexible Implant Arthroplasty in the Hand and Extremities, p. 275. CV Mosby, St Louis, 1973

124. Swanson AB: Implant arthroplasty for disabilities of the distal radioulnar joint. Use of a Silicone Rubber Capping Implant Following Resection of the Ulnar Head. Orthop Clin North Am 4:373–382, 1973

125. Taleisnik J: The ligaments of the wrist. J Hand Surg 1:110–118, 1976

126. Taleisnik J: Symposium on distal ulnar injuries. Contemp Orthop 7:81–116, 1983

127. Taleisnik J: Personal communication re: Report on the results of the Sauve-Kapandji procedure. J Bone Joint Surg (in press) 1987

128. Taylor GW, Parsons CL: The role of the discus articularis in Colles' fracture. J Bone Joint Surg 20:149–152, 1938

129. Taylor JL: An operation for chronic dislocation of the inferior radioulnar articulation. Texas State J Med., 35:278–280, 1939

130. Tsai T, Stillwell JH: Repair of chronic subluxation of the distal radioulnar joint (ulna dorsal) using flexor carpi ulnaris tendon. J Hand Surg 9B:289–293, 1984

131. Van Lannep GA: Dislocation forward of the head of the ulna at the wrist joint. Fracture of the styloid process of the ulna. Hahnemannian Monthly 32:350–354, 1897

132. Vesely DG: The distal radio-ulnar joint. Clin Orthop 51:75–91, 1967

133. Vergoz and Choussat: Luxation palmaire isolee de l'extremite inferieure du cubitus, traitee par la nouvelle technique de Sauve et Kapandji: Memoires de l'Academy de Chirurgie 63:992, 1937

134. Weigl K, Spira E: The triangular fibrocartilage of the wrist joint. Reconstr Surg Traumatol 11: 139–153, 1969

Fractures of the Distal Radius

22

Andrew K. Palmer

Fractures of the distal radius represent the most common fractures of the upper extremity. Beginning with the works of Pouteau (1783), then Colles (1814) and later Dupuytren (1847), physicians have thought of distal radius fractures as a homogenous group of injuries with a relatively good prognosis, irrespective of the treatment given.[25,26,48,67,109,110,111,112,115] Today, however, distal radius fractures are recognized as very complex injuries with a variable prognosis that depends upon the fracture type and the treatment given.[4–7,13,16,19,21,24,27,30,40,44,54,56,59,60,62,66,70,71,74,78,81–84,95,110,117,129,130,139,145]

Traditionally, hand surgeons have been called upon to manage some of the problems associated with distal radius fractures, such as carpal tunnel syndrome, ruptured tendons, and reflex sympathetic dystrophy, but not for the management of acute fractures.[44,69,86,91,103,105,118,119,149] Nevertheless, as more subtle late problems associated with distal radius fractures, such as midcarpal instability, incongruity of the distal radioulnar joint, the ulnar impaction syndrome, and pain syndromes secondary to small degrees of radial malalignment have come to be recognized, the hand surgeon has become more involved in not only the care of problems following fracture healing, but also in dealing with the acute fracture in hopes of lessening the number and/or severity of late problems.[10,54,56,77,] [83,85,86,118,128,135,146] Keeping in mind that some who read this chapter will be inexperienced in dealing with even the most straightforward distal radius fracture, I will review in depth the traditional concepts of classification and treatment, as well as our preferred method for treating these fractures and their associated complications, both acute and late, in the adult and pediatric populations.

ANATOMY

The distal radius functions as an articular plateau upon which the carpus rests (Fig. 22-1), and from which the radially based supporting ligaments of the wrist arise (Fig. 22-2A and B).[10,13,42,88,107,108] The hand and radius, as a unit, articulate with and rotate about the ulnar head via the sigmoid notch of the radius (Fig. 22-3).[1,10] This latter relationship is maintained primarily by the ulnar-based supporting ligaments of the wrist: the triangular fibrocartilage complex (Fig. 22-2B).[108]

The distal radius has three concave articular surfaces, the scaphoid fossa, the lunate fossa, and the sigmoid notch for articulation with the scaphoid,

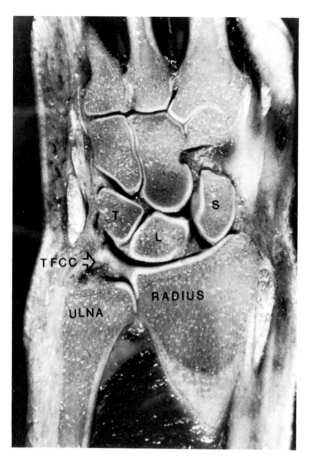

Fig. 22-1. The scaphoid and lunate articulate with the distal articular surface of the radius and the ulnar head with the sigmoid notch. The triangular fibrocartilage complex is interposed between the ulnar carpus and the ulnar head. (*S*, scaphoid; *L*, lunate; *T*, triquetrum; *TFCC*, triangular fibrocartilage complex.)

lunate, and ulnar head, respectively (Fig. 22-4).[42,88] The scaphoid fossa is basically triangular in shape with its apex forming the radial styloid. An anterior/posterior ridge separates this fossa from the smaller lunate fossa. Both fossae are concave in the anterior/posterior plane and the medial lateral plane. The sigmoid notch is concave, with a poorly defined proximal margin and well-defined dorsal, palmar, and distal margins (Fig. 22-5).

The metaphyseal flare of the distal radius begins approximately 2 cm above the distal articular surface. As the radius flares, the thickness of the cortical bone decreases and the amount of cancellous bone increases. The distal articular surface of the

distal radius has a radial inclination or slope of an average 22 degrees and tilts palmarly an average of 11 degrees (Fig. 22-6).[42,45,76,98,104,127,128,142] Radial inclination is measured by the angle drawn between a line tangential to the distal radial articular surface on a PA x-ray and perpendicular to the shaft of the radius. Palmar tilt is measured by the angle between the plane of the distal articular surface as seen on the lateral x-ray and a perpendicular to the longitudinal axis of the radius. The sigmoid notch angles distally and medially an average of 22 degrees to form the "seat" for the ulnar head (Fig. 22-3).[1]

The palmar radial aspect of the radius is flat, with vascular foramen (Fig. 22-4). From this surface arise the major radial supporting ligaments of the wrist: the radial collateral, radiocapite, and radiotriquetral ligaments (Fig. 22-2B). At the palmar aspect of the anterior/posterior midradial ridge is a tubercle for origin of the very important radioscapholunate ligament or Ligament of Testut (Fig. 22-2B). The dorsal aspect of the distal radius is somewhat convex, acting as a fulcrum for extensor tendon function (Fig. 22-4). The radial styloid area, at times, has a groove for the tendon of the first dorsal compartment and ulnar to this, a dorsal longitudinal prominence, Lister's tubercle, which acts as a fulcrum for the extensor pollicis longus tendon. Relatively weak and unimportant supporting ligaments arise from the dorsal radial aspect of the radius; these are the radioscaphoid and radial triquetral ligaments (Fig. 22-2A). Along the entire ulnar aspect of the distal articular surface of the radius, at the distal margin of the sigmoid notch, the triangular fibrocartilage complex arises.[106] This ligamentous complex, the major stabilizer of the distal radioulnar joint and ulnar carpus, extends ulnarly to insert into the base of the ulnar styloid and distally to insert into the lunate (the ulnolunate ligament), triquetrum (the ulnotriquetral ligament), hamate, and finally into the base of the fifth metacarpal (Fig. 22-2B).

Normally the wrist is an extremely mobile joint, capable of 120 degrees flexion and extension and 50 degrees of radial and ulnar deviation. Forearm rotation of up to 150 degrees occurs at the distal radioulnar joint as the distal radius and its fixed member (the hand), rotate about the ulnar head.[10]

Studies have shown that the radius, through its

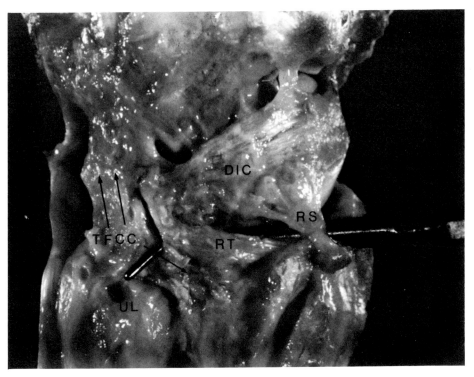

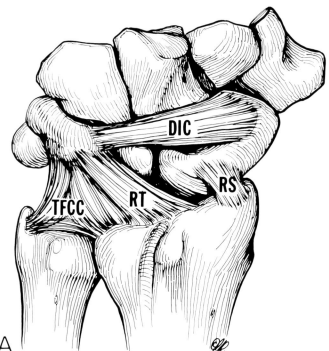

Fig. 22-2. (A) A dissection and illustration composite showing the dorsal ligaments of the wrist. (*RS*, radioscaphoid; *RT*, radiotriquetral; *TFCC*, triangular fibrocartilage complex; *DIC*, dorsal intercarpal ligaments.) (*Figure continues.*)

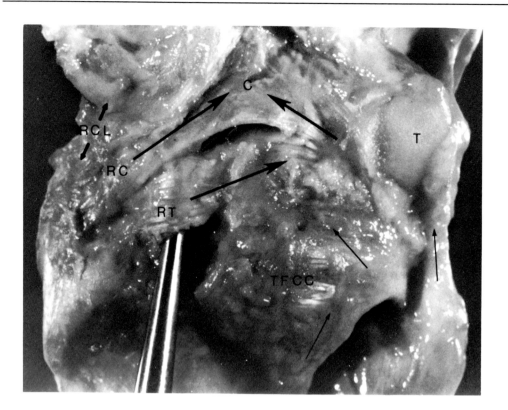

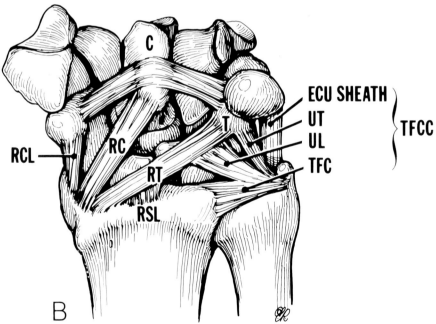

Fig. 22-2 *(Continued).* (B) A dissection and illustration composite showing the complex volar ligaments of the wrist. (*RCL*, radial collateral ligament; *RC*, radiocapitate; *C*, capitate; *RT*, radiotriquetral, *T*, triquetrum; *RSL*, radioscapholunate; *TFCC*, triangular fibrocartilage complex; *ECU sheath*, extensor carpi ulnaris sheath; *UT*, ulnotriquetral; *UL*, ulnolunate; *TFC*, triangular fibrocartilage.)

Fig. 22-3. The ulnar head articulates with the sigmoid notch of the radius at the "seat" of the distal radioulnar joint. The TFCC is the distal restraint of the distal radioulnar joint arising from the most ulnar border of the radius and inserting into the base of the ulnar styloid process (*TFCC*, triangular fibrocartilage complex).

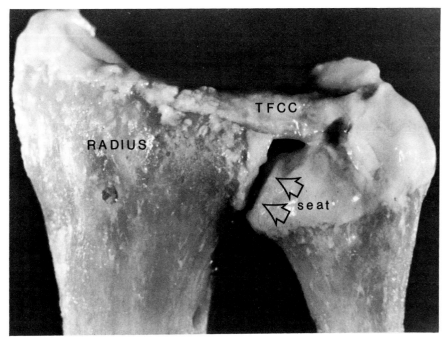

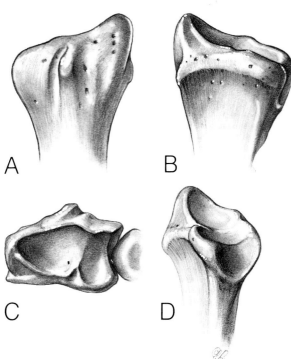

Fig. 22-4. An artist's drawing of the distal radius. **(A)** Dorsal view illustrating Lister's tubercle. **(B)** Palmar view illustrating the scaphoid and lunate fossae distally, as well as the sigmoid notch ulnarly. Vascular foramina can be noted on the palmar and dorsal aspects of the distal radius. **(C)** An end-on view of the distal radius and radioulnar joint showing the scaphoid fossa, lunate fossa, and ulnar head resting in the sigmoid notch. **(D)** A view of the sigmoid notch from the ulnar aspect.

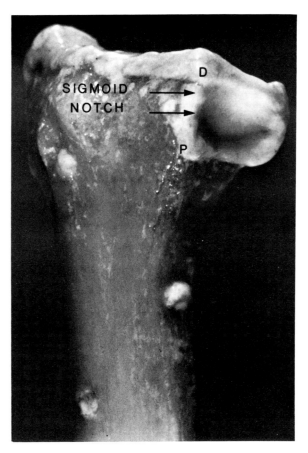

Fig. 22-5. The sigmoid notch showing distinct dorsal, palmar, and distal borders and an indistinct proximal border (*D*, distal; *P*, proximal).

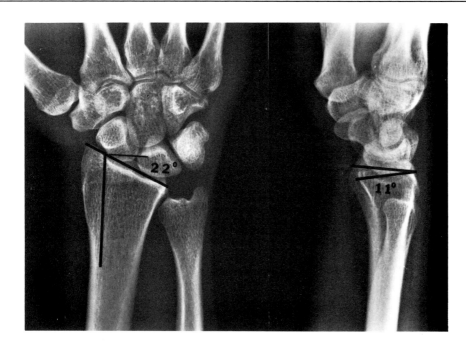

Fig. 22-6. The AP film on the left illustrates normal radial inclination of approximately 22 degrees. The lateral film on the right illustrates normal volar tilt of the distal articular surface of approximately 11 degrees.

articulation with the lateral carpus, carries approximately 80 percent of the axial load of the forearm and that the ulna, through its articulation with the medial carpus, via the TFCC, about 20 percent.[108] Changes in the forearm unit length ratio, as seen with a settled distal radius fracture, increase radial loading beyond physiological limits.

Despite the loads borne by the distal radius and the wide range of motion to which the wrist is subjected, a precise relationship is normally maintained among the various components of the wrist joint. This intrinsic stability is the result of the inherent geometry of the distal radial articulations and their surrounding ligamentous supports.

My preferred method of treatment of all distal radial injuries is one that attempts to restore as closely and quickly as possible these normal anatomic relationships within the obvious constraints of the patient's age and general medical condition.

CLASSIFICATION

Beginning with the classic description of an extraarticular distal radius fracture by Abraham Colles in 1814, many authors have described fractures about the distal radius.[7,25,26,33,34,36–39,48,49–]

[51,95,141] In some instances, an author's name has come to be identified with a particular fracture. In other instances, authors have purposely avoided eponyms, and instead numerically classified fractures based upon whether they were open or closed, displaced or nondisplaced, comminuted or noncomminuted, intra- or extraarticular, or adult or pediatric.[20,59,120]

Some commonly used eponyms for fractures about the distal radius are discussed here.

Colles' Fracture

"This fracture takes place at about an inch and a half above the carpal extremity of the radius. . . . The carpus and base of the metacarpus appear to be

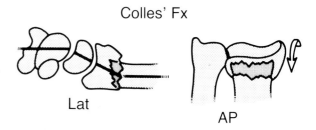

Colles' Fx

Lat

AP

Fig. 22-7. Diagrammatic representation of the typical deformity seen in a Colles' fracture, showing dorsal comminution and displacement with shortening of the radius relative to the ulna.

thrown backward so much as on first view, to excite a suspicion that the carpus is dislocated." Abraham Colles, 1814[25,26]

Figure 22-7 illustrates the typical features of a Colles' fracture, that is, a distal radius fracture with dorsal comminution, dorsal angulation, dorsal displacement, and radial shortening.

Barton's Fracture

"Subluxation of the wrist, consequent to a fracture through the articular surface of the carpal extremity of the wrist." John Rhea Barton, 1838[7]

Barton's fracture is a displaced, unstable articular fracture-subluxation of the distal radius with displacement of the carpus with the articular fracture fragment. Barton's fracture may be either dorsal or volar as shown in Figure 22-8.

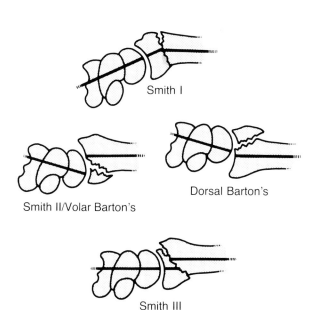

Smith I

Smith II/Volar Barton's

Dorsal Barton's

Smith III

Fig. 22-8. Thomas' classification of Smith's fractures. Type I Smith's fracture: An extraarticular fracture with palmar angulation and displacement of the distal fragment. Type II Smith's fracture: An intraarticular fracture with volar and proximal displacement of the distal fragment along with the carpus. Type III Smith's fracture: An extraarticular fracture with volar displacement of the distal fragment and carpus. (In Type III, the fracture line is more oblique than in Type I fracture.) Smith's Type II fracture is essentially a volar Barton's fracture. A dorsal Barton's fracture is illustrated for comparison, showing the dorsal and proximal displacement of the carpus and distal fragment on the radial shaft.

Smith's Fracture

"A fracture of the lower end of the radius, ½ to 1 inch from the articular surface, in which the lower fragment and the carpus were displaced forwards in relationship to the forearm." "A reverse Colles' fracture." Robert William Smith, 1847

Figure 22-8 illustrates three types of fractures of the distal radius with volar displacement, classified as Smith's Type I, II, and III by Thomas in 1957.[140] Types I and III are in essence reversed Colles' fractures, and Thomas' Type II Smith's fracture is the same as a volar Barton's fracture.

Chauffeur's or Backfire Fracture

Originally, it was felt that "many and varied are the types of fracture which result from a backfire. It appears that anything may happen."[51] Over the years, however, most have come to accept that "the chauffeur's fracture is an oblique fracture of the lower end of the radius by which a triangular portion of bone, including the styloid process, is separated from the main bone." Harold C. Edwards, 1910[51]

Figure 22-9 illustrates a chauffeur's fracture with displacement of the carpus and attached radial styloid avulsion.

Lunate Load or Die-Punch Fracture

An intraarticular fracture with displacement of the medial articular surface of the radius as described by Rutherford in 1891 and Frederic J. Cotton in 1900.[33,34]

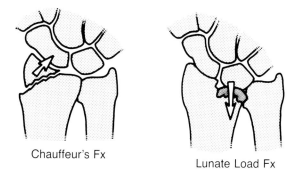

Chauffeur's Fx

Lunate Load Fx

Fig. 22-9. A chauffeur's fracture is illustrated with the carpus displaced ulnarly by the radial styloid fracture. A lunate load (die-punch) fracture is shown with a depression of the lunate fossa of the radius that allows proximal migration of the lunate and/or proximal carpal row.

Scheck[124] coined the term "die-punch" fracture, and Figure 22-9 illustrates this fracture, which usually represents a depression of the dorsal aspect of the lunate fossa.

Frykman's Classification

Of the many classifications suggested for distal radius fractures, the one proposed by Frykman in 1937 is perhaps the most useful.[59] His classification

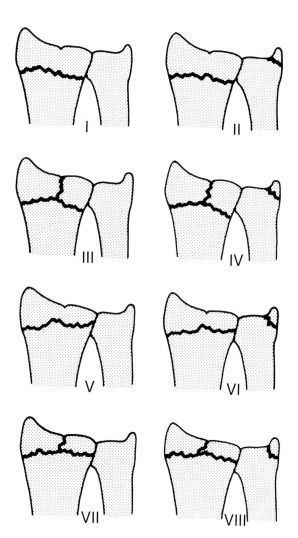

Fig. 22-10. Frykman's classification of distal radius fractures. Types I, III, V, and VII do not have an associated fracture of the distal ulna. Fractures III through VIII are intraarticular fractures. Higher classification fractures have worse prognoses.

was based upon a biomechanical and clinical study, distinguishing between extraarticular and intraarticular fractures of the distal radius and the presence or absence of an associated distal ulnar fracture. With this classification, the more complex fractures are assigned a higher number. The higher number classification a fracture is assigned, the more complicated fracture healing and the worse the overall prognosis become (Fig. 22-10). The use of such a classification eliminates much of the confusion associated with eponyms, for example, the controversy as to whether a Smith's II fracture is a Barton's fracture or a reversed Barton's fracture.[7,52,81,140] Rather than using an eponym, it is far easier to classify this fracture as an intraarticular fracture with dorsal or palmar displacement of the minor fragment.

Frykman's classification has drawn much-needed attention to the importance of the distal ulna and the distal radioulnar joint in the evaluation and treatment of distal radius fractures.[1,73,76,108,138] All too often, the reduction of a distal radius fracture is evaluated in terms of the congruence of the radiocarpal joint only, with little attention paid to the ulnocarpal joint (i.e., radial length) and the distal radioulnar joint, only to have patients end up with a painful or incongruous distal radioulnar joint or ulnocarpal articulation.

Although we have found Frykman's classification to be very useful, we agree with Milch[96,97] that "no one of the displacements seems entitled to a special consideration and the objective should be a complete restitution of the normal anatomic configuration for, all other factors being equal, the best functional results will be obtained in those instances in which the most satisfactory anatomical alignment has been achieved."

ASSOCIATED INJURIES

Distal radius fractures are usually the result of significant trauma to the entire upper extremity.[3,87,89,90,125] Because of this, when evaluating a patient with an acute distal radius fracture or a patient with a problem following a distal radius fracture, a complete exam of the entire upper extremity should always be undertaken. One must not overlook associated injuries, such as shoulder dislocation, elbow fracture or dislocation, carpal or metacarpal fracture, median nerve injury, or vascular injury.[9,12,14,37,47,55,86,100,102,118,136,142] The associated injuries often lead to more problems than the distal radius fracture itself. Once the other problems have been dealt with, the physician's attention may be directed to the distal radius fracture itself.

TREATMENT OF ACUTE FRACTURES IN ADULTS

Fractures of the distal radius in patients with closed epiphyses represent adult fractures. The principles of dealing with fractures in this very large age group are similar; however, the aggressiveness with which we approach the fracture must be tempered by the patient's age, functional demands, and general medical condition.

Acute distal radius fractures may present in a practitioner's office or in an emergency room. Each patient should be expeditiously evaluated to determine whether the fracture is open or closed, that is, compound or simple; whether neurovascular compromise is present; the degree of displacement of the fracture fragments; and whether the fracture is intra- or extraarticular.

Open Fractures

Most fractures of the distal radius are closed injuries, but I consider any fracture that communicates with the external environment to be an open fracture. The associated skin injury may be massive or it may be a pinpoint, with the only real indication that the wound communicates with the fracture being a small amount of fatty fluid exuding from the wound. All open fractures should be treated as surgical emergencies. My treatment plan for open distal radius fractures calls for emergency room clinical and radiographic evaluation followed by a wound culture. Appropriate IV antibiotics are then begun while the patient is prepared for the operating room. As soon as possible, the patient is transported to the operating room where a general or regional anesthetic is administered. The open wound is enlarged, the wound margins and fracture margins debrided, and the wound irrigated with 10 liters of normal saline. The fracture itself is then dealt with in terms of immobilization. If the wound has been suitably cleaned, and the fracture is unstable, I prefer to insert internal fixation using an AO plate or a combination of internal fixation with K-wires and an external fixator. If the fracture is stable, the wound is simply closed and the fracture immobilized in plaster. If the wound cannot be suitably cleaned, or if the wound has been open for more than 12 hours, the wound is left open and closed secondarily at 48 hours, either directly or with a split-thickness skin graft.

Associated Median Nerve Injury

Patients presenting with acute distal radius fractures quite frequently have neurovascular compromise, that is, median nerve symptoms to a greater or lesser extent. My treatment plan for such individuals calls for a closed reduction of the fracture in the emergency room. If a satisfactory reduction is obtained, the nerve compression syndrome is treated with observation alone. In most instances, if the reduction can be maintained, the nerve compression syndrome will resolve, or at least improve substantially over the subsequent 24 to 48 hours. If the nerve compression syndrome worsens or shows little or no sign of improvement over the first 24 to 48 hours following reduction, or if the reduction cannot be obtained or maintained in the presence of median nerve compression, I favor early open reduction, carpal tunnel release, and if necessary, skeletal stabilization of the fracture. A carpal tunnel release is not routinely performed at the time of open reduction of a distal radius fracture unless significant median nerve symptoms were present preoperatively.

Timing of Reduction

Reduction of displaced distal radius fractures is usually most easily accomplished if performed acutely. In this regard, my treatment plan calls for an attempted closed reduction of the distal radius fracture in the emergency room at the time of presentation. If the fracture requires skeletal stabilization to maintain the reduction or an open reduction to gain a desirable reduction, the patient is admitted to the hospital, evaluated medically, and electively operated upon.

Nondisplaced Distal Radius Fractures

All would agree that nondisplaced distal radius fractures should be immobilized for a minimal period of time and that a good result is to be expected. All forms of immobilization have been used for distal radius fractures ranging from a wooden splint to a long arm cast to internal fixation with plates and screws. [4,7,8,9,11,17,18,22,24,28,29,31,32,35,39,41,43,45,46,51,57,58,61,63–65,68,79,83,84,93–95,106,114,116,121–124,126,132,133,137,142,147] All authors have emphasized the need for the fingers to be free. Most have applied devices that allow elbow motion. The period of immobilization has ranged from days to months.

Author's Preferred Method of Treatment

For a stable, undisplaced, distal radius fracture, I prefer a short arm cast for 4 weeks followed by a removable prefabricated splint (Fig. 22-11). For a potentially unstable, yet nondisplaced distal radius fracture, I prefer a long arm cast for 3 weeks followed by a short arm cast for 3 weeks and then a removable prefabricated splint.

I treat all patients with distal radius fractures with a removable prefabricated splint following immobilization, whether they had a nondisplaced fracture requiring a minimal degree of immobilization or a markedly displaced fracture requiring an open reduction. The splint is removed for bathing and range of motion exercises daily. The patient is asked to gradually wean himself or herself from the splint over a 2 to 3 week period of time, as seen fit. I have found this policy to be extremely helpful for my patients. Following plaster immobilization, all patients seem concerned that they will fall and refracture the wrist. By providing them with a removable splint that they can wean themselves from as they regain wrist motion and upper extremity strength, much of this anxiety is relieved and their rehabilitation process shortened.

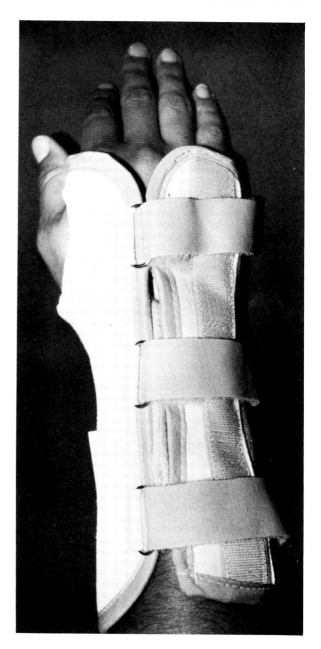

Fig. 22-11. A prefabricated splint is recommended following discontinuation of plaster immobilization.

During the period of immobilization and weaning from the splint, all patients are instructed to keep their fingers mobile by performing, at least three times a day, the "six-pack" exercises as popularized by Dobyns (JH Dobyns, personal communication) and illustrated in Figure 22-12. Steps 1 through 6 illustrate finger extension, MP flexion,

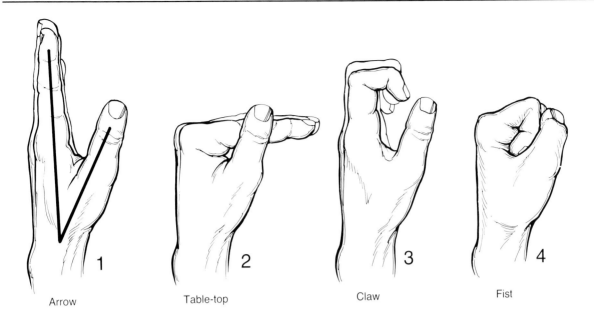

1 Arrow 2 Table-top 3 Claw 4 Fist

"Six-Pack" Exercises

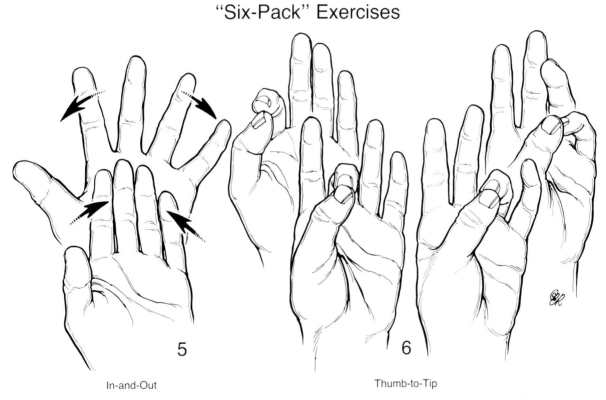

5 In-and-Out 6 Thumb-to-Tip

Fig. 22-12. "Six-pack" exercises. 1 through 6 illustrate the position that the patient's hand should assume when performing these exercises. It is helpful to illustrate to the patient that full MP extension makes his hand look like an arrow; full MP flexion makes his hand look like a table top; full MP extension combined with PIP and DIP flexion creates a claw; complete finger flexion, a fist; abduction and adduction of the fingers, an in and out motion; and finally, to complete the exercises, the individual touches the tip of his thumb to the tip of fingers 2 through 5.

PIP flexion, full finger flexion, finger abduction and adduction, and thumb motion, respectively. Although the services of hand therapists are used for the recalcitrant patient, most of our patients prefer to perform their own therapy. They have found the "six-pack" exercises easy to remember and perform.

Displaced Distal Radius Fractures

IS FRACTURE REDUCTION NECESSARY?

Over 170 years ago, Abraham Colles, in discussing treatment of the fracture that now bears his name, suggested that closed reduction of a distal radius fracture is usually easily accomplished but that "the distortion of the limb instantly returns on the extension being removed."[25] He went on, however, to state that "the limb will at some remote period again enjoy perfect freedom in all its motions and be completely exempt from pain. The deformity, however, will remain undiminished throughout life."[25] Although I am sure that some would agree with this statement, most physicians today believe that few patients with a malunited distal radius fracture "enjoy perfect freedom in all motions and are exempt from pain."[6,30] Yet there is no real agreement among physicians as to which patients require a reduction or the extent to which a fracture must be reduced to achieve a functional result.

DePalma, in contrast to Colles, has written that every attempt should be made to restore normal anatomy. He suggested that a poor result was inevitable if "a residual dorsal tilt of the radius of more than 5 degrees and loss of the inward tilt of the articular surface of the radius exceeding 3 mm" was found.[41] Biomechanical studies done on cadaver forearms in our lab support this clinical observation. It has been shown that shortening the distal radius by small amounts (2.5 mm) (Fig. 22-13) and/or the residual dorsal tilt of the distal radial articular surface results in a significant increase in the axial load transmitted to the ulnar shaft (Fig. 22-14).[108,128] Theoretically, this increased ulnar load leads to degenerative arthritis and pain on the ulnar aspect of the wrist. Further biomechanical studies have shown that as the distal radius tilts dorsally, the contact area of the distal articular surface with the scaphoid and the lunate decreases in size and shifts dorsally (Fig. 22-15A and 15B).[128] This finding also suggests, theoretically, that loss of the volar tilt of distal radius fractures is biomechanically unsound and will lead to post-traumatic arthritis and pain.

Malunions of the distal radius may be associated with decreased range of motion, wrist pain, sublux-

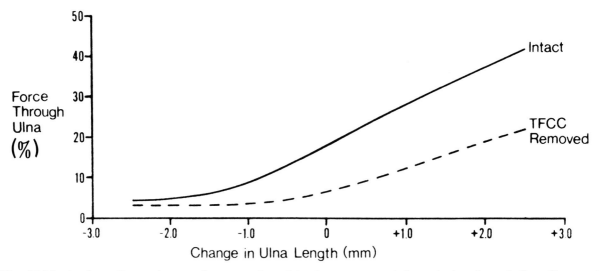

Fig. 22-13. As the radius is shortened, increased axial load is transmitted through the ulnar shaft as illustrated graphically. As the radius is shortened approximately 2.5 mm, the load transmitted through the ulna doubles.

Axial Load

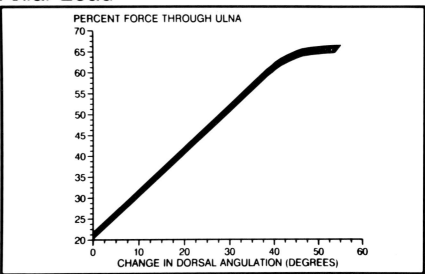

Fig. 22-14. This graph summarizes the results of a laboratory study, indicating that as the distal articular surface of the radius inclines more dorsally, the percent of force transmitted through the ulna increases respectively.

ation of the distal radioulnar joint, midcarpal instability, and post-traumatic arthritis. Of the many complications associated with distal radial fractures, post-traumatic arthritis is perhaps the most serious and disabling to the patient.[30,128,135] Ghormley stated in 1932 that "any injury to the articular surface of the radius is bound to set up active traumatic arthritis in the radiocarpal joint."[62] Frykman has shown this to be true for not only the radiocarpal, but the distal radioulnar joint as well.[59] More recently, Jupiter and Knirk found that intraarticular distal radius fractures that healed with a depression of an articular component of greater than 1 mm resulted in symptomatic post-traumatic arthritis in more than 90 percent of patients reviewed.[82]

Despite this accumulating wealth of knowledge indicating the need for an anatomic reduction, some have felt that extensive treatment to achieve such a reduction is not warranted. Instead, they have advocated immediate excision of the distal ulna allowing the radius to settle primarily.[39,58,116] Others have recommended immobilization of the distal radius fracture without great attempts at reduction, and secondary excision of the distal ulna if symptomatic.[10,39,43,44]

Based on the large body of clinical and experimental evidence, I believe that an attempt at an anatomic reduction of a distal radius fracture is warranted. The patient's functional demands and general medical condition should always be considered when developing a treatment program for distal radius fractures. I therefore recommend that all displaced distal radius fractures be treated with reduction and stabilization as necessary to maintain reduction of the fracture in functionally active, otherwise healthy individuals.

CLOSED REDUCTION TECHNIQUES

Ford and Key stated "there are as many methods of reduction as there are fracture surgeons" (Lidstrom).[89] In the 1920s, Böhler introduced the concept of manual traction being applied to the limb and countertraction being applied to the arm.[8,15] Although this method of reduction proved reliable, many times the assistant tired out or his fingers slipped before the plaster could be applied and the reduction was lost. In 1931, Caldwell introduced "finger-trap" traction as a mechanical means of obtaining the traction that Böhler had popularized.[15] Since 1931, many means of and devices for applying traction to the hand and arm have been introduced.

Most methods of reduction have emphasized that once the fracture fragments are disimpacted,

11 Degrees of Volar Tilt (Original Position)

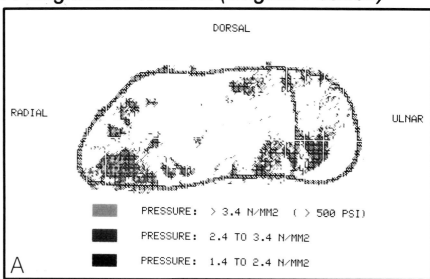

A

28 Degrees of Dorsal Tilt

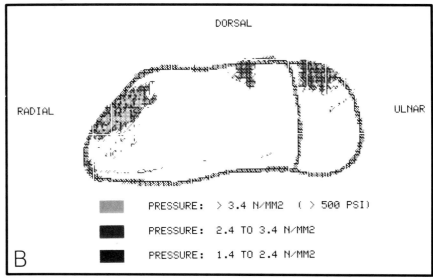

B

Fig. 22-15. **(A)** A pressure-sensitive film plot showing the concentration of pressures on the distal radius and TFCC area in the resting position in a normal distal radial articular surface with 11 degrees of volar tilt. Pressure is concentrated in the scaphoid fossa, lunate fossa, and triangular fibrocartilage complex–ulnar head area. **(B)** A pressure-sensitive film with the distal radial articular surface experimentally tilted to a position of 28 degrees dorsal tilt, showing a dramatic shift in the load to the dorsal lip of the radius in the scaphoid fossa, lunate fossa, and triangular fibrocartilage complex–ulnar head.

each component of the fracture displacement should be reduced.[96] As an example, in a Colles' fracture, the distal fragment is angulated dorsally, displaced proximally and radially, and supinated. To effect reduction of a Colles' fracture, traction is applied to the hand, the fracture disimpacted and the distal fragment flexed, translated palmarly, and pronated on the radial shaft. For a Smith's fracture, with palmar displacement and angulation of the distal fragment, the fracture would be first disim-pacted and then the distal radial fragment extended, dorsally translocated, and supinated upon the radial shaft.

Author's Preferred Method of Reduction

In dealing with displaced acute fractures of the distal radius, my first step is a gentle, sterile, 5-minute preparation of the fracture area. The hematoma associated with the fracture is then infiltrated with 1 percent Xylocaine without epinephrine,[23] and the anesthesia is allowed to diffuse about the fracture site for approximately 5 minutes. (Brachial block or general anesthesia is preferred by some surgeons, and is certainly satisfactory.) The arm is gently suspended with finger-traps attached to the thumb, index, and long fingers (Fig. 22-16). The

patient is asked to relax. The weight of the arm usually provides enough countertraction to disimpact an acute fracture. After allowing the arm to hang from the finger-traps for 5 to 10 minutes, pressure is applied by the treating physician's thumb to the distal fracture fragment in a direction that will reduce the displacement (Fig. 22-16). For a displaced Colles' fracture, the distal fragment is manipulated with the treating physician's thumb into a flexed, palmarly translocated and pronated position on the radial shaft. With the hand still suspended from the finger-traps, an x-ray is taken to evaluate the reduction obtained.

POSITION OF IMMOBILIZATION

In an attempt to prevent displacement in splints or plaster of a reduced radius fracture, the position of acute flexion, extreme pronation, and ulnar deviation (the Cotton-Loder position) has been advocated.[33,34] This position, however, is no longer popular because of problems encountered with median nerve compression and finger and wrist stiffness as a result of an inability to use one's fingers.[30] Most physicians now recommend immobilization in slight flexion and ulnar deviation for a Colles' fracture. Most authors also recommend immobilization of the forearm in neutral forearm rotation or slight pronation. Sarmiento is currently the only strong advocate of immobilization of a distal radius fracture in supination,[121-123] a technique originally espoused by Fahey.[54] Sarmiento's work has recently been questioned by Gibson.[63]

Author's Preferred Position for Plaster Immobilization

My recommended position of immobilization for a Colles' fracture is that of slight palmar flexion, ulnar deviation, and neutral forearm rotation. All other distal radius fractures should be immobilized based on a similar logic to that used in recommending the position to immobilize a Colles' fracture, that is, adapt the position of the hand and wrist to a position that is directly opposite to the displacement that occurred in producing the original deformity. Although theoretical arguments can be made for immobilization of distal radius fractures in full supination or full pronation, I favor neutral forearm rotation, as it seems to lead to less long-term prob-

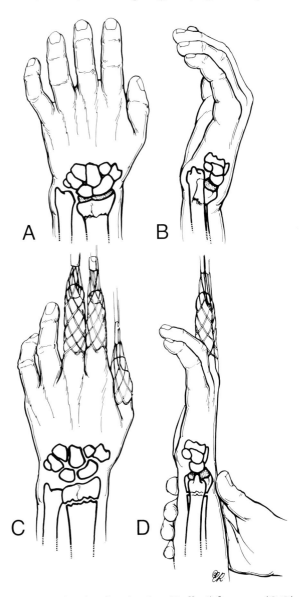

Fig. 22-16. **(A,B)** A distal radius (Colles') fracture. **(C,D)** The author's recommended reduction of this fracture. After suspending the arm from finger-traps and allowing for fracture disimpaction, pressure is applied with the thumb over the distal fragment.

lems in regaining forearm rotation while still maintaining fracture reduction.

METHODS OF IMMOBILIZATION

Milch has stated that "the reduction of a Colles' fracture represents no difficulty but the application of a plaster cast, which is tight enough to prevent displacement and not so tight as to interfere with circulation, demands skill and expertise."[96,97] All would agree that it requires "skill and expertise" to apply a cast that will maintain a reduction of an unstable fracture. Frequently, however, even the most skilled practitioner cannot maintain a reduction with plaster alone. External fixation devices, internal fixation devices, or both may be required to maintain the reduction. A desire on the part of the treating physician to maintain an anatomic reduction either with closed or open methods has lead to a deluge of literature on how to best immobilize a distal radius fracture. The problem has been to devise a method of immobilization that will maintain the reduction with a minimum of complications associated with both the fracture and its treatment, while allowing maximum mobilization of surrounding joints.

Originally, wooden or prefabricated splints were used (Colles).[25] Splints that were molded or conformed to the arm, however, rapidly became popular, and to this day, sugar tong splints that allow for some soft tissue swelling while immobilizing the wrist and forearm in a functional position are very popular (Fig. 22-17). Also very popular are long arm casts. Although it has been recognized that there are potential complications associated with a circular plaster used for an acute fracture, many believe that a circular plaster provides sufficiently better maintenance of reduction than a sugar tong splint to warrant its use.[30]

Author's Preferred Method of Immobilization

I prefer to immobilize an acute distal radius fracture in a sugar tong splint. This splint is applied while the arm is suspended from finger-traps fol-

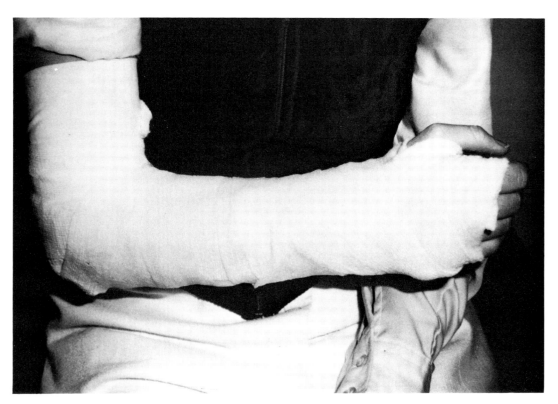

Fig. 22-17. A sugar tong splint in place for a distal radius fracture.

lowing the reduction. As the plaster dries, the fracture is manipulated into the desired position; for example, for a Colles' fracture, the wrist is manipulated into slight flexion and ulnar deviation. This splint allows for some swelling while maintaining good maintenance of reduction. As the swelling decreases, the splint can be tightened by simply overwrapping it with a 4-inch Kling bandage, thus eliminating the need for a cast change and possible associated loss of fracture reduction. The sugar tong splint is changed to a long arm cast at 2 weeks and then to a short arm cast at 4 weeks. Plaster immobilization is usually discontinued at 8 weeks and a removable splint applied, from which the patient weans himself or herself.

SKELETAL FIXATION

In spite of the expertise of the treating physician in performing a reduction and applying a plaster, and regardless of the position of immobilization, the reduction of some distal radius fractures cannot be predictably maintained with the use of splints or circular plasters alone. For this reason, many have advocated skeletal immobilization. Böhler first popularized this technique with his introduction of the pins and plaster technique in 1929.[65] Since then, many have advocated the use of this technique with pins placed in the skeleton at sites distal and proximal to the fracture, that is, the metacarpals and the radius and/or ulna.[11,21,24,36,61,65,93,124,125]

In 1944, Roger Anderson and Gordon O'Neil[4] introduced the concept of external fixation using an external frame to hold the skeletal fixation pins rather than plaster as had Böhler. This technique has become very popular today; it is used for comminuted, unstable distal radius fractures, both with and without internal fixation of the fracture fragments themselves.[28,31,64,65,75,106,126,145]

Many other forms of internal skeletal fixation have been advocated for the maintenance of reduction of distal radius fractures. These include percutaneous pins, compression screws, tension band wires, Rush rods, and plate fixation. Of these, only plate fixation enjoys wide popularity today.[8,22,41,45,46,79,84] This technique, as outlined by the Swiss, is well suited for unstable fractures with large distal fragments when early discontinuation of immobilization is desired.[70,128]

Methods of Skeletal Fixation

Operative Technique — Closed Reduction and Percutaneous Pin Fixation. Displaced fractures of the distal radius, even those that are not particularly comminuted, have a great propensity for "slipping" in casts, and for this reason, some surgeons (including the Editor, DP Green, personal communication, 1986) prefer percutaneous pin fixation for the treatment of displaced, relatively noncomminuted extraarticular fractures of the distal radius. The main prerequisite for this technique is that the radial styloid fragment be fairly large.

The procedure is done in the operating room, usually under brachial block anesthesia. A pneumatic tourniquet is not necessary, but the image intensifier greatly facilitates and shortens the time required for the procedure. After a satisfactory level of anesthesia has been achieved, the affected hand is suspended in finger-traps as previously described, with 5 to 10 pounds of counterweight across the upper arm. Closed reduction is performed in the manner described on page 1004, adequacy of reduction is confirmed radiographically, and the arm is scrubbed with a routine surgical prep. (An alternative sequence is to prep the hand first and then apply sterile finger-traps, which eliminates the problem of possible contamination on unsterile finger-traps during the actual pinning.) Pinning of the fracture is done with the hand suspended in finger traps. The largest size K-wires (0.054 or 0.0625 inch) are preferred because these can be inserted with the 3-M mini-driver using only one hand, leaving the surgeon's other hand free to stabilize the fracture. Steinmann pins must be inserted with a Jacobs' chuck, which requires both hands or an assistant to make adjustments on the pin.

Under radiographic guidance, one K-wire is inserted from the tip of the radial styloid obliquely across the fracture site to engage the ulnar cortex of the radius proximal to the fracture. A second pin is then inserted in a slightly more longitudinal direction to engage the ulnar cortex of the radius proximal to the first pin. If may be desirable to insert one pin dorsal and one pin volar to the first dorsal compartment tendons. The K-wires do *not* enter the ulna, contrary to the technique described by De-Palma.[41] If radiographs show satisfactory purchase of the pins in both the proximal and distal fragments, the finger-traps are removed and the pins are cut off approximately 2 cm above the skin and bent at right angles to facilitate later removal in the office. Generous incisions are made in the skin only (no deeper, to avoid the superficial branch of radial nerve) around the pins to prevent skin tethering. A well-padded, short-arm volar plaster splint is applied and changed a few days later in the office to a short arm cast with a window to allow the patient to care for the pins himself (application of alcohol, hydrogen peroxide, or Betadine to the skin around the pins once or twice daily). Full forearm rotation is allowed in the cast, and the cast and pins are removed at 6 weeks following reduction.

Operative Technique—AO Plating. I prefer the palmar approach because (1) less contouring of the plate is necessary; (2) the plate is well protected by soft tissue; and (3) there is less problem with tendon adherence postoperatively (Fig. 22-18). However, I do use the dorsal approach when the angle of the fracture is such that there is inadequate bone stock distally for purchase of the plate or when the fracture is semi-acute, such that an elevator will be needed to free the distal fragment from the proximal fragment (see Fig. 22-22). For a description of the operative technique of the dorsal approach to the radius, the reader is referred to the section entitled Operative Technique—Distal Radial Osteotomy on page 1018.

Under tourniquet control, the sterile-prepped and draped arm is approached through a palmar incision. The incision is centered over the flexor carpi radialis tendon sheath beginning at the palmar flexion crease and coursing proximal for 8 to 10 cm. If the patient has exhibited preoperative evidence of median nerve injury, the incision is carefully extended over the palmar cutaneous branch of the median nerve to the level of the superficial arch and the carpal canal is decompressed. The flexor carpi radialis sheath is opened, and the flexor tendons are retracted ulnarly and the radial artery radially. The pronator quadratus and flexor pollicis longus are sharply elevated from the radius and retracted. The fracture is thus exposed.

An assistant then applies traction to the fingers, disimpacting the distal fragment from the proximal fragment. Unless the bone is markedly osteoporotic, I use a periosteal elevator to lever the distal

fragment back on to the proximal radius while the fracture fragments are being distracted. Once the reduction has been obtained in this manner, an AO distal radial plate is applied. Two distal screws and one proximal screw are then inserted. If a radiograph at this time reveals an anatomic reduction, the remainder of the screws are applied. If the reduction cannot be confirmed, the one proximal screw can be removed and a better reduction obtained.

For closure, the pronator quadratus is gently sutured back into position over the plate, and the subcutaneous tissue and skin closed. A large bulky dressing is applied, incorporating a sugar tong splint. At 5 days, this is converted to a short arm cast or splint, depending upon the fixation obtained. The period of immobilization varies from 2 to 6 weeks, depending upon the degree of stability obtained at the time of open reduction. If the fracture involved the distal radioulnar joint, a long arm cast rather than a short arm cast is applied in neutral forearm rotation for the first 2 weeks.

Occasionally, traction applied to the hand and fingers by an assistant does not disimpact the fracture fragments, and because of suspected comminution of the distal fragment or osteoporosis, I am reluctant to disimpact the fragments with an elevator. In these instances, a 3-mm external fixation pin is inserted into the radial border of the second metacarpal at its base, and another percutaneously into the radial border of the radius, 12 to 15 cm proximal to the fracture. An external fixation device is then applied to the pins and distraction applied. This nicely disimpacts the fragments so that a manual reduction can be performed and an AO plate applied. Once the plate is in place, the external fixation device is removed.

Operative Technique—External Fixation. The anesthetized upper extremity is sterilely prepped from the fingertips to the lower arm, just below a pneumatic tourniquet that has been applied to the arm. Sterile finger-traps are applied to the thumb, index, and long finger. The arm is abducted from the side, the hand is suspended with finger-traps, and 5 pounds of countertraction is applied to the arm. The arm is then sterilely draped and the pneumatic tourniquet inflated.

AP and lateral radiographs of the wrist are then

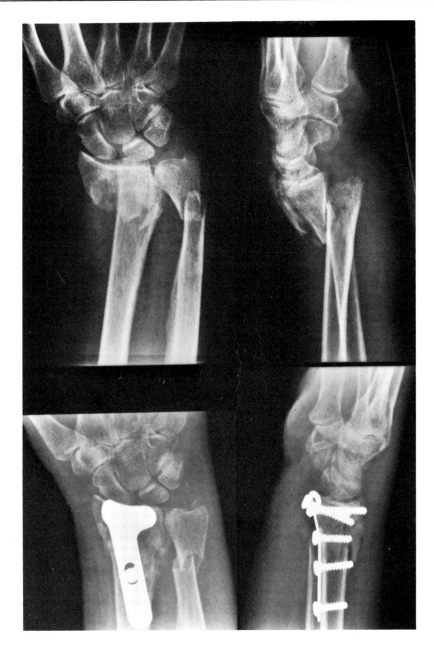

Fig. 22-18. The top two radiographs are of a dorsally displaced, open, comminuted distal radius fracture. The lower two radiographs show this fracture following open reduction and internal fixation through a volar approach.

obtained. (I have found the use of a sterilely draped C-arm most helpful in evaluating fracture reduction and placement of pins for external fixation.) The time taken in draping the C-arm and obtaining the radiographs is usually long enough to allow the fracture fragments to disimpact. If necessary, however, the wrist is gently flexed and extended to disimpact the fracture fragments. Manual reduction is then accomplished by applying pressure in the appropriate direction to restore normal anatomy (Fig. 22-16). In this manner, it should be possible to restore radial inclination and length. The dorsal tilt, however, can usually only be reduced to neutral.

If the radiographs show satisfactory reduction, 3-mm half pins are inserted under fluoroscopic control and the external fixation frame applied. For relatively stable fractures, a simple frame with a single distraction rod is used. In this instance, two parallel pins are inserted into the base of the second metacarpal on its radial aspect and two parallel pins into the radial border of the radius proximal to the fracture. These latter two pins are inserted percutaneously, just proximal to the outcropper muscle bellies. The simple frame is then applied.

For comminuted, unstable fractures a complex external fixation frame is applied incorporating two 3-mm half pins inserted into the bases of the second and third metacarpals at 60 degrees to one another and two 3-mm half pins inserted into the radial shaft proximal to the fracture, also at 60 degrees to one another; a quadrilateral frame is used.

Postoperatively, only a light bandage is applied to the wrist and early finger motion begun. If moderate radiograpic healing is present at 8 weeks, the fixator is removed and the patient is given a removable splint. This splint, however, is not removed except for bathing for the next 2 weeks. Following that, the patient removes the splint for exercises of the wrist. Immobilization is usually complete by 3 months.

Operative Technique—Combined External and Internal Fixation (Fig. 22-19). A tourniquet is applied, and, with the arm resting on a hand table, the external fixation device using a single distraction rod is applied as described above. The wrist joint is then approached through a dorsal longitudinal midline incision. The skin flaps are elevated and retracted radialward and ulnarward. The proximal portion of the extensor retinaculum is divided as far distally as the level of the radiocarpal joint. This preserves enough extensor retinaculum distal to the wrist joint to prevent later bow-stringing of the extensor tendons with wrist dorsiflexion. The retinaculum is then reflected radialward and ulnarward and the extensor pollicis longus freed from about Lister's tubercle. The wrist extensors and extensor pollicis longus are retracted radialward and the finger extensors ulnarward. The wrist joint capsule is opened transversely at the level of the radiocarpal joint. This allows excellent visualiza-

tion of the depressed fracture fragments. The fragments are manually elevated with a Freer elevator and percutaneously fixed with 0.035-inch K-wires introduced from the radial aspect of the wrist. The wires usually pass through the radial styloid and into the elevated fragment, but do not enter the distal radioulnar joint.

If the defect left in the radius from elevation of the depressed fragment is larger than 3 to 4 mm in diameter, bone graft is harvested from the iliac crest (Fig. 22-20) and packed in the defect.

The wound is then closed by reapproximating the wrist capsule and placing the divided portion of the extensor retinaculum deep to the extensor tendons. I have found it helpful postoperatively to immobilize the arm in a sugar tong splint for 3 weeks followed by an orthoplast palmar wrist splint for an additional 3 weeks. After 6 weeks, the percutaneous pins are removed; at 8 weeks the external fixator is removed; and at 10 weeks, wrist motion is begun.

If there is joint incongruity involving the sigmoid notch of the radius, every attempt is made to achieve an anatomic reduction there also. If an anatomic reduction cannot be achieved, I prefer not to proceed with immediate distal ulna excision, but instead to leave this procedure until such time as when and if the patient becomes symptomatic.

Operative Technique — Harvesting of Bone Graft (Fig. 22-20). Whenever there is the remotest chance that bone graft will be necessary, the patient is apprised of this preoperatively and the iliac crest is prepped at the time of surgery. After a rolled towel has been placed under the ipsilateral gluteal area, the iliac crest region is sterilely prepped and draped. A 5-cm long incision is made over the iliac crest beginning 2 cm posterior to the anterior superior iliac spine and coursing posteriorly. Using an osteotome, a section of the iliac crest, 3 cm in length and 1 cm thick, is reflected on its medial periosteum. This exposes an abundant area of cancellous bone, between the two cortical wings. Cancellous bone is harvested. The flap of iliac crest if then turned back down into its bed and sutured in place. (This technique leaves virtually no cosmetic defect either to the eye or touch along the iliac crest.) The wound is then closed in layers over a suction catheter drain.

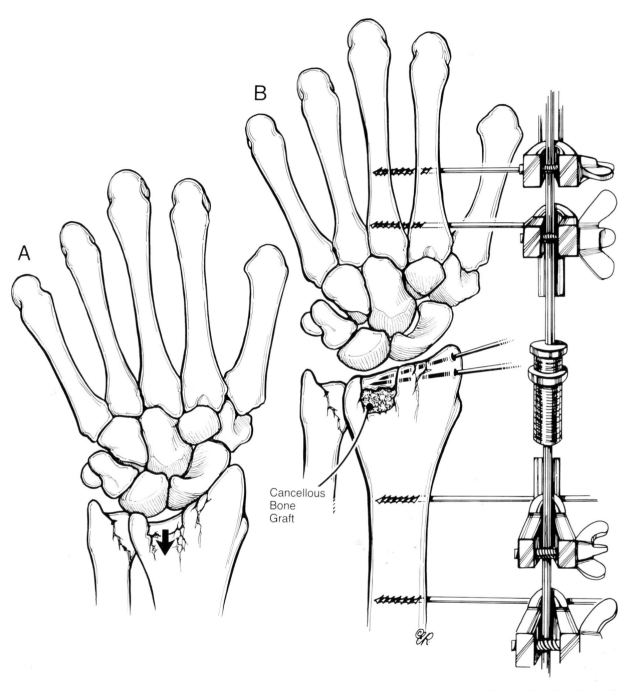

Cancellous
Bone
Graft

Fig. 22-19. A depressed fracture of the distal radius with a portion of the lunate fossa of the radius dorsally and proximally displaced is shown in (**A**). The author prefers to treat this fracture with the application of an external fixation device, carpal distraction, elevation of the depressed fragment, and fixation with two K-wires and cancellous bone grafting of the bony defect left behind by elevation of the depressed fracture fragment.

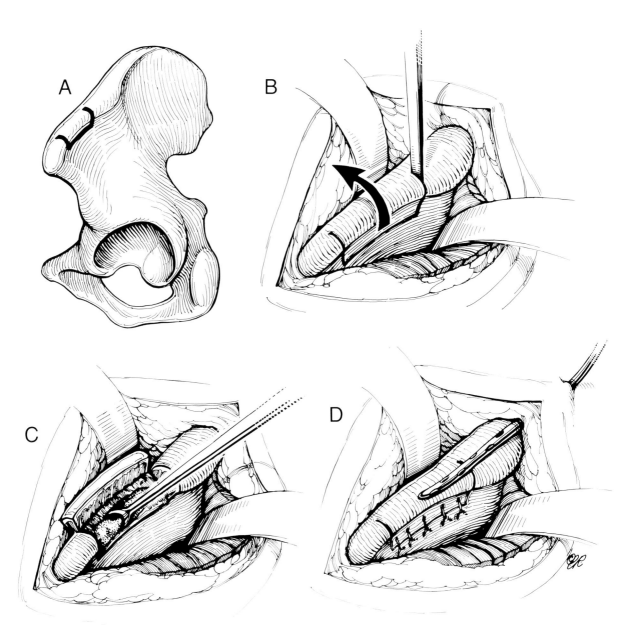

Fig. 22-20. The author's preferred method for harvesting an iliac crest bone graft. (**A**) The area of iliac crest exposure posterior to the anterior superior iliac spine. (**B**) An osteotome is used to cut through the lateral, anterior, and posterior aspects of the iliac crest, with medial reflexion of the cortical window. (**C**) A cortical window has been reflected medially, exposing abundant cancellous bone that can be easily harvested with a curette. (**D**) The cortical window has been returned to its anatomic position and sutured in place. A suction catheter for drainage is placed external to the fascial closure.

AUTHOR'S PREFERRED METHODS OF TREATMENT FOR SPECIFIC DISTAL RADIUS FRACTURES

Colles' Fracture

All distal radius fractures deserve an attempt at closed reduction or immobilization. Although an anatomic reduction is desirable, I will accept up to 2 mm of shortening and 15 degrees loss of palmar

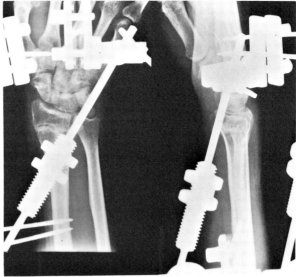

Fig. 22-22. AP and lateral radiographs showing treatment of a comminuted distal radius fracture with an external fixation device.

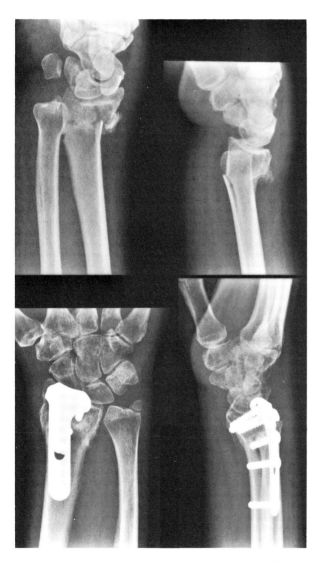

Fig. 22-21. The top two radiographs are AP and lateral views of a typical comminuted distal radius fracture with some dorsal displacement. The lower two films show the same wrist following open reduction and plating through a dorsal approach.

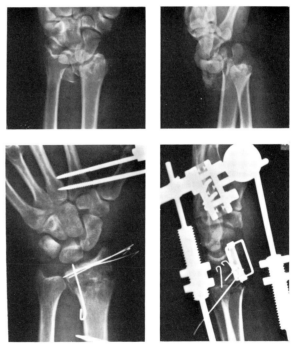

Fig. 22-23. The top two radiographs are AP and lateral views of a severely comminuted distal radius fracture. The lower two radiographs show the application of an external fixation device for treatment of this fracture, combined with open reduction and internal fixation with K-wires and bone grafting for restoration of the distal radial articular surface.

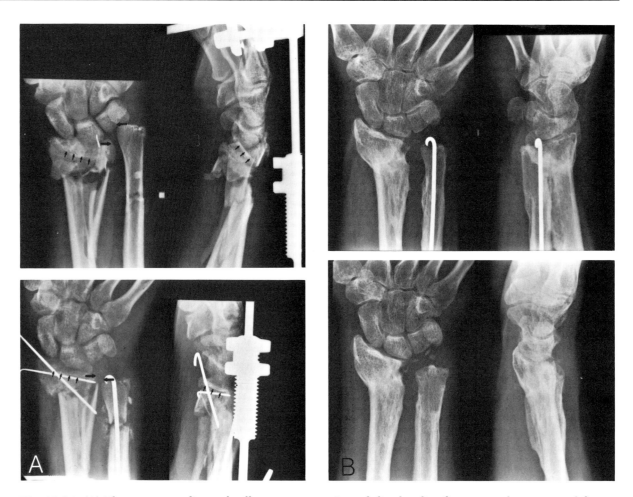

Fig. 22-24. (A) The top two radiographs illustrate a comminuted distal radius fracture with an external fixation device having been applied. In this instance, external fixation did not restore radial length or congruence of the radiocarpal joint. The lower two radiographs show the addition of elevation and pinning of the articular surfaces combined with ulnar shortening. (B) A one year follow-up of the patient in A showing healing of the radius with good reduction of the radiocarpal joint space. In the lower two radiographs, the Rush rod has been removed from the distal ulna; the patient was able to regain full pronation and supination.

tilt (in an otherwise healthy, active individual).[128] I try to accept no incongruity of either the radiocarpal or distal radioulnar articular surface (again, in an otherwise healthy and active individual). To assess the adequacy of reduction, special imaging studies, such as CT scans and hypocycloidal tomography (polytomes), are sometimes necessary.[98,99] When an acceptable reduction of a distal radius fracture cannot be obtained or maintained with closed techniques, operative treatment is recommended. The surgical approach and technique

of skeletal fixation used depend upon the specific fracture type.

If an acceptable reduction was not obtained or cannot be maintained with my plaster regimen as outlined above, surgery is undertaken. If the distal fragment is large enough to support screw fixation with a plate (i.e., the distal fragment is at least 1 cm wide and without comminution) I favor the use of an AO plate (Fig. 22-21). If the distal fragment is comminuted, I prefer external fixation (Fig. 22-22). If depression or incongruity of the articular surface of any of the distal radial articular surfaces exists, I prefer external fixation combined with reduction or elevation of the depressed fragment, fixation with K-wires and when necessary, iliac crest bone grafting of the defect below the elevated fragment (Figs. 22-23 and 22-24A and B).

Smith's Fracture

As with all fractures of the distal radius, the treatment of a volarly displaced distal radial fracture should begin with an attempt at closed reduction and plaster immobilization. If open reduction and internal fixation are needed to obtain or maintain a reduction, I prefer the palmar approach and use of a buttress plate.[14,52,55,140,147]

Barton's Fracture

Displaced Barton's fractures nearly always require open reduction and internal fixation to achieve and maintain congruous reduction.[5,7,14,40,52,81] These fractures are best fixed acutely with interfragmentary screws or pins.

Chauffeur's Fracture

In this fracture, the displaced radial styloid process remains attached to the displaced carpus, via the radial collateral ligament, radiocapitate, and occasionally the radiotriquetral ligaments. This fracture is an ideal indication for closed reduction and precutaneous pin fixation, but if anatomic alignment of the articular surface cannot be achieved by closed reduction, then open reduction and fixation with a K-wire or screw is indicated. Either method generally restores complete stability to the carpus,[50,51,57,90] and extensive ligamentous reconstruction of the wrist is seldom necessary (Fig. 22-25).

Lunate Load Fracture (Die Punch Fracture)

Depression fracture of the lunate fossa of the radius results from severe axial loading of the forearm unit. Although the severity of the original injury may predispose to a poor result, I believe that the best way to minimize the chances of this is with an anatomic reduction.[13,33,34,95] As the depressed

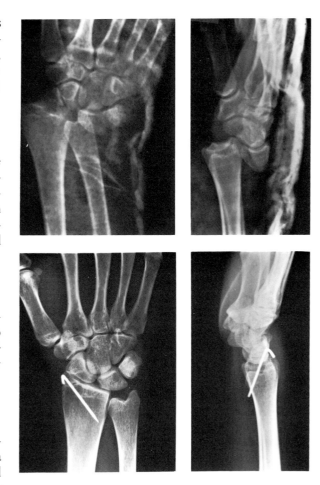

Fig. 22-25. The top two radiographs depict a chauffeur's-type fracture with marked dorsal and ulnar displacement of the radial styloid and entire carpus. The lower two radiographs show restoration of the radiocarpal articulation with simple fixation of the radial styloid process.

fragment is frequently depressed dorsally only, the wrist should usually be approached dorsally. The fragment is elevated, fixed with K-wires, and the defect left below the elevated fragment filled with bone graft (Fig. 22-26). External fixation of the wrist in conjunction with K-wire fixation of the fragment is seldom necessary, as the patient's bone stock is usually sufficient to support K-wire fixation. I believe that the displaced die-punch fracture should be reduced anatomically whether it is an isolated fracture (as illustrated in Fig. 22-26) or part of a comminuted distal radius fracture.

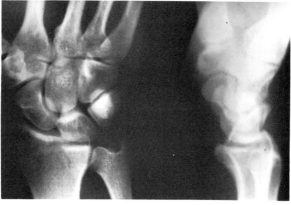

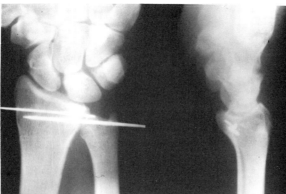

regardless of age, adequacy of treatment or severity of fracture was 24 percent permanent loss of function of the hand."[6]

The complications associated with Colles' fracture that result in these surprisingly high unsatisfactory results are persistent neuropathy, radiocarpal or radioulnar arthrosis, malposition/malunion, nonunion, tendon ruptures, reflex sympathetic dystrophy, finger stiffness, and Volkmann's ischemia.[6,16,19,44,60,69,71,81,84,85,91,105,119,135]   An understanding that these problems exist and are in fact,

Fig. 22-26. The top two radiographs illustrate an isolated depressed lunate load (die-punch) fracture. The lower two radiographs show the fracture following open reduction of the lunate fossa and fixation with K-wires.

COMPLICATIONS

Although it was once believed by many that all patients with distal radius fractures did relatively well, regardless of treatment, it is now well recognized that distal radius fractures are associated with a high complication rate. Fractures involving the radiocarpal or distal radioulnar articular surface are especially prone to complications.

Cooney et al, in an excellent review of 565 fractures, found a complication rate of 31 percent.[30] Gartland and Werley, in reporting "surprisingly good results" found unsatisfactory results in 31.7 percent of their patients.[60] Bacorn and Kurtzke reported a series of 2,132 cases of Colles' fracture recorded by the New York Compensation Board in which only 2.9 percent were judged to have no permanent disability and "the average disability

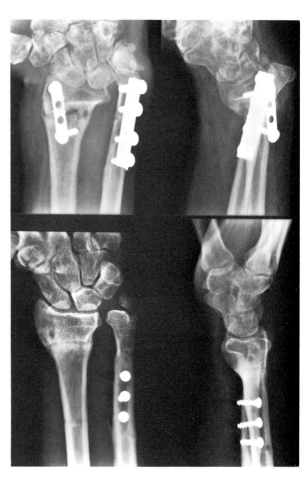

Fig. 22-27. The top two radiographs show a distal radius fracture treated with a small fragment fixation device that led to a nonunion of the distal radius and a malunion of the distal ulna. The lower two radiographs show the same wrist following removal of the hardware, osteotomy of the radius and ulna, external fixation and bone grafting of the distal radius, shortening of the ulna, and eventual union of the radius and ulna.

relatively common sequelae of distal radial fractures should, in my opinion, lead us to be more aggressive in the original care of such fractures.

Acute Median Nerve Compression

As mentioned on page 999, acute nerve compression or injury should be dealt with by an immediate reduction of the fracture. However, in considering nerve decompression, it should always be remembered that an injured nerve that does not improve with fracture reduction seldom improves completely with nerve decompression.

Reflex Sympathetic Dystrophy

Although complete reflex sympathetic dystrophy is a relatively uncommon problem, milder variants are surprisingly common in conjunction with distal radius fractures. Early attention to pa-

tients with an inordinate amount of pain, finger stiffness, or paresthesias may prevent many of the problems of this serious complication. Early splinting or immobilization to alleviate pain, removal or splitting of a dressing or cast to relieve pressure, elevation of an edematous hand, and/or intensive hand therapy are frequently very helpful in preventing the development of complete sympathetic dystrophy. Recognition and treatment of acute median nerve compression may also abort the development of dystrophy. For the patient who does not respond to early local measures, sympathetic blocks, even while the cast is in place, should be considered (see Chapter 15).

Nonunion

Nonunions of distal radius fractures are extremely rare, but they do occur and are usually symptomatic. In contrast, nonunions of ulnar styloid process fractures in conjunction with distal

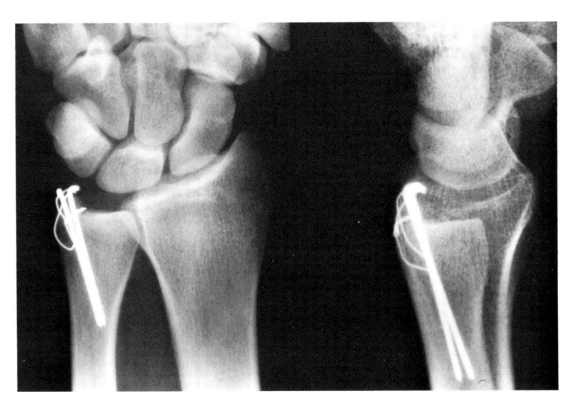

Fig. 22-28. Fixation of a large ulnar styloid fracture that was associated with instability of the distal radioulnar joint prior to being repaired.

radius fractures are quite common, yet are rarely symptomatic (Fig. 22-27).[44] Treatment for distal radius nonunions must be individualized and based on the patient's symptoms, functional deficit, and bony substance. Basically, however, one should strive to achieve union with rigid internal fixation and iliac crest bone grafting. Symptomatic nonunions of the ulnar styloid are best treated with styloid excision unless the ulnar styloid fragment is quite large, in which case the fragment should be treated with open reduction and internal fixation (Fig. 22-28). If the styloid nonunion is accompanied by distal ulnar instability, the TFCC should be reattached to the fovea at the time of fragment excision or fixation (see Chapter 21).

Malunion

Reduction and maintenance of reduction of the fracture remains the single most important factor in the overall outcome of a distal radius fracture. Malunions of distal radius fractures, as one might expect, are quite common. Based upon comments in the literature, one would not expect that many of these malunions would be symptomatic, but in my experience they are frequently found to cause significant symptoms. Malunions result in wrist pain (radiocarpal, radioulnar, and/or ulnocarpal), decreased range of motion, and/or midcarpal instability. To treat a malunion of the distal radius, one may excise the distal ulna, osteotomize the malunited radius, or both. Distal ulna resection (Fig. 22-29) (Darrach procedure) or a limited distal ulna resection (Fig. 22-30) (Bowers' hemiresection interposition arthroplasty) may be appropriate treatment for problems of the ulnocarpal or distal radioulnar joint in older individuals (see Chapter 21).[10,39] In younger individuals with a cosmetic or functional disability or individuals with problems restricted to the radiocarpal or midcarpal joint secondary to a malunited distal radius fracture, a distal radial osteotomy with iliac crest bone graft is advised (Fig. 22-31).[16,54,71,128,131,135]

Operative Technique — Distal Radial Osteotomy

Under tourniquet control, the wrist is approached through a dorsal midline incision (Fig. 22-32). The skin flaps are elevated and retracted

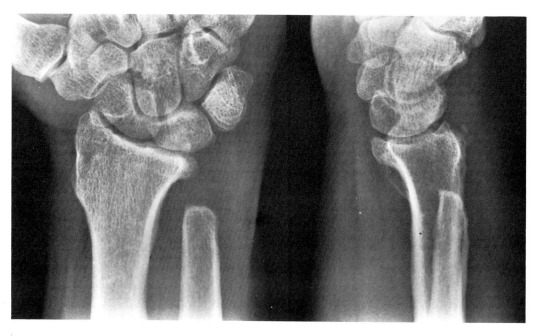

Fig. 22-29. The typical appearance following a Darrach procedure for distal radioulnar joint incongruity.

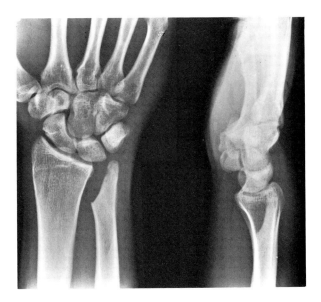

Fig. 22-30. The typical appearance following a HIT procedure (Hemi-resection interposition arthroplasty) procedure as described by Bowers for distal radioulnar joint incongruity (see Chapter 21).

until the radiocarpal articular surface is at the same level as the distal surface of the ulnar head, thus restoring radial length. If correction in two planes is required, it is necessary to cut the volar periosteum (at least on the radial aspect) to allow the gap to be widened on the radial side as well as dorsally. A 0.045-inch K-wire is then inserted percutaneously through the ulnar head into the distal radial fragment. This pin will maintain radial length while an x-ray of the reduction is taken. If the correction is satisfactory, Lister's tubercle is removed with a rongeur or osteotome, and an AO distal radial plate is applied, screwed in place, and the temporary transfixing K-wire removed. The distal radioulnar joint is then manually stressed. If it is unstable, the

radially and ulnarly. The proximal portion of the extensor retinaculum is opened as far distally as the level of the radiocarpal joint. This preserves enough extensor retinaculum distal to the wrist joint to prevent later bowstringing of the extensor tendons with wrist extension. The retinaculum is then reflected radialward and ulnarward and the extensor pollicis longus tendon freed from about Lister's tubercle. The wrist and finger extensors are retracted radialward and the extensor digiti quinti and extensor carpi ulnaris ulnarward.

The wrist joint capsule is then opened in a T-shaped fashion with the longitudinal limb over the ulnar border of the radius and the transverse limb at the level of the radiocarpal joint. The capsule and radial periosteum are elevated as one. This exposes the distal radioulnar joint but leaves intact the TFCC origin from the distal radius and insertion into the ulnar styloid base.

Using a power saw, the radius in then divided 1.5 cm proximal to the radiocarpal joint, leaving intact the volar periosteum. Using manual pressure or a lamina spreader, the distal fragment is palmar flexed, opening up the dorsal cortex. The distal fragment is displaced distally and flexed palmarly

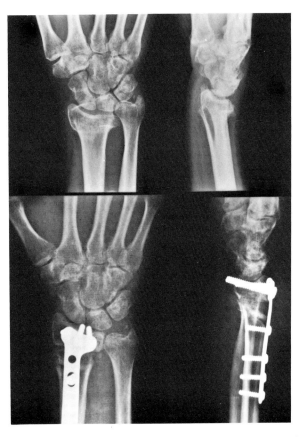

Fig. 22-31. The top two radiographs show a malunited distal radius fracture with marked radial shortening and dorsal tilt of the distal radial fragment. The lower two films illustrate the same wrist following osteotomy, distraction, plating, and bone grafting of the distal radius with restoration of the normal volar tilt and radial length.

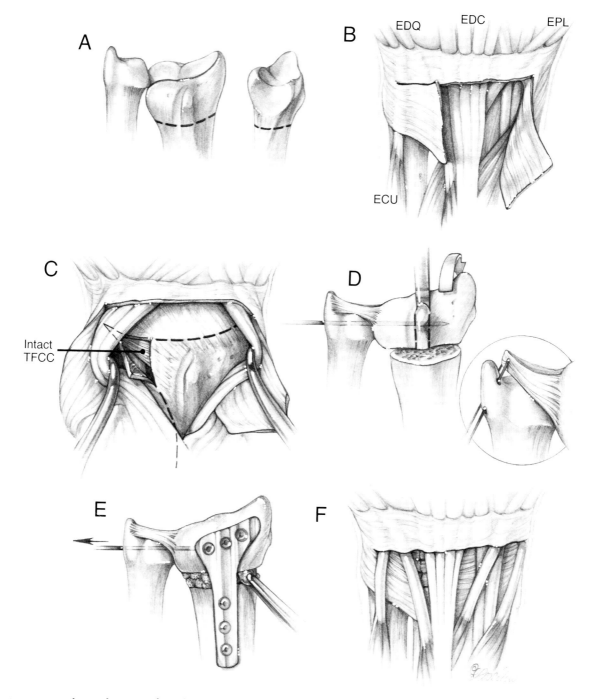

Fig. 22-32. The author's preferred technique for distal radial osteotomy and bone grafting. (**A**) The level of cut through the radius. (**B**) The extensor retinaculum is preserved distal to the radiocarpal joint and opened in a T-shaped fashion proximal to the radiocarpal joint. (**C**) The capsule is opened in a T-shaped fashion over the distal radioulnar and radiocarpal joints, preserving the TFCC origin from the radius and insertion into the ulnar styloid. (**D**) After the osteotomy of the radius is completed, the distal articular fragment of the radius is distracted and rotated palmarly to open a wedge dorsally. A pin is passed through the ulnar head into the distal radial fragment once the radial fragment has been elevated to the proper level. Detail illustrates reattachment of the TFCC to the base of the ulnar styloid following plating of the radius if the distal radioulnar joint is unstable. (**E**) A plate has been applied to the dorsal radius, and cancellous bone graft is being packed beneath the plate into the osteotomy site. (**F**) Closure of the wrist with the proximal retinaculum placed deep to the extensor tendons to cover the plate and reinforce the capsular closure. The distal extensor retinaculum is still in place, preventing bowstringing of the tendons.

TFCC insertion into the ulnar styloid is tightened by passing a nonabsorbable suture through the styloid base, through the TFCC, and back out through the styloid base. Tying this suture down tight over the ulnar border of the ulna tightens the TFCC and stabilizes the distal ulna in the sigmoid notch. Iliac crest bone graft is then harvested in the manner previously described. Cancellous bone is firmly packed into the osteotomy site. No cortical bone is used.

The capsule of the wrist joint and distal radioulnar joint are then closed with nonabsorbable suture material over the plate. The previously divided extensor retinaculum is closed deep to the extensor tendons to reinforce the capsular closure.

Postoperatively, the fracture is immobilized in a long arm cast for 4 weeks followed by a short arm cast for an additional 2 weeks. Radiographic union is usually complete at 4 to 8 weeks.

TREATMENT OF FRACTURES IN CHILDREN

Distal radial epiphyseal injuries are the most common epiphyseal injury, accounting for about 50 percent of all epiphyseal injuries.[2,72,120,134]

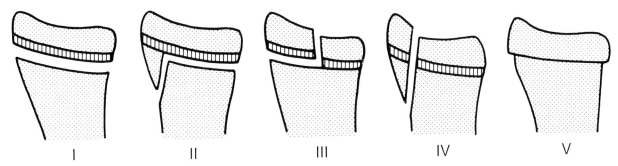

Fig. 22-33. Salter-Harris classification of distal radial epiphyseal fractures in children. Type V is a crush injury.

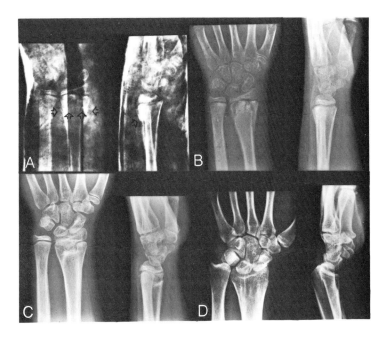

Fig. 22-34. (A) Films illustrate a Type II epiphyseal fracture of the distal radius as seen through plaster at age 10. (B) Films reveal early healing of the fracture. (C) These films reveal partial epiphyseal closure at age 13, with some early ulnar overgrowth and increased volar tilt of the distal radius. (D) Radiographs at age 22 reveal marked ulnar overgrowth and volar tilt of the radius, 12 years after this Type II fracture of the distal radius with partial epiphyseal closure occurred.

They usually occur in children between the ages of 6 and 10. The physeal injury is usually a Type II fracture in the Salter-Harris classification (Fig. 22-33).[2,120,134] Treatment consists of a gentle attempt at closed reduction followed by immobilization in a long arm cast for 4 to 6 weeks.[92]

Repeated attempts at reduction should be avoided, for even if the reduction is poor, remodeling is usually such that no functional deficit is noted. As with all epiphyseal fractures, occasionally what appears to be a Type I or II fracture is really a Type V fracture, that is, a crushing injury of the germinal cells of the epiphysis. When this happens, premature closure of all or part of the epiphyseal plate results and deformity of the distal radius develops as the patient grows (Fig. 22-34). The treatment of choice for premature epiphyseal closure must be individualized. Treatment options include epiphyseodesis of the distal ulnar epiphysis, distal radial osteotomy, epiphyseal bar resection and insertion of a spacer such as fat, or a combination thereof (Fig. 22-35). All treatment decisions should be predicated not only upon the patient's cosmetic and functional desires, but upon any future deformities that might develop as a result of abnormal epiphyseal growth.

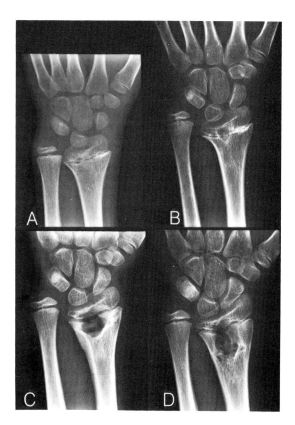

Fig. 22-35. (A) This radiograph reveals early distal radial epiphyseal closure one year after a Type II fracture (partial Type V) of the distal radius has occurred. In (**B**), marked ulnar overgrowth 2 years later is revealed as a result of partial distal radial epiphyseal closure; (**C**) shows the same wrist 3 months following resection of the distal radial bar and insertion of an abdominal fat graft. (**D**) The same wrist 1½ years later with the distal radial epiphysis completely open, the fat still in place, and some early correction of the discrepancy in relative radioulnar lengths.

REFERENCES

1. AF Ekenstam F, Hagert CB: Anatomical studies on the geometry and stability of the distal radio ulnar joint. Scand J Plast Reconstr Surg 19:17–25, 1985
2. Aitken AP: Further observations on the fractured distal radial epiphysis. J Bone Joint Surg 17:922–927, 1935
3. Alffram PA, Bauer GCH: Epidemiology of fractures of the forearm. A biomechanical investigation of bone strength. J Bone Joint Surg 44A:105–114, 1962
4. Anderson R, O'Neil G: Comminuted fractures of the distal end of the radius. Surg Gynecol Obstet 78:434–440, 1944
5. Aufranc OE, Jones WN, Turner RH: Anterior marginal articular fracture of distal radius. JAMA 196:788–791, 1966
6. Bacorn RW, Kurtzke JF: Colles' fracture: A study of two thousand cases from the New York State Workmen's Compensation Board. J Bone Joint Surg 35A:643–658, 1953
7. Barton JR: Views and treatment of an important injury to the wrist. Med Examiner 1:365, 1838
8. Bate JT: Apparatus for use in reduction and fixation of fractures of distal radius. Clin Orthop 63:190–195, 1969
9. Bilos ZJ, Pankovinch AM, Yelda S: Fracture-dislocation of the radiocarpal joint. A clinical study of five cases. J Bone Joint Surg 59A:198–203, 1977
10. Bowers WH: The distal radioulnar joint. pp. 743–769. In: Green DP (ed): Operative Hand Surgery Vol. 1. Churchill Livingstone, New York, 1982

11. Brady LP: Double pin fixation of severely comminuted fractures of the distal radius and ulna. South Med J 56:307–311, 1963

12. Brindley H: Wrist injuries. Clinical Orthop Rel Research 83:17–23, 1972

13. Buterbaugh G, Palmer A: Lunate load fractures — An anatomical and biomechanical study. Presented at the American Society for Surgery of the Hand Annual Meeting, New Orleans, February, 1986

14. Caldwell JA: Manuel of the treatment of fractures. Charles C Thomas, Springfield, IL, 1947

15. Caldwell JA: Device for making traction on the fingers. JAMA 96:1226, 1931

16. Campbell WC: Malunited Colles' fracture. JAMA 109:1105–1108, 1937

17. Carothers RG, Berning DN: Colles' fracture. Am J Surg 80:626–629, 1950

18. Carothers RG, Boyd FJ: Thumb traction technique for reduction of Colles' fracture. Arch Surg, 58:848–852, 1949

19. Cassebaum WH: Colles' fracture: A study of end results. JAMA 143:963–965, 1950

20. Cautilli RA, Joyce MF, Gordon E, Juarez R: Classifications of fractures of the distal radius. Clin Orthop 103:163–166, 1974

21. Chapman DR, Bennett JB, Bryan WJ, Tullos HS: Complications of distal radial fractures: Pins and plaster treatment. J Hand Surg 7:509–512, 1982

22. Clancey GJ: Percutaneous Kirscher wire fixation of Colles' fractures. A prospective study of thirty-five cases. J Bone Joint Surg 66A:1008–1014, 1984

23. Cobb AG, Houghton GR: Comparison of local anesthetic infiltration and intravenous regional anesthesia in patients with Colles' fractures. J Bone Joint Surg 67B:845, 1985

24. Cole JM, Obletz BE: Comminuted fractures of the distal end of the radius treated by skeletal transfixion in plaster cast: An end result study of thirty-three cases. J Bone Joint Surg 48A:931–945, 1966

25. Colles A: On the fracture of the carpal extremity of the radius. Edinburgh Med Surg J 10:182–186, 1814

26. Colles A: The classic: On the fracture of the carpal extremity of the radius. (Reprinted from the original 1814 article) Clin Orthop 83:3–5, 1972

27. Conwell HE, Vesely DG: Fractures of the distal radius in adults. Clin Orthop 83:13–16, 1972

28. Cooney WP, III: External mini-fixators: Clinical applications and techniques. pp. 155–171. In Johnston RM (ed): Continuing Education Course on External Fixation. Year Book Publishers, Chicago, 1980

29. Cooney WP: External Fixation of distal radius fractures. Clin Orthop 180:44–49, 1983

30. Cooney WP, III, Dobyns JH, Linscheid RL: Complications of Colles' fractures. J Bone Joint Surg 62A:613–619, 1980

31. Cooney WP, III, Linscheid RL, Dobyns JH: External pin fixation for unstable Colles' fractures. J Bone Joint Surg 61A:840–845, 1979

32. Cornell NW: Fractures of the base of the radius in adults. Arch Surg 31:897–916, 1935

33. Cotton FJ: The pathology of fracture of the lower extremity of the radius. Ann Surg 32:194–218, 1900

34. Cotton FJ: The pathology of fractures of the lower extremity of the radius. Ann Surg 32:388–415, 1900

35. Cozen L: Colles' fracture: A method of maintaining reduction. Calif Med 75:362–364, 1951

36. Darrach W: Colles' fracture. N Engl J Med 226:594–596, 1942

37. Darrach W: Forward dislocations at the inferior radioulnar joint fracture of the lower third of the radius. Ann Surg 56:801, 1912

38. Darrach W: Fractures of the lower extremity of the radius: Diagnosis and treatment. JAMA 89:1683–1685, 1927

39. Darrach W: Partial excision of the lower shaft of ulna for deformity following Colles' fracture. Ann Surg 17:764–765, 1913

40. DeOliveira JC: Barton's fractures. J Bone Joint Surg 55A:586–594, 1973

41. DePalma AF: Comminuted fractures of the distal end of the radius treated by ulnar pinning. J Bone Joint Surg 34A:651–662, 1952

42. Destot E: Injuries of the wrist: A radiological study. (Translated by Atkinson FRB.) Ernest Benn, London, 1925

43. Dingman PVC: Resection of the distal end of the ulna (Darrach Operation): An end-result study of twenty-four cases. J Bone Joint Surg 34A:893–900, 1952

44. Dobyns JH, Linscheid RL: Complications of treatment of fractures and dislocations of the wrist. pp. 271–352. In Epps CH Jr (ed): Complications in Orthopaedic Surgery. JB Lippincott, Philadelphia, 1978

45. Dobyns JH, Linscheid RL: pp. 411–510. In Rockwood CA, Green DP (eds): Fractures in Adults 2nd. Ed. JB Lippincott, Philadelphia, 1984

46. Dowling JJ, Sawyer B: Comminuted Colles' fractures—Evaluation of a method of treatment. J Bone Joint Surg 43A:657–668, 1961

47. Dunn AW: Fractures and dislocations of the carpus. Surg Clin North Am 52:1513–1538, 1972

48. Dupuytren B: On the injuries and diseases of bones. The Sydenham Society, London, 1847

49. Edwards H, Clayton EB: Colles' fractures. (Correspondence) Br Med J 1:523, 1929

50. Edwards H, Clayton EB: Fractures of the lower end of the radius in adults (Colles' fracture and backfire fracture). Brit Med J 1:61–65, 1929

51. Edwards HC: The mechanism and treatment of backfire fracture. J Bone Joint Surg 8:701–717, 1926

52. Ellis J: Smith's and Barton's fractures: A method of treatment. J Bone Joint Surg 47B:724–727, 1965

53. Fahey JH: Fractures and dislocations about the wrist. Surg Clin North Am 37:19–40, 1957

54. Fernandez DL: Correction of post-traumatic wrist deformity in adults by osteotomy, bone grafting and internal fixation. J Bone Joint Surg 64A:1164–1178, 1982

55. Fernandez DL: Irreducible radiocarpal fracture-dislocation and radioulnar dissociation with entrapment of the ulnar nerve, artery and flexor profundus II-V—Case Report. J Hand Surg 6:456–461, 1981

56. Fisk GR: An overview of injuries of the wrist. Clin Orthop 149:137–144, 1980

57. Fitzsimons RA: Colles' fracture and chauffeur's fracture. Br Med J 2:357–360, 1938

58. Freese CF: Treatment of comminuted Colles' fracture by ulnar styloid resection. NYS J Med 49:2540, 1949

59. Frykman G: Fracture of the distal radius including sequelae—Shoulder-hand-finger syndrome, disturbance in the distal radio-ulnar joint and impairment of nerve function. Acta Orthop Scan (Suppl.) 108:1–153, 1967

60. Gartland JJ, Werley CW: Evaluation of healed Colles' fractures. J Bone Joint Surg 33A:895–907, 1951

61. Geckeler EO: Treatment of comminuted Colles' fracture. J Int Col Surg 20:596–601, 1953

62. Ghormley RK, Mroz RJ: Fractures of the wrist—A review of one hundred seventy-six cases. Surg Gynecol Obstet 55:377–381, 1932

63. Gibson AGF, Bannister GC: Bracing or plaster for Colles' fractures? A randomized prospective controlled trial. J Bone Joint Surg 65B:221, 1983

64. Grana WA, Kopta JA: The Roger Anderson device in the treatment of fractures of the distal end of the radius. J Bone Joint Surg 61A:1234–1238, 1979

65. Green DP: Pins and plaster treatment of comminuted fractures of the distal end of the radius. J Bone Joint Surg 57A:304–310, 1975

66. Green JT, Gay FH: Colles' fracture—residual disability. Am J Surg 91:636–646, 1956

67. Gurd FB: The Colles-Pouteau fracture of the lower end of the radius. Am J Surg 38:526–538, 1937

68. Heim U, Pfeiffer KM: Small fragment set manual. 2nd Ed. pp. 119–161. Springer-Verlag, New York, 1982

69. Helal B, Chen SC, Iwegbu G: Rupture of the extensor pollicis longus tendon in undisplaced Colles' type of fracture. Hand 14:41–47, 1982

70. Hitzrot JM, Murray CR: The factors that influence the prognosis in fractures at the base of the radius. Am J Surg 35:17–29, 1921

71. Hobart MH, Kraft GL: Malunited Colles' fracture. Am J Surg 53:55–60, 1941

72. Hoffman BP: Fractures of the distal end of the radius in the adult and in the child. Bull Hosp Joint Dis 14:114–124, 1953

73. Hollingsworth R, Morris J: The importance of the ulnar side of the wrist in fractures of the distal end of the radius. Injury 7:263–266, 1976

74. Hudson OC, Rusnack TJ: Comminuted fractures of the lower end of the radius. Am J Surg 95:74–80, 1958

75. Huiskes R, Chao ES: Guidelines for external fixation frame rigidity and stress. J Orthop Res 4:68–75, 1986

76. Hulten O: Ober Anatomische variationen der handgelenkknocken: ein beitrag zur kenntnis der genese zwei verschiedener mondbeinveranderungen. Acta Radiol 9:115–168, 1928

77. Hyman G, Martin FR: Dislocation of the inferior radio-ulnar joint as a complication of fracture of the radius. Brit J Surg 27:481–491, 1939

78. Jones KG: Colles' fracture. J Arkansas Med Soc 73:244–247, 1976

79. Katznelson A, Volpin G, Lin E: Tension band wiring for fixation of comminuted fractures of the distal radius injury 12:239–242, 1984

80. King RE: Barton's fracture-dislocation of the wrist. Curr. Pract Orthop Surg 6:133–144, 1975

81. Knapp ME: Treatment of some complications of Colles' fracture. JAMA 148:825–827, 1952

82. Knirk JL, Jupiter JB: Intraarticular fractures of the distal end of the radius in young adults. J Bone Joint Surg 68A:647–659, 1986.

83. Knirk JL, Jupiter JB: Intraarticular distal radial fractures in young adults. Orthop Trans 9:456–457, 1985

84. Kristiansen A, Gjersoe E: Colles' fracture: Operative treatment, indications and results. Acta Orthop Scand 39:33–46, 1968

85. LeBreton P: Arthritis of the joints of the hand following Colles' fracture. Surg Gynecol Obstet 20:450–455, 1915

86. Lewis MH: Median nerve decompression after Colles' fracture. J Bone Joint Surg 60B:195–196, 1978

87. Lewis RM: Colles' fracture—Causative mechanism. Surg 27:427–436,1950

88. Lewis OJ, Hamshere RJ, Bucknill TM: The anatomy of the wrist joint. J Anat 106:539–552, 1970

89. Lidstrom A: Fractures of the distal radius. A clinical and statistical study of end results. Acta Orthop Scand (Suppl.) 41:1–95, 1959

90. Lund FB: Fractures of the radius in starting automobiles. Boston Med Surg J 151:481–486, 1904

91. Lynch AC, Lipscomb PR: The carpal tunnel syndrome and Colles' fractures. J Am Med Assn 185:363–366, 1963

92. Manoli A: Irreducible fracture-separation of the distal radial epiphysis. A case report. J Bone Joint Surg 64A:1095–1096, 1982

93. Marsh HO, Teal SW: Treatment of comminuted fractures of the distal radius with self-contained skeletal traction. Am J Surg 124:715–719, 1972

94. Mayer JH: Colles' fractures of the distal radius. Brit J Surg 27:629–642, 1940

95. Melone CP: Articular fractures of the distal radius. Orthop Clin North Am 15:217–236, 1984

96. Milch H: Colles' fracture. Bull Hosp Joint Dis 11:61–74, 1950

97. Milch H: Treatment of disabilities following fracture of the lower end of the radius. Clin Orthop 29:157–163, 1963

98. Mino D, Palmer AK, Levinsohn EM: The role of radiology and computerized tomography in the diagnosis of subluxation and dislocation of the distal radioulnar joint. J Hand Surg 8:23–31, 1983

99. Mino DE, Palmer AK, Levinsohn EM: Radiography and computerized tomography in the diagnosis of incongruity of the distal radioulnar joint. J Bone Surg 67A:247–252, 1985

100. Mital MA, Patel UH: Fractures and dislocations about the distal forearm, wrist, and hand. Progress in treatment in the last decade. Am J Surg 124:660–665, 1972

101. Moberg E: Shoulder-hand-finger syndrome, reflex dystrophy, causalgia. (Abstract) Acta Chir Scand 125:523, 1963

102. Moore EM: Three cases illustrating luxation of the ulna in connection with Colles' fracture. Med Record 17:305–308, 1880

103. Morrissy RT, Nalebuff EA: Distal radial fracture with tendon entrapment. A Case Report. Clin Orthop 124:205, 1977

104. Morton R: A radiographic survey of 170 cases clinically diagnosed as "Colles' fracture." Lancet 1:731–732, 1907

105. Murakami Y, Todani K: Traumatic entrapment of the extensor pollicis longus tendon in Smith's fracture of the radius—Case Report. J Hand Surg 6:238–240, 1981

106. Nakata RY, Chand Y, Matiko JD, Frykman GK, Wood VE: External fixators for wrist fractures: A biomechanical and clinical study. J Hand Surg 10A:845–851, 1985

107. Palmer AK, Skahen JR, Werner FW, Glisson RR: The extensor retinaculum of the wrist: An anatomical and biomechanical study. J Hand Surg 10B:11–16, 1985

108. Palmer AK, Werner FW: The triangular fibrocartilage complex of the wrist—Anatomy and function. J Hand Surg 6:153–162, 1981

109. Peltier LF: Eponymic fractures: Abraham Colles and Colles' fracture. Surgery 35:322–328, 1954

110. Peltier LF: Eponymic fractures: John Rhea Barton and Barton's fractures. Surgery 34:960–970, 1953

111. Peltier LF: Eponymic fractures: Robert William Smith and Smith's fracture. Surgery 45:1035–1042, 1959

112. Peltier LF: Fractures of the distal end of the radius. An historical account. Clin Orthop 187:18–22, 1984

113. Pilcher LS: Fractures of the lower extremity or base of the radius. Ann Surg 65:1–27, 1917

114. Plewes LW: Colles' and Smith's fractures. J Bone Joint Surg 44B:227, 1962

115. Pouteau, p. 310. In Stimson, LA (ed): Fractures and Dislocations. 7th Ed., Lea & Febriger, New York, 1912

116. Reeves B: Excision of the ulnar styloid fragment after Colles' fracture. Int Surg 45:46–52, 1966

117. Rogers SC: An analysis of Colles' fracture. Brit Med J 1:807–809, 1944

118. Rychak JS, Kalenak A: Injury to the median and ulnar nerves secondary to fracture of the radius. A case report. J Bone Joint Surg 59A:414–415, 1977

119. Sadr B: Sequential rupture of extensor tendons after a Colles' fracture. J Hand Surg 9A:144–145, 1984

120. Salter RB, Harris WR: Injuries involving the epiphyseal plate. J Bone Surg 45A:587–622, 1963

121. Sarmiento A: The brachioradialis as a deforming force in Colles' fractures. Clin Orthop 38:86–92, 1965

122. Sarmiento A, Pratt GW, Berry NC, Sinclair WF: Colles' fractures: Functional bracing in supination. J Bone Joint Surg 57A:311–317, 1975

123. Sarmiento A, Zagorski JB, Sinclair WF: Functional bracing of Colles' fractures: A prospective study of immobilization in supination vs pronation. Clin Orthop 146:175–183, 1980

124. Scheck M: Long term follow-up of treatment of

comminuted fractures of the distal end of the radius by transfixation with Kirschner wires and cast. J Bone Joint Surg 44A:337–351, 1962

125. Schurmeier HL: Mechanics of fractures at the wrist. JAMA 77:2119, 1921

126. Scott IH: Comminuted Colles' fractures: Their treatment by skeletal pinning and external fixation. J Int Col Surg 41:521–526, 1964

127. Sever JW: Colles' fracture: A study of x-ray films before and after reduction. New Engl J Med 226:790–794, 1942

128. Short W, Palmer A, Werner F: Distal radial fractures: A clinical and biomechanical study. Presented at the American Society for Surgery of the Hand Annual Meeting, New Orleans, February, 1986

129. Smaill GB: Long-term follow-up of Colles' fracture. J Bone Joint Surg 47B:80–85, 1965

130. Snodgrass LE: Fractures of the carpal bones. Am J Surg 38:539–548, 1937

131. Speed JS, Knight RA: Treatment of malunited Colles' fractures. J Bone Joint Surg 27:361–367, 1945

132. Speed K: Traumatic injuries of the carpus, including Colles' fracture. Appleton, New York, 1925

133. Stevens JH: Compression fractures of the lower end of the radius. Ann Surg 71:594–618, 1920

134. Tachdjian M: Pediatric orthopedics. p. 1643. WB Saunders, Philadelphia, 1972

135. Taleisnik J, Watson HK: Midcarpal instability caused by malunited fractures of the distal radius. J Hand Surg 9A: 350–357, 1984

136. Tanzer TL, Horne JG: Dorsal radiocarpal fracture dislocation. J Trauma 20:999-1000, 1980

137. Taylor GW, Parsons CL: Fractures of the lower end of the radius. Surg Gynecol Obstet 67:249–252, 1938

138. Taylor GW, Parsons CL: The role of the discus articularis in Colles' fracture. J Bone Joint Surg 20:149–152, 1938

139. Testut JL, Laterjet A: Traite d'Anatomie Humaine Vol. 1. 8th Ed. Doion, Paris, 1928

140. Thomas FB: Reduction of Smith's fracture. J Bone Joint Surg 39B:463–470, 1957

141. Thomas NP, Ferris BD, Simpson D, Dewar M: The Roehampton brace. J Bone Joint Surg 67B:493, 1985

142. Toft P, Bertheussen K, Otkjaer S: Translunate, transmetacarpal, scapho-radial fracture with perilunate dislocation — A case report. J Hand Surg 10B:382–384, 1985

143. Van der Linden W, Ericson R: Colles' fracture: How should its displacement be measured and how should it be immobilized? J Bone Joint Surg 63A:1285–1288, 1981

144. Wahlstrom O: Treatment of Colles' fracture. A prospective comparison of three different positions of immobilization. Acta Orthop Scan 53:225, 1982

145. Weber SC, Szabo RM: Severely comminuted distal radial fracture as an unsolved problem. Complications associated with external fixation and pins and plaster techniques. J Hand Surg 11A:157–165, 1986

146. Weiss C, Laskin RS, Spinner M: Irreducible radiocarpal dislocation — A case report. J Bone Surg 52A:562–564, 1970

147. Woodyard JE: A review of Smith's fractures. J Bone Joint Surg 51B:324–329, 1969

148. Younger CP, DeFiore JC: Rupture of flexor tendons to the fingers after a Colles' fracture. A case report. J Bone Joint Surg 59A:828, 1977

Infections

23

Robert J. Neviaser

GENERAL PRINCIPLES

Until the advent of antibiotics, infections of the hand often resulted in severe disabilities, including stiffness, contracture, and amputation. Although such unfortunate results are now less common, they still can and do occur. Improper treatment, as well as delay in instituting appropriate therapy, can result in a disastrous outcome. It is important, therefore, to recognize the general principles that apply to management of hand infections before embarking on a detailed operative approach to a specific condition.

Although the use of antibiotics in these infections is extremely valuable, these agents alone will effect a cure in only a very few cases and only under specific conditions. If the problem is diagnosed within the first 24 to 48 hours of onset, high doses of systemic antibiotics—with appropriate splinting to rest the affected part—can arrest the condition. Beyond this time, such success is unlikely because of thrombosis of the local small vessels and certain anatomic peculiarities in many areas of the hand. Many closed spaces and compartments in the hand permit early and rapid walling off of any infection, thus preventing systemic antibiotic agents from reaching the area. The selection of an antibiotic is usually based on empirical evidence. Cultures of drainage are taken when the patient is first seen or at the time of surgical drainage. Since the most common infecting organism is *Staphylococcus aureus*, the choice of agent should be based on this fact. Once culture and sensitivity results are known, the antimicrobial agent can be changed. It need not be continued for more than 7 to 10 days, except in those cases where osteomyelitis is present. Although initially it is best given intravenously, the oral route can be used after 2 or 3 days. The prolonged use of intravenous or oral antibiotics in soft tissue infections cannot be justified.

Infections begin as cellulitis. At this early stage there is no place for incision and drainage. Such an approach is useful, however, when an abscess is formed. Therefore, surgical drainage must be undertaken when the condition is seen late or when the nonoperative approach does not produce rapid resolution in the first few days. Systemic antibiotics and splinting with plaster of Paris are integral parts of the postoperative regimen in all surgically treated infections.

If the surgeon undertakes the responsibility of draining an infection, he must also carry out preoperative planning. The type and placement of incisions must not only allow direct access to the abscess but follow accepted surgical principles of hand surgery. All incisions should permit easy extension in any direction in case the magnitude of the problem is greater than anticipated. Correlatively, the incision or its extension should not traverse any flexion crease at or approaching a right angle (Fig. 23-1), lest a contracture develop. The approach should avoid injuring the vessels, nerves, or tendons. It should be planned to avoid compromising the blood supply to an adjacent area or leaving a sensitive scar, especially in an important tactile area.

It has been advocated that excision and primary closure can yield a better result when strict criteria are followed.[24] These include excision of all necrotic tissue by specific incisions and direct closure of the wounds after instilling antibiotics. Postoperative care includes immobilization for 10 days, after which the sutures are removed. This approach carries substantial risk of contributing to a much worse infection. Although it may yet secure a proper place in the treatment of infections, it

should not be adopted for use until its role has been more carefully defined.

All procedures should be carried out under tourniquet control. Before inflating the tourniquet, the arm should be elevated for several minutes; however, forceful exsanguination using an elastic wrapping is contraindicated since this can force bacteria into the circulatory system and seed other areas of the body.

Throughout this chapter, repeated reference is made to irrigation via catheters. Although the wounds are closed around the catheter and an exit drain, there is an avenue for egress of the fluid and drainage, i.e., around the small Penrose drain. This technique differs from that of excision and complete closure mentioned above. In other techniques the incisions are left open and are allowed to close by secondary intention. When allowed to do this, all wounds are managed in virtually the same manner, including packing for 48 to 72 hours, followed by saline soaks and exercises. The term *standard* (or *routine* or *usual*) *aftercare* is used throughout this chapter to refer to this regimen.

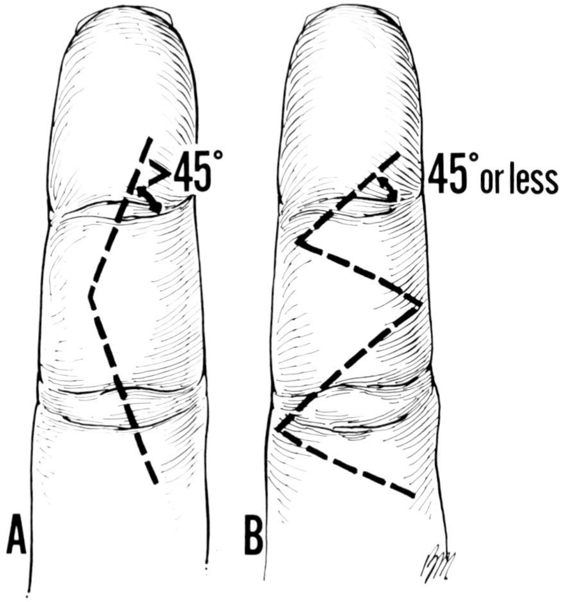

Fig. 23-1. (A) Improper location of a zigzag volar incision. If the incision approaches the flexion creases at an angle greater than 45 degrees, a contracting scar can result. (B) Correct placement of a volar zigzag incision, i.e., approaching the flexion creases at an angle of 45 degrees or less.

ACUTE INFECTIONS

Paronychia

This infection involves the soft tissue fold around the fingernail. It usually results from introduction of *Staphylococcus aureus* into the paronychial tissue by a sliver of nail or hangnail, a manicure instrument, or a tooth. Because of the continuity of this fold with the eponychial tissue overlying the base of the nail, the infection often extends into this region and may continue around to the fold on the opposite side of the fingernail. This rather unusual occurrence is called a *run-around infection*. Paronychia is the most common infection in the hand.

In the very early stages, this process can be aborted by soaks in warm saline solution, systemic oral antibiotics, and rest of the affected part. If the abscess is very superficial, treatment can be carried out without anesthesia and should consist of opening the thin layer of tissue over the abscess with a sharp blade directed away from the nail bed and matrix.

In larger, more extensive lesions there are two approaches available, depending on the extent of the lesion. Both procedures are best carried out under digital block anesthesia at the level of the metacarpal head with plain lidocaine (no epinephrine). If the paronychial fold and the adjacent part of the eponychium are involved, one-fourth of the nail on the appropriate side is bluntly separated from the underlying nail bed with the flat part of a metal probe (Fig. 23-2A). The elevated portion of the nail is then cut from the remainder with sharp-pointed scissors. If this does not allow drainage of the pus, an incision is made in the fold with a # 11 blade, with the point directed away from the nail bed and matrix (Fig. 23-2B). After the cavity is irrigated to evacuate the purulence, it is packed with a plain gauze wick. The packing is removed 48 to 72 hours later, and intermittent warm saline soaks are instituted. These can be discontinued when the inflammatory reaction has receded.

If the infection involves the entire eponychium, as well as one lateral fold, it is known as an *eponychia*. It is extremely rare to see both lateral folds and the dorsal tissue infected in the same digit. An eponychia usually presents with a collection of pus beneath the proximal portion of the nail in the region of the lunula. This effectively separates this portion of the nail from the underlying bed. Although there are options to surgical drainage, all procedures emphasize certain points. The entire nail does not need to be removed unless it is floating free, a most unusual circumstance. Removal of all the nail leaves an exposed, sensitive nail bed. In placing an incision, the scalpel blade should always be directed away from the nail bed to avoid scarring and producing a ridge later, as well as away from the nail matrix to prevent subsequent growth deformity.

Operative Methods.

No Incision. The eponychial fold is elevated from the nail gently by a flat, blunt instrument such as the flat portion of a malleable or metal probe or a Freer elevator. This separation is carried far enough proximally to permit the proximal edge of the nail to be seen (Fig. 23-3A). The proximal one-third of the nail is removed by transecting it with scissors. The pus is then evacuated, and a gauze packing is inserted beneath the fold to keep the cavity open. After 48 hours the wick is removed, and warm saline soaks are begun.

Single Incision. An incision is made in the paronychial fold, starting at its midpoint and extending proximally into the eponychium as far as the base of the nail (Fig. 23-3B). The blade is directed away from the bed and matrix. The eponychium is elevated gently, and the proximal one-third of the nail is separated bluntly from the bed and matrix and excised with scissors. A gauze wick is inserted under the fold and removed after 48 hours. Warm saline soaks are then begun.

Double Incisions. Incisions are made on each side of the nail, starting at the midpoint of each paronychial fold and continuing proximally as far as the base of the nail (Fig. 23-3C). With the use of the flat end of a malleable metal probe or Freer elevator, the entire eponychial fold is gently elevated as a flap to expose the base of the nail (Fig. 23-3D). The proximal one-third of the nail is removed with scissors after separating it from the bed and matrix. Gauze packing is inserted under the flap of eponychium (Fig. 23-3E) and is removed 48 hours

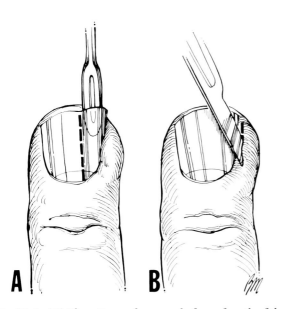

Fig. 23-2. (A) Elevation and removal of one-fourth of the nail to decompress the paronychium. (B) Incision of the paronychial fold with the blade directed away from the nail bed and matrix.

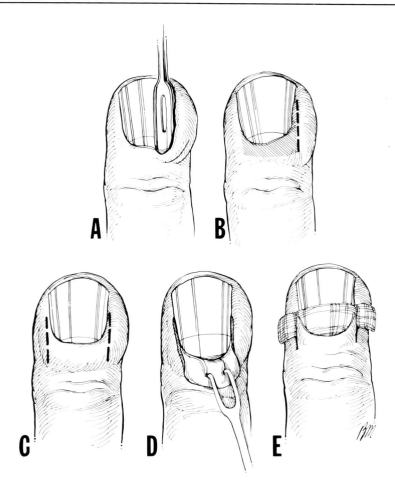

Fig. 23-3. (**A**) Elevation of the eponychial fold with a flat probe to expose the base of the nail. (**B**) Placement of an incision to drain the paronychium and to elevate the eponychial fold for excision of the proximal one-third of the nail. (**C–E**) Incisions and procedure for elevating the entire eponychial fold with excision of the proximal one-third of the nail. A gauze pack prevents premature closure of the cavity.

later at which time warm saline soaks can be started.

Author's Preferred Method. None of the techniques described above should be used exclusively as there are cases in which each is applicable. When the abscess has separated the entire proximal portion of the nail, drainage can be easily achieved by unroofing the nail without making incisions, minimizing the risk to the bed and matrix. If the infection is limited to one-half of the eponychium, a single incision is useful to aid in separating the nail base. In those cases where the entire eponychium is involved and the nail is at least partially adherent, it is necessary to make two incisions. An adequate number and length of incisions must be used but can be kept to a minimum.

Felon

A felon is a subcutaneous abscess of the distal pulp of a finger or thumb. It differs from other types of subcutaneous abscesses because of the multiple vertical fibrous trabeculae or septa that divide the pulp into several small compartments. There is often, but not always an injury preceding a felon. The pain and swelling usually develop rapidly. The expanding abscess breaks down the septa and can extend toward the phalanx, producing an osteitis or osteomyelitis, or toward the skin, causing necrosis and a sinus somewhere on the palmar surface of the digital pulp. If such spontaneous, although inadequate, decompression does not occur, it is possible that the digital vessels will be obliterated and a slough of the tactile pulp will result. Other complications of the untreated felon include sequestration of the diaphysis of the distal phalanx, pyogenic arthritis of the DIP joint, and a flexor tenosynovitis from proximal extension, although the latter is quite rare.

Surgical drainage is indicated when there is fluctuance in the pulp. Although this may be difficult to assess, it is usually present if the process has been going on for more than 48 hours. The basic tenets of all approaches are (1) to avoid injury to the digital nerve and vessels, (2) to use an incision that will not leave a disabling scar, (3) to keep exploration distal enough so that the flexor tendon sheath is not violated and a tenosynovitis is not produced iatrogenically, and (4) to produce adequate drainage. In the index, middle, and ring fingers, the lateral incisions are on the ulnar side; in the thumb and small finger, they are on the radial border.

Operative Methods.

Fish-Mouth Incision.[5] An incision is made beginning in line with the most proximal visible portion of the nail, on the side of the digit dorsal to the apex of the interphalangeal joint flexion crease (Fig. 23-4A). It is continued distally, staying parallel to the volar edge of the underlying phalanx as it curves around the fingertip onto the opposite side, ending at a point identical to the starting one. The entire volar flap is carefully raised from the phalanx with a knife until the abscess is encountered. A clamp is then inserted into the cavity, and the vertical septa are ruptured bluntly to ensure that no pocket of pus has been missed. After debridement of the necrotic tissue and irrigation of the cavity, the wound is packed open with a gauze wick. Two days later the pack can be removed and soaks started. The wound will eventually close by secondary intention.

Although this incision has been recommended for severe infections, it has virtually no place in the treatment of this lesion. It often leaves an unsightly, tender scar, and it can produce a slough of the tactile pad, if not performed precisely as described, or a bulbous mobile pad, making it difficult for the patient to pick up objects.

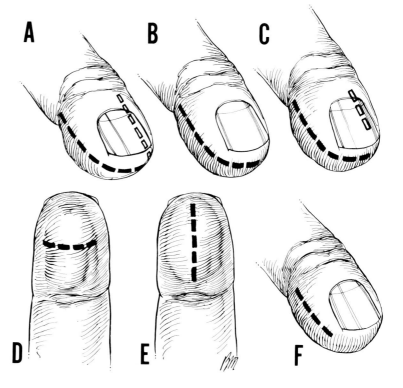

Fig. 23-4. Incisions for drainage of felons. (**A**) Fish-mouth incision. This approach has significant complications and should be avoided. (**B**) Hockey stick or J incision should be reserved for extensive or severe abscess or felon. The incision should be more dorsal at the tip than shown, i.e., at the junction of the skin and nail bed. (**C**) Incision for through-and-through drainage of a felon is rarely, if ever, necessary. Again, the distal incision should be at the junction of the skin and nail bed. (**D**) Volar drainage. Useful if the abscess points volarward but this incision risks injury to digital nerves. (**E**) Alternative volar approach. Less risk to digital nerves but should not touch or cross the DIP flexion crease. (**F**)Unilateral longitudinal approach. Most felons should be drained via this incision.

J, or Hockey Stick, Incision.[23,33] An incision is made just dorsal to the midlateral line on the ulnar side of the finger, starting at a point 1 cm distal to the level of the flexion crease of the DIP joint. The incision is extended distally, following a plane close to the junction of the pad and the nail bed, around the fingertip to the corner of the nail on the opposite side of the digit (Fig. 23-4B). The pulp tissue and septa are separated from the periosteum of the phalanx, thus allowing all septa to be opened for drainage. After irrigation, the wound is kept open with a gauze wick. The pack is removed and soaks are begun at 48 hours.

The best indication for using this incision is an extensive or severe abscess. Because it crosses the fingertip, it is too elongated for routine use; it can produce a sensitive, disabling scar at the fingertip.

Through-and-Through Drainage.[6] An incision is made just distal and dorsal to the DIP joint flexion crease on the ulnar aspect of the finger. It is continued distally halfway around the fingertip, incising at the pulp–nail bed junction in the tip itself (Fig. 23-4C). A 1-cm counterincision is made on the radial side to establish through-and-through drainage. This is achieved by rupturing the vertical trabeculae in the pulp by spreading with a pointed clamp. A wet gauze wick is extended through both incisions and is removed after 2 or 3 days to permit commencement of warm saline soaks.

This approach is rarely needed since adequate drainage can be achieved by a single incision. Therefore, a second or counterincision is usually superfluous.

Volar Drainage.[4] After the site of greatest tenderness and tension has been localized by palpation with the tip to a probe, a transverse incision 4 to 5 mm long is made over the side of a central abscess (Fig. 23-4D). If the point of the abscess is lateral, the incision should be longitudinal but not across the flexion crease. If a volar sinus is present, an elliptical incision is made at its location to excise the necrotic edges of the tract. Occasionally a collar button effect will be present, with an intact epidermis containing the pus that has leaked through a sinus in the dermis; in such cases this should be the site of incision. The knife should only be allowed to penetrate the dermis while a clamp is used to spread the subcutaneous tissue. This minimizes the risk to the digital nerves.

An alternative volar approach[19] is to place a longitudinal incision in the midline of the tactile pad (Fig. 23-4E), extending from a few millimeters distal to the interphalangeal joint flexion crease to the end of the palmar surface of the underlying bone. The blade is gently inserted deeper until the abscess is encountered; then the opening is enlarged to the limits of the abscess.

Proponents of the volar approach maintain that the use of wicks is not necessary and that petrolatum gauze or zinc oxide ointment over the wound, with a dressing change every 3 days, is sufficient postoperative care.

The volar approach is most appropriate in the face of an existing sinus. The major disadvantage of such volar incisions is the risk of a sensitive scar on the tactile surface of the digit. With the use of a transverse incision, injury to the digital nerves can occur.

Unilateral Longitudinal Incision.[27] An incision is made on the ulnar side of the digit (radial side in the thumb and small finger), dorsal to and 0.5 cm distal to the DIP joint flexion crease. It is continued distally in a straight line to within 0.5 cm of the medial edge of the nail, ending at a point slightly beyond the start of the free, unattached distal part of the nail (Fig. 23-4F). It does not cross over the fingertip. The incision is deepened along a plane just volar to the palmar cortex of the phalanx until the abscess is entered. The opening in the cavity is enlarged until adequate evacuation is achieved. A gauze pack is placed in the cavity for 2 days; then it is removed and soaks are begun.

Author's Preferred Method. There are two preferred methods. If there is a draining sinus, incision of the sinus longitudinally, with excision of the necrotic skin edges, is effective. If no sinus is present, the unilateral longitudinal approach is used; this has the least potential for untoward sequelae and provides satisfactory drainage. In those cases in which the infection is severe enough to warrant close observation by hospitalization, the use of catheter irrigation is helpful. After the appropriate incision is made, a 16- or 18-gauge polyethylene catheter is placed along the digit up to, but not into, the wound and secured with appropriate sutures. After the hand and fingers are enclosed in a compression dressing with a plaster splint, the proximal end of the catheter is brought out through the dressing and connected to a bottle of sterile saline solution. The saline is permitted to run onto the wound and dressings at a rate that will keep the dressings wet, usually 100 ml/hour for 48 hours. This promotes drainage and egress of the pus. The catheter irrigation can then be discontinued and the routine postoperative regimen started.

Herpes Simplex

An important differential diagnosis to either a pyogenic paronychia or felon is the herpetic whitlow. The whitlow is a viral infection caused by the herpes simplex virus, seen frequently in medical or dental personnel and sometimes in small children. It is important that it be treated nonoperatively, unlike the surgical drainage approach to pyogenic infections.[7,20,36]

The affected digit initially becomes painful and then erythematous. Tenderness is present but is noticeably less than that seen with bacterial infections. Small vesicles appear early and may coalesce to form bullae. The fluid in the vesicles may be clear or turbid but not purulent. Occasionally hemorrhagic areas are seen. The lesions then become encrusted and desquamate. The process runs a self-limited course, resolving in 3 to 4 weeks.

The diagnosis can be made clinically by history and physical examination. The vesicles can be cultured if seen early, but one usually does not have that opportunity. Immunofluorescent titers of serum antibodies to herpes simplex antigens can be of assistance if early and late titers are compared. Generally one is forced to rely on a clinical impression.

It is extremely important to consider this diagnostic possibility. Incising this aseptic area is contraindicated, for secondary bacterial infection can ensue with prolonged, disabling fingertip problems arising.

Deep Space Infections in the Palm

There are four confined spaces in the palm of the hand that are subject to infection. Each presents its own characteristic picture and problems.

WEB SPACE ("COLLAR BUTTON") ABSCESS

An infection in the web space (collar button or collar stud abscess) usually occurs through a fissure in the skin between the fingers, from a distal palmar callus or from extension of an infection in the subcutaneous area of the proximal segment of a finger. The pain and swelling are localized to the web space and distal palm. The adjacent fingers lie abducted from each other. The swelling may be more prominent on either the palmar or dorsal aspect, depending on the nature of the infection. The term *collar button* is derived from the hourglass configuration of the abscess, which can develop in one of two ways. One process involves a superficial subepidermal collection of pus within a palmar callosity; a sinus forms through the dermis, leaking pus to a second collection point in the fatty tissue of the volar surface of the distal palm. The other way is through a hole in the palmar fascia distally in the region of the superficial transverse metacarpal ligaments; this creates palmar and dorsal abscesses that are connected through the fascia. Even though the greater swelling often occurs on the dorsal side, one should not be misled into overlooking the more important volar component of this infection.

There are two important concepts to bear in mind when draining such abscesses. One is that the incision should not be placed transversely across the web space, since this will create a contracting scar that will restrict spreading of the fingers. The other is to be alert for the double-abscess configuration.

Operative Methods.
Curved Longitudinal Incisions.[5,9] The incision is begun just proximal to the ulnar end of the proximal flexion crease of the radial digit of the two involved fingers (Fig. 23-5A). It is continued proximally and ulnarward, stopping just distal to the midpalmar crease overlying the metacarpal of the ulnar digit involved. After the skin is divided, the subcutaneous tissue is spread with a clamp until pus is encountered. The opening in the abscess is enlarged longitudinally. Compression is applied to the dorsum of the webspace by the surgeon while the wound is retracted. Increased drainage can be seen in the depth of the wound if there is a deep

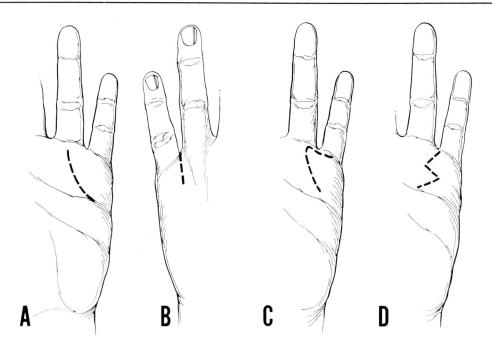

Fig. 23-5. (A) Curved longitudinal volar incision for drainage of a web space abscess. (B) Dorsal incision to be used in conjunction with (A). (C) Volar transverse incision. This incision can cause a web space contracture due to the transverse limb near the margin of the web. (D) Volar exposure. Used with the dorsal incision shown in (B).

collar button abscess. A second incision is then made on the dorsum. It begins at the level of the MP joints but lies between the metacarpals, and is extended distally in a straight line to end at the base of the involved web, a distance of 1 to 1.5 cm (Fig. 23-5B). The deep tissues are divided in a plane toward the palmar abscess. When the dorsal collection is entered, the opening is enlarged in the direction of the wound. After the pus has been evacuated and the wound irrigated, drains are placed into both wounds; these are gauze wicks. The hand is dressed in a compressive dressing with a plaster splint; this is removed in 48 to 72 hours and soaks are started. Active motion is encouraged.

A modification of this approach is a longitudinal volar incision between the metacarpals. This provides a less adequate exposure to the volar aspect of the abscess.

Volar Transverse Approach.[2,4,36] A transverse incision is made in the proximal flexion crease of the more ulnar of the two involved fingers. A longitudinal extension may be added between the metacarpal heads of the two digits (Fig. 23-5C). The

deep dissection is as previously described. The dorsal approach may be needed as well.

The disadvantage of this incision is the placement of the transverse limb at the flexion crease. If this part of the incision is inadvertently carried too far into the web, a web space contracture can result.

Volar and Dorsal Drainage with Irrigation. This is the technique preferred by the author. A zigzag incision is made on the palmar surface, starting just proximal to the web and stopping just distal to the midpalmar crease (Fig. 23-5D). The flaps are reflected and the deep tissues dissected in the web while the digital arteries and nerves are retracted to either side. The superficial transverse metacarpal ligament and other fibers of the palmar fascia are divided to allow ample exposure of the volar and dorsal compartments of the dumbbell-shaped abscess. A 1.5-cm dorsal longitudinal incision is made between the bases of the proximal phalanges. Generous communication between the two incisions is established. A 16-gauge polyethylene catheter is placed into the palmar wound and sutured to the skin to prevent accidental removal. The volar wound is sutured around the catheter. A small Penrose drain is placed into the dorsal wound. Manual irrigation with saline is done to be certain that the irrigating solution exists dorsally. The hand is dressed in a compressive dressing and supported with a plaster splint. Continuous irrigation with sterile saline at the rate of 100 ml/hour is maintained for 48 hours. The outflow spills onto the dressing. The hand is then inspected, and if it is found to be free of infection, the catheter and drain are removed. Exercises are started in a dry dressing.

PALMAR SPACE INFECTIONS

The thenar and midpalmar compartments are potential spaces in which infections can occur; therefore, the anatomy of these spaces is pertinent[18] (Fig. 23-6). The midpalmar space is deep to the flexor tendons, extending dorsally to the fascia over the second and third volar interossei and the third and fourth metacarpals. It is bordered radially by the vertical septum between the third metacarpal and the sheath of the long finger profundus and ulnarly by the fascia of the hypothenar muscles. The distal margins of this space are the vertical septa of the palmar fascia, which are approximately 2 cm short of the webs. It is limited proximally by a thin fascial layer at the distal end of the carpal canal.

The thenar space is located radial to the vertical septum between the third metacarpal and the long finger profundus and extends to the lateral edge of the adductor pollicis. For clinical purposes, it can involve the subcutaneous thenar region volarly and extend to the adductor pollicis as well as over its distal margin to the first web space. The hypothenar space contains the hypothenar muscles and is enveloped by their fascia. It is bordered radially by a fibrous septum from the fifth metacarpal to the palmar fascia.

Midpalmar Space Infections

These can result from a penetrating wound, from rupture of a flexor tenosynovitis of the middle, ring, or small finger, or from distal palmar abscesses extending proximally through the lumbrical canal. The hand loses its normal palmar concavity, and there is tenderness over the midpalmar space. As with all palmar infections, there is swelling dorsally. This must not be mistaken for the area of infection; the dorsum will not be tender, fluctuant, or erythematous in these cases. Motion of the middle and ring fingers is painful and limited.

Operative Methods.

Transverse Incision in the Distal Crease.[3,13,17,36] An incision is made in or parallel to the distal palmar crease overlying the third and fourth metacarpals (Fig. 23-7A). The nerves and arteries are protected, and the flexor tendons of the ring finger are used as a guide to the midpalmar space. The dissection is continued on either side of these tendons

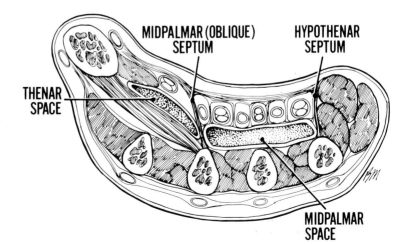

Fig. 23-6. The potential midpalmar spaces.

MIDPALMAR (OBLIQUE) SEPTUM

HYPOTHENAR SEPTUM

THENAR SPACE

MIDPALMAR SPACE

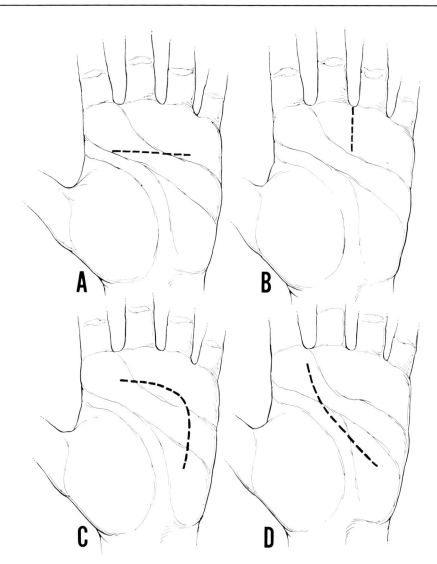

Fig. 23-7. (**A**) Transverse distal palmar exposure of the midpalmar space. (**B**) Approach to the midpalmar space through the lumbrical canal. (**C**) Combined longitudinal and transverse approach. (**D**) Longitudinal approach to the midpalmar space.

until the abscess is opened. After the purulence is evacuated, a drain is brought from the space through the skin. This drain is removed 48 to 72 hours later, and soaks and exercises are begun. Active motion of the fingers is emphasized.

Distal Palmar Approach Through the Lumbrical Canal.[13,17] A longitudinal incision is made on the palmar surface of the third web space (between the middle and ring fingers) (Fig. 23-7B). It extends from just proximal to the web itself and ends just distal to the midpalmar crease but does not touch or cross it. A clamp is inserted into the wound and directed proximally down the canal of the third lumbrical, dorsal to the flexor tendons, until the

midpalmar space is entered and pus is encountered. After adequate evacuation of the space, a drain is placed for 48 hours. Aftercare is the same as that already described.

Combined Transverse and Longitudinal Approach.[5] An incision is made parallel to the distal palmar crease between the second and third metacarpal heads. It is extended transversely to the fourth metacarpal and then continued proximally just radial to the hypothenar eminence (Fig. 23-7C). The palmar fascia is divided, and the digital nerves and arteries, as well as the superficial palmar arch, are protected. With the use of the flexor tendons of the ring finger as a guide, the surgeon obtains access to the space by passing on either side of the tendons. After the abscess is evacuated, a drain is left in place for 48 hours. The routine aftercare is then begun.

Longitudinal Approach.[23,27] A slightly curved incision is made in the midpalm, beginning just proximal to the distal palmar crease in line with the third ray. This extends proximally and slightly ulnarward, paralleling the thenar crease (Fig. 23-7D). After the palmar fascia is split and the superficial palmar arch and the digital arteries and nerves are protected, the surgeon identifies the flexor tendons to the ring finger. The space is entered by going on either side of these tendons. After the cavity is evacuated, a drain is placed into the wound for 48 hours. Aftercare is as outlined earlier.

Author's Preferred Method. The author's preferred technique is the longitudinal approach with one modification. Instead of using a drain, a large-bore (16-gauge) polyethylene catheter is placed through the proximal end of the incision into the space. In the distal portion, a Penrose drain is brought out of the space. Both are sutured in place, the incisions around them are closed, and the hand is encompassed in a compressive dressing with a dorsal plaster splint. The catheter is connected to a bottle of sterile isotonic saline, and the cavity is irrigated at the rate of 100 ml/hour for 48 hours. The fluid is allowed to drain onto the dressings. After 48 hours, the irrigation is stopped and the catheter and drain are removed. Active finger motion is encouraged.

The advantages of this modification are the improved mechanical lavage of the infected space and the primary wound healing. The other techniques described require healing by secondary intention. The transverse and distal palmar incisions give less exposure than the others, while the combined transverse and longitudinal incision is unnecessarily extensive. Another complication of the distal palmar incision is that a contracting scar may result if the surgeon is not careful to avoid touching or crossing the distal palmar crease longitudinally.

Thenar Space Infections

This process can arise from a penetrating injury, a subcutaneous abscess of the thumb or index finger, a tenosynovitis of the thumb or index finger,

or extension of an infection of the radial bursa or midpalmar space. It presents as a marked swelling of the thenar eminence and first cleft, which forces the thumb into abduction. Surgically, this space can be drained from dorsal as well as volar approaches.

Operative Methods.

Volar Transverse Approach.[3] An incision is made parallel to and 2 cm proximal to the MP joint flexion crease of the thumb, in the distal third of the thenar eminence (Fig. 23-8A). It is placed toward the web. The digital nerves are directly subcutaneous in this region and must not be injured. The dissection is deepened bluntly toward the space between the first and second metacarpals, toward the proximal third of the palm. After the volar compartment has been decompressed, a clamp is directed dorsally over the distal margin of the adductor pollicis into the space between it and the first dorsal interosseous muscle. When both spaces have been irrigated thoroughly, one Penrose drain is placed into the dorsal space and another into the palmar compartment. Both drains exit through the incision and are removed after 48 hours. The standard aftercare is then started.

Thenar Crease Approach.[23,24,27,35] An incision is made on the palmar surface of the hand just adjacent and parallel to the thenar crease on its side (Fig. 23-8B). Great care must be exercised to avoid damaging the palmar cutaneous branch of the median nerve, which lies subcutaneously in the proximal part of the incision, and the motor branch of the median nerve, which lies somewhat deeper near the juncture of the proximal and middle thirds of the approach. The deeper dissection is performed bluntly toward the adductor pollicis until pus is encountered. After the area has been drained adequately, the dissection is extended over the distal edge of the adductor to decompress the first dorsal interosseous space. Two Penrose drains are placed as previously described and are removed after 48 hours. The standard program is then undertaken.

Dorsal Transverse Approach.[17] An incision is made on the dorsum of the first web at the middle of a line between the distal ends of the metacarpals of the thumb and index finger (Fig. 23-8C). Pus is usually encountered once the incision divides the skin. The approach is deepened between the first dorsal-adductor interval and volarly over the distal

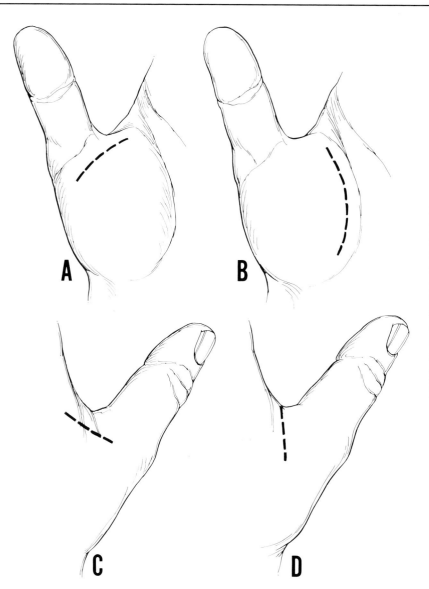

Fig. 23-8. (A) Volar transverse approach to the thenar space. Nerve injury is a potential complication. (B) Thenar crease approach. Nerve injury can result from this approach. It has the added disadvantage of limited drainage of the space behind the adductor pollicis. (C) Dorsal transverse approach. A contracture of the web space can result if this incision is placed too close to the edge of the web. (D) Dorsal longitudinal approach to the thenar space.

edge of the adductor (if necessary). A single drain is usually adequate for 48 hours before the routine postoperative regimen is begun.

Dorsal Longitudinal Approach.[6,13,23,27] A straight or slightly curved longitudinal incision is made in the dorsum of the thumb cleft, starting near the web and extending proximally along the radial margin of the first dorsal interrosseous muscle (Fig. 23-8D). The dissection is continued deeper into the interval between the first dorsal interosseous and the adductor pollicis, at which point pus should be encountered. After thorough

irrigation and debridement of the abscess, a drain is brought out through the skin incision. This is removed after 48 hours and the postoperative regimen begun.

Combined Dorsal and Volar Approach.[5] Two incisions are made: one dorsally, which is the slightly curved longitudinal approach described above, and one volarly, which parallels the thenar crease. Each approach is used to drain the corresponding half of the space. A separate drain is used for each incision, but through-and-through drains are not employed.

Author's Preferred Method. The preferred approach is one that uses the combined dorsal and volar approach just described. A 16-gauge polyethylene catheter is sutured into the palmar wound and the wound closed around it; a drain is sutured into the dorsal wound, which in turn is nearly closed around it (some opening must be left around the drain to permit egress of the irrigating fluid). The hand is dressed in a compressive dressing with a plaster splint. The catheter is brought out of the dressing and connected to a bottle of sterile isotonic saline. The irrigating fluid runs continuously at the rate of 100 ml/hour for 48 hours. After 2 days, the dressing is removed, and, if the infection seems to have resolved clinically, the catheter and drain are removed. Active exercise is emphasized. Sutures are removed after 10 to 14 days.

The advantages of this technique are the thorough mechanical lavage of the space and the primary wound healing provided.

Hypothenar Space Infections

This is an extremely rare entity. It is so unusual that there is virtually no mention of it in the literature. The infection can result from a penetrating injury or a local subcutaneous abscess. It presents as a fullness with considerable tenderness of the hypothenar eminence.

Operative Methods. An ulnar approach is used, with the incision made on the most ulnar aspect of the palm, starting just proximal and medial to the ulnar end of the midpalmar crease (Fig. 23-9). This is continued in a straight line proximally, to end 3 cm distal to the wrist flexion crease. The incision is deepened to the level of the hypothenar fascia. This layer is divided in the line of the incision, and the abscess should be directly beneath it. After the purulence has been evacuated, a drain is placed in the wound for 48 hours, after which time the routine postoperative regimen begins.

Pyogenic Flexor Tenosynovitis (Flexor Tendon Sheath Infection)

Although most significant infections in the hand can result in severe disability if not treated expeditiously and properly, none raises more fear than the purulent flexor tendon sheath infection. The purulence within the sheath destroys the gliding mechanism, rapidly creating adhesions that lead to marked limitation of tendon function and severe loss of motion. It also destroys the blood supply, thus producing tendon necrosis.

These infections usually are caused by a penetrating injury but can also be of hematogenous origin. The ring, middle, and index fingers are the most commonly involved digits. The most common offending organism is *Staphylococcus aureus*.[28]

Kanavel[17] described the four classic findings of pyogenic flexor tenosynovitis: (1) a flexed position of the finger, (2) symmetric enlargement of the whole finger, (3) excessive tenderness over the course of the sheath but limited to the sheath, and (4) excruciating pain on extending the finger passively, most marked at the proximal end. The latter is the most valuable of these signs and may be the only one present very early in the process.

If the patient is seen within the first 24 to 48 hours of onset of the infection, it is possible to abort the process. Treatment includes parenteral antibi-

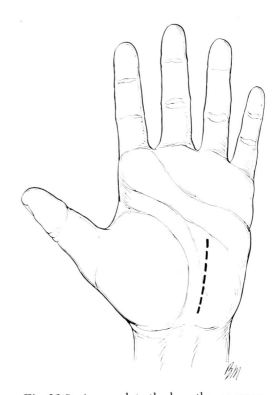

Fig. 23-9. Approach to the hypothenar space.

otics in high doses, rest of the affected part by immobilization of the entire hand and all digits in a compressive dressing with a plaster splint, elevation of the hand, and close observation (the patient should be seen twice daily). The findings should be well resolved within 2 days for this treatment to be considered successful. If this course is not successful, or if the patient is seen more than 48 hours after onset, surgical drainage should be undertaken at once.

Operative Methods.

Open Drainage.[5,11,13,14] A midaxial incision is made in the finger, usually on the ulnar side; in the thumb and small finger, the radial side is used. The incision begins dorsal and distal to the distal flexion crease of the finger and extends proximally to the web space (Fig. 23-10A). The digital artery and nerve are kept with the volar flap. The dissection proceeds toward the tendon sheath dorsal to the neurovascular structures. When the tendon sheath is visualized, the synovium between the A3 and A4 pulleys is incised. Cloudy serosanguinous fluid or frank purulence is encountered. Another incision is made in the palm over the tendon to drain the cul-de-sac. It is either longitudinal between the proximal flexion crease of the finger and midpalmar crease, or curved. A transverse incision in the palmar crease is an acceptable alternative. The tenosynovium between the pulleys is excised from the palm to the distal phalanx, but the annular pulleys are left undisturbed. The wound is irrigated thoroughly with saline or an antibiotic solution. The wounds are kept open with drains, and a compressive dressing and plaster splint are applied. After 48 hours, the wounds are inspected. The drains are removed, and saline soaks with active exercise are started.

Single Incision for Antibiotic Instillation.[2] A transverse incision is made in the palm over the involved finger, just distal to or in the transverse midpalmar crease (Fig. 23-10B). It is similar to the incision used for a trigger finger release. A 16-gauge polyethylene catheter is introduced into the sheath at its proximal end and passed far enough distally to prevent its being dislodged during the postoperative treatment. The wound is closed around the catheter. Over the next 48 to 72 hours, 0.2 ml of an antibiotic solution is introduced into

the sheath every 1 to 2 hours. After this time if the signs of infection have resolved, the catheter is removed and an exercise program started, emphasizing active motion to prevent loss of tendon function.

Distal Drainage with Proximal Instillation of Antibiotics.[24] The tendon sheath is inspected via a short transverse incision over its distal end just proximal to the distal flexion crease (Fig. 23-10C). The sheath is opened and the purulence evacuated. A needle is introduced into the proximal end of the sheath in the palm, and, when there is no resistance to its advance, an antibiotic solution is flushed from proximal to distal until the fluid comes through clear. The wound is closed and the needle withdrawn. The hand is immobilized for a few days; then active exercises are begun.

Through-and-Through Intermittent Antibiotic Irrigation.[8,32] An incision is made near and parallel to the distal flexion crease (Fig. 23-10D). The tendon sheath is visualized by retracting both neurovascular bundles to their respective sides. A transverse incision in the sheath allows the fluid to drain. A transverse counterincision is made in the distal palm over the proximal end of the sheath. A polyethylene catheter with holes cut along its length is inserted well into the sheath. The sheath and its contents are then flushed with antibiotic solution until there is no more pus. The catheter is sutured in place so that a repeat irrigation can be done on the following day. In severe infections a continuous drip is attached to the catheter and run at one drop per second for 24 to 48 hours. Then the catheters are removed and exercises started.

Closed Tendon Sheath Irrigation.[28-30] The author prefers this method over all the others. A zigzag incision is made in the distal palm over the proximal end of the sheath. The sheath is opened at the proximal margin of the A1 pulley. A second incision is made on the ulnar midaxial side of the finger in the middle and distal segments. Access to the distal end of the sheath is obtained through a plane dorsal to the digital artery and nerve. The sheath is resected distal to the A4 pulley. A 16-gauge polyethylene catheter with a single opening at its end is inserted under the A1 pulley in the palm for a distance of 1.5 to 2 cm (Fig. 23-10E). The catheter is sutured to the skin and the wound closed around it. The sheath is irrigated copiously

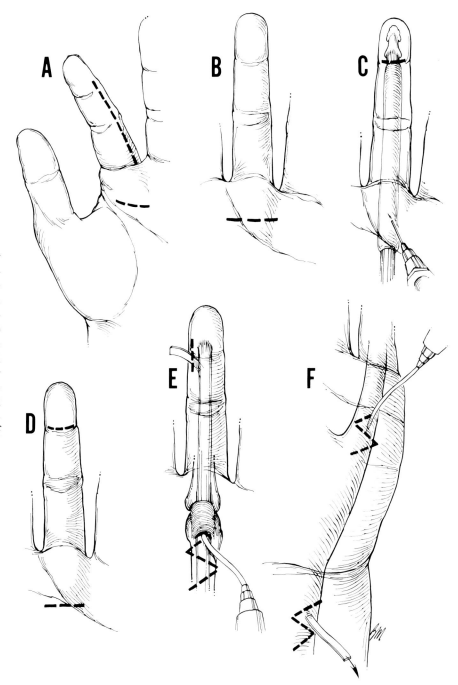

Fig. 23-10. Incisions for drainage of tendon sheath infections. (**A**) Open drainage incisions. (**B**) Single incision for instillation therapy of tendon sheath infection. (**C**) Sheath irrigated via needle proximally and single distal incision. (**D**) Incisions for through-and-through intermittent irrigation. (**E**) Closed tendon sheath irrigation technique. (**F**) Closed irrigation of ulnar bursa.

with saline. A small drain is brought from the tendon through the skin distally and sutured to the skin. The wound is closed around the drain. The system is flushed again to test its patency. The hand is dressed and splinted, with the catheter brought out of the dressing and connected to a 50-ml syringe. The dressing is arranged so that the drain can be seen distally. The system is tested just prior to the patient's leaving the operating suite. Postoperatively, the sheath is flushed manually with 50 ml of sterile saline every 2 hours for 48 hours. At this time the digit is inspected. If signs of infection have abated, the catheter and drain are removed, the wounds dressed lightly to avoid impeding motion, and exercises started. If any doubt exists, the irrigation may be continued for an additional 24 hours. Complete motion can be expected in a week.

In the thumb, the proximal part of the sheath is exposed through a thenar crease incision. The distal centimeter of the transverse carpal ligament is incised to allow access to the passage of the flexor pollicis longus through the wall of the canal into the thenar eminence. The catheter is placed in this opening.

The advantages of this method are: (1) primary wound healing (not provided by the others — especially open drainage); (2) thorough mechanical irrigation of the sheath (not accomplished with a single incision); (3) relief from concern about empirical selection of an effective antibiotic solution; (4) accurate placement of the catheter rather than blind probing with a needle; and (5) rapid return of function with minimal inconvenience to the patient, as opposed to the prolonged morbidity associated with healing by secondary intention.

Ulnar and Radial Bursal Infections

The radial bursa is a proximal extension of the tendon sheath of the flexor pollicis longus. It extends through the carpal canal into the distal forearm. The ulnar bursa is a comparable extension of the sheath of the flexor digitorum profundus of the little finger. There is often an hourglass constriction at the proximal end of the respective tendon sheaths in the palm; this can act as a temporary barrier to the spread of infection into these bursae. If the tendon sheath infection is not treated promptly, however, it will spread into the bursae, and this infection must be treated in addition to the distal one. In each case, the digital portion of the tenosynovitis is managed as described above.

Operative Methods — Ulnar Bursa.

Open Drainage.[5] The distal portion of the ulnar bursa is exposed through the incision used to visualize the proximal end of the tenosynovium of the small finger. It can be extended proximally along the radial margin of the hypothenar eminence. The proximal end of the bursa is exposed through a 5-cm incision at the ulnar aspect of the wrist proximal to the wrist flexion crease at the dorsal margin of the flexor carpi ulnaris. This tendon is retracted volarward along with the ulnar artery and nerve and the dorsal branch of the latter. The bursa is found between the flexor tendons on the volar side and the pronator quadratus on the dorsal side; it is opened at both ends and irrigated thoroughly. Drains are placed in the bursa and brought out through the skin; they are removed after 48 hours so that exercises can be started.

Through-and-Through Irrigation.[28,30] The distal end of the bursa is exposed through a short extension of the zigzag incision used as the palmar approach to the tendon sheath of the small finger. The bursa is opened, and a second 16-gauge polyethylene catheter is introduced into the wound, directed proximally into the bursa (Fig. 23-10F). Another incision, either straight or zigzag, is made in the volar ulnar surface of the wrist just radial to the flexor carpi ulnaris. The tendon and ulnar artery and nerve are retracted medially and the flexor superficialis and profundus retracted laterally to expose the bursa. The bursa is incised and saline flushed through it from the distal end. A rubber drain is brought out from the bursa through the skin in the proximal wound. The wounds are sutured around the implants. The irrigating system is managed the same as, and in conjunction with, the system in the finger as described earlier.

Operative Methods — Radial Bursa. As with the ulnar bursal infection there are two means of treating the radial bursal infection. In both cases, the palmar incision is made adjacent to the thenar crease, while the proximal incision is placed just ulnar to the flexor carpi radialis. The respective ends of the bursa are opened and the sac is irrigated thoroughly. With the open technique, a drain is placed in each wound for 48 hours prior to starting rehabilitation. For closed irrigation, the catheter is placed in the palmar wound and a drain in the forearm. Irrigation is done from distal to proximal for 48 hours.

The author's preferred approach in both bursal infections is by closed irrigation. The reasons for this choice have already been enumerated. It is possible for pyogenic ulnar bursitis to rupture into the radial bursa, or vice versa, creating a "horse-shoe" abscess. This can be treated by combining the approaches to the individual bursae.

Gangrenous Infections

Various anaerobic organisms can cause gas-producing infections in the hand. Anaerobic or microaerophilic *Streptococcus* is thought to cause Meleney's infection, a rapid swelling and gangrenous change in a digit following an insignificant puncture wound.[23] Classic gas gangrene from clostridial infections can occur after a variety of open wound injuries.

Such problems require immediate opening of the affected part, adequate debridement, and thorough irrigation of the wound. An initial culture prior to administration of antibiotics is essential. The wound must be left open. Appropriate antibiotic therapy must begin immediately. Amputation of the affected part may be required to save the life of the patient.

Bites

Bites of the hand can be caused by humans or other animals. Those inflicted by humans are often over the metacarpophalangeal joints and may communicate with the joint. The mechanism of injury usually is a clenched-fist blow to another person's mouth. Although oral flora contains a variety of organisms,[26] cultures from human bites have been reported with increasing frequency to grow *Eikenella corrodens*,[15] an anaerobic gram-negative rod. Although *Eikenella* is not sensitive to most of the penicillinase-resistant penicillins, penicillin and ampicillin are effective against it.[15,21]

Domestic animal bites or scratches can produce acute cellulitis and lymphangitis. These conditions frequently develop very rapidly and with particular virulence. Cultures usually identify *Pasturella multicida*,[1] a small gram-negative coccus, as the pathogen. The antibiotic of choice in treating this organism is penicillin, but the cephalosporins are also effective. *Pasturella* infections caused by cat bites can be particularly difficult to control.

No bite should be sutured primarily. If small or punctate, the wound may require extension. Thorough debridement and irrigation should be undertaken; use of a WaterPik has been recommended. The wound should be left open. If closure is necessary, it should be done only when all evidence of infection has disappeared. All wounds should be cultured for both aerobic and anaerobic organisms.

Osteomyelitis

This process is almost always the result of the direct involvement of bone from an adjacent wound infection, adjacent joint infection, or tenosynovial infection. Injuries that penetrate directly into the bone can also cause osteomyelitis. Hematogenous osteomyelitis is rare in the hand, probably because of the widespread use of antibiotics to treat the kinds of infections elsewhere in the body that might produce a bacteremia. The most common of these organisms is *Staphylococcus aureus*.

The incisions or approaches depend on the location of the bone involved. In the phalanges a midaxial incision is preferred, whereas in the metacarpals dorsal approaches work best. The infected areas are curetted if they are soft enough, but cortical drill holes may be needed so that a small window can be removed from the cortex to allow decompression of the infection. All infected bone, as well as any sequestra, must be removed. Postoperatively, the wound can be packed open and allowed to heal by secondary intention after removal of the packing. An alternative regimen that is preferred whenever possible is constant irrigation of the site with sterile saline through a 16-gauge polyethylene catheter. The wound is closed over the catheter while a Penrose drain is placed at the opposite end of the incision to allow egress of the fluid. The catheter and drain are removed after 1 week. For severe, extensive involvement in a digit, amputation may be the most expeditious treatment and may prevent stiffness and major disability of the uninfected parts.

Pyogenic Arthritis

Joint infections usually result from penetrating trauma, such as a bite or wound from a tooth. They also can arise from extension of an adjacent bony or soft tissue infection. The joint is usually swollen, warm, and tender. Passive motion is markedly restricted and very painful.

Drainage is imperative as soon as the diagnosis is made to prevent extensive articular cartilage destruction by lysozymal activity. The interphalangeal and MP joints are entered through a longitudinal dorsolateral incision. Access to the joint is obtained by incising dorsal to the cord portion of the collateral ligament. The joint is debrided and irrigated. It can be packed open for 48 to 72 hours. When the packing is removed, motion is started and the wound granulates closed. A preferable postoperative course is to place a 20- or 18-gauge catheter into the joint to irrigate it for 48 to 72 hours. The wound is sutured over the catheter, but a small drain is placed at the other end of the incision to allow the fluid to escape. Motion is begun at the time of catheter and drain removal.

Septic Boutonnière

Septic boutonnière is a complication of a pyogenic arthritis of the PIP joint. It arises in those cases that have undergone delayed treatment; intraarticular collection of purulence has reached a volume that can no longer be retained within the joint, and the path of least resistance for escape is dorsally. The joint is well supported by the volar plate palmarly, which blends with the accessory collateral ligaments and collateral ligaments on the sides. All these structures are thick and unyielding; therefore, the pus escapes dorsally through the thin dorsal capsule. It subsequently destroys the extensor mechanism over the dorsum of the joint, producing a boutonnière deformity as the lateral bands slip volarward away from the attenuated or eroded central slip. The management of this problem is difficult, but the first priority is that the joint infection must be drained and cured before dealing with the boutonnière deformity.

If the boutonnière is due to attenuation of the mechanism, joint function is often salvageable. In these cases, the extensor tendon can be reefed or tightened to bring the lateral bands more dorsal. The PIP joint should be kept splinted in full extension for 6 to 8 weeks postoperatively, allowing free motion at the MP and DIP joints.

If, however, the joint, along with the extensor mechanism, is significantly damaged, it can be treated in the same way as a joint destroyed by rheumatoid disease with a fixed boutonnière.[29] In each instance there is virtually no tissue to use to reconstruct an extensor mechanism; therefore, implant arthroplasty would be a poor choice for treating the joint. It is better to fuse the PIP joint and tenotomize the extensor tendon over the midportion of the middle segment of the finger[10] (Fig. 23-11). If necessary, the DIP joint is manipulated into flexion after the tenotomy, and motion of the distal joint is allowed postoperatively. A mallet finger does not result because the oblique retinacular ligaments are intact; yet flexion of the distal joint is now possible. If the tenotomy is made too far distally, the oblique retinacular ligaments will be divided and active extension of the DIP joint will be impaired.

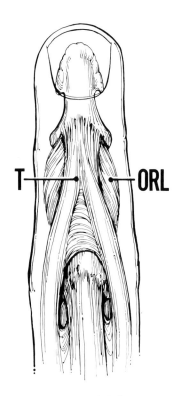

Fig. 23-11. Tenotomy site (T) for treatment of septic boutonnière, distal to the triangular ligament but proximal to the oblique retinacular ligament (ORL).

CHRONIC INFECTIONS

There are several causative agents for chronic infections, including atypical mycobacteria, tuberculosis, and various fungi. In many of these conditions, recognizing the disease is more difficult than treating it properly. The mycobacteria, both tuberculous and atypical, show a predilection for synovial tissue of either joints or tendon sheaths. They are often mistakenly diagnosed as gout, rheumatoid arthritis, or low-grade pyogenic infections.

Atypical Mycobacterial Infections

There are several types of mycobacteria; although they have been classified, it is not germane to this discussion to delve into the various groups or subtypes. The most common offending organism is *Mycobacterium marinum*. The only others seen in the hand are *M. kansasii*, *M. avium*, and *M. intracellularis.*[16]

The patient presenting such a condition often has a history of a penetrating wound in a marine environment, usually in the region of the eastern or southern coast of the United States, from warm freshwater lakes, or from tropical fish tanks. There is usually a prolonged, relatively nonpainful swelling of the finger, palm, or wrist that may have responded briefly to injections of steroids.

The diagnosis is established by culturing a synovial biopsy on Lowenstein-Jensen medium at 30° to 32°C rather than the usual cultures at 37°C. Microscopically, one sees noncaseating granulomas and acid-fast bacilli.[37]

Operative Methods. The surgical treatment, of course, depends on the location of the infection. If a joint is involved, a midaxial approach is best. The joint is entered dorsally between the collateral ligament and the extensor. At the MP level this is accomplished easily, but at the PIP joint, the collateral ligament may need to be detached to allow access to the joint and then repaired. A thorough joint synovectomy should be carried out. After a week of rest in a dressing and splint, exercises should be started. If there is a great deal of joint damage, the finger should be rested until the infection is believed to be cured before undertaking reconstructive surgery. The associated drug therapy will be discussed subsequently.

When the tenosynovium is involved, it is usually in the finger although it can be in the carpal canal or on the extensor aspect of the wrist. A finger is best approached through a volar zigzag incision, extending from the distal flexion crease to the midpalm (Fig. 23-12A). The involved synovium is thick, infected, and hypertrophic. It surrounds the tendon and erodes the pulleys. Tendon erosion or ischemia can occur, but is a late complication. All involved synovium should be removed, with every effort made to save all the pulleys. This is usually possible except in very advanced cases.[16] The operative incisions are closed primarily.

The carpal tunnel is approached through the standard incision parallel to the thenar crease, with an ulnar extension at the wrist flexion crease (Fig. 23-12B). The extensor tenosynovitis can be exposed through a longitudinal or oblique incision over the dorsum of the wrist (Fig. 23-12C). In each case, thorough excision of the involved tenosynovium should be done. The extensor retinaculum should be retained or, if reflected, repaired to prevent bowstringing of the tendons later. With any tenosynovectomy, active motion should be started within a few days to minimize tendon adherence.

Antituberculous medication is an important part of the treatment of these processes. Since cultures take up to 6 weeks to produce an organism, therapy should be started at the time of synovectomy on a presumptive basis. Currently the drugs for treatment include isoniazid, ethambutol, and rifampin; these should be continued for 18 to 24 months.

Tuberculosis

This infection is less common now than it was several decades ago. It presents in many of the same ways as the atypical mycobacterial infections. Synovectomy is appropriate for synovial involvement of tendons or joints.[22] Tuberculosis can produce a dactylitis that is not commonly seen with the atypical infections. Tuberculosis dactylitis causes enlarged fingers that, on radiographs, show proliferation of subperiosteal reaction of the phalanges (or metacarpals) and can involve adjacent joints.[34]

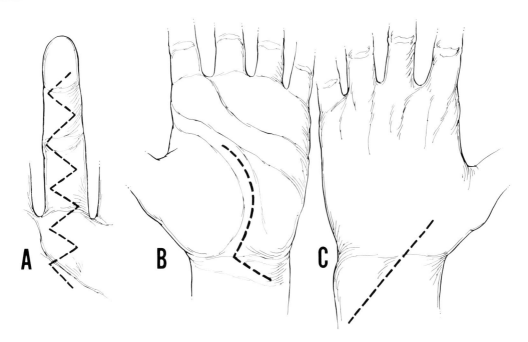

Fig. 23-12. (**A**) Volar zigzag approach for digital and palmar flexor tenosynovectomy. (**B**) Incision for exposure of flexor tenosynovium in the carpal canal, wrist, and distal forearm. (**C**) Incision for extensor tenosynovectomy of the wrist. S-shaped or lazy-S incisions usually present problems with skin slough at the margins and leave an unsightly scar.

Surgical treatment includes excision and curettage of the involved areas. Antituberculous drugs are also mandatory in the treatment regimen.

Leprosy

Mycobacterium lepraemurium demonstrates a predilection for the cooler areas of the body. It commonly affects the hands, usually by producing a neuropathy that most frequently involves the ulnar nerve. The hands are seen to have intrinsic atrophy, clawing, and weakness in pinch. Surgical procedures are usually confined to various types of reconstruction for the neurologic deficits.[31]

Fungal Infections

Although fungal infections may involve the hands, they are properly treated by systemic or local antifungal agents. Except for biopsy for diagnostic purposes, surgical treatment per se is virtually never necessary.

Occasionally coccidioidomycosis may produce a tenosynovitis or blastomycosis, and brucellosis can cause a septic arthritis or osteomyelitis. Under such circumstances appropriate debridement is required, but the mainstay of treatment remains the appropriate antifungal agent.

REFERENCES

1. Arons MS, Fernando L, Polayes IM: *Pasturella multicida* — The major cause of hand infections following domestic animal bites. J Hand Surg 7:47–52, 1982

2. Besser MIB: Digital flexor tendon irrigation. Hand 8:72, 1976

3. Bingham DIC: Acute infections of the hand. Surg Clin North Am 40:1285–1298, 1960

4. Bolton H, Fowler PJ, Jepson RP: Natural history and treatment of pulp space infection and osteomyelitis

of the terminal phalanx. J Bone Joint Surg 31B:499–504, 1949

5. Boyes JH: Bunnell's Surgery of the Hand, 5th Ed. pp. 613–642. JB Lippincott, Philadelphia, 1970

6. Brown H: Hand infections. Am Fam Physician 18:79–84, 1978

7. Cahill JM: Special infections. p. 839. In Flynn JE (ed): Hand Surgery. Williams & Wilkins, Baltimore, 1966

8. Carter SJ, Burman SO, Mersheimer WL: Treatment of digital tenosynovitis by irrigation with peroxide and oxytetracycline. Ann Surg 163:645–650, 1966

9. Crandon JH: Lesser infections of the hand. pp. 803–814. In Flynn JE (ed): Hand Surgery. Williams & Wilkins, Baltimore, 1966

10. Dolphin JA: Extensor tenotomy for chronic boutonniere deformity of the finger. J Bone Joint Surg 47A:161–164, 1965

11. Entin MA: Infections of the hand. Surg Clin North Am 44:981–993, 1964

12. Farmer CB, Mann RJ: Human bite infections of the hand. South Med J 59:515–518, 1966

13. Flynn JE: The grave infections. pp. 815–832. In Flynn JE (ed): Hand Surgery. Williams & Wilkins, Baltimore, 1966

14. Flynn JE: Modern considerations of major hand infections. N Engl J Med 252:605–612, 1955

15. Goldstein EJC, Barones MF, Miller TA: *Eikenella corrodens* in hand infections. J Hand Surg 8:563–567, 1983

16. Gunther SF, Neviaser RJ: Tenosynovial infections in the hand; Part II: Chronic tenosynovial infections. pp. 117–128. AAOS Instructional Course Lectures, Vol. 29. CV Mosby, St Louis, 1980

17. Kanavel AB: Infections of the Hand. A Guide to the Surgical Treatment of Acute and Chronic Suppurative Processes in the Fingers, Hand, and Forearm. 7th Ed. Lea & Febiger, Philadelphia, 1943

18. Kaplan EB: Functional and Surgical Anatomy of the Hand. 2nd Ed. JB Lippincott, Philadelphia, 1965

19. Kilgore ES Jr, Brown LG, Newmeyer WL, Graham WP, Davis TS: Treatment of felons. Am J Surg 130:194–197, 1975

20. LaRossa D, Hamilton R: Herpes simplex infections of the digits. Arch Surg 102:600–603, 1971

21. Leddy JP: Infections of the upper extremity. J Hand Surg 11A:294–297, 1986

22. Leung PC: Tuberculosis of the hand. Hand 10:285–291, 1978

23. Linscheid RL, Dobyns JH: Common and uncommon infections of the hand. Orthop Clin North Am 6:1063–1104, 1975

24. Loudon JB, Miniero JD, Scott JC: Infections of the hand. J Bone Joint Surg 30B:409–429, 1948

25. Louis DS, Silva J Jr: Herpetic whitlow: Herpetic infections of the digits. J Hand Surg 4:90–94, 1979

26. Mann RJ, Hoffeld TA, Farmer CB: Human bites of the hand: Twenty years experience. J Hand Surg 2:97–104, 1977

27. Milford LW: The hand. Pyogenic infections. pp. 390–397. In Crenshaw AH (ed): Campbell's Operative Orthopaedics. 5th Ed. CV Mosby, St Louis, 1971

28. Neviaser RJ: Closed tendon sheath irrigation for pyogenic flexor tenosynovitis. J Hand Surg 3:462–466, 1978

29. Neviaser RJ, Adams JP: Complications of trauma surgery and reconstructive surgery of the hand. pp. 366–402. In Epps CH Jr (ed): Complications in Orthopaedic Surgery. JB Lippincott, Philadelphia, 1978

30. Neviaser RJ, Gunther SF: Tenosynovial infections of the hand; Part I: Acute pyogenic tenosynovitis of the hand. pp. 108–117. AAOS Instructional Course Lectures, Vol. 29. CV Mosby, St Louis, 1980

31. Neviaser RJ, Wilson JN, Gardner MM: Abductor pollicis longus transfer for replacement of first dorsal interosseous. J Hand Surg 5:53–57, 1980

32. Pollen AG: Acute infection of the tendon sheaths. Hand 6:21–25, 1974

33. Robins RHC: Infections of the hand. A review based on 1000 consecutive cases. J Bone Joint Surg 34B:567–580, 1952

34. Robins RHC: Tuberculosis of the wrist and hand. Br J Surg 54:211–218, 1967

35. Scott JC, Jones BV: Results of treatment of infections of the hand. J Bone Joint Surg 34B:581–587, 1952

36. Shamblin WR: The diagnosis and treatment of acute infections of the hand. South Med J 62:209–212, 1969

37. Williams CS, Riordan DC: *Mycobacterium marinum* (atypical acid-fast bacillus) infections of the hand. J Bone Joint Surg 55A:1042–1050, 1973

Principles of Microvascular Surgery

24

William E. Sanders

The use of the microscope in repair and reconstruction has increased dramatically in recent years in many surgical specialities, but especially in surgery of the hand.[22,26,28,29,54] Microsurgical repair of vessels was first reported by Jacobson in 1960,[52] and in the short span of time since, multiple applications of this technique have been developed, including digital replantation[55] and free tissue transfer.[33] More applications lie in the future.[28,54,69] At the time the first edition of this book was written, there were few publications, courses, or training programs offering instruction in microvascular techniques, and this chapter dealt almost exclusively with the mechanics of laboratory vessel anastomosis. That is certainly not the case at the present time, with complete texts[45,61] meetings, symposia, fellowships, and journals now devoted entirely to microsurgery. A bibliography limited to the microsurgical literature listing over 2000 references has been published.[15]

The emphasis of this chapter has therefore changed, and an attempt has been made here to provide a foundation of basic knowledge in this rapidly expanding field. To this end, sections dealing with clinical microvascular techniques, physiology and pharmacology of the microcirculation, and potential applications of current research in microsurgery have been added to an expanded discussion of the fundamental techniques of microvascular anastomosis.

BASIC MICROVASCULAR TECHNIQUES

To the uninitiated, the perceived difficulty in anastomosing vessels with a diameter of 1 mm or less is monumental. This feeling arises from frustration experienced during surgical procedures on small structures without the aid of magnification. In fact, anyone with reasonable technical ability can perform microsurgery, given three prerequisites: (1) suitable magnification; (2) appropriately sized instruments and suture material; and (3) initial training and subsequent practice to establish the hand-eye coordination and experience needed to handle delicate tissues, instruments, and suture in a variety of laboratory and clinical situations.

Magnification

LOUPES

Loupes or surgical telescopes are widely used for magnification, and the quality of these has improved dramatically in recent years. "Wide-field" versions are now available from several manufacturers, and numerous combinations of magnification, focal length, depth, and size of field are available.

These can be mounted to glasses or headbands, and a custom prescription can be ground into the lenses. In the "wide-field" versions, slightly higher magnification of $3.2\times$ to $4.5\times$ can be used comfortably, with working distances of 10 to 20 inches available. These are useful for any dissection in the hand, especially for exposure of neurovascular structures prior to repair or reconstruction. The microscope should be used for the actual repair because of the higher magnification available. For the surgeon who does microsurgery on a routine basis, the expense is easily justified (Fig. 24-1).

OPERATING MICROSCOPE

The operating microscope has evolved rapidly to keep pace with developments in the field of microsurgery; complex, tedious, and lengthy procedures demand an instrument that is "user-friendly" and versatile. Several manufacturers now produce top quality instruments designed for extremity microsurgery to include the following essentials (Fig. 24-2A):

1. A double headed system allowing the surgeon and assistant to share the operating field;
2. Foot or voice controlled magnification (zoom) and focusing;
3. Interchangeable eyepiece and objective lenses to match the working distance and magnification range to the clinical situation; and
4. A fiber optic light source—updated versions are available to provide constant illumination to the field as magnification changes.

Although not essential, motorized X-Y axis control is an extremely helpful and time-saving fea-

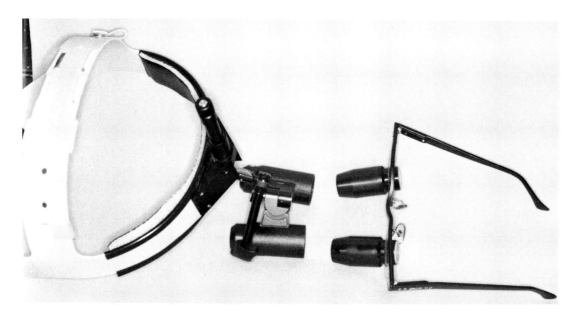

Fig. 24-1. Surgical telescopes. On the left is an adjustable 4.0 power headband version. On the right, a pair of 4.5 power loupes, fixed to the surgeon's prescription eyeglasses. These units are expensive, but the adjustable type has the advantage of use by different members of the microsurgical team.

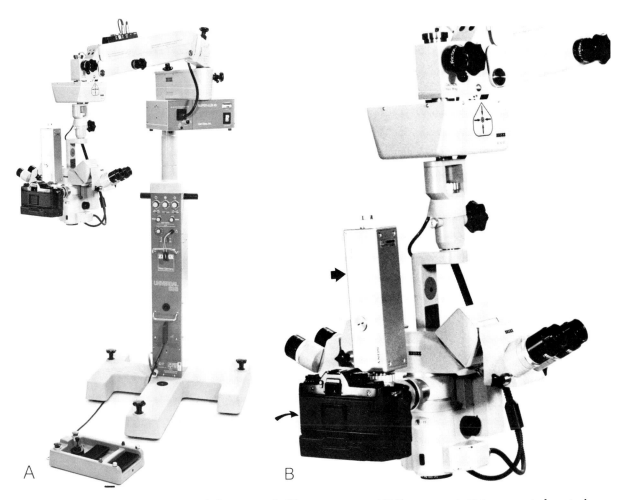

Fig. 24-2. (**A**) A Zeiss microscope with foot control of focus, zoom, and X-Y movement. Voice-operated controls are also available. (**B**) Double heads for the surgeon and assistant with eyepieces that can be inclined and attachments for video *(straight arrow)* and still photography *(curved arrow)* documentation are optimum; simpler versions will certainly suffice. (Courtesy of Zeiss, Inc.)

ture, especially during long procedures. This allows the surgeon to move the microscope over the operative field without moving the patient or having to look away from the field. Beam splitters for attachment of a third viewing post and/or photographic equipment are available. Cameras and color video systems can be attached and operated remotely; the latter is especially useful for teaching and for allowing the operating room personnel to observe the procedure (Fig. 24-2B).

Ceiling and floor mounts are available. The latter allows more mobility, but the microscope is a fragile instrument and movement should be kept to a minimum. Trained service personnel and a second, simpler backup microscope in case of failure must be available.

Arm, Table, and Chair Positioning

As pointed out by Acland and others, the most important factors in avoiding fatigue, frustration, and tremor are positioning and comfort.[7,47] To that end, multiple (and often conflicting) recommendations have been made in the literature regarding types of seating, table design and height, and microscope design. In fact, they are all interrelated, and each surgeon will need to devise a system that matches his needs and personal desires to the clinical situation. This can be accomplished by experimentation and an understanding of equipment interrelations (Fig. 24-3).

The most comfortable position for sitting for long periods is with the feet flat on the floor, and the hips and knees at approximately right angles. The height of the chair is therefore determined by the habitus of the surgeon. Chairbacks and arm rests are at the discretion of the surgeon.

The most effective *working height* is one that places the surgeon's elbows at or near 90 degrees when the forearm and hands are supported to minimize tremor. This implies that the *table height* should be less than the *working height* by a distance

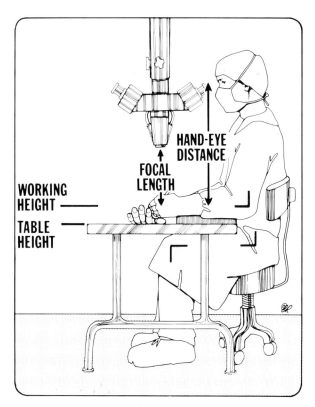

Fig. 24-3. In the optimum situation, the surgeon is comfortably seated over a stable hand table. The comfort level of the surgeon is dependent upon his own habitus, the focal length of the objective lens, and the height of the hand table, as described in the text.

equal to the table padding, drapes, and thickness of the extremity being operated on. A bit of experimentation will show that this leaves a relatively short distance between the thighs and the forearm in which to place the hand table. It should therefore be thin, and free of large braces projecting downward, yet it must be very stable to minimize vibration. I find that many of the standard, commercially available hand tables are not suitable for microvascular surgery for various reasons, including (1) inadequate stability, (2) working surface too small, and (3) inability to lower the table to an acceptable working height.

Once these factors are determined, the distance from the working height to the microscope eyepieces should be equal to the vertical distance from the surgeon's eyes to his hands (hand–eye distance). The surgeon can vary this distance by flexing or extending the spine from its most comfortable position, or by bending the elbows; the former quickly leads to fatigue, but the latter is useful within a limited range (Fig. 24-4).

The distance from working height to eyepieces can be varied easily in only two ways. First, if adjustable-incline (versus inclined) eyepieces are available, the angle can be adjusted to meet the surgeon's eye level. Second, the *focal length of the objective lens* can be changed. There is a common misconception that focusing will vary this distance, but focusing merely places the objective lens at the correct distance above the working height. Selecting the appropriate focal length objective lens will therefore place the eyepieces at the correct height.

Magnification is determined by the combination of objective lens, magnification changer, and eyepieces, as shown in the formula:

$$Mt = \frac{Fb}{Fo} \times Me \times Mc$$

where Mt is total magnification, Fb is the objective tube focal length, Fo is the objective lens focal length, Me is the eyepiece magnification, and Mc is the magnification factor of the zoom apparatus.[12]

Various objective lens focal lengths are available depending on the manufacturer; these range between 125 mm and 450 mm in most instances. I find a 175 or 250 mm objective lens most useful for hand surgery. Eyepieces of $10\times$ or $12.5\times$ are most commonly used, but $20\times$ eyepieces are occasion-

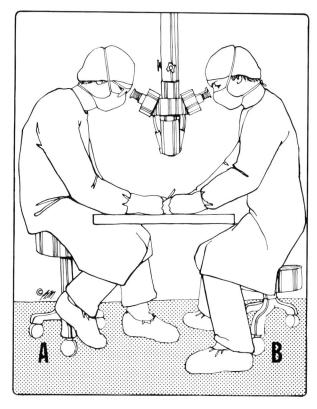

Fig. 24-4. Incorrect position rapidly leads to fatigue, poor co-ordination, and poor results. In (**A**) the chair is too high, causing back and arm strain; in (**B**), the seat is too low and the arms are unsupported.

ally needed for repair of small digital vessels in children and for microlymphatic surgery, even though this means a resultant decrease in field size. The size of the field is inversely proportional to magnification, and one should use the zoom control freely. Intimal inspection and suture placement are done under maximum magnification, while dissection and suture tying require less magnification and a wider field of view.

A few words of caution:

1. The working height can vary significantly between a digital vessel repair and a free flap anastomosis on an obese lower extremity, and may require a change in the objective lens.
2. Contamination of the surgical field by contact with the microscope during use is more likely with a short focal length objective lens, and

practice is required to avoid this problem. The microscope can be draped or sterilized, but the lens cannot.[77] The microscope should be draped to allow positioning over the field without contamination.

3. Eyepieces on some microscopes have an annoying habit of "backing out" slightly from the eyepiece holder, leading to focusing difficulties. This is a common cause of calls to the repair service, but is easily corrected by the surgeon. Always check to assure that the eyepieces are firmly seated.
4. Most microscopes will remain in focus at all magnifications (parfocality), but only if the diopter setting of each eyepiece matches the surgeon's vision. A simple instrument is available from the manufacturer to determine this setting, or the surgeon may have his correction determined by an ophthalmologist or optometrist.

For further in-depth information regarding the field of microsurgery, the history and development of the microscope, and correction of problems arising with its use, the reader is referred to the pertinent literature.[7,21,51,60,61,69,77]

Microsurgical Instruments and Suture Material

ESSENTIAL FEATURES

A confusing array of instruments and supplies for microsurgery is now available, and choosing instruments is difficult for the beginner. Experience is required to select features that will be of value, or to justify the cost of a special instrument. Essential features in all microsurgical instruments include fine tips to spread, hold, or cut delicate tissue and suture; a nonreflective surface; and comfortable handles that close easily to prevent fatigue.[60] Combined and double-ended instruments may decrease operative time, but require increased closing pressure and may be tiring.[46,63] A storage and sterilization case to protect these delicate instruments during use is mandatory.

The best way to clean micro-instruments is submersion for 30 minutes in a hemolytic enzyme solution (Hemosol). Saline solutions used in the operating suite will rust even resistant metals; water should therefore be used to rinse the instruments and they should be dried completely before storage. Only specially trained operating room personnel should clean and handle the instruments to prevent damage.[5–7]

FORCEPS

Forceps of varying designs are always used during microsurgical procedures. Adventitia forceps having a small toothed end are useful during the initial dissection of small vessels and nerves, and for repair of tendons under loupe magnification.

Smooth-tipped jeweler's forceps are available in varying sizes from #2 (most coarse) to #5 (most delicate) and are used under the microscope to handle the vessel and suture material. Only the tips meet, and they are easily damaged. Several pair should be available, as frequent replacement is needed.

Tying forceps have a broader grasping area and more blunt tips than jeweler's forceps. Angled tying forceps are recommended for the beginning microsurgeon to use as needle holders because there is less potential for vessel damage and there are no hinges to snag the suture.[23] Forceps do not grasp the needle as firmly, and excessive force applied by the novice will cause the needle to slip rather than tear the vessel wall (Fig. 24-5A).

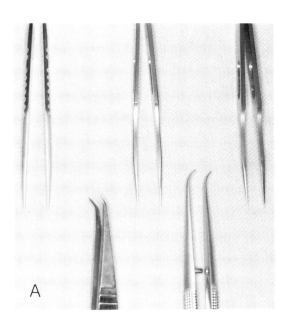

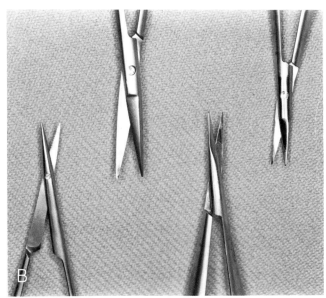

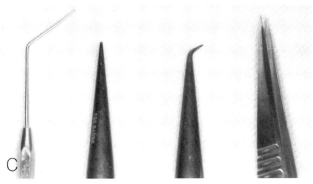

Fig. 24-5. (A) Types of microsurgical forceps (left to right): adventitia; angled tying; coarse jeweler's (#3); angled tying with different tip plane relative to handle; fine jeweler's (#5). (B) Microsurgical scissors (left to right): serrated straight blades for sectioning nerves; larger straight blades for dividing vessels and cutting suture; small straight blades for trimming adventitia; small curved blades for vessel dissection. (C) Dilators (left to right): lacrimal dilator useful to relieve spasm; straight and curved graduated dilators; forceps-type dilator used once the vessel has been clamped.

SCISSORS

Straight and curved scissors are available, both with blunt or sharp tips. Blunt, curved designs are most useful for dissection of vessels and nerves. Straight scissors are used for circumcision of adventitia and freshening the ends of vessels and nerves. Straight scissors with serrated blades for sectioning nerves are also available (Fig. 24-5B).

DILATORS

Dilators are available in several styles. Spring-type dilators are similar to forceps, but have externally polished jaws for dilation of the vessel end prior to anastomosis. They are especially useful once clamps have been applied to the vessel where the longer straight dilators cannot be used.

Straight constant-diameter (lacrimal) dilators can be used to relieve spasm occurring along a vessel, and tapering dilators are used to enlarge a vessel to correct size discrepancy (Fig. 24-5C).

Small Fogarty catheters can be used to dilate and clear vessels of larger diameter proximal to the midpalm. Hydrostatic dilation is not recommended.[64]

CLAMPS

In order to perform an anastomosis, blood flow through the vessel must be temporarily occluded. Vascular clamps accomplish this, and selection of

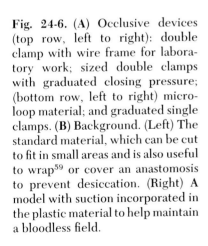
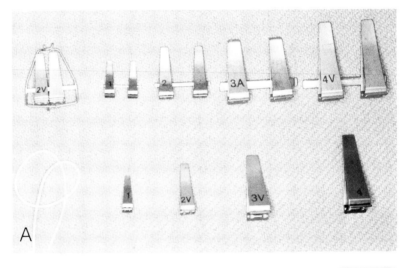
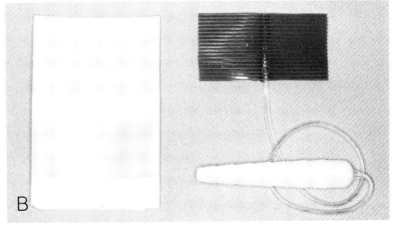

Fig. 24-6. (A) Occlusive devices (top row, left to right): double clamp with wire frame for laboratory work; sized double clamps with graduated closing pressure; (bottom row, left to right) micro-loop material; and graduated single clamps. (B) Background. (Left) The standard material, which can be cut to fit in small areas and is also useful to wrap[59] or cover an anastomosis to prevent desiccation. (Right) A model with suction incorporated in the plastic material to help maintain a bloodless field.

the correct clamp is important to minimize damage to the vessel wall. Sets of clamps are available that match the closing pressure to the size of the vessel. Less traumatic clamp design is important in achieving high patency rates.[36,49,74,75,78] Dual clamps allow tension-free approximation of the vessel edges prior to anastomosis.[3,50] Single clamps are necessary where space is limited and in other special situations.[1] Microsized rubber vessel loops are also available and useful in areas where clamp application is difficult (Fig. 24-6A).

BACKGROUND

Thin sheets of plastic background material (available in several colors) are helpful to enhance the surgeon's view of the vessel and sutures and to iso-

late the vessel from the surrounding tissue and blood.[59] Models with a mechanism for suction incorporated into the sheets have been introduced (Fig. 24-6B).

IRRIGATION

Frequent irrigation of the vessel with heparinized saline or Ringer's lactate is necessary during anastomosis to remove small clots from the lumen. Ringer's appears to be the least damaging to the vessel. Heparinized solutions also prevent sticking of the suture to the tissue.[8,20,57,72] Irrigation tips should be blunt; these are commercially available or can be made by modifying 25- to 30-gauge needles. Other syringes and tips should be available for irrigation of the vessel with lidocaine or other phar-

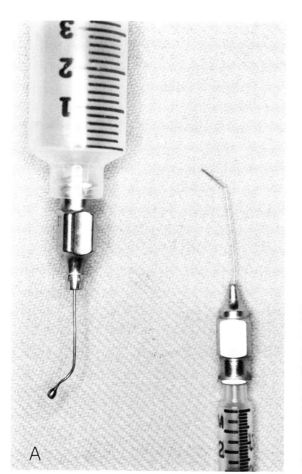

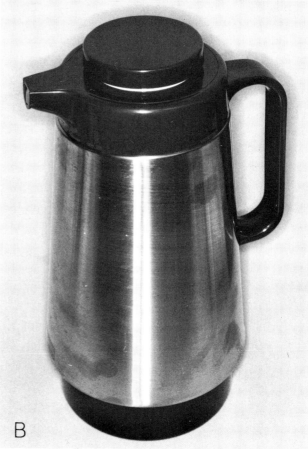

Fig. 24-7. Irrigation. **(A)** A large syringe and blunt tip for heparinized Ringer's solution is shown on the left; on the right, a modified 30-gauge needle and tuberculin syringe for lidocaine irrigation. **(B)** A gas-sterilized thermos for maintaining warmed irrigating solutions.

macologic substances to decrease spasm. Warming these topical solutions is important to prevent vasospasm,[11] and maintaining a warm solution in a cold operating suite is difficult. We have solved this problem by gas sterilization of inexpensive plastic thermos bottles, using these to keep the solutions warm until they are needed (Fig. 24-7).

NEEDLE DRIVERS

Needle drivers are available with straight or curved tips, and once the surgeon has mastered the gentle placement of sutures with tying forceps, a simple, curved nonlocking needle holder will be most often used. Special designs with tips in various planes relative to the handle are helpful in performing end-to-side anastomoses, and in difficult situations encountered in free tissue transfer. Although some surgeons prefer locking needle holders, most find the force necessary to lock and unlock the instrument difficult to apply without tearing the vessel. The ultimate choice of needle holder will depend on the anastomotic technique used, the presentation of the vessels to the surgeon, and the choice of straight or curved needle (Fig. 24-8).

ACCESSORY INSTRUMENTS

Several other types of instruments are helpful, including (1) small Weck hemoclips for clamping vessel branches during initial dissection; (2) a bipolar coagulator with both standard and microtips; (3) small cellulose sponges (Wexcel) for removing blood and irrigation fluid from the field; and (4) an instrument demagnetizing coil, which is necessary to prevent attraction of the needle and suture to the instruments (Fig. 24-9).

Suction is occasionally helpful, but must be used with extreme caution to prevent damage to vessels, suture, and surrounding structures.

Suture ligation is safe at any distance from the parent vessel, and bipolar coagulation as close as 2 mm. Although widely used clinically, hemoclips have a high experimental failure rate due to loosening.[31,65]

SUTURE

Microsuture is available from several manufacturers in multiple combinations of material, suture size, and needle configuration. Unsterilized suture

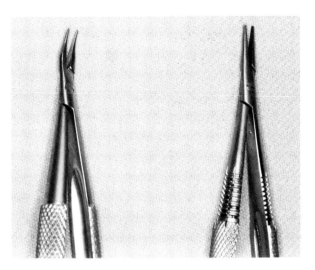

Fig. 24-8. Needle drivers are available with curved or straight jaws.

can be obtained at less expense for laboratory work. The most widely used suture is 10–0 monofilament nylon on a 75-μ curved or straight needle. Smaller suture and needle combinations (10–0 and 11–0 on 30- and 50-μ needles) are useful for children's digital vessels, but require proportionately higher magnification. For repair of larger vessels and nerves, larger combinations are available. Less reactive absorbable suture material has been recently introduced in appropriate sizes (Fig. 24-10A).

Microsurgical needles are either tapered or have cutting edges only at the tip to prevent damage to the fragile vessel wall. Needles are designated as straight or curved, by wire diameter in microns, and by chord length (Fig. 24-10B).

Straight needles have the advantage of being more easily picked up in a position ready for use and are preferred by some microsurgeons in situations where they can be used.[25]

INSTRUMENT SOURCES

ASSI and Moria both offer a wide range of affordable instruments designed by practicing microsurgeons. Complete sets of "state of the art" microinstruments are sold by several manufacturers, but are usually more expensive.

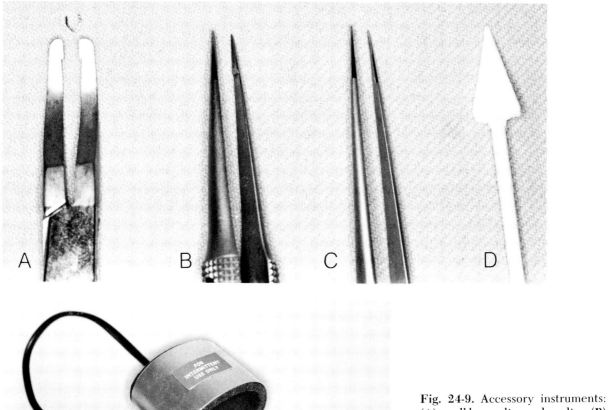

Fig. 24-9. Accessory instruments: (**A**) small hemoclips and applier; (**B**) standard bipolar coagulator; (**C**) microbipolar coagulator; (**D**) Wexcel sponges; and (**E**) instrument demagnetizer.

Laboratory

Microsurgery cannot be learned without a practice laboratory.[40] The surgeon who is forced to do so alone will have to acquire a microscope, instruments, lab space, animal models, and someone to care for them.[35] Many hospitals have older operating microscopes suitable for animal use that are sitting about unused. Drug companies, veterinary schools, research facilities, and medical schools may have lab space and animal care facilities. A mini-laboratory may be constructed in the office or home.[76] In some cases a microsurgery lab may be already in operation and permission may be obtained to use the facility. Physicians trained in microsurgical techniques may be willing to instruct the neophyte, and may have access to practice facilities. Several basic laboratory manuals have been published.[7,9,12,13,23,70]

Probably the best way to begin is to register for

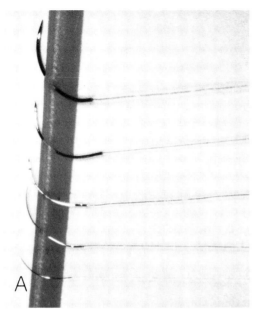

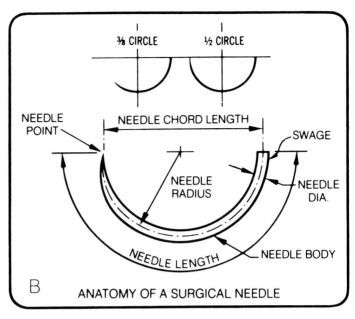

Fig. 24-10. **(A)** Suture material (top to bottom): 9–0 nylon, 130 μ needle; 10–0 nylon, 100 μ needle; 10–0 nylon, 75 μ needle; 10–0 nylon, 50 μ needle; 11–0 nylon, 30 μ needle. **(B)** Microsurgical needles. Microsurgical needles are designated by diameter and chord length. (Courtesy of Ethicon, Inc.)

one of the many short, intensive training programs offered.° These vary in length from a few days to a few weeks, and have many advantages. Everything needed is provided, there are few outside distractions, and "one-to-one" instruction is available so that good habits and techniques are learned from the start. The student also has the opportunity to observe the setup of the lab, which will facilitate organizing his own lab for continued maintenance and improvement of acquired skills.

The first step is to become familiar with the microscope and to adjust the table, chair, and microscope to one's comfort. For those with refractive errors, the eyepieces can be set so that glasses are not needed. I find that removal of the protective eye cups provides a much wider field of vision; they can be replaced after use to protect the eyepieces.

The interpupillary distance is adjusted, and coordinated use of zoom, focus, and X-Y axis control is then mastered. It is important to adjust the microscope so that it remains parfocal (in focus throughout the entire magnification range) according to the manufacturer's instructions. Once comfortable with the microscope, the student should practice holding and manipulating the instruments without tremor and then master the handling of fine suture material. This is an important step that if well learned will make later exercises much easier. Acland and others have described the intricacies in minute detail, and these references should be read carefully.[4,7,12] For the sake of brevity, they are not reproduced here. Once these are learned, the student is ready for a nonanimal model.

NONANIMAL MODELS

The initial exercise is to suture a slit in a thin piece of rubber or latex. These practice cards can be constructed easily or bought commercially.[10,12,14,56] A fresh leaf can also be used in a similar manner. It is friable and nonelastic, and technical errors

---

° In preparing this chapter, I found that a comprehensive list of short courses and microsurgery fellowships was not available. An updated list may be obtained from the author by request, and I would ask anyone who offers such programs to notify me in order to keep the list current.

will become readily apparent. This model best demonstrates the tissue damage produced by crude technique.[12,53] Small silicone tubing can be used to simulate vessel anastomosis, and umbilical vessels, easily obtained from obstetric or pathology departments, are a challenging model.[38,58]

ANIMAL MODELS

Arterial and venous anastomosis and neurorrhaphy are then learned on animal models. Several are available, with the rat being most widely used for study of basic techniques.[39] The rat femoral and carotid arteriovenous systems are easily accessible with the animal anesthetized and pinned supine to a board. These animals are relatively inexpensive and easy to maintain.

The rabbit ear has been used as a model for digit revascularization and replantation.[41] Larger animals (cats, dogs, and primates) are useful for research in free tissue transfer. Models of free flap and free bone transfer have been devised in several species.[39,66,67,71] End-to-side and size discrepancy models have been developed.[34,42,44]

The exact mechanics for animal model anesthesia and preparation are beyond the scope of this chapter, as some attention to detail is required to assure survival during the procedure. The most complete description of these techniques is that by Seaber.[68] Several laboratory manuals also include abbreviated descriptions of animal models.[7,12,13,23]

Basic Techniques

ESSENTIALS FOR A PATENT ANASTOMOSIS

Once the animal has been prepared and the vascular structures have been exposed, the microscope is then positioned. There are several essential requirements to ensure an anastomosis with long-term patency, whether in the laboratory or clinical situation, and they are listed below.

1. Meticulous atraumatic dissection and handling of the vessel, with tying or coagulation of branches.[31]
2. The vessel wall and intima at the site of anasto-

mosis *must* be normal when visualized under high power magnification; if not, it is imperative that the vessel be resected back to normal tissue.
3. Adequate flow must then be demonstrated from the proximal vessel.
4. The anastomosis must be done without tension, and vessel mobilization or grafting may be needed to ensure a tension-free anastomosis. The incidence of early and late failure is increased by tension on the anastomosis.[79]
5. Meticulous attention to detail is required in completing the anastomosis. Adequate removal of local overhanging adventitia (which is intensely thrombogenic),[30] followed by suture placement, without grasping the intima, to produce a nearly leak-proof anastomosis is required. The most common technical error is inadvertent suturing of the backwall, and this may be prevented by several techniques described later in this chapter.

Figure 24-11 illustrates these principles in the preparation of rat femoral vessels.

END-TO-END ANASTOMOSIS TECHNIQUE

Once the vessel has been prepared and adequate proximal flow ensured, the anastomosis is performed. If proximal flow is impaired, gentle dilatation with a lacrimal dilator and application of local vasodilating agents (lidocaine, etc.) may improve flow. Allowing the vessels to rest undisturbed for several minutes and warming of the tissue may also aid in decreasing spasm.

The basic anastomosis procedure described next is a summation of the techniques most widely recommended by several noted authors.[7,12-14,17-19,23,45,48,51,61,62,70]

The clamps are adjusted so that no tension exists on the anastomosis site (Fig. 24-12A – C). The artery is divided cleanly, and the adventitia trimmed (Fig. 24-12D – F). The lumen is gently dilated (Fig. 24-12G and H).

The vessel is now ready for anastomosis (Fig. 24-13). Only the adventitia is picked up in the forceps, and the sutures are placed atraumatically. Intraluminal counterpressure with the forceps is use-

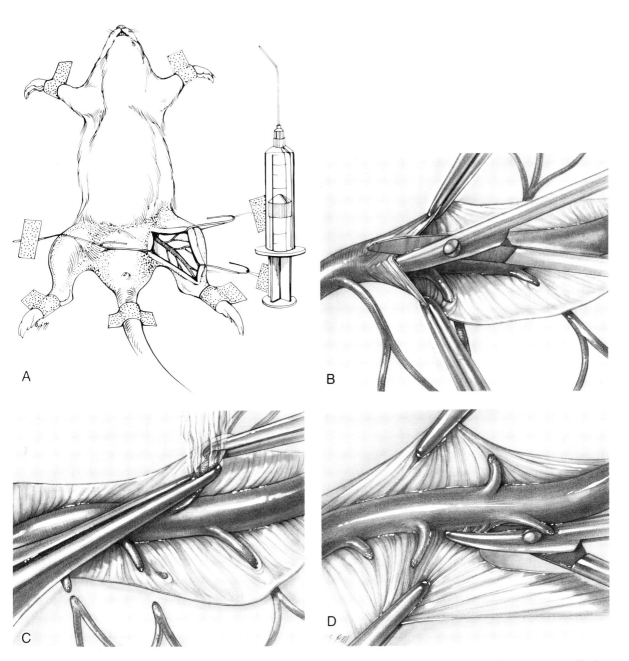

Fig. 24-11. Animal preparation (rat femoral vessels). (**A**) Nembutal (50 mg/cc) is administered intraperitoneally (0.6 to 1.0 cc/100 g body weight). The groin is shaved with clippers, and the animal is taped on a board with all four legs secured. The skin is prepped with Betadine and the groin incised longitudinally. Sutures or bent paper clips secured to the board with tape can be used to provide self retaining skin retractors. Blunt dissection can be used through the fat layer. The irrigation setup uses a blunt-tipped needle and heparinized Ringer's lactate (200 units/cc). (**B**) After dissecting through the fat layer, the adventitia is sharply divided using traction-countertraction and blunt-nosed scissors, keeping close to the femoral artery. (**C**) Branches of the artery are cauterized with the bipolar coagulator. Large branches should be cauterized and divided several millimeters from the main vessel, while smaller vessels can be transected closer to the main vessel. (**D**) The artery is dissected from surrounding tissue by pulling the adjacent tissue slightly and sharply cutting with scissors close to the artery. The artery is supported by surrounding tissue; the wall of the artery is never grasped directly with forceps. The basic principles of microdissection include traction and countertraction to place moderate tension on the structure, and then sharp dissection of the layers under direct visualization.

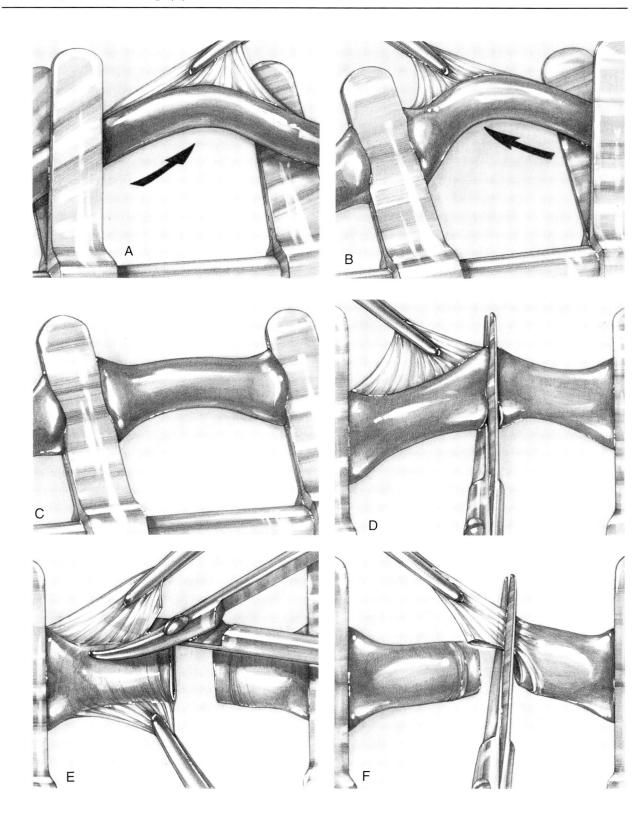

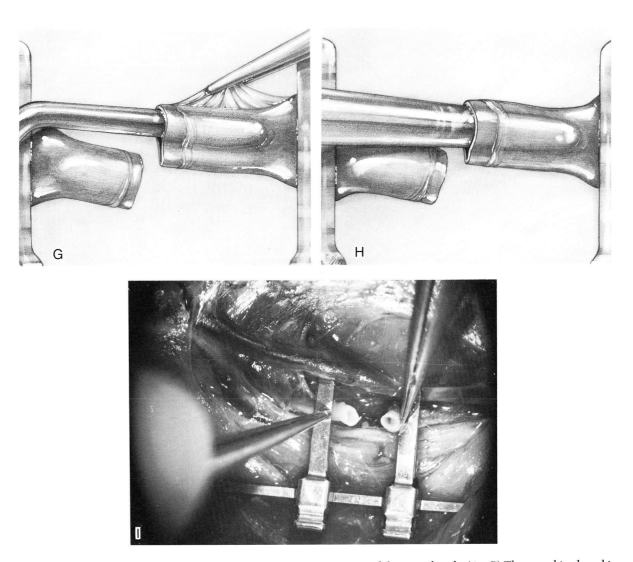

Fig. 24-12. Technique of arterial anastomosis. Steps in preparation of the vessel ends. (**A–C**) The vessel is placed in the clamps so there is moderate slack. (**D**) The artery is cut cleanly with sharp scissors in a single motion. (**E**) There will be adventitia in and around the lumen. This must be carefully removed without touching the vessel itself. Only the loose adventitia should be grasped; it is cut cleanly, close to the artery. (**F**) The adventitia is pulled and sharply trimmed along the cut edge of the artery ("circumcised"). The extent of adventitia removed should be confined to all loose strands around the end to provide a clear view of the vessel wall and keep any material out of the lumen. Both ends should be thus prepared, switching instruments to accomplish this. (**G**) The lumen is gently dilated first with a small, angled dilator and (**H**) then with a pencil dilator. The intima is carefully inspected under high power for any loose material or defects. (**I**) The vessel is now ready to be sutured. The adventitia has been cleaned off and the vessel dissected sharply back to good intima. Normal intima can be seen in the lumen of the vessel, and over-hanging adventitia has been sharply dissected.

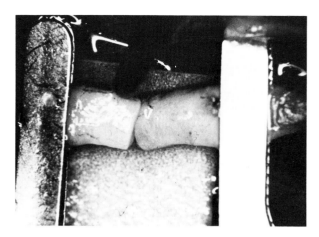

Fig. 24-13. Close-up of an 0.8-mm vessel showing the vessel in the clamp. The ends come together easily without tension, even with no sutures. Note that the adventitia has been trimmed back so that there is no adventitia overhanging the lumen.

ful, but the intima and vessel edge should never be grasped by the forceps.

Corner sutures 120 to 180 degrees apart (Fig. 24-14A) are first placed. In arteries, the suture bite should be 1 to 2 times the thickness of the vessel wall. In veins, a width of 2 to 3 times the wall thickness is used (Fig. 24-15A).

If a surgeon's knot is used for the first throw, the suture can be gently tightened until the vessel walls just meet. Over-tightening the suture will invert, evert, or tear the vessel wall, exposing thrombogenic surfaces to the lumen.[16,61,73] Over-tightening also results in direct narrowing of the lumen as the tissue is distorted. A square knot and third throw are then completed, again avoiding over-tightening. As the suture is pulled through the vessel wall, care should be taken to guide the leading and following suture with the instruments such that the suture is pulled smoothly through the vessel wall. Suture forcibly pulled through the wall against resistance will tend to "cut through," leading to endothelial damage.

There are two options for retrieving the needle. First, it may be carefully placed in the field of view prior to tying the knot, and then picked up for the next stitch. The second method is to pull the needle and attached suture out of the field, tie the knot, cut the suture, and then pull on the trailing end while guiding the suture with forceps to retrieve the needle. I prefer the latter method, as less suture material is present in the field to interfere with tying the knot. The surgeon must always hold the suture near the vessel with forceps when releasing the needle from the needle driver. If this is not done, the needle or suture may stick to the instrument and be pulled out of the vessel.

One or more sutures are then placed between the corner sutures. The last suture placed in either the front or back wall is critical, as it is difficult to visualize the lumen and prevent inadvertent suturing of the opposite wall. If the corner sutures are placed 120 degrees apart, the back wall will tend to fall away and thus be protected (asymmetric biangulation technique).[62] The vessel is then rotated 180 degrees by flipping the vessel clamp. The back wall is then sutured, and as each suture is placed, the lumen is irrigated and gently dilated with the forceps to assure that the back wall is not caught up in one of the sutures.

Placement of the final suture is critical, and several techniques can be used to avoid suturing of the opposite wall.

1. The neighboring two sutures can be left long, and traction placed on them to isolate the intervening vessel wall for placement of the final suture.

2. The needle can be passed through one side of the anastomosis, brought out through the defect, and then used to gently pick up and evert the adjacent wall as it is placed.

3. A two suture technique can be used in which the first needle is passed through both sides, but not pulled through. The second stitch is then placed and tied and the first suture then pulled through and tied.[27,37]

4. I prefer a modification of the Harashima procedure.[43] The last two sutures are placed as if one were performing a continuous running suture. The loop between the sutures is left large instead of being tightened down, and is then cut with the suture scissors, leaving two sutures in place and ready for tying. This conserves suture and motion, and minimizes the number of needles, instruments, and sutures in the operative field. It is also the best alternative for the microsurgeon working alone (Fig. 24-16).

The "lathe-rest" principle of supporting one instrument with the other is often useful to control tremor.[51] The frustration that can be experienced in dealing with fine suture and tenacious tissues in vivo defies description. Acland has addressed the handling of suture material in these circumstances, and his article is required reading for the microsurgeon who wishes to minimize his or her frustration.[4]

The clamp is then released, and the flow is observed under the microscope. Oozing from the anastomosis is normal, but pulsatile bleeding must be controlled by placement of additional sutures. Brisk flow usually occurs through a well-performed anastomosis, but occasionally vessel spasm severely limits flow. If this appears to be the case, apply local vasodilating agents, warm the area if possible, and avoid manipulating the vessel for 15 to 20 minutes.

PATENCY TEST

Assessment of anastomotic patency may be done in several ways.[2,32] In clinical situations, return of color to and capillary oozing or venous bleeding from the revascularized tissue signal a competent arterial anastomosis. Engorgement of the tissue indicates compromise of venous drainage.

Direct inspection of both arterial and venous anastomoses under the microscope may reveal signs of patency. Arterial patency is indicated by nicely dilated vessels showing pulsatile elongation ("wriggling") or expansile pulsation. Gently lifting the vessel distal to the anastomosis by placing forceps underneath it will demonstrate the "flicker" of blood flowing across this area, but is easily visible only in thin-walled vessels.

The empty and refill patency test is traumatic and should be performed as gently and infrequently as possible.[48] Two pair of smooth forceps are used to occlude the vessel distal to the anastomosis. The more "downstream" forceps is then moved gently about 1 cm down the vessel, creating an empty segment between the two forceps. The proximal compression is then released, and rapid filling of the empty segment indicates patency of the anastomosis. This test is useful for either arteries or veins, and for any size vessel (Fig. 24-17).

VEINS

Rat vein anastomosis is very difficult because: (1) these vessels are extremely friable and thin walled; (2) it is difficult to separate the adventitia from the vessel without damage; and (3) the lumen tends to collapse. Performing the anastomosis under fluid or with copious irrigation to "float" the lumen open is often necessary. Clamps tend to tear the vein and must be used with extreme care or not at all (Fig. 24-18).

Fortunately, veins encountered in replantation and free tissue transfer in humans are more substantial, but they still retain some of the characteristics mentioned above, and require more careful handling and additional sutures to prevent intraluminal collapse of segments of the vessel wall.

CLINICAL MICROVASCULAR TECHNIQUES

The ability to perform a technically adequate vessel anastomosis in the laboratory does not guarantee success in clinical situations such as replantation and free tissue transfer. Many other factors may influence the eventual outcome, and the surgeon will need to favorably influence as many of these as possible (Table 24-1). This section and the following one on physiology and pharmacology will address these problems.

Presentation, Access, and Size Discrepancy

Many difficulties may be encountered in moving from a totally controlled laboratory setting to a clinical situation, including:

1. Difficulty in orienting the vessels for ease of anastomosis;[201]
2. Limited access to the vessels in a deep wound;
3. Vessel size discrepancy; and
4. Inability to rotate the clamp holding the vessel for suturing of the back wall.

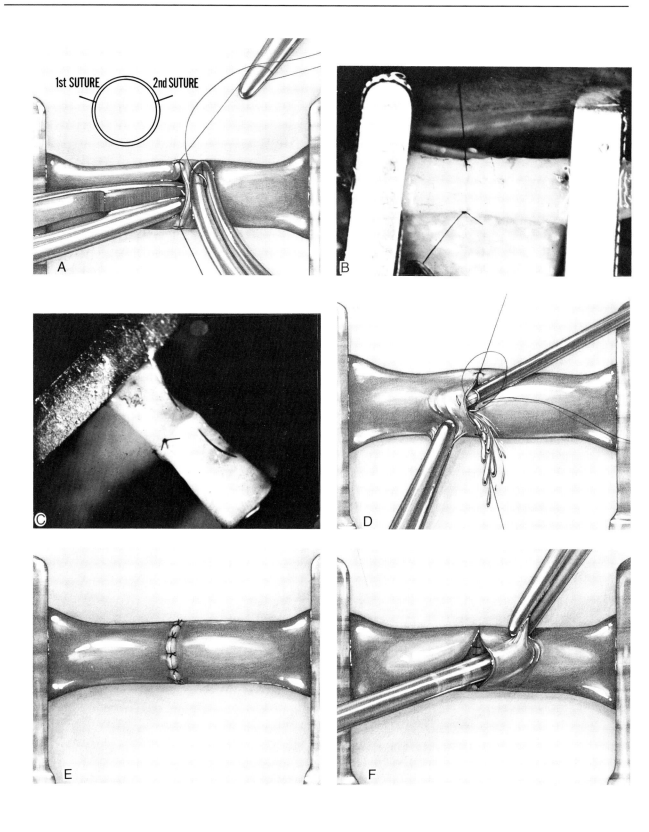

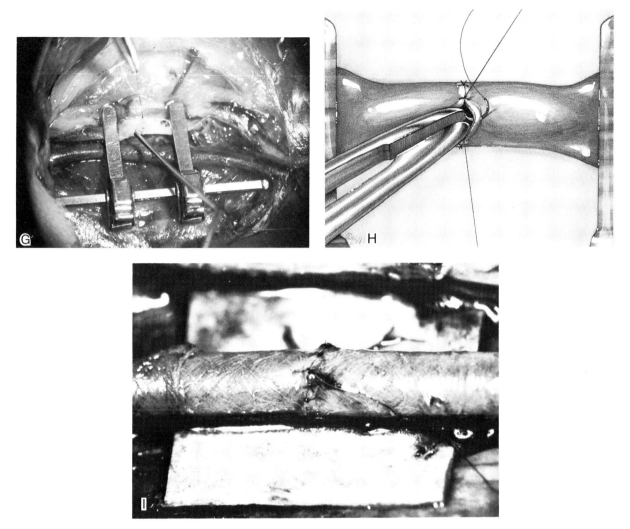

Fig. 24-14. Suture placement. A minimum of four sutures are placed for 0.5-mm vessels or less and 6 to 8 sutures for 1.0-mm vessels. The number of sutures also depends on the thickness of the wall; more sutures are needed for thin-walled vessels and veins. **(A)** Sutures should be evenly placed with the initial two corner sutures placed 120 degrees apart. This allows the back wall to fall away from the front wall, minimizing the tendency to catch the back wall with the front wall sutures. **(B)** The ends of previously placed sutures are used to elevate the front wall of the anastomosis. **(C)** The needle is placed through one side of the vessel and visualized in the gap to assure that the back wall has not been penetrated. **(D)** The needle can then be put through the other wall separately or passed through both the vessel ends simultaneously. The correct maneuver in each case is the one that is least traumatic and gives the greatest view of the needle at all times. Angled probes or the irrigating tip can be used to visualize the vessel during placement. **(E)** The front wall completed. **(F)** The clamp is turned and inspection is made of the lumen to make sure that none of the anterior wall sutures have caught the posterior wall. **(G)** The sutures are well placed around the anterior wall, and the vessel will come together nicely. There is no tension. **(H)** The final suture. Care must be taken not to catch the back wall. The best way to prevent this is to show the tip of the needle in the gap. Alternate methods for last suture placement are described in the text. When the clamps are released, no major gaps allowing blood to squirt more than 1 to 2 inches should exist. If gaps are present, additional sutures should be added. An ooze of blood is normal and will cease. **(I)** A completed anastomosis.

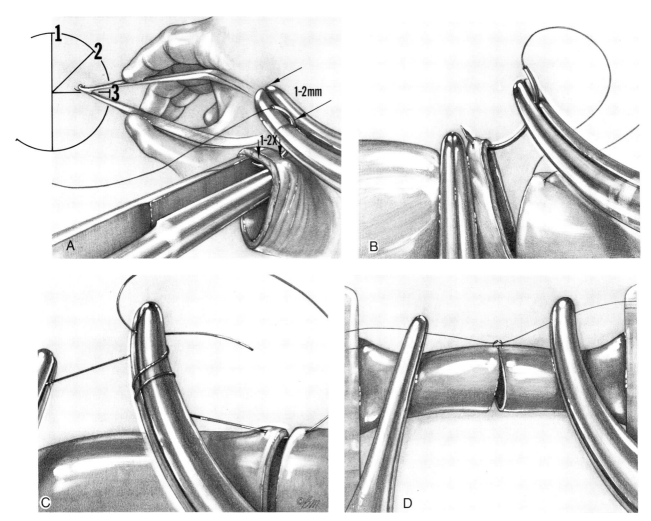

Fig. 24-15. Suture technique. (**A**) The needle driver is held like a pencil, resting comfortably on the long finger and held gently with the thumb and index finger. If one draws a circle with a bisecting line, the straightest line usually gives the most comfortable needle-passing direction (most commonly, position 3 or 2). The needle is passed parallel to the vessel axis, with the forearm perpendicular to the axis of the vessel. The needle is held 1 to 2 mm from the tip of the needle driver. Needle bites should be placed back from the cut edge a distance equal to 1 to 2 times the wall thickness in arteries and 2 to 3 times that in veins. The tip should pass perpendicular (at right angles) to the surface of the vessel. Care should be taken to pass the needle cleanly, without any pulling or trauma to the vessel wall. The needle is pushed into the wall, using the forceps inside the vessel to provide counterpressure to complete penetration. (**B**) In passing through the second wall, the forceps are used outside the wall to provide counterpressure. The suture is pulled carefully through the vessel until 1 to 2 cm of suture material is left on the short end. (**C**) The needle is carefully laid either in the microscopic field or on a white lap pad directly in front of the operator. Under the microscope, a surgeon's knot is laid squarely, using the needle driver and tying forceps or two pairs of tying forceps. (**D**) The knot is tightened carefully under the microscope to bring the edges together without the suture cutting through. The first tie alone should bring the edges together; if not, then excessive tension on the vessel exists. A total of three knots are laid squarely. One end is cut 1 mm from the knot and the other left long for retraction.

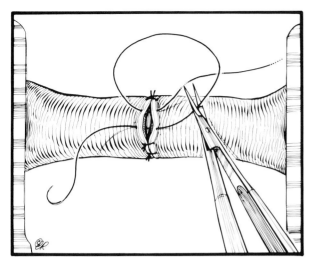

Fig. 24-16. Modified Harashima procedure. Both sutures are placed as for a running technique, and the loop is then cut as shown, leaving two sutures ready to be tied.

It is frequently impossible to significantly change the presentation of the vessels. Anticipating such situations, one should practice anastomoses in the laboratory with the vessels oriented at various angles between horizontal and vertical. In difficult situations in the hand and upper extremity an additional assistant may be required to hold or rotate the extremity, or an alternative method of revascularization may have to be used. A prime example is thumb revascularization or replantation. To approach the volar vessels the extremity must be severely pronated or supinated, and it is extremely difficult to maintain this position and perform the anastomosis. Other options include repair or grafting of the volar vessels prior to bone fixation[96] or interpositional vein grafting to a more accessible dorsal vessel (e.g., the radial artery).

Limited access to deeply placed structures may be improved by extension of the surgical incision to provide a more open wound, or by placing moist sponges beneath the vessels, lifting them out of the wound. Alternative anastomosis techniques (end-to-side or backwall-first) are often useful in this situation.

Several solutions have been proposed for vessel size discrepancy. A difference of 2:1 or less may be handled by gently dilating the smaller vessel and not dilating the larger one. Above 2:1, however, alternate techniques are preferred. Vein grafts are more distendable than arteries and are very useful to match vessels of varying diameters.[90]

End-in-end and spatulation techniques have been described for differences in size up to 3:1.[92,99,117,131,193,212-214] If the smaller vessel empties into the larger one, the smaller end may be telescoped inside the larger vessel (end-in-end technique). Cutting one or both vessel walls longitudinally and repair by triangulating the corners as is often used by vascular surgeons may be helpful (spatulation technique). Cutting the vessel ends obliquely at varying angles may also be used to change the effective diameter. This method has been described with mathematical precision.[92] In my experience, these techniques are infrequently required. End-to-side anastomosis can be used for virtually any size discrepancy problem. When using all of these techniques, it must be remembered that *any rapid change in size or direction of the vessel will produce turbulence and increase the chance of thrombosis.*[131,170]

Excessive tension at the suture line is a common cause of both immediate and delayed anastomotic failure. The surgeon should anticipate this problem and utilize an interpositional vein graft rather than attempt an end-to-end anastomosis that is under tension. This technique is addressed more fully in the section on vein grafting.

Alternative Anastomosis Techniques

Three alternative techniques are frequently used clinically in situations where presentation of the vessels is not optimum for standard end-to-end anastomosis. These are: (1) the backwall-first technique; (2) "flipping" of a mobile vessel; and (3) end-to-side technique.

BACKWALL-FIRST TECHNIQUE

The backwall-first technique is most useful with vessels of approximately equal size where one or both presenting ends cannot be rotated within a double clamp. This most commonly occurs when the repair is made close to a parent trunk or large

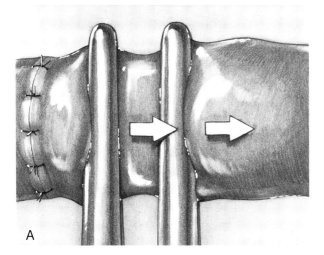

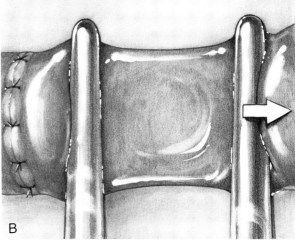

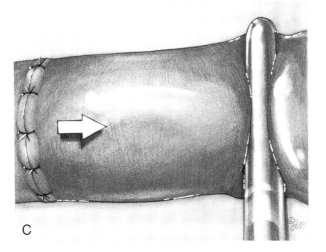

Fig. 24-17. The patency test is performed using two blunt-tipped tying forceps distal to the anastomosis. (**A**) The proximal forceps remain stationary while the second forceps push the blood distally and stop, remaining closed. (**B**) The proximal forceps are then opened while the distal remain closed. (**C**) If the anastomosis is good, there will be immediate filling of the segment. Any delay in filling usually means that there is a problem with the anastomosis.

branch that cannot be sacrificed. With some practice this "free hand" anastomosis is not difficult and has the added advantage that one is not likely to suture both walls together. In performing any anastomosis, the most difficult suture should always be placed first, and so I prefer to begin the anastomosis on the posterior wall at the point farthest away from the surgeon. Interrupted sutures are placed sequentially toward the surgeon until the back wall is completed, and then the front wall is repaired. The knots are, of course, placed outside the lumen. The initial suture is left long to aid in traction and rotation of the vessel (Fig. 24-19). Backwall-first

repair can also be done by adding sutures alternatively to either side of the first suture until the anastomosis is completed.[132,145,168,220]

"FLIPPING" TECHNIQUE

In many situations, one vessel end is freely mobile and can be "flipped" end-over-end to repair the backwall. Examples include:

1. Vein grafting, where the first anastomosis can be completed in this manner and the second by standard technique; and

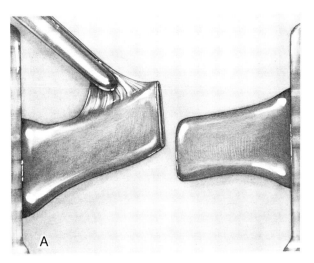

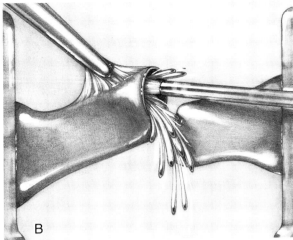

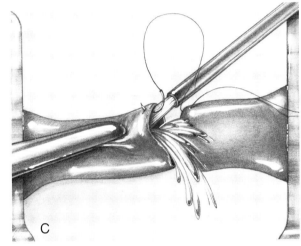

Fig. 24-18. Technique of vein anastomosis. (**A**) Veins are thinner, flatter, and more difficult to anastomose. Although the basic technique is somewhat similar to that for arteries, there are some differences. (**B**) Veins can be more easily sutured by using Ringer's solution to float or irrigate the vessel open. Special care must be taken to prevent adventitia from blocking the lumen while suturing and to avoid catching the back wall. (**C**) Somewhat deeper bites must be taken equal to 2 to 3 times the thickness of the vessel wall. Generally, more sutures must be taken to prevent large gaps and to prevent collapse of the wall.

2. Free tissue transfer where the flap may be freely mobile if it is revascularized prior to insetting. Extreme care must be used when handling and insetting the flap to avoid damage to the anastomosis by tension or kinking of the pedicle when using this technique.

This technique is useful when a vessel presents for anastomosis in such a manner that double clamp placement and rotation are difficult. I have found this useful in vein grafting patients with retrocarpal thrombosis of the radial artery[182] where the distal anastomosis is done on a vessel presenting "end-up" toward the surgeon between the two heads of the first dorsal interosseus. A single clamp is placed on the distal vessel and the vein graft, and the front wall is completed. The vein graft is then flipped end-over-end and the back wall repaired (Fig. 24-20).

END-TO-SIDE TECHNIQUE

The end-to-side technique is a standard one that is taught in all microsurgical laboratory courses,[81, 87,95] and has been studied experimentally.[83,105, 130,167] If only a single vessel maintains the viability

Table 24-1. Major Factors that Influence Failure After Microsurgery in Experimental Animals

Technical
  Both walls sutured together
  Traumatic vessel handling
  Apposition of vessel edges
  Disproportional vessel size
  Tension at suture line
  Excessive clamp pressure
  Kinking of vessels

Reperfusion
  No reflow
  Blood turbulence
  Spasm
  Hypercoagulability
  Acidosis
  Cold
  Hypovolemia
  Circulating constrictors

Postoperative Care
  Infection
  Acidosis
  Environmental factors
  Transplantation
  Cold
  Limb position

(Seaber AV: Laboratory design preparing for elective microvascular surgery. Hand Clinics, 1:233–45, 1985.)

of an extremity it cannot be sacrificed as the donor vessel for an end-to-end anastomosis, and an end-to-side repair must be used. Marked size discrepancy also demands this method. Improvement in patency rates over end-to-end anastomosis has been reported with this technique.[83,123] Theoretically, this is because of the propensity of the arterial wall to retract when cut, thus effectively "holding open" the anastomotic site.

The arteriotomy into the donor vessel is the most critical (and irreversible) step in the procedure. One should master the technique in the laboratory on vessels of varying diameter and wall thickness before using it in clinical practice.

The arteriotomy may be done by excising a "wedge" of vessel wall with straight scissors, as described by Godina,[153] or begun with a micro-knife and enlarged carefully to an elliptical or circular defect with microscissors. Special arteriotomy clamps are available, but these also require practice to achieve consistent results. The arteriotomy should match the size of the vessel to be anas-

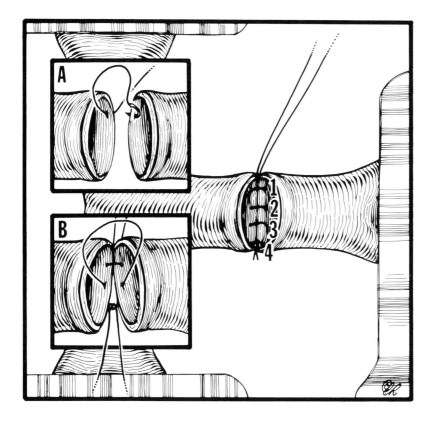

Fig. 24-19. The back-wall-first technique. Suturing begins at the point farthest away from the surgeon, and progresses toward the surgeon. The knots are placed outside the lumen. This method is useful when rotation of the vessel is limited.

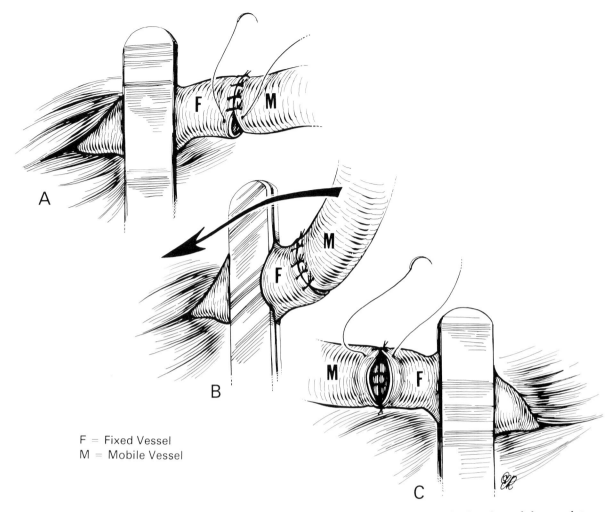

F = Fixed Vessel
M = Mobile Vessel

Fig. 24-20. "Flipping" a mobile vessel. When the free flap, digit, or vein graft is attached to the mobile vessel, it can be "flipped" to expose the back wall for repair if rotation of the vessel is difficult.

tomosed. A 90-degree angle of take-off is preferred, as the angle of take-off does not seem to significantly influence the flow.[105,167] Also, oblique cuts through a vessel wall produce a fragile tip of tissue with the intima and media at different levels, which is weak because of interruption of the circular fibers of the vessel wall.[123] In most cases, the front wall is first repaired, and then the backwall is sutured (Fig. 24-21). Using one of the techniques mentioned for placement of the last suture is especially important in completing the anastomosis. An end-to-side anastomosis can also be easily performed using the backwall-first technique if the

donor vessel is deeply placed and mobilization of the recipient vessel is difficult (Fig. 24-22).

Research is ongoing to improve the patency rate and decrease the time required for microvascular anastomoses. Methods currently under investigation are covered in the final section of this chapter.

Revision of the Failed Anastomosis

Failure of blood to flow across an anastomosis is usually due to one of three factors: (1) technical errors with the anastomosis; (2) poor flow from the

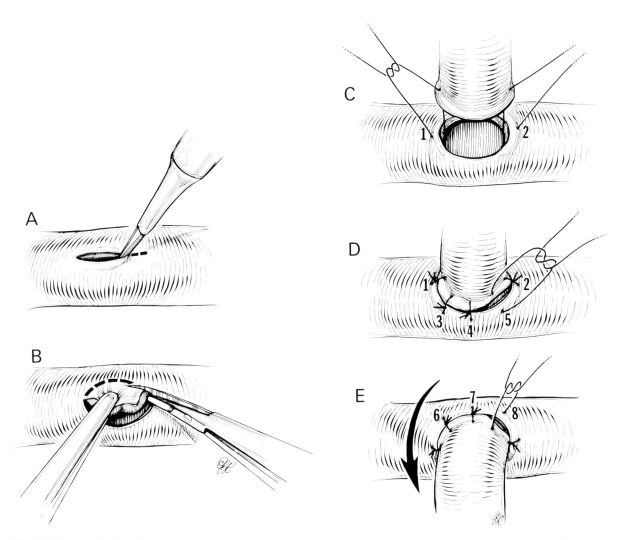

Fig. 24-21. Standard end-to-side technique. (**A, B**) The creation of the arteriotomy is critical and irreversible. (**C, D**) The near side is sutured first, the recipient vessel is mobilized, and (**E**) the far side then sutured. Care must be taken not to suture the opposite wall of the donor vessel.

proximal vessel due to undetected damage more proximally or vasospasm; or (3) a clot or thrombus at the anastomotic site, or in an area where a clamp was applied.

One should attempt to discern the cause of failure and proceed accordingly. If there is sufficient vessel length, reanastomosis can be performed; if not, a vein graft is inserted. Poor proximal flow that does not respond to local vasodilators and warming may require proximal exploration of the vessel, dilatation along a proximal length of vessel sufficient to relieve vasospasm, and/or treatment with local or intraarterial vasodilators.[142,217] In some cases, a vein graft from an adequate donor vessel more proximally may be required.

Small nonoccluding platelet thrombi occur at every anastomosis and are necessary to seal the suture line. If blood flow is allowed to continue undisturbed, these will usually not progress to occlude the lumen. Damage to the endothelium from excessive clamp pressure, poor technique, or contamination of the intraluminal blood with throm-

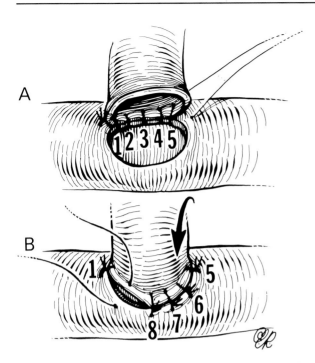

Fig. 24-22. An optional end-to-side technique. The far side can be sutured using the "back-wall-first" technique, and the near side then completed.

boplastins from the wound area may, however, result in an occluding thrombus. If blood flow across an anastomosis must be occluded for any reason, the suture line should be bombarded with heparinized solution immediately following occlusion and before flow is restored. Systemic heparin will also protect the anastomosis if reapplication of clamps is necessary.[81,111,116]

Vein Grafts

One of the most critical essentials of microvascular surgery is that there not be excessive tension on the anastomosis.[184] Experimental studies have shown a high incidence of aneurysm formation and thrombosis in vessels sutured under tension.[89,184,199,215] Veins and arteries have both been used for interpositional grafts in microsurgery, but venous grafts are the most readily available and appear to have the highest patency rate.[91,97,165,171,189] Although dorsal hand veins are commonly used in digital replantation and revascularization, they are

larger than the digital vessels. The small volar subcutaneous veins just proximal to the wrist are long and straight with matching diameter and have few major side branches. The dorsal hand veins and the cephalic vein near the wrist are appropriately sized for palmar and forearm vessels, as is the lower saphenous vein above the ankle for several free flap pedicles. All vein grafts should be marked and reversed when used in arterial reconstruction, as it has been shown that even the smallest digital vessels contain valves.[90,164] Most authors recommend completion of both anastomoses prior to removal of the clamps to prevent thrombosis at the site of the first repair. The anastomoses should be briskly irrigated with heparinized solution before removal of the clamps. Vein grafts always seem to elongate after reperfusion, and a determination of the required length of vein graft to bridge a defect requires considerable experience. If the graft is too short, tension will be present at the anastomoses; if too long, retraction of the arterial ends with concomitant narrowing, or kinking of the elongated graft may occur.[83,189] When possible (i.e., in elective procedures), the defect to be grafted should be measured before excision, and the vein graft measured and marked before harvesting. Frozen sections of the margins of the resected segment may be necessary to insure adequate removal of the diseased segment, as in grafting an ulnar artery thrombosis. Clinical failure may occur even with a patent graft if microembolization occurs from remaining areas of abnormal intima.

Clinically, it seems difficult to stretch the graft enough, and some elongation always seems to occur. Experimentally, the graft can be up to 35 percent longer than the replaced segment without kinking.[189]

Venous Drainage

Inadequate venous drainage is a common problem in digital replantation and is occasionally seen in free tissue transfer as well. Venous drainage of the digits has been studied in great detail, and an understanding of venous anatomy may allow location of additional veins for anastomosis.[156,164,219] Transfer of veins dissected from adjacent areas or digits may be helpful. In situations in which adequate venous drainage cannot be established, or congestion appears late, several means of augmentation of venous drainage have been described.

Leeches are widely used in European countries, but rarely in the United States because of psychological aversion and fear of transmitting serious infection.[107,119,128,211] They are quite effective in removing venous blood by feeding, and by oozing that occurs later from the powerful anticoagulant (hirudin) they inject locally.[88,119,138,153,158,178] Medical grade leeches are available within 24 hours from New York,° or from Europe, but the services of a customs broker will be required to arrange shipment into this country.

Survival of replanted digits without venous anastomosis has been reported by anticoagulation with heparin and allowing open drainage of the part.[118,185,219] Blood loss with this technique can be substantial.[144] The risks of transfusion must be weighed against the functional need for the amputated part. Venous drainage can also be augmented by removal of the nail and heparinization as reported by Gordon et al.[125] Blood loss is less with this technique and survival rates above 70 percent have been reported. Others, including myself, have been unable to achieve even the reasonable success rates reported using these techniques; my failure rate approaches 100 percent.

Milking the replanted digit of venous blood may also be effective, and an automatic milking apparatus has been constructed from readily available parts.[152] In replantation, Smith et al reported that if both digital arteries are available, one may be used to construct an arteriovenous anastomosis to decompress the digit if venous drainage is absent.[197] Despite the method used, if the part survives, venous congestion usually disappears between the fifth and seventh day. The exact mechanism for this is unknown, but presumably some type of collateral vascular channel is re-established.[125] The time required for re-establishment may vary by the type of tissue (skin, subcutaneous, muscle), and late loss of pedicle and free tissue transfers has been reported.[115]

° See appendix.

Maintaining Flow

Once the anastomoses are completed, what additional steps can be taken to improve or maintain blood flow? Both pharmacologic and nonpharmacologic methods have been suggested, but none will substitute for a technically adequate anastomosis of normal vessel ends without tension. Measures used empirically often have some basis, and others have been studied clinically or in the laboratory.[124,216] The first opportunity to protect the anastomosis is during the procedure. Meticulous hemostasis will prevent hematoma formation.[183,186] Fasciotomy following a long ischemic interval in limb replantation will prevent constriction due to postoperative swelling. Warming the amputated part or flap will reduce vasospasm and increase flow.[86] The wound is closed in such a way that the vessels are not kinked or compressed, and so that later swelling or hematoma does not compromise the lumen. Veins, being low pressure systems, are more prone to these problems, and many clinical failures have been attributed to venous compromise. The wound may be left partially open as in the midlateral incision used for replantation, or loosely closed over drains if adequate skin is available. If not, local flaps, primary skin grafting, or other biologic dressings may provide coverage without constriction. Scheker et al reported monitoring the revascularized part during closure to avoid pedicle compression.[188] Drains should be soft and pliable (Penrose or silicone) and should not be placed directly against the vessels so that their suction or removal does not cause vasospasm. They may be sutured in place with 6–0 plain suture to prevent migration but still allow later removal.

The dressing has several functions: it protects and immobilizes the extremity, and should provide gentle compression to control edema. Soft padding is placed between digits after wound coverage with noncircumferential dressings. Dressing removal may cause pain and secondary vasospasm. Therefore, in cases where dressing change is required in the early postoperative period because of excessive bleeding (usually seen with heparinization), the possibility of infection, or for secondary skin grafting, I remove the dressing in a warmed operating suite under long-acting axillary block or general anesthesia.

As venous congestion seems more common than problems with adequate arterial inflow, elevation is usually prescribed. Less elevation or even a dependent position will help arterial inflow, but increases the risk of edema and venous congestion.[139]

Postoperative Measures

Once the dressing is applied, most measures are directed toward prevention of vasospasm. Of the factors influencing blood flow through a revascularized part, several are under sympathetic control (Fig. 24-23).[175] The following measures appear to be widely recommended by most microvascular surgeons:

1. Bedrest or limited moving of the patient for 3 to 5 days
2. Room warmed above 78°

3. Private room; limiting of visitors and phone calls to decrease emotional stress
4. Adequate analgesia
5. Smoking, caffeine, and chocolate are prohibited as they may cause vasoconstriction.[110,133,163,179,218]

Fluid administration will lower blood viscosity and maintain cardiac output to provide adequate arterial inflow.[85,106,201] Vasopressor agents are contraindicated. Oxygen administration during periods of postanesthesia respiratory depression, and transfusion to maintain adequate hemoglobin levels will improve oxygenation of the revascularized part.[94] Although endothelial regeneration begins immediately, experimental studies have shown that as many as 7 days may be required for complete regeneration at the site of repair.[192,206] Therefore, these measures should be continued for at least that period, and I continue to recommend a

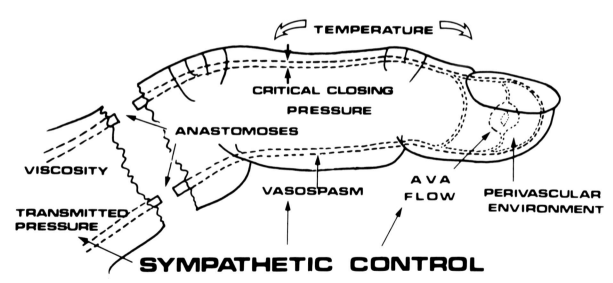

Fig. 24-23. Factors influencing flow through replanted or revascularized tissues include (1) technical perfection of microvascular anastomoses; (2) intraarterial pressure transmitted to the distal tissues (which falls with decreasing vessel size and extremity elevation); (3) vasospasm, which may be neurogenic (mediated through sympathetic pathways that control vessel caliber and status of arteriovenous anastomoses) or autonomous (mediated by vessel wall catecholamines); (4) alterations in the perivascular environment (pH, electrolyte concentration, blood outside vessel wall, etc.); (5) ambient temperature (direct vessel effect as well as neurogenic influence); and (6) blood viscosity. The influence of soft tissue edema is significant in the critical closing pressure, i.e., an intravascular pressure lower than vessel wall tension and extramural pressure. Note the factors that are under sympathetic control. (Phelps DB, Rutherford RB, Boswick JA: Control of vasospasm following trauma and microvascular surgery. J Hand Surg 4:109–117, 1979.)

warm environment and abstinence from smoking and caffeine for 3 weeks.

Pharmacologic measures designed to protect the microcirculation and prevent or reduce vasospasm are discussed in the next section.

Failure of Reperfusion

CRUSH AND AVULSION INJURIES

Failure of blood flow through an anastomosis may be immediate or delayed. If proximal blood flow was verified, the repair was technically well-performed, and vasospasm has been treated, brisk flow usually occurs. If not, the problem is probably to be found in the revascularized part. Immediate failure of flow may be due to unrecognized vessel damage more distally, which should be identified and corrected with a vein graft. It is also important to make sure that the anastomosis was not made distally to a vein instead of an artery.

In replantation, injury to the amputated part may be of such severity and extent that, perhaps, disseminated coagulation occurs in the distal vessels and capillary network. Crush and avulsion injuries may produce sufficient intimal damage to massively activate the cascade mechanism by activation of Factor XII.[102,122,205] If this occurs, significant flow does not occur into the revascularized part. Milking the amputated part prior to revascularization, or perfusion with fibrinolytic agents, free radical scavengers, or oxygenated blood substitutes, might help (theoretically), but in my experience these digits are usually not salvageable.

REPERFUSION INJURY (NO REFLOW PHENOMENON)

Occasionally, following a well-performed anastomosis, arterial inflow can be demonstrated by initial bleeding from the revascularized part, and patency tests may indicate patency, but venous return is sluggish or absent.[160] Gradual cessation of flow then occurs, the distal bleeding ceases, and the arterial anastomosis fails. This is termed no reflow phenomenon, which was first described following revascularization in the cerebral circulation,[84] and later in experimental flaps by May.[109,160] Experi-

mental studies have shown a 50 percent incidence of failure due to no reflow after 4 hours of warm ischemia time in rat hindlimbs; ongoing arterial obstruction, arteriovenous shunting, and alterations of the clotting mechanism were suggested as possible factors.[221] Other more likely possibilities include: (1) edema and swelling of the vascular endothelium and parenchymal cells with resultant narrowing of the capillary lumen; (2) disseminated intravascular thrombosis; and (3) loss of physiologic integrity of the venule or capillary wall.[109,160]

Whether prior perfusion with various solutions significantly affects the rate of ultimate survival in experimental situations is as yet unanswered.[98,150,161] However, perfusion with either oxygenated fluorocarbon, Collins solution, or hemoglobin perfusion solution, combined with hypothermia, has been shown experimentally to markedly lengthen the allowable ischemic interval.[204,207] Also, raising a flap some time prior to the actual transfer (flap delay) increases the time it may remain devascularized without demonstrating the no reflow phenomenon.[209] Alpha receptor hypersensitivity to circulating catecholamines may play a role,[100] and the delay phenomenon may some day be explained by a better understanding of no reflow problems.[100,140,208]

Other research has implicated reperfusion injury and the production of free radicals as the cause of the no reflow phenomenon. During prolonged ischemia, adenosine triphosphate is broken down to hypoxanthine, and xanthine oxidase is formed by the action of a protease in response to the low oxygen tension produced by ischemia.[151] When reperfusion occurs, the presence of molecular oxygen allows hypoxanthine conversion to xanthine and superoxide radicals (oxygen free radicals). The oxygen free radical may react further with water to produce hydrogen peroxide, and hydrogen peroxide may then also react with other oxygen radicals to form highly reactive hydroxyl radicals (OH⁻) (Fig. 24-24). During normal metabolism, superoxide dismutase (SOD) is present in sufficient quantities to scavenge these free radicals and prevent damage, but following long periods of ischemia, this system is overloaded by excess free radicals.

Pharmacologic manipulation to prevent or reverse this injury is being explored.[129,140,141,143,151,157,160,166,174,187,195,210] Tissue damage from reperfusion may be decreased by blocking the conversion of hypoxanthine to xanthine or by providing excess superoxide dismutase to scavenge the oxygen free radicals. Allopurinol blocks the former reaction, and has been shown experimentally to exert a protective effect.[143] SOD and other free radical scavengers are still investigational drugs, and not available for clinical use.

Unfortunately, at the present time there is no satisfactory treatment for failure of reperfusion, and these digits or flaps are usually lost. Treatment of the revascularized part with fibrinolytic agents (urokinase, streptokinase) has been suggested in these situations.[101,177,205] Improvement in flow has been demonstrated in ischemic flaps[103,177] and in hand ischemia secondary to distal arterial occlusion.[146] However, an experimental study designed to test the effect of intravascular fibrinolysis on small-vessel thrombosis showed no effect in vessels with an internal diameter of 0.8 to 1.5 mm.[104]

Monitoring Techniques

Loss of the revascularized tissue may occur in the postoperative period due to loss of the arterial inflow and/or venous drainage. Following replantation, there is a failure rate of 15 to 25 percent. In free tissue transfer, in order to achieve a 90 to 95 percent success rate, up to 20 percent of patients will have to be reoperated for revision of the anastomosis.[154] Considering the investment of time, surgical risk, and money in microsurgical procedures, an objective means of monitoring is highly

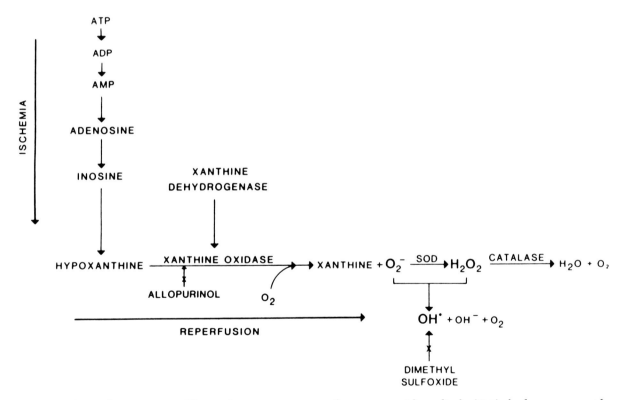

Fig. 24-24. Reperfusion injury. Tissue damage may occur from superoxide radicals (O_2^-), hydrogen peroxide (H_2O_2), and hydroxyl radicals ($OH\cdot$). Allopurinol and superoxide dismutase (SOD) may exert a protective effect by blocking the reaction, as shown. (Korthuis RJ, Granger DN, Townsley MI, Taylor AE: The role of oxygen-derived free radicals in ischemia-induced increases in canine skeletal muscle vascular permeability. Circ Res 57:599–609, 1985. Reprinted by permission of The American Heart Association, Inc.)

Table 24-2. Microvascular Monitoring Techniques

Method	Description	Advantages	Disadvantages	Comments
1. Temperature See Refs. 155, 200	Measures the surface or deep temperature (depending on probe used)	Inexpensive and simple to use; baseline values for survival well established in digital replantation; noninvasive and continuous	Good only for end-organ systems (replanted parts); flaps may remain warm due to environmental factors, but be nonviable	Very adequate and most widely used for monitoring of replants
2. Doppler ultrasound probe See Ref. 198	Measures blood flow in larger caliber vessels	Readily available and can determine direction of flow; can distinguish arterial from venous flow	Doesn't given quantitative value or measure capillary flow; may read adjacent vessels and give a false negative reading; of limited use with deeply buried anastomoses	Occasionally useful for intermittent check of flow, but difficult to adapt for continuous monitoring; hard to position probe over pedicle consistently
3. Pulsed Doppler cuff See Refs. 173, 203	Measures blood flow directly through small vessels by implanted cuff	Continuous with instantaneous response; waveform analysis possible; inexpensive; quantitative	Invasive; infection, vascular thrombosis or anastomosis disruption possible; requires removal	May be useful for buried flaps
4. Laser Doppler See Refs. 112–114, 137, 147, 176, 202	Measures movement of red cells in the capillary network by Doppler shift of laser light	Continuous & noninvasive; detects either arterial or venous obstruction; probes to monitor buried transfers are available; can monitor all types of tissue transfers	Expensive; requires calibration to establish baseline (intraoperatively); no absolute flow value is obtained; clotted blood and exudate interfere with recording; measures only 1–2 mm in depth	Either this method, PPG, or pH measurement will probably be most commonly used in the future
5. Transcutaneous O$_2$ See Refs. 80, 149, 159, 181, 191, 196	Measures tissue PO$_2$ diffusing through the skin	Continuous; baseline easily established; can test flow by having patient inhale O$_2$; rapid response time for loss of arterial inflow	Useful on skin only and requires heating the tissue to obtain local hyperemia; cannot monitor deep flaps; halothane, N$_2$O$_2$, and fluothane interfere with TcO$_2$ measurements; probe is large	Probe must be fixed to the skin; requires frequent calibration; effects of venous occlusion not known
6. Photoplethysmography (PPG) See Refs. 82, 108, 134–136, 188	Uses reflected light to measure minute changes in tissue volume associated with pulsatile blood	Noninvasive; waveform can predict venous obstruction	Requires experience to interpret waveform; no definite zero level	Useful with replants, skin, and muscle flaps
7. Tissue pH See Refs. 180, 181	Measures pH of tissue	Continuous; possibly more sensitive in evaluating survival of distal or marginal flap tissue	Slower detection than laser Doppler; requires inserted probe (invasive); normal values vary widely	May not indicate loss of perfusion for 3 hours or more
8. Fluroscein See Refs. 127, 194	Measures fluroscein in the tissue following intravenous injection	Relatively inexpensive and useful for skin flaps; minimally invasive; will detect problems earlier than clinical evaluation only, and can detect venous obstruction by fluroscein buildup	Venous obstruction may lead to fluroscein buildup in the tissue; requires repeated injections; not yet adapted for continuous monitoring.	Useful for replants and skin flaps but not for deep flaps, muscle, etc; must compare to control area for baseline
9. Radioisotope scanning or clearance	Measures flow of radioactive substance ''into'' (scanning) or ''out of'' (clearance) the tissue	Helpful in deeply placed osseous flaps (e.g., free fibular transfer)	Not continuous and cannot be repeated frequently due to radiation hazard and accumulation	Limited usefulness
10. Hydrogen washout See Ref. 121	Measures hydrogen concentration in the revascularized part after inhalation of hydrogen gas	Sensitive; repeated measurements possible	Requires special gas mixtures and electrodes; not continuous	

desirable.[201] The ideal monitor should:

1. Be safe, reliable, inexpensive, and noninvasive;
2. Provide continuous monitoring and rapid indication of impaired perfusion;
3. Distinguish between arterial and venous obstruction;
4. Be able to monitor all types of tissues; and
5. Be easily interpreted by nursing personnel.[82,134,136,137,148]

Biomedical technology has produced several instruments for monitoring the vascularity of tissue, but unfortunately no one instrument is optimum for all clinical situations.

End organ systems such as replanted digits can be adequately monitored using temperature probes, and this technique is widely used. The equipment is relatively inexpensive, the minimum temperature associated with viability has been established, and interpretation by nursing personnel is straightforward.[155,200]

Monitoring free tissue transfers surrounded by or buried in other well-vascularized tissue cannot be done adequately by temperature measurement. The transfer will assume the temperature of its surroundings and thus may remain warm even if nonviable. More sophisticated monitors are therefore required.[134–137,147] The methods currently available or under investigation are shown in Table 24-2, and a brief summary of the advantages and disadvantages of each is given. Transcutaneous oxygen, laser Doppler, pH monitoring, and photoplethysmography appear most promising at this time.

Organizing a Microsurgical Service

Replantations and free tissue transfer can be tedious and demanding procedures, and for many reasons are best performed using a team concept. As the team members work together and learn their respective tasks, less time will be wasted and frustration will be minimized. Guidelines for organizing a microsurgical team will be helpful to the reader contemplating such an undertaking.[93,120, 126,162,169,172]

PHYSIOLOGY AND PHARMACOLOGY OF THE MICROCIRCULATION

Physiology of the Microcirculation

BASIC MECHANISMS

Decremental changes in pressure occur with decreasing vessel size. Extremity elevation also decreases pressure distally by a hydrostatic effect. Pouiselle's law states that fluid flow through a vessel (F) is proportional to the pressure gradient ($\Delta P/L$, change in pressure over length), the radius (r), and the fluid viscosity (η), as shown below:[259,269]

$$F \propto \left(\frac{\Delta P}{L} \right) \left(\frac{r^4}{\eta} \right)$$

Therefore, to increase flow we must: (1) increase vessel radius (diameter); (2) decrease the viscosity, and/or (3) increase $\Delta P/L$. This is a factor that can be increased by: (1) increasing the perfusion pressure, and/or (2) decreasing the vessel resistance.

Smooth muscle in the walls of arteries, arterioles, and temperature regulating arteriovenous anastomoses (A-V shunts) is under sympathetic control.[226,268] Sympathetic stimulation reduces skin and digital flow, while sympathectomy markedly increases flow. Other than agents affecting the clotting mechanism, most adjunctive drug therapy is aimed at producing a chemical sympathectomy, which increases the vessel diameter and decreases the peripheral resistance.[269,291]

In addition, local mechanical factors are important. External pressure on the vessel wall from tight dressings, hematoma, or edema may exceed the "critical closing pressure," especially in the venous system (see Fig. 24-24).[269,277] Tissue anoxia and decreased perfusion lead to increased capillary permeability and tissue edema, and a vicious cycle akin to that seen in compartment syndromes may occur. Both Dextran and heparin appear to lower viscosity; Dextran by hemodilution and its "antiplatelet clumping effect," and heparin as a result of surface binding to red blood cells. Adequate hydration of the patient is also important not only in preventing peripheral vasoconstriction, but also to lower blood viscosity.[225,241] Maintenance of cardiac output and prevention of shunting to the central circulation will keep the perfusion pressure adequate. Although not a substitute for a perfect anastomosis of undamaged vessel, pharmacologic manipulation of the microcirculation may at times be an important adjunct. Its importance increases in traumatic situations where imperfect anastomoses and damaged vessels may be present. The reader in this area will be confused by the multitude of postoperative regimens advocated by various authors, and only through an understanding of the physiology of the microcirculation and clotting mechanisms can one critically assess these recommendations.

HEMOSTATIC MECHANISMS

Three major mechanisms function to repair vascular injury. Eventual vessel patency or lack thereof is determined by the net result of the interaction of these three mechanisms: (1) formation of a platelet clot, (2) formation of a fibrin clot, and (3) fibrinolysis.

Drugs commonly used following microvascular surgery may affect one or more of these mechanisms and be helpful or detrimental, occasionally both, as we shall see when discussing aspirin. Several feedback systems prevent extension of the repair process beyond the site of injury.

Platelets

Formation of a platelet clot at a site of vessel injury occurs before a fibrin clot, and is most likely to block a small vessel repair.[232,264,276] Endothelial damage exposes collagen and subendothelial Factor VIII: von Willebrand factor polymers (synthesized by endothelial cells), which attract and bind platelets. Once platelets adhere, they change in shape from discs to spheres and release their granule contents locally and into the vessel lumen (release phenomenon). These granule contents are rich in adenosine diphosphate (ADP), a potent platelet aggregating agent that causes further platelet aggregation and absorption of fibrinogen

from plasma.[271,293] The result is a platelet plug, rich in fibrinogen and ready for conversion into a fibrin thrombus by the action of thrombin (see Fig. 24-27). Both thrombin (from the cascade coagulation pathway) and epinephrine (stress hormone) enhance platelet aggregation and the release phenomenon. Epinephrine is also a potent vasoconstrictor.

Endothelial cells also synthesize and release into the vessel lumen prostaglandin I_2 (PGI_2), a vasodilator that exerts a protective effect by limiting excess accumulation of platelets on damaged subendothelial structures. PGI_2 synthesis from arachidonic acid requires the enzyme cyclooxygenase. Aspirin inhibits formation of PGI_2 by acetylating the active site on this enzyme, and thus may have a negative effect on patency, but this effect is dose related[232,248,271,272] (Fig. 24-25).

Platelets are derived from megakaryocytes that surround bone marrow sinuses. There are 150,000 to 350,000 platelets in a microliter of blood, and the average platelet survives for up to 10 days. Platelets have no nucleus or DNA, and therefore no metabolic means to synthesize proteins. If they are altered biochemically by drug treatment that renders them incapable of aggregation, they remain ineffective during their life span. The blood level of aspirin attained from a single dose as low as 3 mg/kg (2.5–3.5 grains a day) will acetylate the cyclooxygenase present in the platelet wall, preventing formation of endoperoxides PGG_2 and PGH_2, and thus thromboxane A_2. Drugs containing an imidazole group block thromboxane production more directly. Thromboxane A_2 potentiates release of platelet granules, induces further platelet aggregation, and is locally vasoconstrictive. Blocking thromboxane A_2 production will limit platelet aggregation and release phenomena[248,249,272] (Fig. 24-26). Therefore, many microsurgeons recommend a low dose of aspirin following microvascular repair to inhibit thromboxane A_2–induced platelet aggregation. Higher doses may be harmful however, as they block the beneficial effects of PGI_2.

Figures 24-25, 24-26, and 24-27 should be referred to as an aid in understanding the mechanism and/or site of action of any drug that has an anticoagulant effect on the microcirculation. As new drugs are reported, one should attempt to place them appropriately in this scheme as well.

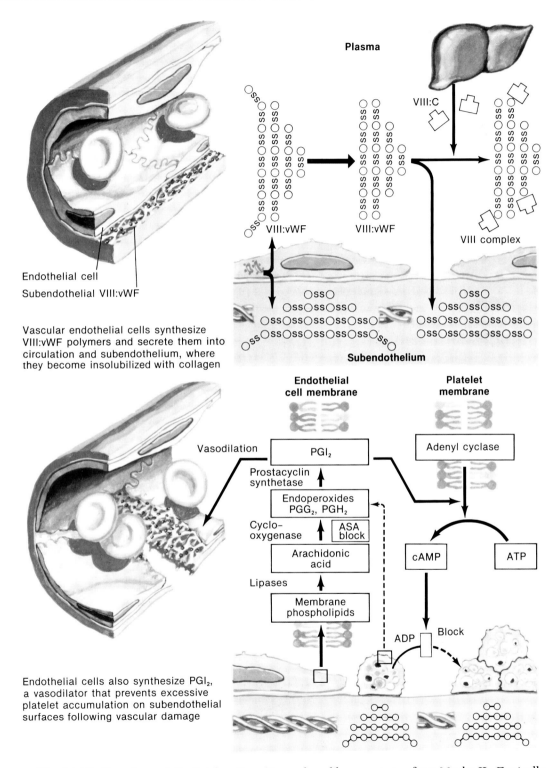

Endothelial cell

Subendothelial VIII:vWF

Vascular endothelial cells synthesize
VIII:vWF polymers and secrete them into
circulation and subendothelium, where
they become insolubilized with collagen

Plasma

VIII:C

VIII:vWF

VIII:vWF

VIII complex

Subendothelium

**Endothelial
cell membrane**

**Platelet
membrane**

Vasodilation

PGI₂

Adenyl cyclase

Prostacyclin
synthetase

Endoperoxides
PGG₂, PGH₂

Cyclo-
oxygenase

ASA
block

cAMP

ATP

Arachidonic
acid

Lipases

Membrane
phospholipids

ADP

Block

Endothelial cells also synthesize PGI₂,
a vasodilator that prevents excessive
platelet accumulation on subendothelial
surfaces following vascular damage

Fig. 24-25. Vascular endothelial function. (Reproduced by permission from Moake JL, Funicella
T: Common bleeding problems. CIBA Clinical Symposia 35(3):2–32, 1983.)

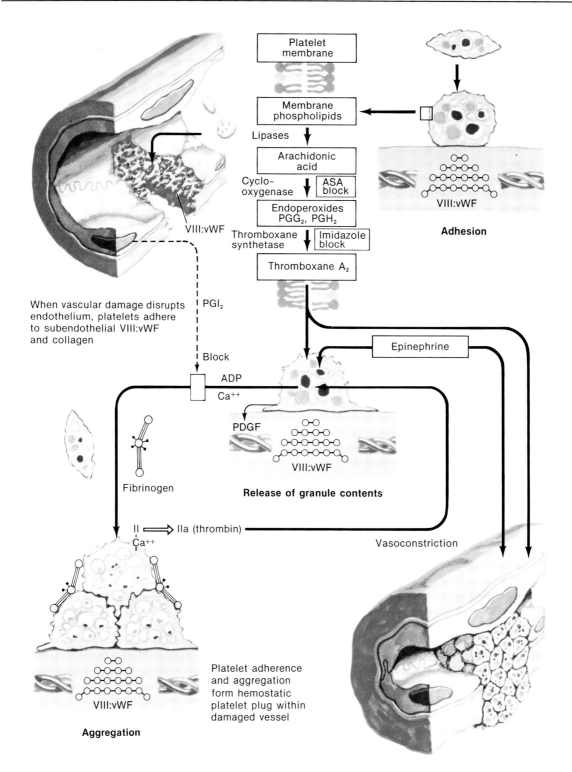

Fig. 24-26. Platelet adhesion, release, and aggregation. (Reproduced by permission from Moake JL, Funicella T: Common bleeding problems. **CIBA Clinical Symposia** 35(3):2–32, 1983.)

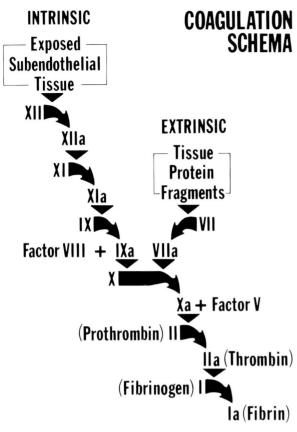

INTRINSIC

COAGULATION SCHEMA

Exposed Subendothelial Tissue

XII

XIIa

XI

XIa

IX

EXTRINSIC

Tissue Protein Fragments

VII

Factor VIII + IXa   VIIa

X

Xa + Factor V

(Prothrombin) II

IIa (Thrombin)

(Fibrinogen) I

Ia (Fibrin)

Fig. 24-27. Cascade pathway.

Cascade Pathway

The coagulation proteins in the classic cascade clotting mechanism are labeled with Roman numerals; Factors I (fibrinogen), II (prothrombin), and VII through XIII. Activated forms are indicated by the additional suffix "a" (e.g., cleavage of prothrombin [Factor II], to the active enzyme thrombin [Factor IIa]). The liver synthesizes and secretes all the coagulation proteins. Endothelial cells (including the vascular endothelium) also synthesize and secrete a polymer of Factor VIII, bound to von Willebrand factor (vWF).[271] The net result of activation of the cascade system is the generation of thrombin, which converts soluble fibrinogen into insoluble fibrin, forming a "red clot." Thrombin is generated by two different sequences known as the intrinsic and the extrinsic pathways (Figure 24-27).

In the intrinsic pathway, all needed coagulation factors are present (intrinsic) in normal blood. Vascular endothelial disruption exposes charged subendothelial molecules, and Factor XII is attracted to the site of damage where it is activated. The coagulation cascade is then locally activated.[271]

The extrinsic pathway is initiated by leakage into the blood stream of phospholipoprotein membranes from disrupted tissue cells, which are normally extrinsic to the circulation. These substances activate Factor VII, and initiate the cascade. The extrinsic path is probably more rapid in vivo.

Once formed, thrombin splits fibrinogen into fibrin polymers, which link with each other and with aggregated platelets to form a thrombus at the site of injury. When a thrombus is formed, the portions of the thrombus projecting into the vessel lumen that are not necessary for repair of the endothelial injury may be degraded by fibrinolysis, restoring the vessel lumen.

Excessive formation of intravascular thrombin is prevented by inhibition of various coagulation factors and thrombin itself by antithrombin and protein C, which are present both in blood and on endothelial cells. Thrombus formation is normally restricted in this way to the site of vascular injury and does not progress to completely occlude the lumen.

Fibrinolysis

Once bleeding is controlled and repair of the vessel wall has begun, the fibrin meshwork is lysed by plasmin. Plasminogen is absorbed onto fibrin from the blood plasma and activated to plasmin by hydrolytic enzymes derived from disrupted tissue lysosomes. In addition, the endothelium has inherent fibrinolytic activity that decreases progressively during ischemia, reaching a minimum following 6 hours of ischemia. After restoration of flow, up to 96 hours is required before this inherent fibrinolytic activity returns to normal levels.[258]

Urokinase (of renal origin) and streptokinase (a bacterial enzyme) do not directly lyse fibrin polymers, but instead activate circulating plasminogen by exposing active enzyme sites.[235,237,238,260,264] Their possible clinical use will be discussed later.

Pharmacology of Selected Drugs

The timing and route of administration of pharmacologic agents are important to achieve maximum benefit. The stress of anesthesia and surgery cause epinephrine to be released into the circulation, thus increasing the possibility of thrombosis. Prophylactic adjunctive drug treatment should therefore be considered. Although re-endothelialization begins immediately, some form of anticoagulant therapy should be continued for at least 3 to 5 days until the endothelium regenerates and covers the anastomotic site.[234,273,288] Diurnal variations in coagulability also occur, and may affect the outcome of microvascular procedures.[253] The reader should be aware that the recommendations that follow regarding individual drugs are in most cases based on firm *theoretical* considerations, but supporting experimental data or controlled clinical trials are in most cases lacking.

ANTICOAGULANTS

Heparin

Heparin is a complex substance with multiple actions in vivo. Most important to the microvascular surgeon is the preferential binding to vascular endothelial cells that replaces the normal negative charge lost in areas of endothelial damage. This high concentration in the area of damage also inhibits platelet aggregation, decreases fibrinogen clotting, and activates local antithrombin III. Systemic heparin also has two direct effects on the blood itself; activation of serum antithrombin III, and lowering of blood viscosity.[242,244,253,264,285] When sharply divided vessels are repaired, the patency rate using systemic heparin as an adjunct is probably no greater than that of untreated controls.[242,264] However, another laboratory study designed to test the efficacy of systemic heparin following crush and avulsion injuries showed dramatic improvement in the patency rate following repair of traumatized vessels.[236] Also, in a retrospective study of replantation failures, 20 percent occurred within 4 hours of discontinuing systemic heparin.[253] This same study suggested that full heparinizing doses were required, and that "low dose" regimens were ineffectual. However, low dose regimens and heparin analogs with less effect on overall clotting are attractive from the standpoint of bleeding complications, and further research in this area is needed. Full heparinizing doses will usually require transfusion and repeated dressing changes.[257]

Although heparinization is probably not needed in replantation of sharp amputations or uncomplicated free tissue transfer, it should be strongly considered in problem cases such as avulsion or crush injury which would be expected to expose multiple areas of endothelial injury.[236,250,290] Patients demonstrating a tendency to hypercoagulability and thrombosis requiring anastomotic revision should also be protected.[245] In these instances, a full heparinizing dose of 40 units/kg of body weight should be given prior to completion of the anastomosis and release of the clamps. Heparin is also important as a local anticoagulant in irrigating solutions.[289]

Acetylsalicylic Acid (Aspirin)

Aspirin is widely used following microvascular procedures because of its antiplatelet effect. Administration of a single dose as low as 3 mg/kg will inactivate circulating platelets by acetylating the enzyme cyclooxygenase present in the platelet wall.[248] Arachidonic acid cannot be metabolized to PGG_2 and PGH_2, and thromboxane A_2 cannot be formed. Thromboxane A_2 is necessary for the release phenomenon that leads to platelet aggregation (Fig. 24-26). However, aspirin also blocks the synthesis of PGI_2 in the vessel wall. PGI_2 has several beneficial effects including local vasodilatation and blockage of platelet aggregation[272] (Fig. 24-25). Fortunately, vascular endothelium has the ability to resynthesize cyclooxygenase (the platelet cannot). Also, the effect of aspirin is dose related. The average dose required to inhibit 50 percent of platelet aggregation is 3.2 mg/kg, but 4.9 mg/kg is needed to inhibit PGI_2 production by the vessel wall.[232] Because of this differential effect, a small dose of aspirin is theoretically indicated. The recommended dose is 3 mg/kg (2.5–3.5 grains) daily. A secondary platelet release phenomenon (which is not blocked by aspirin) may be stimulated by thrombin and high collagen concentrations, and may explain the lack of bleeding problems noted when aspirin is given following trauma.[264,293]

Persantine is an aspirin analog, also with anti-prostaglandin effects. Its metabolism has not been as well studied, and it probably does not offer any significant advantage over aspirin, except possibly a concomitant vasodilatory effect. It appears to be rarely used by microsurgeons at this time.

Dextran

The mechanism of action of Dextran is not well understood, but it appears to have both antiplatelet and heparinlike effects. Although more widely used than heparin because of its lower incidence of side-effects, good statistical evidence to support its use is lacking. Pharmacologically, it is classified as a plasma expander, and it is indicated for prophylaxis of deep vein thrombosis and pulmonary embolism in patients undergoing procedures known to be associated with a high incidence of thromboembolic complications. Rare allergic reactions caused by hypersensitivity to Dextran have been reported, and infrequent fatal anaphylactic reactions have also been reported. Most of these reactions occur in patients not previously exposed to IV Dextran, and occur early in the infusion period. Recently, a solution known as Dextran I has been introduced as a pretreatment to decrease the incidence of adverse reactions. The indication for its use is prophylaxis of severe anaphylactic reactions associated with IV infusion of clinical Dextran solutions. This drug binds to polysaccachride reacting antibodies that cross-react with clinical Dextran, and thus prevents the allergic reaction. The dosage in adults is 20 cc (150 mg/cc) IV over 1 to 2 minutes, given 1 to 2 minutes before the IV infusion of clinical Dextran solutions. The dose in children is 0.3 cc/kg. The administration of clinical Dextran should then be started within 15 minutes.[261]

Many surgeons, including myself, use Dextran following elective or traumatic microvascular procedures. The recommended dose in the adult is 500 cc of Dextran 40 in normal saline given over 5 to 6 hours once daily for 3 to 5 days. Other microsurgeons instead administer the 500 cc of Dextran slowly over a 24-hour period. Since the peak antithrombotic effect of Dextran is present 4 hours after infusion, the initial dose should be started prior to beginning the anastomosis for maximum effect.[230,261,264]

Prostaglandins

As we have seen, certain prostaglandins might be useful for preventing primary platelet aggregation. They have been studied experimentally both as local and systemic agents, but are not readily available at this time for clinical use.[232,243,264,266,272,287]

In summary, the most widely used drug regimen seems to be aspirin and Dextran. In situations where damaged vessels are presumed or known to be present such as crush and avulsion injuries, heparin is often added and continued until the endothelium regenerates. Endothelial regeneration begins very early, and for small areas coverage may be completed quickly. In cases with more severe trauma such as the crush and avulsion type, as long as 5 to 7 days may be required to seal the endothelium and the anastomotic site. The complications of heparinization, including bleeding and hematoma formation, have been previously discussed.[257]

VASODILATORS

Topical and Intraarterial Agents

Vasodilatation may be accomplished by topical, intraarterial, or systemic drug administration. Topical vasodilators are applied directly onto the vessels during dissection or following repair. Lidocaine is the most commonly used agent, but probably in strengths too low to have much beneficial effect. Concentrations of 4 to 20 percent are recommended based on experimental studies, and will probably have to be specially prepared in the hospital pharmacy.[228,229,252,270,277,284,295] Magnesium sulfate, chlorpromazine, sodium nitroprusside, and certain prostaglandins have also been used as local agents.[222–224,231,266,267,270,275] In rare instances, pathologic vasoconstriction that threatens viability of the revascularized tissue may occur, and be refractory to methods previously mentioned. Intraarterial injection of Priscoline (tolazoline hydrochloride), nitroglycerin, reserpine, or guanethedine may be helpful in these situations.[256,264] Reports of clinical use of these agents are sparse, and these reports should be referred to regarding the dosages and method of administration.

Pharmacology of Systemic Agents

The terminal arteries and arterioles of the peripheral circulation contain significant smooth muscle in their walls, and are innervated by adrenergic fibers of the sympathetic nervous system. These adrenergic fibers release norepinephrine, which acts on the alpha receptors of vascular smooth muscle. Cutaneous (skin) vessels of the extremities only respond to changes in the basal tone of the sympathetic system; there are no direct vasodilatory fibers. Therefore, vasodilatation of skin vessels can be accomplished only by a reduction of sympathetic nervous system discharge. Skeletal muscle, on the other hand, also has beta-receptors and, thus, sympathetic dilator control. Lowered body or blood temperature and anxiety can both cause pronounced vasoconstriction mediated through the hypothalamic axis.[226,268,269,277,291,292]

There are several levels at which sympathetic tone can be blocked or decreased (Table 24-3). The site of action of the various vasodilators is shown in Figure 24-28. A warm, calm environment will decrease central stimulation and the level of norepinephrine released,[226,269,277] as will a stellate block, peripheral nerve block, or sympathectomy. Inhibition of the amine pump and depletion of the norepinephrine precursors will also decrease production of this neurotransmitter. Reserpine blocks the storage granule transport system, and guanethidine replaces norepinephrine in the storage vesicles.[264,268] Bretylium prevents release of the neurotransmitter.[268] Phenoxybenzamine and Prasozin bind to receptor sites, and nifedipine blocks the effect of norepinephrine on the smooth muscle by blocking the calcium channels.[240,265,291]

Several systemic vasodilator agents have been tried in microsurgical situations to improve tissue perfusion. No clear indications exist stating when to employ these agents or whether their effect is statistically significant.[247,251,253–255,262,263,277] Isoxsuprine, Terbutaline, and Prazosin have each been discussed in the literature, and in some instances recommended for use as peripheral vasodilators. However, these drugs do not appear to be widely used by microsurgeons at the present time. For further information about their effects and possible use in these situations, the reader is referred to

Table 24-3. Methods of Decreasing Sympathetic Tone[265,268,292]

1. Stop production of neurotransmitter
   a. Decrease central stimulation (warm and calm environment)
   b. Proximal stellate block or sympathectomy
   c. Inhibit amine pump
   d. Deplete precursors
2. Block storage granule transport system (reserpine) or displace transmitter from axon terminal (quanethidine)
3. Block vesicle release (Bretylium)
4. Block receptor uptake or effect of neurotransmitter
   a. Block alpha receptor (Prazosin, Phenoxybenzamine)
   b. Block calcium channels of vascular smooth muscle (Nifedipine)

the pertinent literature.[233,246,247,253,278–280,286,291]

Phenoxybenzamine (Dibenzyline) is a long-acting alpha-blocking agent that increases cardiac output. It increases blood flow to the skin, and has been used to treat vasospastic disorders such as Raynaud's syndrome and frostbite sequelae, and to improve the survival of marginal tissue of pedicle flaps.[246,262,274,294] Orthostatic hypotension is the most common side-effect. The initial dose is 10 mg p.o. daily, and may be increased as tolerated. In the supine patient following flap transfer or replantation, 10 or 20 mg p.o. b.i.d. to t.i.d. is usually well tolerated.[268,283,291]

Nifedipine (Procardia) is a calcium channel blocker which is probably the drug of choice for cold intolerance following successful digit or extremity replantation. It is often effective if taken just before cold stress. An initial dose of 20 mg p.o. daily should be tried, but up to 60 mg/day may be required to relieve symptoms.[281]

Chlorpromazine (Thorazine) has a wide variety of actions including alpha blockade, anti-inflammatory properties, anti-platelet effects, and cell membrane stabilization. All of these actions aid in increasing the tolerance of tissue to ischemia.[231,239,264] In extremely large doses, chlorpromazine consistently prevents or diminishes flap necrosis in experimental animals.[227] However, no clinical studies following replantation or free tissue transfer are available. The recognized sedative effect of chlorpromazine is probably also beneficial; the recommended dose is 50 mg orally or IM every 6 to 8 hours.[282]

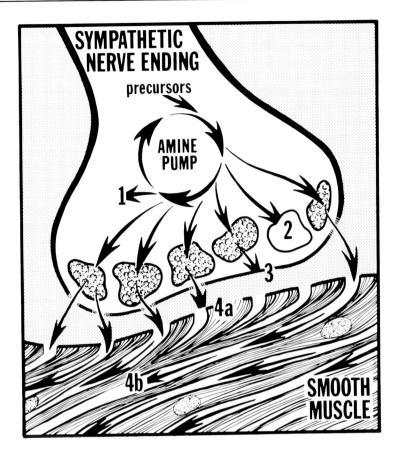

Fig. 24-28. Methods of decreasing sympathetic tone. *(1)* Stop production of neurotransmitter; *(2)* decrease neurotransmitter available in vesicles; *(3)* block release; *(4)* block alpha receptor *(4a)* or calcium channel *(4b)*.[265]

FIBRINOLYTIC AGENTS

Urokinase and streptokinase have been recommended as being possibly beneficial in salvaging a failing replant or tissue transfer. Life-threatening allergic reactions and bleeding complications may occur, and an experienced hematologist should probably be consulted for management of these medications. Treatment must be administered early if it is to be effective, and salvage of failing replants has been reported using these techniques. (Russell RC: Personal communication, 1987.) These drugs must be administered by intraarterial catheterization, and the literature should be consulted regarding the dose and route of administration.[235,237,238,258,260,264]

Research is being done to identify drugs that are more specific in their effects on the microcircula-

tion. This may some day allow protection of the anastomosis without the threat of bleeding complications.[232,263,264]

RESEARCH AND NEW TECHNIQUES IN MICROVASCULAR SURGERY

As one might expect in such a rapidly expanding area, today's laboratory experiment often becomes tomorrow's clinical technique. Many imaginative ideas have been published that fall into this category. Mentioning these will hopefully prevent this chapter from being outmoded before it is even published.[347]

Several major areas of research are evident in a review of the recent literature, and each seeks to address a current clinical problem. Alternative anastomotic techniques attempt to decrease operative time and provide a more "perfect" anastomosis. Chemical and fibrin glues,[297,304,317,349] circular anastomotic clips,[303] external ring techniques,[308,345,357,358] cuffing the repair with adventitia or a vein graft segment,[300,332,348,352] end-in-end techniques,[348,360-363] and vessel repair using laser coagulation[298,340,341,343,346] have been reported. Synthetic grafts may obviate the need for harvesting autogenous grafts.[302,312,319,320,325,333,335] Other factors influencing the patency rates of anastomoses, such as suture material, clamp pressure, and suture and needle size, have been studied experimentally and microscopically.[299,310,311,321,327-330,334,336] Arguments over continuous versus interrupted suture technique continue.[301,309,314,315,318,323,325,326,351,356,359]

Flaps vascularized by arteriovenous anastomosis or venous blood only have been investigated.[316,322,344,350,355] Prolonging tissue survival by hypothermia and various perfusion solutions is being studied.[305,324,331,353,354]

Vascularized allografting of various tissues and transplantation of extremity parts may someday be feasible when immunologic responses can be more predictably controlled with less toxic drugs and if problems associated with nerve regeneration can be overcome.[296,306,307,313,337-339,342]

ACKNOWLEDGEMENTS

I would like to thank Robert Russell, M.D. and Allen Roth, Ph.D. for their invaluable assistance and suggestions regarding the pharmacology and physiology of the microcirculation.

My appreciation is also extended to Robert Acland, M.D., Ivan Turpin, M.D., and Leonard Gordon, M.D. for their suggestions and help with the section on monitoring devices.

APPENDIX

Listed below are two reliable overnight sources for medical-grade leeches. Keep in mind that each of these sources is closed over the weekend; orders cannot be placed between Friday night and Monday morning (of the local time).

United States:
ASSI
300 Shames Drive
Westbury NY 11590
1-800-645-3569 (between 9 and 5 NY time)

Europe:
Biofarm, Ltd.
2-8 Morfa Road
Swansea, West Glam
SA1 2ET UNITED KINGDOM
(0792) 467-536 (between 9 and 5 Wales time, which is NY time +5 hours)

REFERENCES

1. Acland R: New instruments for microvascular surgery. Br J Surg 59:181–184, 1972
2. Acland R: Signs of patency in small vessel anastomosis. Surgery 72:744–748, 1972
3. Acland RD: Microvascular anastomosis: A device for holding stay sutures and a new vascular clamp. Surgery 75:185–187, 1974
4. Acland R: Notes on the handling of ultrafine suture material. Surgery 77:507–511, 1975
5. Acland R: Instrumentation and technique. pp. 8–20. In Daniller AI, Strauch B (eds): Symposium on Microsurgery. CV Mosby, St Louis, 1976
6. Acland RD: Instrumentation for microsurgery. Orthop Clin North Am 8:281–294, 1977
7. Acland RD: Microsurgery Practice Manual. CV Mosby, St Louis, 1980
8. Acland RD, Lubbers LL, Grafton RB, Bensimon R: Irrigating solutions for small blood vessel surgery —A histologic comparison. Plast Reconstr Surg 65:460–465, 1980
9. American Academy of Orthopaedic Surgeons: Mi-

crosurgical Skills Development Laboratory Manual. American Academy of Orthopaedic Surgeons, 1985

10. Awwad AM: A training card for microsurgery. Microsurgery 5:160, 1984

11. Awwad AM, White RJ, Webster MHC, Vance JP: The effect of temperature on blood flow in island and free skin flaps: An experimental study. Brit J Plast Surg 36:373–382, 1983

12. Ballantyne DL, Chin DTW, Razaboni RM, Harper AD, Chen L: Introduction to Microsurgery: A Microvascular and Microneurological Laboratory Manual. University Park Press, Baltimore, 1985

13. Ballantyne DL, Razaboni RM, Harper AD: Microvascular Surgery. A Laboratory Manual. Institute of Reconstructive Plastic Surgery, New York University Medical Center, New York 1980

14. Ballantyne DL, Reiffel RS, Harper AD: A systematic learning program for microvascular technique. Plast Reconstr Surg 65:80–82, 1980

15. Ballantyne DL, Rosenburg BB: Organized bibliography of the microsurgical literature. Aspen Systems Corporation, Rockville, MD, 1985

16. Baxter TJ, O'Brien BMcC, Henderson PN, Bennett RC: The histopathology of small vessels following microvascular repair. Brit J Surg 59:617–622, 1972

17. Bright DS: Microsurgical techniques in vessel and nerve repair. pp. 1–15. AAOS Instructional Course Lectures. Vol. 27, CV Mosby, St Louis, 1978

18. Bright DS: Techniques of microsurgery. pp. 40–52. AAOS Symposium on Microsurgery: Practical Use in Orthopaedics, CV Mosby, St Louis, 1979

19. Bright DS: Principles of microvascular surgery. pp. 793–810. In Green DP (ed): Operative Hand Surgery. Churchill Livingstone, New York, 1982

20. Buchler U, Phelps DB, Winspur I, Boswick JA: The irrigation jet: An aid in microvascular surgery. J Hand Surg 2: 24–28, 1977

21. Buncke HJ: The development of microsurgery. pp. 3–7. In Daniller AI, Strauch B (eds): Symposium on Microsurgery. CV Mosby, St Louis, 1976

22. Buncke HJ: The role of microsurgery in hand surgery. Int J Microsurgery 2:5, 1980

23. Buncke HJ, Chater NL, Szabo Z: The manual of microvascular surgery. Davis & Geck, Pearl River, NY, 1975

24. Buncke HJ, Furnas DW (eds): Symposium on Clinical Frontiers in Microvascular Surgery. CV Mosby, St Louis, 1984

25. Buncke HJ, McLean DH: The advantage of a straight needle in microsurgery. Plast Reconstr Surg 47:602–603, 1971

26. Buncke HJ: ASSH report of the microsurgical committee. J Hand Surg 8:727–730, 1983

27. Cassel J, Alpert BS, Buncke HJ, Gordon L: The Tweener Maneuver. J Reconstr Microsurgery 1:287–289, 1985

28. Chase RA: The development of tissue transfer in hand surgery. ASSH presidential address. J Hand Surg 9:463–477, 1984

29. Chase RA: Historical review of skin and soft tissue coverage of the upper extremity. Hand Clinics 1:599–608, 1985

30. Chow SP: A comparison of five methods of dealing with the adventia in microvascular anastomosis. Intl J Microsurgery 4:47–50, 1982

31. Chow SP, Zhu JK, So YC: Effect of bipolar coagulation and occlusion clamping on the patency rate in microvascular anastomosis. J Reconstr Microsurgery 2:111–115, 1986

32. Curtis LM, Loftis JW, Wissinger HA: Objective signs of patency following microvascular arterial anastomosis: A controlled study. J Hand Surg 2:22–23, 1977

33. Daniel RK, Taylor GI: Distant transfer of an island flap by microvascular anastomoses. A clinical technique. Plast Reconstr Surg 52:111–117, 1973

34. de Carolis V, Sepulveda S: A new experimental model for microanastomosis between vessels of different diameter. Microsurgery 6:151–154, 1985

35. Derman GH, Schenck RR: Microsurgical technique — Fundamentals of the microsurgery laboratory. Orthop Clin North Am 8:229–248, 1977

36. Dujovny M, Kossovsky N, Kossowsky R, Perlin A, Gatti EF, Segal R, Diaz FG: Mechanical and metallurgical properties of vascular clips designed for temporary use. Microsurgery 4:124–133, 1983

37. Foucher G, Schwind F: A new trick for end-to-end anastomosis in microvascular surgery. J Reconstr Microsurgery 1:49–51, 1984

38. Goldstein M: Use of fresh human placenta for microsurgical training. Journal of Microsurgery 1:70–71, 1979

39. Gordon L, Buncke HJ: Models and techniques for microsurgery research. Orthop Clin North Am 8:273–280, 1977

40. Gould SH: The role of the microsurgical laboratory in orthopedic training programs. Orthopedics 9:881–882, 1986

41. Haines P, Nichter LS, Morgan RF, Horowitz JH,

Edgerton MT: A digit replantation model. Microsurgery 6:70–72, 1985

42. Hall EJ: End-to-side anastomosis: A model and a technique with clinical application. J Microsurgery 2:106–112, 1980

43. Harashina T: Use of the untied suture in microvascular anastomosis. Plast Reconstr Surg 59:134–135, 1977

44. Harashina T, Takaki JL: A new anastomosis technique for large-calibered vein grafts. Microsurgery 4:171–175, 1983

45. Hariri K: Microvascular tissue transfer. Fundamental Techniques and Clinical Applications. Igaku-Shoin, Tokyo, 1983

46. Hariri RJ, Goldstein M: Dual-ended, multi-function tools for microsurgery. Microsurgery 6:251–252, 1985

47. Harwell RC, Ferguson RL: Physiologic tremor and microsurgery. Microsurgery 4:187–192, 1983

48. Hayhurst JW, O'Brien BMcC: An experimental study of microvascular technique, patency rates and related factors. Brit J Plast Surg 28:128–132, 1975

49. Huang G-K, Hu R-Q, Pan G-P: Influence of vessel clips on vascular patency in microarterial grafts less than 0.5 mm in external diameter. J Hand Surg 10A:538–541, 1985

50. Ikuta Y: Microvascular double clamp Type A-II. J Reconstr Microsurgery 1:41–43, 1984

51. Jacobson JH: Microsurgery. Curr Prob Surg 2:56, 1971

52. Jacobson JH, Suarez EI: Microsurgery in anastomosis of small vessels. Surg Forum 11:243–245, 1960

53. Kaufman T, Hurwitz DJ, Ballantyne DL: The foliage leaf in microvascular surgery. Microsurgery 5:57–58, 1984

54. Kleinert HE: A quarter century personal perspective of microsurgery. Founder's Lecture presented at the 2nd Annual Meeting of the American Society for Reconstructive Microsurgery, New Orleans, 1986

55. Komatsu S, Tamai S: Successful replantation of a completely cut-off thumb: Case Report. Plast Reconstr Surg 42:374, 1968

56. Lee S, Coppersmith WJ: A microvascular surgical practice disc for beginners. Microsurgery 4:67–69, 1983

57. Mazer N, Barbieri CH, Goncalves RP: Effect of different irrigating solutions on the endothelium of small arteries: Experimental study in rats. Microsurgery 7:9–28, 1986

58. McGregor JC, Wyllie FJ, Grigor KM: Some anatomical observations on the human placenta as applied to microvascular surgical practice. Brit J Plast Surg 36:387–391, 1983

59. McLean DH, Buncke HJ: Use of the saran wrap cuff in microsurgical arterial repairs. Plast Reconstr Surg 51:624–627, 1973

60. Nunley JA: Microscopes and microinstruments. Hand Clinics 1:197–204, 1985

61. O'Brien BMcC: Microvascular Reconstructive Surgery. Churchill Livingstone, Edinburgh, 1977

62. O'Brien BMcC, Henderson PN, Bennett RC, Crock GW: Microvascular surgical technique. Med J Aust 1:722–725, 1970

63. Owen ER: The microneedle holder scissors and the microforceps. Microsurgery 5:213–217, 1984

64. Richards RR, Mercer N: Effect of hydrostatic dilation on the structure and patency of small arteries. J Reconstr Microsurgery 2:97–102, 1986

65. Roth JH, Urbaniak JR, Boswick JM: Comparison of suture ligation, bipolar cauterization, and hemoclip ligation in the management of small branching vessels in a rat model. J Reconstr Microsurgery 1:7–9, 1984

66. Ruby LK, Greene M, Risitano G, Torrejon R, Belsky M: Experience with epigastric free flap transfer in the rat: Technique and results. Microsurgery 5:102–104, 1984

67. Schoots M, Cariou JL, Amarante J, Panconi B, Bovet JL, Baudet J: Microvascular free bone transfer: Experimental technique on rat's femur. Microsurgery 5:19–23, 1984

68. Seaber AV: Laboratory design in preparing for elective microvascular surgery. Hand Clinics 1:233–245, 1985

69. Serafin D: Microsurgery: Past, present, and future. Plast Reconstr Surg 66:781–785, 1980

70. Serafin D, Georgiade NG, Morris RL, Mullen RY: A laboratory manual of microvascular surgery. Division of Plastic, Reconstructive and Maxillofacial Surgery, Duke University Medical Center, Durham, NC, 1978

71. Shaffer JW, Field GA, Goldberg VM, Zdeblick TA: A vascularized fibula model to study vascularized canine bone grafts. Microsurgery 5:185–190, 1984

72. Sinclair S: The importance of topical heparin in microvascular anastomoses: A study in the rat. Brit J Plast Surg 33:422–426, 1980

73. Spaet TH, Rhee CY, Gaynor E: Delayed occlusion of anastomosed blood vessels: Pathogenetic mechanisms. pp. 30–31. In Danniller AI, Strauch B (eds): Symposium on Microsurgery. CV Mosby, St Louis, 1976

74. Stamotopoulos C, Biemer E, Duspiva W, Blumel G: Microvascular damage caused by the application of surgical microclips: The effects of pressure and tissue. Int J Microsurgery 2:181–186, 1980

75. Stark R, Sanger JR, Matloub HS: A new microvascular clamp for the production of experimental ischemia. Microsurgery 5:202–206, 1984

76. Sukoff MH, Salibian A, Arick TP: A portable microvascular laboratory for the office. Microsurgery 4:71–74, 1983

77. Thomson JR: Operating under magnification. Aust NZ J Surg 41:160–165, 1971

78. Thurston JB, Buncke HF, Chater NL, Weinstein PR: A scanning electron microscopy study of micro-arterial damage and repair. Plast Reconstr Surg 57:197–203, 1976

79. Wilber RG, Shaffer JW, Field GA: The effect of redundancy and tension on microvascular vein grafts. J Hand Surg 9A:649–652, 1984

Clinical Microvascular Techniques

80. Achauer BM, Black KS: Transcutaneous oxygen: Past, present and future. pp. 420–424. In Buncke HJ, Furnas DW (eds): Symposium on Clinical Frontiers in Reconstructive Microsurgery. CV Mosby, St Louis, 1984

81. Acland RD: Microsurgery Practice Manual. CV Mosby, St Louis, 1980

82. Acland R, Banis JC, Ulfe EE, Thoma A, Hildreth D: The usefulness of the PPG in monitoring free flaps — Results of a critical prospective study in 56 consecutive cases (unpublished).

83. Albertengo JG, Rodriguez A, Buncke HJ, Hall EJ: A comparative study of flap survival rates in end-to-end and end-to-side microvascular anastomosis. Plast Reconstr Surg 67:194–199, 1981

84. Ames A, Wright RL, Kowada M, Thurston JM, Majno G: Cerebral ischemia: II. The no-reflow phenomenon. Am J Path 52:437–447, 1968

85. Awwad AM, White RJ, Lowe GDO, Forbes CD: The effect of blood viscosity on blood flow in the experimental saphenous flap model. Brit J Plast Surg 36:383–386, 1983

86. Awwad AM, White RJ, Webster MHC, Vance JP: The effect of temperature on blood flow in island and free skin flaps: An experimental study. Brit J Plast Surg 36:373–382, 1983

87. Ballantyne DL, Chin DTW, Razaboni RM, Harper AD, Chen L: Introduction to Microsurgery: A Microvascular and Microneurological Laboratory Manual. University Park Press, Baltimore, 1985

88. Batchelor AGG, Davison P, Sully L: The salvage of congested skin flaps by the application of leeches. Brit J Plast Surg 37:358–360, 1984

89. Baxter TJ, O'Brien BMcC, Henderson PN, Bennett RC: The histopathology of small vessels following microvascular repair. Brit J Surg 59:617–622, 1972

90. Biemer E: Vein grafts in microvascular surgery. Brit J Plast Surg 30:197–199, 1977

91. Blair WF, Chang L, Pedersen DR, Gabel RH, Bell LD: Hemodynamics after autogenous interpositional grafting in small arteries. Microsurgery 7:84–86, 1986

92. Brener BJ, Raines JK, Darling RC: The end-to-end anastomosis of blood vessels of different diameters. Surg Gynecol Obstet 138:249–251, 1974

93. Brunelli G: The organization of a microsurgical service. Int Surg 65:489–490, 1980

94. Buchler U, Phelps DB, Boswick JA Jr: The influence of experimentally induced anemia on the patency of microvascular anastomoses. J Hand Surg 2:29–30, 1977; Letter to the Editor — AS Earle. J Hand Surg 2:412, 1977; Reply — DB Phelps and JA Boswick, Jr. J Hand Surg 2:412–413, 1977

95. Buncke HJ, Chater NL, Szabo Z: The manual of microvascular surgery. Davis & Geck, Pearl River, NY, 1975

96. Caffee HH: Improved exposure for arterial repair in thumb replantation. J Hand Surg 10:416, 1985

97. Carmignani G, Belgrano E, Puppo P, Cichero A, Sanna A: Long term results with autogenous microvascular grafts in various experimental models in rats. J Microsurgery 2:189–194, 1981

98. Chait LA, May JW Jr, O'Brien BM, Hurley JV: The effects of the perfusion of various solutions on the no-reflow phenomenon in experimental free flaps. Plast Reconstr Surg 61:421–430, 1978

99. Choi HK, Stowe N, Novick AC: Comparison of end-to-end and telescoped arterial anastomoses in renal transplantation in rats. J Microsurgery 3:85–88, 1981

100. Clothiaux PL, Wood MB, Van Houtte P: The effects of progressive ischemia on the vasoreactivity of the isolated canine tibia. Presented at the 2nd annual meeting of the American Society for Reconstructive Microsurgery, New Orleans, 1986

101. Cooley BC, Jones MM, Dellon AL: Comparison of efficacy of thrombolysin, streptokinase, and urokinase in a femoral vein clot model in rats. Microsurgery 4:1–4, 1983

102. Cooley BC, Hansen FC: Microvascular repair following local crush and avulsion vascular injury. Microsurgery 6:46–48, 1985

103. Cooley BC, Morgan RF, Dellon AL: Thrombolytic

reversal of no-reflow phenomenon in rat free flap model. Surg Forum 34:638–640, 1983

104. Cooney WP, Wilson MR, Wood MB: Intravascular fibrinolysis of small-vessel thrombosis. J Hand Surg 8:131–138, 1983

105. Crawshaw HM, Quist WC, Serrallach E, Valeri R, LoGerto FW: Flow disturbance at the distal end-to-side anastomosis. Effect of patency of the proximal outflow segment and angle of anastomosis. Arch Surg 115:1280–1284, 1980

106. Dell PC, Seaber AV, Urbaniak JR: Effect of hypovolemia on perfusion after digit replantation. Surg Forum 31:503–504, 1980

107. Dickson WA, Boothman P, Hare K: An unusual source of hospital wound infection. Brit Med J 289:1727–1728, 1984

108. Doyle DF: A microminiature photoplethysmograph probe for microvascular surgery. Microsurgery 5:105–106, 1984

109. Eriksson E, Anderson WA, Replogle RL: Effects of prolonged ischemia on muscle microcirculation in the cat. Surgical Forum, 25:254–255, 1974

110. Falcone RE, Ruberg RL: Pharmacologic manipulation of skin flaps: Lack of effect of barbituates or nicotine.Plast Reconstr Surg 66:102–104, 1980

111. Fernandes EJ, Nadal RD, Gonzalez SM, Caffee HH: The effect of stasis on a microvascular anastomosis. Microsurgery 4:176–177, 1983

112. Fischer JC, Parker PM, Shaw WW: Comparison of two laser Doppler flow meters for the monitoring of dermal blood flow. Microsurgery 4:164–170, 1983

113. Fischer JC, Parker PM, Shaw WW: Laser Doppler flowmeter measurements of skin perfusion changes associated with arterial and venous compromise in the cutaneous island flap. Microsurgery 6:238–243, 1985

114. Fischer JC, Parker PM, Shaw WW: Waveform analysis applied to laser Doppler flowmetry. Microsurgery 7:67–71, 1986

115. Fisher J, Wood MB: Late necrosis of a latissimus dorsi free flap. Plast Reconstr Surg 74:274–278, 1984. Serafin D: Discussion. Plast Reconstr Surg 4:278–281, 1984

116. Fossati E, Harashina T, Fujino T: The reapplication of microvascular clamps after venous anastosmosis: An experimental study. J Microsurgery 3:239–241, 1982

117. Fossati E, Asurey N, Irigaray A: Application of Kunlin's technique in vascular micro-anastomosis: Experimental and clinical study. Microsurgery 6:53–55, 1985

118. Fossati E, Irigaray A: Successful revascularization of an incompletely amputated finger with serious vascular congestion — A case report. J Hand Surg 8:356–358, 1983

119. Foucher G: Use of leeches in microvascular surgery. ASSH Correspondence Newsletter 1985–82, 1985

120. Furnas DW: Microsurgery and the community based plastic surgeon. Clin Plast Surg 10:145–148, 1983

121. Gelogovac SV, Bitz DM, Whiteside LA: Hydrogen washout technique in monitoring vascular status after replantation surgery. J Hand Surg 7:601–605, 1982

122. Glover MG, Seaber AV, Urbaniak JR: Arterial intimal damage in avulsion and crush injuries in rat limbs. J Reconstr Microsurgery 1:247–251, 1985

123. Godina M: Preferential use of end-to-side arterial anastomosis in free flap transfers. Plast Reconstr Surg 64:673–682, 1979

124. Goldner RD: Symposium on microvascular surgery: Post-operative management. Hand Clinics 1:205–215, 1985

125. Gordon L, Leitner DW, Buncke HJ, Alpert BS: Partial nail plate removal after digital replantation as an alternative method of venous drainage. J Hand Surg 10A:360–364, 1985

126. Gould SH, Gould JS: The microsurgical assistant. J Reconstr Microsurgery 1:113–115, 1984. Buncke HJ: Discussion. Microsurgery 1:117, 1984

127. Graham BH, Gordon L, Alpert BS, Walton R, Buncke HJ, Leitner DW: Serial quantitative skin surface fluorescence: A new method for post-operative monitoring of vascular perfusion in revascularized digits. J Hand Surg 10A:226–230, 1985

128. Green C, Gilby JA: The medicinal leech. J Roy Soc Health 103:42–44, 1983

129. Greenwald RA (ed): CRC Handbook of Methods for Oxygen Radical Research. CRC Press, Boca Raton, 1985

130. Hall EJ: End-to-side anastomosis: A model and a technique with clinical application. J Microsurgery 2:106–112, 1980

131. Harashina T, Takaki JL: A new anastomosis technique for large-calibered vein grafts. Microsurgery 4:171–175, 1983

132. Harris GD, Finseth F, Buncke HJ: Posterior-wall-first microvascular anastomotic technique. Brit J Plast Surg 34:47–49, 1981

133. Harris GD, Finseth F, Buncke HJ: The hazard of cigarette smoking following digital replantation. J Microsurgery 1:403–404, 1980

134. Harrison DH, Girling M, Mott G: Experience in monitoring the circulation in free-flap transfers.

Plast Reconstr Surg 68:543–553, 1981. Acland RD: Discussion. Plast Reconstr Surg 68:554–555, 1981

135. Harrison DH, Girling M, Mott G: Monitoring the circulation in the free flap transfer. pp. 399–407. In Buncke HJ, Furnas DW (eds): Symposium on Clinical Frontiers in Reconstructive Microsurgery. CV Mosby, St Louis, 1984

136. Harrison DH, Girling M, Mott G: Methods of assessing the viability of free flap transfer during the post-operative period. Clin Plast Surg 10:21–36, 1983

137. Heden PG, Hamilton R, Arnander C, Jurell G: Laser Doppler surveillance of the circulation of free flaps and replanted digits. Microsurgery 6:11–19, 1985

138. Henderson HP, Matti B, Laing AG, Morelli S, Sully L: Avulsion of the scalp treated by microvascular repair: The use of leeches for post-operative decongestion. Brit J Plast Surg 36:235–239, 1983

139. Holling HE, Verel D: Circulation in the elevated forearm. Clinical Sci 16:197–213, 1957

140. Howell ST, Seaber AV, Urbaniak JR: Innervation and the blood flow response to superoxide anion. Presented at the 2nd Annual Meeting of the American Society for Reconstructive Microsurgery, New Orleans, 1986

141. Huber W, Menander-Huber KB: Orgotein. Clin Rheumatic Dis 6:465–498, 1980

142. Hurst LN, Evans HB, Brown DH: Vasospasm control by intra-arterial reserpine. Plast Reconstr Surg 70:595–599, 1982

143. Im MJ, Manson PN, Buckley GB, Hoopes JE: Effects of superoxide dismutase and allopurinol on the survival of acute island skin flaps. Ann Surg 201:357–359, 1985

144. Isaacs IJ: The vascular complications of digital replantation. Aust NZ J Surg 47:292–299, 1977

145. Jacobson JH: Microsurgery. pp. 2–56. In Current Problems in Surgery 1971

146. Jelalian C, Mehrhof A, Cohen IK, Richardson J, Merritt WH: Streptokinase in the treatment of acute arterial occlusion of the hand. J Hand Surg 10A:534–538, 1985

147. Jones BM: Predicting the fate of free tissue transfers. Master of Surgery Thesis, University of London, 1982

148. Jones BM: Monitors for the cutaneous microcirculation. Plast Reconstr Surg 73:843–850, 1984

149. Keller HP, Lanz U: Objective control of replanted fingers by transcutaneous partial O_2 (PO_2) measurement. Microsurgery 5:85–89, 1984

150. Ketchum LD, Wennen WW, Masters FW, Robinson DW: Experimental use of pluronic F68 in microvascular surgery. Plast Reconstr Surg 53:288–292, 1974

151. Korthuis RJ, Granger DN, Townsley MI, Taylor AE: The role of oxygen-derived free radicals in ischemia-induced increases in canine skeletal muscle vascular permeability. Circ Res 57:599–609, 1985

152. Kotani H, Kawai S, Doi K, Kuwata N: Automatic milking apparatus for the insufficient venous drainage of the replanted digit. Microsurgery 5:90–94, 1984

153. Lim CL: Successful transfer of "free" microvascular superficial temporal artery flap with no obvious venous drainage and use of leeches for reducing venous congestion. Case Report. Microsurgery 7:87–88, 1986

154. Lineaweaver WC, Buncke HJ: Complications of free flap transfer. Hand Clinics 2:347–351, 1986

155. Lu S-Y, Chin H-Y, Lin T, Chen M-T: Evaluation of survival in digital replantation with thermometric monitoring. J Hand Surg 9A:805–809, 1984

156. Lucas GL: The pattern of venous drainage of the digits. J Hand Surg 9A:448–450, 1984

157. Manson PN, Anthenelli RM, Im MJ, Bulkley GB, Hoopes JE: The role of oxygen-free radicals in ischemic tissue injury in island skin flaps. Ann Surg 198:87–90, 1983

158. Markwardt F: Pharmacology of Hirudin: One hundred years after the first report of the anticoagulant agent in medicinal leeches. Biomed Biochem Acta 44:1007–1013, 1985

159. Matsen FA III, Bach AW, Wyss CR, Simmons CW: Transcutaneous PO_2: A potential monitor of the status of replanted limb parts. Plast Reconstr Surg 65:732–737, 1980. JW May Jr: Discussion. Plast Reconstr Surg 65:746, 1980

160. May JW, Chait LA, O'Brien BM, Hurley JV: The no-reflow phenomenon in experimental free flaps. Plast Reconstr Surg 61:256–267, 1978

161. Mazer N, Barbieri CH, Goncalves RP: Effect of different irrigating solutions on the endothelium of small arteries: Experimental study in rats. Microsurgery 7:9–28, 1986

162. Mirza MA, Korber KE: Organization and implementation of a community hospital microsurgical service for the management of amputation injuries. Microsurgery 5:136–139, 1984

163. Mosely LH, Nigro CAL, McKee NH: Lack of effect of nicotine on replanted rabbit ears. J Microsurgery 3:200, 1982

164. Moss SH, Schwartz KS, von Drasek-Ascher G,

Ogden LL, Wheeler CS, Lister GD: Digital venous anatomy. J Hand Surg 10A:473–482, 1985

165. Musella RA, Willey EN: Evaluation of patency of synthetic and autogenous venous and arterial micrografts in rats. Microsurgery 6:85–91, 1985

166. Myers MB, Bolli R, Lekich RF, Hartley CJ, Roberts R: Enhancement of recovery of myocardial function by oxygen free-radical scavengers after reversible regional ischemia. Circulation 72:915–921, 1985

167. Nam DA, Roberts TL III, Acland RD: An experimental study of end-to-side microvascular anastomosis. Surg Gynecol Obstet 147:339–342, 1978

168. Nathan PA, Rose MC: An alternative technique for microvascular suture. Plast Reconstr Surg 58:635–637, 1976

169. O'Brien BMcC: Organization of a microsurgery unit. pp. 243–246. In Daniller AI, Strauch B (eds): Symposium on Microsurgery. CV Mosby, St Louis, 1976

170. O'Brien BMcC: Microvascular Reconstructive Surgery. pp. 40–48. Churchill Livingston, Edinburgh, 1977

171. O'Brien, BMcC: Microvascular Reconstructive Surgery. pp. 102–118. Churchill Livingston, Edinburgh, 1977

172. O'Brien BMcC: Microvascular Reconstructive Surgery. pp. 29–39. Churchill Livingstone, Edinburgh, 1977

173. Parker PM, Fischer JC, Shaw WW: Implantable pulsed Doppler cuff for long-term monitoring of free flaps: A preliminary study. Microsurgery 5:130–135, 1984

174. Parks DA, Bulkley GB, Granger DN: Role of oxygen free radicals in shock, ischemia, and organ preservation. Surgery 94:428–432, 1983

175. Phelps DB, Rutherford RB, Boswick JA Jr: Control of vasospasm following trauma and microvascular surgery. J Hand Surg 4:109–117, 1979

176. Powers EW, Frager WW: Laser Doppler measurement of blood flow in the microcirculation. Plast Reconstr Surg 51:250–255, 1973

177. Puckett CL, Misholy H, Reinisch JF: The effects of streptokinase on ischemic flaps. J Hand Surg 8:101–104, 1983

178. Rao P, Bailie FB, Bailey BN: Leechmania in microsurgery. The Practitioner 229:901–905, 1985

179. Rao VK, Morrison WA, O'Brien BMcC: Effect of nicotine on blood flow and patency of experimental microvascular anastomosis. Ann Plast Surg 11:206–209, 1983

180. Raskin DF, Erk Y, Spira M, Melissinos EG: Tissue pH monitoring in microsurgery: A preliminary evaluation of continuous tissue pH monitoring as an indicator of perfusion disturbances in microvascular free flaps. Ann Plast Surg 11:332–338, 1983

181. Raskin DJ, Nathan R, Erk Y, Spira M: Critical comparison of transcutaneous PO_2 and tissue pH as indices of perfusion. Microsurgery 4:29–33, 1983

182. Richards RR, Urbaniak JR: Spontaneous retrocarpal radial artery thrombosis: A report of two cases. J Hand Surg 9A:823–827, 1984

183. Roth JH, Urbaniak JR, Boswick JM: Comparison of suture ligation, bipolar cauterization, and hemoclip ligation in the management of small branching vessels in a rat model. J Reconstr Microsurgery 1:7–9, 1984

184. Russell RC: Effects of tension on microvascular anastomoses. Chirurgia Plastica 5:223–233, 1980

185. Sadahivo T, Endoh H: Continuous blood-letting for congestion in replantation of the amputated finger. Br J Hand Surg 9B:83–88, 1984

186. Sadove R, Cline C, Buncke HJ: The effects of artificial postoperative hematoma on patency of microvascular anastomoses in rat femoral vessels. J Microsurgery 1:50–55, 1979

187. Sagi A, Ferder M, Levens D, Yu H-L, Strauch B: The role of superoxide dismutase and different pH medium perfusates in improving survival of island skin flaps after prolonged ischemia. Presented at the 2nd Annual Meeting of the American Society for Reconstructive Microsurgery, New Orleans, 1986

188. Scheker LR, Slattery PG, Firrell JC, Lister GD: The value of the photoplethysmograph in monitoring skin closure in microsurgery. J Reconstr Microsurgery 2:1–4, 1985

189. Schneider P, Pribaz F, Zook EG, Russell RC: Microvenous graft determination for arterial repair. Surgical Forum 34:631–634, 1983

190. Seaber AV: Laboratory design in preparing for elective microvascular surgery. Hand Clinics, 1:233–245, 1985

191. Serafin D, Lesene CB, Voci VE, Mullen RY, Georgiade NG: Assessing skin flap viability and predicting survival using the transcutaneous PO_2 monitor. pp. 408–419. In Buncke HJ, Furnas DW (eds): Symposium on Clinical Frontiers in Reconstructive Microsurgery. CV Mosby, St Louis, 1984

192. Servant J-M, Ikuta Y, Harada Y: A scanning electron microscope study of microvascular anastomoses. Plast Reconstr Surg 57:329–334, 1976

193. Siemionow M: Evaluation of different microsurgical techniques of arterial anastomosis of vessels of diameter less than one millimeter. Presented at the 2nd Annual Meeting of the American Society for Reconstructive Microsurgery, New Orleans, 1986

194. Silverman DG, LaRossa DD, Barlow CH, Bering TG, Popky LM, Smith TC: Quantification of tissue fluroscein delivery and prediction of flap viability with the fiberoptic dermofluorometer. Plast Reconstr Surg 66:545–553, 1980

195. Simmons K: Defense against free radicals has therapeutic implications. JAMA 251:2187–2192, 1984

196. Smith AR, Sonneveld GJ, Kort WF, vander Meulen JC: Clinical application of transcutaneous oxygen measurements in replantation surgery and free tissue transfer. J Hand Surg 8:139–145, 1983

197. Smith AR, Sonneveld GF, vander Meulen JC: AV anastomosis as a solution for absent venous drainage in replantation surgery. Plast Reconstr Surg 71:525–530, 1983

198. Solomon GA, Yaremchuk MJ, Manson PN: Doppler ultrasound monitoring of both arterial and venous flow in clinical free tissue transfers. Presented at the 2nd Annual Meeting of the American Society for Reconstructive Microsurgery, New Orleans, 1986

199. Spaet TH, Rhee CY, Gaynor E: Delayed occlusion of anastomosed blood vessels: Pathogenetic mechanisms. pp. 30–31. In Danniller AI, Strauch B (eds): Symposium on Microsurgery. CV Mosby, St Louis, 1976

200. Stirrat CR, Seaber AV, Urbaniak JR, Bright DS: Temperature monitoring in digital replantation. J Hand Surg 3:342–347, 1978

201. Strauch B, Greenstein B, Goldstein R, Liebling RW: Problems and complications encountered in replantation surgery. Hand Clinics 2:389–399, 1986

202. Svensson H, Svedman P, Holmberg J, Wieslander JB: Detecting changes of arterial and venous blood flow in flaps. Ann Plast Surg 15:35–40, 1985

203. Swartz WM, Jones NF, Klein A, Moosa HH, Rogers VCF, Cherup L: Direct monitoring of microvascular anastomoses: Experimental and clinical experiences in 40 patients. Presented at the 2nd Annual Meeting of the American Society for Reconstructive Microsurgery, New Orleans, 1986

204. Takahashi F, Tsai T-M, Fleming PE, Ogden L: The ability of oxygenated fluorocarbon solution to minimize ischemic skeletal muscle injury. Presented at the International Society of Reconstructive Microsurgery, Paris, 1985

205. Tamai S, Tatsumi Y, Shimizu T, Hori Y, Okuda H, Takita T, Sakamoto H, Fukui A: Traumatic amputation of digits: The fate of remaining blood. J Hand Surg 2:13–21, 1977

206. Thurston JB, Buncke HF, Chater NL, Weinstein PR: A scanning electron microscopy study of micro-arterial damage and repair. Plast Reconstr Surg 57:197–203, 1976

207. Tsai T-M, Jupiter JB, Serratoni F, Seki T, Okubo K: The effect of hypothermia and tissue perfusion on extended myocutaneous flap viability. Plast Reconstr Surg 70:444–452, 1982 Schlender JID: Discussion. Plast Reconstr Surg 70:453–454, 1982

208. Weinberg H, Song Y, Silverman DG, Baek SM, Brousseau DA, Norton KJ: Vascular island skin-flap tolerance to warm ischemia: An analysis by perfusion fluorometry. Plast Reconstr Surg 73:949–952, 1984. Walton RL: Discussion. Plast Reconstr Surg 73:953–955, 1984

209. Weinberg H, Song Y, Douglas B: Enhancement of blood flow in experimental microvascular flaps. Microsurgery 6:121–124, 1985

210. Weiss A-PC, Wang ES, Moore JR, Randolph MA, Weiland AJ, Riley LH: The role of oxygen free radicals in the reperfusion injury of ischemic revascularized bone grafts. Presented at the 2nd Annual Meeting of the American Society for Reconstructive Microsurgery, New Orleans, 1986

211. Whitelock MR, O'Hare PM, Sanders R, Morrow NC: The medicinal leech and its use in plastic surgery: A possible cause for infection. Brit J Plast Surg 36:240–244, 1983

212. Weislander JB, Aberg M: Blood flow in small arteries after end-to-end and end-in-end anastomoses: An experimental quantitative comparison. J Microsurgery 2:121–125, 1980

213. Weislander JB, Aberg M: Stenosis following end-in-end microarterial anastomosis: An angiographic comparison with the end-to-end technique. J Microsurgery 3:151–155, 1982

214. Weislander JB, Aberg M: Blood flow in end-to-end versus end-in-end anastomosis. Letter to the Editor, Microsurgery 4:75, 1983

215. Wilber RG, Shaffer JW, Field GA: The effect of redundancy and tension on microvascular vein grafts. J Hand Surg 9A:649–652, 1984

216. Wilgis EFS: Complications of vascular conditions in the hand. Hand Clinics 2:383–388, 1986

217. Winters RRW, Puckett CL: Evaluation of pathologic vasoconstriction (vasospasm) in microvascular operation. Surgical Forum 34:636–638, 1983

218. Yaffe B, Cushin BF, Strauch B: Effect of cigarette smoking on experimental microvascular anastomoses. Microsurgery 5:70–72, 1984

219. Yamano Y: Replantation of the amputated distal part of the fingers. J Hand Surg 10A:211–218, 1985

220. Yu H-L, Sagi A, Ferder M, Strauch B: A simplified

technique for end-to-end microanastomosis. J Reconstr Microsurgery, 2:191–194, 1986

221. Zdeblick TA, Shaffer JW, Field GA: An ischemia-induced model of revascularization failure of replanted limbs. J Hand Surg 10A:125–131, 1985

Physiology & Pharmacology of the Microcirculation

222. Acland R: Thrombus formation in microvascular surgery: An experimental study of the effects of surgical trauma. Surgery 73:766–771, 1973

223. Acland RD: Does the topical use of magnesium sulfate improve the results in microvascular anastomosis? Plast Reconstr Surg 56:440–441, 1975

224. Acland R: Prevention of thrombosis in microvascular surgery by the use of magnesium sulfate. Brit J Plast Surg 25:292–299, 1972

225. Awwad AM, White RJ, Lowe GDO, Forbes CD: The effect of blood viscosity on blood flow in the experimental saphenous flap model. Brit J Plast Surg 36:383–386, 1983

226. Awwad AM, White RJ, Webster MHC, Vance JP: The effect of temperature on blood flow in island and free skin flaps: An experimental study. Brit J Plast Surg 36:373–382, 1983

227. Bibi R, Ferder M, Strauch B: Prevention of flap necrosis by chlorpromazine. Plast Reconstr Surg 77:954–959, 1986

228. Blair WF, Greene ER, Eldridge M, Cipoletti R: Hemodynamics after microsurgical anastomosis: The effects of topical lidocaine. J Microsurgery 2:157–164, 1981

229. Blair WF, Greene ER, Eldridge M, Cipoletti R: Hemodynamic response of small arteries to topical lidocaine. J Surg Res 31:77–81, 1981

230. Bryant MF, Bloom WL, Brewer SS: Study of the anti-thrombotic properties of dextrans of large molecular weight. J Cardiovasc Surg 5:48–52, 1964

231. Buncke HJ, Blackfield HM: The vasoplegic effects of chlorpromazine. Plast Reconstr Surg 31:353–362, 1963

232. Chang WHJ, Petry JJ: Platelets, prostaglandins, and patency in microvascular surgery. J Microsurgery 2:27–35, 1980

233. Cherry GW: The differing effects of isoxsuprine on muscle flap and skin flap survival in the pig. Plast Reconstr Surg 64:670–672, 1979

234. Chow SP: The histopathology of microvascular anastomosis: A study of the incidence of various tissue changes. Microsurgery 4:5–9, 1983

235. Cooley BC, Jones MM, Dellon AL: Comparison of efficacy of thrombolysin, streptokinase, and uro-kinase in a femoral vein clot model in rats. Microsurgery 4:1–4, 1983

236. Cooley BC, Hansen FC: Microvascular repair following local crush and avulsion vascular injury. Microsurgery 6:46–48, 1985

237. Cooley BC, Morgan RF, Dellon AL: Thrombolytic reversal of no-reflow phenomenon in rat free flap model. Surg Forum 34:638–640, 1983

238. Cooney WP, Wilson MR, Wood MB: Intravascular fibrinolysis of small-vessel thrombosis. J Hand Surg 8:131–138, 1983

239. Copeland JG, Puckett CL: Dimethyl sulfoxide (DMSO) as an adjunct to combat ischemia in microvascular surgery. Presented at the 2nd Annual Meeting of the American Society for Reconstructive Microsurgery, New Orleans, 1986

240. Couraud JY, Di Giamberardino L: Axonal transport of the molecular forms of acetylcholinesterase in normal and regenerating peripheral nerves. Intl J Microsurgery 3:133–137, 1981

241. Dell PC, Seaber AV, Urbaniak JR: Effect of hypovolemia on perfusion after digit replantation. Surg Forum 31:503–504, 1980

242. Elcock HW, Fredrickson JM: The effect of heparin on thrombosis at microvenous anastomotic sites. Arch Otolaryngology 95:68–71, 1972

243. Emerson DJM, Patel CB, Krishna BV, Sykes PJ: The use of prostacyclin in preventing occlusion of microvascular anastomoses by platelet thrombus: An experimental study in rats. Brit J Plast Surg 34:35–37, 1981

244. Erdi A, Thomas DP, Kakkar VV, Lane DA: Effect of low-dose subcutaneous heparin on whole-blood viscosity. Lancet 2(7981):342–344, 1976

245. Fernandes EJ, Nadal RD, Gonzalez SM, Caffee HH: The effect of stasis on a microvascular anastomosis. Microsurgery 4:176–177, 1983

246. Finseth F, Adelberg MG: Prevention of skin flap necrosis by a course of treatment with vasodilator drugs. Plast Reconstr Surg 61:738–743, 1978

247. Finseth F, Buncke HJ: Improvement of tissue blood flow by vasodilator therapy with isoxsuprine: Direct measurement by Xenon washout. pp. 438–443. In Buncke HJ, Furnas DW (eds): Symposium on Clinical Frontiers in Microvascular Surgery. CV Mosby, St Louis, 1984

248. Flower RJ, Moncada S, Vane JR: Analgesic-antipyretics and anti-inflammatory agents; Drugs employed in the treatment of gout. pp. 682–698. In Goodman LS, Gilman AG (eds): The Pharmacological Basis of Therapeutics, 6th Ed. McMillian, London, 1980

249. Furr WS, Seaber AV, Urbaniak JR: The role of

thromboxane in post-ischemic microcirculatory blood flow. Presented at the 2nd Annual Meeting of the American Society for Reconstructive Microsurgery, New Orleans, 1986

250. Glover MG, Seaber AV, Urbaniak JR: Arterial intimal damage in avulsion and crush injuries in rat limbs. J Reconst Microsurgery 1:247–251, 1985

251. Griffiths RW, Hobby JAE, Humphries NL, Trengove-Jones G: The influence of post-operative pharmacological vasodilator agents on the pattern of necrosis in a standardized rat skin flap. Brit J Plast Surg 34:441–445, 1981

252. Haines P, Nichter LS, Morgan RF, Horowitz JH, Edgerton MT: A digit replantation model. Microsurgery 6:70–72, 1985

253. Hendel PM: Pharmacologic agents in microvascular surgery. pp. 427–437. In Buncke HJ, Furnas DW (eds): Symposium on Clinical Frontiers in Microvascular Surgery. CV Mosby, St Louis, 1984

254. Hendel PM, Lilien DL, Buncke HJ: A study of the pharmacological control of blood flow to acute skin flaps using xenon washout. Part I. Plast Reconstr Surg 71:387–398, 1983. Myers B: Discussion. Plast Reconstr Surg 71:408, 1983. Edstrom LE: Discussion. Plast Reconstr Surg 71:409–410, 1983

255. Hendel PM, Lilien DL, Buncke HJ: A study of the pharmacologic control of blood flow to delayed skin flaps using xenon washout. Part II. Plast Reconstr Surg 71:399–407, 1983. Myers B: Discussion. Plast Reconstr Surg 71:408, 1983. Edstrom LE: Discussion. Plast Reconstr Surg 71:409–410, 1983

256. Hurst LN, Evans HB, Brown DH: Vasospasm control by intra-arterial reserpine. Plast Reconstr Surg 70:595–599, 1982

257. Isaacs IJ: The vascular complications of digital replantation. Aust NZ J Surg 47:292–299, 1977

258. Jacobs GR, Reinisch JF, Puckett CL: Microvascular fibrinolysis after ischemia: Its relation to vascular patency and tissue survival. Plast Reconstr Surg 68:737–741, 1981

259. Jacobson JH: Microsurgery. pp. 2–56. Current Problems in Surgery. 1971

260. Jelalian C, Mehrhof A, Cohen IK, Richardson J, Merritt WH: Streptokinase in the treatment of acute arterial occlusion of the hand. J Hand Surg 10A:534–538, 1985

261. Kastrup EK, Olin BR (eds): Drug Facts and Comparisons. pp. 238–244. JB Lippincott, Philadelphia, 1987

262. Kerrigan CL, Daniel RK: Pharmacologic treatment of the failing skin flap. Plast Reconstr Surg 70:541–548, 1982. Cherry CW: Discussion. Plast Reconstr Surg 70:549, 1982

263. Ketchum LD, Wennen WW, Masters FW, Robinson DW: Experimental use of pluronic F68 in microvascular surgery. Plast Reconstr Surg 53:288–292, 1974

264. Ketchun LD: Pharmacological alterations in the clotting mechanism: Use in microvascular surgery. J Hand Surg 3:407–415, 1978

265. Koman LA, Poehling GG, Pollock FE, Hoppers SC, Renn JA: Alterations in thermoregulatory response in reflex sympathetic dystrophy. (unpublished)

266. Leung PC, Chan MY, Roberts MB: The use of prostaglandins as local anti-thrombotic agents in microvascular surgery. Brit J Plast Surg 34:38–40, 1981

267. Mathews WS, Mote PS: The topical use of sodium nitroprusside for relief of intra-operative arterial spasm. Anesthesiology 61:776–777, 1984

268. Mayer SE: Neurohumoral transmission and the autonomic nervous system. pp. 56–90. In Goodman LS, Gilman AG (eds): The Pharmacological Basis of Therapeutics, 6th Edition, McMillian, London, 1980

269. McGrath MA, Penny R: The mechanisms of Raynaud's phenomenon: Part I. Med J Australia 2:328–333, 1974

270. Milling MAP, Patel CB: Topical vasodilators: A controlled trial. Intl J Microsurgery 3:219–220, 1981

271. Moake JL, Funicella T: Common bleeding problems. CIBA Clinical Symposia 35(3):2–32, 1983

272. Moncada S, Flower RJ, Vane JR: Prostaglandins, prostacyclin, and thromboxane A_2. pp. 668–681. In Goodman LS, Gilman AG (eds): The Pharmacological Basis of Therapeutics, 6th Ed. McMillian, London, 1980

273. Morecraft R, Blair WF, Chang L: Histopathology of microvenous repair. Microsurgery 6:219–228, 1985

274. Myers MB, Cherry G: Enhancement of survival in devascularized pedicles by the use of phenoxybenzamine. Plast Reconstr Surg 41:254–260, 1968

275. Nomoto H, Bunke HJ, Chater NL: Improved patency rates in microvascular surgery when using magnesium sulfate and a silicone rubber vascular cuff. Plast Reconstr Surg 54:157–160, 1974

276. O'Brien BMcC: Microvascular Reconstructive Surgery. pp. 40–48. Churchill Livingstone, Edinburgh, 1977

277. Phelps DB, Rutherford RB, Boswick JA: Control of vasospasm following trauma and microvascular surgery. J Hand Surg 4:109–117, 1979

278. Physicians' Desk Reference: Isoxsuprine. p. 1569. Barnhart, Oradell, NJ, 1986

279. Physicians' Desk Reference: Terbutaline. p. 889. Barnhart, Oradell, NJ, 1986

280. Physicians' Desk Reference: Prazosin. p. 1420. Barnhart, Oradell, NJ, 1986

281. Physicians' Desk Reference: Nifedipine. p. 1423. Barnhart, Oradell, NJ, 1986

282. Physicians' Desk Reference: Chlorpromazine. p. 872. Barnhart, Oradell, NJ, 1986

283. Physicians' Desk Reference: Phenoxybenzamine. p. 1713. Barnhart, Oradell, NJ, 1986

284. Puckett CL, Winters RRW, Geter RK, Goebel D: Studies of pathologic vasoconstriction (vasospasm) in microvascular surgery. J Hand Surg 10A:343–349, 1985

285. Rosenberg RD: Actions and interactions of antithrombin and heparin. N Engl J Med 292:146–151, 1975

286. Sasaki A, Harii K: Lack of effect of isoxsuprine on experimental random flaps in the rat. Plast Reconstr Surg 66:105–108, 1980

287. Sasaki GH, Pang CY: Experimental evidence for involvement of prostaglandins in viability of acute skin flaps: Effects on viability and mode of action. Plast Reconstr Surg 67:335–340, 1981

288. Servant J-M, Ikuta Y, Harada Y: A scanning electron microscope study of microvascular anastomoses. Plast Reconstr Surg 57:329–334, 1976

289. Sinclair S: The importance of topical heparin in microvascular anastomoses: A study in the rat. Brit J Plast Surg 33:422–426, 1980

290. Tamai S, Tatsumi Y, Shimizu T, Hori Y, Okuda H, Takita T, Sakamoto H, Fukui A: Traumatic amputation of digits: The fate of remaining blood. J Hand Surg 2:13–21, 1977

291. Weiner N: Drugs that inhibit adrenergic nerves and block adrenergic receptors. pp. 176–210. In Goodman LS, Gilman AG (eds): The Pharmacological Basis of Therapeutics, 6th Ed. McMillian, London, 1980

292. Weiner N: Norepinephrine, epinephrine, and the sympathomimetic amines. pp. 167–168. In Goodman LS, Gilman AG (eds): The Pharmacological Basis of Therapeutics, 6th Ed. McMillian, London, 1980

293. Weiss HJ: Platelet physiology and abnormalities of platelet function. N Engl J Med 293:531–540, 1975

294. Wexler MR, Kalisman M, Yeschua R, Neuman Z: The effect of Phenoxybenzamine, Phentolamine and 6-Hydroxydopamine on skin flap survival in rats. J Surg Res 19:83–87, 1975

295. Winters RRW, Puckett CL: Evaluation of pathologic vasoconstriction (vasospasm) in microvascular operation. Surg Forum 34:636–638, 1983

Research and New Techniques in Microvascular Surgery

296. Aebi M, Regazzoni P, Perren SM, Harder F: Microsurgically revascularized bone allografts with immunosuppression with Cyclosporine. Transplantation, 42:564–568, 1986

297. Aksik IA, Kikut RP, Apshkalne DL: Extracranial anastomosis performed by means of biological gluing materials: Experimental and clinical study. Microsurgery 7:2–8, 1986

298. Bailes JE, Quigley MR, Kwaan HC, Cerullo LJ, Brown JT: Fibrinolytic activity following laser-assisted vascular anastomosis. Microsurgery 6:163–168, 1985

299. Baxter TJ, O'Brien BMcC, Henderson PN, Bennett RC: The histopathology of small vessels following microvascular repair. Brit J Surg 59:617–622, 1972

300. Bell LD, Blair WF, Pedersen DR, Gabel RH: A hemodynamic evaluation of cuffed microarteriorrhaphy. Microsurgery 6:106–112, 1985

301. Blair WF, Pedersen DR, Joos K, Green ER, Bondi D: Microarteriorrhaphy: Blood flow after wound healing. Microsurgery 6:116–120, 1985

302. Caffee HH: Microvascular synthetic grafts. Plast Reconstr Surg 66:380–382, 1980. Also, J Microsurgery 2:140–142, 1980

303. Carton CA, Kessler LA, Seidenberg B, Hurwitt ES: Experimental studies in the surgery of small blood vessels. IV. Nonsuture anastomosis of arteries and veins, using flanged ring prosthesis and plastic adhesive. Surg Forum 11:238–239, 1960

304. Casanova MD, Vasconez MA, Herrera G, Lemons V, Vasconez L: Microarterial sutureless anastomoses using a polymeric adhesive: An experimental study. Presented at the 2nd Annual Meeting of the American Society for Reconstructive Microsurgery, New Orleans, 1986

305. Chait LA, May JW Jr, O'Brien BM, Hurley JV: The effects of the perfusion of various solutions on the no-reflow phenomenon in experimental free flaps. Plast Reconstr Surg 61:421–430, 1978

306. Chase RA: The development of tissue transfer in hand surgery. ASSH Presidential Address. J Hand Surg 9:463–477, 1984

307. Chase RA: Historical review of skin and soft tissue coverage of the upper extremity. Hand Clinics 1:599–608, 1985

308. Cheema TA, Schenck RR, Weinrib HP: The external ring technique for end-to-side microvascular anastomosis. J Hand Surg 10:151, 1985

309. Chen L, Chin DTW: Spinal interrupted suturing technique for microvascular anastomosis: A comparative study. Microsurgery 7:72–78, 1986

310. Chow SP: The histopathology of microvascular anastomosis: A study of the incidence of various tissue changes. Microsurgery 4:5–9, 1983

311. Cook AF, Azar CA, Dinner MI: The short-term effects of Dexon and nylon in experimental microvascular surgery—A quantitative comparison. J Hand Surg 8:299–301, 1983

312. Cuadros CL: One hundred percent patency of one millimeter polytetrafluoroethylene (Gore-Tex) grafts in the carotid arteries of rats. Microsurgery 5:1–11, 1984

313. Daniel RK, Egerszegi EP, Samulack DD, Skanes SE, Dykes RW, Rennie WR: Tissue transplants in primates for upper extremity reconstruction: A preliminary report. J Hand Surg 11A:1–8, 1986

314. Firsching R, Terhaag PD, Muller W, Frowein RA: Continuous- and interrupted-suture technique in microsurgical end-to-end anastomosis. Microsurgery 5:80–84, 1984

315. George PT, Creech BJ, Bunke HJ: A rapid new technique for microvascular anastomosis (the loop technique). Plast Reconstr Surg 56:99–100, 1975

316. Graf P, Biemer E, Ascherl R: Viability of surrounding tissue attached to vein graft. J Reconstr Microsurgery 1:119–122, 1984

317. Green AR, Milling MAP, Green ART: Butylcyanoacrylate adhesives in microvascular surgery: An experimental pilot study. J Reconstr Microsurgery 2:103–105, 1986

318. Hamilton RB, O'Brien BMcM: An experimental study of microvascular patency using a continuous suture technique. Brit J Plast Surg 32:153–154, 1979

319. Hess F: History of (micro) vascular surgery and the development of small-caliber blood vessel prosthesis (with some notes on patency rates and reendothelialization). Microsurgery 6:59–69, 1985

320. Hess F, Jerusalem C, Braun B, Grande P: Three years experience with experimental implantation of fibrous polyurethane microvascular prosthesis in the rat aorta. Microsurgery 6:155–162, 1985

321. Huang G-K, Hu R-Q, Pan G-P: Influence of vessel clips on vascular patency in microarterial grafts less than 0.5 mm in external diameter. J Hand Surg 10A:538–541, 1985

322. Ji SY, Chia SL, Cheng HH: Free transplantation of venous network pattern skin flap: An experimental study in rabbits. Microsurgery 5:151–159, 1984

323. Joos KM, Blair WF, Maynard JA: A histologic comparison of continuous and interrupted microarteriorrhaphy. Microsurgery 6:141–146, 1985

324. Ketchum LD, Wennen WW, Masters FW, Robinson DW: Experimental use of pluronic F68 in microvascular surgery. Plast Reconstr Surg 53:288–292, 1974

325. Kon ND, Martin MB, Meredith JW, Meredith JH: Comparison of suture technique on patency of polytetrafluoroethylene-microarterial anastomosis. Microsurgery 5:12–14, 1984

326. Lee BY, Brancato RF, Shaw WW, Browne S, Thoden WR, Madden JL: Effect of suture technique on blood velocity waveforms in the microvascular anastomosis of autogenous vein graft. Microsurgery 4:151–156, 1983

327. Longa EZ, Weinstein PR, Chater G: Scanning electron microscopy studies of needle and suture damage in rat carotid and femoral arteries. Microsurgery 5:169–174, 1984

328. Lourie GM, Seaber AV, Urbaniak JR: Microanastomotic response to needle and suture size. J Reconstr Microsurgery 1:135–138, 1984

329. Lourie GM, Seaber AV, Urbaniak JR: Growth and microanastomotic response in the repair of the growing artery. Presented at the 2nd Annual Meeting of the American Society for Reconstructive Microsurgery, New Orleans, 1986

330. Mallon WJ, Seaber AV, Urbaniak JR: A comparison of absorbable and nonabsorbable sutures to vascular response in immature arteries. J Reconstr Microsurgery 2:87–92, 1986

331. Mazer N, Barbieri CH, Goncalves RP: Effect of different irrigating solution on the endothelium of small arteries: Experimental study in rats. Microsurgery 7:9–28, 1986

332. Merrell JC, Zook EG, Russell RC: Cuffing techniques in microarterial surgery. J Hand Surg 9A:76–82, 1984

333. Miyake H, Handa H, Yonekawa Y, Taki W, Naruo Y, Yamagata S, Ikada V, Iwata H, Suzuki M: New small-caliber antithrombotic vascular prosthesis: Experimental study. Microsurgery 5:144–150, 1984

334. Morecraft R, Blair WF, Chang L: Histopathology of microvenous repair. Microsurgery 6:219–228, 1985

335. Musella RA, Willey EN: Evaluation of patency of synthetic and autogenous venous and arterial micrografts in rats. Microsurgery 6:85–91, 1985

336. O'Brien BMcC: Microvascular Reconstructive

Surgery. pp. 79–101. Churchill Livingstone, Edinburgh, 1977

337. Paskert JP, Yaremchuk MJ, Randolph MA, Weiland AF: The role of cyclosporine in experimental vascularized bone allografting. Presented at the 2nd Annual Meeting of the American Society for Reconstructive Microsurgery, New Orleans, 1986

338. Paskert JP, Yaremchuk MJ, Randolph MA, Weiland AF: Prolonging survival in vascularized bone allograft transplantation without chronic immunosuppression: Developing specific immune unresponsiveness. Presented at the 2nd Annual Meeting of the American Society for Reconstructive Microsurgery, New Orleans, 1986

339. Press BHJ, Sibley RK, Shons AR: Experimental limb allotransplantation: Modification of rejection with cyclosporine and prednisone. Surg Forum 34:591–594, 1983

340. Quigley MR, Bailes JE, Kwaan HC, Cerullo LJ, Brown TJ, Sprague B: Laser-assisted end-to-side anastomosis. Presented at the 2nd Annual Meeting of the American Society for Reconstructive Microsurgery, New Orleans, 1986

341. Quigley MR, Bailes JE, Kwaan HC, Cerullo LJ, Brown TJ, Sprague B, Fitzsimmons J: Comparison of bursting strength between suture—and laser—anastomosed vessels. Microsurgery 6:229–232, 1985

342. Randolph MA, Robinson RA, Coleman RA, Nettleblad H, Weiland AJ: Electron microscopic observations in revascularized bone allografts immunosuppressed with cyclosporine. Presented at the 2nd Annual Meeting of the American Society for Reconstructive Microsurgery, New Orleans, 1986

343. Sartorius CF, Shapiro SA, Campbell R, Klatte EC, Clark SA: Experimental laser-assisted end-to-side microvascular anastomosis. Microsurgery 7:79–83, 1986

344. Sasa M, Xian W, Breidenbach W, Tsi T-M, Shibata M, Firrell J: Experimental venous flaps. Presented at the 2nd Annual Meeting of the American Society for Reconstructive Microsurgery, New Orleans, 1986

345. Schenck RT, Weinrib HP, Labanauskas IG: The external ring technique for microvascular anastomosis. J Hand Surg 8:105–108, 1983

346. Serure A, Withers EH, Thomsen S, Morris J: Comparison of carbon dioxide laser-assisted microvascular anastomosis and conventional microvascular sutured anastomosis. Surg Forum 34:634–636, 1983

347. Shaw WW: Editorial: Microsurgery versus reconstructive microsurgery. Microsurgery 4:15–16, 1983

348. Siemionow M: Evaluation of different microsurgical techniques of arterial anastomosis of vessels of diameter less than one millimeter. Presented at the 2nd Annual Meeting of the American Society for Reconstructive Microsurgery, New Orleans, 1986

349. Sugiura K, Nakatsuchi Y, Yagi R, Sugimoto Y: A new method for venous interposition grafts using fibrin glue. Microsurgery 6:125–128, 1985

350. Smith AR, Sonneveld GF, vander Meulen JC: AV anastomosis as a solution for absent venous drainage in replantation surgery. Plast Reconstr Surg 71:525–530, 1983

351. Stoll AW, Chater N, Phillips M: Arterial anastomosis and autogenous interposition grafts in growing rats. Microsurgery 4:245–249, 1983

352. Sully L, Nightingale MG, O'Brien BMcC, Hurley JV: An experimental study of the sleeve technique in microarterial anastomoses. Plast Reconstr Surg 70:186–192, 1982

353. Takahashi F, Tsai T-M, Fleming PE, Ogden L: The ability of oxygenated fluorocarbon solution to minimize ischemic skeletal muscle injury. Presented at the International Society of Reconstructive Microsurgery, Paris, 1985

354. Tsai T-M, Jupiter JB, Serratoni F, Seki T, Okubo K: The effect of hypothermia and tissue perfusion on extended myocutaneous flap viability. Plast Reconstr Surg 70:444–452, 1982. Schlender JD: Discussion. Plast Reconstr Surg 70:453–454, 1982

355. Tsai T-M, Matiko J, Breidenbach W, Kutz J: Clinical venous flaps. Presented at the 2nd Annual Meeting of the American Society for Reconstructive Microsurgery, New Orleans, 1986

356. Urbaniak JR, Soucacos PN, Adelaar RS, Bright DS, Whitehurst LA: Experimental evaluation of microsurgical techniques in small artery anastomoses. Orthop Clin North Am 8:249–263, 1977

357. Weinrib HP, Cook JQ, Penn RD: The ring technique for end-to-side microvascular anastomosis. Microsurgery 5:76–79, 1984

358. Weinrib H, Schenck RR, Sadr B: The external ring method of microvenous anastomosis: A new experimental concept. Microsurgery 4:134–139, 1983

359. Wheatley MJ, Mathes SJ, Hassett C: Comparison of continuous and interrupted suture techniques in microvascular end-to-side anastomosis. J Reconstr Microsurgery 2:93–96, 1986

360. Weislander JB, Aberg M: Blood flow in small arteries after end-to-end and end-in-end anasto-

moses: An experimental quantitative comparison. J Microsurgery 2:121–125, 1980

361. Weislander JB, Aberg M: Stenosis following end-in-end microarterial anastomosis: An angiographic comparison with the end-to-end technique. J Microsurgery 3:151–155, 1982

362. Weislander JB, Aberg M: Blood flow in end-to-end versus end-in-end anastomosis. Letter to the Editor, Microsurgery 4:75, 1983

363. Weislander JB, Rausing A: A histologic comparison of experimental microarterial end-in-end (sleeve) and end-to-end anastomoses. Plast Reconstr Surg 73:279–285, 1984. Lauritzen C: Discussion. Plast Reconstr Surg 73:286–287, 1984

Replantation

25

James R. Urbaniak

Although experimental replantation of amputated limbs of animals was successfully performed at the turn of this century,[8,20] clinical accomplishment of limb replantation was not realized until the 1960s. In Boston in 1962, Malt successfully replanted a completely amputed arm of a 12-year-old boy.[29] In 1965 Komatsu and Tamai of Japan reported the first successful replantation of an amputated digit by microvascular technique.[24] During the following 20 years several microsurgical centers around the world reported impressive series of successful replantation with viability rates greater than 80 percent.[3,21,23,25,28,32,33,43,46,48,51–53,64,67] Developments in the field of microsurgery (operating microscope, ultrafine nonreactive suture material, and precisioned microcaliber needles) have made successful replantation of digits and hands possible.[1,4,10,36,59,60]

DEFINITIONS

A knowledge of certain terminology concerning amputation is essential for surgeons who perform replantations so that universal comparison of results may be possible. *Replantation* is defined as reattachment of the part that has been *completely amputated*; there is no connection between the severed part and the patient. *Revascularization* of a limb is defined as reconstructing a limb that has been *incompletely amputated*, that is, some of the soft tissue (e.g., skin, nerves, or tendons) is intact. Vascular repair is necessary to prevent necrosis of the partially severed extremity. The distinction between replantation and revascularization is important when discussing the methods and especially the results of reattachment of amputated parts. Revascularization procedures are much easier to manage than replantations since less surgical time is required and higher success rates are expected, as adequate venous drainage is usually present. The viability results of revascularizations are generally better than those of replantations, because a small amount of drainage system (venous and/or lymphatic) may be intact. However, in some instances revascularizations are extremely difficult, especially the avulsing type, and even longer hours of surgery may be necessary because individual teams cannot prepare the parts simultaneously since they are not separate.

PATIENT SELECTION

Our criteria for proper patient selection for replantation are based on our team's experience of over 1200 parts. Even with this knowledge, the decision to replant an amputated part is not always easy. Nearly any amputated part can be reattached by an experienced replantation service and remain viable. However, success in viability should not be misconstrued as success in useful function of the replanted body part. Certainly patients with guillotine-type amputations are ideal candidates; however this type of amputation is uncommon. Most limbs are amputated by crushing or avulsing injuries, which makes the surgical repair more difficult and lowers the percentage of viability.

Good candidates for replantation are those with the following amputations: (1) thumb, (2) multiple digits, (3) partial hand (amputation through the palm), (4) almost any body part of a child, (5) wrist or forearm, (6) elbow and above elbow (only sharply or moderately avulsed), and (7) individual digit distal to the flexor superficialis insertion.

All of the above are not necessarily strict indications for replantation. However, if all other factors are favorable, an attempt at reattachment should be performed. The prime parts for replantations are the thumb, multiple digits and the complete hand (Fig. 25-1 and 25-2). In some instances of multiple digit amputations, only the least damaged digits may be replanted. The digits that are the

least damaged may be shifted to the most useful or least injured stumps. For example, if both the thumb and index finger have been completely amputated in a crushing injury and the distal thumb has irreparable distal vessels, the amputated index finger should be attached to the thumb stump. This shifting will result in excellent thumb function and cosmetic acceptability.

The *level* of the digital amputation is an important determinate for deciding on replantation. Amputations distal to the interphalangeal joint of the thumb or the DIP joint of the fingers can be successfully replanted if dorsal veins can be located in the amputed part. In general, at least 4 mm of dorsal skin proximal to the nail plate must be present on the amputated digit for realistic venous reconstruction to be possible. If replantation is elected in more distal amputations, then volar veins may be successfully anastomosed. Other salvage methods to achieve venous outflow in replantations distal to the distal digital joints will be discussed in the section on technique.

An effort should always be made to salvage the amputated thumb, even as far distal as the nail base, if vessels for revascularization can be located.

Replantation of amputated digits distal to the superficialis insertion function well (Fig. 25-3). We like to replant amputations at this level because the operative time is short (less than 4 hours), and the motor and sensory function and cosmetic results are all good.[58,65] In addition, no painful neuromas occur in replanted digits, whereas they are often dilemmas in amputated finger stumps.

Successful replantations at the level of the palm, wrist, and *distal* forearm result in good hand function[23,33,46,51] (Fig. 25-4). Amputations proximal to this level are usually of the severe avulsing type with considerable muscle trauma. Muscle necrosis and subsequent infection are a frequent problem with these replantations at the elbow level or more proximal; therefore, the surgeon must be very selective at these levels.

In a child, an attempt should be made to replant almost any amputated body part, for if the part survives, useful function can be anticipated.

Types of injuries that are not considered to be favorable for replantation are: (1) severely crushed or mangled parts; (2) amputations at multiple levels; (3) amputations in patients with other seri-

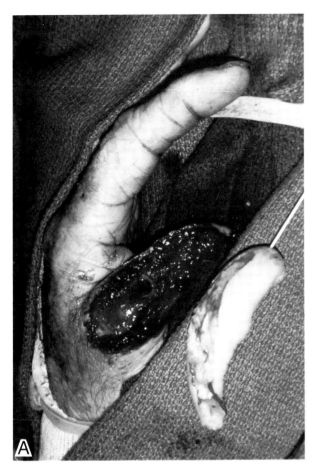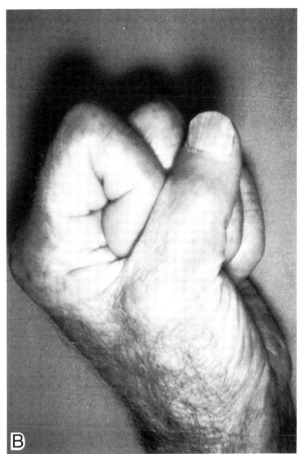

Fig. 25-1. (**A**) An oblique complete amputation of the thumb of a 66-year-old man. An intramedullary pin has been inserted in the amputated thumb for skeletal fixation. Vein grafts were necessary to salvage this thumb because of the oblique injury along the entire neurovascular bundle. (**B**) The thumb 4 months after replantation with good range of motion of the MP joint and protective sensation.

ous injuries or diseases; (4) amputations in which the vessels are arteriosclerotic; (5) amputations in mentally unstable patients; (6) individual finger amputations in the adult at a level proximal to the flexor superficialis insertion; and (7) amputations with prolonged warm ischemia time.

These contraindications to replantation are not absolute. In severe crushing or avulsing injuries, some parts can be successfully salvaged with the use of vein grafts to replace the injured vessels, but there is no method of replacing the most distal vessels in an amputated part. In older patients, the arteries at the amputated site should be examined for arteriosclerosis, which frequently precludes

functional patency following reanastomosis in the small vessel.[50]

If the patient has multiple injuries, the amputated part may be preserved at 4°C for at least 24 hours and delayed replantation performed.[62] Of course, this applies only to digital amputations where preservation of muscle tissue is not necessary.

Mentally unstable patients are not uncommon in the group of patients who have their upper extremities severed. However, a patient's stability is frequently difficult to ascertain during the limited preoperative evaluation period.

In general, in the adult the isolated finger ampu-

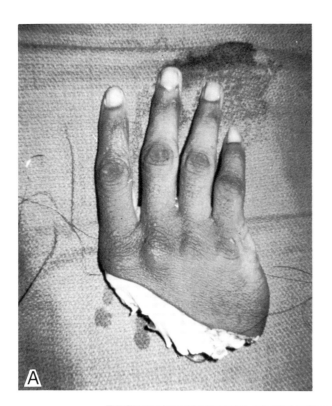

Fig. 25-2. (A) A complete amputation through the midpalm of the hand of an 18-year-old boy. Nine months following successful replantation the amount of (B) flexion and (C) extension is seen. This young man eventually obtained 8-mm two-point discrimination in all replanted digits.

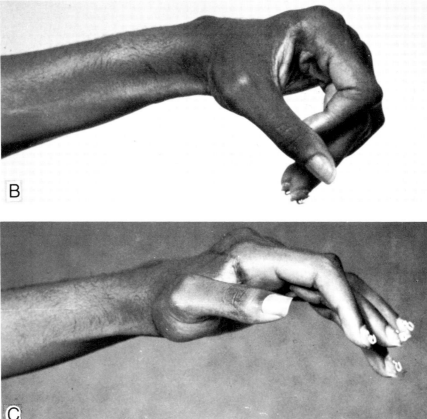

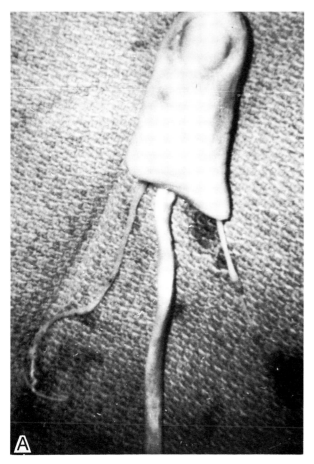

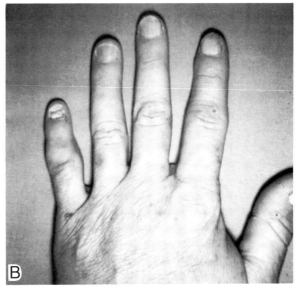

Fig. 25-3. (A) A complete amputation by an avulsion injury to the small finger in a 35-year-old man. The amputation was distal to the superficialis insertion. The avulsed digital nerves are apparent as well as the flexor profundus tendon. (B) Six months postreplantation, the little finger has full extension at the PIP and MP joints. (C) Full flexion enables the patient to touch the palm. The patient obtained 14-mm two-point discrimination.

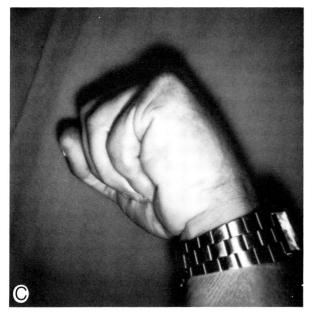

tation proximal to the flexor superficialis tendon insertion should *not* be replanted. Special considerations (e.g., a young woman, violinist, pianist) do influence the decision. However, our long-term evaluations have demonstrated that useful function will usually not occur.[58] Even with the replanted index finger at the base, the patient will usually bypass the replanted digit.

Usually the patient and his family desire a replantation and expect a miraculous result. The surgeon must explain to the patient the chances of success of viability, anticipated function, length of operation and hospitalization, and amount of time lost from work compared with time lost by a simple amputation revision.

Age is not necessarily a barrier; we have performed replantations in patients who were 10 weeks to 76 years old. Oftentimes the decision cannot be made until the status of the vessels of the amputated part is carefully studied under the operating microscope.

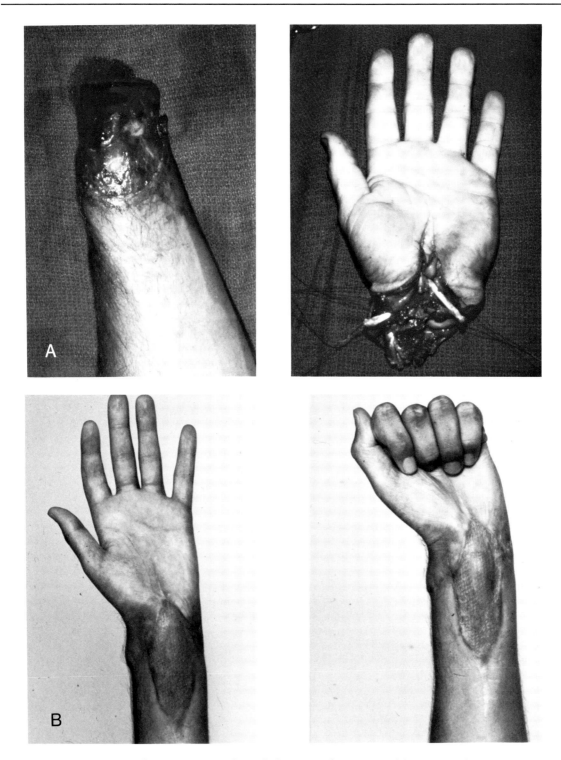

Fig. 25-4. (A) A complete amputation through the wrist of a 21-year-old man. **(B)** Three years following successful replantation, the amount of digital flexion and extension is seen. *(Figure continues.)*

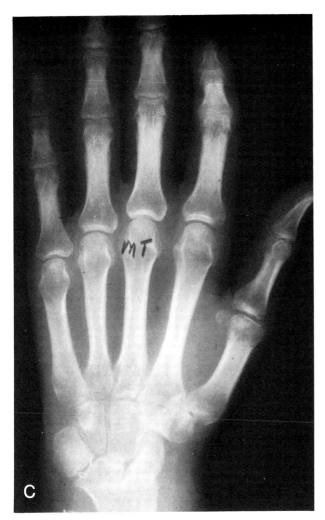

Fig. 25-4 *(Continued)*. **(C)** Postoperative radiograph shows complete healing of the radioscapholunate fusion at the site of replantation.

INSTRUMENTS

The microsurgical instruments and materials are described in detail in Chapter 24; thus only the essential equipment for replantation surgery will be emphasized here. The replantation surgeon need not have a vast amount of expensive equipment, but he must have the proper instruments and they must be maintained in fine functioning order, which is not always easy.[5,36]

Surgical loupes or telescopes of 3.5 × to 4.5 × are used for the initial exploration and dissections of the amputated parts and the injured extremity. An operating microscope, preferably a diploscope, with magnification at least to 20 × is essential. The ideal scope should have a beam splitter in the double head that allows the surgeon and the first assistant to see the same microfield, and foot control for zoom magnification, focusing, and horizontal XY movement. The microscope should be used for repair of any vessels distal to the elbow.

To a degree the choice of the microsurgical instuments depends on the individual surgeon's preferences. All of the instruments should be at least 10 cm long to allow the handles to rest comfortably in the thumb-index web space. Fine spring-loaded (noncatching handles) needle holders and scissors are helpful. Jeweler's forceps, small-tipped tying forceps, a microtipped dilator (lacrimal duct dilator), and a microirrigator (30-gauge needle attached to a plastic syringe) are other essentials. The microclips should have less than 30 g of closing pressure to minimize intimal damage. Two clips mounted on a sliding bar provide a convenient method of approximating the vessel ends without undue tension. The less complex, the better the microclip.

Small silver vascular clips (hemoclips) are used to tag the microvessels and nerves in the initial debridement. A small-tipped bipolar cautery is essential in isolating and mobilizing the vessels to be repaired. A small piece of blue or yellow rubber balloon serves as background material to diminish eye fatigue in the longer cases. Actually, yellow background is preferred, particularly when the lighting is diminished.

The level of the amputation determines the choice of suture and needle size for the vascular repair. Table 25-1 provides suggestions for needle and suture size at the various levels of the hand and

Table 25-1. Appropriate Needle and Suture Size for Microvascular Repairs in the Hand

Location	Needle Size (μ)	Suture Size
Wrist and forearm	130	9–0
Palm	100	10–0
Proximal digit	50–75	10–0
Distal digit	50	11–0

wrist.[52] The most commonly used suture is 10–0 nylon on a 75μ needle. The use of smaller suture and needle is more difficult and fatiguing. 8–0 nylon may be used proximal to the elbow.

Monofilament nylon is preferred over polypropylene and polyglycolic material, since nylon is easier to handle and knot. Naturally, smaller sizes of needles and sutures are used in children.

surgical schedule of the surgeon. The availability of an adequate number of proficient microsurgeons enables relatively rested surgeons to perform in a platoon fashion and lessens fatigue. In addition, many replants survive because of meticulous and intelligent postoperative management, which may mean returning some patients to the operating room for reexploration and revision, possibly as time-consuming as the original procedure.

WHO SHOULD PERFORM REPLANTATIONS

Achievement of survival and useful function in replantation of upper extremity amputations is difficult. Of course, the initial survival of the replanted part depends on patent microvascular anastomes and immediate postoperative care, but the ultimate function and acceptability is dependent on the total performance of the tendon, nerve, bone, and joint repairs. Therefore the replantation surgeon must first be a thoroughly trained and accomplished hand surgeon, second a competent microsurgeon, and third have the knowledge for a predictable outcome of the part selected for reattachment.

The surgeon who engages in microvascular replantation should be able to consistently achieve a 90 percent patency rate in 1-mm vessels in the animal laboratory. The operating theater is not the setting for practicing.[44] Although possible, it is very difficult for a microvascular surgeon functioning independently to maintain a high success rate in replantations. The concept of a well-integrated team seems to be essential if a continued high degree of viability and ultimate function is to be realized.[38,51] A replantation team should be available around the clock everyday. Retattachment of a single uncomplicated digit may be performed within 3 or 4 hours by an experienced microsurgeon or team, but reattachment of multiple digits may require 15 hours. Such emergency procedures may be extremely disquieting to the routine clinical or

PREPARATION OF THE AMPUTATED PART FOR TRANSPORTATION

There are basically two methods of preserving the amputated part: wrapping the part in a cloth moistened with Ringer's lactate solution or saline solution and placing the bundle on ice, or immersing the part in one of these solutions in a plastic bag and placing the bag on ice. Whichever method the replantation surgeon selects, he must give clear and concise instructions about the management of the amputated part to the referring physician. I prefer the immersion method for the following reasons: (1) the part is less likely to become frozen ("frostbitten"); (2) the part is less likely to be strangled by the wrapping; (3) the instructions are easier to explain to the primary care physician; and (4) maceration secondary to immersion is not a problem. In our laboratory we have proved that by using either method of preserving amputated animal parts for 24 hours, equal viability rates of replantation can be achieved.[60]

The tissues will survive for approximately 6 hours if the amputated part is not cooled. If the part is cooled, it may survive 12 hours, or even longer if it is a digit, because the digit has no muscle tissue. Transportation of the amputated part and patient should be as rapid as possible, but successful replantation of digits may be achieved in those that have been without blood supply for 24 to 30 hours if they are properly cooled.[62]

INITIAL SURGICAL MANAGEMENT

When the patient with an amputated part arrives in the emergency room, the replantation team divides into two subteams in an effort to save time. One team immediately transports the amputated part to the operating room where it is cleansed with Hibiclens° and sterile Ringer's lactate solution. The amputated part is placed on a bed of ice covered with a sterile plastic drape. If there are multiple digits, these are cooled by keeping them in the refrigerator or under ice packets until they are required for reattachment.

Using operating loupes or an operating microscope (depending on the size of the amputated part), the part is carefully debrided and the nerves and vessels are identified and tagged with small silver vascular clips (hemoclips). The tagging of the vessels and nerves will prove to be very helpful and timesaving when working in a bloody field later. Failure to label these structures, particularly in multiple amputations, can result in extreme frustration to the surgeon in the later stages of reconstruction where the fatigue factor influences the surgeon's proficiency.

Longitudinal midlateral incisions on each side of the digit provide the most rapid and best exposure of the nerves and vessels (Fig. 25-5). The digital nerves and vessels should be dissected free under magnification for 1.5 to 2.0 cm and then labeled. The dorsal veins are easily identified by reflecting the entire dorsal fold of skin and searching in the subdermal tissue (Fig. 25-5). In the amputated part, the searching for veins may be delayed until after one arterial anastomosis, which makes veins easier to identify by good back bleeding. Further debridement is continued after the neurovascular bundles have been isolated.

Appropriate bone trimming and shortening are performed on the amputated part. Retrograde insertion of one or more intramedullary K-wires in the amputated part is performed so that the part is ready for immediate reattachment.

During this initial period, the other subteam as-

° Stuart Pharmaceuticals, Wilmington, DE.

sesses the patient with a routine physical examination, radiographs of the injured extremity and chest, electrocardiogram, blood chemistries, complete blood count, urinalysis, blood type and crossmatch, and activated partial thromboplactin time. Intravenous fluids are begun, and the patient is given intravenous antibiotics and tetanus prophylaxis. An indwelling urethral catheter is inserted if a long procedure is anticipated.

Most replantations should be performed under axillary block with bupivacaine (Marcaine), a long activating local anesthetic.[18] General anesthesia is usually required for children under 10 years of age.

Peripheral blood flow to the injured limb is enhanced by the sympathetic block provided by regional anesthesia and by maintaining a *warm body temperature.*

Under tourniquet ischemia and magnification while one team prepares the amputated part, the

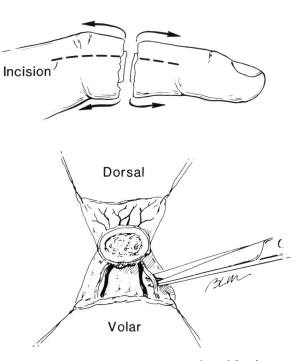

Fig. 25-5. Midlateral incisions are preferred for the amputated digit and stump. The incisions are slightly toward the dorsal side so that both the dorsal and volar skin can be reflected to locate the arteries and veins with ease.

other team debrides the stump and identifies and tags the nerves and vessels in a manner similar to that used on the amputated part. The veins on the stump are often particularly difficult to locate in the digit. Their identification requires patience, experience, and meticulous dissection, since successful replantation depends on a skillful anastomosis of an adequate number of veins.

It is useful to find one good vein in the subdermal layer and then use this vein as a guide to the others by reflecting the incised skin and searching in the same subdermal plane of the initially located vein. Another method is to continue to dissect the initial vein proximally until branches to other veins are located.

TECHNIQUE AND SEQUENCE OF SURGERY

The operative sequence of replantation varies slightly with the level of the amputation (digit and hand versus areas proximal to the wrist) and the type of injury (clean cut, crush, or avulsion). As digital, partial hand, and hand replantations are much more common than more proximal replantations, the sequence of the surgery will be described for digit and hand replantation first, and variations in the technique will be described later.

The operative sequence for digital and hand replantation is as follows.

1. Locate and tag the vessels and nerves.
2. Debride.
3. Shorten and fix the bone.
4. Repair the extensor tendons.
5. Repair the flexor tendons.
6. Anastomose the arteries.
7. Repair the nerves.
8. Anastomose the veins.
9. Obtain skin coverage.

Location and tagging of the vessels were described in the section on initial management. It is extremely important to carefully isolate these vital structures prior to any debridement. Magnification

is essential to obtain optimal debridement. The surgeon's haste to reestablish blood flow must not result in neglect of proper wound cleansing. A pulsating jet lavage is useful in severely contaminated wounds. Any potentially necrotic tissue must be excised, particularly the muscle tissue.

All severed structures that can possibly be repaired are reconnected during the replantation procedure. In addition to the tissues mentioned above, periosteum, joint capsule, ligaments, and the lateral bands are repaired when possible. I am convinced that accurate and complete primary repair results in optimal hand function. Total repair of all structures provides effective stabilization and allows early mobilization of the reconstructed hand. It is much easier to repair these tissues primarily, rather than subject the patient to additional surgery at a later date. In delayed repairs, there is always the concern of injuring the repaired major vessels.

Bone Shortening and Fixation

Bone shortening and fixation are critical aspects of replantation.[57] Sufficient bone must be resected to ensure the approximation of normal intima in the vascular anastomoses. The connection of arteries, veins, and nerves must never be performed under tension. Therefore, the bone ends must be sufficiently shortened to obtain easy approximation of these vital structures. In addition, bone shortening allows easier and important dorsal skin coverage of anastomosed veins. The amount of bone resected depends on the type of injury. In an avulsion or crush injury, a greater amount of bone must be resected until normal intimal coaptation is possible without tension. In the digit, it is usually necessary to resect 0.5 to 1.0 cm of bone, and in amputations proximal to the hand, it is frequently necessary to resect 2 to 4 cm of bone. Even more bone may need to be resected in the avulsion injury.

Some replantation surgeons have emphasized that bone shortening is rarely necessary and recommend vein grafting when there is considerable intimal damage.[49] However, it is our opinion that bone shortening should generally be chosen over vein grafting, for one easy anastomosis is more favorable than two. Also, in an injury where vessels require vein grafting because of extensive damage, there is frequently concomitant damage to the nerves and other soft tissue structures that likewise need to be shortened. In addition, the shortened replanted digit, which usually has a restricted active range of motion, is generally less obvious and less likely to "get in the way." We hasten to add, however, that we do not hesitate to perform vein grafts when they are indicated, for example, when bone shortening may result in loss of a potentially functional joint. Certainly it is easier, quicker, and less frustrating to perform a vein graft than it is to redo a difficult anastomosis several times, or even one time. Again, any difficult anastomosis when performed under tension is unlikely to remain patent.

In thumb amputations, the major portion of the bone shortening should be on the detached part, so that a maximal amount of bone is preserved on the stump to ensure good bone stock should the replantation fail. However, sometimes this is not possible if an attempt is made to save joint function.

Numerous methods of bone stabilization have been suggested[19]: (1) one or two longitudinal intramedullary K-wires; (2) a longitudinal intramedullary K-wire plus a short oblique K-wire to prevent rotation; (3) crossed K-wires; (4) intraosseous wiring;[26] (5) intramedullary screw or peg; and (6) small plate with screws.

All of these methods may be used to stabilize amputations through the diaphyseal or metaphyseal areas and the joints (Fig. 25-6). Certain methods of fixation are preferred at different areas.

We prefer the single or double axial K-wire fixation when possible in digital bone fixation. This is

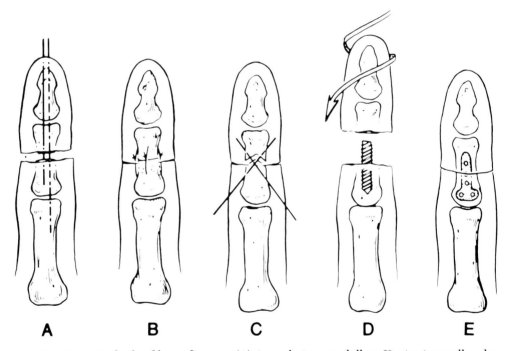

A   B   C   D   E

Fig. 25-6. Methods of bone fixation. (A) A single intramedullary K-wire is usually adequate. A second K-wire (*dotted line*) may be inserted if the amputation is close to the joint or if rotation is a problem. The second, longer K-wire may be removed early to begin motion at the joint that it previously crossed. (B) Intraosseous wiring may be used to allow early motion. This method is more often used in a metaphyseal region. (C) A chevron-type fusion is most often used for primary fusion at an amputation through a joint. (D) A bone screw is inserted into the amputation stump, the screw head cut off, and the digit literally "screwed on." (E) Mini-plate and screws provide stability to allow early joint motion. The mini "H" plate is preferred by the authors when this type of fixation is used.

the most universal and easiest method. A *motorized* drill is paramount for accurate and careful pin placement. A nasal speculum is frequently useful as a retractor of the surrounding soft tissue near the bone ends. We have experimented with all of the above methods of bone fixation in more than 1000 replantations, but usually prefer single or double axial K-wire fixation for the following reasons: (1) simplicity and speed of technique, (2) less bone exposure is required, (3) less skeletal mass is needed for fixation, (4) rotational deformity of the replanted digit is easily corrected if needed, and (5) ease of reshortening after fixation if further shortening is indicated for nerve, vessel, or skin approximation.[19,57]

A second axial intramedullary pin is frequently used for better stability. We have been reluctant to use crossed pins for fear of damaging a repaired neurovascular bundle by tethering of the vessel or the protective retaining ligaments over the protruding ends of the pins.

Crossed K-wires are our preferred choice for arthrodesis at a joint level. We prefer a chevron type of bone cut for stabilization (Fig. 25-6). Intramedullary screw fixation is ideal for thumb MP stabilization in the complete amputation at this level (Fig. 25-6). The technique is easy and rapid and provides immediate stability.[46] Since joints other than the thumb MP joint are usually arthrodesed in some flexion, the screw method has limited use. This method can be used quite effectively with immediate fixation in the phalangeal or metacarpal shafts if bone screws of appropriate size are available. Herbert screw fixation has been used for replantations at the distal joint level. The disadvantage of intramedullary screws or pegs is that they are difficult to remove from the replanted finger that becomes infected. Therefore their use is not advisable in contaminated wounds.

Intraosseous wiring or circular wiring through drill holes (Fig. 25-6B) is suggested for metaphyseal fractures so that immediate or early motion can be started.[26] However, this method requires more bone exposure and precise technique; it may be time-consuming and frequently does not give immediate stabilization. Supplementation with a crossed K-wire for increased stability may be used.

Plate and screw fixation seems to be an "overkill" and is seldom indicated since nonunion is rarely a significant problem in replantation of digits. With the development of increased proficiency in the application of minifragment screws and plates, this technique is gaining popularity in replantation. We have often employed the mini "H" plate for immediate stability. These methods require more time and bone exposure, with possible further soft tissue damage. In major limb replantation we prefer plates and screws because of the rigid fixation.

Even the experienced hand and replantation surgeon has a difficult time obtaining proper alignment when reattaching multiple digits. The relationship of the digits must be frequently checked in flexion, and, in general, the tips should point to the scaphoid bone. Since most replantations survive, great care should be taken to achieve anatomic alignment and correct rotation of the replanted parts.

There are special indications for primary implant arthroplasty in replantation. An example might be replantation of one or more fingers that have been cleanly amputated through the PIP joint in a piano player. Since the hazard of infection is increased, only the plain silicone implants should be used. Actually, the experienced hand surgeon will find that it is technically easier and quicker to perform a silicone implant arthroplasty than a primary fusion. However, the indications for this implant are not common.

In addition to bone fixation, it is wise to repair the periosteum, capsule, and ligamentous structures when possible to allow for better gliding surface and joint stability.

Extensor Tendon Repair

After bone fixation, the extensor tendon should be repaired for further stabilization. Usually two horizontal mattress sutures of 4–0 polyester are sufficient. In amputations through the proximal phalangeal region, repair of the lateral bands of the extensor tendon is extremely important if optimal extension of the distal joints is to be expected.

In some instances of severe avulsion injuries, no extensor tendons are available for repair. In these situations, interphalangeal joint arthrodesis or extensor tendon grafting as secondary procedures are necessary.

Flexor Tendon Repair

Primary flexor tendon surgery should be attempted in most replantations since secondary repair involves returning to areas of tremendous scarring about repaired nerves and vessels. Secondary flexor tendon surgery in replanted digits usually requires two-stage silicone rod procedures in digits other than the thumb. In ragged or avulsion injuries, we do not advocate extensive dissection or lengthy incisions to retrieve or reconstruct the avulsed tendon as a primary procedure.

We prefer to use the Tajima suture method for primary flexor tendon repair in replantation[45] (Fig. 25-7). If the flexor tendon transection occurs in the proximal portion of the digit, it may be expeditious to insert the sutures into the free flexor tendon ends (Tajima's method) but to not coapt the tendon ends until after the vascular and nerve repairs have been accomplished in the flexor surface. This sequence of repairs has the advantage of allowing the digit to be easily held in full extension for better exposure for nerve and vascular repairs on the flexor surface of the hand. When multiple tendons, such as in the palm or wrist, are to be repaired, the sutures are placed in all of the proximal and distal

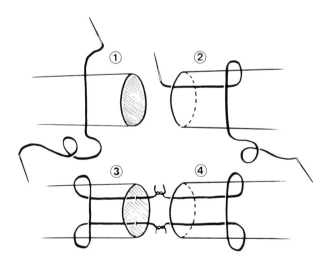

Fig. 25-7. The Tajima-type flexor tendon suture is preferred since the suture may be inserted in both ends of the tendon and the actual connection of the tendons may subsequently be performed at the ideal time, depending on the level and neurovascular structures involved.

tendon stumps prior to any knot tying. After an appropriate matchup is ensured, the tendon ends are all connected by securing the knots.

Some of the primary repairs of flexor tendons in replantation may require subsequent tenolysis. If secondary repair of the flexor tendons is necessary, it can be safely performed 3 months after replantation. As mentioned, the two-stage silicone rod method is then usually indicated. Delayed Z-lengthening of the flexor pollicis longus at the wrist and advancement distally has been successfully used in some of our thumb replantations,[56] but primary repair is the rule if possible.

Vascular Repair

The microvascular techniques have been thoroughly described in Chapter 24, so only important related points will be emphasized in this section. The arteries are anastomosed following bone fixation and extensor and, usually, flexor tendon repair. In a digit, we always attempt to repair both digital arteries when possible, and in a partial hand or wrist amputation, we repair all arteries that can possibly be restored. Some microsurgeons recommend repairing only one digital artery to save time; however, we stress repairing both, even in multiple digit amputations, to increase survival rate.

The arterial repair should not be attempted until *spurting* blood flow occurs from the proximal vessel. If a pulsating proximal arterial flow is not evident, steps to induce flow include: (1) relief of vascular tension or compression; (2) proximal resection to healthy vessel walls; (3) warming of the operating room and patient; (4) adequate hydration of the patient; (5) elevation of the patient's blood pressure; (6) irrigation of the proximal vessel with warm Ringer's lactate solution; (7) external application or gentle intraluminal flushing with Papavarine solution (1 : 20 dilution); (8) checking with the anesthesiologist about a metabolic problem that could incite vasospasm (e.g., acidosis[12]); (9) being certain that the tourniquet is not inflated; and (10) wait!

The severed artery must be resected until normal intima is visualized under high-power magnification; only *normal intima is reconnected* (Fig. 25-8). If this cannot be achieved, an interpositional

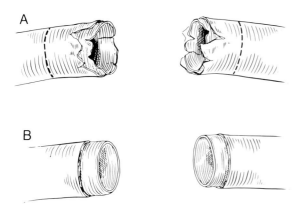

Fig. 25-8. The damaged microvessel must be sharply incised back to completely normal intima. The intima should be evaluated under the highest possible magnification through the operating microscope.

vein graft is used (Fig. 25-9) or futher bone shortening may be performed. The two most critical factors in achieving successful microvascular anastomoses are the skill and expertise of the microsurgeon and easy coaptation of normal intima to normal intima.

In many avulsion or crushing injuries, undamaged arteries may be shifted. For example, in a ring finger avulsion injury, the proximal ulnar digital artery may be attached to the distal radial digital artery if these are the ends that are least traumatized. This shifting principle is most often used when one of the distal vessels is nonsalvageable. In the past, in replantation of an avulsed thumb we often shifted the radial digital artery of the index finger to replace the severely damaged princeps pollicis artery. This practice has been discontinued for three reasons: (1) scar contracture of the thumb

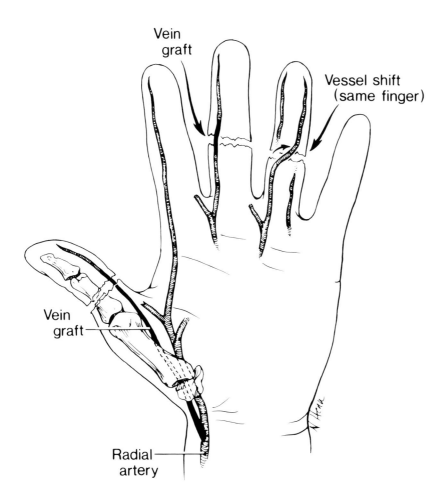

Fig. 25-9. Three methods of making up a gap in the microvessels. (1) In the completely amputated thumb, an *interposition vein graft* may be used from the ulnar digital artery of the amputated thumb end-to-side into the radial artery at the wrist. (2) A *vein graft* may be used to bridge the gap. (3) The proximal radial digital vessel has been *shifted* to the distal ulnar digital vessel in the complete replantation. This method is particularly useful in ring avulsion injuries.

index web space; (2) frequent small size of the radial digital artery; and (3) concomitant damage of the radial digital artery of the index finger and the princeps pollicis artery.

Some authors have recommended the transposition of vascular pedicles[25,50] and even neurovascular pedicles[29] to replant avulsed thumbs, but we believe that the use of vein grafts is easier, quicker, and more reliable.

For replantation of thumbs we prefer to use an *interposition vein graft* from the ulnar digital artery of the amputated thumb to the first dorsal metacarpal artery on the dorsum of the hand or end-to-side into the radial artery at the wrist (Fig. 25-9). For expediency, the reversed vein graft is often anastomosed to the ulnar digital artery of the detached thumb prior to the bone fixation.[7]

Interposition vein grafts are used in approximately 20 percent of our replantations to obtain reapproximation of the healthy arteries and veins. The volar aspect of the wrist contains several veins, 1 to 2 mm in diameter, which are ideal for replantation of digits. In fact if there is any indication that vein grafts may be needed, one of our initial steps is to harvest the veins from the wrist and store them in a Ringer's lactate and Papaverine solution. This preparatory procedure is done with loupe magnification, prior to using the operating microscope, requires only a few minutes, and will save time and eliminate potential frustration later. Two easy anastomoses are quicker and more likely to be successful than one difficult anastomosis under tension.

A pneumatic tourniquet may safely be used for each vascular anastomosis. If the technique of the microvascular anastomosis is skillfully performed, tourniquet ischemia will not diminish patency rate. The tourniquet should be released at the conclusion of each anastomosis. The tourniquet may be inflated and deflated many times during the procedure to allow considerable decrease in operating time and blood loss. If hemorrhage is not excessive nor obscuring the visual field, then a tourniquet is not used.

Since all available microclips do produce some amount of vessel wall damage, their application time should not exceed 30 minutes. Just prior to beginning the first anastomosis, we recommend a bolus of 3000 to 5000 units of intravenous heparin.

Subsequent doses of 1000 units of heparin every hour or so may be repeated in lengthy procedures or in crushed or avulsed injuries. The dosage is adjusted for children and the clinical appraisal of the bleeding tendency of the patient.

An attempt should be made to anastomose two veins for each artery. It may be necessary to mobilize or "harvest" veins to achieve this ratio (Fig. 25-10). *The greatest error in vein repair is attempting the anastomosis under tension.* This is never necessary. If harvesting of veins does not allow coaptation without undue tension, the surgeon should proceed immediately with a *vein graft.* The surgeon's time and frustration will be diminished and the patency rate elevated.

Many recognized replantation surgeons repair veins prior to arteries to decrease the blood loss and maintain a bloodless field for better vision.[10,33,38] However, by judicious use of the tourniquet, the artery may be repaired first and a dry field maintained. This provides the advantages of earlier revascularization and allows easier location

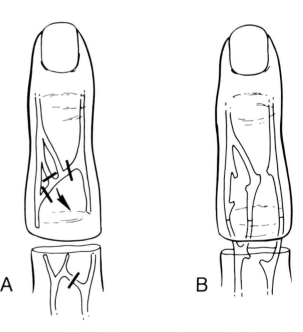

Fig. 25-10. The mobilization or "harvesting" of veins is a very useful method of obtaining ease of approximation for vein reconstruction in the complete amputation. An attempt should be made to repair three veins on each digit replantation.

of the most functional veins detected by their spurting backflow. In addition, if the veins are first repaired, especially in an avulsion injury, and subsequent arterial anastomosis fails to show adequate arterial inflow, the surgeon has wasted valuable time on a nonsalvable part.

If replantations are attempted at the level of the base of the nailplate or even more distal, the location of dorsal veins in the distal stump is usually not possible. If surgical reattachment of the distal amputation is believed to be indicated (e.g., a musician's fingertip or the tip of a dominant thumb), adequate venous drainage may be achieved by at least four methods: (1) repair of volar veins, although these are smaller with thinner walls and more difficult to repair than dorsal veins; (2) anastomosis of one distal digital artery (which has backflow) to a proximal vein (creation of A-V fistula); (3) removal of the nail plate and subsequent scraping of the raw nail bed with a cotton applicator every 2 hours to encourage bleeding, with a heparin soaked pledget applied afterwards; and (4) use of medical-grade leeches (difficult to acquire and store in the United States).

Nerve Repair

Since the bone has usually been shortened in replantation, nerve repair is generally not difficult, for there is no tension at the suture line. The microscope is used for careful fascicular (or bundle) alignment of the freshly injured nerve. Even with the aid of the microscope, it is sometimes difficult to determine how much nerve to resect in severe avulsion injuries. However, in almost all replantations, primary nerve repair should be done.

Primary nerve grafts are performed when end-

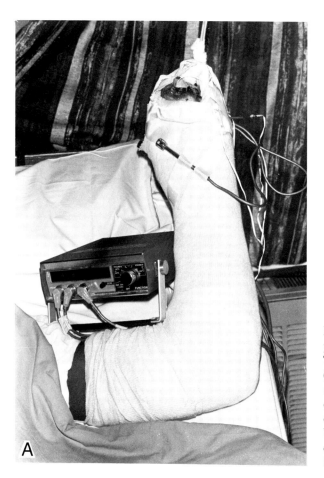

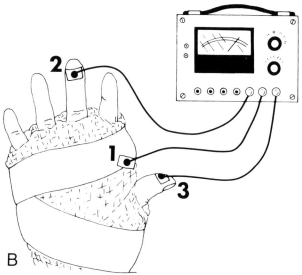

Fig. 25-11. (A) The postoperative dressing extends proximal to the elbow to prevent slippage. The YSI-Tele-thermometer with the connected probes is shown. (B) Temperature probes are inserted on the dressing for (1) the ambient temperature, (2) on a nonamputated digit for a control temperature, and (3) on the replanted digit for monitoring. (B reproduced by permission from Urbaniak JR: Replantation of amputated hands and digits. p. 15. AAOS Instructional Course Lectures, Vol. 27. CV Mosby, St Louis, 1978.)

to-end repair is not possible. The medial ante-brachial cutaneous nerve is ideal as a donor for digital nerve grafting because most replantations are performed under regional anesthesia. This nerve is located one fingerbreadth medial and two fingerbreadths distal to the medial epicondyle of the elbow and lies superficial to the muscle fascia. In multiple digital amputations, nerve grafts may be obtained from discarded digits.

We have noted no statistical difference in nerve recovery in our replants with secondary or primary repair.[15]

The peripheral nerves are repaired with 8 – 0 to 10 – 0 monofilament nylon or Prolene by epineurial repair after fascicular alignment is determined. In the digital nerves only two or three sutures are necessary; more sutures are used in proximal injuries.

Skin Coverage and Dressing

Meticulous hemostasis is obtained after all the structures have been repaired and revascularization of the replanted part has been assured. The skin is loosely approximated with a few interrupted nylon sutures. All damaged skin that may become necrotic is excised, and no tension should be placed on the skin during closure. Frequently the midlateral incisions of the digit are *not closed* to allow for decompression of the digital vessels. The vessels should be covered without constriction from the overlying skin or sutures. A local flap or split-thickness skin graft may be necessary, even for digital vessel coverage. Fasciotomies are indicated if the slightest indication of compression or constriction is present. The wounds are covered with small strips of gauze impregnated with petrolatum. Care must be taken in the placement of these strips so that they are not continuous in a circumferential manner.

The upper extremity is immobilized in a bulky compression hand dressing that extends above the elbow to prevent slippage (Fig. 25-11). Each step of the dressing is carefully designed to prevent circumferential constriction. In general, the plaster splints should be placed only on the volar aspect of the dressing to permit ease of exposure if a problem arises postoperatively. However, when flexor ten-dons are repaired, a dorsal splint only is applied to eliminate flexor tendon contraction against a fixed resistance.

POSTOPERATIVE CARE

Postoperative management is extremely important in achieving a high success rate in replantation. Despite a technically successful replantation, postoperatively the replanted part may develop vascular insufficiency that can be frequently corrected if detected early. The postoperative care may be categorized into three segments: (1) routine precautions, (2) procedures for difficult replantation, and (3) reversal of a failing replant.

Routine Postoperative Precautions

The hand in the bulky compression dressing is usually elevated by a rope attached to the dressing. The elbow should rest on the bed. If arterial inflow is diminished, the hand may be lowered. If venous outflow is slow, the hand needs elevation.

The use and type of anticoagulants is certainly a controversial topic (see Chapter 24). Some surgeons use none (or perhaps only aspirin and Persantine), and some use all or various combinations of those discussed here.[10,23,32,38,46,47,51] We prefer the use of some type of anticoagulation in all of our patients. In clean-cut amputations and in replantations where the anastomoses are technically easy and the blood flow immediately brisk, heparin is generally not indicated. In these patients, we use dipyridamole (Persantine) 50 mg twice a day. Additional medication includes Dextran 40 (500 cc a day), aspirin (300 g twice a day), and chlorpromazine (Thorazine) (25 mg four times a day), all for 1 week. The chlorpromazine is useful as a peripheral vasodilator and tranquilizer to diminish vasospasm secondary to anxiety.

If the injury is of the crushed or avulsed type, intravenous heparin 1000 units hourly is used for 1 week. The dosage of heparin is regulated according to the activated partial thromboplastin time, which is maintained at 1½ times normal. If bleeding into the dressing occurs, the dosage is diminished and the dressing is changed immediately to prevent constriction by a "blood cast." Heparin prophylaxis is not used in amputations proximal to the wrist level.

Color, pulp turgor, capillary refill, and warmth are all useful aids in monitoring the replant, but quantitative skin temperature measurements have proved to be the most reliable indicators.[15] The digital temperature is monitored with a YSI Tele-Thermometer and small surface probes° (Fig. 25-11). If the skin temperature of the replanted part drops below 30°C, poor perfusion of the replanted part is certain, and a cause for the compromised circulation must be found and corrected if possible. Of course, the ambient temperature influences the interpretation of the recordings. Other methods of monitoring include transcutaneous oxygen measurements,[43] hydrogen washout technique,[16] and flourescein perfusion.[9] These methods are sensitive indicators, but are more complex and expensive and require more technical expertise by the nursing personnel then does temperature monitoring.

The patient's room should be maintained comfortably warm, and cool drafts should be avoided. The patient is not permitted to smoke. The patient is kept at bed rest for 2 to 3 days, and then activity is permitted in accordance with the patient's course, desires, and personality. Antibiotics are administered for 1 week.

Procedures for Difficult Replantations

Oftentimes the surgeon can predict which replantation is going to have postoperative problems of circulatory perfusion with a lesser chance of survival. Examples are replantations in children under 10 years of age, crush and avulsion injuries, ring

° Yellow Springs Instrument Company, Yellow Springs, Ohio.

avulsions, poor proximal flow evident prior to the anastomosis, and intermittent or inconsistent distal flow despite a technically good anastomosis. In these situations, extra postoperative efforts are advisable to enhance the survival rate.

Intravenous heparin in the dosage previously advised is particularly beneficial in these difficult replants. Insertion of a silicone catheter (No. 5 silicone urethral stent) adjacent to the median or ulnar nerve (depending on the digits replanted) will permit a regional block to be administered with ease.[39] We recommend 5 cc bupivacaine (Marcaine) (0.025 percent) every 6 to 8 hours to provide a continuous sympathetic block for vasodilation. This obviates the use of stellate or brachial blocks, which are anxiety provoking to the patient, especially children, and are somewhat hazardous in heparinized patients. The regional block also alleviates pain, which may be present in the incomplete replantation. We recommend the use of the indwelling silicone catheter in most of the children in whom our success rate of viability is lower than adults.

Reversal of the Failing Replant

If the reattached part appears in jeopardy (detected by skin temperature, color, pulp turgor, and/or capillary refill), immediate rectifying action must be taken. The dressing should be inspected for any constriction. Depression or elevation of the hand may improve the vascular flow, depending on whether the problem is arterial or venous. A stellate block or brachial block (if no regional indwelling catheter is present) should be given immediately to relieve vasospasm. If the patient complains of pain, intramuscular narcotics are helpful, and, in fact, should be given prior to the dressing inspection. An intravenous bolus of heparin (3000 to 5000 units) will frequently incite a recovery. Chlorpromazine may be given to allay anxiety and decrease vasospasm. The surgeon should be certain that the patient is adequately hydrated. There is no conclusive evidence that the microvessel patency rate is influenced by a normal or low hematocrit, but a near-normal hematocrit is suggested.[30]

The environment of the patient's room may need to be altered; for example, increase the temperature or remove smokers or other agitating factors. All efforts should be made to calm the patient, especially a child, as pain, fear, and anxiety may instigate unwanted vasospasm.

If a careful and intelligent postoperative program is employed, it is rarely necessary to return the patient to the operating room for reexploration. If this decision is made, however, it must be carried out within 4 to 6 hours of the loss of adequate perfusion. Seldom have we found reexploration of benefit if the exploration occurs more than 1 or 2 days after the replantation. Reexploration with correction of the problem (redoing the anastomosis, removal of a thrombus, or vein grafting a previously unrecognized damaged vessel segment) is most effective when acute cessation of arterial inflow is diagnosed.

MAJOR LIMB REPLANTATION

Most amputations of the upper extremity occur at the digit or hand level, so the emphasis on replantation has described the reattachment at these levels. Replantation of limbs amputated at or proximal to the wrist level employs similar principles with minor modifications. Because more muscle mass is involved, the duration of avascularity of the detached part is more critical.

Whereas a digit may be successfully replanted 24 hours after amputation, an arm amputated at the elbow is in jeopardy if it has been avascular for 10 to 12 hours, even if it has been properly cooled. Extensive muscle debridement, both on the detached part and the stump, is essential to prevent myonecrosis and subsequent infection, which is a problem in major limb replantation, but infrequent in digital reattachment.

In replantations proximal to the metacarpal level, immediate arterial inflow is necessary to prevent or diminish myonecrosis. Therefore, after initial debridement and rapid bone stabilization, at least one artery must be anastomosed and then the surgical sequence is similar to digital replantation.

A Sundt shunt or a ventriculoperitoneal shunt (Fig. 25-12) is used to obtain rapid arterial inflow from the proximal vessel to the amputated part.° This connection is performed prior to bone fixation if the duration from amputation to arrival in the operating room is longer than 4 to 6 hours.

Stable fixation is necessary, but the method must be rapid. We prefer rigid plate and screw fixation of the long bones and crossed Steinmann pin fixation at the joint level. Adequate bone shortening must be carefully planned relative to the type of injury and tissue damage. *The working premise is to convert the revascularized limb to a fractured extremity with peripheral nerve injury.*

Arterial repair should always be performed prior to the venous repair because a rapid systemic return of lactic acid and other noxious catabolities can be detrimental to the patient. We have found it beneficial to give intravenous sodium bicarbonate to the patient prior to the venous anastomoses.

Extensive fasciotomies are always indicated in major limb replantation. *The two most common causes of failure in major limb replantation are myonecrosis with subsequent infection and failure to provide adequate decompression of the restored vessels.* Any exposed vessels may be safely covered by meshed split-thickness skin grafts. Other areas may be covered in a few days.

In replanted digits we usually do not change the dressing for at least 2 weeks for fear of producing harmful vasospasm. However, in major limb replantation, the limb must be examined in the operating room under anesthesia (regional or general) within 48 to 72 hours to evaluate the condition of the muscle tissue. Any necrotic tissue must be further debrided to prevent infection.

Anticoagulants are not used in major limb replantation. Postoperative temperature monitoring is reliable in these replants also.

° Sundt and loop carotid endarterectomy shunts for 3- to 4-mm vessels and ludenz peritoneal shunts for 2.5- to 3-mm vessels (Heyer Shulte Corporation, Goleta, California).

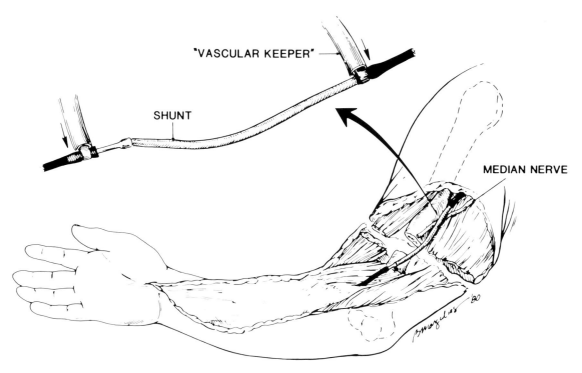

Fig. 25-12. A Sundt shunt or a ventriculoperitoneal shunt is used to obtain rapid arterial inflow from the proximal vessel to the amputated part.

EXPECTATIONS FOLLOWING REPLANTATION

By applying the principles described in this chapter, the experienced and proficient microsurgeon should be able to achieve at least an 80 percent viability rate in complete replantations. The results, based on reports from major replantation centers, should be as follows.[6,48,52,53]

1. Nerve recovery — comparable to that of repair of an isolated severed peripheral nerve.
2. Active range of joint motion — approximately 50 percent of normal (related to level of injury).
3. Cold intolerance — a definite problem that is usually resolved by 2 years.
4. Cosmetic acceptability — usually better than any amputation revision or prosthesis.
5. The best results are obtained in replantation of the thumb, hand at the wrist or distal forearm level, and in the finger distal to the insertion of the flexor superficialis.

REFERENCES

1. Acland RD: Microsurgery Practice Manual. CV Mosby, St Louis, 1980
2. Belsky MR, Ruby LK: Double level amputation: Should it be replanted? J Reconstr Microsurg 2:159–162, 1986
3. Biemer, E: Replantation von Fingern und Extremitatenteilen: Technik und Ergebnisse. Chirurgie, 48:353, 1977
4. Bright DS: Microsurgical techniques in vessel and nerve repair. pp. 1–15. AAOS Instructional Course Lectures, Vol. 27. CV Mosby, St Louis, 1978
5. Bright DS: Techniques of microsurgery. p. 40. AAOS Symposium on Microsurgery Practical Use in Orthopaedics. CV Mosby, St Louis, 1979
6. Buncke HJ, Alpert BS, Johnson-Giebink R: Digital replantation. Surg Clin North Am 61:383–394, 1981
7. Caffee, HH: Improved exposure for arterial repair in thumb replantation. J Hand Surg 10A:416, 1985
8. Carrel A, Guthrie CC: Results of a replantation of a thigh. Science 23:393, 1906

9. Chow JA, Bilos ZJ, Chunprapaph B: Thirty thumb replantations. Plast Reconstr Surg 64:626–630, 1979

10. Daniel R, Terzis J: Reconstructive Microsurgery. Little, Brown, Boston, 1977

11. Dell, PC, Seaber AV, Urbaniak JR: Effect of hypovolemia on perfusion after digit replantation. Surg Forum 31:503, 1980

12. Dell PC, Seaber AV, Urbaniak JR: The effect of systemic acidosis on perfusion of replanted extremities. J Hand Surg 5:433–442, 1980

13. Earley MJ, Watson JS: Twenty-four thumb replantations. J Hand Surg 9B:98–102, 1984

14. Ferreira MC, Marques EF, Azze RJ: Limb replantation. Clin Plast Surg 5:211, 1978

15. Gelberman RH, Urbaniak JR, Bright DS, Levin LS: Digital sensibility following replantation. J Hand Surg 3:313–319, 1978

16. Goldner RD: Postoperative management. Hand Clinics 1:205–215, 1985

17. Hamilton RB, O'Brien BMcC, Morrison A, MacLeod AM: Survival factors in replantation and revascularization of the amputated thumb—10 years experience. Scand J Plast Reconstr Surg 18:163–173, 1984

18. Harmel MH, Urbaniak JR, Bright DS: Anesthesia for replantation of severed extremities. pp. 161–166. Anaesthesiologie und Intensivmedizin, Band 138, Neue Aspekte in der Regional-anaesthesia 2. Wust HJ, Zindler M (eds), Springer-Verlag, Berlin

19. Hayes MG, Urbaniak JR: Management of bone in microvascular surgery. p. 96. AAOS Symposium on Microsurgical Practical Use in Orthopaedics. CV Mosby, St Louis, 1979

20. Hopfner E: Uber Gefassnaht, Gefasstransplantation und Reimplantation von amputierten Extremitaten. Arch Klin Chir 70:417, 1903

21. Ikuta Y: Microvascular Surgery. p. 42. Lens Press, Hiroshima, 1975

22. Jones JM, Schenck RR, Chesney RB: Digital replantation and amputation—Comparison of function. J Hand Surg 7:183–189, 1982

23. Kleinert HE, Juhala CA, Tsai T-M, Van Beek A: Digital replantation—selection, technique, and results. Orthop Clin North Am 8:309–318, April 1977

24. Komatsu S, Tamai S: Successful replantation of a completely cut-off thumb: Case report. Plast Reconstr Surg 42:374–377, 1968

25. Lendvay PG: Replacement of the amputated digit. Br J Plast Surg 26:398, 1973

26. Lister G: Intraosseous wiring of the digital skeleton. J Hand Surg 3:427–435, 1978

27. Lobay GW, Moysa GL: Primary neurovascular bundle transfer in the management of avulsed thumbs. J Hand Surg 6:31–34, 1981

28. MacLeod AM, O'Brien BMcC, Morrison WA: Digital replantation: Clinical experiences. Clin Orthop 133:26–34, June 1978

29. Malt RA, McKhann C: Replantation of severed arms. JAMA 189:716, 1964

30. Morris HB, Seaber AV, Urbaniak JR: The effect of acute limited normovolemic hemodilution on pH and temperature recovery of ischemic rat extremities. Presented at the 27th Annual Meeting of the Orthopaedic Research Society, Las Vegas, Feb 1981

31. Morris HB, Sylvia AL, Seaber AV, Urbaniak JR: Effect of acute normovolemic Dextran 70 hemodilution on post-ischemic skeletal muscle respiration and perfusion. Surg Forum 32:536–538, 1981

32. Morrison WA, O'Brien BMcC, McLeod AM: Evaluation of digital replantation—A review of 100 cases. Orthop Clin North Am 8:295–308, April 1977

33. Morrison WA, O'Brien BMcC, McLeod AM: Digital replantation and revascularization: A long term review of one hundred cases. Hand 10:125–134, 1978

34. Morrison WA, O'Brien BMcC, McLeod AM: The surgical repair of amputations of the thumb. Aust NZ J Surg 50:237–243, 1980

35. Murakami T, Ikuta Y, Tsuge K: Relationship between the number of digital nerves sutured and sensory recovery in replanted fingers. J Reconstr Microsurg 1:283–286

36. Nunley JA: Microscopes and microinstruments. Hand Clinics 1:197–204, 1985

37. Nunley JA, Koman LA, Urbaniak JR: Arterial shunting as an adjunct to major limb revascularization. Ann Surg 193:271–273, 1981

38. O'Brien BMcC: Microvascular Reconstructive Surgery. Churchill Livingstone, London, 1977

39. Phelps DB, Rutherford RB, Boswick JA Jr: Control of vasospasm following trauma and microvascular surgery. J Hand Surg 4:109–117, 1979

40. Schlenker JD, Kleinert HE, Tsai T-M: Methods and results of replantation following traumatic amputation of the thumb in sixty-four patients. J Hand Surg 5:63–69, 1980

41. Seyfer AE, Seaber AV, Dombrose FA, Urbaniak JR: Coagulation changes in elective surgery and trauma. Ann Surg 193:210–213, 1981

42. Shafiroff BB, Palmer AK: Simplified technique for replantation of the thumb. J Hand Surg 6:623–624, 1981

43. Sixth People's Hospital, Shanghai: Replantation of

severed fingers: Clinical experience in 162 cases involving 270 severed fingers. (pamphlet) July 1963

44. Stirrat CR, Seaber AV: The microsurgery laboratory. p. 12. AAOS Symposium on Microsurgery Practical Use in Orthopaedics. CV Mosby, St Louis, 1979

45. Tajima T: History, current status, and aspects of hand surgery in Japan. Clin Orthop Rel Res 184: 41–49, 1984

46. Tamai S: Digit replantation: Analysis of 163 replantations in an 11-year period. Clin Plast Surg 5:195, 1978

47. Tamai S, Hori Y, Tatsumi Y, Okuda H, Nakamura Y, Sakamoto H, Takita T, Fukui A: Microvascular anastomosis and its application on the replantation of amputated digits and hands. Clin Orthop 133:106–121, 1978

48. Tamai S: Twenty years experience of limb replantation—Review of 293 upper extremity replants. J Hand Surg 7:549–556, 1982

49. Tupper JW: Vascular defects and salvage of failed vascular repairs. p. 111 AAOS Symposium on Microsurgery Practical Use in Orthopaedics. CV Mosby, St Louis, 1979

50. Urbaniak JR: Replantation of amputed hands and digits. pp. 15–26. AAOS Instructional Course Lectures, Vol. 27. CV Mosby, St Louis, 1978

51. Urbaniak JR: Digit and hand replantation: Current status. Neurosurgery 4:551–559, 1979

52. Urbaniak JR: Replantation of amputated parts—Technique, results and indications. p. 64. AAOS Symposium on Microsurgery Practical Use in Orthopaedics. CV Mosby, St Louis, 1979

53. Urbaniak JR: To replant or not to replant? That is not the question. (Editorial) J Hand Surg 8:507–508, 1983

54. Urbaniak JR: Replantation in children. p. 1168. Pediatric Plastic Surgery. CV Mosby, St Louis, 1984

55. Urbaniak JR, Evans JP, Bright DS: Microvascular management of avulsion injuries. J Hand Surg 6:25–30, 1981

56. Urbaniak JR, Goldner JL: Laceration of the flexor pollicis longus tendon: Delayed repair by advancement, free graft or direct suture. A clinical and experimental study. J Bone Joint Surg 55A:1123–1148, 1973

57. Urbaniak JR, Hayes MG, Bright DS: Management of bone in digital replantation: Free vascularized and composite bone grafts. Clin Orthop 133:184–194, 1978

58. Urbaniak JR, Roth JH, Nunley JA, Goldner RD, Koman LA: The results of replantation after amputation of a single finger. J Bone Joint Surg 67A:611–619, 1985

59. Urbaniak JR, Soucacos PN, Adelaar RS, Bright DS, Whitehurst LA: Experimental evaluation of microsurgical technniques in small artery anastomoses. Orthop Clin North Am 8:249–263, 1977

60. Urbaniak JR, Steichen JB, Weiland AJ, Wood MB, Seaber AV: Microsurgical skills development. Laboratory manual. AAOS, 1985

61. Van Giesen P, Seaber AV, Urbaniak JR: Hypothermic preservation prior to replantation. Presented at AAOS Course—Microsurgery in reconstruction of the Upper and Lower Extremities. Durham, NC, May 1979

62. Van Giesen PJ, Seaber AV, Urbaniak JR: Storage of amputated parts prior to replantation. An experimental study with rabbit ears. J Hand Surg 8A:60–65, 1983

63. Vlastou C, Earle AS: Avulsion injuries of the thumb. J Hand Surg 11A:51–56, 1986

64. Weiland AJ, Villarreal-Rios A, Kleinert HE, Kutz J, Atasoy E, Lister G: Replantation of digits and hands: Analysis of surgical techniques and functional results in 71 patients with 86 replantations. J Hand Surg 2:1–12, 1977

65. Yamano Y: Replantation of the amputated distal part of the fingers. J Hand Surg 10A:211–218, 1985

66. Yamauchi S, Nomura S, Yoshimura M, Ueno T, Iwai Y, Shimamura K: A clinical study of the order and speed of sensory recovery after digital replantation. J Hand Surg 8:545–549, 1983

67. Yoshizu T, Katsumi M, Tajima T: Replantation of untidy amputated finger, hand and arm: Experience of 99 replantations in 66 cases. J Trauma 18:194–200, 1978

Emergency Free Flaps

26

Graham Lister

Emergency free flaps have been defined as those flaps transferred for coverage of soft tissue defects at the first surgical procedure after injury.[28] This definition places an upper limit of 24 hours on the term "emergency."

Godina[17] defined another, similar, group of "early" free flaps as those done within 3 days of injury and initial debridement. In comparing a group of early free flaps with another that satisfied the definition of "emergency," he found no difference "provided that the wounds are closed in the first 72 hours and a proper debridement is done immediately after the injury."

The writing of this chapter commenced in Ljubljana, Yugoslavia, on February 12, 1986, the day of the memorial service for Marko Godina. The concept of emergency free tissue transfer belongs solely to Godina, who practiced it routinely before others first attempted it. I learned it from him, as I, and others throughout the world, learned countless things from him. Surgical progress has been slowed by the death of this unique man at the age of 42.

THEORETICAL DISADVANTAGES OF EMERGENCY FREE FLAPS

Especially following high energy injuries, fear of infection has long dictated delayed wound closure. The Vietnam experience with high velocity gunshot wounds demonstrated the safety of such an approach in the hand.[8] In contrast to this established practice, Godina[17] showed an infection rate of 1.5 percent in 134 patients, all with Grade 3 extremity injuries, treated with early free flaps as opposed to 17.5 percent in 167 to whom similar flaps were applied after a delay of anywhere from 72 hours to 3 months. In 31 emergency free flaps for various defects of the upper extremity, Lister and Scheker[28] had one mild cellulitis and one severe infection in a flap that failed. These figures compare favorably with those of Nylen and Carlsson,[39] who reported 52 percent infection with delayed treatment. Both the reports from Godina and

1127

from Lister and Scheker emphasize the paramount importance of radical debridement, which is described below.

Free tissue transfer in its early years was a lengthy, unpredictable undertaking. In Ljubljana between 1976 and 1983, only 12 of the first 100 free flaps took less than 6 hours to complete.[17] By contrast, 92 of the last 100 were finished in less than 6 hours, 24 of them in less than 4. The failure rate in the first 100 was 26 percent, in the last 100, 4 percent. It appears that free tissue transfer is now a relatively swift and reliable undertaking when performed by an experienced team.

Some of those well versed in free tissue transfer suggest that it should remain an elective procedure, arguing that it is more likely to fail when undertaken as an emergency, and that it adds unacceptable time to the initial surgery. In the Louisville series of emergency free flaps,[28] the failure rate was 6.5 percent. This is not as good as Godina's 0.75 percent failure rate in 134 early free flaps, but is comparable to the Ljubljana failure rate of 4 percent in 100 flaps in 1983, and superior to their 12 percent failure of flaps used in the delayed treatment of complex trauma.[17] The entire initial procedure in the Louisville patients, which always included debridement and frequently bone fixation, tendon repair, revascularization and even nerve graft, averaged under 5 hours for small defects, under 8 hours for medium defects, and under 12 hours for large defects. It would appear that in those centers with replantation teams available at all hours there is no reason why emergency free tissue transfer should not be done. Nevertheless, these are long operations, which should be undertaken only after thorough assessment of the patient's fitness for them.

Age is not a factor in selected patients. The youngest patient on whom the author has performed an early free flap was 2.5 years old; the oldest was 76. Both have done well, with no complications attributable to age.

Free flaps will not help unsuitable limbs. Especially in crush injuries, the wound may be so ill-defined that indisputably radical debridement might needlessly destroy structures that may survive to give irreplaceable function. In such cases, debridement of unquestionably dead and contaminated tissue should be followed by the application of wet dressings or, perhaps better, a copious application of a petrolatum based ointment such as Neosporin. At a second look within 72 hours, it may be possible to create a good wound by further excision to which an "early" flap can be applied. If doubt remains beyond 72 hours and further debridement is necessary, the chance of infection beneath the flap rises twelvefold.[17] Split-thickness skin grafts should therefore be employed wherever possible after the later, final debridement. Flap reconstruction is left until the wounds are healed. There is a corollary to this approach. The initial injury or necessary debridement may expose tissues that it is known will not or should not support a skin graft: bare bone, cartilage, ligament or tendon; exposed vessels or nerves. A flap will be required at some stage. We know from personal observation that with the best nursing in the world and with the wettest of wet dressings, exposed bone and tendon desiccate, die, and have to be excised. It follows that in exposure of such important but poorly vascularized structures, emergency or early flap cover is mandatory.

Free tissue transfer should not be used to salvage a limb with insufficient potential for eventual function. Such function can only be attained by an acceptably sensate hand with mobile joints controlled by sufficient musculotendinous units. In complex injuries, the potential of a limb can often only be assessed by an experienced hand surgeon. This may be the ultimate disadvantage of emergency free tissue transfer: if it is to be performed judiciously, senior staff must be present when it is being considered.

ADVANTAGES OF EMERGENCY FREE FLAPS

Provided that nonviable or contaminated tissue has been eliminated from the wound, that the free flap survives and that the patient has been well selected, there are many self-evident advantages of immediate microvascular skin cover.

Knowing that immediate skin cover is to be applied, the surgeon can proceed with whatever reconstruction is necessary or desirable.[11] Necessary reconstruction includes the placement of a vein graft to restore flow to an avascular extremity. Desirable reconstruction may, in appropriate circumstances, include plate fixation, cancellous bone graft, joint replacement, tendon repair, graft or transfer, and nerve repair or graft. Many will not concede the need for any such complex primary procedures and this is not the place to debate the issue fully. However, let us take two examples. A patient has lost dorsal skin from the hand and sustained multiple fractures of the metacarpals with some bone loss as a result of a car roll-over (Fig. 26-1). It is decided to provide a stable skeleton and soft tissue cover with an immediate intercalated bone graft and a combination of plate and wire fixation covered with a partial latissimus dorsi muscle flap to which skin grafts can later be applied. Has the extensor digitorum to all fingers been avulsed? Put in immediate tendon grafts. Is the princeps pollicis damaged? Use an arterial graft[18] to restore it. A second patient has a large soft tissue defect of the antecubital fossa, with an open elbow joint, an avascular hand, and no median nerve function, but intact ulnar and radial nerves (Fig. 26-2). A long saphenous vein graft from brachial to ulnar and radial arteries restores flow but a latissimus dorsi flap is required to cover the joint and the graft. In the case illustrated, the median nerve was exposed and contused, but in continuity. In a similar case, there was a high median nerve defect of 12 cm, which required an interfascicular sural nerve graft. By doing bioassay[13,15] immediately, one can identify motor and sensory fascicles both proximally and distally, theoretically giving a better chance of median nerve recovery. Done electively, only proximal identification would be possible — and worthless — and the dissection would be difficult and the graft consequently longer. The decision to use an immediate free flap gives the surgeon the freedom to do what he has long known is needed,[11] but which has been ill-advised or impossible because the skin cover was not available, not reliable, or not suitable.

With immediate reconstruction, all necessary operative procedures are often completed at the first encounter following injury. Apart from the psychological benefit to the patient, the timesaving factor has economic considerations. The patient will return to his original occupation or commence retraining at an earlier date after injury. His total hospital time will be reduced. This was dramatically shown in patients undergoing extremity reconstruction in Ljubljana. Those having early flaps stayed for a total of 27 days, those having delayed flaps stayed for 130 days, and those having late flaps for 256 days.[17]

Why a free flap? Local or regional flaps to the hand have the distinct advantage that they are of similar skin and they require no wounds elsewhere in the body. However, they are limited in their availability. The larger the primary defect, the less local skin remains to provide flap cover. Even when there is sufficient area, the thickness required to fill a defect is often lacking. Further, the raising of a local flap inflicts additional injury on the traumatized limb. The resultant compound wound may impair hand function more than would the first soft tissue defect. In localized injury of the thumb pulp, the neurovascular island can provide sensate, glabrous skin, but it is not appropriately oriented cortically. Distant pedicle flaps, most commonly from the groin, can provide sufficient tissue in all but the most massive defects. However, the hand must be dependent during attachment, the position may be uncomfortable, lack of exercise may result in joint stiffness, the flap may be avulsed by the young or the incompetent, the thickness of the tube presents a later problem in certain defects, and circumferential defects are difficult to cover. Most important in the long term is the fact that an axial pedicle flap ceases to have that vascular axis from the time of division. It becomes something of a parasite, seeking supply from the underlying scarred bed. By contrast, the free flap has a permanent pedicle. While the contention that a flap brings new blood supply to relatively avascular tissue is fallacious, certainly at the time when it is applied and probably in the long term, there is merit in the fact that it will never place vascular demands on the already compromised limb. There is a strong similarity between tissues adjacent to a major wound and those that have been irradiated, and the advantages of a "permanent pedicle, blood-carrying flap" in covering radiation ulcers was shown many years ago.[6] By contrast to these limitations of conventional

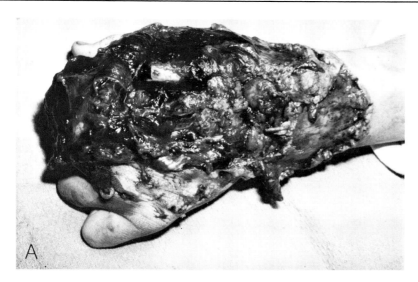

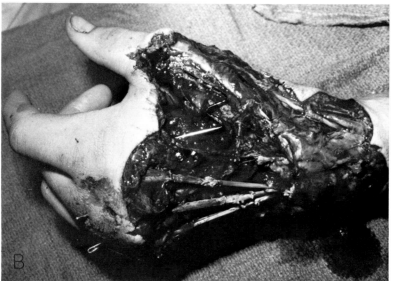

Fig. 26-1. (**A**) This patient sustained open fractures of the metacarpals together with loss of extensor tendons and dorsal skin and damage to the princeps pollicis artery in a roll-over injury. (**B**) Immediate reconstruction was performed using an intercalated bone graft, plate, and wire fixation with maintenance of the first web space using a "W" wire. The extensor tendons were grafted. (**C**) The entire reconstruction was covered with the transfer of the anterior half of the latissimus dorsi as a free flap. (*Figure continues.*)

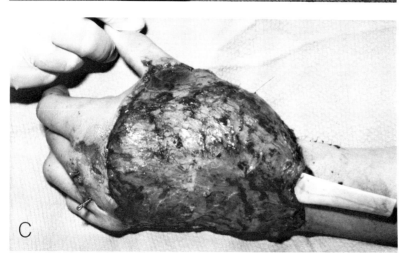

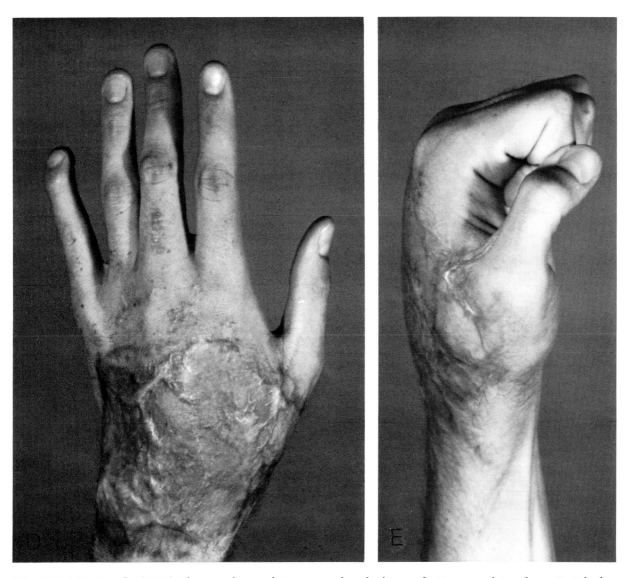

Fig. 26-1 (*Continued*). (**D, E**) The muscle was later covered with skin graft. One year later the patient had a satisfactory range of motion without further reconstruction.

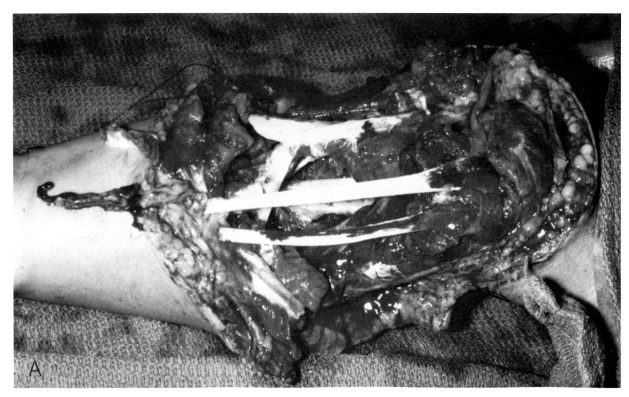

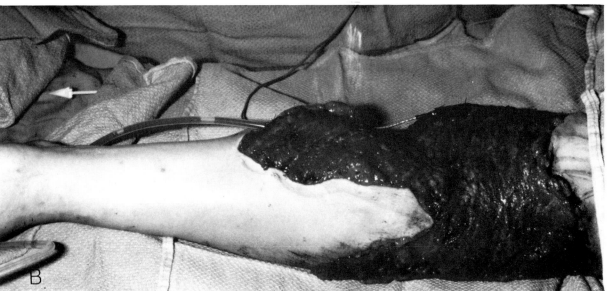

Fig. 26-2. (A) This patient sustained an open injury of the elbow joint with devascularization of the hand and exposure and contusion of the median nerve. Vascularity was restored with a saphenous vein graft. (B) The entire reconstruction was covered with a latissimus dorsi free flap. (*Figure continues.*)

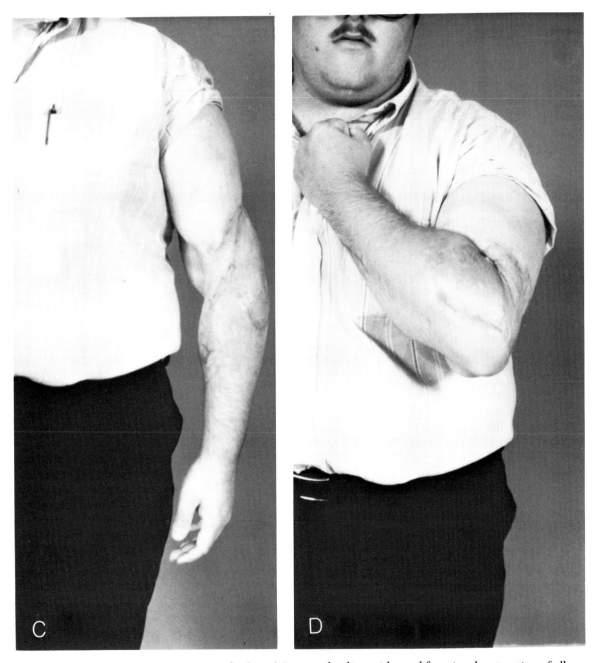

Fig. 26-2 (*Continued*). (**C, D**) Primary healing with good functional restoration of elbow motion was achieved, and median nerve function was restored.

methods of skin cover, free flaps offer an attractive alternative. They are now available in virtually any size. They can provide correctly oriented sensate glabrous skin. They can be cut to fit the defect with incomparable precision. They permit elevation of the limb and early mobilization. They permit random movement by the infant and the disorientated patient.

The natural responses of the body to a major wound, which occur in the adjacent tissues during the days following injury, create increasing difficulties for the surgeon. Bone and tendon become desiccated and die. Soft tissues become edematous, indurated, and difficult to handle. Granulation commences, with its inevitable infection,[7] the bacterial cause of which is relatively inaccessible to systemic antibiotics.[45] Fibrosis follows,[43] not only close to the wound surface but also along the tissue planes between longitudinal structures, bone, tendon, nerve, and vessel. Vessels adjacent to the wound, initially manageable, become narrowed and friable. If an artery was divided at the time of the original injury, it becomes unsuitable as a recipient for flap transfer. If it was not, the fibrosis, narrowing, and friability dictate that any anastomosis must be made far from the wound. These problems are so significant after 72 hours that Godina recommended the use of temporary skin grafts where possible to avoid the 12 percent flap failure and 17.5 percent infection that he encountered in delayed flap transfers to open wounds.[17]

A new free flap is introduced almost monthly. Experience has shown the limitations of the established flaps and taught how to evaluate the new. As a result, there is now an almost limitless choice as to size, thickness, and special properties, as detailed below. It is possible to cover defects small and large, thick and thin. They avoid the additional damage to an already injured limb inflicted by a local flap. They offer the bulk to fill a defect which the local flap cannot provide. In replacing pulp skin, a free toe flap can be innervated by the original digital nerves with greater ease than can a pedicle neurovascular island.[14,36] Flaps can be tailored[19] to fit the defect in a manner not possible with conventional distant flaps, in which the pedicle must be preserved. The injured limb to which a free flap has been applied can be elevated and exercised as necessary. In the infant, the confused, or the epileptic, much less restraint need be applied. This early exercise, unencumbered by attachment to a distant site and reinforced by the robust circulation, promises superior motion. When considered in conjunction with the fact that all tissues of reduced perfusion, which are prone to heavy scar formation, have been excised, the possibilities of improved hand function with emergency free tissue transfer are evident.

WOUND PREPARATION

To apply a free flap, the wound should be over a stable skeleton. It should contain no contamination and no tissue of compromised blood supply. It should present as flat a surface as possible to the flap. These prerequisites are achieved by rigid fixation and radical debridement.[24] Such debridement may be performed with confidence only in the knowledge that good soft tissue cover is available. A parallel with tumor surgery exists. Resection of a malignancy with adequate clear margins is best achieved by the surgeon who knows he can close the resulting defect. As with cancer ablation, true debridement demands incision through normal tissue. Thus, in efficient debridement, all doubtful tissue is excised back to bleeding margins. This should be done under tourniquet control, for otherwise the briskness of the bleeding will obscure the viability or ischemia of tissues incised thereafter. Where major vessel repair is intended, tissue distal to that repair will be better perfused thereafter. In some such cases, debridement distally should follow that repair. In others, where adequate bone shortening can approximate muscle and soft tissue, as in macroreplantation, the debridement must precede the vessel anastomosis. Those parts that will be viable can be demonstrated by cannulating the distal end of the vessel to be repaired and perfusing the ischemic part with heparinized Ringer's lactate. "Weeping" of the fluid from cut tissue will indicate its potential viability. After debridement the wound may be uneven. Additional excision of vital but nonessential tissue is justified to create a flat wound surface. Close contact between flap and bed is thus assured, eliminating dead spaces that may become the site of later infection or fibrosis. The only exceptions to the rule of radical debridement are longitudinal structures that carry promise of function: intact tendons or nerves; or major vessels carrying flow. These should be retained and cleansed with the help of magnification. Provided always that immediate flap cover is intended, contaminated bone can also be retained, by scrubbing vigorously and using burrs and rongeur to remove contamination. Even free fragments can be so treated and used as bone grafts, but only if they are to be covered with well-vascularized soft tissue. With the exception of highly specialized areas, such as fingertip or palm, all marginally viable skin should be removed. If retained, such skin may harbor infection and will certainly heal with profuse scarring. When excision appears adequate, tissue samples are taken from several points in the wound for rapid Gram stain and quantitative cultures.[46]

Once debridement is complete, rigid skeletal fixation should be applied. Plates are used for long bones and Type A intraosseous wiring[27] for phalanges. Where bony defects exist, external fixation is employed. Small defects are filled with cancellous bone grafts and large defects either with a projection of the flap cover or with a block of silicone, pending later reconstruction.

The skin margins are considered next. Already debrided, they should be made even by excising any promontories and peninsulas of no functional importance. They are marked with ink and a pattern is taken with suitable material (e.g., a portion of rubber cut from an Esmarch bandage that has been moistened with alcohol).

FLAP SELECTION

In choosing a free flap, the surgeon should consider eight factors: the health, comfort, and cosmetic demands of the patient; the size, thickness, and special needs of the defect; and his own skill and experience along with that of his team. Patients with respiratory problems require full lung expansion after long surgical procedures. Flaps from the chest wall should therefore be avoided. If the upper extremity wound is only one of several, other injuries may dictate a period of prolonged bed rest. Flaps from the back of such a patient would create a nursing problem. In these patients the forearm flap[5,12,29,30,37,50] may be an appropriate substitute for medium-to-large defects. Girls in particular are likely to be distressed enough by the primary wound without adding a disfiguring scar

on the upper arm, forearm, or over the scapula. For them, the free groin flap[4,23,33,49] has no rival (Fig. 26-3).

Large defects, involving for example the entire anterior or posterior surface of the forearm (Fig. 26-4), require a latissimus dorsi flap.[2,26,32,38,51,54] Whether or not this should be taken with skin is a matter of debate.[20] Godina believed that perfusion of the distal part of the flap was superior when skin was taken. He also showed that the latissimus dorsi musculocutaneous flap could be tailored accurately to fit virtually any defect.[19]

Medium-sized defects can be covered with such a tailored latissimus, which offers a long pedicle without the disadvantage of the bulky portion of the muscle close to the insertion that was previously taken with such flaps. The scapular flap[3,16,22,29,47] offers remarkably tough skin with no underlying muscle (Fig. 26-5). The flap is therefore well suited to large palmar defects in which split-thickness skin grafts will not suffice. The exception is the overweight patient, where the necessary plane of dissection of the pedicle would dictate the transfer of an excessive quantity of subcutaneous fat.

Small defects for which no local flap is available or suitable are most often covered with a lateral arm flap.[26,48] This can be made small enough to provide cover for one phalanx of one finger (Fig. 26-6). It can also be made thick or thin in the slim or the obese. Thickness is achieved by taking a larger area of fascia than of skin and folding it into the primary defect; thinness is achieved by taking fascia without skin and later applying a split-thickness graft. Defects that are double can be covered by splitting the latissimus flap longitudinally between its two feeding vessels, or by dividing a fascial flap transversely, preserving intact the intermuscular septum that contains the pedicle (Fig. 26-7).

Special needs of the defect that may be met by flap selection include bone, tendon, nerve, artery, and sensation. Bone that can be vascularized by an overlying free flap includes segments of ilium with the groin flap,[21,52] of radius with the forearm flap,[30] of metatarsal with the dorsalis pedis flap,[40] and of humerus with the lateral arm flap.[25] With the exception of the first, I have no experience with such transfers. Fashioning bone that is attached to a flap

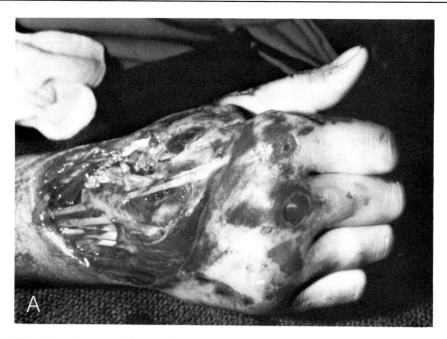

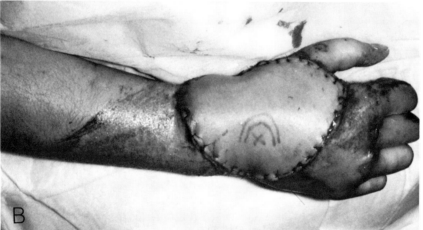

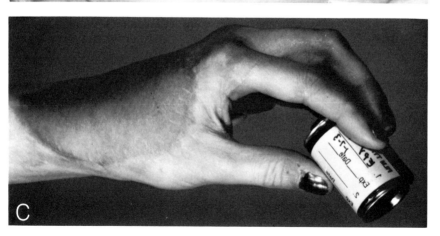

Fig. 26-3. (A) This patient abraded the dorsum of her hand against the road surface. The extensor pollicis longus was disrupted, as were the wrist extensors, and the carpus was opened. A primary transfer of extensor indicis proprius to extensor pollicis longus was performed. The wrist extensors were restored and the carpus was closed. **(B)** The entire reconstruction was covered with a free groin flap. **(C)** No further reconstruction was required and full function was achieved.

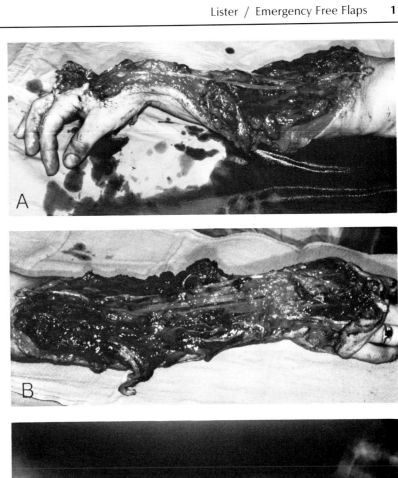

Fig. 26-4. (A, B) This patient sustained avulsion of the dorsal aspect of his forearm in a roller machine. The extensor muscles were entirely absent and there was a defect in the median nerve. The hand was viable and the ulnar nerve and long flexor tendons were intact. (C) X-ray examination revealed that the skeleton also was intact, although there were long grooves cut on the radius by the rollers. (D) Primary bone grafting of the metacarpal fracture was undertaken and the defect was covered with a total latissimus dorsi muscle flap. (*Figure continues.*)

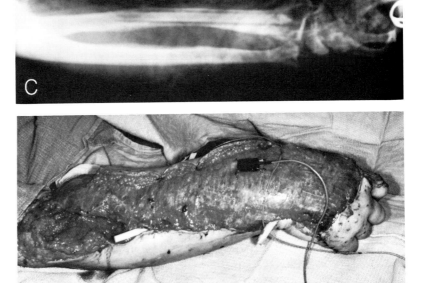

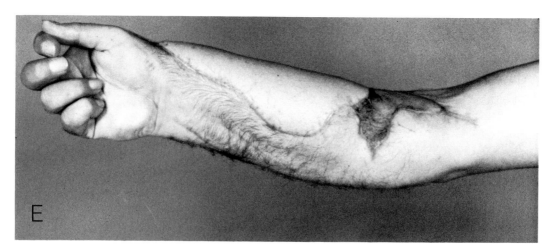

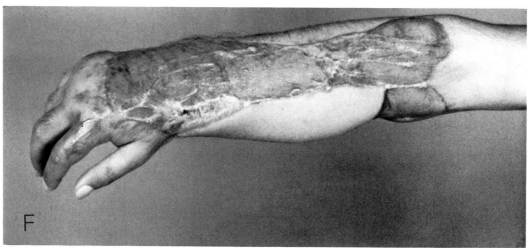

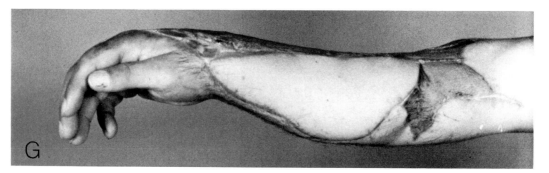

Fig. 26-4 (*Continued*). (**E–G**) The patient achieved primary healing of the soft tissues. Median nerve interfascicular grafting with bioassay of the proximal end and dissection of the distal end has been undertaken since these last photographs were made, and the patient is scheduled for extensor tendon grafts using flexor carpi ulnaris via the Silastic rods that were placed at the time of the initial injury.

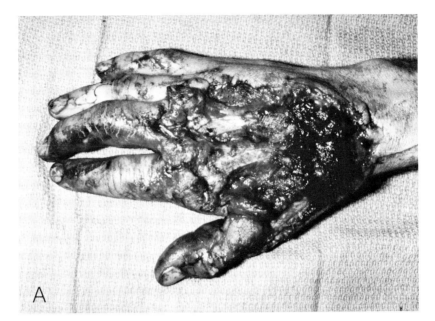

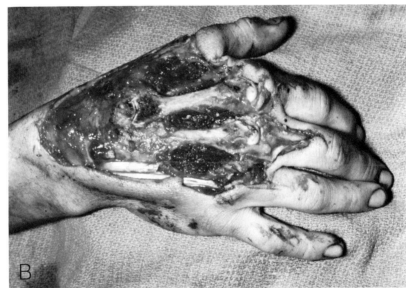

Fig. 26-5. (A) This patient sustained loss of skin and extensor tendons with associated fractures when he was thrown from a motorcycle. **(B)** Thorough debridement with bone excision that exposed the carpus and metacarpus was undertaken. **(C)** Silastic rods were placed primarily and the entire defect covered with a scapular flap. (*Figure continues.*)

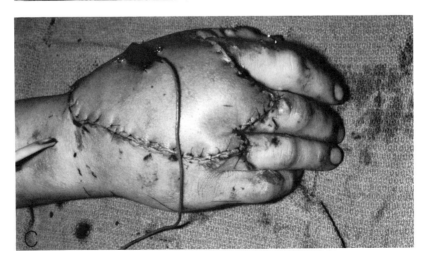

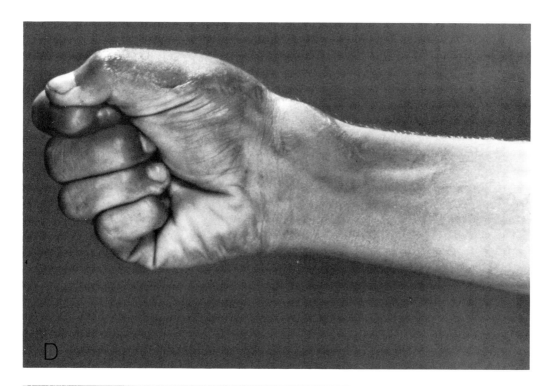

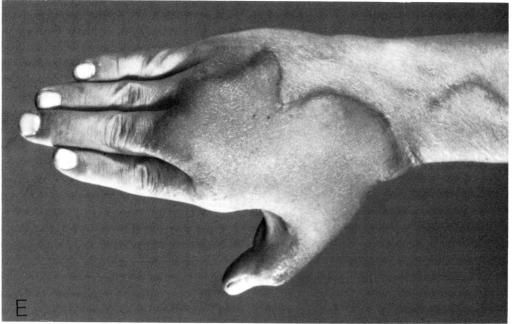

Fig. 26-5 (*Continued*). (**D**) This healed satisfactorily without complication, and (**E**) the Silastic rods have been replaced with extensor tendon grafts.

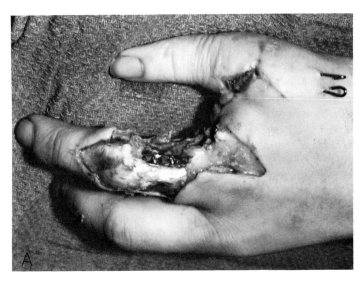

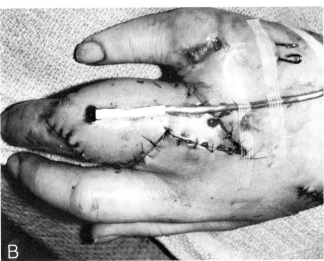

Fig. 26-6. Here, in a delayed reconstruction, the use of a lateral arm flap to cover a small defect over the proximal phalanx is illustrated. (**A**) Following a gunshot wound, this patient has loss of skin over a plate placed primarily on the proximal phalanx. (**B**) This was covered with a lateral arm flap, the pedicle of which was anastomosed to the radial artery in the snuffbox. (**C**) Satisfactory healing was achieved.

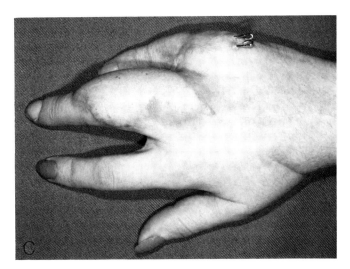

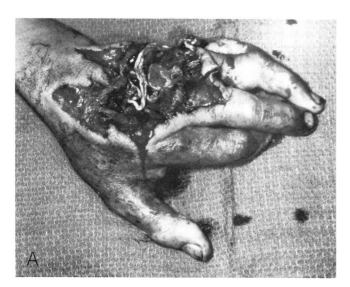

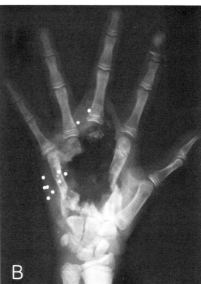

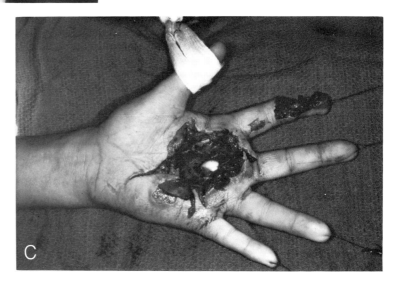

Fig. 26-7. (A) A 14-year-old right hand dominant youth sustained this close range shotgun injury to his left hand. (B) X-ray evaluation showed total disruption with significant loss of metacarpal substance. Distraction displayed the (C) palmar and (D) dorsal defects. (*Figure continues.*)

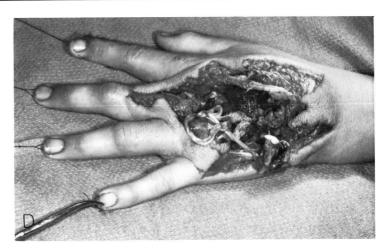

Fig. 26-7 (*Continued*). (**E, F**) The middle finger was nonviable and had no metacarpal. It was therefore amputated and the index finger was translocated to the position of the middle metacarpal. Length was restored by inserting the middle phalanx from the middle finger as an intercalated bone graft. The long defect in the ring metacarpal was restored by using the proximal phalanx of the middle finger in a similar fashion. Significant palmar and dorsal defects remained. Patterns were taken and placed end-to-end in designing a lateral arm flap taken from the same arm. (*Figure continues.*)

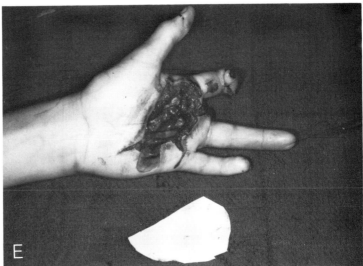

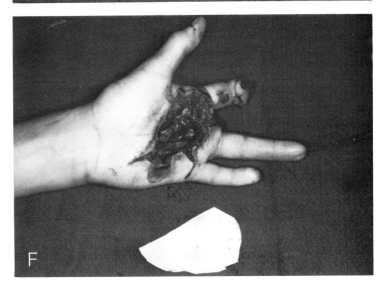

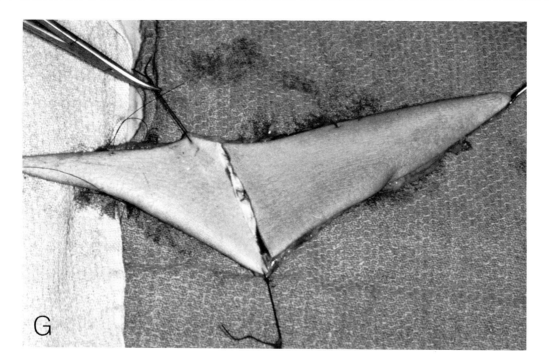

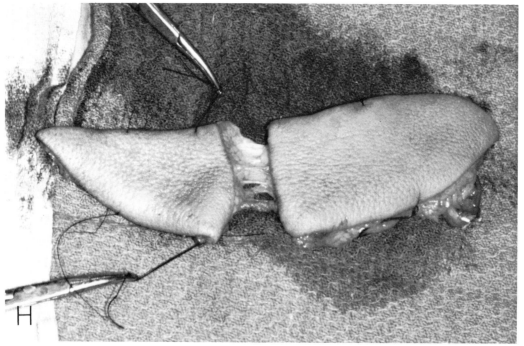

Fig. 26-7 (*Continued*). (**G, H**) The lateral arm flap after it was raised was divided transversely through skin and subcutaneous tissue down to the level of the intermuscular septum containing the pedicle. The vessels of the flap were then anastomosed to the radial and cephalic veins, placing the proximal portion of the flap on the dorsal defect and the distal portion of the flap on the palmar defect. The intervening pedicle was accommodated between the heads of the ring and now translocated index finger. (*Figure continues.*)

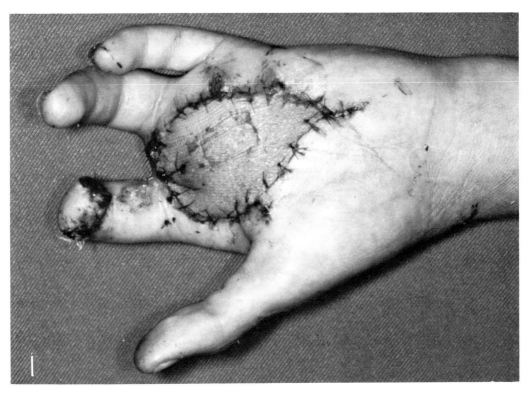

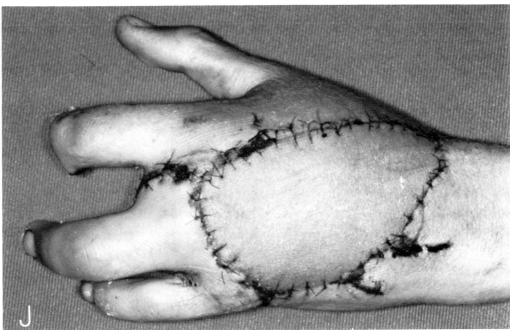

Fig. 26-7 *(Continued).* (**I, J**) Complete viability of the flap was maintained as seen here at day 14 when the patient started on a passive and active exercise program.

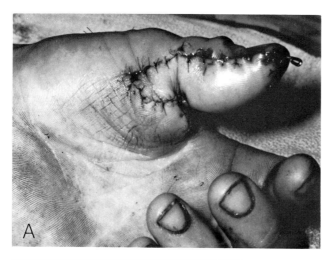

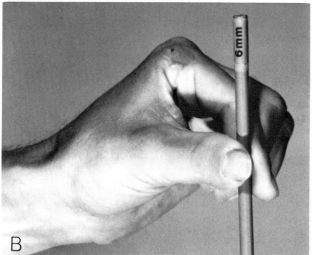

Fig. 26-8. (A) Following avulsion of the entire pulp of the left thumb with a table saw, a flap from the fibular aspect of the right great toe was transferred as an emergency. (B) Two years later there is good healing of the pulp with 6-mm two-point discrimination, correctly oriented. (C) The defect on the foot presents no problems.

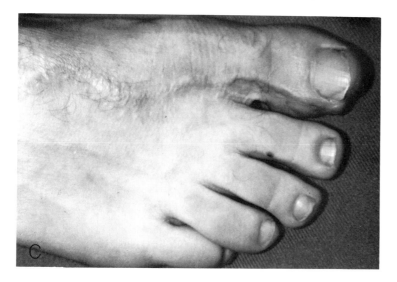

is difficult if devascularization of the bone is to be avoided. My attempts usually result in disappointing compromise. Small bone defects can be well filled with cancellous bone, either as a block for structure or as chips. Large defects in long bones are best reconstructed with a vascularized fibula,[1,9,10,44, 55] although I am not aware of any emergency transfers of this tissue. Vascularized tendon and nerve can both be transferred with the dorsalis pedis flap.[34,35,41,53] The resultant defect is troublesome and there is no evidence that function is better than with conventional tendon and nerve grafts beneath a good skin flap. Arterial reconstruction in the limb can be undertaken with the same vessel as supplies the free flap. Thus the subscapular artery has been used to restore flow to the foot via the posterior tibial artery while the thoracodorsal branch supplied the overlying latissimus flap. The radial artery has been used with the forearm flap in similar fashion in both the upper and lower extremities.[42] In both these examples the flap is supported by branches of a major artery, a portion of which is used to replace a segment of another major vessel. The distal end of the artery of the flap can also be anastomosed to a vessel of similar caliber. This has been described in restoring flow to a thumb with the continuation of the posterior radial collateral artery supplying a lateral arm flap covering a defect over the anatomic snuffbox and the first metacarpal.[49] Sensation can be restored to essential pulp by transfer of tissue from the great toe on the first dorsal metatarsal artery[14,36] (Fig. 26-8).

AUTHOR'S PREFERRED METHODS

This brief chapter is a statement of my preferred methods and my reasons. I now use local and regional flaps only for small defects, where I am confident that raising the flap will not further impair function. Where significant pulp is lost I use tissue from the toe rather than a neurovascular island flap. For the reasons discussed above, I rarely use distant pedicle flaps, random or axial, to cover medium or large defects of the upper extremity. The exception would be where I anticipated the later need for skin additional to that required simply to provide cover; that is, where elective pollicization or toe transfer seems indicated. In those cases I use a pedicle groin flap (see Chapter 48). This is now such an infrequent operation in my practice that I find more interested observers attend during its execution than during a free tissue transfer.

The free flaps I select in differing circumstances are also indicated. In practice I use three flaps more than all other flaps for provision of skin cover immediately following injury. Defects of the pulp are covered with transfers from the great toe. I replace small soft tissue defects with the lateral arm flap; medium and large defects with a latissimus dorsi flap tailored accurately to fit the defect. In those likely to be especially distressed by the secondary defect, I consider the groin flap.

TECHNIQUES AND POSTOPERATIVE CARE

The detailed operative techniques of the free flaps favored for emergency transfer are described in Chapters 27 and 28, and the methods of postoperative care and monitoring are described in Chapter 24.

REFERENCES

1. Allieu Y, Gomis R, Yoshimura M, Dimeglio A, Bonnel F: Congenital pseudarthrosis of the forearm—Two cases treated by free vascularized fibular graft. J Hand Surg 6:475–481, 1981
2. Bailey BN, Godfrey AM: Latissimus dorsi muscle free flaps. Br J Plast Surg 35:47–52, 1982
3. Barwick WJ, Goodkind DJ, Serafin D: The free scapular flap. Plast Reconstr Surg 69:779–785, 1982
4. Baudet J, LeMaire JM, Guimberteau JC: Ten free groin flaps. Plast Reconstr Surg 57:577–595, 1976
5. Braun FM, Hoang Ph, Merle M, Van Genechten F, Foucher G: Technique and indications of the forearm flap in hand surgery. A report of thirty-three cases. Ann Chir Main 4:85–97, 1985

6. Brown JB, Fryer MP, McDowell F: Application of permanent pedicle blood-carrying flaps. Plast Reconstr Surg 8:335–340, 1951

7. Burke JF: Effects of inflammation on wound repair. J Dent Res 50:296, 1971

8. Burkhalter WE, Butler B, Metz W, Omer G: Experiences with delayed primary closure of war wounds of the hand in Vietnam. J Bone Joint Surg 50A:945–954, 1968

9. Dell PC, Sheppard JE: Vascularised bone grafts in the treatment of infected forearm non-unions. J Hand Surg 9A:653–658, 1984

10. Donski PK, Buechler U, Tschopp HM: Surgical dissection of the fibula for free microvascular transfer. Chir Plast 6:153–164, 1982

11. Edgerton MT: Immediate reconstruction of the injured hand. Surgery 36:329–343, 1954

12. Emerson DJM, Sprigg A, Page RE: Some observations on the radial artery island flap. Br J Plast Surg 38:107–112, 1985

13. Engel J, Ganel A, Melamed R, Rimon S, Farine I: Choline acetyltransferase for differentiation between human motor and sensory nerve fibers. Ann Plast Surg 4:376–380, 1980

14. Foucher G, Merle M, Maneaud M, Michon J: Microsurgical free partial toe transfer in hand reconstruction: A report of 12 cases. Plast Reconstr Surg 65:616–626, 1980

15. Ganel A, Engel J, Luboshitz S, Melamed R, Rimon S: Choline acetyltransferase nerve identification method in early and late nerve repair. Ann Plast Surg 6:228–230, 1981

16. Gilbert A, Teot L: The free scapular flap. Plast Reconstr Surg 69:601–604, 1982

17. Godina M: Early microsurgical reconstruction of complex trauma of the extremities. Plast Reconstr Surg 78:285–292, 1986

18. Godina M: Arterial autografts in microvascular surgery. Plast Reconstr Surg 78:293–294, 1986

19. Godina M: The tailored latissimus dorsi flap. Plast Reconstr Surg (August 1987)

20. Gordon L, Buncke HJ, Alpert BS: Free latissimus dorsi muscle flap with split-thickness skin graft cover: A report of 16 cases. Plast Reconstr Surg 70:173–178, 1982

21. Gordon L, Buncke HJ, Alpert BS, Wilson C, Koch RA: Free vascularized osteocutaneous transplants from the groin for delayed primary closure in the management of loss of soft-tissue and bone in the hand and wrist. J Bone Joint Surg 67A:958–964, 1985

22. Hamilton SGL, Morrison WA: The scapular free flap. Br J Plast Surg 35:2–7, 1982

23. Harii K, Ohmori K, Torii S, Murakami F, Kasai Y, Sekiguchi J, Ohmori S: Free groin skin flaps. Br J Plast Surg 28:225–237, 1975

24. Haury B, Rodeheaver G, Vensko J, Edgerton MT, Edlich RF: Debridement: An essential component of traumatic wound care. Am J Surg 135:238–242, 1978

25. Katsaros J, Schusterman M, Beppu M, Banis JC, Acland RD: The lateral upper arm flap: Anatomy and clinical applications. Ann Plast Surg 12:489–500, 1984

26. Lassen M, Krag C, Nielsen IM: The latissimus dorsi flap. Scand J Plast Reconstr Surg 19:41–51, 1985

27. Lister G: Intraosseous wiring of the digital skeleton. J Hand Surg 3:427–435, 1978

28. Lister GD, Scheker LR: Emergency free flaps to the upper extremity. J Hand Surg (in press)

29. Mahaffey PJ, Tanner NSB, Evans HB, McGrouther DA: The degloved hand: Immediate complete restoration of skin cover with a contralateral forearm free flap. Br J Plast Surg 38:101–106, 1985

30. Matthews RN, Fatah F, Davies DM, Eyre J, Hodge RA, Walsh-Waring GP: Experience with the radial forearm flap in 14 cases. Scand J Plast Reconstr Surg 18:303–310, 1984

31. Mayou BJ, Whitby D, Jones BM: The scapular flap—An anatomical and clinical study. Br J Plast Surg 35:8–13, 1982

32. Maxwell GP, Manson PN, Hoopes J: Experience with thirteen latissimus dorsi myocutaneous free flaps. Plast Reconstr Surg 64:1–8, 1979

33. McConnell CM, Hyland WT, Neale HW: Microvascular free groin flap for soft-tissue coverage of the extremities. J Trauma 20:593–598, 1980

34. McCraw JB: On the transfer of a free dorsalis pedis sensory flap to the hand. Plast Reconstr Surg 59:738–739, 1977

35. McCraw JB, Furlow LT: The dorsalis pedis arterialized flap. Plast Reconstr Surg 55:177–185, 1975

36. Minami A, Usui M, Katoh H, Ishii S: Thumb reconstruction by free sensory flaps from the foot using microsurgical techniques. J Hand Surg 9B:239–244, 1984

37. Muhlbauer W, Herndl E, Stock W: The forearm flap. Plast Reconstr Surg 70:336–342, 1982

38. Nielsen IM, Lassen M, Gregersen BN, Krag C: Experience with the latissimus dorsi flap. Scand J Plast Reconstr Surg 19:53–63, 1985

39. Nylen S, Carlsson B: Time factor, infection frequency and quantitative microbiology in hand injuries. Scand J Plast Reconstr Surg 14:185–189, 1980

40. O'Brien BM, Morrison WA, Dooley BJ: Microvascular osteocutaneous transfer using the groin flap and

iliac crest and the dorsalis pedis flap and second metatarsal. Br J Plast Surg 32:188–206, 1979

41. Ohmori K, Harii K: Free dorsalis pedis sensory flap to the hand, with microneurovascular anastomoses. Plast Reconstr Surg 58:546–554, 1976

42. Partecke BD, Buck-Gramcko D: Free forearm flap for reconstruction of soft tissue defects concurrent with improved peripheral circulation. J Reconstr Microsurg 1:1–6, 1984

43. Peacock EE: Wound Repair. 3rd Ed. WB Saunders, Philadelphia, 1984

44. Pho RWH: Free vascularised fibular transplant for replacement of the lower radius. J Bone Joint Surg 61B:362–365, 1979

45. Robson MC, Edstrom LE, Krizek TJ, Groskin MG: The efficacy of systemic antibiotics in the treatment of granulating wounds. J Surg Res 16:299–306, 1974

46. Robson MC, Heggers JP: Delayed wound closures based on bacterial counts. J Surg Oncol 2:379–383, 1970

47. Santos LF: The scapular flap: A new microsurgical free flap. Rev Brasileria Cirurgia 70:133–141, 1980

48. Scheker LR, Kleinert HE: The ipsilateral lateral arm flap. J Hand Surg (submitted)

49. Shah KG, Garrett JC, Buncke HJ: Free groin flap transfer to the upper extremity. Hand 11:315–320, 1979

50. Song R, Gao Y, Song Y, Yu Y, Song Y: The forearm flap. Clin Plast Surg 9:21–26, 1982

51. Stern PJ, Neale HW, Gregory RO, McDonough JJ: Functional reconstruction of an extremity by free tissue transfer of the latissimus dorsi. J Bone Joint Surg 65A:729–737, 1983

52. Swartz WM: Immediate reconstruction of the wrist and dorsum of the hand with a free osteocutaneous groin flap. J Hand Surg 9A:18–21, 1984

53. Takami H, Takahashi S, Ando M: Use of the dorsalis pedis free flap for reconstruction of the hand. Hand 15:173–178, 1983

54. Watson JS, Craig RDP, Orton CI: The free latissimus dorsi myocutaneous flap. Plast Reconstr Surg 64:299–305, 1979

55. Yoshimura M, Shimamura K, Iwai Y, Yamauchi S, Ueno T: Free vascularized fibular transplant: A new method for monitoring circulation of the grafted fibula. J Bone Joint Surg 65A:1295–1301, 1983

Free Skin and Composite Flaps

27

Stephen J. Mathes
Bernard S. Alpert

Two factors have greatly influenced the hand surgeon's approach to wound coverage. First, a clear understanding of the anatomy of skin and muscle circulation has altered the entire concept of flap design. Flap selection is no longer limited to the random flap with its classic 2:1 length-width ratio or the axial flap based on longitudinally oriented cutaneous vessels. The addition of the muscle flap and the skin–fascial flap have immensely expanded flap selection. The second factor relates to the technique of microsurgery. Flaps are no longer limited to a specific arc of rotation determined by the length and location of the flap's vascular pedicle. The hand surgeon may now select the best source of tissue, regardless of location, to restore form and function to the upper extremity. This composite of tissue is then transplanted in one stage to the extremity, with restoration of circulation by microanastomosis of the flap and extremity vasculature.[2,5,11] The composite of tissue may include skin, subcutaneous tissue, fascia, tendon, sensory and motor nerves, bone, and muscle transplanted separately or as a unit. These two factors have allowed an explosion of both new flaps and

unique methods for their utilization in reconstructive surgery in the upper extremity.

SKIN CIRCULATION—IMPACT ON FLAP DESIGN

Skin circulation is provided by a series of vascular connections from the regional source of deep vessels ultimately supplying the subdermal plexus. With the identification of musculocutaneous perforating vessels, the use of the muscle as a carrier of skin was made possible.[8,9] Muscles with a single major or dominant pedicle may be transposed locally or transplanted by microvascular surgery.[6] Between muscle bellies, direct vascular communications to the fascia have been identified. Vascular pedicles within these intermuscular septa provide circulation to the skin–fascial flap.[4,10,12] Vascular connections to bone, nerves, and tendons allow use of specialized flaps containing these unique structures with intact circulation. The "axial flap" is no longer limited to a few privileged sites on human skin topography; it now includes skin–fascial and musculocutaneous vessels coursing in all body regions capable of providing reliable circulation to skin and deeper structures.

FREE SKIN AND MUSCLE FLAPS FOR COVERAGE

Indications

Despite this explosion in the number of available flaps, coverage of congenital or acquired defects in the upper extremity is not readily accomplished by use of local flaps. All tissue in the upper extremity is unique, and its use for reconstruction results in some donor site morbidity. Obviously, skin grafts readily solve most coverage problems without the need for sacrifice of local tissue. Distant flaps transferred by conventional staged techniques have proven reliability. Transplantation by microsurgical techniques requires specialized instrumentation and training; specific indications for microsurgical transplantation of flaps for upper extremity coverage have been identified. The following paragraphs outline the advantages of free vascularized flaps.

Reliability

In distant tubed-flap transfer, the flap must be vascularized by the hand before flap division and inset can be accomplished. When circulation to the injured hand is marginal, the transferred skin may either have marginal vascularity or undergo subsequent avascular necrosis. Free transplantation of a distant skin flap allows immediate vascularization of the flap via receptor vessels proximal to the injury site. With the identification of muscle and skin–fascial flaps with long vascular pedicles, the microsurgeon is almost always able to reach a normal receptor artery and vein in the upper extremity. Free flap failure rates below 5 percent are now standard for hand centers using microsurgical techniques for flap transplantation.

Wound Access

Wound care and prevention of prolonged edema are problems associated with staged distant flap transfer to the upper extremity (e.g., groin flap transfer to the hand). Microsurgical flap transplantation allows immediate placement of the hand in an optimal position, which minimizes the formation of edema and allows early hand therapy.

Contaminated and Infected Wounds

Early complete wound coverage with well-vascularized tissue avoids prolonged exposure of tendon and bone and decreases the potential for infection. The large size and reliability of flaps suitable for microsurgical transplantation allows the surgeon to perform aggressive wound debridement followed by immediate coverage with microvascular flap transplantation.

Established infections in bone and soft tissue are frequently associated with poor local wound circulation. Debridement of nonviable infected bone and soft tissue followed by immediate or staged microsurgical flap transplantation provides both stable coverage and well-vascularized tissue to restore local circulation.[7]

Number of Operations

The distant tubed-flap transfer requires a minimum of two operative procedures to accomplish skin coverage. Free composite tissue transplantation requires one procedure and may allow earlier attention both to hand rehabilitation and reconstruction of associated hand injuries (e.g., tendon graft).

Immediate Heterotopic Transplantation (Salvage of Nonreplantable Parts)

In extensive injuries with multiple amputations, replantation of parts in their normal position may not be feasible. However, parts of structures with an intact vascular pedicle may be utilized at different sites for immediate reconstruction. In multiple finger amputations, the finger with minimal injury may be placed in the index ray position. Parts of a nonreplantable foot may be useful for coverage of an associated upper extremity reconstruction. Immediate heterotopic transplantation allows salvage of specialized structures not easily replaced in subsequent reconstructive procedures.

Specialized Reconstructive Requirements

By using special donor flaps, composite tissue transplantation may include bone, joint, epiphyses, tendon, and motor or sensory nerves. The tissues may either be transplanted separately or all be vascularized by one pedicle (e.g., toe-digital transplantation), thus satisfying multiple requirements in one operation.

General Considerations

Flap Design

When microvascular flap transplantation is elected as a technique to provide upper extremity coverage, certain general considerations are applicable regardless of donor flap selection. The surgeon should practice the dissection in the anatomy laboratory prior to clinical use of the techniques described here for donor flap elevation. Since flap transplantation of skin–fascial and muscle or musculocutaneous flaps is not impeded by donor site–recipient site connections, the surgeon can precisely tailor the transplanted structure to fit the reconstructive requirements of the defect. Therefore, a precise calculation of the donor area allows modifications in the design and operative technique for each reconstructive procedure.

Vascular Assessment

Normal receptor arteries and veins in proximity to the reconstructive site are an absolute requisite for successful microvascular transplantation. Use of palpation and the Doppler probe may provide inaccurate information about the status of these vessels in the upper extremity. An arteriogram is routinely obtained to evaluate the status of the arterial vasculature if proposed recipient vessels are located in the zone of trauma prior to free flap transplantation. The role of donor site arteriography varies with the donor flap, and indications are discussed for each flap in this chapter. If the vascu-

larity of the donor flap is questionable due to trauma or prior surgery in proximity to the pedicle of the flap, an arteriogram for the donor region is also advisable.

The Microvascular Anastomoses

A thorough knowledge of microvascular techniques is an obvious requisite for microvascular transplantation of composite tissue.[1] The actual microvascular phase of the procedure is started only after the free flap is fully dissected and appropriate receptor vessels adjacent to the defect are exposed. The vascular pedicles to the free flaps are then divided, and the free flap is brought to the recipient defect. The flap is placed over the defect to again confirm the relationships of the flap to the defect and the donor vessels of the flap to the proposed recipient vessels. This maneuver should not be time-consuming if adequate planning has preceded this phase of the procedure. Failure of the vascular pedicle to reach the recipient vessels because of inadequate length should have been determined by measuring the pedicle length before the actual division of the free flap from its donor region. Interposition vein grafts are mandatory when tension will result from stretching of the vascular pedicle at the site of either arterial or venous repairs. If this situation appears likely, vein grafts should be prepared before the flap is actually divided for inset into the recipient defect.

Recipient Site Preparation

Chronic scar tissue and nonviable tissue should be debrided from the recipient site before the microvascular phase has been started. This debridement is generally accomplished using a separate set of instruments to avoid contamination of the donor flap region and the area of microvascular anastomoses. It is also helpful to establish hemostasis in the area of wound debridement prior to actual vascularization of the flap by the microvascular anastomosis. Use of Avatene may be helpful if diffuse bleeding at the recipient site is observed.[13]

Sequence of Repairs

The donor free flap is loosely sutured over the prepared recipient site. The correct position for alignment of the donor vessels with the recipient vessels is confirmed. The operating microscope is brought into place, and the microvascular repairs are accomplished. (The techniques of microvascular anastomoses are discussed in detail in Chapter 24.) Both arterial and venous repairs are generally completed before microclips are removed, allowing perfusion of the flap. If two venous repairs are to be made, perfusion is started before the second venous repair is completed. Once perfusion is noted to be adequate within the transplanted flap, the flap is carefully inset to provide coverage of the recipient area. Meshed skin grafts are used where direct closure of the flap to the recipient site in the region of the vascular pedicles might result in constriction of the vascular pedicles.

Adjunctive Procedures

If any adjunctive procedures are to be performed, such as bone grafting, tendon repairs, or tendon transfers, they should not be done until after the flap has been successfully vascularized. If flap perfusion is not possible because of either technical or logistical problems and the surgeon has not already performed other procedures, a skin graft may still be used to provide at least temporary coverage at this point in the operation.

Postoperative Management

Low molecular weight Dextran is started intraoperatively prior to the onset of flow into the transplanted flap. Low molecular weight Dextran (500 cc/24 hours) and aspirin (325 mg/day) are used for the initial postoperative period (5 days). If either arterial inflow or venous outflow is questionable, the patient should be immediately returned to the operating room and the appropriate repair sites inspected. Since we began following this aggressive approach in our institution, all elective free flaps with questionable circulation have been successfully salvaged.

Specific Flap Selection

A variety of factors warrant consideration in selection of a specific flap for composite tissue transplantation. Almost any segment of skin or muscle with an identified vascular pedicle can be transplanted to the upper extremity. Futhermore, each flap is readily tailored to meet local reconstructive requirements in the upper extremity. In general, hand centers extensively using microvascular flap transplantation in upper extremity reconstruction have developed specific preferences in flap selection.

Wound coverage can be accomplished by three techniques using microsurgery: (1) skin–fascial flap, (2) musculocutaneous flap, and (3) fascial or muscle flap with an overlying skin graft. Specific advantages and comparisons of each method are discussed below.

Ease of Dissection

The muscle flap is readily located between its bony origin and insertion. Variation in the location of its vascular pedicle is uncommon.[6] The skin–fascial flap is centered over an intermuscular septum containing its vascular pedicle. The specific site of origin of the skin–fascial vascular pedicle is associated with greater variation than the muscle flap.[1]

Quality of Skin Coverage

The skin–fascial flap provides durable coverage with skin and subcutaneous tissue. Subsequent elevation of the flap for delayed procedures (i.e., tendon or bone grafts) is readily accomplished. Although the thickness of the subcutaneous tissue is variable in the skin–fascial flap, the addition of this flap to the upper extremity does not alter the normal contour in the majority of available skin–fascial flaps. In contrast, the thickness of the musculocutaneous flap is usually excessive when used for upper extremity reconstruction. Use of skin grafts over vascularized fascia provides the thinnest coverage and is often desirable over certain defects (i.e., the dorsal and palmar surfaces of the hand). Likewise, using muscle plus skin grafts eliminates the subcutaneous tissue, which may be excessive in the obese patient. Secondary reconstructive procedures beneath the fascia and muscle flap with skin graft coverage is less desirable than beneath a flap containing normal skin and subcutaneous tissue.

Donor Site Morbidity

If skin is not included with a flap, direct closure of the donor site is easily accomplished. There is minimal contour deformity in the donor site. Functional disability after use of only fascia in the fasciocutaneous flap has not been reported. Use of a large skin–fascial flap may preclude direct donor site closure. Conversely, a large muscle flap (i.e., latissimus dorsi) is possible without the additional difficulty of donor site skin closure. In general, synergistic muscles are available to preserve normal function. Segmental muscle transplantation is also possible with use of only part of the muscle as a flap while preserving the origin, insertion, and motor innervation of the muscle.

Each flap has specific advantages that ultimately determine its usefulness in upper extremity reconstructive surgery. Factors such as vascular anatomy, flap design, and technique of elevation warrant careful consideration. Flaps with established reliability in upper extremity reconstruction are discussed here.

Skin – Fascial Flaps

GROIN FLAP

This skin–fascial flap, described by McGregor and Jackson,[16] has become the standard distant tubed-flap for reconstruction of upper extremity wounds. After its successful microvascular transplantation by Daniel and Taylor,[15] the groin flap has been commonly used as a free flap for upper extremity reconstruction. With the addition of other fasciocutaneous flaps and the deep groin modification (see the section under vascularized bone), this flap is less commonly selected now that other fasciocutaneous flaps and the deep groin modification are available (see Chapter 48 for a discussion of the groin flap used as a distant flap).

Vascular Anatomy

The groin flap is vascularized by the superficial circumflex iliac artery, a branch of the common femoral artery. The superficial inferior epigastric artery may originate as a common branch with the superficial circumflex iliac artery. Occasionally, the superficial inferior epigastric artery is the more dominant artery to the area of the groin flap.

Venous drainage of the groin flap is maintained by two systems. The superficial system consists of the superficial epigastric vein and superficial iliac veins draining into the saphenous system. The deep system consists of paired venae comitantes located adjacent to the artery and draining into the femoral vein. The variability of the arterial and venous systems generally does not preclude the use of the groin flap for microsurgical transplantation, but it does warrant a careful analysis of the vascular anatomy of the groin flap before completing elevation and planned transplantation.

Technique of Elevation of the Superficial Groin Flap

Distal Approach. The groin flap may be elevated either proximally or distally in preparation for its microvascular transplantation. The distal approach (Fig. 27-1) requires incision of the planned skin island centered over the course of the superficial circumflex iliac artery as determined by the use of the Doppler probe. Flap elevation then begins distally with the skin overlying the iliac crest superficial to the deep fascia. At the lateral border of the sartorius muscle, the fascia of the muscle is included with the flap. At the medial edge of the sartorius muscle, the superficial circumflex iliac artery and deep venous system are identified, and the donor vessels are elevated to their junctions with the femoral artery, femoral vein, and saphenous vein, respectively. This approach allows a rapid flap elevation but assumes normal vascular anatomy in the femoral triangle. If the vessels have an anomalous course or are not suitable for microvascular transplantation, the surgeon may be forced to discard the flap.

Proximal Approach. The second, and our preferred, approach is the proximal technique as described by Acland[13] (Fig. 27-2). A transverse incision is made in the groin between the medial edge of the sartorius muscle and the femoral vessels. The superficial circumflex iliac artery and the deep and superficial venous systems are identified (Fig. 27-2B and C). The design of the cutaneous terri-

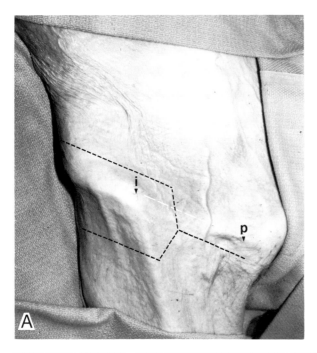

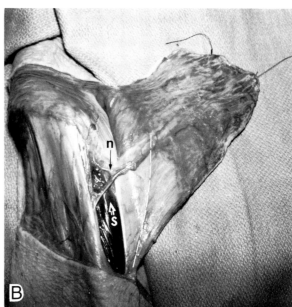

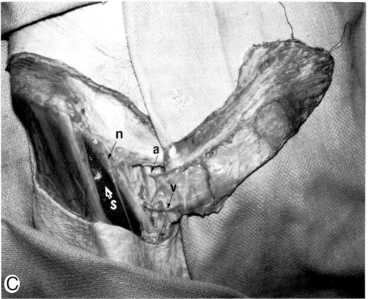

Fig. 27-1. (A) Groin flap design. The long axis of the flap parallels the inguinal ligament. (*i*, anterior superior iliac spine; *p*, pubic tubercle.) (B) Groin flap — distal approach technique of elevation. The fascia of the sartorius muscle (dotted white line) is elevated with the flap. The lateral femoral cutaneous nerve (*n*) is released from the deep aspect of the flap (*s*, sartorius muscle). (C) The dissection proceeds medially to expose the origins of the flap donor vessels in the femoral triangle. (*n*, lateral femoral cutaneous nerve; *a*, superficial circumflex iliac artery; *v*, superficial circumflex iliac vein.)

tory of the axial flap is then based precisely on the location of the superficial circumflex iliac vessels or on anomalous vessels, if encountered. After determining the flap design, the distal to proximal dissection is performed as described in the distal approach. Although the proximal approach requires a longer operating time, it has several advantages:

(1) a long vascular pedicle is developed; (2) the skin island can be centered more superiorly if there is a dominant superficial epigastric artery (see Superficial Inferior Epigastric Artery Flap on page 1184) or anomalous superficial circumflex iliac artery; (3) if there are multiple arterial pedicles, the incision can be closed and the opposite groin explored as a

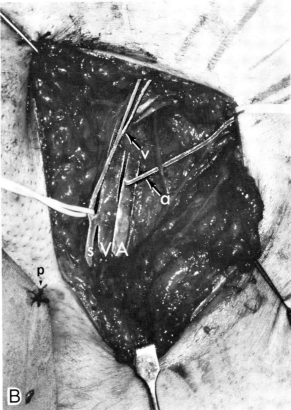

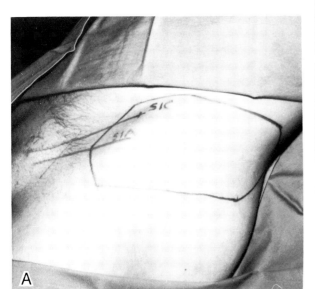

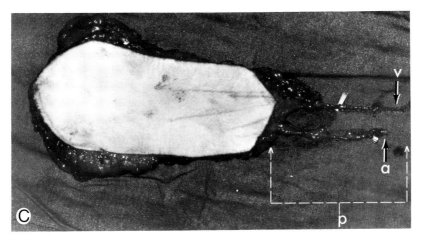

Fig. 27-2. Groin flap—proximal approach technique of elevation. (**A**) The design of the flap is centered over the course of the superficial circumflex artery as determined by the Doppler probe. (*SIC*, superior iliac crest; *SIA*, course of superficial circumflex iliac artery.) (**B**) Initial exposure of the donor vessels is between the pubic tubercle and the medial border of the sartorius muscle. (*A*, femoral artery; *V*, femoral vein; *s*, saphenous vein; *a*, superficial circumflex iliac artery; *v*, superficial circumflex iliac vein; *p*, pubic tubercle; *i*, iliac crest.) (**C**) The flap dissected completely free. The donor pedicles are exposed from the femoral vessels to the medial border of sartorius muscle. (*p*, donor pedicle length of 5 to 8 cm; *a*, superficial circumflex iliac artery; *v*, superficial circumflex iliac vein.)

potential donor source for free groin flap (Taylor[19] noted that only one-third of anatomic groin dissections are symmetrical in their vascular configurations); and (4) if the superficial epigastric artery is the dominant artery, the surgeon may design the skin–fascial flap in its territory over the inferior abdominal wall.

The distal portion of the free flap lateral to the fascia of the sartorius muscle may be thinned after the flap is detached. The superficial veins are identified for microvascular repair into suitable receptor veins in the recipient site. It is not necessary to repair the deep venous system (venae comitantes) to recipient vessels in the upper extremity.

Flap Design

The skin territory of the superficial circumflex iliac artery and associated veins is centered over the lateral groin and iliac crest (Fig. 27-2A). A line connecting the anterior superior iliac spine and pubic tubercle delineates the axis of the flap. The skin territory is generally designed between the medial border of the sartorius muscle medially, 5 to 10 cm beyond the anterior superior iliac spine laterally, 2 cm above the inguinal ligament superiorly, and 6 cm below the inguinal ligament inferiorly. Obviously, the advantage of microsurgical transplantation is that the skin may be precisely designed to fit the defect, so these measurements function only as guidelines (Fig. 27-3).

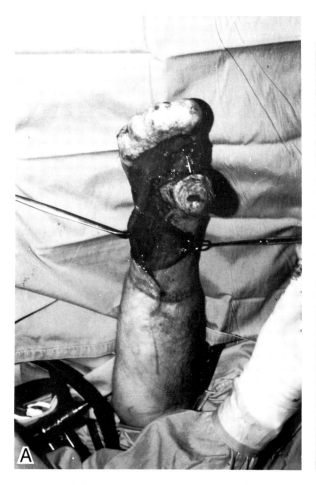
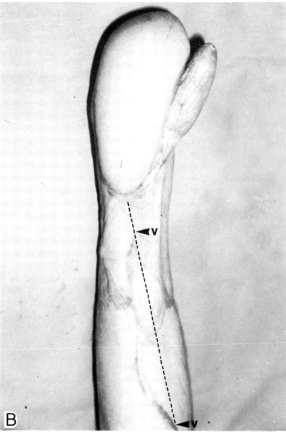

Fig. 27-3. (A) Avulsion-burn amputation of digits with resultant unstable skin, with wrist and first web space contractures. **(B)** Groin flap transplantation to the volar hand and wrist. An 18-cm vein graft *(v)* was required due to distal arterial injuries.

Nerve

The sensory branch of T12 is located at the lateral margin of the flap. Inclusion of this sensory nerve at the distal end of the flap may result in a sensory flap if a suitable recipient nerve is available at the distal portion of the flap recipient site. Since location of a sensory nerve in close proximity to the vascular pedicle is generally required, the groin flap is rarely used as a neurosensory free flap.

Bone

The iliac crest provides an excellent source for vascularized bone grafting to the upper extremity (Fig. 27-4). A segment of the iliac crest may be transplanted either as an isolated vascularized bone graft or as an osteocutaneous flap. Taylor has described and demonstrated the blood supply of the bone graft from the deep circumflex iliac vascular system.[17,18] The cutaneous portion of the osteocutaneous flap may also be vascularized by the deep circumflex iliac vessels. However, the blood supply to the skin portion of the flap from the deep system may be both variable and unreliable. When using the flap as an osteocutaneous flap, the superficial circumflex iliac vascular system is a more reliable blood supply to the skin portion of the flap. Both vascular systems may be repaired by a double

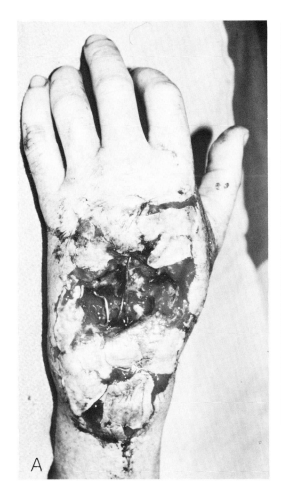
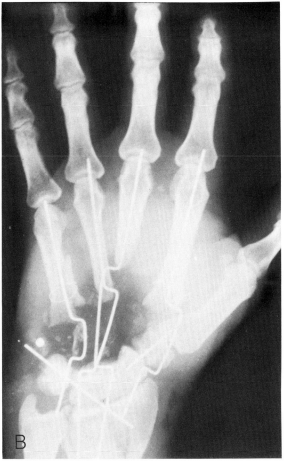

Fig. 27-4. Groin osteocutaneous flap. **(A)** Preoperative view. Gunshot wound to the hand with loss of dorsal skin and carpal bones. **(B)** Preoperative radiograph. Traumatic absence of the distal carpal row and lateral four metacarpal bases. K-wires have been used as temporary spacers to maintain bone position. *(Figure continues.)*

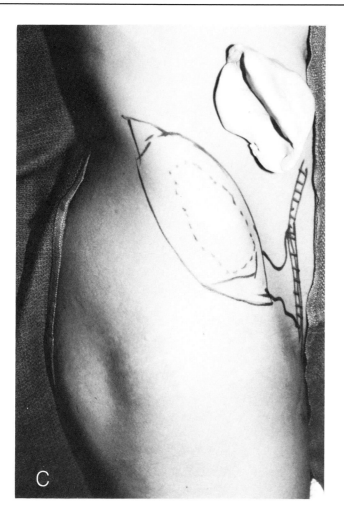

Fig. 27-4 *(Continued).* (**C**) Flap design. Preoperative planning includes skin island location and a template of the vascularized bone graft. (**D**) Flap elevation completed. Note the dual circulation to the flap from the superficial circumflex iliac artery *(sa)* and deep circumflex iliac artery *(da)* (*f*, femoral artery). *(Figure continues.)*

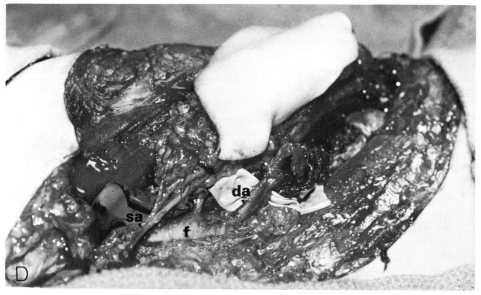

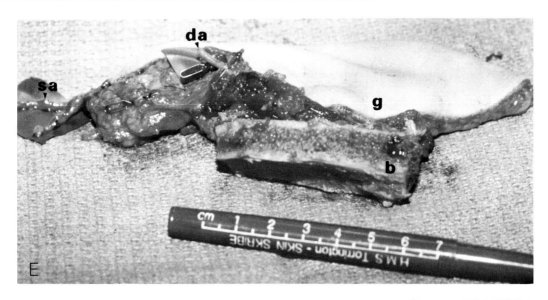

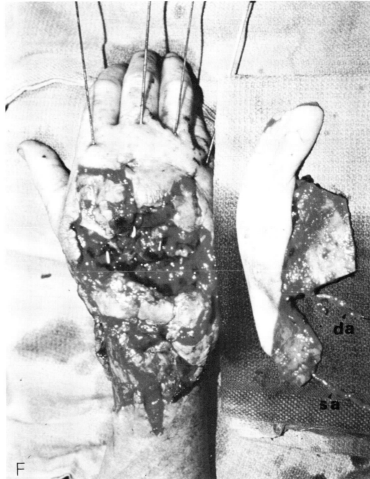

Fig. 27-4 *(Continued).* **(E)** The deep circumflex iliac flap is ready for transplantation. (*b*, iliac bone; *g*, groin skin; *sa*, superficial circumflex iliac artery pedicle; *da*, deep circumflex iliac artery.) **(F)** The vascularized bone prior to its insertion to replace the segmental defect. (*sa*, superficial circumflex iliac artery; *da*, deep circumflex iliac artery.) *(Figure continues.)*

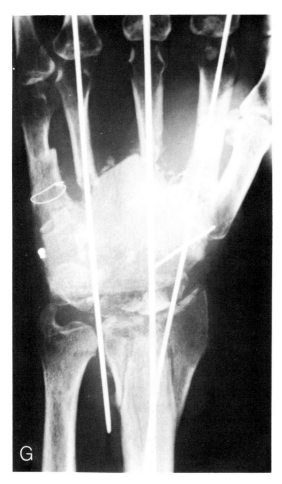

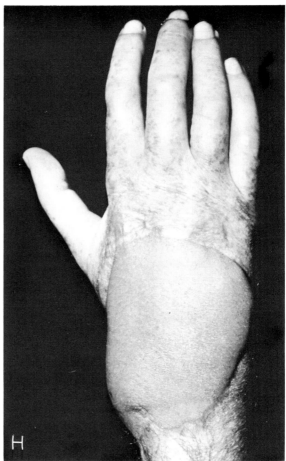

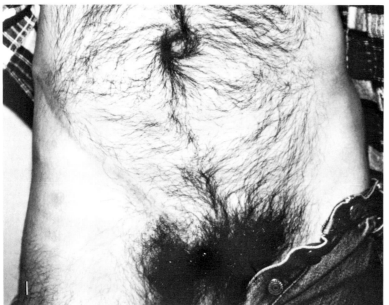

Fig. 27-4 *(Continued).* **(G)** A postoperative radiograph demonstrates the position of the vascularized iliac bone graft. **(H)** The flap has provided both vascularized bone and skin coverage in a single procedure. **(I)** Direct closure of the donor site with acceptable contour.

system microvascular anastomotic technique or by reconstruction of an internal shunt between the two vascular pedicles (Fig. 27-4F).

It has been demonstrated that, on occasion, the superficial circumflex iliac vascular system may support both the bone and skin portions of this osteocutaneous flap. However, this is much less reliable for the bone circulation than the deep system. In summary, the deep circumflex iliac vascular system alone should be used when transplanting the vascularized iliac bone itself; both the deep and superficial circumflex iliac systems are recommended when the osteocutaneous flap is transplanted. When no receptor vessels are available adjacent to the defect, vein grafts should be considered (Fig. 27-3).

Technique of Elevation of DCIA* Flap (Deep Groin Flap)

The technique of elevation of the deep circumflex iliac vascularized flap has been well described by Taylor.[17,18] Initially, a superior medial groin incision is made with a transinguinal approach to identify the external iliac artery and the origins of the deep circumflex iliac artery and vein. The vessels are then dissected from their origin to the inner surface of the iliac wing. In performing the dissection, the vessels should be kept under direct vision, with a muscular cuff preserved around the vessels to ensure preservation of attachments to both the bone and the perforator branches to the cutaneous portion of the flap. This muscle cuff will include portions of the external oblique, internal oblique, and transversus abdominis muscles. The periosteum over the iliac bone is preserved as the dissection proceeds in the iliac fossa after sweeping away the overlying portions of the iliacus muscle. Laterally, the origins of the sartorius, tensor fascia lata, and portions of the gluteus musculature are separated from their attachments to the iliac bone. The bone is cut according to a premade template, depending upon the requirements of the reconstruction (e.g., a bone block for replacement of lost metacarpals and carpals) (Fig. 27-4C). The vascular pedicle, which is immediately adjacent to the

° DCIA = Deep circumflex iliac artery.

deep surface of the iliac wing, must always be kept in view during the osteotomy. As the bone becomes detached, care must be taken to avoid lateral traction on the bone graft to prevent tension on the vessels.

If an osteocutaneous flap is planned, it is preferable to also include the superficial circumflex iliac vascular system with the flap. The origin of this vascular pedicle is dissected in a fashion similar to that described in the section on Elevation of the Superficial Groin Flap Proximal Approach on page 1155. The preferable venous system for the skin portion of the flap is through branches to the greater saphenous vein entering near the saphenous femoral bulb. When dissecting the osteocutaneous flap, care must be taken to preserve the perforators from the deep circumflex iliac vascular system through the fascia to the skin to provide cutaneous circulation through the deep system.

Injection studies have demonstrated that the lateral portion of the cutaneous skin flap is supplied more reliably by the deep system than is the medial portion of the skin flap.[14] During elevation of the osteocutaneous flap, the adequacy of the deep vascular system as the blood supply to the entire flap may be assessed, after completing the entire flap and vascular pedicle dissections, by placing a microvascular clamp on the superficial circumflex iliac vascular system. The cutaneous portion of the flap is then observed. Caution should be used in this technique, however, as a significant delay may be necessary to observe the true effects of temporary occlusion of the superficial circumflex iliac vascular systems. The inclusion of the superficial circumflex iliac vessels in the use of the osteocutaneous flap should be considered to ensure adequate circulation to the skin portion of the flap.

If both the superficial and deep vascular systems are to be used when transplanting the osteocutaneous flap, separate system microvascular anastomoses may be accomplished. However, an alternative to this is the microvascular connection of an internal arterial shunt between the deep and superficial systems. In this technique, the ascending vascular branch from the deep circumflex iliac artery to the flat muscles of the abdomen is preserved. This artery is repaired to the proximal end of the superficial circumflex iliac artery. An internal shunt is therefore established that will then be

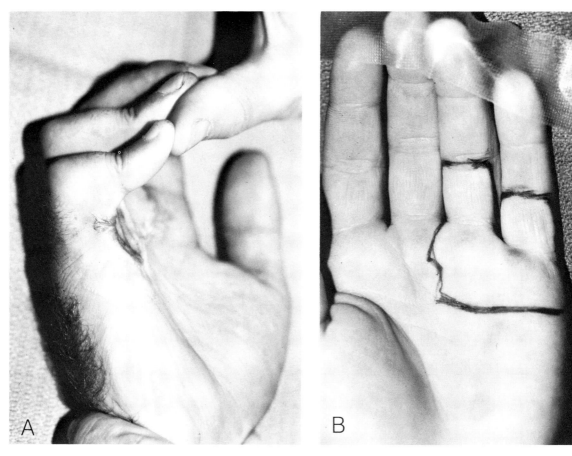

Fig. 27-5. Dorsalis pedis flap. **(A)** A burn scar contracture involving skin of the distal palm and proximal segments of the little and ring fingers. **(B)** The contralateral hand is used to determine the skin requirements for flap design. *(Figure continues.)*

in use when the proximal deep circumflex iliac artery is repaired to the recipient artery in the recipient area. The advantage is that dual arterial supply for the flap components is provided here while still only one recipient artery in the area of reconstruction is required. It is also possible for the deep circumflex iliac vein to provide satisfactory venous egress for the entire flap, obviating the need for a secondary venous anastomosis from the superficial system. If there is any question regarding the venous drainage, a second venous repair, using the superficial branches of the saphenous system, is recommended.

Donor Site

Superficial Groin. The donor site closure following elevation and transplantation of the groin flap generally can be accomplished by direct closure, although flexion of the hip is often necessary. A closed suction drainage system is required to avoid seroma formation. If the flap dimensions exceed 7 cm in width, skin grafts may be required in the donor site.

Deep Groin. The donor site closure for the deep circumflex iliac artery flap or osteocutaneous flap must be performed carefully to avoid a hernia (Fig.

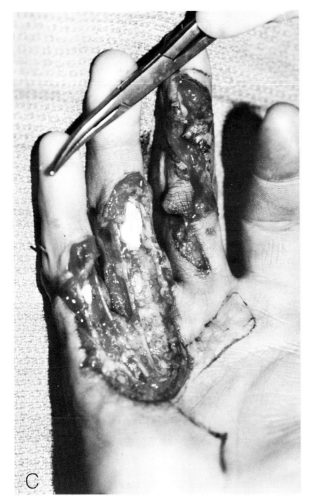

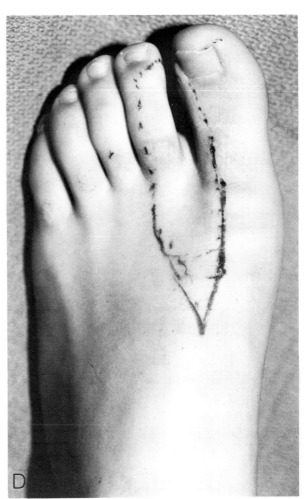

Fig. 27-5 *(Continued).* **(C)** The scarred skin is resected. **(D)** Flap design includes skin of the lateral side of the great toe and medial side of the second toe. *(Figure continues.)*

27-4I). The fascia of the iliacus and its muscle should be repaired to the transversalis fascia. The remnants of the internal and external oblique muscles are repaired in layers to the dissected ends of the tensor fascia lata and gluteus muscles. Transosseous sutures from the flat muscles of the abdomen to the remaining iliac bone may be placed for additional security. Reattachment of the inguinal ligament laterally also may be accomplished. Suction drainage is recommended.

DORSALIS PEDIS FLAP

The dorsalis pedis flap is now well accepted as a useful skin–fascial flap for microvascular transplantation. Initially described by both O'Brien and Shanmugan[40] and Furlow,[36] the flap was originally used as a local transposition flap and is now widely used as a reliable donor flap for transplantation to distant sites by microvascular techniques. The flap has two distinct advantages as a donor flap source in

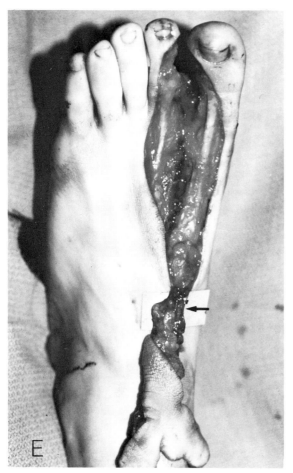 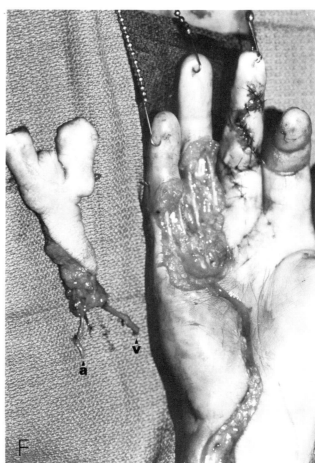

Fig. 27-5 *(Continued).* (**E**) Dorsalis pedis flap elevation is completed based on the dorsalis pedis artery and superficial vein. (The arrow indicates the pedicle location.) (**F**) The flap is ready for inset and revascularization. (*a*, dorsalis pedis artery; *v*, superficial vein.) *(Figure continues.)*

upper extremity reconstruction: its thinness (Fig. 27-5) and its potential as a sensory flap (Fig. 27-6). The major disadvantage in this flap is possible donor site disability. The flap size is limited to the dorsum of the foot, which is another disadvantage for coverage of large defects.[22–35,37–39,41–50]

Vascular Anatomy

This axial flap receives its arterial blood supply from the dorsalis pedis artery proximally, and distally from the continuation of this artery as the first dorsal metatarsal artery (Fig. 27-7). After the anterior tibial artery passes beneath the extensor retinaculum of the ankle, it is located between the ex-

tensor digitorum longus tendon laterally and the extensor hallucis longus tendon medially, beneath the extensor hallucis brevis muscle and superficial to the tarsal bones. At this level, the artery becomes the dorsalis pedis artery. The medial and lateral tarsal arteries, which are branches of the dorsalis pedis artery, provide cutaneous branches to the proximal skin of the dorsum of the foot. This portion of the skin also receives circulation from musculocutaneous perforators from the extensor hallucis brevis muscle. Immediately distal to the heads of the first and second metatarsals, the dorsalis pedis artery bifurcates into the first metatarsal artery and a deep branch into the plantar aspect of the foot. At this level, arterial branches are di-

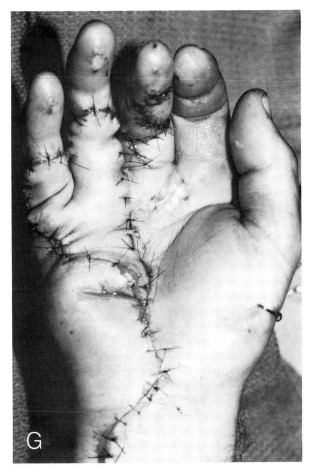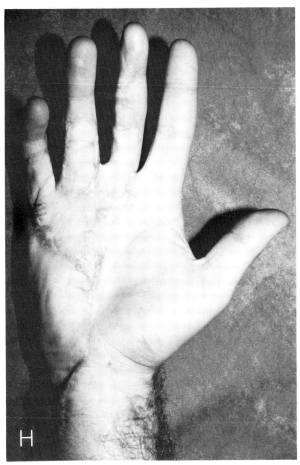

Fig. 27-5 *(Continued).* **(G)** The flap is inset after the microsurgical anastomoses have been completed. **(H)** Stable skin with release of scar contracture after single-staged flap transplantation.

rected into the dorsal skin, second metatarsal, and interosseous muscles. The first metatarsal artery continues into the first web space. At the level of the first transverse metatarsal ligament, the first and second dorsal digital arteries are branches of the first metatarsal artery. The artery then continues as a distal communicating artery that joins the plantar metatarsal arteries.

Variations in the arterial anatomy of this flap occur at the level of the bifurcation of the dorsalis pedis artery and at the level where the dorsal digital arteries arise from the first metatarsal artery. In anatomic studies, May and colleagues[34] noted that the first dorsal metatarsal artery may arise deep within the first dorsal metatarsal space. In this situ-

ation, the dorsal metatarsal artery courses beneath or through the interosseous muscle.

The venous drainage of the flap is via a superficial and deep system. Robinson[45] has noted three potential superficial venous systems: the greater saphenous vein, the median dorsal vein, and the lesser saphenous vein. The dorsalis pedis artery has paired venae comitantes that also provide for venous drainage via the deep system.

Flap Design

The flap is centered over the dorsum of the foot (Fig. 27-8A). Proximally, the flap is located below the extensor retinaculum, and distally it may be

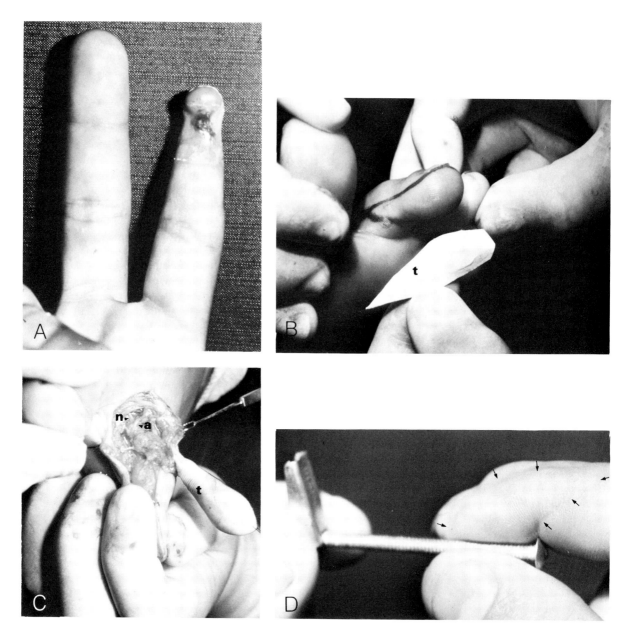

Fig. 27-6. Partial second toe–volar finger neurosensory flap. **(A)** Preoperative view. The index finger has complete loss of the distal digital nerve with very poor skin coverage. **(B)** Preoperative flap design on the medial plantar aspect of the second toe. A template *(t)* determines the exact dimensions of skin required to resurface the index finger defect. **(C)** Intraoperative view. The medial web space of the second toe *(t)* is elevated based on the first dorsal metatarsal artery *(a)*, superficial vein, and deep peroneal nerve *(n)*. **(D)** A postoperative view demonstrates greatly improved skin coverage on the volar aspect of the distal index finger (arrows denote flap inset site), with restoration of fine touch.

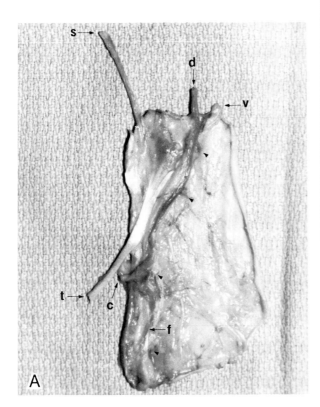
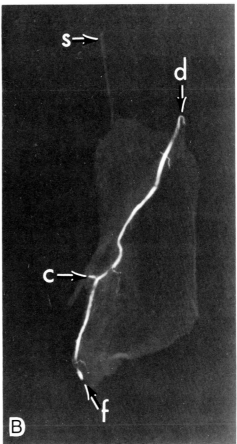

Fig. 27-7. Vascular anatomy of dorsalis pedis flap. (**A**) The deep surface of a dorsalis pedis flap. The small arrows denote cutaneous vascular communications from the pedicle. (*s*, superficial peroneal nerve; *d*, dorsalis pedis artery; *v*, venae comitantes; *f*, first dorsal metatarsal artery; *c*, deep communicating artery at first interosseous space; *t*, tendon of extensor hallucis brevis.) (**B**) Selective arteriogram of a dorsalis pedis flap. (*s*, superficial peroneal nerve; *d*, dorsalis pedis artery; *f*, first dorsal metatarsal artery; *c*, deep communicating artery at first interosseous space.)

extended either several centimeters above the web space or may include the first web space. The medial border of the flap is located along the course of the extensor hallucis longus tendon. Although the flap may be extended more medially, donor site problems can be avoided by preserving as much medial skin as possible. Laterally, the flap border is generally located at the level of the fifth metatarsal. Here, the flap may also be extended, but this skin is a random portion of the flap and is, therefore, less reliable in its circulation.

Bone

The second metatarsal is vascularized by the first dorsal metatarsal artery. The bone may be included within the flap where a composite of bone and overlying skin may be useful in upper extremity reconstruction.

Joint

The second metatarsophalangeal joint is also vascularized by the first dorsal metatarsal artery. Thus, for pediatric joint replacement, both skin

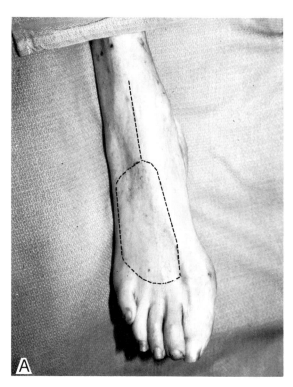
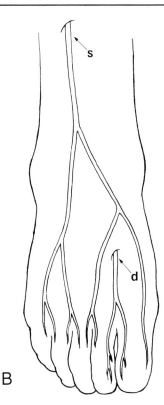

Fig. 27-8. Dorsalis pedis flap design. (**A**) Skin markings for a standard dorsalis pedis flap. (**B**) Preservation of sensory nerves allows skin coverage with potential as neuro-sensory flaps. (*s*, superficial peroneal nerve; *d*, deep peroneal nerve.)

and joint and associated epiphyses may be transplanted in one operation. In this specialized use of this skin–fascial flap, a joint with skin coverage can be transplanted with bone growth potential remaining intact (Fig. 27–9). See Chapter 30 for a more detailed discussion of the indications and techniques of free vascularized joint transplants.

Tendon

The extensor hallucis brevis tendon is generally included with the flap. The tendons of the extensor digitorum brevis may also be included with the flap as vascularized tendon grafts for reconstruction of upper extremity defects requiring both short tendon grafts and coverage.

Nerve

The superficial peroneal nerve provides sensory fibers for the proximal portion of the dorsalis pedis flap (Fig. 27-8B). After piercing the fascia on the lateral distal leg, it branches into the medial and intermediate dorsal cutaneous nerves. The individual nerves or the entire superficial peroneal nerve may be incorporated with the free flap as potential donor sensory nerves.

The deep peroneal nerve pierces the deep fascia of the foot at the first interosseous space. Distal to this level, the nerve provides sensory fibers to the first web space and lateral hallux and medial second toe. This nerve is only useful for dorsalis pedis flap transplantation if the first web space extension has been included with the flap (Fig. 27-6). When dorsal skin and bone are transplanted, the deep peroneal nerve should be included if sensation and flap coverage are required.

Technique of Elevation of the Dorsalis Pedis Flap

Preoperative palpation and the Doppler probe are used to locate the course of the dorsalis pedis artery. If there is evidence of prior trauma or vascular disease, arteriography is used to evaluate the

Fig. 27-9. Dorsalis pedis flap with joint transplantation. **(A)** 4-year-old child with traumatic loss of the long finger and the ring finger MP joint. Reconstructive requirements include dorsal skin and metatarsophalangeal joint with growth potential. **(B)** A radiograph of the hand demonstrates absence of the ring MP joint. **(C)** Structural similarity of the MP and metatarsophalangeal joints (arrows denote pertinent joint epiphyses). Ring finger — absence of MP joint (at left); ring finger (contralateral hand) MP joint (at center); second toe metatarsophalangeal joint (at right). *(Figure continues.)*

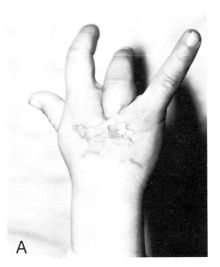

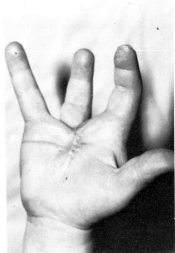

A

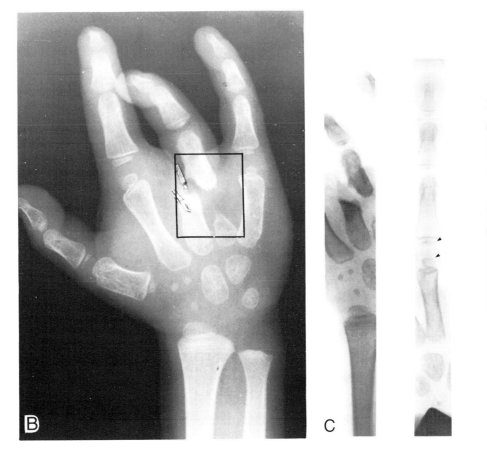

B

C

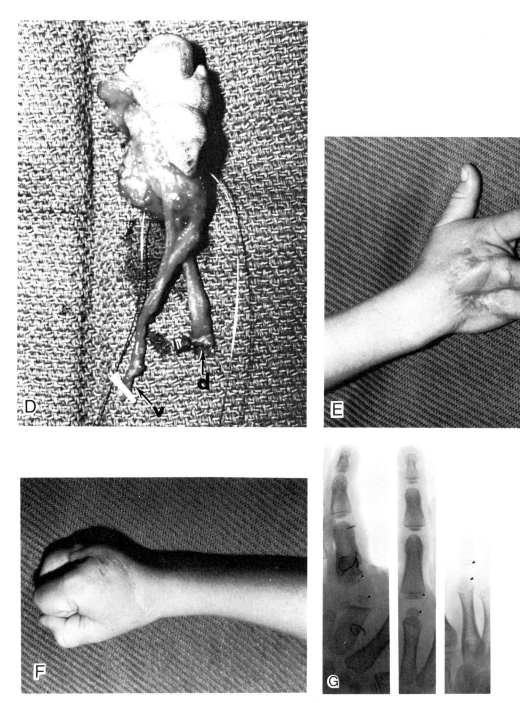

Fig. 27-9 *(Continued).* **(D)** The donor second metatarsophalangeal joint (note wires to the proximal phalanx and metatarsal for fixation). (*d*, dorsalis pedis artery; *v*, dorsal vein.) **(E)** Three years following microvascular joint transplantation (dorsal skin, extensor tendon, and joint). **(F)** The transplanted second joint provides functional joint space and growth of both epiphyses 3 years postoperatively. **(G)** Two and one-half years following free joint transplantation. Comparison of epiphyseal growth in the second metatarsophalangeal and second MP joints (arrows denote pertinent epiphyses). Ring finger — transplanted second metatarsophalangeal joint (at left); ring finger (normal contralateral hand) MP joint (at center); second toe (contralateral foot) second metatarsophalangeal joint (at right). *(Figure continues.)*

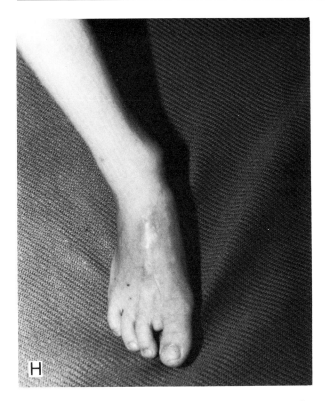

Fig. 27-9 *(Continued).* **(H)** Three years postoperatively, donor site closure provides stable coverage and no functional disability. (**A–D,G** from Mathes SJ, Buchanan R, Weeks PM: Microvascular joint transplantation with epiphyseal growth. J Hand Surg 5:586–589, 1980.)

common extensor tendons (Fig. 27-10B). The dissection proceeds medially at the level of the second metatarsal; the bifurcation of the dorsalis pedis artery into the first metatarsal artery and communicating branch must be identified. This is a critical area of the dissection. After the surgeon has identified the continuation of the dorsalis pedis artery as the first dorsal metatarsal artery, the deep branch is divided (Fig. 27-10C). The dissection is then continued distally, carefully staying beneath the first dorsal metatarsal artery. The medial flap incision is then made, and this portion of the dissection is performed superficial to the paratenon of the extensor hallucis longus tendon. The dissection again enters into the first interosseous space until communication with the lateral dissection is completed. The extensor hallucis brevis tendon is divided as the distal first interosseous space is entered. The distal first dorsal metatarsal artery and its venae comitantes are divided at the distal end of the flap. If the first web space is included with the flap, the dissection should stay plantar to the first and second dorsal digital arteries. Finally, in this situation, the distal digital arteries and distal communicating artery at the level of the transmetacarpal ligament are divided.

The initial flap elevation may begin with the incision along the medial flap border. With this approach, the proximal flap dissection again is started beneath the dorsalis pedis artery. The interosseous space is entered and the deep branch is located at the level of the first metatarsal head. The entire borders of the flap are generally not incised until the deep branch is divided and the dorsalis pedis artery and the first metatarsal artery are seen correctly and located within the flap. Then, the lateral flap is elevated as previously described, completing flap elevation.

During proximal flap elevation, the previously noted superficial veins are preserved. With completion of flap elevation, the superficial veins are dissected proximally, depending on required pedicle length. In a similar manner, the arterial pedicle can be lengthened by proximal dissection until the desired length is achieved. By proximal dissection in the distal leg, the dorsalis pedis–anterior tibial pedicle length may reach 6 to 8 cm. The superficial peroneal nerve for the dorsal foot skin and the deep peroneal nerve for the web space may be preserved with the flap when a sensory flap is indicated. This

donor vessels. In rare instances, the anterior tibial artery will be absent. A tourniquet above the ankle is used to occlude venous flow, allowing mapping of the superficial venous system through the flap. The leg is not wrapped with an Esmarch bandage before the thigh tourniquet is inflated. This allows a bloodless field for the flap elevation but does not completely empty the veins. In this manner, the delicate veins can be readily identified and preserved. A vertical incision proximal to the base of the flap is made between the extensor hallucis longus and extensor digitorum longus tendons (Fig. 27-10A). The extensor retinaculum is incised, allowing visualization of the proximal dorsalis pedis artery and its associated venae comitantes. The distal belly of the extensor hallucis brevis muscle is divided at the base of the flap. The lateral aspect of the flap is then incised and the lateral flap elevated immediately superficial to the paratenon of the

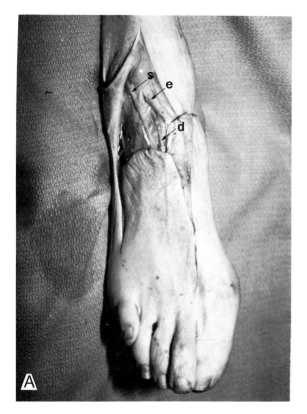

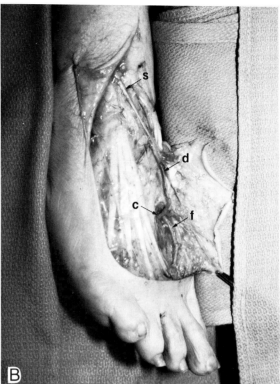

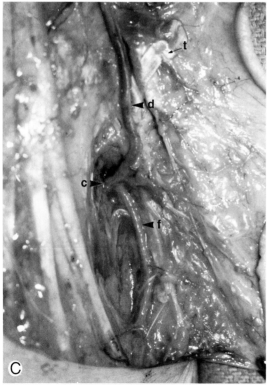

Fig. 27-10. Dorsalis pedis flap — technique of elevation. (**A**) A proximal vertical incision allows exposure of the dorsalis pedis artery, superficial dorsal veins, and superficial peroneal nerve. (*s*, superficial peroneal nerve; *d*, dorsalis pedis artery and venae comitantes; *e*, extensor hallucis longus.) (**B**) A critical phase of dissection occurs between the first and second metatarsals. (*s*, superficial peroneal nerve; *d*, dorsalis pedis artery and venae comitantes; *c*, deep communicating artery; *f*, first dorsal metatarsal artery.) (**C**) The first dorsal interosseous space with the dorsalis pedis flap retracted medially. Flap dissection must remain deep to the dorsalis pedis artery and first dorsal metatarsal artery at this level. (*t*, tendon of extensor hallucis brevis; *d*, dorsalis pedis artery; *c*, deep communicating artery at site of its division for flap elevation; *f*, first dorsal metatarsal artery.)

is especially useful in upper extremity reconstruction.

Transplantation of a composite flap incorporating the second metatarsal or second metatarsophalangeal joint requires slight modification of the operative technique (Fig. 27-9). At the level of the deep branch of the dorsalis pedis artery, the second metatarsal is divided. The distal dissection then remains beneath the periosteum of the second metatarsal. The metatarsophalangeal joint is disarticulated or the proximal phalanx is divided if transplantation of the joint is intended. If the MP joint is removed with the flap, the plantar skin of the second toe is used as a flap to assist in closure of the donor defect.

Donor Site

The donor site following dorsalis pedis flap elevation requires skin graft coverage. The skin graft is meshed 1.5 : 1 and placed on the donor defect. Although not expanded, the mesh graft contours nicely to the irregular surface on the dorsum of the foot. This results in rapid graft vascularization and acceptable graft appearance. A compressive dressing immobilizing both the ankle and knee joints is worn for 7 days. At the time of discharge, the patient is instructed to wear a Jobst compressive stocking for 3 to 6 months to minimize hypertrophic scar formation on the dorsum of the foot. Although donor site coverage problems are a recognized complication of the dorsalis pedis flap operation, this approach to the standard dorsalis pedis free flap has provided successful stable coverage in patients in whom it has been used.

With both extended dorsalis pedis flap into the first web space and the composite dorsalis pedis flap and second metatarsal, distal donor site coverage often requires a local plantar flap. Closure following metatarsophalangeal joint removal has been accomplished by removal of the distal phalanx and use of the plantar skin of the second toe to assist in donor site coverage (Fig. 27-9H).

SECOND TOE–TO–DIGIT TRANSPLANTATION

Using the entire second toe as a composite free flap is a natural extension of the dorsalis pedis flap, and therefore a discussion of this flap is presented here.

Indications

In patients requiring opposable digits for use with a thumb, the second toe–to–digit transplant provides an opposable structure with good sensation that does not require cortical reorientation. The pulp surface of the second toe is quite usable for opposition and pinch with the thumb. Both congenital and traumatic deformities are potential indications for second toe–to–digit transplantation (Fig. 27–11). Where a single opposable digit is available in the hand, second toe transplantation to an adjacent position provides excellent three-finger pinch and grasp. In patients where there are no opposable digits for the thumb, double second toe transplantation, performed simultaneously, may accomplish a tremendous reconstructive goal in one operation.[54,57] The two second toe transplants may also be performed in separate operations. If the appropriate level of microvascular expertise is available in the surgical team, there should be no difference in the success rate of simultaneous double toe transplantations as opposed to sequential operations. The time and cost effectiveness of the double toe procedure in one operation versus two is obvious.

The second toe is also useful in toe-digital transplantation for thumb reconstruction[55] (Fig. 27-12). The complexity of the procedure is similar to great toe transplantation, so the decision to use great or second toe is based both on donor and recipient site factors. The great toe generally looks more natural as a thumb than the second toe. In a very large great toe, a second debulking procedure is frequently required. There are several features about the biomechanics of the second toe that differ from the fingers, thumb, or great toe. The metatarsophalangeal joint of the second toe is a hyperextensile joint. It is extremely difficult to obtain any useful flexion at this joint in reconstruction. In addition, the interphalangeal joints of the second toe have a tendency to assume a flexed posture. This is an advantage in obtaining flexion postoperatively; however, this may be a disadvantage if excessive flexion results in a hooked position. The problem is avoided by pinning the interphalangeal joints of the second toe transplant in extension for 3 weeks.

Although no significant difference in foot function is observed after use of either the great or second toe, the foot appearance is better after sec-

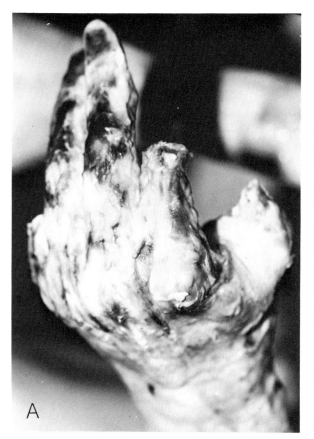
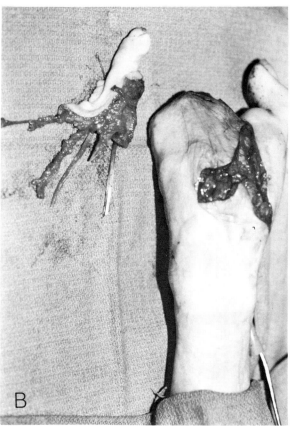

Fig. 27-11. Second toe — digital transplantation. **(A)** Preoperative view: The left hand presented with deep circumferential full thickness burns. Initial reconstruction required wound debridements and skin grafts. **(B)** The patient has already had a hallux-thumb transplantation. The second toe is ready for transplantation to index finger position. *(Figure continues.)*

ond toe transplantation. If the metatarsal bone is required with the toe transplantation, the second toe is preferred since loss of the second metacarpal does not impair foot function, in contrast to isolated absence of the first metatarsal.

Generally, distal finger amputation sites provided with stable, nonpainful coverage are well accepted by the patient in terms of function and appearance. However, Yoshimura[63] has demonstrated excellent reconstruction of the distal half of digits with toe-digital transplantation, and when either cosmetic appearance or finger length is essential, this procedure warrants consideration.

Restoration of sensation to the volar aspect of the thumb and opposing digits has traditionally been accomplished by transposition of a neurovascular island flap from an adjacent digit, or the use of a radial sensory-innervated cross-finger flap. Both techniques require cortical reorientation to adapt to sensory input from an alternate digit. Furthermore, the donor digit, especially in the volar digital neurovascular island flap, has an area of sensory loss. The innervated cross-finger flap, using the stump of the digital nerve from the injured digit as a proximal source of sensory axons, has addressed the problem of cortical re-education. All of these techniques require availability of local vascularized tissue with an expendable intact sensory nerve.

An alternate method of reconstruction that provides the ability to restore native sensation to the injured digit is the microsurgical transplantation of

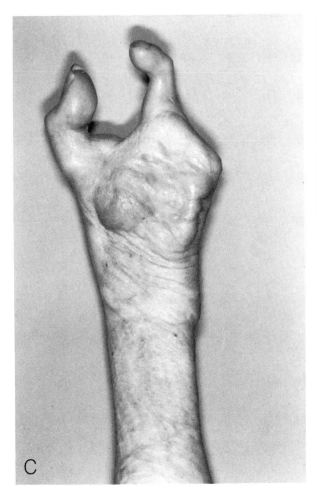

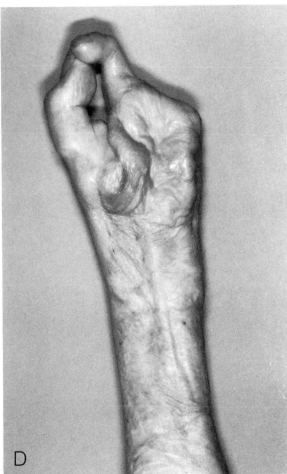

Fig. 27-11 *(Continued).* **(C)** Postoperative view. Hallux and second toe transplanted digits to the hand. **(D)** Postoperative view. Pinch between the transplanted hallux and second toe has been restored. **(E)** Staged hallux and second toe transplants can provide useful function in a severely injured hand.

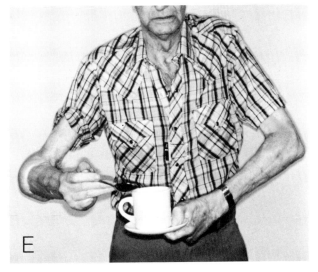

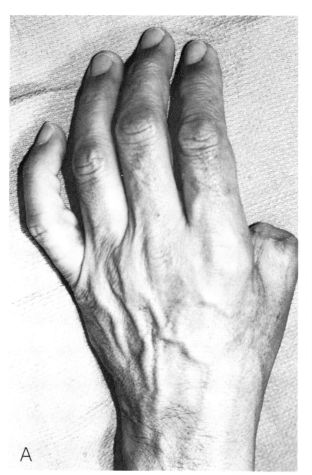

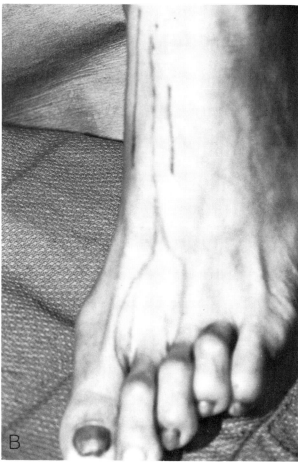

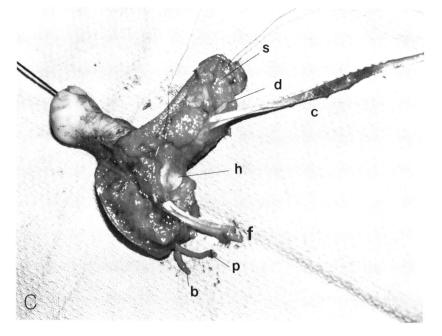

Fig. 27-12. Second toe— thumb transplantation. **(A)** Pre- operative view showing trau- matic loss of the thumb. **(B)** Preoperative design of the sec- ond toe composite flap. **(C)** The second toe is ready for transplan- tation to thumb position. (Note: the plantar arterial system was used to revascularize the second toe in this patient.) (*s*, superficial vein; *c*, extensor tendon; *d*, deep peroneal nerve; *h*, proximal pha- lanx; *f*, flexor tendon; *p*, plantar nerve; *b*, plantar artery. (*Figure continues.*)

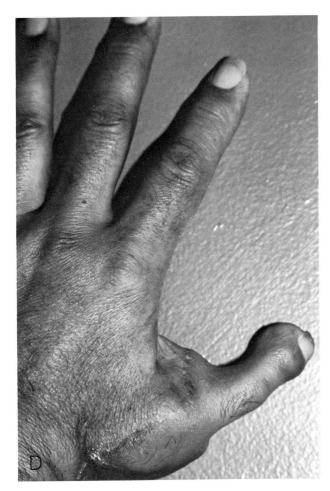

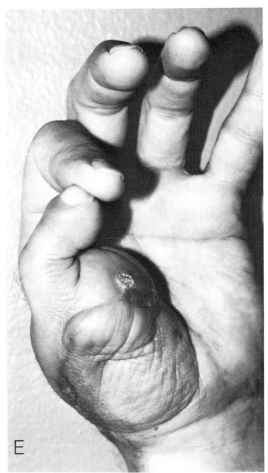

Fig. 27-12 *(Continued).* **(D)** Two years postoperative, dorsal view. The thumb was revascularized by microvascular anastomosis between the plantar artery and the deep volar arterial arch and between the superficial vein and the dorsal hand vein. **(E)** The second toe provides opposition between the reconstructed thumb and the normal index finger.

neurovascular island flaps of either toe pulp or a small distal dorsalis pedis flap.[59,61] The use of a distant source for the neurovascular flap eliminates the necessity of using local tissue in an already impaired upper extremity.

A small, distally designed dorsalis pedis flap may include branches of the superficial or deep peroneal nerves or both as they enter and exit the flap to provide two vascularized nerve grafts, along with a full-thickness skin flap for resurfacing small defects in the hand and using the proximal sensory nerves of the area as recipient sensory axons.

Maximum rehabilitation of the hand should be completed before the use of toe-digital transplantation for hand reconstruction is considered. The techniques described for toe-digital transplantation will vary, depending on the extent of the hand injury and reconstructive requirements. The donor dissection must correspondingly be tailored to these requirements. Donor site closure in the foot must be considered in order to avoid future functional impairment of the foot. With careful preoperative planning, the medial foot and its terminal phalanges provide the hand surgeon knowledgeable in microsurgical techniques a means to restore useful function to the injured hand.

Vascular Anatomy

The second toe is vascularized by both the first and second dorsal metatarsal arteries via the dorsalis pedis artery and the first and second plantar metatarsal arteries via the deep plantar arch (Fig. 27-13). In most instances, the dominant arterial source for the second toe is via the first metatarsal artery. As previously noted in the description of the vascular anatomy for the dorsalis pedis flap, the first dorsal metatarsal artery courses in the first web space. Here it bifurcates into the dorsal plantar arteries, entering into the hallux and second toe. The plantar or deep branch of the dorsalis pedis artery courses between the first and second metatarsals, joining the lateral plantar artery to form the deep plantar arch. The first and second plantar metatarsal arteries, branches from the deep plantar arch, course beneath the head of the flexor hallucis brevis muscle. At the plantar aspect of each web space, the plantar artery bifurcates and forms digital vessels to adjacent toes. In the first web space, the digital vessels supply the great and second toes. The second toe is transplanted based on either the first dorsal metatarsal artery from the dorsalis pedis artery or the plantar digital artery from the deep plantar arch.

The technique for second toe transplantation to

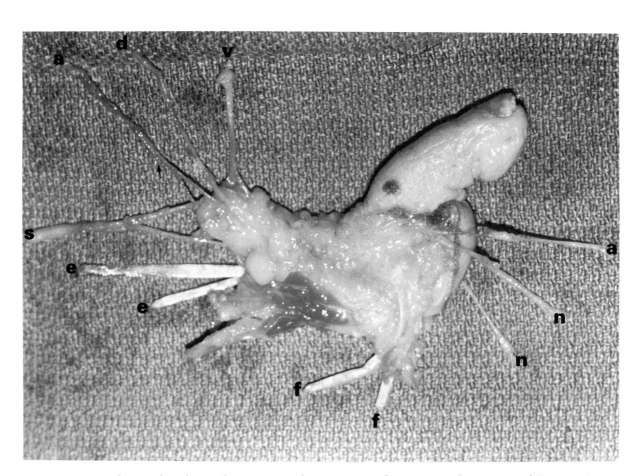

Fig. 27-13. Second toe — digital transplantation. A cadaver specimen demonstrates the anatomy of the second toe as a composite tissue for transplantation to thumb or digital position in the hand. Dorsal structures: *v*, superficial vein; *d*, deep peroneal nerve; *a*, dorsalis pedis artery (arrow denotes divided branch of first dorsal metatarsal artery to hallux); *s*, superficial peroneal nerve; *e*, extensor tendons. Plantar structures: *f*, flexor tendons; *n*, plantar sensory nerves; *a* plantar artery.

the thumb or digit position is quite similar to the operative sequence used in the great toe transplantation (see Chapter 31). Either the dorsal arterial system, using the first dorsal metatarsal artery from the dorsalis pedis artery or the plantar system (if the first dorsal metatarsal artery is not the dominant vessel in the toe) may be used. The medial plantar artery is the one vascular pedicle most readily used when the plantar arterial system is required. Division of the intermetatarsal ligament between the great and second toes facilitates dissection of the plantar arterial system. Whichever arterial arcade is used, the branch of that system to the great toe must by necessity be divided. If both systems are to be preserved in the transplant, as an insurance policy, vessels to the great toe from both systems must then be divided. Management of the tendons and nerves is similar to great toe transplantation.

Unlike the great toe transplant, the metatarsal is readily elevated in second toe transplantation. An osteotomy at the appropriate level, depending upon the amount of length required in the hand, is accomplished. This also facilitates donor site closure. The donor site is closed in layers. The intermetatarsal ligament is reapproximated with care taken to establish a balanced relationship with the remaining metatarsal heads.

In toe-to-digit transplantation, use of a common volar digital arterial system as the recipient vasculature in the hand is often indicated. Venous drainage is again established through the dorsal venous system.

Technique for Second Toe – Thumb Transplantation

The technique for toe-thumb transplantation can be divided into three phases: (1) toe dissection, (2) hand dissection, and (3) toe fixation in the thumb position and microvascular repair. The first two phases may be performed simultaneously by two operating teams. As the microvascular repair and associated bone and tendon repairs are accomplished, the second team may close the foot donor area.

Toe Dissection. Unless the foot shows evidence of arterial disease, absent dorsalis pedis pulse, or prior injury, preoperative arteriography is not required. The design for the skin incision should

allow for direct closure of the plantar aspect of the donor area by preservation of plantar skin to close over the preserved second metatarsal (Fig. 27-12B). The operative procedure is performed with an arterial tourniquet in place to obtain a bloodless field. A vertical incision between the first and second metatarsals is connected to a circumferential incision around the toe. Medial and lateral dorsal skin flaps are elevated superficial to the dorsal veins of the foot. The dorsal veins draining the toe are dissected proximally where they unite to form the greater saphenous vein. The tendon of the extensor hallucis brevis is divided, preserving the dorsal veins, and the muscle is retracted laterally. At this level, the deep peroneal nerve and the dorsalis pedis artery and its paired venae comitantes are located, and the dissection proceeds distally into the first web space. In the course of this dissection, the deep branch of the dorsalis pedis artery is also identified. With the dissection proceeding along the first metatarsal artery, the branches of the first metatarsal artery and the deep peroneal nerve to the great toe are divided. A plantar flap is elevated proximally to the level of the metatarsophalangeal joint. The plantar digital arteries and the plantar nerves are identified. The medial plantar artery to the great toe is divided, and the lateral plantar artery is preserved for later assessment of its role in second toe arterial circulation.

The long flexor to the second toe is identified at the level of the metatarsophalangeal joint. An incision is made in the medial plantar foot, extending between the abductor hallucis and flexor digitorum brevis muscles. The flexor tendon is divided at this level. The tendon is then pulled into the distal operative field at the level of the metatarsophalangeal joint. The flexor tendon must be of adequate length so that this tendon repair can be performed at wrist level following toe transplantation in the thumb position.

Following identification and division of the extensor tendon proximal to the metatarsophalangeal joint, the joint is disarticulated. The toe is now completely mobilized with the exception of its nerve, arterial, and venous proximal communications.

The tourniquet is released, allowing assessment of the relative role of the first metatarsal artery and the lateral digital plantar artery in the toe circulation. A microclip is placed on the lateral plantar digital artery, and toe circulation is evaluated. In most instances, the dominant arterial source is via the first metatarsal artery, so this maneuver should not adversely affect the arterial circulation of the toe. If arterial inflow is adversely affected by this maneuver, the microclip is removed and placed on the first dorsal metatarsal artery. If the dominant arterial source to the toe is from the plantar digital artery, proximal dissection of the plantar metatarsal artery beneath the flexor hallucis brevis muscle is required to increase the pedicle length. The second toe is now ready for transplantation based on either the dorsal or plantar metatarsal artery. The dominant of these two arteries is selected for the arterial repair. The arterial and venous pedicles are, however, not divided until the hand dissection is completed and appropriate receptor vessels and nerves have been identified.

Hand Dissection. In general, the princeps pollicis artery and dorsal hand veins are available as receptor vessels on the dorsum of the hand. These vessels are located by use of the Doppler probe for the artery and venous tourniquet for the veins. In extensive hand injuries, preoperative arteriography is required to locate an appropriate receptor artery in the hand. A hand radiograph is required to evaluate the location for bony fixation for the transplanted toe. The following structures are located in the hand during this dissection: (1) dorsal receptor veins; (2) princeps pollicis artery or other appropriate receptor arteries (deep volar arch for plantar artery); (3) extensor pollicis longus tendons or other suitable extensor tendon for use as thumb extensor; (4) flexor pollicis longus tendon or other suitable tendon for use as thumb flexor; (5) dorsal sensory branch of the radial nerve; (6) volar digital nerve to the thumb (in thumb avulsion amputations, the stumps of these nerves can generally be located volar to the adductor pollicis muscles); and (7) first metacarpal or remaining portion of proximal phalanx. (The site of bony fixation of the transplanted toe will obviously vary, depending on the nature of the injury resulting in thumb loss.) Since the flexor tendon repair is generally performed in the wrist, the flexor pollicis longus tendon is also identified at the wrist level through a volar incision

proximal to the transverse carpal ligament. The stump of the flexor pollicis longus tendon is connected to a tendon rod or rubber catheter and then pulled into the wrist. Later the transplanted flexor of the toe will be connected to the silicone rod and also pulled into the wrist, maintaining its correct position in the flexor tendon sheath.

In the severely injured hand, variables in hand dissection may include location of the receptor artery, appropriate receptor site for bony fixation, and appropriate tendons to provide the thumb with flexion and extension and abduction, if the thenar muscles are absent. Careful preoperative assessment should include these considerations to expedite the hand dissection.

Toe Fixation in Thumb Position and Microvascular Repairs. If they are required, vein grafts should be prepared before the vasculature to the toe is divided. Proximal dissection of the deep peroneal nerve and plantar nerves of the toe may be required if appropriate sensory nerves in the hand are located at some distance from the thumb position. Careful measurements will avoid nerve repairs under tension or the need for nerve grafts.

The dorsal vein and dorsalis pedis artery and its paired venae comitantes and sensory nerves are divided. The deep branch of the dorsalis pedis artery and the lateral plantar digital artery (unless this is the dominant blood supply to the thumb) are divided and ligated.

There are now many options for the technique of osteosynthesis in toe-to-thumb transplantation. These techniques will work very well as long as solid bony fixation and contact are achieved. When the stump of the proximal phalanx of the thumb is long enough, an excellent technique is to fashion a bony spike out of this proximal phalangeal stump and to core out a mirror image receptacle pocket in the proximal phalanx of the toe. Excellent bony contact can then be achieved by inserting the proximal phalangeal spicule of the thumb into the cored-out proximal phalanx of the toe, establishing a large area of bony surface contact, as well as a tight junction. Fixation with this technique is then provided by K-wires.

Interosseous wires are also a satisfactory way to achieve fixation. These may be oriented in a perpendicular fashion to each other or in a solid tetrahedral design. The combination of one K-wire, along with interosseous wires, is also quite satisfactory. Other techniques, such as figure-of-8 tension band wiring, screws, and small plates are all additional ways to achieve fixation.

Step-cut osteotomies are an alternative method of providing an extensive area of bony contact. This technique is frequently used when the amputation site in the hand is proximal to the MP joint.

In the special situations where the thumb amputation site is at the level of the MP joint, reconstruction of this joint is possible. If the articular surface of the head of the first metacarpal is in satisfactory condition, mobilization of the distally based soft tissue flaps around the base of the head of the metacarpal may be accomplished to achieve a capsular ligament framework. The concave cartilaginous surface of the proximal phalanx of the toe may be articulated with the thumb metacarpal and the collateral ligaments, volar plate, and dorsal capsule of the toe itself used in reconstructing the new capsule of the MP joint. This joint reconstruction has proved to be very satisfactory, achieving significant stable and painless motion at the newly reconstructed joint.

After completion of osteosynthesis or joint reconstruction, the actual repair of nerve, vascular pedicles, and tendon is started. The long flexor of the toe is connected to a silicone rod or rubber catheter and pulled into the wrist for later repair. Volar digital – plantar digital nerve and radial sensory – deep peroneal nerve repairs are accomplished by using the operating microscope. The dorsal vein – saphenous vein, dorsal vein – venae comitantes, and princeps pollicis or deep volar arch – dorsalis pedis or plantar artery microanastomoses are completed. After adequate profusion of the hallux is confirmed, the extensor and flexor tendon repairs are performed.

Skin closure should be done so as to avoid tension in the region of the arterial and venous repairs. Skin grafts are commonly used over the dorsal first web space directly covering the arterial and venous repair sites if tension is likely, following direct closure.

The donor site closure on the foot is performed simultaneously with hand closure. Preserved plantar skin is reflected over the distal metatarsal. Skin grafts are often used to complete skin closure over the dorsum of the foot.

Immediate and Late Postoperative Management

Postoperatively, patients are given low molecular weight Dextran, 500 cc/day, and aspirin, 325 mg/day, for 5 days. The patient's room is kept warm postoperatively to facilitate vasodilitation and to prevent spasm. Products containing nicotine and caffeine are avoided. During the immediate postoperative period, the hand is immobilized in a plaster splint. A custom orthoplast splint is fashioned at approximately 1 week by the hand therapy department. Active and passive range of motion exercises are instituted within 3 weeks with careful supervision by the hand therapist. A close line of communication between the surgeon, therapist, and patient is mandatory to achieve the optimal functional result.

This early motion regimen may be modified depending upon local conditions involved in each specific case. Factors dictating such modifications would include extensive skin grafts, position and type of osteosynthesis, and the overall quality of the tissue in the hand. Supervised passive motion of isolated joints is instituted early in essentially all patients. At 8 weeks, the patients are allowed to resume normal daily activities using the hand. Heavy and stressful activities are allowed at 3 months postoperatively.

PULP TRANSPLANTATION

The transplantation of a neurovascular island flap from the great toe lateral plantar pulp or second toe medial pulp is a very useful operation to reconstruct the distal volar portions of thumb or index finger.[61] The tremendous advantage of this technique is in providing innervated pulp tissue that is similar to the missing tissue in these critical pinch and grasp areas. The hand digital nerves are used to reinnervate the neurovascular island flap so that no cortical reorientation by the patient is required to adapt to alternative sensory sources. Donor site morbidity is negligible and limited to a minor aesthetic deformity. A skin graft may be required for closure of the defect in the toe.

JOINT TRANSPLANTATION

Microvascular joint transplantation from the foot to the hand in both MP and PIP joint positions has been reported for both congenital and traumatic indications.[58] The results in large numbers of cases are not available as yet, and the candidacy for these cases must be highly individualized. Obviously, the restoration of joint function in a damaged or missing joint, without the use of allogeneic material, is a desirable goal. See Chapter 30 for a more detailed discussion of the indications, techniques, and limitations of free vascularized joint transfers.

SUPERFICIAL INFERIOR EPIGASTRIC ARTERY FLAP

The skin located between the umbilicus and pubis represents an excellent donor site since closure of the donor defect, especially in the parous female, is accomplished at the pubic crease. This region of skin was initially utilized as a pedicle flap by Wood[62] in 1863. Shaw and Payne[60] in 1964 and Barfred[52] in 1976 described use of the superficial inferior epigastric pedicled flap for hand coverage. This area was frequently utilized for staged transfer for coverage of hand defects prior to the description of the groin flap. In 1971, Antia and Burk[51] successfully transplanted this skin–fascia flap to the face. Subsequently, Boeckx and colleagues[54] demonstrated the reliability of this flap in microvascular composite tissue transplantation.

The location of the donor site on the lower abdominal wall allows simultaneous flap elevation and preparation of the upper extremity recipient site (Fig. 27-14). In the thin patient, the flap is reasonably thin. Furthermore, fat located deep to Scarpa's fascia can be safely excised. The ideal location of the donor site scar has made this flap useful in upper extremity reconstruction (Fig. 27-15).

Vascular Anatomy

The superficial epigastric artery originates from the common femoral artery 2 to 3 cm below the inguinal ligament (Fig. 27-14B). The artery has been noted to have a common origin with the superficial circumflex iliac artery in 48 percent of dissections in anatomical studies. Although Taylor and Daniels[19] noted complete absence of this vessel in 35 percent of their dissections, Hester and his colleagues[56] found the vessels inadequate for free flap transplantation in only one of 16 patients (10 percent). The artery and its venae comitans course superior and lateral deep to Scarpa's fascia over the inguinal ligament. Midway between the pubic tubercle and anterior superior iliac spine, the vascular pedicle courses superiorly onto the abdominal wall. Immediately superior to the inguinal ligament, the pedicle perforates Scarpa's fascia and branches within the anterior inferior abdominal wall subcutaneous tissue. The pedicle supplies circulation to the entire ipsilateral hemiabdomen skin and will support skin across the midline.

The venous drainage of this flap is provided by both a superficial and deep system. The superficial inferior epigastric vein accompanies the artery. A large medial epigastric vein, which drains into the saphenous vein, is located medial to the superficial inferior epigastric artery and is most commonly utilized as the draining vein for flap transplantation.

Flap Design

A Doppler probe is used to locate the course of the superficial inferior epigastric artery as it courses over the inguinal ligament midway between the pelvis and anterior superior iliac spine. The flap is designed either vertically or horizontally on the inferior abdominal wall. Transverse orientation of the skin island between the pubis and umbilicus is preferred since direct closure by advancement of the superior abdominal skin is possible (Fig. 27-14A). The skin island extends from the midline to the anterior superior iliac spine. The contralateral skin is often excised and discarded to allow closure as a standard abdominoplasty in the parous female.

Technique of Elevation of the Inferior Epigastric Flap

The inferior border of the flap is incised to the level of Scarpa's fascia with a vertical incision extending across the inguinal ligament over the femo-

Fig. 27-14. Superficial inferior epigastric flap. (**A**) Preoperative flap design (cadaver specimen). The inferior skin incision is located 2 to 3 cm superior to the inguinal ligament (*p*, pubic tubercle; *s*, anterior superior iliac spine). Vertical incision (a–b) is used to locate the vascular pedicle. The flap may extend across the midline with transverse orientation or extend to the costal margin with vertical orientation. (**B**) Vascular anatomy. Cadaver specimen demonstrates the vascular pedicle to skin fascial flap, with superficial inferior epigastric artery branch of femoral artery (*a*), and superficial branch of saphenous vein (*v*).

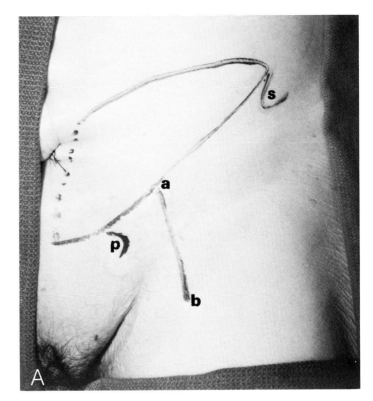

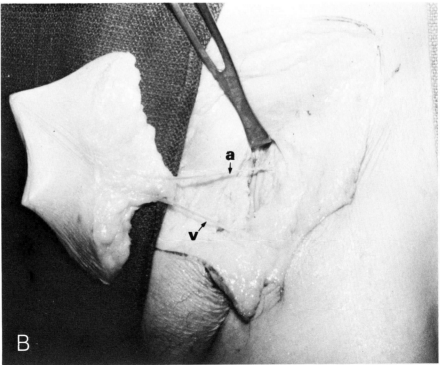

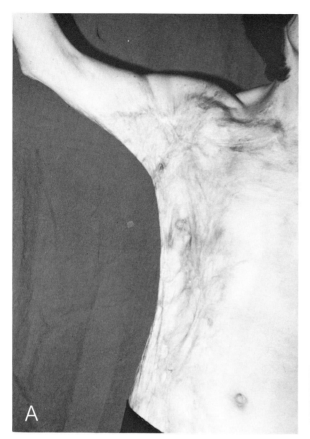

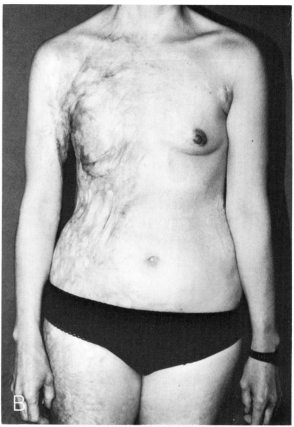

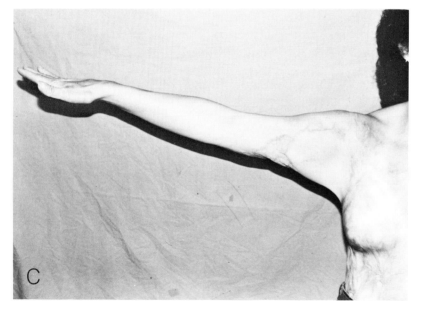

Fig. 27-15. Superficial inferior epigastric flap. **(A)** A preoperative photograph demonstrates severe axillary burn contracture in a young woman. **(B)** The left inferior abdominal wall contains normal skin without excessive subcutaneous tissue. This area was selected as the donor site for the flap, since direct closure will avoid a severe donor site scar. **(C)** A postoperative photograph demonstrates the site of axillary release with transplanted lower abdominal skin–fascial flap.

ral vessels. Below the inguinal ligament, the superior epigastric artery and vein are located. The artery and vein are then followed to their origins from the femoral vessels, depending on required pedicle length. The pedicle vessels are then dissected superiorly to the level of the skin island. If an inadequate or absent inferior epigastric artery is noted, the incision is closed with dissection of the contralateral flap, or the surgeon may locate the superficial circumflex iliac artery and switch to a superficial groin flap (see the section Groin Flap — Proximal Approach on page 1155). If the pedicle is adequate, the remainder of the skin borders are incised and the flap is completely elevated immediately superficial to the anterior rectus sheath medially and external oblique fascia laterally. Immediately after division of the vascular pedicle, excessive fat deep to Scarpa's fascia is excised as required to reduce flap thickness, avoiding injury to the pedicle at the inferior flap edge.

Donor Site

Closure is accomplished directly, either in a transverse or vertical direction, depending on flap design. A suction catheter is placed in the donor site.

SCAPULAR FLAP

The scapular flap represents the largest of the fasciocutaneous flaps presently available for upper extremity reconstruction. This flap was initially described by dos Santos[65] in 1978, and is now frequently used in reconstructive surgery.[65,66,67,69] The vascular pedicle to the scapular flap, the circumflex scapular artery and veins, has direct branches into the periosteum of the lateral scapula, allowing design as an osseous-cutaneous flap. Although the flap dimensions are great, 14×28 cm, the subcutaneous fatty layer often results in excessive flap thickness. Since flap elevation is performed in the lateral decubitus or prone position, simultaneous preparation of the upper extremity recipient site is not always possible. This flap, however, is excellent for coverage of large defects in the upper extremity (Fig. 27-16).

Vascular Anatomy

Vascularization of the scapular flap is through the cutaneous branches of the circumflex scapular artery. This vessel, along with the thoracodorsal artery, comprises the two major branches of the subscapular arterial system. The subscapular artery is the major arterial source for the latissimus dorsi muscle and musculocutaneous flaps, the serratus anterior muscle and musculo-osseous flaps, and the scapular fasciocutaneous and osteocutaneous flaps. A thorough knowledge of the vascular anatomy of this important region is a prerequisite for the surgeon using microvascular tissue transplantation.

The circumflex scapular artery originates from the subscapular artery and passes through the triangular space to reach the posterior axillary region and trunk. The space is formed by the long head of the triceps laterally, the teres major inferiorly, and the teres minor superiorly. This anatomic space is the key to the dissection of the scapular flap. The artery passes through the triangular fossa and gives off multiple branches to the lateral border of the scapula and its investing musculature. A cutaneous scapular artery then provides cutaneous branches to essentially all of the skin over the scapula from an area encompassing the medial to lateral scapular borders and from the spine of the scapula superiorly to the tip of the scapula inferiorly. The circumflex scapular artery has two venae comitantes that are intimately associated with the vessel throughout its course proximally in the triangular fossa and superiorly to the subscapular artery and vein. The vessels have an external lumen diameter of 2 mm, making them ideal for microvascular anastomoses. A pedicle length from 4 to 6 cm is consistently available. The vascular arrangement of separate branches of this vascular pedicle to the bone of the lateral border of the scapula and the skin gives the scapular osteocutaneous flap the unique advantage of having the bone and skin separate on a Y-shaped pedicle. Both limbs of the Y originate from the circumflex scapular artery. This separation of the vascularized bone and skin allows great versatility in flap design and facilitates the inset in the recipient site.

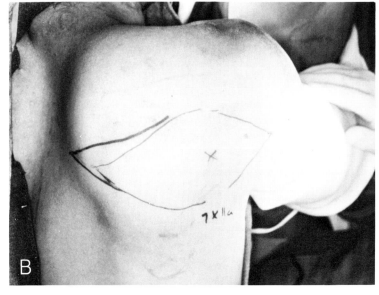

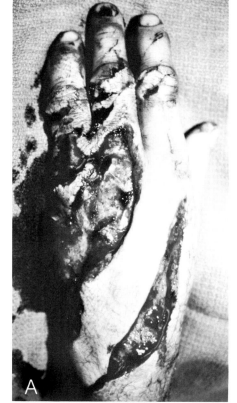

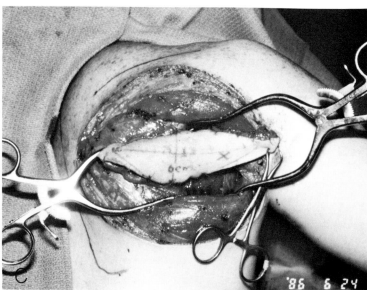

Fig. 27-16. Scapular flap. (A) Preoperative view. An industrial injury with avulsion of the little finger and fifth metatarsal and associated skin and soft tissue loss. (B) Preoperative flap design. (C) Flap elevation completed. *(Figure continues.)*

Flap Design

The cutaneous territory of the circumflex scapular artery encompasses essentially all of the skin from the medial to the lateral border of the scapula with 2 to 3 cm extensions on each side. The superior margin of the territory is the scapular spine, and the inferior margin is the tip of the scapula. Specific transverse and descending cutaneous branches may be located preoperatively with the use of the Doppler. Such preoperative mapping of the fasciocutaneous vasculature allows increased versatility in flap design with the use of a bilobed

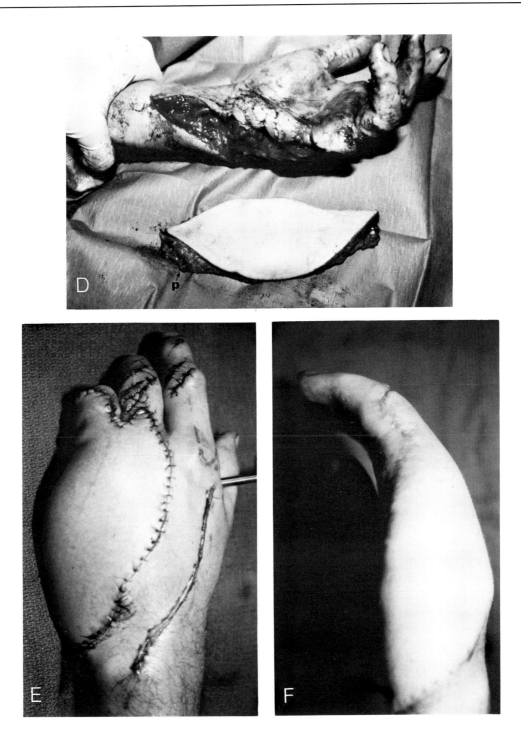

Fig. 27-16 *(Continued).* **(D)** The flap is ready for inset into the lateral hand defect. (*p*, circumflex scapular artery and vein). **(E)** The flap is inset and revascularized by microanastomoses between the circumflex scapular artery and vein and the ulnar artery (end-to-side) and a superficial wrist vein (end-to-end). **(F)** The postoperative result with stable hand coverage after flap transplantation.

flap, with one limb oriented transversely and the other obliquely or inferiorly.

The most common pattern for scapular flap design is that of a transverse ellipse, which allows direct closure of the donor site and avoids the need for a skin graft to achieve wound closure. The width of the ellipse is usually determined by skin laxity in the posterior trunk. It is not uncommon for flaps of 8 cm in width by 12 or 15 cm in length to be used without any difficulty in donor site closure. Wider flaps often require skin grafts for donor site closure.

The flap is easily outlined and dissected with the patient in the lateral decubitus position. It is helpful to have the arm included in the operative field. Manipulation of the extremity between abduction and adduction assists flap dissection. The lateral extent of the flap is located over the triangular fossa, just above the posterior axillary fold. After palpation of the notch at the inferior border of the glenoid, use of a Doppler immediately below this bony landmark allows the surgeon to locate the circumflex scapular artery (Fig. 27-17). In a thin person, with the arm abducted, it is often possible for one to palpate the triangular fossa by placing the thumb and index finger around the teres major into the triangular fossa.

Bone

The lateral border of the scapula, from below the glenoid notch all the way to the tip, is consistently supplied by branches of the circumflex scapular artery. These branches are adherent to the bone and its investing musculature. Care must be taken during dissection to preserve these branches when elevation of the osteocutaneous flap is planned. A straight segment of corticocancellous bone of 10 to 14 cm in length and 3 cm in width may be safely included as vascularized bone in the scapular osteocutaneous flap.[68] As noted above, the Y-shaped vascular arrangement of the skin and bone portions of this flap greatly enhances its versatility (Fig. 27-18). A common limitation that most osteocutaneous flaps have is the predetermined spatial orientation required in flap design, necessitated by the intimate association of vascular branches to the bone and the skin.

Technique of Elevation of the Scapular Skin Flap

The scapular cutaneous flap elevation may be carried out either from the superior lateral or inferior lateral approach to the triangular fossa. If the superior incision is made initially, then the deltoid muscle will be the first muscle identified. Proceeding with dissection inferior to the deltoid toward the triangular space, the next muscle encountered will be the teres minor. Dissection proceeds along the edge of the teres minor until the triangular fossa is identified and entered. In this space the circumflex scapular vascular pedicle will be identified.

The inferior incision allows initial identification of the latissimus dorsi and teres major muscles. Dissection proceeds superiorly over the teres major muscle until the triangular fossa is entered. The circumflex scapular pedicle is quite predictable and reliable in its location in the fatty areolar tissue of the triangular fossa, and dissection of the pedicle proximally may proceed to its junction with the thoracodorsal artery. If a larger pedicle is required, the subscapular artery is dissected superior to the thoracodorsal arterial branch to the latissimus dorsi muscle.

After identification of the vascular pedicle, the medial to lateral portion of elevation of the flap goes quite easily with the flap dissected beneath the fascia of the underlying musculature. Care is taken to preserve the fasciocutaneous branches of the circumflex scapular artery. As the dissection proceeds toward the lateral border of the scapula, multiple branches, intimately adherent to this border and its investing musculature on both sides, are encountered. These are divided if a cutaneous flap is planned. This is the single portion of the dissection where great care must be taken not to injure the transversely oriented cutaneous branches of the flap. The distance between the branching points of these vessels and their entrance into the adjacent scapula is very short. After the flap is detached from the scapula, dissection proceeds between the teres major and minor muscles into the triangular fossa, where the proximal portion of the vascular pedicles, the circumflex scapular artery, and associated veins have been previously identified.

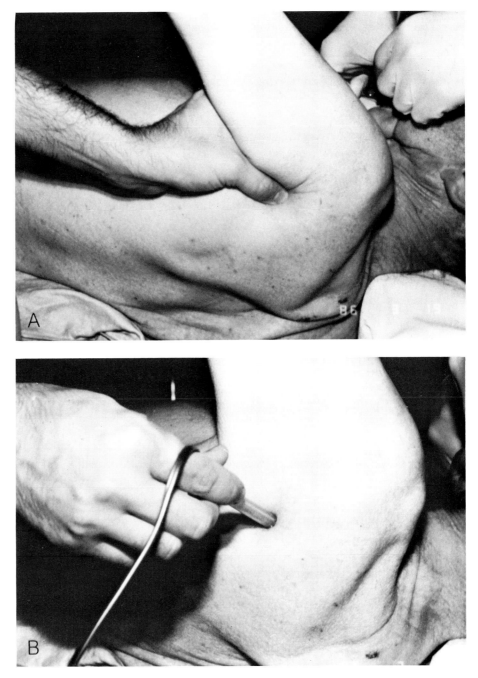

Fig. 27-17. Scapular flaps—vascular anatomy. (**A**) Location of the triangular space between the long head of triceps laterally, teres major inferiorly, and teres minor superiorly. (**B**) Doppler probe confirms the location of the circumflex scapular artery in the triangular fossa.

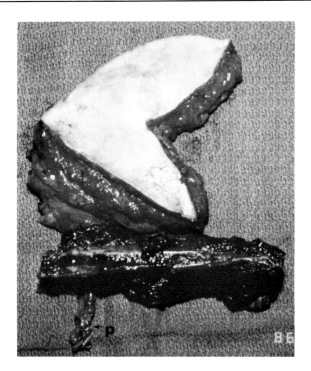

Fig. 27-18. Scapular osteocutaneous flap. Operative view of skin and scapular bone based on the circumflex scapular artery and vein *(p)*.

Technique of Elevation of the Scapular Osteocutaneous Flap

The dissection for the osteocutaneous scapular flap is exactly the same as that for the skin flap alone, with the exception that the above-mentioned branches to the bone and investing musculature on the lateral border of the scapula are not divided. Instead, once this point is reached, the overlying musculature of the scapula is incised and the osteotomy sites are exposed. An osteotomy may be performed from just below the glenoid notch in a transverse fashion for several centimeters, and then, turning vertically, extending down to the tip of the scapula. Care must be taken both to protect the vascular pedicle during the osteotomy and to avoid injury to the glenoid fossa. The bone cuts are made from the posterior approach. Once the full-thickness osteotomy of the scapula has been performed, the anterior musculature is peeled off the opposite side, which results in free mobility between the cutaneous and bony portions of the osteocutaneous flap. The remainder of the dissection proceeds exactly as described above for the skin flap, following the circumflex scapular artery and its two venae comitantes into the triangular fossa and proximally, depending on the required length of the vascular pedicle, to the subscapular artery. Four to six centimeters of additional proximal pedicle may be obtained with division of the thoracodorsal vessels. The potential for a massive flap, including latissimus dorsi (with or without skin), serratus anterior (with or without rib), and scapular flap (with or without bone) based on one vascular pedicle from the subscapular artery, is theoretically possible based on the vascular anatomy of this region.

Donor Site—Skin Flap

Linear closure of the scapular cutaneous flap is done without difficulty. Use of flaps in which the width precludes direct close are avoided since skin grafts on the back increase donor site morbidity.

Donor Site—Osteocutaneous Flap

Closure of the investing musculature of the scapula (teres major, infraspinatus, subscapularis) is important in managing the donor site of the osteocutaneous flap. The remainder of the closure is the same as for the skin flap alone. Suction drainage is important, particularly for the osteocutaneous flap. Shoulder immobilization is recommended for 7 to 10 days postoperatively. This is followed by a program of gradual progressive range of motion exercises for shoulder mobilization.

TEMPORAL PARIETAL FASCIA FLAP

The superficial temporal artery and associated vein provide circulation to the temporal fascia and the overlying hair-bearing scalp. Although transplantation of scalp has no application in upper extremity surgery, it is possible to elevate the fascia with its fasciocutaneous vascular pedicle as a flap, leaving the overlying scalp skin in place. Microvascular transplantation of the vascularized fascia represents a unique technique to provide very thin tissue to support skin grafts for palmar and dorsal hand and finger defects (Figs. 27-19 and 27-20).[71] Direct closure of the scalp leaves the donor site scar completely covered with scalp hair.

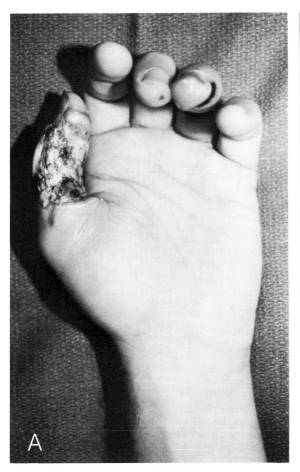

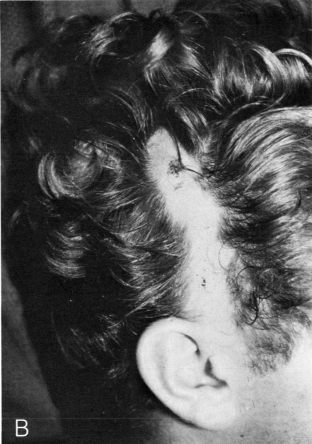

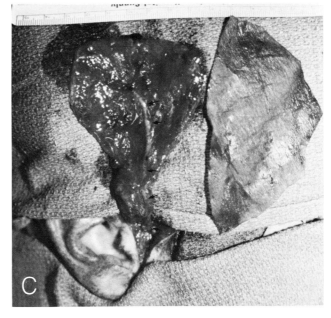

Fig. 27-19. Temporal parietal fascia flap. (A) Pre-operative view. An electrical injury with loss of proximal phalangeal skin and soft tissue. The ulnar digital nerve was intact. (B) Donor site preparation. Three centimeters of scalp hair shaved along the course of the superficial temporal artery and vein. (C) A template was made to delineate the tissue required for wound coverage and to determine the dimensions of the flap. Arrows indicate the course of the vascular pedicle in this vascularized fascial flap. *(Figure continues.)*

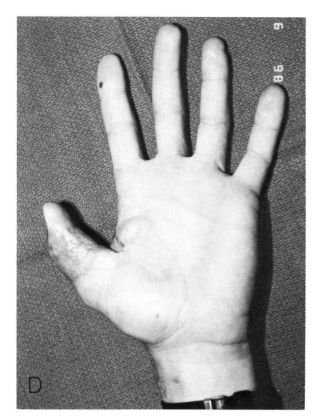

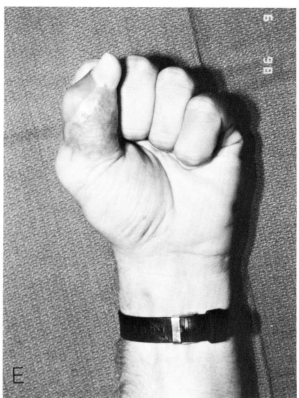

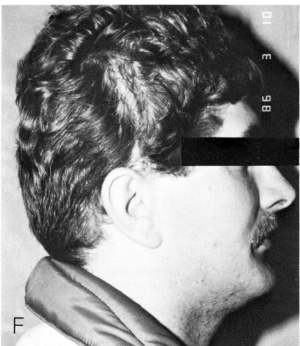

Fig. 27-19 *(Continued).* **(D)** Postoperative view. Transplanted fascia covered with skin grafts provides stable coverage for the thumb. **(E)** Postoperative view. The fascia flap with skin grafts avoids excessive bulk and provides excellent contour for palmar surface of the digits and hand. **(F)** Postoperative view. Hair growth will cover the donor-site scar.

Fig. 27-20. Temporal parietal flap. **(A)** Preoperative view of a thermal injury with exposed carpal bones and tendons on the dorsum of the hand, including index and middle fingers. **(B)** The palmar aspect of the hand has viable intrinsic muscles, allowing direct skin graft coverage. The median nerve and flexor tendons are exposed at the wrist. **(C)** Preoperative flap design. Doppler probe is used to trace the course of the superficial temporal artery. *(Figure continues.)*

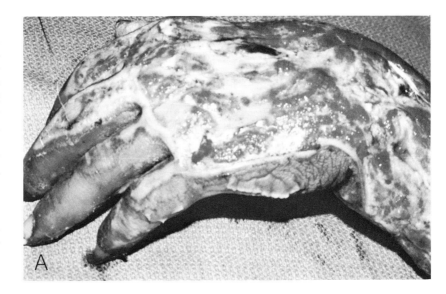

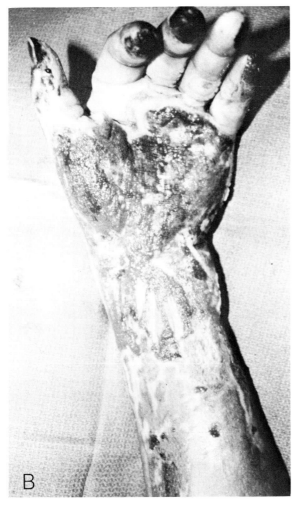

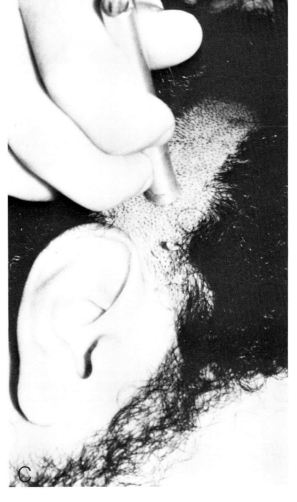

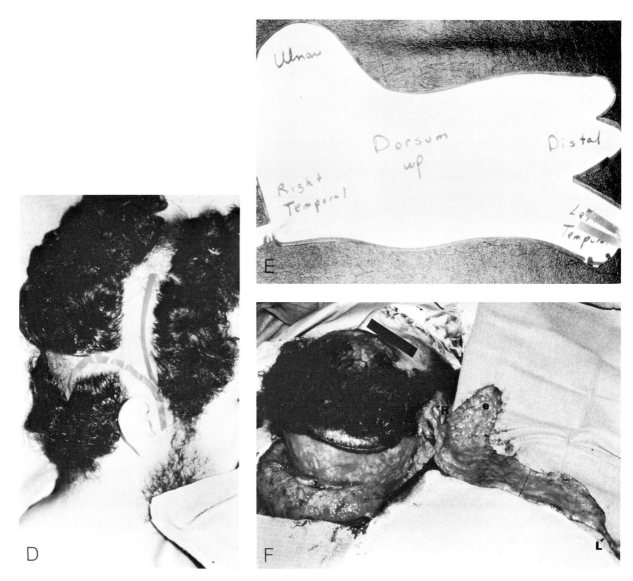

Fig. 27-20 *(Continued).* **(D)** Preoperative flap design. A fascial flap will be designed on the temporal and occipital branches of the right superficial temporal artery and vein. Occipital extension will be used for volar vein coverage. **(E)** Preoperative flap design. A template is used to determine an exact flap design based on the size of the defect and the relationship to the planned site of the microvascular repair of flap and recipient vessels. In order to obtain length to cover both the dorsal wrist and hand defects, the fascia is extended across the midline to the contralateral ear to include the opposite left superficial temporal vessels. **(F)** Flap elevation. The left superficial temporal artery and vein have been divided *(L)*. Entire left fascia is elevated to the right side with intact right superficial temporal artery and vein *(R)*. Occipital extension *(e)* will be used for volar wrist coverage. Dotted lines indicate the midline of scalp fascia. *(Figure continues.)*

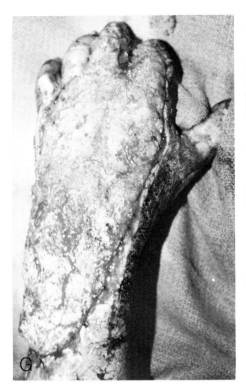
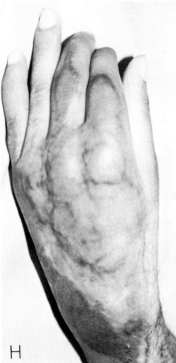
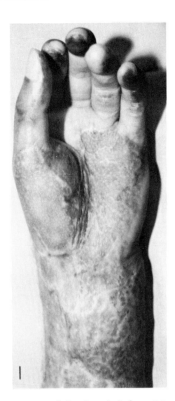

Fig. 27-20 *(Continued).* **(G)** Vascularized fascia inset over both dorsal and volar aspects of the hand defect. No acceptable recipient vessels were available to repair the left superficial temporal artery and vein. With the exception of that portion of the flap across the midline used on the fingers, the entire fascial unit was well vascularized by repair of the right superficial temporal artery and right vein into the ulnar artery and vein. **(H)** Postoperative dorsal view. Vascularized fascia with skin grafts provided stable wound coverage in a single-stage procedure. **(I)** Postoperative volar view. Fascia plus skin grafts avoids excessive bulk and contour deformity in the hand.

Vascular Anatomy

The temporal parietal fascia is supplied by the superficial temporal artery and its single venae comitans.[70] These vessels are easily identified and palpated in front of the ear as they emerge from the parotid gland (Fig. 27-21). As the vessels pass from their position in front of the ear in a superior direction onto the temporal and parietal scalp, they become invested by the galea or fascial layer of the scalp. The vessels are located within the galea, whose thickness is barely more than the diameter of the vessels themselves. This relationship persists throughout the entire length of the flap. This unusual anatomic relationship results in a very thin flap, whose ratio of vascular axis to gram of tissue is probably higher than any other flap used. This relationship also dictates that a very meticulous dissection must be accomplished in order to avoid any injury to the delicate vessels that supply this flap.

Just above the ear, there is a frontal branch of the artery that courses anteriorly toward the forehead. This branch must always be divided during elevation of this flap. The main parietal portion of the artery continues in a cephalic direction toward the center of the scalp. An occipital branch is also often found that may be used to vascularize a small posterior extension of fascia.

The venae comitans with the superficial temporal artery is usually just posterior and superficial to the artery. This relationship continues through the course of the pedicle into the scalp. Multiple branches from this vein that enter the subcutaneous tissue of the scalp are encountered during flap dissection, and great care must be taken to bipolarly coagulate them without injuring the dominant

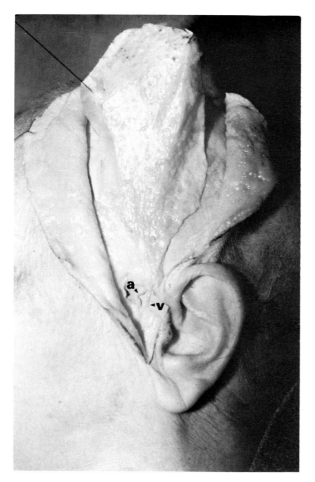

Fig. 27-21. Temporal parietal fascial flap. Vascular anatomy. Cadaver dissection demonstrates the position of the superficial temporal artery *(a)* and vein *(v)* in the preauricular region.

fascial flap. This allows safe dissection and preservation of the frontalis muscle and the frontal branch of the facial nerve. The region of the fascia included with the flap is located posterior to the course of the superficial temporal artery.

A 1 to 1.5 cm strip of scalp is shaved over the vascular axis into the temporal parietal scalp (Fig. 27-19B). This may start from just above the ear all the way to the midsagittal plane of the scalp if necessary. If a wide flap is desired, a posterior limb is added to the skin incision producing a Y-type of configuration (Fig. 27-20D). Narrower flaps may be easily elevated with one simple linear incision.

In preoperative planning the head and neck region must be carefully examined for evidence of previous surgery. Previous operations in this region, such as rhytidectomy, parotidectomy, or radical neck dissection, may preclude the use of this flap due to prior ligation of the superficial temporal vessels.

Nerve

The auriculotemporal nerve runs along the same course as the superficial temporal vessels and is seen during exposure of the primary pedicle anterior to the ear. This nerve courses primarily in this flap and is divided in the flap dissection. The potential for sensory innervation of an overlying skin graft placed on this flap is possible if the proximal nerve end is sutured to a regional sensory nerve in the recipient area.

Bone

Vascularization of the outer table of the calvarium through the superficial temporal arterial system and the investing galea and overlying periosteum has been demonstrated.[72-76] Regional pedicled osseofascial reconstructions using this flap have been performed in the head and neck region.[75] The use of this membranous bone as a vascularized fascial and bone graft for the upper extremity has yet to be reported. However, success in using this bone in other areas where membranous bone is present, such as the facial skeleton, has been demonstrated.[77]

vein. The ipsilateral superficial temporal artery system will not reliably supply flap extension across the midline of the scalp.

Flap Design

The area of the temporal parietal fascial flap is located beneath the temporal parietal scalp. A flap of 6 cm by 14 cm may be elevated, based on the fasciocutaneous circulation of the superficial temporal artery and vein. The flap is designed so that the vascular axis from the superficial temporal artery is located close to the anterior edge of the

Technique of Elevation of the Temporal Parietal Fascia Flap

Preoperative shaving, as described above, is accomplished and a standard head drape is applied. For use in the upper extremity, the contralateral side of the head is used to allow simultaneous donor and recipient site dissection. The supine position with the patient's head turned to the side provides a very satisfactory exposure for flap dissection. Preoperative markings are made along the line of the proposed incision in the temporal parietal scalp, immediately posterior to the vascular axis of the superficial temporal artery as determined by Doppler probe. The preauricular portion of the incision may extend either anterior or posterior to the tragus, according to the surgeon's preference.

The preauricular incision is made, using high power loupe magnification, and the superficial temporal artery and its venae comitans are identified in this region. The vessels are quite small, and there may be multiple branches that must be divided. The bipolar cautery is used to coagulate small vessels located superficial and posterior to the artery.

After the vascular pedicle has been identified, the remainder of the incision is made superiorly into the scalp. The initial plane of dissection is superficial to the galeal-fascial layer and deep to the subcutaneous tissue. There is no need to leave fat on the flap. In most inferior portions of the dissection, hair follicles may be seen in the scalp. As one proceeds superiorly, the subcutaneous layer is thicker. The proper plane is located precisely between the subcutaneous tissue with associated hair follicles and the fascia of the flap. Dissection continues both anterior and posterior to the incision until the preoperatively determined amount of fascia has been exposed. Care is taken not to extend the dissection too far anterior from the axis of the superficial temporal artery, as injury to the frontalis muscle or frontal branch of the facial nerve may result.

After complete exposure of the superficial surface of the temporal parietal scalp and the superficial temporal artery and vein in the preauricular region, the incision through the fascia into the loose areolar plane above the periosteum of the skull is made. The entire posterior portion of the incision may be safely made to this level from just in front of the ear all the way up to the most superior portion of the flap. The anterior part of the incision through the fascia is made to the site where the frontal branch of the temporal artery courses anteriorly. At this point, this branch should be divided and dissection carefully done just at the anterior margin of the superficial temporal artery inferiorly to its origin just in front of the ear. By proceeding in this fashion, injury to the frontal branch of the facial nerve will be avoided.

Dissection in the loose areolar plane below the galea on top of the periosteum proceeds quite easily. The flap is easily raised in a distal to proximal fashion. The inferior dissection proceeds immediately superficial to the temporalis muscle to the level of the vascular pedicle, as described previously. The flap pedicle is not divided until the recipient site, including appropriate receptor vessels, is prepared for the microanastomosis.

Bone. If an osseofascial flap is to be elevated, the outline of the appropriate amount of bone superior to the temporalis muscle is made. Care is taken to avoid the sagittal region of the skull. The fascia is raised, as previously described, until the borders of the osseous flap are reached. Power burrs are then used to mark the limits of the bone flap and osteotomes appropriately used to elevate the outer table of calvarium. These osteotomies are performed with great care in order to avoid penetration through the inner table of the skull and dura. The remainder of the flap is elevated in the same fashion as for the fascia alone with the fascial and periosteal attachments of the galea to the bone left intimately associated.

Donor Site

Meticulous hemostasis is accomplished in the scalp. Closure is performed with one layer of nonabsorbable suture. A small suction drain is placed in the depths of the wound. If bone is harvested with the flap, no special attention is taken for the outer table calvarial defect as long as there is no inner table penetration. The preauricular incision is closed with fine nylon sutures that are removed within the first 5 days to avoid suture marks. Alopecia is a potential complication with this donor site. Careful handling of the scalp flaps and precise dissection in the proper layer will prevent this complication and produce one of the best donor sites for any flap used in microvascular transplantations.

LATERAL ARM FASCIOCUTANEOUS FLAP

Song[83] in 1982 described a fasciocutaneous flap located in the upper lateral arm. Subsequently, both Schusterman[82] and Matloub[81] in 1983 demonstrated successful microvascular transplantation of this flap. Further anatomic studies with clinical reports by Katsaros and colleagues[79] demonstrated the reliable vascular anatomy and vast potential for clinical use of this flap. The flap is ideally suited for upper extremity reconstruction, especially for defects in the hand and forearm, since the dissection of both donor and recipient sites is confined to the involved extremity. This fasciocutaneous flap can be modified for use as a neurosensory flap, a cutaneous flap with vascularized bone, and a fascial flap with a vascularized nerve graft.

Vascular Anatomy

The profunda brachii artery arises from the proximal brachial artery and courses posteriorly around the humerus in the spiral groove. It maintains a close association with the humerus, passing through the lateral intermuscular septum just distal to the insertion of the deltoid muscle. Immediately distal to the deltoid insertion, the profunda brachii artery divides into two arteries, the anterior and posterior radial collateral arteries. These branches are located posterior and anterior to the origin of the brachioradialis from the lateral intermuscular septum. The posterior branch, the posterior radial collateral artery, is accompanied by the posterior cutaneous nerve of the arm and the lateral cutaneous nerve of the forearm. The smaller anterior branch of the profunda brachii artery courses with the radial nerve and eventually communicates with the radial recurrent artery.

The posterior radial collateral artery has consistent branches that perforate the fascia overlying the triceps and brachioradialis muscles, providing cir-

culation to the fascia and its overlying skin (Fig. 27–22E). The most proximal fasciocutaneous perforator is always the largest, usually measuring 1 mm in diameter. Distal to these perforators, the artery either terminates as a cutaneous vessel or continues around the lateral epicondyle to anastomose with the interosseous recurrent artery. The distal arterial end of the flap is usually too small to be routinely used as a distally based flap.

Veins

The posterior radial collateral artery has two large venae comitantes, each approximately 2 mm in diameter. If one vein has a larger lumen diameter, repair of the second vein may not be necessary.

Nerve

The radial nerve has two sensory branches entering into the lateral intermuscular septum, both originating more proximally in the spiral groove. The posterior cutaneous nerve of the arm supplies the skin territory of the flap in addition to skin in the lateral epicondyle area. This nerve is always included with the skin flap. The posterior cutaneous nerve occasionally enters the territory of the flap posterior and superior to the intermuscular septum where the nerve penetrates the posterior aspect of the triceps muscle (Fig. 27-22C). Its origin can be separated from the radial nerve, providing a long proximal nerve if a neurosensory flap is planned.

The second sensory nerve, the posterior cutaneous nerve of the forearm, is located within the intermuscular septum and innervates the radial aspect of the proximal forearm. Although this nerve is generally included with the flap, Katsaros and Webster described dissection within the intermuscular septum to separate the posterior cutaneous nerve of the forearm from the vascular pedicle of the flap, thus preserving its innervation to the forearm. If the nerve is retained in the flap, an anesthetic area results over the brachioradialis muscle belly. Also, the posterior cutaneous nerve of the forearm may be utilized as a vascularized nerve graft either separately with the vascularized fascia or included within the skin–fascial flap for combined skin, soft tissue, and segmental nerve loss in the upper extremity.

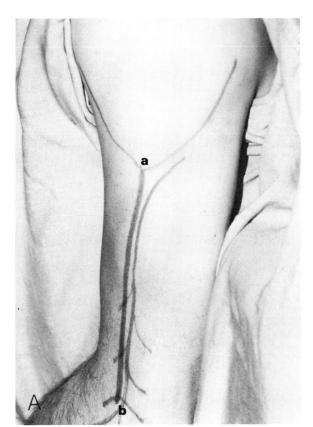

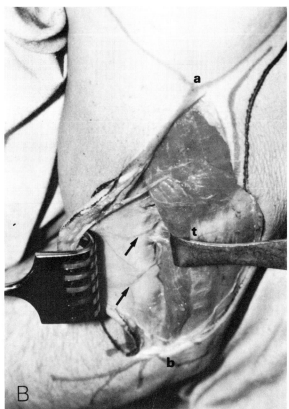

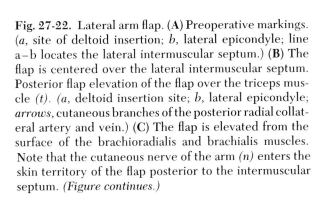

Fig. 27-22. Lateral arm flap. (A) Preoperative markings. (a, site of deltoid insertion; b, lateral epicondyle; line a–b locates the lateral intermuscular septum.) (B) The flap is centered over the lateral intermuscular septum. Posterior flap elevation of the flap over the triceps muscle (t). (a, deltoid insertion site; b, lateral epicondyle; arrows, cutaneous branches of the posterior radial collateral artery and vein.) (C) The flap is elevated from the surface of the brachioradialis and brachialis muscles. Note that the cutaneous nerve of the arm (n) enters the skin territory of the flap posterior to the intermuscular septum. (Figure continues.)

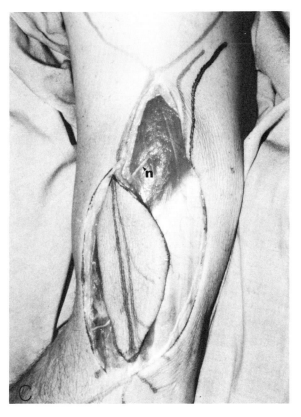

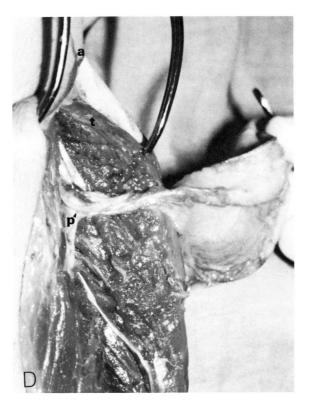

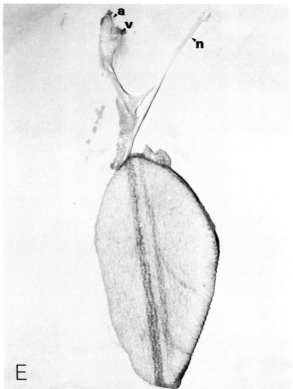

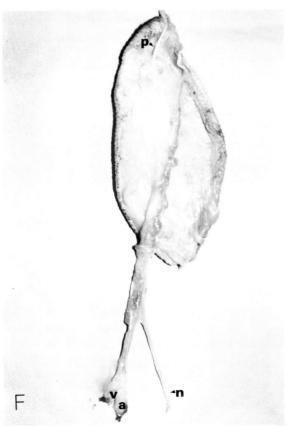

Fig. 27-22 (Continued). (D) Proximal dissection of the posterior radial collateral artery and vein (p) requires an incision into the lateral head of the triceps muscle (t) (a, site of deltoid insertion). (E) Flap anatomy. Lower lateral cutaneous nerve of the arm (n) and posterior radial collateral artery (a) and vein (v) are labeled. (F) Flap anatomy. Deep surface. Note that the flap includes the investing fascia of muscles. Lower lateral cutaneous nerve of arm (n), posterior radial collateral artery (a) and vein (v), and posterior cutaneous nerve of forearm (p) are labeled.

Bone

The posterior radial collateral artery supplies periosteal branches to a region of humerus along the intermuscular septum, supplying a strip of cortex approximately 1 cm in width and 10 cm in length. These periosteal vessels course through the borders of the triceps and brachioradialis and brachialis muscles before entering the periosteum. Therefore, the portions of muscle immediately overlying the long strip must be included with the flap. Care must be taken to identify and protect the radial nerve during its course between the brachioradialis and brachialis muscle before resecting bone. An osteotomy is performed along the humerus to obtain the vascularized posterior cortex, preserving the remaining portion of the humerus. The supracondylar ridge is the most reliable donor site, extending proximally along the intermuscular septum.

Flap Design

The use of a tourniquet greatly facilitates dissection and is used during the initial flap dissection. The flap is elevated with the arm positioned in internal rotation and the forearm pronated. If the flap requires dimensions larger than 7 cm in width, the dissection is started with the arm draped across the patient's chest with the elbow flexed.

A line is drawn from the insertion of the deltoid to the lateral epicondyle. This marks the longitudinal midline axis for the flap (Fig. 27-22A). This axis is deceptively located more posterior than would seem apparent on first glance at the lateral arm, particularly in young muscular males, where the biceps muscle occupies the majority of the lateral surface of the arm.

The proximal end of the flap is located immediately distal to the deltoid insertion on the humerus. The length of the flap can extend to the distal end of the lateral epicondyle. Flaps have extended past the epicondyle, including skin over the origin of the extensor musculature and proximal brachioradialis, but closure of this portion of the donor site results in a donor site crossing the elbow joint, with the resulting potential for joint contracture. This extended flap design is distal to the fasciocutaneous branches and depends on a random blood supply.

Technique of Elevation of the Lateral Arm Fasciocutaneous Flap

The flap is centered over the lateral intermuscular septum located between the triceps muscle posteriorly and the brachioradialis and brachialis muscles anteriorly. The vascular pedicle, the posterior radial collateral artery, and associated veins enter the intermuscular septum superiorly at the level of the deltoid insertion. An incision is made along the posterior edge of the flap located over the triceps muscle (Fig. 27-22B). The flap includes the superficial investing fascia of the muscle. The fascia and overlying subcutaneous tissue and skin are elevated until the intermuscular septum is reached. It is possible to see the cutaneous branches of the flap pedicle located superficial to the fascia (Fig. 27-22C). After the triceps muscle is separated from the intermuscular septum, the vascular pedicle is identified within the superior aspect of the intermuscular septum at the level of the deltoid insertion. The deltoid and triceps muscles are separated, and the posterior fibers of the triceps are divided to enter the spiral groove (Fig. 27-22D). The junction of the posterior and anterior radial collateral arteries with the profunda brachii artery is seen, and the vascular pedicle is dissected proximally until adequate pedicle length is achieved (Fig. 27-22E). Muscular branches to the triceps muscle are divided. The two sensory nerves associated with the flap are also identified. Both the superficial cutaneous nerve to the arm and the deeper cutaneous nerve to the forearm are identified. These nerves are divided and included within the flap. Proximal dissection of the nerves to their junction with the radial nerve is important if a neurosensory flap is planned to ensure adequate nerve length to reach suitable sensory nerves at the flap recipient site (Fig. 27-22E and F). The distal end of the posterior cutaneous nerve of the forearm will be identified later if a vascularized nerve graft is planned.

The anterior flap edge is now incised through investing fascia over the surface of the brachioradialis and brachialis muscles. A subfascial dissection is performed until the lateral intermuscular septum is reached (Fig. 27-22C). The radial nerve and the anterior radial collateral artery are identified as they pass between the brachioradialis and the brachialis muscles. The radial nerve is protected while the posterior radial collateral artery, veins, and sensory nerves are dissected from the periosteum of the humerus. The anterior radial collateral artery is divided at its origin from the profunda brachii artery to increase the pedicle length. The distal end of the pedicle at the inferior edge of the flap is divided, completing the flap elevation.

Donor Site

Direct donor site closure is generally performed if a muscle flap is designed. Skin grafts over exposed muscle will heal nicely.

Muscle and Musculocutaneous Flaps

The value of muscle and musculocutaneous flaps as standard transposition flaps for wound coverage is well recognized. Any muscle with a dominant vascular pedicle located close to either its origin or insertion may be transposed to adjacent defects to provide coverage.[63] Although muscles located in the upper extremity have potential as transposition flaps for use in coverage problems, these muscles are generally not expendable. In the injured extremity, expendable muscles are generally reserved for functional transfers.

The skin overlying superficial muscles may be included with the muscles to provide a musculocutaneous flap. In upper extremity reconstructive surgery, the muscle is generally transplanted without its overlying skin to reduce excessive flap bulk. Exposed portions of the muscle are covered with skin grafts. The muscle flap is particularly useful in coverage of contaminated wounds.[7] Experimental and clinical studies have demonstrated superior resistance to infection in the muscle flap when compared with a skin–fascial flap.[78] In treatment of infected bone, the muscle flap provides safe coverage after aggressive bone debridement in combination with culture-specific antibiotic therapy.[80]

Muscle and musculocutaneous flaps for both coverage and motor function are described in Chapter 28. The serratus anterior flap is not included in that chapter and therefore is described here.

SERRATUS ANTERIOR FLAP

The serratus anterior muscle may be transplanted for small upper extremity defects (Figs. 27–23 and 27–24).[85] The inferior half of the muscle is elevated as a flap, preserving the superior half to maintain its function. The exposed portion of the muscle at the recipient site is covered with a skin graft. This flap has potential use as an osseous-muscular flap based on vascular connections to the underlying ribs. This flap has a long vascular pedicle and a well-located donor site scar, located in the axilla and lateral superior chest wall.

Vascular Anatomy

The serratus anterior muscle originates by nine slips from the first nine ribs. It inserts into the entire medial border of the scapula. The muscle has a dual blood supply that facilitates its use as tissue for microvascular transplantation.[84] The lowest three slips of the muscle, arising from the 7th, 8th, and 9th ribs, are vascularized through the subscapular-thoracodorsal arterial system. A large branch from the thoracodorsal artery supplies these slips and may easily be elevated from the first six slips of the serratus without disturbing the blood supply. The superior six slips of the serratus anterior are primarily supplied by branches of the lateral thoracic artery. This dual vascular arrangement allows elevation of the lowest one, two, or three slips of the serratus while still preserving the vascular integrity of the rest of the muscle to avoid a winged scapula as a sequela of using the entire muscle as donor tissue (Fig. 27-25A).

It is possible to obtain a section of serratus anterior muscle with a 15 cm vascular pedicle by dividing the thoracodorsal artery and vein and dissecting the subscapular arterial system superiorly into the axilla. Obviously, this long vascular pedicle has tremendous potential when recipient vessels are not available adjacent to an upper extremity defect and vein grafts are required for a flap with a short vascular pedicle. The proximal pedicle also has the same advantages as the latissimus dorsi flap, with large vessel lumen diameters of 2 to 3 mm, which facilitates the microvascular repair.

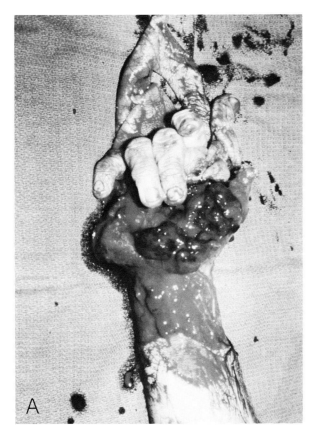

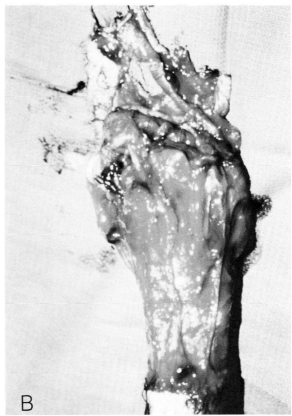

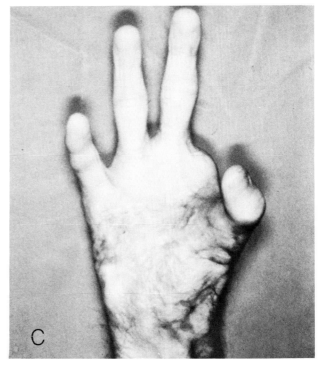

Fig. 27-23. Serratus anterior muscle flap. **(A)** Preoperative view. This is the result of an industrial press injury. Initial treatment included thumb replantation, fracture stabilization, and skin graft coverage of the hand. **(B)** Preoperative view of the dorsum of the hand. **(C)** Skin grafts provide initial wound coverage. A contracture on the palmar aspect of the hand and thumb exists. *(Figure continues.)*

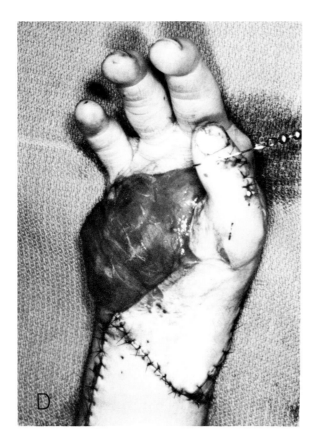

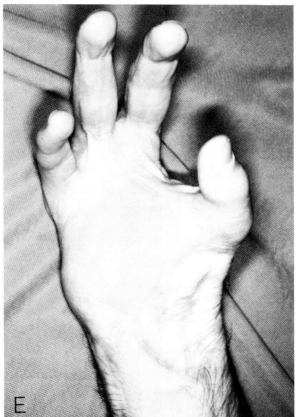

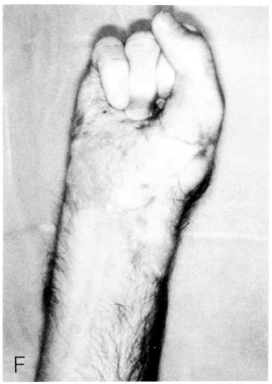

Fig. 27-23 *(Continued).* **(D)** The inferior three slips of the serratus anterior were transplanted into the palmar defect, with contracture release. **(E)** Postoperative view (extension). The transplanted muscle is covered with skin grafts. **(F)** Postoperative view (flexion) demonstrates stable coverage with thumb flexion.

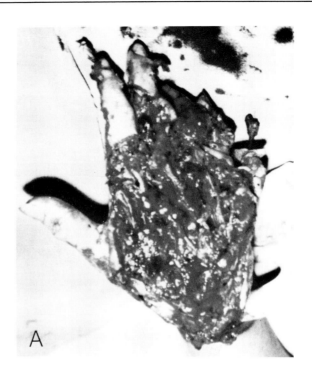

Fig. 27-24. Serratus anterior muscle flap. (**A**) Preoperative view. A motor vehicle accident caused this severe crush injury of the palmar and dorsal surfaces of the hand. Initial treatment included stabilization of fractures, index amputation, and skin graft coverage. (**B**) A serratus anterior muscle flap transplanted to the dorsum of hand with skin graft coverage. Initially, a tissue expander was placed under the muscle flap to increase the region of flap coverage. A thumb web space release has been performed. (**C**) The tissue expander ready for removal. *(Figure continues.)*

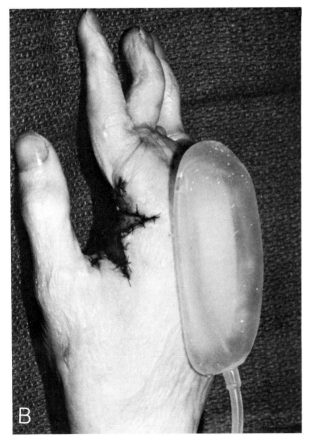

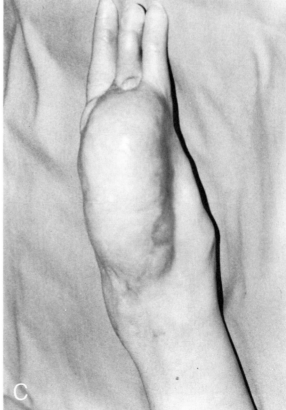

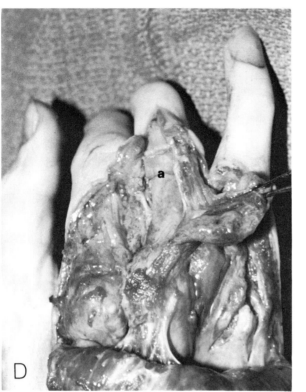

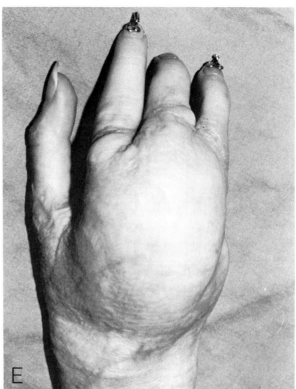

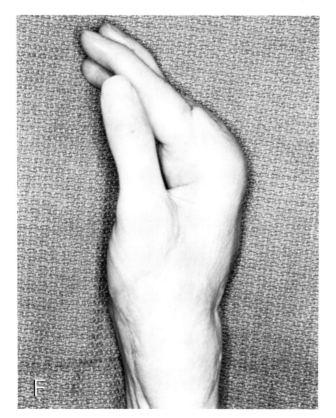

Fig. 27-24 *(Continued).* (**D**) The serratus anterior muscle flap was secondarily elevated after expansion. An MP joint arthroplasty *(a)* was performed. (**E**) Postoperative dorsal view. Stable coverage on the dorsum of the hand was provided by the transplanted muscle flap with skin. (**F**) Postoperative lateral view: A muscle flap with skin grafts provides minimal bulk and will tolerate secondary elevation or expansion for later reconstructive procedures.

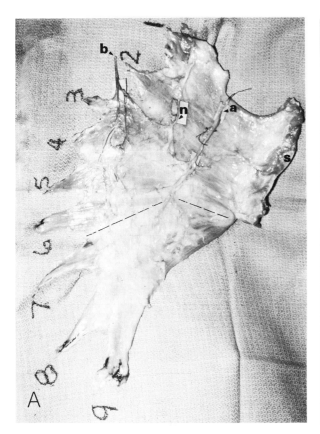

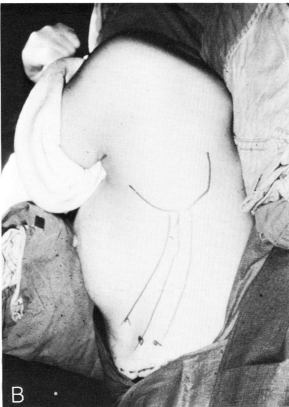

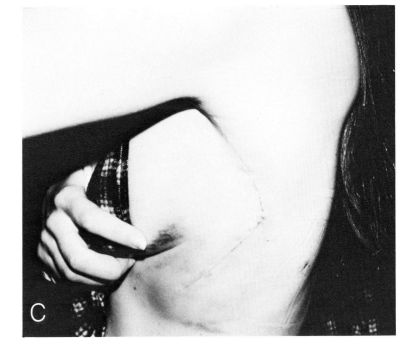

Fig. 27-25. Serratus anterior muscle flap. (**A**) Vascular anatomy. Cadaver specimen demonstrates serratus anterior sites of origin from ribs 1–9 and insertion into the scapula *(s)*. Dotted lines indicate flap design based on the serratus branch of the subscapular artery *(a)*. Preserved lateral thoracic artery *(b)* and long thoracic nerve *(n)* maintain remaining muscle circulation and motor innervation. (**B**) Technique of elevation. Preoperative markings showing the location of the inferior three muscle slips of the serratus anterior. (**C**) Postoperative view. The donor site closure is well concealed beneath the left arm in the superior lateral chest wall.

Motor Nerve

The motor nerve of the serratus anterior muscle is the long thoracic nerve. Using high power magnification, the branches of the motor nerve to the bottom three slips are divided while preserving the innervation of the superior six slips. This requires interfasicular dissection but may be accomplished by using the operating microscope. The ability to preserve both circulation and motor innervation to the upper six slips of the serratus muscle while using only the lower one, two, or three slips minimizes potential donor problems. The muscle is quite useful for coverage problems of the palm. Since these motor nerve branches to the inferior three slips may be repaired at the donor site at the same time, the potential exists for use of this muscle for both function and coverage.

Bone

The vascular attachments of the muscle with the rib periosteum allow transplantation of an osseous-muscular flap.

Flap Design and Technique of Elevation of the Serratus Anterior Flap

The patient is placed in the lateral decubitus position with the arm included in the operative field. One to three of the inferior slips of the serratus anterior muscle are elevated, depending upon the size of the donor defect. The muscle is exposed through a midaxillary incision, extending from the axilla to the level of the 9th rib (Fig. 27-25B). The anterior border of the latissimus dorsi is identified and elevated. Beneath the anterior edge of the latissimus dorsi, the branch of the thoracodorsal artery to the serratus anterior muscle is identified. The long thoracic nerve lies on the chest wall directly anterior to the vascular pedicle to the serratus anterior muscle.

The muscular branches of the vascular pedicle to the superior muscle slips of the serratus are divided, preserving all the vascular branches to the 7th, 8th, and 9th muscle slips. Care is taken during this dissection to avoid injury to motor nerve branches from the long thoracic nerve to the upper six slips. Magnification is required for this portion

of the dissection. The vascular pedicle is lifted off the top six slips of the muscle up to the level of the thoracodorsal artery and vein. If a longer pedicle is required, the thoracodorsal vessels to the latissimus dorsi muscle may be divided. If a longer pedicle is not required, the serratus pedicle may be dissected to just distal to the take-off of the thoracodorsal vessels, preserving the major blood supply to the latissimus dorsi muscle.

The deep dissection of the inferior slips of the muscle is started inferiorly below the 9th slip in the loose aerolar plane between the muscle and the chest wall. The inferior muscle slips are then divided at the level of their insertions into the scapula. The muscular origin from the 7th, 8th, and 9th ribs are divided, taking care not to penetrate the intercostal muscles and pleura. If the motor nerve is required, an interfasicular dissection is performed to preserve the nerve supply from the long thoracic nerve to the superior six slips of the serratus anterior muscle. The flap is allowed to perfuse only on its major vascular pedicle until the recipient site has been completely prepared.

Donor Site

The remaining slips of the serratus are sutured to the inferior portion of the scapula to re-establish a broad muscle insertion. The wound is then closed directly, leaving a suction drain in place. Since the scar is located at the midaxillary line, it is well concealed by the arm (Fig. 27-25C). A small Z-plasty is occasionally used in the axilla to avoid a tight scar.

CONCLUSION

With the rapid identification of many types of skin–fascial and muscle flaps, the hand surgeon has a wide selection of tissue for use in reconstructive hand surgery. The reliability of microsurgical techniques has started a new era in hand surgery in which form and function can be restored in both congenital and acquired upper extremity deformities.

REFERENCES

Upper Extremity Reconstruction

1. Acland RD: Microsurgery Practice Manual. CV Mosby, St Louis, 1980
2. Cobett JR: Small vessel surgery in the hand. Hand 1:57, 1969
3. Cohen L, Mathes SJ: The use of microcrystalline collagen in microsurgery and its effect on anastomotic patency. Ann Plast Surg 9:471–474, 1982
4. Cormack GC, Lamberty BGH: Fasciocutaneous vessels in the upper arm: Application to the design of new fasciocutaneous flaps. Plast Reconstr Surg 74:244–249, 1984
5. Jacobsen JH, Suarez EL: Microsurgery in anastomosis of small vessels. Surg Forum 11:243–245, 1960
6. Mathes SJ, Nahai F: Classification of the vascular anatomy of muscles: Experimental and clinical correlation. Plast Reconstr Surg 67:177–187, 1981
7. Mathes SJ, Feng LJ, Hunt TK: Coverage of the infected wound. Ann Surg 198:420–429, 1983
8. McGraw JB, Dibbell DG, Carraway JH: Clinical definition of independent myocutaneous vascular territories. Plast Reconstr Surg 60:341–352, 1977
9. Orticochea M: The musculocutaneous flap method: An immediate and heroic substitute for the method of delay. Br J Plast Surg 25:106–110, 1972
10. Ponten B: The fasciocutaneous flap: Its use in soft tissue defects of the lower leg. Br J Plast Surg 34:215–220, 1981
11. Tamia S, Komatsu S, Sakamoto H, Sano S, Sasauchi N, Hori Y, Tatsumi Y, Okuda H: Free muscle transplants in dogs, with microsurgical neurovascular anastomoses. Plast Reconstr Surg 46:219–225, 1970
12. Tolhurst DE, Haeseker B, Zeeman RJ: The development of the fasciocutaneous flap and its clinical applications. Plast Reconstr Surg 71:597–605, 1983

Groin Flap

13. Acland RD: The free iliac flap: A lateral modification of the free groin flap. Plast Reconstr Surg 64:30–36, 1979
14. Baudet J, LeMaire JM, Guimberteau JC: Ten free groin flaps. Plast Reconstr Surg 57:577–595, 1976
15. Daniel RK, Taylor GI: Distant transfer of an island flap by microvascular anastomoses: A clinical technique. Plast Reconstr Surg 52:111–117, 1973
16. MacGregor IA, Morgan G: Axial and random pattern flaps. Br J Plast Surg 26:202–213, 1973
17. Taylor GI: Reconstruction of the jaw with free composite iliac bone grafts. pp. 106–122. In Buncke HJ,

Furnas DW (eds): Symposium on Clinical Frontiers in Reconstructive Microsurgery. Ch. 14. CV Mosby, St Louis, 1984
18. Taylor GI, Corlett R: Refinements of the free iliac osteocutaneous flap designed on the deep circumflex iliac vessels. Plast Surg Forum 111:185, 1980
19. Taylor GI, Daniel RK: The anatomy of several free flap donor sites. Plast Reconstr Surg 56:243, 1975
20. Taylor GI, Townsend P, Corlett R: Superiority of the deep circumflex iliac vessels as the supply for free groin flaps: Experimental work. Plast Reconstr Surg 64:595–604, 1979
21. Taylor GI, Townsend P, Corlett R: Superiority of the deep circumflex iliac vessels as the supply for free groin flaps: Clinical work. Plast Reconstr Surg 64:745–759, 1979

Dorsalis Pedis Flap

22. Bilmer E, Dispiera W: Coverage of defects with free flaps by means of microvascular anastomoses. MMW 119:587, 1977
23. Buncke HJ, Rose EH: Free toe-to-fingernail neurovascular flaps. Plast Reconstr Surg 63:607–612, 1979
24. Caffee HH, Hoefflin SM: The extended dorsalis pedis flap. Plast Reconstr Surg 64:807–810, 1979
25. Daniel RK, Terzis J, Midgley RD: Restoration of sensation to an anaesthetic hand by a free neurovascular flap from the foot. Plast Reconstr Surg 57:275–280, 1976
26. Daniel RK, Terzis J, Schwarz G: Neurovascular free flaps. Plast Reconstr Surg 56:13–20, 1975
27. Gilbert A: Composite tissue transfers from the foot: Anatomic basis and surgical technique. In Strauch B, Daniller A (eds): Symposium on Microsurgery. Vol. 14. CV Mosby, St Louis, 1976
28. Gilbert A, Morrison W: First web space neurovascular free flap transfer. Groupe Adv Microchir 3:1, 1976
29. Gilbert A, Morrison W, Tubiana R, Lisfranc R, Firmin F: Transfert sur la main d'un lambeau libre sensible. Chirurgie 101:691–694, 1975
30. Hurwitz, PJ: Experimental transplantation of small joints by microvascular anastomoses. Plast Reconstr Surg 64:221–231, 1979
31. Man D, Acland RD: The microarterial anatomy of the dorsalis pedis flap and its clinical applications. Plast Reconstr Surg 65:419–423, 1980
32. Mathes SJ, Buchannan R, Weeks PM: Microvascular joint transplantation with epiphyseal growth. J Hand Surg 5:586–589, 1980
33. Mathes SJ: The role of microsurgery in acute hand

injuries. In Weeks PM, Wray RC (eds): Management of Acute Hand Injuries: A Biological Approach. 2nd Ed. CV Mosby, St Louis, 1978

34. May JW Jr, Chait LA, O'Brien BM, Hurley JV: The no-flow phenomenon in experimental free flaps. Plast Reconstr Surg 61:256–267, 1976

35. May JW, Chait LA, Cohen BE, O'Brien BMcC: Free neurovascular flap from the first web of the foot in hand reconstruction. J Hand Surg 2:387–393, 1977

36. McCraw JB, Furlow LT Jr: The dorsalis pedis arterialized flap: A clinical study. Plast Reconstr Surg 55:177–185, 1975

37. Minami A, Usui M, Katoh H, Ishii S: Thumb reconstruction by free sensory flap from the foot using microsurgical techniques. J Hand Surg 9(B):239–244, 1984

38. Morrison WA, O'Brien BMcC, MacLeod AM, Gilbert A: Neurovascular free flaps from the foot for innervation of the hand. J Hand Surg 3:235–242, 1978

39. Morrison WA, O'Brien BMcC, Hamilton RB: Neurovascular free foot flaps in reconstruction of the mutilated hand. Clin Plast Surg 5:265–272, 1978

40. O'Brien BMcC, Shanmugan N: Experimental transfer of composite free flaps with microvascular anastomoses. Aust NZ J Surg 43:285–288, 1973

41. Ohmori K: Application of microvascular free flaps to burn deformities. World J Surg 2:193–202, 1978

42. Ohmori K, Harii K: Free dorsalis pedis sensory flap to the hand, with microneurovascular anastomoses. Plast Reconstr Surg 58:546–554, 1976

43. Ohmori K, Harii K, Sekiguchi Y, Torii S: The youngest groin flap yet? Br J Plast Surg 30:273–276, 1977

44. Robinson DW: Dorsalis pedis flaps. pp. 257–284. In Serafin D, Buncke HJ Jr (eds): Microsurgical Composite Tissue Transplantation. CV Mosby, St Louis, 1978

45. Robinson DW: Microsurgical transfer of the dorsalis pedis neurovascular island flap. Br J Plast Surg 29:209–213, 1979

46. Strauch B, Tsur H: Restoration of sensation to the hand by a free neurovascular flap from the first web space of the foot. Plast Reconstr Surg 62:361–367, 1978

47. Taylor GI, Townsend P: Composite free flap and tendon transfer: An anatomical study and a clinical technique. Br J Plast Surg 32:170–183, 1979

48. Tamai S, Fukui A, Shimizu T, Yamaguchi T: Thumb reconstruction with an iliac bone graft and a dorsalis pedis flap transplant including the extensor digitorum brevis muscle for restoring opposition in a case report. Microsurgery 4(2):81–86, 1983

49. Takai H, Takahashi S, Ando M: Use of the dorsalis pedis free flap for reconstruction of the hand. Hand 15:173–178, 1983

50. Zuker RM, Manktelow RT: The dorsalis pedis free flap: Techniques of elevation, foot closure and flap application. Plast Reconstr Surg 77(1):93–104, 1986

Toe-Digital Transplantation

51. Antia NH, Buch VI: Transfer of an abdominal dermo-fat graft by direct anastomosis of blood vessels. Br J Plast Surg 24:15–19, 1971

52. Barfred T: The Shaw abdominal flap. Scand J Plast Reconstr Surg 10:56, 1976

53. Boeckx, WD, DeConinck A, Vanderlinden E: Ten free flap transfers: Use of intra-arterial dye injection to outline a flap exactly. Plast Reconstr Surg 57:716–721, 1976

54. Gordon L, Leitner DW, Buncke HJ, Alpert BS: Hand reconstruction for multiple amputations by double microsurgical toe transplantation. J Hand Surg 10A:218–225, 1985

55. Gordon L, Rosen J, Alpert BS, Buncke HJ Jr: Free microvascular transfer of second toe ray and serratus anterior muscle for management of thumb loss at the carpo-metacarpal joint level. J Hand Surg 9A:642–644, 1984

56. Hester TR Jr, Nahai F, Beegle PE, Bostwick J III: Blood supply of the abdomen revisited, with emphasis on the superficial inferior epigastric artery. Plast Reconstr Surg 74:657–666, 1984

57. Kleinert HE, Manstein CH: Current techniques of limb reconstruction. pp. 213–226. In Buncke HJ, Furnas DW (eds): Symposium on Clinical Frontiers in Reconstructive Microsurgery. Ch. 24. CV Mosby, St Louis, 1984

58. Mathes SJ, Buchanan R, Weeks PJ: Microvascular joint transplantation with epiphyseal growth. J Hand Surg 5:586–589, 1980

59. May JW, Chait LA, Cohen BE, O'Brien BMcC: Free neurovascular flap from the first web of the foot in hand reconstruction. J Hand Surg 2:387–393, 1977

60. Shaw DT, Payne RL: One-staged tubed abdominal flaps. Single pedicle tubes. Surg Gynecol Obstet 83:205–208, 1946

61. Stern PJ, Kreilein JG, Kleinert HE: Neurovascular cutaneous flaps for the management of radiation-induced fingertip dermal necrosis. J Hand Surg 8:88, 1983

62. Wood J: Extreme deformity of the neck and forearm. Med Chir Trans 46:151, 1983

63. Yoshimura M: Toe-to-hand transfer. Plast Reconstr Surg 66:74–83, 1980

Scapular Flap

64. Barwick WJ, Goodkind DJ, Serafin D: The free scapular flap. Plast Reconstr Surg 69:779–785, 1982
65. dos Santos LF: The scapular flap: A new microsurgical free flap. Biol Chir Plast 70:133, 1980
66. Gilbert A, Teot L: The free scapular flap. Plast Reconstr Surg 69:601–604, 1982
67. Hamilton SGL, Morrison WA: The scapular free flap. Br J Plast Surg 35:2–7, 1982
68. Scwartz WM, Banis JC, Newton ED, Ramasastry SS, Jones NF, Acland R: The osteocutaneous scapular flap for mandibular and maxillary reconstruction. Plast Reconstr Surg 77:530–545, 1986
69. Urbaniak J, Koman LA, Goldner RD, Armstrong NB, Nunley JA: The vascularized cutaneous scapular flap. Plast Reconstr Surg 69:772–778, 1982

Temporal Parietal Fascia Flap

70. Abul-Hassan HS, Ascher GVD, Acland RD: Surgical anatomy and blood supply of the fascial layers of the temporal region. Plast Reconstr Surg 77:17–24, 1986
71. Brent B, Upton J, Acland RD, Shaw WW, Finseth FJ, Rogers C, Pearl RM, Heintz VR: Experience with the temporo-parietal fascial free flap. Plast Reconstr Surg 76:177–188, 1985
72. Casanova R, Cavalcante D, Grotting JC, Vasconez LO, Psillakis JM: Anatomic basis for vascularized outer-table calvarial flaps. Plast Reconstr Surg 78:300, 1986
73. Coleman S, Buncke HJ, Alpert BS, Hing DN, Lineaweaver W, Chater N: Reconstruction of the mandible with full thickness cranial bone grafts. Surg Forum 36:556–557, 1985
74. Cutting CB, McCarthy JG, Berenstein A: Blood supply of the upper craniofacial skeleton: The search for composite calvarial bone flaps. Plast Reconstr Surg 74:603–610, 1984

75. McCarthy JG, Zide BM: The spectrum of calvarial bone grafting: Introduction of the vascularized calvarial bone flap. Plast Reconstr Surg 74:10–18, 1984
76. Pensler J, McCarthy JG: The calvarial donor site: An anatomic study in cadavers. Plast Reconstr Surg 75:648–651, 1985
77. Psillakis JM, Grotting JC, Casanova R, Cavalcante D, Vasconez LO: Vascularized outer table calvarial bone flaps. Plast Reconstr Surg 78:309–317, 1986

Lateral Arm Fasciocutaneous Flap

78. Calderon W, Chang N, Mathes SJ: Comparison of the effect of bacterial inoculation in musculocutaneous and fasciocutaneous flaps. Plast Reconstr Surg 77:785, 1986
79. Katsaros J, Schusterman M, Beppu M, Banis JC, Acland RD: The lateral upper arm flap: Anatomy and clinical applications. Ann Plast Surg 12:489–500, 1984
80. Mathes SJ, Alpert BS, Chang N: Use of the muscle flap in chronic osteomyelitis: Experimental and clinical correlation. Plast Reconstr Surg 89:815–828, 1982
81. Matloub HS, Sanger JR, Godina M: The lateral arm flap: A neurosensory free flap. p. 125. In Williams HB (ed): Transactions of the VIII International Congress of Plastic Surgery, Montreal, IPRS, 1983
82. Schusterman M, Acland RD, Banis M, Beppu M: The lateral arm flap, an experimental and clinical study. p. 132. William HB (ed): Transactions of the VIII International Congress of Plastic Surgery, Montreal, IPRS, 1983
83. Song R: One-stage reconstructions. Clin Plast Surg 9(1):27, 1982

Serratus Anterior Flap

84. Mathes SJ, Nahai F: Clinical Atlas of Muscle and Musculocutaneous Flaps. p. 337. CV Mosby, St Louis, 1979
85. Takayanagi S, Tsukie R: Free serratus anterior muscle and myocutaneous flaps. Ann Plast Surg 8:277–283, 1982

Free Muscle Transfers

28

Ralph T. Manktelow

Most of the muscles of the body have been assessed for their usefulness as free tissue transfers, and many have now been identified as readily expendable and suitable for microvascular transfer. These muscles usually have large, long, predictable neurovascular pedicles that provide a vigorous blood supply and are reliable free tissue transfers. Free muscle transfers have been found to be useful both for soft tissue coverage and as functioning contracting muscles for reconstruction of the extremities.

Following a brief discussion of the recipient vessels available for connection to the free muscle transfer, this chapter is divided into three separate sections:
1. Muscles available for free tissue transfer
2. Upper extremity coverage with free muscle transfers
3. Functioning muscle transplantation

Recipient Vessels for Free Muscle Transfers in the Upper Extremity

Arterial anastomoses in the upper extremity may be end-to-end or end-to-side. In the proximal arm, small branches, such as the ulnar recurrent and an-terior interosseous arteries, are available as end-to-end sources of arterial input. Both the radial and the ulnar arteries are available, depending upon the extent of injury, and provide excellent vessels for end-to-side anastomoses. Within the palm, the common digital arteries and the palmar arch are available. On the dorsum of the hand just proximal to the first web space, the radial artery is in a very accessible location. This is often the location of choice for the arterial repair in free tissue transfers to the digits and thumb. When the presence or condition of a suitable artery is unclear from the clinical examination, an arteriogram is required.

Either superficial or deep veins can be used for anastomoses. Superficial arm veins are more useful than superficial leg veins, as there is not the same tendency to spasm in the veins of the arm. However, superficial veins may have been damaged by previous intravenous medication.

In the upper extremity, the surgeon must be particularly careful that all factors affecting peripheral perfusion are being considered. Blood volume and pressure must be maintained and the patient warmed in order to support the peripheral as well as the core body temperature, and to prevent peripheral vasospasm (see also Chapter 24).

MUSCLES AVAILABLE FOR FREE TISSUE TRANSFERS

GRACILIS

The gracilis muscle can be used to cover small- to medium-sized soft tissue defects as well as to provide functioning muscle transfers. Small soft tissue defects are adequately covered by using only a small piece of the muscle centered on the vascular pedicle. The cutaneous flap, based on the gracilis muscle, is quite reliable in the proximal half of the muscle (Fig. 28-1B). A single constant perforator usually exists from the muscle at the level of the dominant vascular pedicle. In some patients, the medial thigh fat is very thick and creates a very thick, bulky cutaneous flap. In many coverage situations, it is preferable to transfer the muscle without a skin paddle and apply a split-thickness skin graft directly to the muscle. The donor site scar is excellent, as it lies in the upper half of the medial aspect of the thigh. For functioning muscle transplantation, this is the preferred muscle for upper extremity reconstruction, and it is also commonly used for facial paralysis reconstruction.

Anatomy

The gracilis is a superficial muscle located on the medial aspect of the thigh. It is a strap muscle that is broad proximally and tapers distally. By a thin aponeurosis, its origin is from the body of the pubis and the adjacent ramus of the ischium. The belly of the muscle lies just posterior to the adductor longus and sartorius muscles and ends in a well-defined tendon that inserts into the medial shaft of the tibia just below the tibial tubercle (Fig. 28-2). In the distal thigh, the tendon lies just posterior to the sartorius tendon and anterior to the semitendinosis.

There are two or three vascular pedicles. The proximal pedicle is the dominant one and will reliably perfuse the muscle. It lies under the adductor longus and takes origin from the profunda femoris artery. This dominant upper artery is 1 to 2 mm in diameter, 6 cm in length, and enters the muscle 8 to 12 cm from the muscle's origin. There are two venae comitantes, each measuring 1.0 to 4.0 mm in diameter (Fig. 28-3). In our clinical experience with 90 gracilis free muscle transfers, all muscles have survived on the single superior vascular pedicle. In one case, the superior pedicle was a double pedicle with two arteries and four venae comitantes, and it appeared that the circulation proximal to the pedicle was dependent on one artery and that distal to the pedicle dependent on the other artery.

There is a single motor nerve, a branch of the obturator, which is composed of two to seven fascicles. The nerve enters the muscle immediately proximal to the vascular pedicle and lies under the adductor longus. With nerve stimulation, the adult gracilis muscle will contract more than 50 percent of its extended length for a functional contraction of 12 to 15 cm (Fig. 28-4). In over 20 operative procedures, the fascicles of the motor nerve were teased apart and each fascicle separately stimulated. Using a nerve stimulator with frequency and voltage control, it was usually possible to separate the muscle into two longitudinal, separately functioning neuromuscular territories. Ninety percent of the time, a single fascicle will control the anterior 20 to 50 percent of the muscle and the remaining portion of the muscle is controlled by the remaining fascicles. This functional separation is quite useful when the muscle is used to provide independent thumb and finger flexion (Fig. 28-5).

The muscle fiber anatomy has been studied by Fish at our institution. In the proximal three-fifths of the muscle belly, the muscle fibers are parallel in a strap muscle configuration. In the distal two-fifths, the muscle fibers insert in sequential fashion into the tendon, which is located in the posterior border of the muscle. The posterior muscle fibers are shorter and insert proximally; the longer anterior muscle fibers insert more distally.

The function of this muscle is to flex, medially rotate, and adduct the thigh. Removal of the muscle results in no apparent functional deficit in the leg.

Technique of Preparing the Gracilis Muscle

The entire thigh and knee is prepped and draped free. The procedure is done with the surgeon standing on the opposite side of the table from the donor leg, with the knee and hip flexed and the hip externally rotated and abducted.[6]

A straight line is drawn between the tendon of

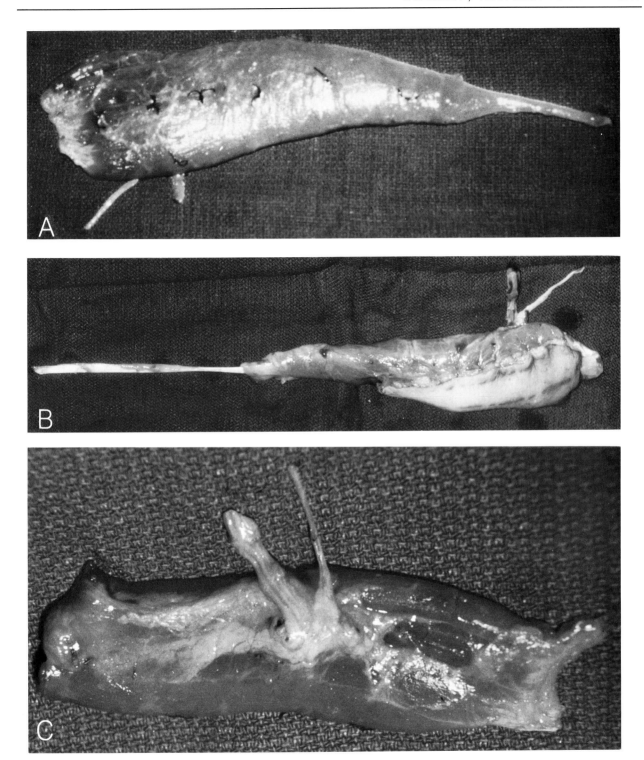

Fig. 28-1. (**A**) Superficial aspect of the gracilis muscle. The motor nerve enters diagonally at the lower left, and the vascular pedicle is adjacent to the nerve. (**B**) A myocutaneous gracilis transfer with skin centered on the proximal "safe" portion of the muscle. Note the long length of available tendon. (**C**) A 2×10 cm segment of the gracilis muscle centered on the neurovascular pedicle, suitable for coverage of small soft tissue defects.

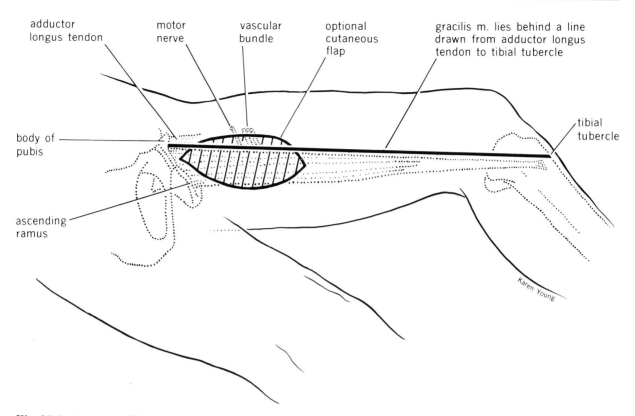

Fig. 28-2. Anatomy of the gracilis muscle and cutaneous flap (see text).

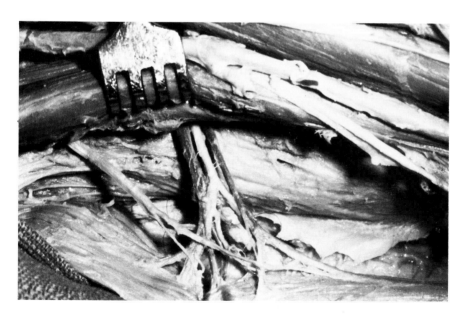

Fig. 28-3. Medial aspect of the left thigh from a cadaver. The adductor longus is elevated by a rake. The dominant artery and venae comitantes enter the gracilis at the bottom of the picture. The motor nerve enters obliquely from the left.

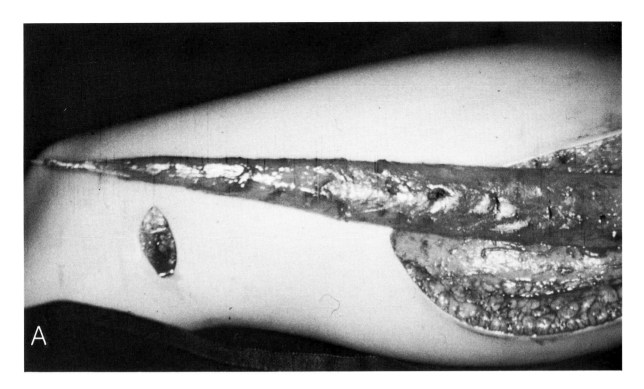

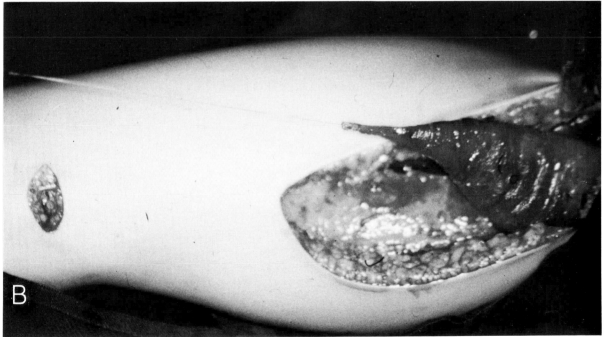

Fig. 28-4. (A) Gracilis muscle dissected free from the right thigh, still attached to its origin and neurovascular bundle. (B) With stimulation of the muscle's motor nerve, the muscle shortens 15 cm (between 50 and 60 percent of its physiological extended length).

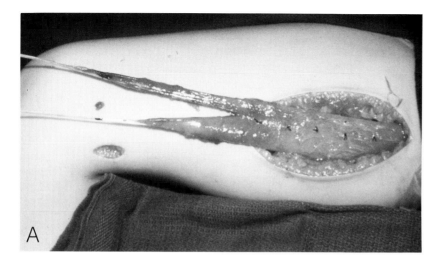

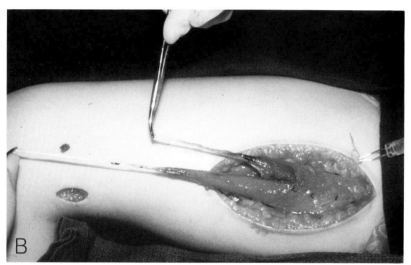

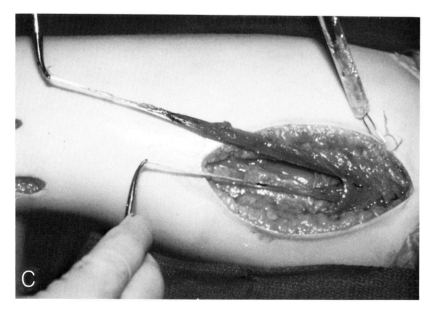

Fig. 28-5. (A) The distal muscle belly and attached portions of tendon of a gracilis muscle are split longitudinally. The location of the split is determined by stimulating each fascicle of the motor nerve and observing the portion of muscle that contracts. This allows the creation of two separately controlled neuromuscular units. (B) Stimulation of one fascicle produces contraction of the anterior portion of the muscle (top part of the picture). (C) Stimulation of the remaining fascicles produces contraction of the posterior portion of the muscle (bottom part of the picture).

the adductor longus and the tibial tubercle. The gracilis muscle lies posterior to this line (see Fig. 28-2).

If the surgeon intends to employ the muscle without a cutaneous flap, an incision is made 2 cm posterior to the upper border of the gracilis in its proximal one-half of the thigh. The dissection is carried through the deep muscular fascia, and the gracilis is separated from the surrounding musculature. The adductor longus is elevated to expose the neurovascular structures that enter the gracilis on the deep aspect of the anterior margin. Arterial and venous side branches to the adductor magnus and longus are ligated in order to develop a long pedicle. Dissection is carried proximally and distally with the dissecting finger. The secondary pedicles to the distal portion of the muscle are located on the anterior margin, and they are divided. The tendon is divided through a transverse incision in the distal thigh. The origin is then divided, and the muscle is now dependent on its single vascular pedicle. It is left intact until the recipient site is prepared for transplantation. The adequacy of muscle perfusion will be apparent from the color of the muscle. On occasion, the distal few centimeters of muscle will not be perfused.

If a myocutaneous flap is required, the skin flap must be outlined over the proximal portion of the muscle. A perforator is always present opposite the dominant pedicle. Our experience with free myocutaneous transfers has shown that the cutaneous portion of the flap is unreliable 15 to 20 cm distal to the pubic tubercle. The flap is quite reliable in the transverse dimension and can be taken a few centimeters wider than the underlying muscle. After the skin flap has been cut, the dermis is tacked anteriorly and posteriorly to the gracilis fascia. This will prevent shearing of the cutaneous flap and damage to the perforating vessels.

LATISSIMUS DORSI

The latissimus dorsi is a very dependable muscle for free tissue transfers. The entire muscle or just a small portion of it can be transferred either with or without a cutaneous paddle. The thoracodorsal artery is a reliable, large diameter, long pedicle. Frequently, only a small strip of the anterior muscle margin is transferred with a larger paddle of over-

lying skin to provide an aesthetic skin coverage. However, if a large skin flap is removed and the donor site cannot be closed directly, the grafted donor site is cosmetically unsatisfactory. For direct closure, a maximum skin-flap width of 10 cm is feasible. For larger soft tissue defects, the muscle is usually used as a muscle-only transfer with a skin graft applied directly to the muscle (Fig. 28-6). Since the thoracodorsal artery also supplies the serratus anterior, both of these muscles can be taken to cover two separate soft tissue defects. Alternately, the latissimus dorsi can be split longitudinally into two separate but attached muscle segments with the expectation of good vascularity in each segment.[15] The thoracodorsal artery usually splits at the vascular hilum into a superior transverse branch and an anterior inferior branch. This muscle can be removed and produce minimal weakness; however, persons who use their arm vigorously in work or for activities such as tennis, skiing, or throwing, notice a decrease in strength.

Anatomy

The latissimus is a fan-shaped muscle that has an aponeurotic origin from the thoracolumbar fascia and the iliac crest, and a muscular origin from the lower three ribs (Fig. 28-7). It inserts by a well-formed tendon into the medial lip of the bicipital groove of the humerus. The primary vascular supply is the thoracodorsal artery, which is a branch of the subscapular artery, and secondarily by a number of posterior perforating vessels. The thoracodorsal artery enters the deep surface of the muscle 8 to 12 cm from its insertion, 2 cm from the anterior margin. The thoracodorsal artery is 1.5 to 3.0 mm in diameter. On its way to supply the latissimus dorsi muscle, it gives off a number of branches to the chest wall, including a branch to the serratus anterior. The two venae comitantes usually join to form a single vein as they approach the axilla. This vein varies in size from 3.0 to 5.0 mm. The nerve to the latissimus dorsi follows the course of the thoracodorsal artery. There are two or three fascicles with a cross-sectional area of approximately 2 mm. The nerve may be separated into two functionally separate divisions in 80 percent of the muscles. One division supplies the lateral portion of the muscle and one the medial portion.[15]

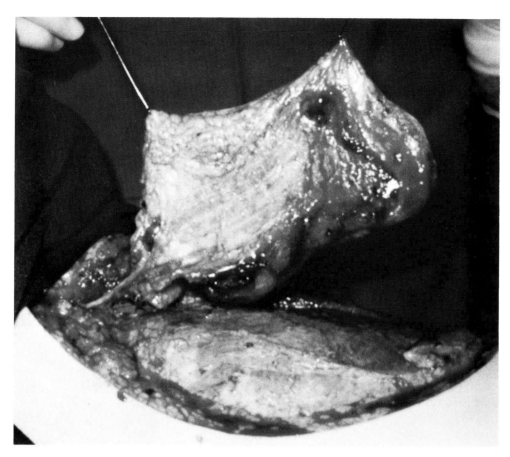

Fig. 28-6. Right latissimus dorsi completely separated except for the pedicle. The muscle has been elevated from its bed with the deep surface exposed.

Technique of Preparing the Latissimus Dorsi Muscle

The patient is placed in the lateral decubitus position, supported on the operating table by a kidney rest, or in the prone position. If only a small piece of muscle is required, the procedure may be done with the patient lying in the supine position. The upper arm is draped free so that the axilla is exposed. The anterior margin of the muscle is marked by drawing a line from the anterior aspect of the posterior axillary fold to a midlateral position on the iliac crest.

A cutaneous flap may be outlined over any portion of the muscle with the expectation that there will be an adequate supply of perforators. However, the skin is particularly well vascularized over the superior and lateral portion of the muscle. (Fig. 28-7).

A curving incision is begun in the axilla along the anterior margin, incorporating the outline of the flap, if desired. The dissection is carried to the muscle's anterior margin, which is followed from the axilla down inferiorly until the required amount of muscle is exposed. Extra muscle is exposed. Extra muscle should be taken beyond that calculated to fill the defect, in order to allow for a margin of error and for muscle shortening. The caudal portion of the muscle is divided transversely toward the spine and is separated from the underlying chest wall. The dissection is carried upward parallel to the spine, where a number of large perforators will be encountered. By separating the distal muscle before dissecting the pedicle, the an-

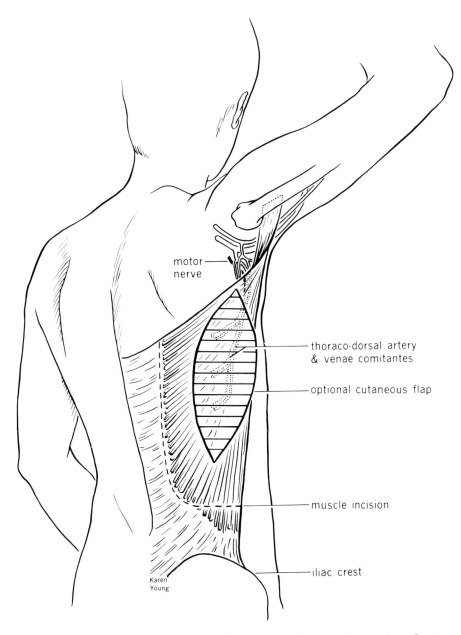

motor
nerve

thoraco-dorsal artery
& venae comitantes

optional cutaneous flap

muscle incision

iliac crest

Karen
Young

Fig. 28-7. Diagrammatic representation of the anatomy of the latissimus dorsi flap (see text).

terior margin of the muscle is relaxed, and the surgeon has a better exposure of the pedicle. The pedicle can be readily palpated 1 to 2 cm under the anterior margin. In dissecting the pedicle, a number of significant branches, including one to the serratus anterior, will be seen passing to the chest wall; these need to be ligated. The long thoracic nerve to the serratus anterior muscle may be seen deep and anterior to the dissection, and this must be spared. The pedicle can be dissected up to the level of the circumflex scapular artery to provide a long pedicle of 8 to 10 cm. The nerve to the latissimus dorsi will be readily identified lying parallel to the pedicle.

RECTUS ABDOMINIS

The application of the rectus abdominis muscle as a muscle-only or musculocutaneous transfer is receiving increasing consideration. The muscle is suitable for defects that are intermediate in size between those covered by the gracilis and the latissimus dorsi, respectively. Because of its shape, the rectus is particularly suitable for long narrow defects on the forearm or lower extremity. Using the deep inferior epigastric artery for its pedicle, the transfer of this muscle is very reliable (Fig. 28-8).

Anatomy

The rectus abdominis is a long muscle that is divided transversely by three tendinous intersections, which are adherent to the anterior rectus sheath. The muscle takes its origin from the symphysis and crest of the pubis and inserts into the cartilages of the fifth, sixth, and seventh ribs. Its function is to support the abdominal viscera and flex the spine. The removal of this muscle does not appear to create a functional problem even for those who are very physically active; however, quantitative testing of patients before and after this operation has not been reported.

The muscle is enclosed in two fascial layers — the anterior and posterior rectus sheaths. These sheaths fuse laterally and medially. The posterior rectus sheath is incomplete below the arcuate line at the level of the anterior superior iliac spines. Inferior to the arcuate line, the muscle is separated from the parietal peritoneum by only the transversalis fascia. The muscle is 7 to 10 cm in width and up to 30 cm in length. The deep inferior epigastric artery is 3 to 4 mm in diameter at its origin from the medial aspect of the external iliac artery. There are one or two venae comitantes that vary from 2.5 to 4.5 mm in diameter.

The cadaver injection studies of Boyd, Taylor and Corlett[1] have defined a concentration of musculocutaneous perforators in the paraumbilical area. A skin flap that is placed in this area is particularly well perfused. However, a flap will survive over the entire length of the rectus abdominis and even survive with a significant extension, either medial or lateral to the muscle.

Technique of Preparing the Rectus Abdominis Muscle

This flap should not be used if there has been previous surgery in the groin, such as a hernia repair, unless an angiogram indicates that the deep inferior epigastric artery is patent. Transverse ab-

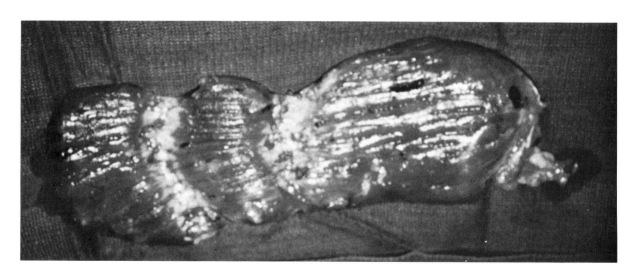

Fig. 28-8. Superficial surface of the right rectus abdominis muscle. The pedicle is seen in the lower right.

dominal scars across the muscle will also preclude its use.

If a cutaneous flap is required, it is usually marked on an axis that passes upward and laterally at about 45 degrees from the umbilicus. The maximum width of this flap depends upon the laxity of the abdominal wall, as the donor site is usually closed directly.

The incision to expose the muscle is usually a longitudinal one, although it can be elevated through a more cosmetically acceptable transverse suprapubic incision. The anterior rectus sheath is incised and the muscle separated from the sheath. Along the lateral margin of the muscle, there are multiple vascular connections with the segmental vessels of the abdominal wall. The muscle can be readily elevated from its sheath with exposure of the deep inferior epigastric artery on the deep surface. This vessel passes laterally to exit from the sheath, just below the arcuate line. To obtain maximum pedicle length, the dissection is carried extraperitoneally to the external iliac artery (Fig. 28-9).

PECTORALIS MAJOR

The pectoralis major muscle has been used more frequently as a pedicled myocutaneous transfer for head and neck intraoral reconstruction. As a free tissue transfer, it suffers from the disadvantage of having a relatively short pedicle and flap that is often removed from a fairly cosmetically visible location. However, for an innervated functioning muscle transfer, it is occasionally useful.

Anatomy

The fan-shaped pectoralis major muscle covers the upper thorax. The superior or clavicular portion arises from the medial half of the clavicle and passes downward and laterally to insert on the humerus lateral to the lip of the bicipital groove. The inferior or sternocostal portion arises from the anterior surface of the sternum, the second to sixth costal cartilages, and the aponeurosis of the external oblique muscle. The sternocostal portion passes laterally and upward to insert on the humerus in such a manner that most of the sternocostal insertion lies behind the clavicular insertion. The sternocostal portion is used for muscle transfers.

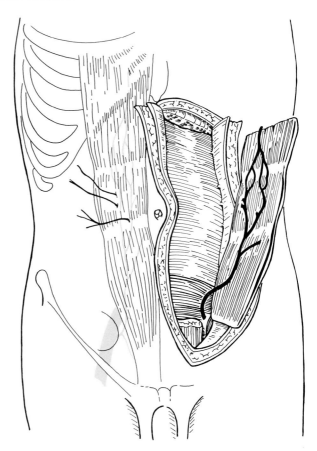

Fig. 28-9. The anatomy of the rectus abdominis showing its pedicle on the deep surface and the connections between the superior epigastric artery and the deep inferior epigastric artery. Periumbilical myocutaneous perforators provide reliable vasculature for a cutaneous flap. (Manktelow RT: Microvascular Reconstruction: Anatomy, Applications and Surgical Techniques. Springer-Verlag, Heidelberg, 1986.)

The pectoral artery, a branch of the thoracoacromial, divides into two constant branches (Fig. 28-10): the superior branch going to the clavicular head and the inferior branch to the sternal head.[10] The sternal head also receives some supply from the superior branch 40 percent of the time. The pectoral branch of the lateral thoracic artery supplies the inferolateral margin of the sternal head and is present 73 percent of the time. The inferior branch of the pectoral artery is the pedicle for transferring the sternal head. The artery is 1.5 to 7.0 cm in length and 1.5 to 2.1 mm in diameter. A venae comitans is always present and is usually slightly larger than the artery. Based on clinical experience in dividing the lateral thoracic branch, it appears that the pectoral artery can reliably supply the entire sternal portion of the pectoralis muscle.

Contrary to classic anatomic descriptions, there are five to seven individual motor branches going to the sternocostal portion of the pectoralis major muscle (Fig. 28-10). Each nerve usually contains only a single fascicle. These branches pass to the muscle from below, through, and above, the pecto-

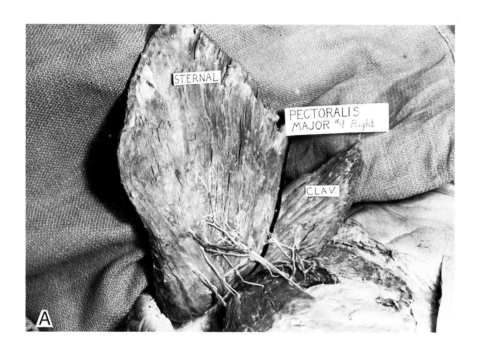

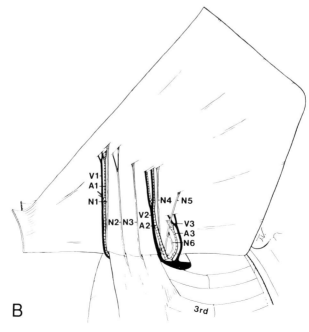

Fig. 28-10. (A) View of a cadaver dissection showing the deep surface of the right pectoralis major muscle. Seven separate motor nerves, passing medial, through, and lateral to the pectoralis major muscle, and three vascular pedicles enter the muscle. (B) Schematic illustration showing the typical pattern and location of neurovascular structures supplying the pectoralis major muscle. (B from Manktelow RT, McKee NH, Vettese T: An anatomical study of the pectoralis major muscle as related to functioning free muscle transplantation. Plast Reconstr Surg 65:610, © 1980 The Williams & Wilkins Co., Baltimore.)

ralis minor muscle. Each nerve supplies an isolated, discreet portion of the pectoralis muscle with very little functional overlap. With a nerve stimulator, the muscle can be separated into five to six separately functioning neuromuscular units. In an adult male, the length of muscle is 20 to 24 cm, with the superior fibers being the shortest.

The function of the muscle is to adduct the humerus and rotate it medially on its long axis. The clavicular portion of the muscle flexes the shoulder, and the sternal portion brings the humerus downward from the flexed position (initiates extension). In our limited experience with removal of the lower four-fifths of the sternocostal head in active young men, there has been no significant loss of shoulder function.

Technique of Preparing the Pectoralis Major Muscle

The chest is prepared with the arm draped free so that the shoulder can be moved during the procedure. If a cutaneous flap is required, it may be outlined over any portion of the muscle. The skin flap is located in a position on the muscle relative to the skin defect that is present on the arm. This cutaneous flap is quite reliable and can be taken down to the distal end of the muscle.

If a portion of the rectus sheath is required for the insertion of the muscle, it can be taken in continuity with the lateral fibers of the muscle. The neurovascular structures may be identified by dividing the muscle inferiorly and medially and elevating the muscle toward the patient's head. The deep surface is exposed, and the pedicle can be seen where it enters on a line drawn between the origin and insertion, about 40 percent of the distance from the humerus to the sternum. This represents the main branch of the inferior pectoral artery and the venae comitantes. The nerves will be seen passing from the chest wall into the muscle. It is extremely easy to damage the motor nerves, particularly the lateral and inferior nerves, when elevating the muscle.

SERRATUS ANTERIOR

The serratus anterior has also been used by some authors as a free muscle flap, and this is described in Chapter 27.

UPPER EXTREMITY COVERAGE WITH FREE MUSCLE TRANSFERS

SELECTION OF A FREE TISSUE TRANSFER FOR SOFT TISSUE COVERAGE IN THE UPPER EXTREMITY

There are many options available for soft tissue coverage in the upper extremity. Most commonly, split-thickness skin grafts or local flaps will provide an adequate solution. When these are not suitable, distant pedicled skin flaps from the chest, abdomen, and groin may be used. A free tissue transfer is useful when there is a major soft tissue defect that cannot be satisfactorily reconstructed with local or pedicled flaps, or when the specific advantages of a free tissue transfer are required.

There are many specific advantages of free tissue transfers. They are done in one stage, which allows early hand rehabilitation. Following a free tissue transfer, the extremity can be elevated immediately after surgery. This controls edema and promotes rapid healing. Mobilization of wrist and finger joints can be carried out without the delay and obstruction that often occurs in a pedicled flap. Some tissues, such as muscle, can be easily transferred by microvascular anastomosis but are difficult to transfer by staged pedicle technique.

The disadvantages of a free tissue transfer are the extra operative time required for the procedure, the technical requirements of obtaining a patent microvascular anastomosis, and the occasional problem of finding a suitable donor site. The success of free tissue transfers in medical centers that are doing large volumes is in excess of 95 percent. This exceeds the reliability of pedicled flaps and is an additional advantage of free tissue transfer.

There are four types of free tissue transfers that are available for hand coverage: skin, muscle, musculocutaneous, and fascial transfers.

A skin-only transfer provides an excellent cosmetic appearance, a durable surface, and the potential for sensibility. The most useful skin-only transfers for relatively small, soft tissue upper extremity defects are the lateral arm flap and the dorsal foot flap. For larger defects, the radial artery–based forearm flap is very useful. This flap may be raised as a pedicled flap based distally, or transferred as a free tissue transfer. (Free skin flaps are discussed in Chapter 27.)

For large defects, particularly those involving the forearm, a muscle-only flap provides excellent coverage. These flaps are covered with a split-thickness skin graft that provides a quite acceptable cosmetic appearance. The muscle contours itself well to complex shapes and cavities and provides a rich blood supply to the defect, which often aids in the control of contamination and may facilitate bony healing and nerve regeneration.

The biologic and aesthetic advantages of a combined skin and muscle flap are supplied by the myocutaneous transfer. In this transfer, the muscle and a portion of the overlying fat and skin are taken as a unit. However, the disadvantages are the limited amount of skin that can be taken and still allow direct closure of the donor site, and the sometimes excessive bulk of the flap itself.

Fascial flaps are just beginning to be developed. They will likely have a place in small soft tissue defects where minimal bulk is required, such as the dorsum or palm of the hand, or fingers. The temporalis fascia flap (described in Chapter 27), covered with a split-thickness skin graft, will provide thin coverage for these defects.

The concept of a myocutaneous flap was first appreciated by Iginio Tansini in the 19th century.[12] He recognized that the blood supply to the skin over the posterolateral chest came from vessels that were carried by the latissimus dorsi muscle. Using this concept, he developed a latissimus dorsi musculocutaneous flap for coverage of radical mastectomy defects.

Using the muscle's pedicle and the muscle as a carrier, the overlying skin can be transferred with considerable reliability. The musculocutaneous transfers that have enjoyed some popularity include the latissimus dorsi, pectoralis major, trapezius, rectus abdominis, gracilis, tensor fascia lata, and gastrocnemius. Many others have been used, both as pedicled and free tissue transfers. The excessive bulk of a myocutaneous flap is often undesirable, however, and the defect produced by a removal of a large myocutaneous flap may not close directly and thus require a split-thickness skin graft (Fig. 28-11). For these reasons, a muscle-only transfer is often more popular (Fig. 28-12). The muscle provides a good bed for a split-thickness skin graft, providing a durable and fairly acceptable appearance.

A muscle is selected for free tissue transfer on the basis of the size and shape of the defect, the recipient vessel size and location, the functional defect produced by removing the muscle, and the technical ease of elevating the muscle. The gracilis and the rectus abdominis are particularly useful, as they can be prepared simultaneously with the forearm preparation to minimize the total operative time.

Following the initial success with the transplantation of skin flaps with microvascular techniques, it became apparent that the transplantation of a muscle with microvascular techniques was not only feasible but usually simpler than the transfer of most cutaneous flaps. As many muscles have relatively large, long, and anatomically reliable vascular pedicles, which facilitate successful microvascular anastomoses, the use of a muscle as a free tissue transfer quickly became popular. Most of the muscles of the body have now been assessed for their possible use as free tissue transfers. If the muscle or portion of muscle to be transferred is reliably perfused by a single pedicle that has an adequate length and size for microanastomoses, and the muscle can be easily removed without leaving a functional deficit, it is suitable for micorvascular transfer. An adequate venous return is always provided through a venae comitans.

THE TECHNIQUE OF UPPER EXTREMITY COVERAGE WITH FREE MUSCLE TRANSFERS

The principles of forearm coverage with a muscle are similar to those in other types of free tissue transfers.

The preoperative preparation involves an estimation of the maximum size of the defect and identification of the likely site of recipient vessels. A pattern of the defect can be taken with the location of the recipient vessels marked. This allows the surgeon to assess various body locations for the most suitable muscle for soft tissue coverage.

The margins of the defect should be excised until undamaged healthy tissue remains. The recipient vessels, after being identified, should be assessed

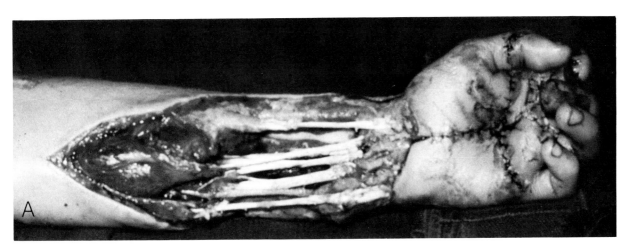

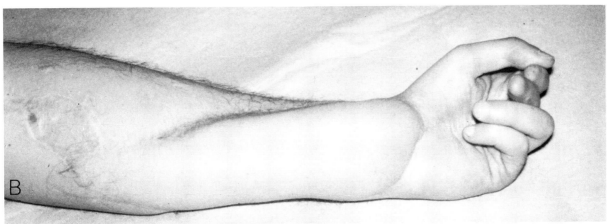

Fig. 28-11. (A) A severe forearm injury with loss of skin and subcutaneous tissue and exposure of the flexor tendons. (B) Six months after application of a latissimus dorsi myocutaneous free tissue transfer. One debulking procedure has been done to the cutaneous flap.

for their condition. If there is a strong tendency to vascular spasm, the arterial repair should be placed at a more proximal level that is further removed from the zone of injury.

After the muscle is removed, it is loosely tacked in the recipient area and the vascular anastomoses are carried out. A successful vascular anatomosis is as much related to careful positioning of the pedicle, so that it is not kinked or obstructed and to the selection of undamaged vessels, as it is to the technique of vascular anastomosis. End-to-side anatomoses are less prone to spasm problems and allow the distal circulation to be maintained.

The muscle should develop good color and epi-

mysial bleeding immediately following the vascular repairs. The muscle is skin grafted immediately and a small window is cut in the skin graft. After the extremity is dressed, a window is created in the dressing to allow direct observation of the color of the muscle. This allows postoperative monitoring and assessment of the muscle's circulation. Nevertheless, the visual observation of the perfusion of a muscle is much more difficult than that of a skin flap. Although numerous devices have been developed and tested, there is no monitoring technique that has been generally accepted (see Chapter 24 for a more detailed discussion of monitoring techniques).

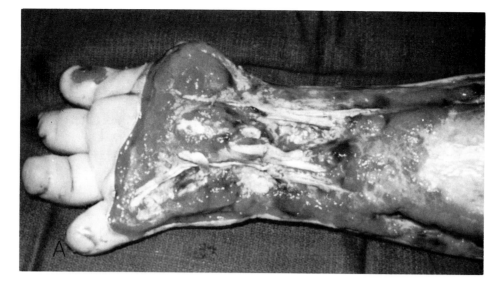

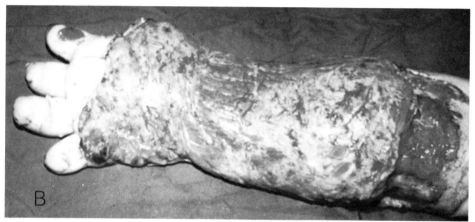

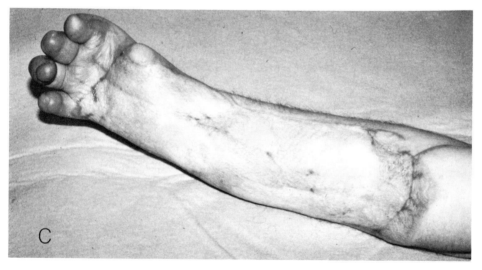

Fig. 28-12. (A) A severe injury of the right forearm with amputation of the thumb, partial amputation of fingers, and loss of all volar skin and subcutaneous tissues over the palm and the distal forearm, exposing nerves and tendons. (B) A latissimus dorsi muscle applied to the defect before application of a split-thickness skin graft to the muscle. (C) Six months after transfer. With muscle atrophy and skin graft maturation, the patient has a durable, non-bulky, cosmetically acceptable coverage.

FUNCTIONING MUSCLE TRANSPLANTATION

Functioning muscle transplantation is a procedure that involves microneurovascular transplantation of a muscle from one location to another. Viability of the transplanted muscle is maintained by microvascular anastomoses between the muscle's artery and vein and a suitable artery and vein in the recipient area. Reinnervation and active muscle contraction is produced by suturing a motor nerve in the recipient area to the motor nerve of the transplanted muscle. When a muscle is transplanted into the flexor aspect of the forearm, it is sutured to the flexor digitorum profundus tendons to produce finger flexion. This operation results in the transfer of a viable muscle that is under voluntary contraction and will provide the patient with a functional grasp and pinch mechanism.

Functional transplantation of skeletal muscle as a free island transfer or flap is a procedure with which there has not been a great deal of experience. In 1970, Tamai and colleagues established the applicability of the procedure in experimental animals.[14] In 1973, Harii, Ohmori, and Torii[3] used the gracilis to replace the muscles of facial expression in a long-standing case of Bell's palsy. In the same year, a surgical team at the Sixth People's Hospital in Shanghai transplanted the lateral portion of the pectoralis major muscle to the forearm to replace finger flexor musculature destroyed in Volkmann's ischemic contracture.[13] We have had experience with 83 functioning muscle transplantations, 32 of which have been to the upper extremity. The technique that has evolved on the basis of this experience is described in this chapter.

INDICATIONS FOR FREE MUSCLE TRANSPLANTATION TO THE FOREARM

This procedure is applicable for a patient who has sustained a major loss of skeletal musculature in the forearm, resulting in a significant functional deficit that cannot be adequately reconstructed by a simpler procedure. Muscle transplantation is a complex procedure and should not be used when simpler satisfactory techniques are available. If a tendon transfer can give an adequate result, it should be employed. The most common causes of

Table 28-1. Guidelines for Patient Selection

1. Available undamaged motor nerve, artery, and vein at the site of muscle transplantation
2. Adequate skin coverage for the distal half of the muscle
3. Supple joints and gliding tendons
4. Good hand sensibility and intrinsic function
5. Good patient motivation
6. No simpler solution for the patient's problem

muscle loss have been direct trauma to the flexor compartment, Volkmann's ischemic paralysis, electrical burns, postreplantation, and gas gangrene.[4,8,11] For a muscle transplantation to provide useful grip function, a number of conditions must be satisfied. A good range of passive joint movement and adequate hand sensibility are prerequisites. There must be a mechanism for finger and thumb extension to enable the grasp mechanism to be usable. Intrinsic muscle function should be present. In addition, the recipient of a muscle transplant must have the patience to wait for reinnervation and the persistence to pursue a post-operative muscle strengthening program (Table 28-1).

The most common application of functioning muscle transplantation has been for the replacement of long flexor muscle function to provide a useful grip. Another useful application has been for the replacement of extensor musculature to provide finger and thumb extension (Fig. 28-13). In the hand itself, small segments of the serratus anterior have been used to reconstruct thenar musculature. In the upper arm, muscle transplantation has been used for biceps and deltoid replacement.

APPLIED MUSCLE PHYSIOLOGY

An individual muscle is made up of many muscle fibers. Each of these fibers or cellular units is 1 to 40 mm in length and is composed of many myofibrils, which lie parallel to each other and are enclosed in sarcolemma. Each myofibril is composed of a hexagonal arrangement of thin actin and thicker myosin fibers that lie adjacent to each other. The configuration of muscle fibers is either strap, pennate, or a combination of the two. In a strap muscle, the fibers lie parallel to the long axis of the muscle. This is important from a functional standpoint. Strap muscles have a potential range of excursion that is directly proportional to the overall muscle length. The maximum potential con-

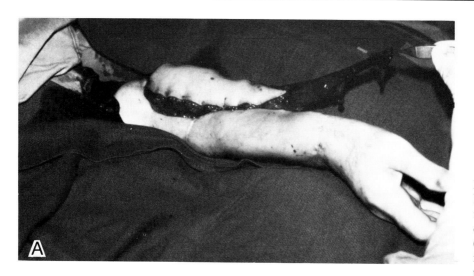

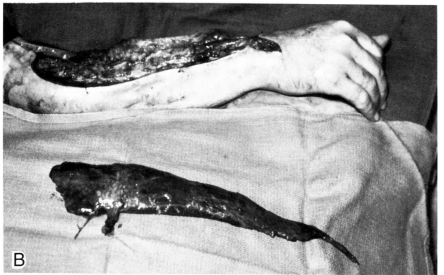

Fig. 28-13. A patient with loss of flexor and extensor musculature secondary to a crush injury of the forearm. (A) A gracilis myocutaneous flap to the flexor digitorum profundus was used to restore flexion. (B) A second gracilis muscle transplantation (done 1 year later), prior to insertion for the extensor digitorum communis, extensor pollicis longus, and abductor pollicis longus. *(Figure continues.)*

tractile force of a strap muscle can be estimated by measuring the cross-sectional area of the entire muscle. In mammals, this maximum tension has been calculated experimentally to be 4 kg/cm².

A pennate muscle has much shorter muscle-fiber units. These muscle-fiber units are attached to a central or lateral tendon. The overall length of muscle contraction is proportional to the length of these short muscle fibers, rather than to the overall length of the muscle itself. If a muscle-fiber unit in a pennate muscle is 6 cm, the overall muscle contraction capability is slightly more than 50 percent of this, or just over 3 cm. Although the overall muscle length may be as long as 30 cm, the entire muscle unit will only shorten a maximum of approximately 3 cm. If this 30 cm muscle unit were a strap muscle, such as the gracilis, the contractile capability would be in excess of 15 cm (Fig. 28-14). However, the pennate muscle is correspondingly more powerful in its contraction, as the aggregate cross-sectional area of the pennate muscle fibers is considerably larger than those in a comparably sized strap muscle. The practical solution to muscle selection for clinical application is provided by selecting a strap muscle with a large cross-sectional area.

Muscle contraction is a dynamic process of sliding the adjacent thick and thin fibers together into

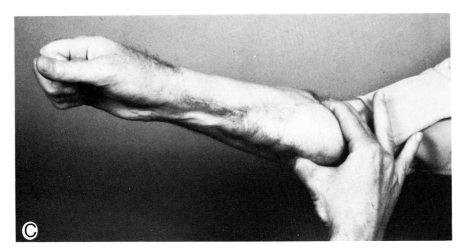

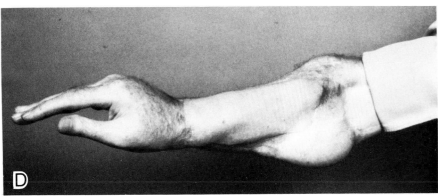

Fig. 28-13 *(Continued).* **(C)** Active flexion. The examiner's fingers demonstrate the bulk of the transferred gracilis muscle to the flexors (innervation by anterior interosseous nerve). **(D)** Active extension through the second gracilis transplant innervated by the radial nerve.

an overlap. The force of muscle contraction is directly proportional to the extent of overlap of the thick and thin fibers. Thus, at maximum extension when there is little overlap, the muscle contraction is weak. With shortening of the muscle and increasing overlap between the actin and myosin fibers, the strength of muscle contraction becomes greater and greater until there is complete overlap. This is the peak of the length-tension curve. With further contraction, there is crumpling of the myosin fibers, less area of overlap, and considerably less force of contraction (Fig. 28-15). The force of contraction is also aided by elasticity within the connective tissue network that surrounds the muscle fibers. This force of elasticity creates a significant tension within the muscle when it is in its fully extended position and plays a significant part in creating the contractile force of the muscle (Fig. 28-16).

In experimental muscle physiology, the total range of contraction of a single muscle fiber is up to 65 percent of its fully stretched length.[3] However, in an intact muscle, this fully stretched fiber length is limited by the connective tissue network that surrounds each muscle fiber and limits its extension.

When a muscle contracts, the force of contraction depends on the number of individual muscle fibers that respond to neural stimulation. The contraction of a muscle fiber is an all-or-none phenomenon. When a weak muscle contraction is required, only a few muscle fibers are activated. However, with strong muscle contraction, most of the fibers respond.

In our laboratory, experimental muscle transplantation in dogs resulted in muscles in which force of contraction varied from 35 to 120 percent of the control muscle in the normal limb.[5] The fac-

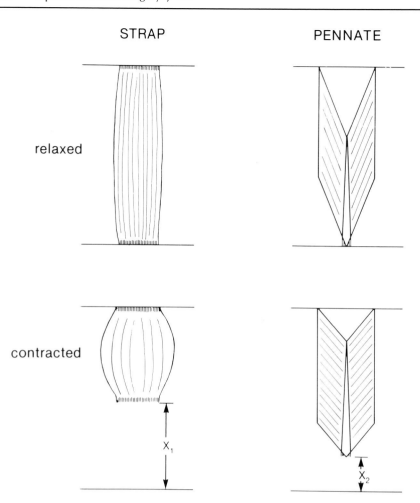

STRAP

PENNATE

relaxed

contracted

X_1

X_2

Fig. 28-14. Schematic representation comparing contraction in strap and pennate muscles. Note the marked difference in muscle excursions X_1 and X_2 with 50 percent of shortening of the muscle fibers in each muscle.

tors responsible for the range in results were not apparent, but we were impressed with the potential of obtaining a normally functioning muscle after transplantation.

Our clinical experience with relatively crude measuring techniques applied to in-vitro testing in the human gracilis muscle has demonstrated a shortening comparable to the experimental findings. The gracilis is mostly a strap muscle, with an average muscle-fiber length of 24 cm. The muscle fibers insert sequentially into its tendon, with the posterior fibers being shortest and the anterior longest. Because of this sequential insertion, the individual fibers in the average muscle have a length of 16 to 30 cm. Adult human gracilis muscles, when stimulated to maximum contraction, shorten 12 to 16 cm when measured from the physiologic fully extended muscle length. In view of the length-tension curve, it would seem reasonable to assume that a useful range of powerful muscle excursion of the gracilis is less than the maximum excursion but likely to be at least 8 to 10 cm.

PREOPERATIVE PLANNING

The optimum muscle for the recipient area is selected on the basis of the anatomic and functional requirements of the recipient area (Fig. 28-17) and the patient's concern about the resulting functional and cosmetic defects (Table 28-2).

A "pure" motor nerve must be selected in order to provide good reinnervation. For replacement of finger long flexor musculature, the preferred motor nerves are the anterior interosseous nerve, branches of the median nerve that had innervated the superficialis muscle, or branches of the ulnar

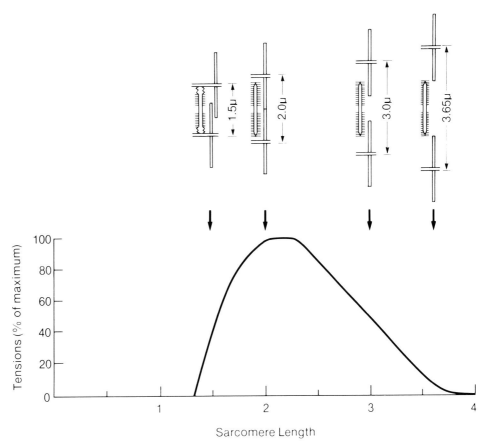

Fig. 28-15. Length-tension curve of a single muscle fiber during active contraction. Above the curve is a schematic representation of the actin and myosin (with bars) fibers at various stages of contraction. At a sarcomere length of 3.65μ there is no overlap of actin and myosin fibers and no active contraction. Note that the maximum overlap occurs at 2.0μ, which represents maximum tension. (Adapted from Carlson FD, Wilkie DR: Muscle Physiology. Prentice-Hall, Englewood Cliffs, NJ, 1974.)

nerve that had innervated the flexor digitorum profundus. For the dorsal (extensor) aspect of the forearm, motor branches of the radial nerve are used. It is important to be sure that there is a healthy, undamaged motor nerve available that has

Table 28-2. Guidelines for Muscle Selection

1. Suitable neurovascular anatomy
2. Adequate strength and range of muscle excursion
3. Suitable gross anatomy to fit the defect (muscle length, location of neurovascular bundle, and tendon availability)
4. Ability to be removed without leaving a significant functional or cosmetic donor defect

a cross-sectional area approximately equal to that of the motor nerve of the muscle to be transplanted. Good muscle function cannot be expected without a technically perfect microneural repair to an undamaged motor nerve.

From the history and physical examination, it is usually possible to make a good guess as to which motor nerve branches in the forearm are likely to be present and undamaged. If there is significant doubt about the availability of a good motor nerve, the surgeon should carry out an exploratory operation and nerve biopsy to assess the status of the motor nerve branches prior to the muscle trans-

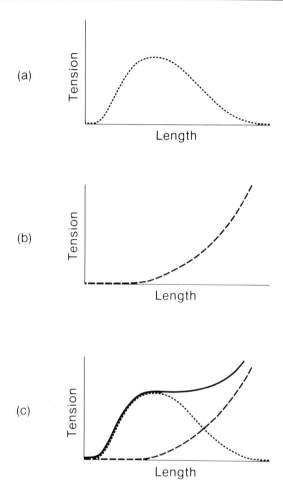

Fig. 28-16. (**A**) Length-tension curve of a single muscle fiber during active contraction. (**B**) Length-tension curve of a resting whole muscle being passively stretched. This resting tension curve varies considerably for different muscles depending upon the extent of the connective tissue framework with the muscle. (**C**) The total tension developed by a whole muscle under tetanic stimulation (solid line) is the sum of the forces produced by active contraction and passive stretching. (Adapted from Carlson FD, Wilkie DR: Muscle Physiology. Prentice-Hall, Englewood Cliffs, NJ, 1974.)

plantation. Neurohistologic examination will indicate the adequacy of the motor nerve branches for neurotization of the muscle.

The forearm is assessed for its ability to accept a free flap. A preoperative angiogram is required when the arterial pattern in the forearm is not clear from the clinical assessment. Either a superficial vein or a venae comitans is used for the recipient vein. The selected artery depends on the vessels that are available and can be determined from the arteriogram. Either end-to-end or end-to-side repairs are suitable.

If local forearm skin is not available for muscle coverage, a skin flap should be provided for the distal half of the forearm. This skin flap can be a local or distant flap, or it can be a cutaneous flap that is carried with the transplanted muscle. Flap coverage must be available for the distal half of the forearm to allow muscle gliding and to cover the flexor tendons.

SURGICAL TECHNIQUE

Preparation of the Forearm

The intended position of the muscle in the forearm is anticipated, and the known location of the neurovascular hilum is matched to the expected position of the neurovascular structures in the forearm. The incision must allow good exposure of the neurovascular structures and flexor tendons and provide flap coverage of the tendon muscle junction in the distal forearm. While one team is raising the muscle, the second team prepares the forearm. This preparation involves the identification and preparation for repair of all of the structures that are involved in the transplantation. For the neurovascular structures, a dissection from proximal to distal, going from undamaged tissues into the damaged areas, is safest. In a scarred forearm, this preparation requires a meticulous dissection to prevent inadvertent damage of the important structures. If exposure of the anterior interosseous artery or nerve is required, the pronator teres, if present, is temporarily separated from its insertion and preserved. The medial epicondyle and its surrounding fascia is exposed in anticipation of suturing the origin of the transplanted muscle. The flexor digitorum profundus tendons are identified, and their gliding capability is tested.

Muscle Transplantation

Following the muscle's separation from the donor site, it is left attached to the vascular pedicle to allow observation of the muscle's perfusion. This can be evaluated by observing the color of the muscle.

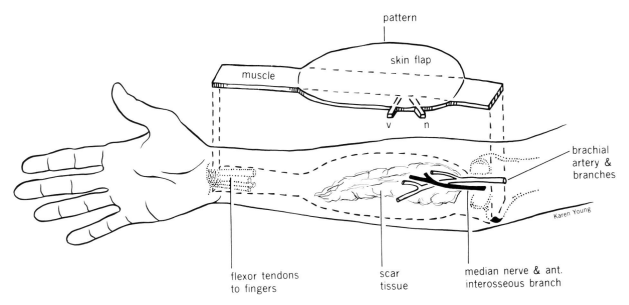

Fig. 28-17. A pattern is taken from the forearm, outlining the size of the required muscle-tendon unit and the expected location of the neuromuscular structures in the forearm. This pattern aids in selecting the most appropriate muscle for the patient. In practice, the gracilis has usually been most suitable for forearm reconstruction.

The muscle is positioned in the arm so that the motor nerve repair can be done as close as possible to the muscle. Tacking sutures are placed between the muscle and its bed so that it will not move during the neurovascular repairs.

The important technical considerations in muscle transplantation are (Fig. 28-18[7]):

1. Revascularization;
2. Nerve repair;
3. Balanced profundus tendon fixation;
4. Positioning of the muscle at optimum tension; and
5. Adequate flap coverage.

Revascularization. While the muscle's origin is held to the medial epicondyle, the insertion is stretched toward the hand and relaxed to simulate finger extension and flexion. The movements of the pedicle are observed, relative to the intended site of anastomosis in order to be sure that with muscle excursion, the anatomosis will not be stretched.

A microvascular anastomosis depends on a technically good repair in a normal vessel. If a vessel is lying in an area of previous trauma, it must be used with caution. The vessel must be examined under the microscope and the wall of the vessel scrutinized for scarring, dissection, or evidence of any other abnormality. Vessels that have been in a zone of inflammation and injury for a prolonged period of time develop a whitish layer of visible scarring in the adventitia. These vessels are very prone to spasm when they are divided in preparation for anatomosis. A good spurt from the cut artery must be present prior to doing the microvascular anastomosis. If the cut vessel tends to go into spasm, it must be resected back to a level where there is a good spurt. The venous return can be adequately handled by one venous anastomosis, if the vein is larger than the artery, or by the anastomosis of two veins, if they are on the small side. It is probably of no consequence whether the artery or the vein is repaired first, although our custom is to anastomose the vein first and then the artery. The muscle will become pink and bleed from all cut areas upon completion of the arterial anastomosis. The distal few centimeters of the gracilis muscle will usually take 5 minutes or more before they completely "pink" up. Any distal musculature that does not pink up should be removed. Often, a short portion of the distal muscle will be removed because the length of muscle is excessive. As the gracilis tendon

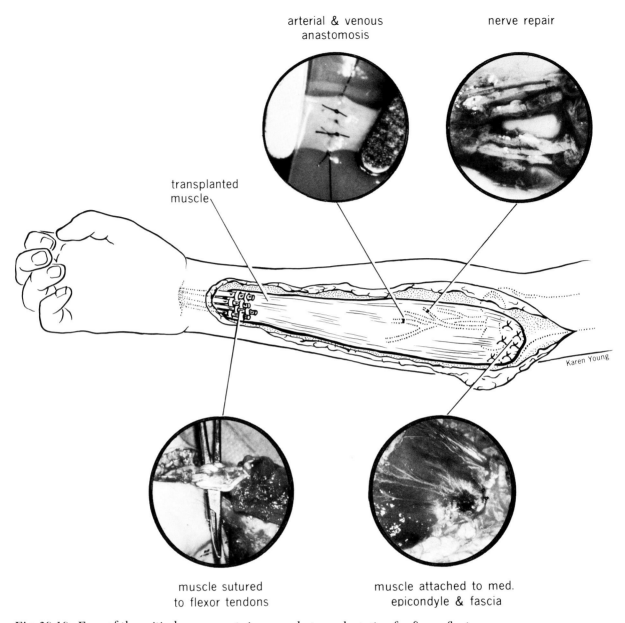

arterial & venous
anastomosis

nerve repair

transplanted
muscle

Karen Young

muscle sutured
to flexor tendons

muscle attached to med.
epicondyle & fascia

Fig. 28-18. Four of the critical components in a muscle transplantation for finger flexion.

extends proximally into the muscle, the excess distal muscle can be removed and cut fibers reattached to the intramuscular portion of the tendon without affecting function.

Reinnervation. The motor nerve repair is placed as close as possible to the muscle's neurovascular hilum to minimize the duration of denervation. Since the gracilis motor nerve has at least 60 per-

cent fatty connective tissue, a fascicular repair is done with 11 – 0 nylon to ensure good apposition of the fascicles.

Balanced Tendon Fixation. When a single muscle is used to provide finger flexion, all of the fingers should flex together to provide even contact with the object being gripped. The profundus tendons are sutured side-to-side to each other in a balanced position, with each digit slightly more flexed than the adjacent radial digit. The transferred tendon will then produce mass flexion of the fingers in a balanced grip position.

When the muscle is going to produce thumb as well as finger flexion, the flexor pollicis longus should be sutured to the finger flexors in a position that has some slack so that the fingers will begin to flex before the thumb moves. In this way, the thumb will come to rest on the radial side of the index, providing useful key pinch, rather than flex into the palm. If the gracilis is going to be used for independent finger and thumb movements, the muscle must be split into two separate neuromuscular territories and innervated with two nerve branches that have separate functions, preferably thumb and finger flexion functions.[7,9]

Muscle Positioning for Optimum Tension. The flexor digitorum profundus tendons are sutured into the distal portion of the muscle or its tendon at a tension that is designed to provide optimal grip strength, a full range of finger flexion, and good muscle balance with the intrinsic and extrinsic extensor musculature. If extensor and intrinsic musculature are intact, the fingers will rest in a position of function when the muscle has been attached to the flexor digitorum profundus tendons. If the extensors are not intact, the following technique is employed to select the optimum muscle tension. This technique is dependent on two assumptions: (1) a muscle's most powerful contraction begins near its maximum range of excursion (Fig. 28-15C); and (2) if a muscle is chosen whose normal physiological range of excursion is greater than that required in the forearm, there is the expectation that a full range of finger movement will be produced.

The technique begins while the muscle is still in its normal site. The muscle is stretched to its maximum physiological extension by moving the appropriate extremity, and markers are placed along the surface of the muscle every 5 cm (Fig. 28-19A). It can be assumed that the muscle can be safely stretched to this resting, extended length when it is transferred. When the muscle is revascularized and

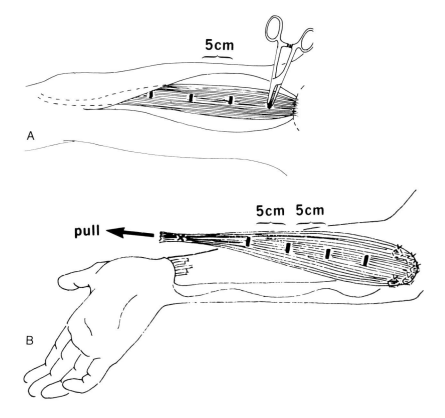

Fig. 28-19. (A) Technique of creating optimal tension in the transplanted muscle. The gracilis is stretched to its physiologic maximum extended length by abducting the thigh and extending the knee. Suture markers are applied every 5 cm on the surface of the muscle.(B) The fingers and wrist are placed in full passive extension and the gracilis is stretched distally until the suture markers are 5 cm apart. Marks are then placed opposite each other on the profundus tendons and the gracilis tendon to locate the points at which the tendons should be sutured together.

the origin attached to the common flexor origin, the muscle is stretched distally so that the markers are spaced 5 cm apart when the fingers and wrist are fully extended (Fig. 28-19B). In this position of maximum finger extension and muscle stretch, the flexor tendon stumps are placed beside the distal portion of the muscle, and adjacent positions are marked on the flexor tendons and on the tendon of the transplanted muscle. This marks the point at which the tendon-to-tendon repair should be done. With the wrist and fingers in flexion, tendon muscle fixation is accomplished without tension on the muscle. The profundus tendons to all four fingers are woven into the transplanted muscle or its tendons at the position marked. In a muscle that does not have a tendinous portion, such as the pectoralis major or the latissimus dorsi, the profundus tendons are inserted into the muscle as shown in Fig. 28-20. This measuring and marking procedure ensures that the muscle will allow full finger and wrist extension and will provide a full range of finger flexion within the most powerful range of excursion of the muscle.

Flap Coverage. Skin flap coverage must be obtained over the musculotendinous junction and the

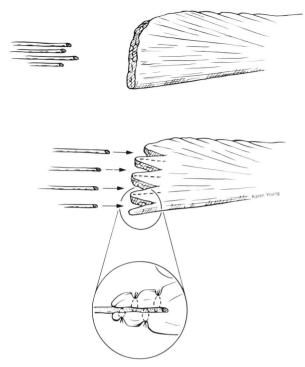

Fig. 28-20. Technique used to attach four profundus tendons to the muscle termination (origin) of the pectoralis or latissimus dorsi muscle.

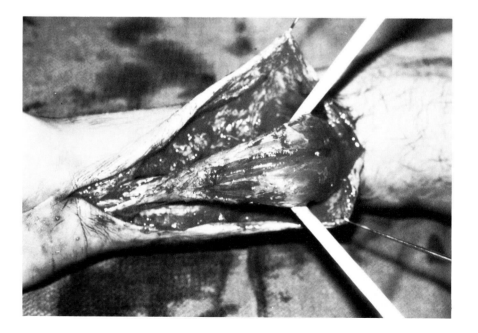

Fig. 28-21. Demonstration of the appearance of a gracilis muscle transplanted to the right forearm, seen 2 years postoperatively during exposure for a flexor tendon tenolysis. The distal third of the muscle is shown under the rubber drain, and the tendon repair to the profundus tendon is seen near the wrist.

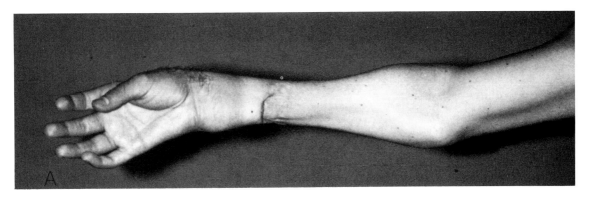

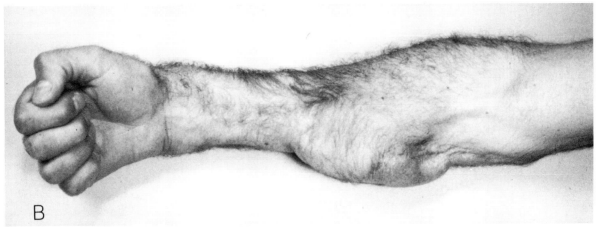

Fig. 28-22. (A) Preoperative view of the right forearm in a 22-year-old man who sustained a crushing injury, with loss of all flexor and extensor forearm musculature except for the extensor carpi radialis longus and the brachioradialis muscles. (B) Flexion of the fingers and thumb after pectoralis major transplantation to motor the flexor digitorum profundus and the flexor pollicis longus. Note the bulging muscle contraction in the proximal forearm. Grip strength is 53 lbs. *(Figure continues.)*

distal portion of the muscle. This may be carried out with a local flap from the forearm, which can be developed by the insertion of tissue expanders prior to muscle transplantation. If a myocutaneous flap is chosen, it is usually too bulky, but it does provide a cutaneous portion that acts as an indicator of vascularity of the underlying muscle. Occasionally, a distant flap, such as an abdominal or groin flap, will be used to cover the forearm. A split-thickness skin graft can be applied directly to the proximal half of the muscle without affecting its function.

POSTOPERATIVE MANAGEMENT

If a thrombosis does occur and is recognized, it is necessary to return the patient to the operating room, revise the anatomosis and obtain an intact circulation within about 3 hours, or severe ischemic damage to the muscle can be expected. However, it is unlikely that the diagnosis of thrombosis can be made quickly enough to enable such a rapid revision to be accomplished. It is thus *imperative* that the vascular anastomoses be done as nearly perfect as technically possible. If a postoperative

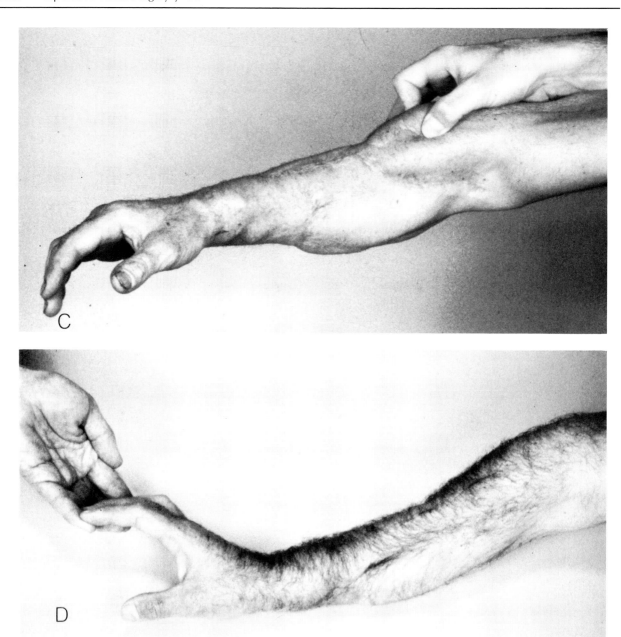

Fig. 28-22 *(Continued)*. **(C)** Extension of the fingers and thumb is provided by a gracilis muscle transplantation to the dorsum of the forearm. Adhesions at the wrist prevent full finger extension. **(D)** Relaxation of the pectoralis muscle allows full passive extension of the wrist and fingers.

thrombosis is recognized, it is preferable to replace the muscle with another one rather than revascularize a muscle that has likely sustained a damaging period of ischemia.

The most important aspect of the immediate postoperative management is to maintain a normal circulation with good peripheral perfusion. An adequate volume of intravenous fluids is given and urine output is monitored. The wrist and fingers are splinted in moderate flexion to relax the junction between the flexor tendons and transplanted muscle. The muscle is flaccid due to its denervation and the amount of tension is not excessive for the tendon repairs.

A program of passive stretching of the wrist and fingers is commenced 3 weeks postoperatively. The program is designed to obtain full passive muscle extension and overcome any tendency to myotonic contracture. Also, it improves tissue gliding at the muscle-tendon junction in anticipation of the development of reinnervation and active contraction. This program has resulted in a low incidence of tendon adhesions requiring subsequent tenolysis. Following the development of spontaneous contraction of the muscle, the patient is encouraged to attempt active flexion frequently throughout the day. When a good range of movement develops, a program of graduated resisted grip exercises is commenced and continued until maximum function is obtained.

RESULTS

Successful muscle transplantation should provide adequate functional restoration of the missing muscles (Fig. 28-21).

A 3-year follow-up review of my first 12 muscle transplantations to the forearm (1984) revealed that one survived partially and 11 survived completely. Ten of the twelve provided a useful range of motion and adequate grip for most of the patients' functional activities. Nine of these provided full finger flexion from the fully extended finger position when the wrist was held in neutral. Five of the nine also provided a nearly full range of finger flexion when the wrist was held in the fully extended or fully flexed position. The maximum grip strength was 50 percent of the patient's normal hand, and ranged from 18 to 60 lbs with the Jaymar dynamometer. All muscles were under precise and voluntary control. Some of the patients were involved in heavy farm or construction labor and did not notice any fatigue in the transplanted muscle (Fig. 28-22).

The most important factors in obtaining a good result after muscle transplantation are proper patient and muscle selection, careful preoperative planning, meticulous surgical technique, and a thorough program of postoperative exercises.

REFERENCES

1. Boyd JB, Taylor GI, Corlett R: The vascular territories of the superior epigastric and the deep inferior epigastric systems. Plast Reconstr Surg 73:1–14, 1984
2. Carlson FD, Wilkie DR: Muscle Physiology. Prentice-Hall, Englewood Cliffs, NJ, 1974
3. Harii K, Ohmori K, Torii S: Free gracilis muscle transplantation with microvascular anastomosis for the treatment of facial paralysis. Plast Reconstr Surg 57:133–143, 1976
4. Ikuta Y, Kubo T, Tsuge K: Free muscle transplantation by microsurgical technique to treat severe Volkmann's contracture. Plast Reconstr Surg 58:407–411, 1976
5. Kuzon WM, Fish JS, Pynn BR, McKee NH: Determinants of contractile function in free muscle transfers. Amer Coll Surg Surgical Forum 35:610, 1984
6. Manktelow RT: Microvascular Reconstruction: Anatomy, Applications and Surgical Techniques. Chap. 6. Springer-Verlag, Heidelberg, 1986
7. Manktelow RT: Microvascular Reconstruction: Anatomy, Applications and Surgical Techniques. Chap. 19. Springer-Verlag, Heidelberg, 1986
8. Manktelow RT, McKee NH: Free muscle transplantation to provide active finger flexion. J Hand Surg 3:416, 1978
9. Manktelow RT, Zuker RM: Muscle transplantation by fascicular territory. Plast Reconstr Surg 73:751–755, 1984
10. Manktelow RT, McKee NH, Vettese T: An anatomical study of the pectoralis major muscle as related to functioning free muscle transplantation. Plast Reconstr Surg 65:610, 1980
11. Manktelow RT, Zuker RM, McKee NH: Functioning free muscle transplantation. J Hand Surg 9A:32, 1984
12. Maxwell GP, Iginio Tansini: Origin of latissimus dorsi musculocutaneous flap. Plast Reconstr Surg 65:686–692, 1980
13. Sixth Peoples Hospital, Microvascular Service,

Shanghai: Free muscle transplantation by microsurgical neurovascular anatomoses. Chin Med J 2(1):47, 1976

14. Tamai S, Komatsu S, Sakamoto H, Sano S, Sasauchi N, Hori Y, Tastsumi Y, Okuda H: Free muscle transplants in dogs with microsurgical neurovascular anastomoses. Plast Reconstr Surg 46:219–225, 1970

15. Tobin GR, Shusterman M, Peterson GH, Nichols S, Bland KI: The intra-muscular neurovascular anatomy of the latissimus dorsi muscle: The basis for splitting the flap. Plast Reconstr Surg 67:637–641, 1981

Vascularized Bone Grafts 29

Andrew J. Weiland
J. Russell Moore

Advances over the past decade in the field of microsurgery have made it possible to provide continuing circulation to bone grafts used in the reconstruction of extremities with massive segmental bone loss following trauma or secondary to tumor resection. To appreciate the significance of transferring segmental autogenous bone grafts on vascular pedicles in reconstructive surgery, the surgeon must have a knowledge of the methods traditionally used and, more importantly, their historical development.

HISTORICAL BACKGROUND

The introduction of bone grafting in the late nineteenth century by Barth[8] led to its use in the treatment of nonunions,[1,16,27,33,46] arthrodesis of joints, the filling of bone cavities secondary to infection, replacement of bone loss secondary to trauma and following tumor reconstruction, and, finally, the replacement of joint surfaces.[5,26,31,37,62,64,65,69,74,83–85,92,98,112] The various techniques employed have evolved into the following: (1) massive autogenous corticocancellous bone obtained from the ilium, tibia, or fibula,[1,16] (2) transfer of whole bone segments,[27,55] (3) allograft bone transplants,[36,66,69,83–85,111] and (4) free vascularized bone grafts.[103,105–108,119–121]

Autogenous Bone Grafts

There is little doubt that autogenous transplants are better tolerated by the host than any other type of bone grafts.[2,41,47,48,56,68,88] The mechanisms involved in bone formation by autogenous grafts are, however, still unresolved. Basically, two concepts have evolved. One theory is that new bone formation results from the functional activity of osteogenic cells that survive in the graft.[43] However, based on observations of bone formation by these grafts, including the fact that only a small percentage of osteocytes and osteoblasts survive transplantation, several authors have proposed another mechanism, which may be referred to as the "metaplasia theory."[9,56,61,62,93,94,111] This theory proposes that bone transformation occurs under the influence of osteogenesis-inducing substances that diffuse from the transplant site into the host's connective tissue.[37] Most investigators now agree that both mechanisms are involved in bone formation.

Since surviving cells in autogenous grafts are entirely dependent on nourishment from the surrounding bed directly after transfer, the superiority of autogenous cancellous bone grafts (directly related to their open structure, which facilitates diffusion of nutrient substances necessary for osteocyte and osteoblast survival) is readily appreciated. In addition, this open structure permits the ingrowth of vessels from the host bed that carry undifferentiated mesenchymal cells. These subsequently differentiate into osteogenic cells.[45] Dense cortical bone acts as a barrier to diffusion, thereby inhibiting cell survival. Since the vast majority of cells in autogenous grafts do not survive transplantation, they must be replaced and repaired by new bone.

The replacement of dead bone by new, living bone was described by Barth in 1895[8] and Marchand in 1900[71] as "creeping substitution" ("schleichender Ersatz"). This process indicates the penetration of newly formed bone directly into the old bone and requires simultaneous removal of the old bone and deposition of new bone at the site of contact. The term "creeping substitution" was introduced into the English-language literature by Phemister in 1914.[86] The ultimate incorporation of autogenous grafts requires adequate circulation in the recipient bed, on which new bone formation can occur in the presence of cells with an osteogenic capacity.

Allograft Bone Transplants

Although it has been shown repeatedly that allografts and xenografts are not as effective in providing an environment conducive to osteogenesis as fresh autogenous bone, the use of autogenous grafts has obvious limitations such as the amount of bone available to reconstruct large defects and limited sources with which to replace articular surfaces.[47] The techniques of massive resection of bone tumors and subsequent reconstruction of large bone defects with allograft transplantations have been reported by Ottolenghi[83]; D'Aubigne, Meary, and Thomine[36]; Mankin and colleagues[69]; Lexer[63–66]; Parrish[84,85]; and Volkov.[112] Complications associated with these procedures include

nonunion between the graft and the recipient bone, resorption, collapse of articular segments, and fracture of the graft, in addition to the prolonged immobilization of 8 to 24 months required for incorporation of the graft.

In an attempt to reduce the immunogenicity of allografts, several investigators have demonstrated a reduction in antigenetic properties in freeze-dried and fresh-frozen allografts.[25,34,47,50,51] This process, however, although resulting in a reduction in the antigenicity of the allograft, kills the osteoprogenitor cells in the graft. Allografts are reported to be inferior to autografts during the early stages of repair due to the cellular response of the host tissue, as well as the impairment of vascularization of the graft.[41]

Pedicle Bone Grafts

As early as 1905, Huntington recognized the advantages of using a bone graft with its own nutrient blood supply intact — a vascularized bone graft — in the reconstruction of large tibial defects.[55] There is little doubt that, in most cases, the ideal bone graft is an autogenous graft that remains organized and alive, defies resorption, and maintains its original size and structural characteristics.

Unimpaired microcirculation is the indispensable basis for the continued life and function of all bone cells; obviously, this can only be achieved by preservation or immediate reconstitution of the primary blood supply to the bone graft. This concept of a vascularized, "living" bone graft is not new. Regional osteomusculocutaneous flaps have been used as vehicles for sections of rib or clavicle, and composite island flaps containing underlying rib have been transferred on long, intact vascular pedicles.

BLOOD SUPPLY OF CORTICAL BONE

Several groups of arteries are usually described as being engaged in the blood supply to cortical bone.[60,89] Well-defined nutrient arteries penetrate the cortex through the nutrient foramen and nutrient canal. After entering the diaphysis, the nutrient artery divides into ascending and descending branches to become the medullary arteries. These vessels have radially oriented branches that supply the diaphyseal cortex by further branching in a longitudinal direction.[109] Epiphyseal and metaphyseal arteries are found at the ends of long bones and supply their respective areas. Finally, the bones are surrounded by a periosteal vascular bed, emerging from the vessels that supply the neighboring muscles.[3] From the studies of Trueta and Caladias,[110] Rhinelander,[91] and Johnson,[59] it is evident that the blood flow through cortical bone depends predominantly on an intact medullary blood supply while the periosteal arteries play a minor role in direct cortical nutrition. Under normal circumstances, arterial blood flow passes centrifugally from the medullary system into the cortical arterioles and into the periosteal system.[17] Venous drainage most likely occurs in a centripetal direction,[109] although this point is somewhat controversial. In pathologic or ischemic situations, blood flow may be reversed; a centripetal periosteal supply then assumes the role of a collateral circulatory system.[17-19]

MICROSURGERY

"The idea of replacing diseased organs by sound ones, of putting back an amputated limb, or even of grafting a new limb on a patient having undergone an amputation is doubtless very old. The performance of such operations, however, was completely prevented by the lack of a method for uniting vessels, and thus, reestablishing a normal circulation through the transplanted structure. The feasibility of these grafts depended on the development of the technique."

Alexis Carrel

This statement, taken from Alexis Carrel's classic paper of 1908,[28] heralded the birth of vascular surgery. Following World War II, the first vascular stapling machine was developed in Russia by Androsov.[6] Various mechanical devices were thereafter designed and tested.[40,55,75] Jacobson and Suarez pioneered microvascular surgery by demonstrat-

ing the value of the operating microscope in 1960.[58] Salmon and Assimacopoulos,[95] Buncke and Schultz,[21-23] Holt and Lewis,[53] and Cobbett[32] were responsible for the improvement in instrumentation and early experimental work in free vascularized tissue transfer. The first clinically successful transfer of an island flap by microvascular anastomoses was reported by Daniel and Taylor in 1973.[35] In the ensuing years, the scope of free tissue transfer has expanded rapidly to include free muscle transfers.[70,100,101]

In 1975, Taylor reported the first clinically successful free bone graft with microvascular anastomoses in which a fibular segment was transferred from the contralateral leg to reconstruct a large tibial defect.[103,105] Since this historic report, many centers have reported on their clinical results with this procedure.[42,54,80,102,113,114,116,122] Similarly, vascularized rib grafts were used for treatment of a nonunion of a mandible following radical resection of a tumor.[96] Free osteocutaneous flaps consisting of the rib and overlying soft tissue have been transferred by Buncke[21] and O'Brien[79] and Taylor and Watson have reported on the one-stage repair of a compound leg defect with an osteocutaneous flap from the groin.[108] Weiland, Daniel, and Riley and other authors have extended the application of free vascularized bone grafts to the treatment of malignant or aggressive bone tumors,[73,119,121] and the technique has been used in the treatment of congenital pseudarthrosis of the tibia.[30,44,117] The advantages of transferring segmental autogenous bone grafts on vascular pedicles for the treatment of upper extremity lesions have also been reported.[4,52,87,99,120]

VASCULARIZED BONE GRAFTS

The preceding sections of this chapter have attempted to point out the traditional methods of bone grafting and to provide some insight into the microcirculation of bone and the emergence of the field of reconstructive microsurgery. In selected patients, free vascularized bone grafts offer significant advantages over conventional methods of treatment, since a massive segment of bone, along with its accompanying nutrient vessels, can be detached from its donor site and transferred to a distant recipient site with preservation of the nutrient blood supply by microvascular anastomoses to recipient vessels. With the nutrient blood supply preserved, osteocytes and osteoblasts in the graft can survive, and healing of the graft to the recipient bone will be facilitated with the usual replacement of the graft by "creeping substitution." This concept has been validated by many authors who have reported experimental studies concerning the various factors affecting the survival of vascularized bone grafts.[7,11–14,38,67,97,115,123] Thus, with vascularized bone grafts the surgeon can achieve more rapid stabilization of bone fragments separated by a large defect without sacrificing viability. This is especially significant when the defect is situated in a highly traumatized or irradiated area with significant scarring and relative avascularity, precluding incorporation of conventional bone grafts.

The surgeon must, however, consider several factors before selecting this obviously difficult technique for the reconstruction of segmental bone defects over more conventional operative procedures. A surgical team that is thoroughly familiar with microsurgical techniques must be available since these procedures are often long and tedious, lasting from 5 to 8 hours. In patients with a history of severe trauma, irradiation, or infection, the likelihood of significant damage to recipient vessels in the extremity must be carefully weighed, since the possibility of failure due to poor arterial inflow and venous outflow is greater in these cases. The extensive dissection and time required for performing the procedure can exacerbate a previously quiescent infection and minimize the chance for success.

Postoperative management does not differ significantly from conventional bone grafting techniques. For the lower extremity, bed rest and elevation of the affected limb are prescribed for 2 weeks, and dressing changes are performed as necessary. Rigid fixation of the graft is usually achieved with plate and screws or an external fixation device allowing free movement of the joints proximally and distally. For upper extremity cases, internal fixation with plate and screws is most often employed. Patients are allowed to ambulate on the donor extremity 3 to 5 days following surgery, and

physical and occupational therapy is instituted to mobilize the upper extremity at that time. We have not used anticoagulants in our series of patients, except for aspirin, which is administered 10 grains, three times a day. The average period of hospitalization has been 10 days. Incorporation of the graft at the proximal and distal juncture sites is usually achieved within 3 to 4 months, and in lower extremity cases partial weight bearing is then allowed, progressing to full weight bearing as the graft undergoes progressive hypertrophy. For upper extremity cases, unrestricted active range of motion of the extremity is permitted as soon as bone union is achieved (3 to 4 months).

Since autografts and allografts employed for massive segmental bone defects greater than 6 cm often require multiple procedures and long-term immobilization of an extremity before healing is achieved, we have used free vascularized bone grafts for segmental defects of 6 cm or more after carefully considering the factors discussed above. Autogenous, nonvascularized cancellous bone grafts have been employed successfully in those situations where defects were 6 cm or less.

The fibula, rib, and iliac crest (with the latter incorporated into a free osteocutaneous flap from the groin) (Fig. 29-1) are the free bone transfers that have been employed most frequently as vascularized bone grafts. The nutrient artery of the fibula (Fig. 29-1A) arises as a branch of the peroneal artery, which in turn originates from the posterior tibial trunk. The peroneal artery gives off several periosteal branches before giving origin to the nutrient artery that supplies the medullary nutrient blood flow to the fibula. Penetration through the fibular cortex usually occurs at the mid-diaphyseal level with a variation of 2.5 cm proximally or distally. The length of the nutrient artery external to the fibula ranges from 5 to 15 mm, and the diameter is from 0.25 to 1.0 mm.[90] The peroneal artery continues distally along the medial and posterior aspect of the fibular diaphysis (Fig. 29-1B) and provides direct musculoperiosteal branches. Preservation of the medullary and periosteal supply to the straight cortical bone is, therefore, possible by isolation of the peroneal artery and its origin from the posterior tibial peroneal trunk. The venous drainage closely parallels the arterial supply and occurs through the venae comitantes of the pero-

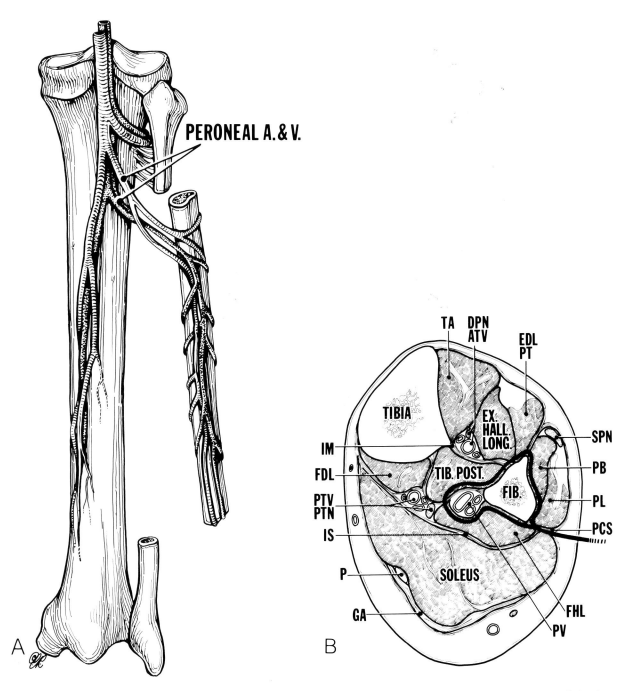

Fig. 29-1. (**A**) The free vascularized fibular graft isolated on the peroneal vessels. (**B**) Cross-section of the leg illustrating the plane of dissection for harvesting a fibular graft *(solid black line)*. (*TA*, tibialis anterior; *DPN*, deep peroneal nerve; *ATV*, anterior tibial vessels; *EDL*, extensor digitorum longus; *PT*, peroneus tertius; *SPN*, superficial peroneal nerve; *PB*, peroneus brevis; *PL*, peroneus longus; *PCS*, posterior crural septum; *FHL*, flexor hallucis longus; *PV*, peroneal vessels; *GA*, gastrocnemius aponeurosis; *P*, plantaris; *IS*, intermuscular septum; *PTV*, posterior tibial vessels; *PTN*, posterior tibial nerve; *FDL*, flexor digitorum longus; *IM*, interosseous membrane.) *(Figure continues.)*

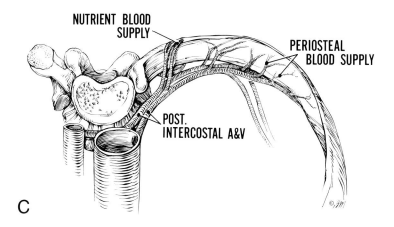

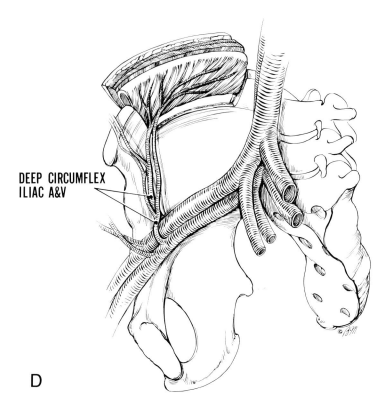

Fig. 29-1 *(Continued)*. (**C**) The free vascularized rib graft demonstrating the nutrient and periosteal blood supply. (**D**) The osteocutaneous groin flap based on the deep circumflex iliac artery and vein.

neal artery and medullary sinusoidal system. The medullary vascular supply to the rib (Fig. 29-1C) arises as a nutrient branch of the posterior intercostal artery, but recent experimental evidence from our laboratory suggests that it is not necessary to preserve the nutrient blood supply to the rib and that vascularized rib transfers will survive equally well on their periosteal or medullary blood supply.[118] While a comparable nutrient blood flow to

the iliac crest does not exist, Taylor and Watson[108] have demonstrated, with injection studies of the superficial circumflex iliac artery, that adequate blood flow to the osseous portion of the osteocutaneous groin flap may be present. However, there is some question as to the validity of these studies. More recently, Taylor has been basing this flap on the deep circumflex iliac artery (Fig. 29-1D), with favorable evidence, experimentally and clinically,

Table 29-1. Free Bone Transfers

Characteristics	Fibula	Rib	Iliac Crest
Bone			
Length (maximum)	22–26 cm	30 cm	10 cm
Shape	Straight	Curved	Slightly curved
Structure	Cortical, straight	Membranous, malleable	Corticocancellous, fixed
Vessels			
Artery	Peroneal (1.5–2.5 mm)	Posterior intercostal (1.5–2.0 mm)	Superficial circumflex iliac (0.8–3.0 mm)
Vein	Two venae comitantes (2.0–3.0 mm)	One intercostal (1.2–2.5 mm)	Superficial inferior epigastric (1.5–3.0 mm)
Vascular stalk	Short (1.0–3.0 cm)	Long (3.0–5.0 cm)	Moderate (1.0–5.0 cm)
Dissection	Superficial, simple, tedious	Deep, difficult, quick	Superficial, meticulous
Options			
Articular surface	Yes	Yes	No
Epiphysis	Yes	No	No
Adjacent muscle	Yes	Yes	No (nonfunctional)
Overlying skin	No	Yes	Yes
Nerve	No	Yes	Yes
Complications	Minimal	Thoracotomy Venous inadequacy and thrombosis	Abdominal wall hernia
Applications	Long bone defects (extremities)	Mandibular reconstruction; composite bone-skin replacement	Composite bone and skin (extremities); mandibular reconstruction

that the nutrient blood flow to the bone is significantly better than with the superficial circumflex iliac artery.[106,107]

A comparison of the characteristics of the fibula, rib, and iliac crest with respect to bone configuration, vessels, and dissection techniques and their applicability in reconstructive procedures is outlined along with their complications in Table 29-1. There is little doubt that the fibula is more suited than the rib to restore long bone defects because of its structural characteristics. The rib is a curved membranous bone that is malleable and may be preferable for reconstructive procedures in the mandible. As originally suggested by Östrup and Frederickson,[81,82] free rib transfers offer rapid reconstruction of the mandible following severe trauma or tumor reconstruction, including those cases that have had postoperative radiation therapy. The experimental validation of this concept was provided by Östrup in his classic monograph.[81]

In situations where skin and bone defects exist, the surgeon may employ a free osteocutaneous flap. Both the intercostal flap incorporating the rib and soft tissue or the groin osteocutaneous flap are available. However, the curvature of the iliac crest usually limits its applicability to bone defects of 10 cm or less, while both the curvature and structural characteristics of the rib may preclude its successful use in long bone defects.

Operative Technique

PREOPERATIVE PLANNING

Multiple cadaver dissections of the donor area to be used in vascularized bone transfers should be carried out in the anatomic laboratory prior to application of these techniques clinically. The surgeon should be totally familiar with the vascular anatomy of the upper and lower extremities. In addition, the surgical team must be thoroughly acquainted with the various techniques of microvascular surgery and must be able to perform multiple types of microvascular anastomoses with facility (see Chapter 24).

Preoperative arteriograms of both donor and recipient sites should be obtained to identify possible vascular abnormalities resulting from congenital malformations or from trauma in the recipient extremity. Clinical experience has taught us that significant problems with arterial inflow may exist in patients with traumatic defects even when preoperative arteriograms appear normal. This finding reflects the fact that the zone of injury to the extremity often extends a significant distance from the obvious bone defect and results in vascular damage that precludes successful microvascular anastomoses.

FREE FIBULAR TRANSFER

In situations where a microvascular surgical team is available to perform free tissue transfer, significant time is saved by using a two-team approach where one team works on the recipient site and the other on the donor site. The operation usually begins at the recipient site where the vessels are identified and isolated. If a tumor is involved, the tumor is excised en bloc, incorporating any biopsy site, and the size of the defect is determined. Where a nonunion or infection exists, the bone ends are debrided and prepared proximally and distally, in order to receive the fibular graft. It is imperative that the bone be resected back to *normal* tissue.

After the recipient vessels are identified, the defect measured, and the technical feasibility of the free fibular transfer determined, the free fibular graft may be harvested from the donor leg.

Dissection of the fibula is performed under general anesthesia with the patient supine and the donor extremity flexed approximately 135 degrees at the knee and 60 degrees at the hip. The surgeon and first assistant stand on the lateral side of the leg with the second assistant positioned medially, supporting the extremity in the flexed position. A tourniquet is used during the course of the dissection, which is performed under 2.5 × to 4.0 × loupe magnification. For descriptive purposes, the procedure can be divided into eight steps. Figure 29-1B illustrates the plane of dissection.

Step I. A longitudinal skin incision is made along the lateral aspect of the fibula extending from the neck as far distally as needed.[49] The incision is carried through the skin and subcutaneous tissue to the superficial fascia overlying the interval between the peroneus longus and soleus muscles. The fascia is then split longitudinally for the length of the graft required.

Step II. The interval between the peroneus longus and soleus muscles is identified and the *deep* fascia incised over the entire length of the incision along this interval. Using a blunt elevator, this interval between the peroneus longus and soleus muscles is developed. The peroneus longus and soleus muscles are then reflected from the fibular diaphysis anteriorly and posteriorly respectively, using an extraperiosteal dissection technique.

Step III. The lateral border of the fibula is now exposed. There are three perforating vessels to the skin lying immediately posterior in the fascia overlying the soleus muscle. If the skin is to be harvested with the fibula, then these branches must be preserved. When the bone alone is to be transferred, these vessels should be ligated.

Step IV. Beginning proximally, the peroneus longus and brevis muscles are elevated from the anterior border of the fibula, using a blunt elevator until the anterior crural septum is reached while staying extraperiosteal. Some preserved muscle tissue is harvested with the fibular graft, but the 1 cm cuff of muscle surrounding the fibula as previously described is no longer used.[117] In the event that the vascularized graft fails, the cuff of muscle will become necrotic and possibly serve as a nidus for infection. In addition, it will delay replacement of the graft by creeping substitution. The anterior crural septum is divided along the length of the graft, and the extensor group of muscles (extensor digitorum longus, peroneus tertius, and extensor hallucis longus) are dissected off of the interosseous membrane. Throughout the course of this portion of the dissection, the anterior tibial artery and nerve should be identified and protected.

Step V. The posterior crural membrane is divided the entire length of the graft. Using careful extraperiosteal dissection techniques, the soleus and flexor hallucis muscles are reflected off the posterior border of the fibula, taking care to preserve the nerve to the flexor hallucis muscle. The dissection continues until the peroneal vessels are encountered. The vessels must be left attached to the posterior surface of the intermuscular septum to prevent separation from the fibular graft. Dissection is continued anteriorly and posteriorly for the length of the graft required. During the posterior dissection, any branches arising from the peroneal artery that will not be taken with the graft must be coagulated. Two or three large branches arising from the peroneal artery will supply a significant portion of the soleus muscle and must be preserved if a composite soleus and fibular graft is desired. Additional branches to the skin can also be preserved if the surgeon desires to monitor circulation to the graft. However, orientation of the skin flap can be difficult, especially when the bone defect is not located in a subcutaneous area. In the distal one-third of the fibula, the peroneal artery lies directly on the posterior surface of the bone, and care should be taken to avoid damage to the artery during the osteotomy.

Step VI. The length of graft needed is measured and marked with methylene blue. The distal 6 cm of the fibula should be preserved to maintain integrity of the lateral aspect of the ankle joint. In children less than 10 years of age, a transfixation screw between the distal fibular segment and tibia is employed, and a formal synostosis of the tibia and fibula is performed distally to preserve the integrity of the ankle mortice and prevent possible proximal migration of the distal fibula, which could lead to valgus instability.

A hole is then made in the intermuscular septum, sufficiently large to allow a 1.5 cm malleable retractor to be placed around the bone, protecting the vessels that lie posterior to the retractor. At this point, a Gigli's saw may be passed, and the distal osteotomy is performed. A similar procedure is carried out at the proximal end of the graft, again taking great care to preserve the peroneal vascular bundle. The peroneal vessels at the distal end of the graft are then ligated with hemoclips.

Step VII. A small bone hook is placed in the medullary canal of the distal portion of the fibular graft. As the graft is retracted posteriorly and laterally, division of the interosseous membrane is performed along the entire length of the graft. The graft is then carefully retracted anteriorly, and the tibialis posterior muscle is dissected off the posterior aspect of the graft in the middle third where it has remained attached to the fibula. On completion of this step, the fibular graft is isolated on its vascular pedicle proximally.

Step VIII. The peroneal artery is traced proximally to its junction with the posterior tibial artery. A vessel loop is placed around the peroneal artery and vein. The fibula is placed back into the bed until the recipient site is prepared. The tourniquet is deflated, permitting circulation to the graft. This portion of the dissection should take about 1½ hours to complete. On completion of the dissection in the recipient bed, the tourniquet is reinflated, and the fibula is harvested and placed in the defect.

We have not established the upper limits of the length of the fibular graft that may be harvested from the donor extremity. Grafts as long as 24 cm have survived completely, and this is not surprising when one considers that the periosteal and medullary blood supply to the bone is preserved. The technique for dissection of the fibula described above is a modification of that employed by Gilbert.[43]

The transferred bone must be rigidly fixed in the recipient site before microvascular anastomoses are begun. We have employed various methods of internal and external fixation. Intramedullary fixation is to be condemned because of the inherent destruction of the medullary blood supply to the bone. A plate spanning the entire length of the graft should be avoided when possible because of possible compromise of the periosteal blood supply to the entire graft under the plate and, more importantly, because of the possible destruction of the vessels by the plate itself. In cases where external fixation is contraindicated, such as in small children or in selected upper extremity cases, the use of two small plates, one over each end of the graft, is preferable. When external fixation devices are indicated, we have used the Wagner apparatus and the AO external fixation device because of their ease of application. The Hoffmann apparatus is also extremely valuable because of the greater control of the proximal and distal fragments afforded, in addition to the extremely rigid fixation provided when compared to the Wagner and AO devices.

Cancellous bone grafts obtained from the iliac crest are placed at the proximal and distal juncture points of the graft with the recipient bone to promote more rapid union. Once the graft is rigidly in place, the operating microscope is positioned, and microvascular anastomoses of one artery and one vein are performed, the latter often representing a confluence of both venae comitantes. Success of the anastomoses is evidenced by bright, red bleeding from the preserved muscle sleeve and good venous return.

FREE OSTEOCUTANEOUS GROIN FLAP

In patients presenting with massive skin and bone loss in an extremity, we have used the free osteocutaneous groin flap. In those cases in which the superficial circumflex iliac artery was used to supply the graft, an inferior-to-superior medial incision was used to identify the vessels.[104] We now believe that the optimal blood supply to the graft is supplied by the deep circumflex iliac system as described by Taylor[106,107] and have used this technique in our most recent cases (Fig. 29-1C).

After identifying the superficial circumflex iliac artery and vein and the inferior epigastric vein, dissection proceeds superior to the inguinal ligament, where the deep circumflex iliac artery and vein are identified arising from the external iliac artery and vein, respectively. Sharp and blunt dissection is used to expose the preperitoneal fascia after incisions are made in the external oblique, internal oblique, and transversus abdominis muscles, thereby allowing the posterior aspect of the inner table of the iliac crest with its iliacus muscle to be seen. The vessel runs approximately two finger breadths below the iliac crest on its internal margin in a fibrous tunnel formed by the line of attachment of the transversalis fascia and iliacus fascia. In men, the spermatic cord and vascular structures are carefully preserved, as well as the genitofemoral branch of the femoral nerve. The size of the flap is then outlined based on the deep circumflex iliac artery. Attention is turned to the lateral margin of the iliac crest where an oscillating saw is used to cut through the crest, preserving a depth of 2.5 cm in the graft. The cut is then continued medially with the osteocutaneous flap finally isolated on its vascular pedicle, consisting of the deep circumflex iliac artery and vein. The attachment of the overlying skin and subcutaneous tissue to the iliac crest must be carefully preserved to avoid accidental shearing of the small nutrient vessels supplying the skin. Due to the curvature of the ilium, grafts larger than 10 cm usually cannot be obtained. A portion of the origin of the tensor fascia lata and gluteus medius can be preserved on the outer table of the iliac crest, but this is not necessary; however, a similar sleeve of iliacus must be retained on the inner table in order to preserve the nutrient blood supply to the bone. The donor site is closed primarily with the hip flexed approximately 30 degrees.[106] (For additional details of the free osteocutaneous groin flap, see Chapter 27.)

Results

We have performed a total of 91 vascularized autogenous bone grafts since 1976. Eighty-two patients underwent free vascularized fibular transfer to reconstruct massive segmental bone defects where adequate soft tissue coverage was present. Nineteen of these patients had free vascularized fibular grafts performed in the upper extremity. In addition, nine osteocutaneous groin flaps were carried out in those instances where combined soft tissue and bone defects existed. All of these cases involved the lower extremity.

There has been no postoperative morbidity at the donor site in any of our patients. The first ten patients had bone scans with[99m]Tc diphosphonate 24 to 48 hours postoperatively and again at 6 weeks following surgery.[91] In each patient, the bone scans revealed uptake in the graft. Because we intended to fully explore the potential of the technique, arteriograms were obtained of the arterial anastomosis 6 weeks postoperatively in the first eight free vascularized fibular transfers. Seven of the arteriograms showed a patent arterial anastomosis, while one case showed partial occlusion between the graft and recipient vessel.

Analysis of the results of vascularized bone grafts in the upper extremity in 19 patients revealed that the average length of the graft was 7.5 cm. Bone union between the graft and recipient bone was obtained in 3 to 4 months. Two patients required secondary grafting procedures for nonunion at one junction site. One patient sustained a fracture of the fibula graft that healed in 6 weeks, and one patient has a persistent nonunion between the graft and distal humerus. There were no postoperative infections in any of the upper extremity cases.

In dealing with upper extremity segmental bone

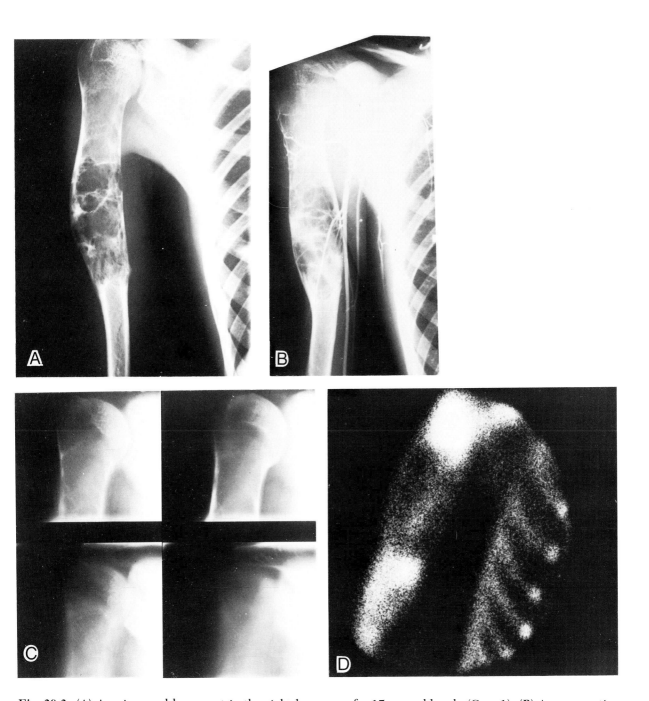

Fig. 29-2. (A) A unicameral bone cyst in the right humerus of a 17-year-old male (Case 1). **(B)** A preoperative arteriogram of the right upper extremity demonstrated the circumflex humeral artery proximally and the profunda brachii artery distally. **(C)** Tomograms revealed that only 1 cm of normal bone was present in the proximal humerus. **(D)** A bone scan demonstrated that sufficient bone stock was present proximally to allow fixation of the humerus with the Wagner apparatus. *(Figure continues.)*

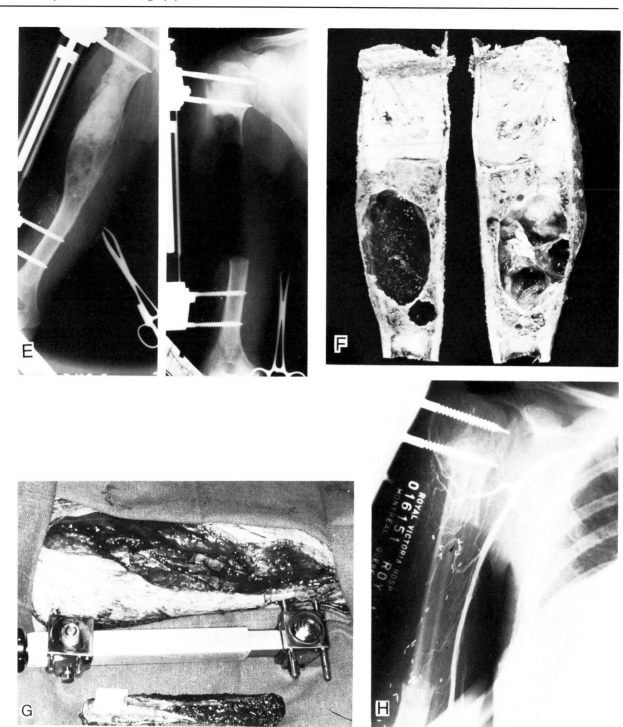

Fig. 29-2 *(Continued).* **(E)** Radiographs showing the Wagner apparatus in place prior to and after resection of the unicameral cyst. **(F)** The resected specimen, with the methylmethacrylate-packed portion of the tumor seen at the top of the picture and the remaining cyst seen distally. **(G)** Intraoperative photograph of the fibular graft just prior to insertion into the humeral defect. **(H)** An arteriogram at 6 weeks revealed a patent arterial anastomosis between the peroneal artery and the profunda brachii artery *(arrow)*; microclips are seen surrounding the graft. *(Figure continues.)*

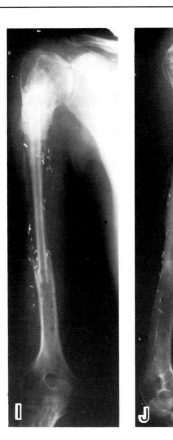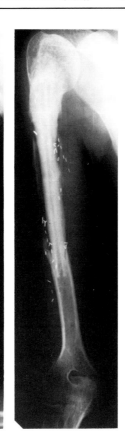

Fig. 29-2 *(Continued)*. Radiographs at (**I**) 6 months and (**J**) 12 months, showing progressive hypertrophy of the free vascularized fibular graft. (Weiland AJ, Daniel RK: Clinical techniques of segmental autogenous bone grafting on vascular pedicles. pp. 646–679. In Mears DC (ed): External Skeletal Fixation. ©1983, The Williams & Wilkins Co, Baltimore.)

defects, the surgeon should be familar with conventional techniques available to achieve skeletal continuity. Shortening of the humerus up to 5 cm and forearm up to 4 cm can result in acceptable function. For forearm bone defects, the option of creating a one-bone forearm should always be kept in mind despite the limitation of loss of forearm rotation.

Illustrative Cases

Case 1

G.R. is a 17-year-old boy who presented with an 8-year history of a unicameral bone cyst of the right humerus. His previous history included multiple pathologic fractures through the lesion and two operative attempts at curettage and bone grafting, each resulting in recurrence of the lesion with subsequent fractures (Fig. 29-2A). Preoperative evaluation included arteriograms of the right upper extremity (Fig. 29-2B) and both legs, in addition to tomograms of the lesion (Fig. 29-2C), which re-

vealed that only 1 cm of normal bone was present proximally in the humeral head. Because of the significant difficulties in obtaining adequate external fixation that would be created by such limited bone stock proximally, a two-stage reconstructive procedure was planned. Stage 1 consisted of meticulous curettage and autogenous cancellous bone grafting of the proximal portion of the humerus from the right iliac crest. In addition, to prevent the tumor from extending proximally into the newly grafted area, methylmethacrylate was packed into the distal aspect of the lesion. The patient recovered uneventfully from this procedure and was followed at regular intervals with serial bone scans to monitor incorporation of the autogenous cancellous bone graft in the proximal humeral segment. Five months postoperatively, it was felt that sufficient bone stock was present to allow adequate external fixation of the humerus with the Wagner apparatus using four Schantz screws, two proximally and two distally (Fig. 29-2D). Resection of 17 cm of humerus was carried out after application of the Wagner apparatus, and immediate reconstruction with a 20.5 cm segment of vascularized fibular graft from the left leg was performed (Fig. 29-2E–G). Microvascular anastomoses of the peroneal artery and venae comitantes of the graft to the profunda brachii artery and its accompanying venae comitantes were performed. Postoperative bone scans revealed excellent uptake in the vascularized graft, and an arteriogram at 6 weeks revealed a patent arterial anastomosis (Fig. 29-2H). At this time, 8½ years after surgery, the graft has united proximally and distally with hypertrophy of the free vascularized graft evident (Fig. 29-2I and J). The patient has full range of motion of the right shoulder, elbow, and forearm and uses the extremity for normal daily activities and participates fully in vigorous athletic events.

Case 2

T.G., a 17-year-old boy, was a victim of a service station robbery, sustaining a shotgun wound to his left, nondominant forearm in 1978, with a resulting 7.5 cm segmental loss of the radius and loss of radial nerve function and significant extensor muscle mass in the extremity. Irrigation and debridement of the wounds were performed initially, in addition to transfixation of the distal radius fragment to the distal ulna to prevent bone shortening (Fig. 29-3A and B).

To preserve pronation and supination of the forearm (since this young man was a ski champion), reconstruction with a vascularized fibular graft was planned rather than creation of a one-bone forearm. A two-stage operation, consisting of tendon transfers to restore radial nerve function, was also formulated.

A 9-cm fibular graft was harvested from the right leg, preserving the nutrient blood supply and a surrounding 0.7 cm muscle cuff as described previously (Fig. 29-3D). The graft was fixed to the proximal and distal radius with two one-third tubular AO plates and 3.5-mm cortical screws to avoid spanning the entire graft with a single plate and possible injury to the nutrient vessels. Microvascular anastomoses of the peroneal artery and its venae comitantes to the radial artery and cephalic vein were performed (Fig. 29-3E and F). Cancellous bone from the right iliac crest was placed at the proximal and distal juncture points (Fig. 29-3G). At

3 months, complete healing of the bone defect was achieved, and all immobilization of the left upper extremity was discontinued (Fig. 29-3H). Approximately 4 months after the initial procedure, tendon transfers were performed to restore radial nerve function. These consisted of transfer of the palmaris longus to the extensor pollicis longus, flexor digitorum sublimis 3 and 4 to the extensor digitorum communis, and the flexor carpi radialis to the extensor carpi radialis longus and brevis. At 1 year postinjury, the patient had returned to his normal activities, including skiing. He has full range of motion of the wrist and fingers but only 20 degrees of pronation and 20 degrees of supination.

Case 3

A.W. is a 54-year-old man who noted pain and swelling of the left wrist in January 1976. One month later, he was seen in our clinic; roentgenograms showed a cystic lesion of the left distal radius compatible with giant cell tumor (Fig. 29-4A), and a biopsy was performed that confirmed the diagnosis. A preoperative arteriogram demonstrated absence of the peroneal artery in the right lower extremity. Because of this, we elected to use the left fibula as a free vascularized bone graft. On March 15, 1976, a free vascularized fibular transfer was performed (Fig. 29-4B). A 10-cm fibular segment was isolated on its vascular pedicle using the technique described previously, and the distal radius incorporating the tumor was resected. The fibular segment was fixed to the proximal and distal carpal bones with a one-third tubular AO compression plate. Proximally, a similar fixation plate was used to secure the fibula and distal radius. After fixation was attained, the peroneal artery was inserted as an interposition graft into the radial artery with proximal and distal anastomoses, thereby maintaining the radial blood supply to the hand. The two venae comitantes were anastomosed to available superficial veins (Fig. 29-4C). The patient's initial postoperative course was uncomplicated. Six weeks after surgery, an arteriogram was performed; this revealed patent anastomoses of the interposition peroneal artery that provided nutrient blood supply to the fibular segment while preserving the radial vascular supply to the hand (Fig. 29-4D). Bone scans were performed 48 hours

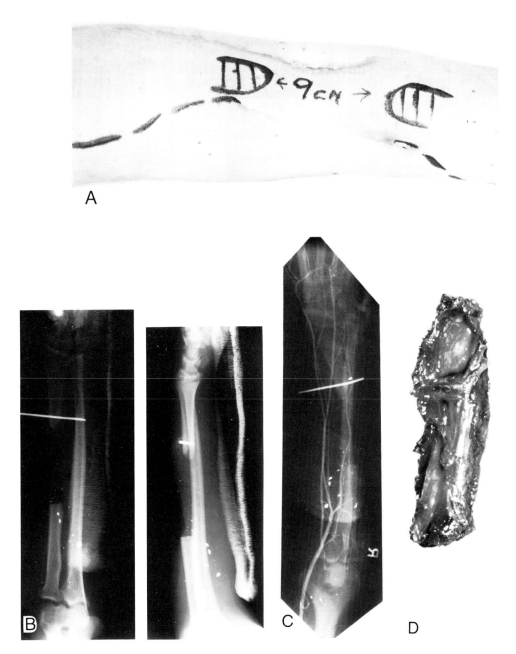

Fig. 29-3. (**A**) The preoperative clinical appearance of the left forearm in a 17-year-old male with a segmental 9-cm bony defect in the radius secondary to a shotgun wound (Case 2). (**B**) Preoperative radiographs of the left forearm. (**C**) Preoperative arteriogram demonstrating normal vascular anatomy supplying the forearm. (**D**) A 9-cm fibular graft with the surrounding 0.7 to 1.0 cm muscle cuff and peroneal vessels preserved. *(Figure continues.)*

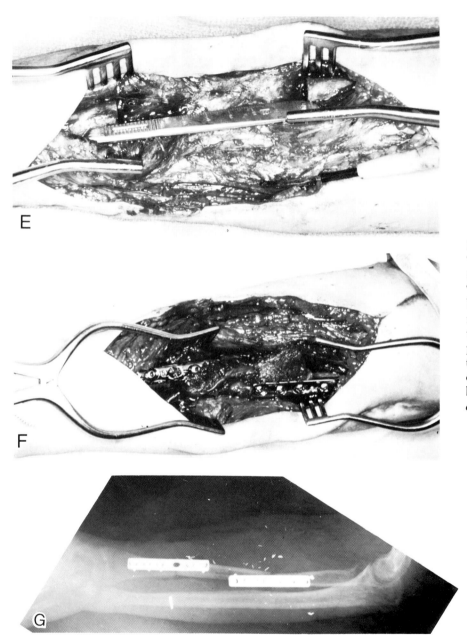

Fig. 29-3 *(Continued).* **(E)** The radial defect as seen at the time of operation. **(F)** The 9-cm fibular graft has been attached to the proximal and distal radius with two one-third tubular plates. **(G)** A radiograph taken immediately after operation, showing the fibular graft in place. *(Figure continues.)*

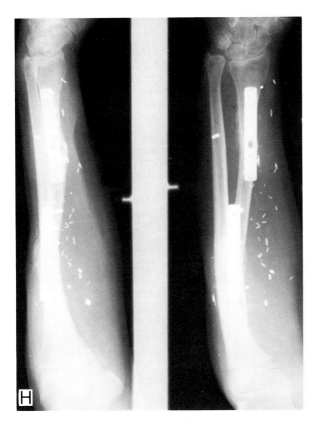

Fig. 29-3 *(Continued).* **(H)** Radiographs at 3 months show solid union of the fibular graft proximally and distally. (Weiland AJ, Daniel RK: Clinical techniques of segmental autogenous bone grafting on vascular pedicles. pp. 646–679. In Mears DC (ed): External Skeletal Fixation. ©1983, The Williams & Wilkins Co, Baltimore.)

after surgery and at 6 weeks, and were interpreted as showing viable, vascularized bone. Six months after surgery, nonunion between the graft and proximal radius became evident. Replating of this nonunion was carried out under axillary block anesthesia, and biopsy of the free vascularized fibular graft was performed. Histologic sections revealed normal cortical bone (Fig. 29-4E). The nonunion subsequently healed uneventfully. Twenty months after the operation, the patient had full range of motion of his elbow, 40 degrees of supination, and 53 degrees of pronation at the wrist (Fig. 29-4F–H).

Present Indications and Future Possibilities

Our experience with microvascular transfer of fibular grafts and composite osteocutaneous groin flaps has shown that massive autogenous bone grafting with an intact vascular pedicle decreases the time for bony union and the immobilization required for functional reconstruction of an extremity. The technique has proven to be reliable for reconstructing bone defects greater than 6 to 8 cm following tumor resection and those defects situated in a fibrotic avascular bed. More importantly, we have employed these techniques in the reconstruction of severely traumatized extremities and in those patients with tumors whom we felt were not candidates for traditional methods of bone grafting. In many patients, amputation would have been the only alternative.[57]

Because the fibular graft is subcutaneous and not available for direct monitoring, immediate postoperative assessment of circulation to the graft is difficult. Although bone scans during the first 24 to 72 hours do afford reasonable assurance that circulation is intact, revision of anastomoses at this stage is not feasible if circulation is not adequate. More effective methods for monitoring patency of anastomoses, such as thermocouples and laser Doppler flowmeters, may provide more accurate evaluation of graft circulation (see Chapter 24). In addition, the surgeon can include a small island of skin with the fibular graft based on the perforating vessels from the peroneal artery.

Trauma is by far the most common cause of segmental bone loss in the upper and lower extremities; however, certain locally aggressive or low-grade malignant tumors of bone are treated by en bloc resection incorporating an adequate margin of normal bone and soft tissue and require reconstruction of the resulting defect. The technique of free vascularized bone grafting for reconstruction of these longer segmental defects would appear to be an excellent surgical technique. In the upper extremity, the vascularized fibular graft may permit correction of nonunions resulting from bone loss and, in the future, may be employed in reconstruction of epiphyseal arrest secondary to trauma or infection and congenital radial club hand. At the

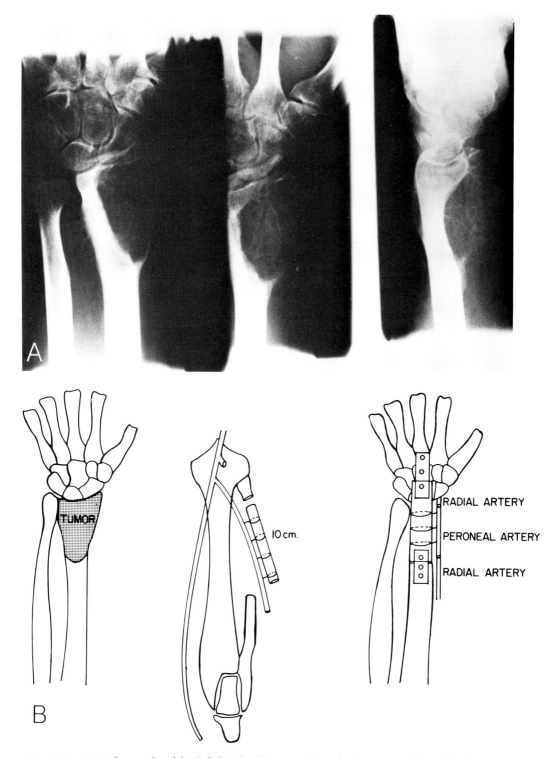

Fig. 29-4. (A) Radiographs of the left distal radius revealing a lesion compatible with giant cell tumor (Case 3). **(B)** Diagram of the free vascularized bone graft transfer. The tumor (left). Isolation of the fibula on its vascular pedicle (center). The free vascularized graft in place with anastomosis of the peroneal artery as an interposition graft between the radial artery proximally and distally (right). *(Figure continues.)*

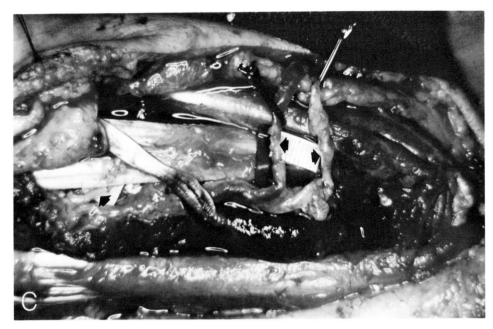

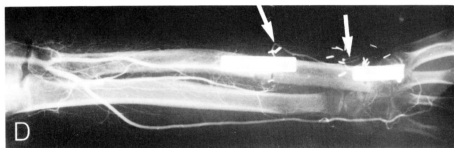

Fig. 29-4 *(Continued).* **(C)** Microvascular anastomosis of the peroneal artery to the radial artery *(left arrow)* and the two venae comitantes *(right arrows).* **(D)** Arteriogram showing patent anatomoses of the peroneal artery and radial artery 6 weeks after operation *(arrows).* **(E)** Bone biopsy of the vascularized graft at 6 months showing viable cortical bone. *(Figure continues.)*

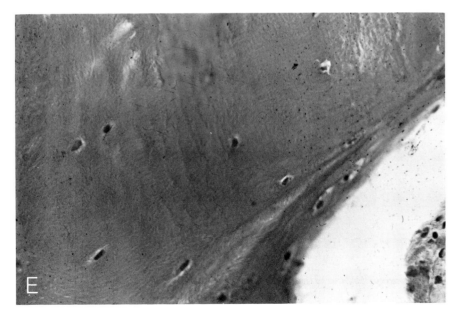

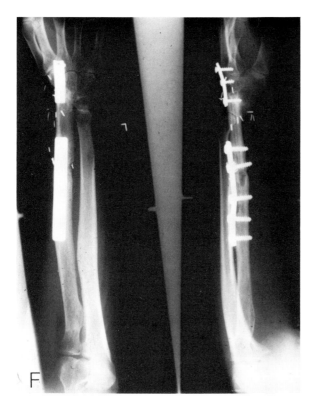

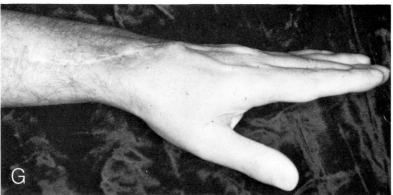

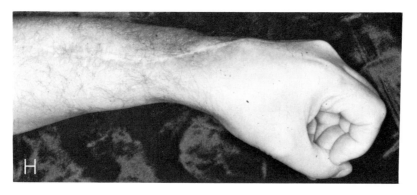

Fig. 29-4 *(Continued).* **(F)** Radiograph at 2 years, showing complete bony healing. **(G,H)** Clinical appearance of the left hand and forearm showing flexion and extension of the wrist and fingers. **(A–F** reproduced with permission from Weiland AJ, Kleinert HE, Kutz JE, Daniel RK: Vascularized bone grafts in the upper extremity. pp. 605–625. In Serafin D, Buncke HJ (eds.): Microsurgical Composite Tissue Transplantation. CV Mosby, St Louis, 1979.)

present time, vascularized epiphyseal transfers cannot be recommended for clinical use. Experimental work on the growth potential of vascularized epiphyseal plate transplantation is in its infancy. While several experimental studies have demonstrated normal or near normal growth with orthotopic° free microvascular epiphyseal plate transplantation,[20,39,76] others have shown significant retardation of growth with heterotopic transfers.[77,78] Further investigation to determine how transplanted growth plates react when transferred to disparate anatomic sites with altered stress loads both longitudinally and transversely and, perhaps, with different normal growth rates are necessary before microvascular transfer of epiphyseal plates can be included in our clinical armamentarium.[72]

Adjacent muscle, including the peroneus longus, can be transferred with the fibula to replace combined muscle and bone loss.[10] The transferred muscle can be innervated in the recipient site by suturing the muscle's dominant nerve supply to the appropriate motor nerve. In situations where skin and bone defects exist, a composite osteocutaneous flap can be employed with a groin flap incorporating the iliac crest based on the deep circumflex iliac system.

Microvascular free bone and soft tissue transfer is a relatively new technique; with more experience, clinically and, more importantly, in the laboratory, its applicability and proper place in the armamentarium of the reconstructive surgeon will become more clearly defined.

REFERENCES

1. Albee FH: Transplantation of a portion of the tibia into the spine for Pott's disease. Clin Orthop 87:5–8, Sept 1972
2. Allgower M, Blocker TG Jr, Engley BWD: Some immunological aspects of auto- and homografts in rabbits tested in vivo and in vitro techniques. Plast Reconstr Surg 9:1–21, 1952
3. Alm A, Stromberg B: Vascular anatomy of the patellar and cruciate ligaments: A microangiographic and histologic investigation in the dog. Acta Chir Scand suppl 445, 1974
4. American Replantation Mission to China: Replantation surgery in China. Plast Reconstr Surg 52:176, 1973
5. Anderssonn GBJ, Gaechter A, Galante JO, Rostoker W: Segmental replacement of long bones in baboons using a fiber titanium implant. J Bone Joint Surg 60A: 31–40, January 1978
6. Androsov PI: New methods of surgical treatment of blood vessel lesions. Arch Surg 73:902, 1956
7. Arata MA, Wood MB, Cooney WP III: Revascularized segmental diaphyseal bone transfers in the canine. An analysis of viability. J Reconstr Microsurg 1:11–19, 1984
8. Barth H: Histologische Untersuchungen über Knochentransplantation. Beitr Path Anat Allg Path 17:65–142, 1895
9. Baschkerzew NJ, Petrow NN: Beitrage zur freien Knochenuberpflanzung. Dtsch Chir 113:490–531, 1912
10. Baudet J: The composite fibula and soleus free transfer. Int J Microsurg 4:10–14, 1982
11. Berggren A, Weiland AJ, Dorfman HD: Free vascularized bone grafts: Factors affecting their survival and ability to heal to recipient bone defects. Plast Reconstr Surg 69:19–29, 1982
12. Berggren A, Weiland AJ, Östrup LT: Bone scintigraphy in evaluating the viability of composite bone grafts revascularized by microvascular anastomoses, conventional autogenous bone grafts, and free nonrevascularized periosteal grafts. J Bone Joint Surg 64A:799–809, 1982
13. Berggren A, Weiland AJ, Östrup LT, Dorfman HD: The effects of storage media and perfusion on osteoblast and osteocyte survival in free composite bone grafts. J Microsurgery 2:273–282, 1981
14. Berggren A, Weiland AJ, Östrup LT, Dorfman HD: Microvascular free bone transfer with revascularization of the medullary and periosteal circulation or the periosteal circulation alone. J Bone Joint Surg 64A:73–87, 1982
15. Bonfiglio M: Repair of bone transplant fractures. J Bone Joint Surg 40A:446–456, 1958
16. Boyd HB: The treatment of difficult and unusual non-unions. J Bone Joint Surg 25:535–552, July 1943
17. Brookes M: The Blood Supply of Bone. Butterworths, London, 1971
18. Brookes M: The vascular architecture of tubular bone in the rat. Anat Rec 132:25–48, 1958

° Orthotopic refers to transplantation to a similar anatomic site; heterotopic implies transfer to another anatomic site.

19. Brookes M: The vascularization of long bones in the human foetus. J Anat 92:261–267, 1958

20. Brown K, Marie P, Lyszakowski T, Daniel R, Cruess R: Epiphyseal growth after free fibular transfer with and without microvascular anastomosis. Experimental study in the dog. J Bone Joint Surg 65B:493–501, 1983

21. Buncke HJ, Furnas DW, Gordon L, Achauer BM: Free osteocutaneous flap from a rib to the tibia. Plast Reconstr Surg 59:799–805, 1977

22. Buncke HJ, Schulz WP: Experimental digital amputation and reimplantation. Plast Reconstr Surg 36:62, 1965

23. Buncke HJ, Schulz WP: Total ear re-implantation in the rabbit utilizing microminiature vascular anastomosis. Br J Plast Surg 19:15, Nov. 1966

24. Burrows HJ, Wilson JN, Scales JT: Excision of tumors of humerus and femur, with restoration by internal prosthesis. J Bone Joint Surg 57B:148–159, May 1975

25. Burwell RG: Biological mechanisms in foreign bone transplantation. In Modern Trends in Orthopaedics, Vol. 4. Butterworths, Washington, DC, 1964

26. Burwell RG: Studies in the transplantation of bone. VII. The fresh composite homograft-autograft of cancellous bone: An analysis of factors leading to osteogenesis in marrow transplants and in marrow-containing bone grafts. J Bone Joint Surg 46B:110–140, 1961

27. Campbell WC: Transference of the fibula as an adjunct free bone graft in tibial deficiency. J Orthop Surg 7:625–631, 1919

28. Carrel A: Results of the transplantation of blood vessels, organs and limbs. JAMA 51:1662–1667, 1908

29. Chalmers J: Transplantation immunity in bone homografting. J Bone Joint Surg 41B:160–179, 1959

30. Chen CW, Yu ZJ, Wang Y: A new method of treatment of congenital tibial pseudarthrosis using free vascularized fibular grafts: A preliminary report. Ann Acad Med Singapore 8:465–473, 1979

31. Clark K: A case of replacement of the upper end of the humerus by a fibular graft: Reviewed after 29 years. J Bone Surg 41B:365–368, 1959

32. Cobbett JR: Microvascular surgery. Surg Clin North Am 47:521–542, 1967

33. Crenshaw AH: Campbell's Operative Orthopaedics. 5th Ed. CV Mosby, St Louis, 1971

34. Curtiss PH Jr, Powell AE, Herndon CH: Immunological factors in homogenous bone transplantation. III. The inability of homogenous rabbit bone to induce circulating antibodies in rabbits. J Bone Joint Surg 41A:1482–1488, 1959

35. Daniel RK, Taylor GI: Distant transfer of an island flap by microvascular anastomoses. Plast Reconstr Surg 52:111–117, Aug 1973

36. D'Aubigne RM, Meary R, Thomine JM: La resection dans le traitement des tumeurs des os. Rev Chir Orthop 52:305–324, 1966

37. DeBruyn PH, Kabisch WT: Bone formation by fresh and frozen autogenous and homogenous transplants of bone, bone marrow, and periosteum. Am J Anat 96:375–417, 1955

38. Dee P, Lambruschi PG, Hiebert JM: The use of Tc-99m MDP bone scanning in the study of vascularized bone implants: Concise communication. J Nucl Med 22:522–525, 1981

39. Donski PK, O'Brien BMcC: Free microvascular epiphyseal transplantation: An experimental study in dogs. Br J Plast Surg 33:169–178, 1980

40. Eadie DGA, DeTakats G: The early fate of autogenous grafts in the canine femoral vein. J Cardiovasc Surg 7:148, 1966

41. Enneking WF, Burchardt H, Puhl JJ, Piotrowski G: Physical and biological aspects of repair in dog cortical-bone transplants. J Bone Joint Surg 57A:237–251, March 1975

42. Gilbert A: Free vascularized bone grafts. Int Surg 66:27–31, 1981

43. Gilbert A: Vascularized transfer of the fibular shaft. Int J Microsurg 1(2):100–102, Apr 1979

44. Hagan KF, Buncke HJ: Treatment of congenital pseudarthrosis of the tibia with free vascularized bone graft. Clin Orthop 166:34–44, 1982

45. Ham A, Gordon S: The origin of bone that forms in association with cancellous chips transplanted into muscle. Br J Plast Surg 5:154–160, 1952

46. Harmon PH: A simplified surgical approach to the posterior tibia for bone grafting and fibular transference. J Bone Joint Surg 27:496–498, 1945

47. Heiple KG, Chase SW, Herndon CH: A comparative study of the healing process following different types of bone transplantation. J Bone Joint Surg 45A:1593–1616, 1963

48. Helsop BF, Zeiss IM, Nesbet NW: Studies on transference of bone. I. A comparison of autologous and homologous bone implants with reference to osteocyte survival, osteogenesis, and host reaction. Br J Exp Pathol 41:269–287, 1960

49. Henry AK: Extensile Exposure. 2nd Ed. pp. 241–276. E & S Livingstone, London, 1966

50. Herndon CH, Chase SW: Experimental studies in the transplantation of whole joints. J Bone Joint Surg 34A:564–578, 1952

51. Herndon CH, Chase SW: The fate of massive autogenous and homogenous bone grafts including ar-

ticular surfaces. Surg Gynecol Obstet 98:273–290, 1954

52. Hirayama T, Suematsu N, Inoue K, Baitoh C, Takemitsu Y: Free vascularized bone grafts in reconstruction of the upper extremity. J Hand Surg 10B:169–175, 1985

53. Holt GP, Lewis FT: A new technique for end-to-end anastomosis for small arteries. Surg Forum 11:242, 1960

54. Hu CT, Chang CW, Su KL, Shen CC, Shen S: Free vascularized bone graft using microvascular technique. Ann Acad Med Singapore 8:459–464, 1979

55. Huntington TW: Case of bone transference. Ann Surg 41:249–256, 1905

56. Hutchinson J: The fate of experimental bone autografts and homografts. Br J Surg 39:552–561, 1952

57. Jackson RW, MacNab I: Fractures of the shaft of the tibia: A clinical and experimental study. Am J Surg 97:543–557, 1959

58. Jacobson JH, Suarez EL: Microsurgery in anastomoses of small vessels. Surg Forum 11:243, 1960

59. Johnson RW Jr: A physiological study of the blood supply of the diaphysis. J Bone Joint Surg 9:153–184, 1927

60. Kelly PJ: Anatomy, physiology and pathology of the blood supply of bones. J Bone Joint Surg 50A:766–783, June 1968

61. Lacroix P: Recent investigations on the growth of bone. Nature 156:576, 1945

62. Levander G: A study of bone regeneration. Surg Gynecol Obstet 67:705–714, 1938

63. Lexer E: Die Entstehung entzundlicher Knochenherde und ihre Beziehung zu den Arterien Versweigungen der Knochen. Arch Klin Chir 81:1, 1903

64. Lexer E: Substitution of whole or half joints from freshly amputated extremities by free plastic operation. Surg Gynecol Obstet 6:601–607, 1908

65. Lexer E: Blutige Vereinigung von Knochenbruchen. Dtsch Z Chir 133: 1970, 1915

66. Lexer E, Kuliga, Turk: Untersuchungen über Knochenarterien. Hirschwold, Berlin, 1904

67. Lukash FN, Zingaro EA, Salig J: The survival of free nonvascularized bone grafts in irradiated areas by wrapping in muscle flaps. Plast Reconstr Surg 74:783–788, 1984

68. Maatz R, Lentz W, Graf R: Spongiosa test of bone grafts for transplantation. J Bone Joint Surg 36A:721–731, 1954

69. Mankin HJ, Fogelson FS, Thrasher AZ, Jaffer F: Massive resection and allograft transplantation in the treatment of malignant bone tumors. N Engl J Med 294:1247–1255, 1976

70. Manktelow RT, McKee NH: Free muscle transplantation to provide active finger flexion. J Hand Surg 3(5):416–426, 1978

71. Marchand: Zur Kenntniss des Knochen-Transplantation. Verh Dtsch Ges Pathol 2:368–375, 1900

72. Mathes SJ, Buchannan R, Weeks PM: Microvascular joint transplantation with epiphyseal growth. J Hand Surg 5:586–589, 1980

73. Metaizeau JP, Olive D, Bey P, Bordigoni P, Plenat F, Prévot J: Resection followed by vascularized bone autograft in patients with possible recurrence of malignant bone tumors after conservative treatment. J Pediatr Surg 19:116–120, 1984

74. Miller RC, Phalen GS: The repair of defects of the radius with fibular bone grafts. J Bone Joint Surg 29:629–636, 1947

75. Nakayama K, Tamiya T, Yamamoto K, Akimoto S: A simple new apparatus for small vessel anastomoses (free autograft of the sigmoid included). Surgery 52:918–931, 1962

76. Nettelblad H, Randolph MA, Weiland AJ: Free microvascular epiphyseal plate transplantation. An experimental study in dogs. J Bone Joint Surg 66A:1421–1430, 1984

77. Nettelblad H, Randolph MA, Weiland AJ: Heterotopic microvascular growth plate transplantation of the proximal fibula: An experimental canine model. Plast Reconstr Surg 77:814–820, 1986

78. Nettelblad H, Randolph MA, Weiland AJ: Physiologic isolation of the canine proximal fibular epiphysis on a vascular pedicle. Microsurgery 5:98-101, 1984

79. O'Brien BM: Microvascular free bone and joint transfer. pp. 267–289. In Microvascular Reconstructive Surgery. Churchill Livingstone, Edinburgh, 1977

80. Osterman AL, Bora FW: Free vascularized bone grafting for large-gap nonunion of long bones. Orthop Clin North Am 15:131–142, 1984

81. Östrup LT: The free, living bone graft — An experimental study. Linkoping University Medical Dissertations, Linkoping, Sweden, 1975

82. Östrup LT, Fredrickson JM: Distant transfer of a free, living bone graft by microvascular anastomoses: An experimental study. Plast Reconstr Surg 54:274–285, Sept 1974

83. Ottolenghi CE: Massive osteo and osteo-articular bone grafts: Technical results of 62 cases. Clin Orthop 87:156–164, Sept 1972

84. Parrish FF: Treatment of bone tumors by total excision and replacement with massive autologous

and homologous grafts. J Bone Joint Surg 48A:968–990, 1966

85. Parrish FF: Allograft replacement of all or part of the end of a long bone following excision of a tumor: Report of twenty-one cases. J Bone Joint Surg 55A:1–22, 1973

86. Phemister DB: The fate of transplanted bone and regenerative power of various constituents. Surg Gynecol Obstet 19:303–333, 1914

87. Pho RWH: Malignant giant-cell tumors of the distal end of the radius treated by a free vascularized fibular transplant. J Bone Joint Surg 63A:877–884, 1981

88. Ray RD, Degge J, Gloyd P, Mooney G: Bone regeneration. An experimental study of bone grafting materials. J Bone Joint Surg 34A:638–647, 1952

89. Reichel SM: Vascular system of the long bones of the rat. Surgery 22:146–157, 1947

90. Restrepo J, Katz A, Gilbert A: Arterial vascularization to the proximal epiphysis and the diaphysis of the fibula. Int J Microsurg 2:49–54, 1980

91. Rhinelander RW: Effects of medullary nailing on the normal blood supply of diaphyseal cortex. AAOS Instructional Course Lectures, Vol. 22. pp. 161–187. CV Mosby, St Louis, 1973

92. Riordan DC: Congenital absence of the radius. J Bone Joint Surg 37A:1129–1140, 1955

93. Rohlich K: Bildung neuer Knochensubstanz in Abgetoteten Knochentransplantation. A Mikrosk Anat Forsch 50:132–145, 1941

94. Rohlich K: Uber die Transplantation Periost-und markloses Knochenstucke. A Mikrost Anat Forsch 51:636–653, 1942

95. Salmon PA, Assimacopoulos CA: A pneumatic needle holder suitable for microsurgical procedures. Surgery 55:446, 1964

96. Serafin D, Villarreal-Rois A, Georgiade NG: A rib-containing free flap to reconstruct mandibular defects. Br J Plast Surg 30:263–266, 1977

97. Shima I, Yamauchi S, Matsumoto T, Kunishita M, Shinoda K, Yoshimizu N, Nomura S, Yoshimura M: A new method for monitoring circulation of grafted bone by use of electrochemically generated hydrogen. Clin Orthop 198:244–249, 1985

98. Starr DE: Congenital absence of the radius. A method of surgical correction. J Bone Joint Surg 27:572–577, 1945

99. Swartz WM: Immediate reconstruction of the wrist and dorsum of the hand with a free osteocutaneous groin flap. J Hand Surg 9A:18–21, 1984

100. Tamai S, Komatsu S, Sakamoto H, Sano S, Sasauchi N, Hori Y, Tatsumi Y, Okuda H: Free muscle transplants in dogs with microsurgerical neurovascular

anastomoses. Plast Reconstr Surg 46:219–225, 1970

101. Tamai S, Sasauchi N, Hori Y, Tatsumi Y, Okuda H: Microvascular surgery in orthopaedics and traumatology. J Bone Joint Surg 54B:637–647, 1972

102. Taylor GI: The current status of free vascularized bone grafts. Clin Plast Surg 10:185–209, 1983

103. Taylor GI: Microvascular free bone transfer. A clinical technique. Orthop Clin North Am 8:425–447, 1977

104. Taylor GI, Daniel RK: The free flap: Composite tissue transfer by vascular anastomosis. Aust NZJ Surg 43:1–3, 1973

105. Taylor GI, Miller GDH, Ham FJ: The free vascularized bone graft. A clinical extension of microvascular techniques. Plast Reconstr Surg 55:533–544, 1975

106. Taylor GI, Townsend P, Corlett R: Superiority of the deep circumflex iliac vessels as the supply for free groin flaps: Clinical work. Plast Reconstr Surg 64:745–759, 1979

107. Taylor GI, Townsend P, Corlett R: Superiority of the deep circumflex iliac vessels as the supply for free groin flaps: Experimental work. Plast Reconstr Surg 64:595–605, 1979

108. Taylor GI, Watson N: One-stage repair of compound leg defects with free revascularized flaps of groin, skin, and iliac bone. Plast Reconstr Surg 61:494–506, 1978

109. Trias A, Fery A: Cortical circulation of long bones. J Bone Joint Surg 61A: 1052–1059, 1979

110. Trueta J, Caladias AX: A study of the blood supply of the long bones. Surg Gynecol Obstet 118:485–498, 1964

111. Urist MR, McLean FC: Osteogenetic potency and new-bone formation by induction in transplants to the anterior chamber of the eye. J Bone Joint Surg 34A:443–470, 1952

112. Volkov M: Allotransplantation of joints. J Bone Joint Surg 52B:49–53, 1970

113. Weiland AJ: Current concepts review: Vascularized free bone transplants. J Bone Joint Surg 63A:166–169, 1981

114. Weiland AJ: Vascularized bone transfers. pp. 446–460. AAOS Instructional Course Lectures, Vol. 33. CV Mosby, St Louis, 1984

115. Weiland AJ, Berggren A, Jones L: The acute effects of blocking medullary blood supply on regional cortical blood flow in canine ribs as measured by the hydrogen washout technique. Clin Orthop 165:265–272, 1982

116. Weiland AJ, Daniel RK: Clinical technique of segmental autogenous bone grafting in vascular pedi-

cles. pp. 646–679. In Mears DC (ed): External Skeletal Fixation. Williams & Wilkins, Baltimore, 1983

117. Weiland AJ, Daniel RK: Congenital pseudarthrosis of the tibia: Treatment with vascularized autogenous fibular grafts. A preliminary report. Johns Hopkins Med J 147:89–95, 1980

118. Weiland AJ, Daniel RK: Microvascular anastomoses for bone grafts in the treatment of massive defects in bone. J Bone Joint Surg 61A:98–104, 1979

119. Weiland AJ, Daniel RK, Riley LH Jr.: Application of the free vascularized bone graft in the treatment of malignant or aggressive bone tumors. John Hopkins Med J 140:85–96, Nov 1977

120. Weiland AJ, Kleinert HE, Kutz JE, Daniel RK: Vascularized bone grafts in the upper extremity. pp. 605–625. In Serafin D, Buncke HJ Jr (eds): Microsurgical Composite Tissue Transplantation. CV Mosby, St Louis, 1979

121. Weiland AJ, Kleinert HE, Kutz JE, Daniel RK: Free vascularized bone grafts in surgery of the upper extremity. J Hand Surg 4:129–144, 1979

122. Weiland AJ, Moore JR, Daniel RK: Vascularized bone autografts. Experience with 41 cases. Clin Orthop 174:87–95, 1983

123. Weiland AJ, Phillips TW, Randolph MA: Bone grafts: A radiologic, histologic, and biomechanical model comparing autografts, allografts, and free vascularized bone grafts. Plast Reconstr Surg 74:368–379, 1984

Vascularized Joint Transfers

30

Guy Foucher

Finger joints play a critical role in the function of the hand. Their function, however, can be absent, disturbed, or destroyed because of congenital malformation, trauma, or disease. Three main levels can be involved: the proximal interphalangeal joint (PIPJ), the metacarpophalangeal joint (MPJ), or the trapeziometacarpal joint (TMJ). Many methods of joint reconstruction have been developed, but all of these fall short of the ideal requirements, which are a painless, stable, strong, durable joint with full range of motion and, in children, potential for growth. The alternatives for treatment of damaged joints include amputation, fusion, prothesis, spacers, nonvascularized joint transfer (NVJT), and vascularized joint transfer (VJT) (free or island).

Finger amputation is rarely indicated for joint damage except in the case of complex associated lesions involving a single finger. Fusion can afford relief of pain with stability, durability, and, usually, good strength, but at the cost of mobility. Arthrodesis must still be thought of as a good operation, at least in adults and in certain joints, such as the thumb MPJ or TMJ, but in other locations fusion may disturb the overall function of the hand, especially with multiple PIPJ or MPJ involvement. Despite constant improvement, prosthetic implants or spacers still present significant problems of stabil-

ity, durability, and mobility, and they remain contraindicated in young patients.

Surgeons have long searched to provide a biologic joint replacement using specialized tissues with a similar anatomic configuration. These attempts fall into three major categories: perichondrial joints grafts, allografts, and autografts (vascularized or nonvascularized half- or whole-joint transfers).

Allograft: A graft of tissue between individuals of the same species but of disparate genotype. Also called *allogeneic graft* or *homograft*.

Autograft: A graft of tissue derived from another site in or on the body of the organism receiving it. Also called *autologous graft*.

In our experience[34] and throughout the literature,[65] results of perichondrial autografts have been quite unpredictable. This operation is applicable only to very limited problems in which damage is confined to the articular cartilage, in the presence of normal bone structure.

Nonvascularized joint autografts and allografts have been extensively studied, but sound clinical series providing long-term results concerning ranges of motion, degenerative changes, and/or percentage of growth in young patients are scarce.

GENERAL PRINCIPLES OF BONE AND CARTILAGE TRANSPLANTATION

There are several basic problems that are common to all biologic reconstructions. Successful transplantation of functioning organs depends upon rapid reestablishment of the circulatory perfusion of their tissues if the transplants are to survive and to function. Curiously, when bone and cartilage are transplanted, difficulties begin when the process of revascularization is established.[51] Ischemic loss of synovium is responsible for poor production of synovial fluid, which is the sole means of nutrition of the articular cartilage.[66] Moreover, the circulation of synovial fluid depends on movement of the joint, and prolonged immobilization causes trophic changes in the articular cartilage.[28,77] The role of denervation in degenerative change in transplanted joints, although poorly documented,[22,72] is probably relatively unimportant.[4]

Allografts

Allografts have been the least successful method experimentally. However, most research with allografts has been concentrated on large weight-bearing joints such as the knee. In 1908, Lexer[74] reported successful cases of homografts of half and whole joints taken from freshly amputated extremities. In 1925,[75] he reviewed the long-term results (knee, shoulder, hip) and concluded that function could remain satisfactory for many years despite obvious degenerative changes in these joints. Subsequent series[6,7,8,58,82,91,107,118] demonstrated a high rate of failure. Whereas bone is strongly antigenic compared to cartilage, *homografts* of the lat-

ter, although antigenic as well, have been shown to survive longer than any tissue except the cornea. It has been demonstrated[106] that in a grafted bone at least 5 mm thick,[7,15,75,90,106] the joint space is relatively well maintained until collapse of subchondral bone occurs. In one study,[58] it was shown that most of the cells (bone and cartilage) in the joints died. Revascularization and active osteogenesis were slow. The transplants functioned for 6 to 8 months and then degenerative changes progressed to complete disintegration of the joint.

Autografts

Nonvascularized replantations or autografts of half and whole joints have also been studied extensively, experimentally as well as clinically. Tietze,[112] in 1902, is thought to have been the first to use a proximal phalanx taken from the big toe, while Goebell[45] reported the substitution of a finger joint by a toe joint in 1913. Since then, many small series with short follow-up have been published. Experimental, radiologic, and histologic studies have demonstrated degenerative changes of cartilage, with survival of only scattered deep layers and progressive replacement with fibrotic tissue.[22–24,58,69–71] Small clinical series have been published concerning whole joint replacement using a toe,[10,11,22,25,49,50,75,83,94] or transposition of a normal joint from an otherwise irreparably damaged digit as a free whole-joint transfer.[22,23,79,92] Technically, several points have been stressed: the smaller the graft, the sooner revascularization takes place. On the other hand, bone periosteum and joint capsule have to be kept intact. Several authors have demonstrated that limited but satisfactory joint motion usually occurs after half- and whole-joint transfer independently of articular cartilage survival.[22,24,58,70,75]

GROWTH POTENTIAL

The growth of such transfers in young patients remains controversial. In experiments several authors have demonstrated some growth,[25,57,61,100] while others have not.[56,57] Clinically, isolated successful cases have been published.[39,40,50,108,117,121] Two short but encouraging series[46,122] stressed that the reasons for success or failure of growth were not apparent. Age (the optimum was 6 months) and technique (conservation of periosteum) seem to be important contributing factors.

VASCULARIZED FREE-JOINT TRANSFERS

Taking into account that most problems in NVJT arise from delay in bone revascularization, it seemed logical in 1966 that preservation or re-establishment of nutrient vessels could be the solution. The technical feasibility of whole, *vascularized free-joint transfer* was demonstrated experimentally in a dog's knee model[107] and in 1968, long-term survival was demonstrated.[67] These findings were soon confirmed by other investigators.[47,48,61,88,97,98,104,105,114] Vascularized grafts are histologically indistinguishable from normal joints[14,61,88,105,114] with viable subchondral bone. Functionally, only slight to moderate hyperplasia of the synovium with some restricted motion[88] was demonstrated. Survival of the epiphyseal plate with growth has been demonstrated experimentally[19,129] and clinically.[18,80,115,125] Vascularized transfers based only on metaphyseal blood supply provide some (but not normal) growth.[19] It seems advisable to use epiphyseal vessels to obtain normal growth.[129] It is necessary to keep in mind that overgrowth may be seen after fractures or in association with inflammatory conditions, and that decreased growth may result in cases of chronic disease or prolonged immobilization.

Clinically, the first island, vascularized joint transfer was performed by Buncke[4] in 1967 and we presented the first free, compound toe-joint transfer in 1976.[30] Since then, few cases have been published.[31,34,72,115,116]

Anatomy

A vascularized transfer can be harvested from either a nonreplantable finger (PIPJ or DIPJ) or from a toe (second and/or third). Two types of toe joints are available: the PIPJ and the metatarsophalangeal joint (MTPJ).

Although its anatomy is similar, the toe PIPJ is rather small compared to the PIPJ of the finger. The mobility in flexion is good, but frequently there is a slight claw deformity that may be reduced by passive flexion of the MTPJ. In the child, only one growth plate is present, located at the base of the middle phalanx.

The MTPJ is larger and quite similar to the MPJ, possessing good lateral stability but a limited range of flexion compared to the range of hyperextension. Two growth plates are present, one on each side of the joint.

The extensor and flexor mechanisms are similar to those of the hand. The innervation of the MTPJ arises from the terminal branch of the peroneal profundus nerve running along the dorsalis pedis artery and from the cutaneous dorsal medial branch of the superficial peroneal nerve.[72]

The vascularization of the second toe has been known for a long time,[43,53,73,81] but only a few studies have been devoted to the vascular pattern of the joints.[72,128] A Chinese study[72] demonstrated that the blood supply of the MTPJ was mainly dependent on the articular branch of the first metatarsal artery. This constant artery presents three different patterns (Fig. 30-1): (1) most commonly (60 percent), the artery branches off the first dorsal metatarsal artery at the distal third of the metatarsal bone; (2) in 18 percent of cases, the articular vessel arises from the origin of the first dorsal metatarsal artery; or (3) in the case of a first dorsal metatarsal artery passing beneath the interosseous muscle, the articular vessel branches off close to the joint. The authors found additional branches emerging from the first plantar metatarsal artery, but they were inconstant and always communicated with the dorsal system. A Japanese study[128] and personal unpublished data stressed that vascularization of the PIPJ and MTPJ of the second toe is provided by both the dorsal and plantar vessels, which do communicate (Fig. 30-2). Furthermore, our study[35,36] underlined the role of a fundamental vessel that has been overlooked in the literature: the second plantar metatarsal artery (Fig. 30-3), which is a constant, reliable vessel passing in close contact to the volar plate of the MTPJ.

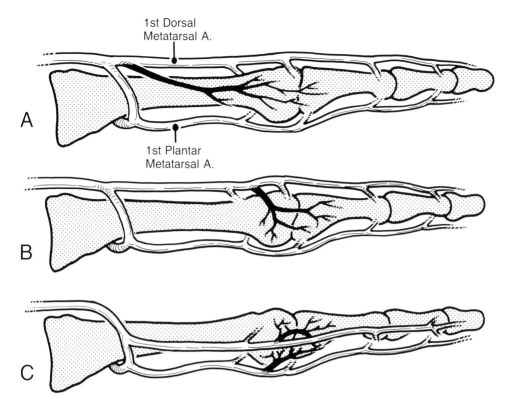

1st Dorsal
Metatarsal A.

A

1st Plantar
Metatarsal A.

B

C

Fig. 30-1. PIP and MTP joint vascularization patterns according to Kuo et al.[72]

Techniques

Several techniques have been described: (1) toe PIPJ transfer for finger MPJ and PIPJ reconstruction; (2) MTPJ transfer for MPJ or TMJ reconstruction; (3) PIPJ or DIPJ "finger bank" transfer (i.e., from an otherwise discarded finger); (4) double transfer for PIPJ[115] for MPJ reconstruction; and (5) "twisted toe flap" technique to add a joint in a "wraparound" thumb reconstruction.[31,33,36]

TOE PIPJ TRANSFER FOR FINGER PIPJ RECONSTRUCTION

There are only a few papers available on this topic.[31,115] The technique as described by Tsai is as follows:

Preoperatively, routine radiographs and selective angiography are performed on the foot and the hand.

Under general anesthesia, the donor and recipient sites are prepared simultaneously by two surgical teams. Through a longitudinal dorsal approach, the dorsalis pedis and first dorsal metatarsal arteries are dissected, along with the dorsal veins. A small skin island over the tibial and dorsal aspect of the PIPJ of the second toe is preserved as a visible monitor of the underlying circulation (Fig. 30-4). The tibial-side digital artery is divided distally at the level of the DIPJ, preserving the articular and metaphyseal branches. The fibular side artery is preserved by ligating its articular and metaphyseal branches. The extensor mechanism is then cut proximally and distally and the joint is isolated by distal disarticulation through the DIPJ and by proximal osteotomy through the first phalanx.

The hand is prepared, the involved PIPJ is excised, and a suitable artery is prepared.

The joint is transferred and stabilized with an

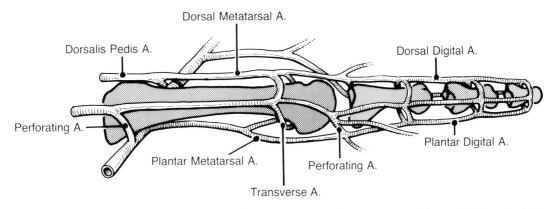

Fig. 30-2. PIP and MTP joint vascularization according to Yoshizu et al.[128]

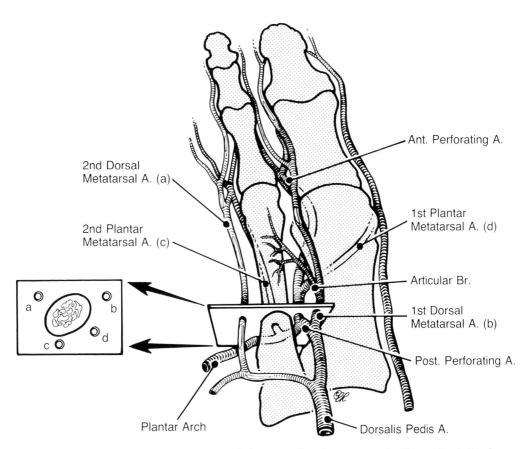

Fig. 30-3. The vascular pattern of the second web space in the foot, which has been overlooked in the literature. The second plantar and/or dorsal artery can frequently be used.

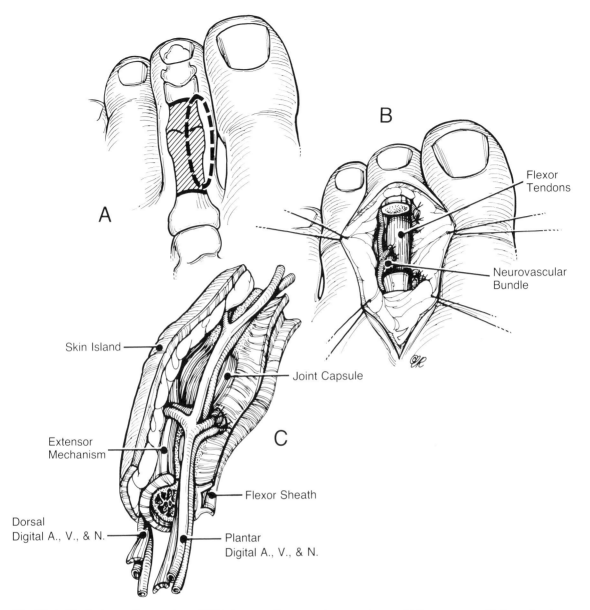

Fig. 30-4. Technique of second toe PIP joint transfer according to Tsai et al,[116] using a small skin island as a visible monitor of viability.

intraosseous wire and longitudinal K-wire. The extensor mechanism is then reconstructed and the arterial suture is done usually by end-to-side anastomosis. At least two veins, including the saphenous vein, are sutured. The foot defect may be managed as a resection arthroplasty or, preferably, by bone graft using the removed joint of the finger.

Nothing was mentioned in their article[114] concerning postoperative management.

The technique described by Yoshizu[128] is similar, except that the second toe PIPJ graft is taken with the medial plantar digital artery or, if necessary, the first dorsal metatarsal artery, which is anastomosed to a common volar digital artery.

TOE MTPJ TRANSFER FOR MPJ RECONSTRUCTION

Under epidural and brachial plexus block anesthesia,[72] this operation is comprised of four steps.

1. The joint is exposed at the recipient site through a curved skin incision. The ulnar side of the extensor hood is incised, retracted and the joint resected. The radial artery and the cephalic vein are approached through a separate incision. A small branch of the superficial radial nerve is dissected at the wrist level to be sutured to the nerve of the transplanted joint.
2. The donor site is prepared by dissection of the great saphenous vein and first dorsal metatarsal artery. The terminal branch of the deep peroneal nerve is also dissected.
3. The graft is turned 180 degrees around its longitudinal axis, that is, dorsal to volar. Bone fixation is done with a K-wire and the vessels are anastomosed: the dorsalis pedis to the radial artery, the great saphenous vein to the cephalic vein and the deep peroneal nerve to the superficial branch of radial nerve. Last, the extensor mechanism is sutured and the skin closed.
4. At the donor site, the defect in the toe is filled either by the finger joint or by a cancellous bone graft.

Postoperative treatment includes prophylactic antibiotics and low molecular Dextran for several days. The K-wires are removed at 4 weeks and functional exercises are then encouraged. The cast on the foot is removed at 4 weeks and walking is allowed.

One of the major shortcomings in this type of MTPJ transfer has been the difficulty with which a skin flap could be incorporated due to the rotation of the transfer. In an effort to solve this problem, Smith and Jones[109] described a technique using an eccentrically placed dorsalis pedis flap (Fig. 30-5). The nondominant lateral digital artery is freed from its attachment to the skin flap. With this maneuver after rotation of the joint, the flap remains dorsal.

Author's Preferred Methods

PIP JOINT RECONSTRUCTION

For PIP joint reconstruction, we continue to use the technique that we described originally[30,31] and which was slightly modified later by Tsai. Specific details must be emphasized.

We do not prescribe any preoperative arteriographic work-up. The operation is performed under general anesthesia by one team only. The one-team approach avoids most of the pitfalls concerning matching of length and size of arteries, veins, nerves, and tendons. The first step is the toe dissection. A cutaneous flap is drawn distally to the DIPJ, and proximally a long tail is taken from the

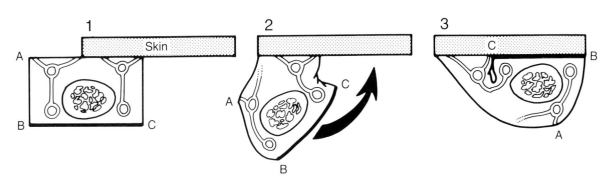

Fig. 30-5. A skin flap can be harvested with the MTP joint after turning the joint upside down (Smith and Jones[109]).

dorsum of the foot. A dorsal approach only is sufficient.[32,33,35,36] After dissection of the venous arch and the great saphenous vein, the dorsalis pedis artery is dissected just beneath the extensor hallucis longus tendon. The field of dissection then moves to the first web, looking for the dorsal metatarsal artery, superficial to the intermetatarsal liga-

ment. If the diameter of this artery is not sufficient, we proceed with extensor tendon section and proximal osteotomy of the second metatarsal, which is then lifted with a bone hook. This osteotomy has two advantages: (1) it provides a wide approach to the plantar arterial system of the first and second space; and (2) it facilitates closure of the donor site.

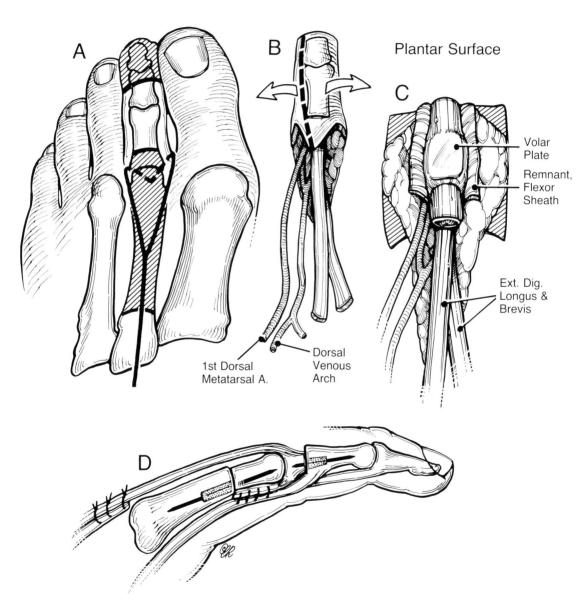

Fig. 30-6. Author's technique for PIP toe joint compound transfer. (A) A large flap is harvested. (B) The plantar skin is split on the midplantar aspect. (C) Two lateral flaps are reflected and the flexor mechanism removed, with preservation of part of the sheath for later repair. (D) Intramedullary bone penetration and suture of the recipient's flexor sheath to the rims of the donor site pulleys. *(Figure continues.)*

When none of the arteries possess a suitable diameter, two (or even three) are taken in continuity with the dorsalis pedis artery. Then the toe is divided distally through the DIPJ. The skin is split on the medial line of the plantar aspect and two lateral flaps are reflected until reaching the vascular bundle (Fig. 30-6). The flexor sheath is then opened longitudinally and medially to remove the flexor mechanism, with care being taken to avoid injuring the retrotendinous vessels and the vascularization of the plantar plate. The first phalanx is osteoto-

mized according to the length needed. A bone peg can be harvested from the discarded metatarsal for bone stabilization either at the donor or recipient sites. When the compound transfer is pedicled only on its artery (or arteries) and vein, the tourniquet is released. Local topic vasodilator (lidocaine 2%) is applied to the artery, and the foot is wrapped with hot wet drapes.

Preparation of the hand is made through a classic longitudinal dorsal incision, but extensive excision of scarred tissue is possible because of the large

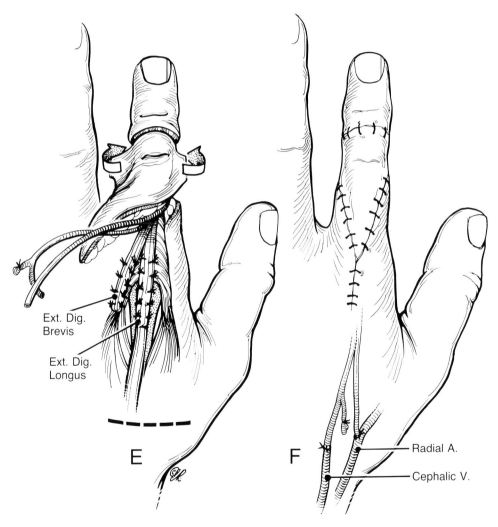

Fig. 30-6 *(Continued).* **(E)** Extensor tendon suture. The extensor brevis is sutured to the intrinsic mechanism, and the longus is sutured to the extrinsic extensor tendon. **(F)** Vessel anastomoses. End-to-side suture with the radial artery and end-to-end suture with the cephalic vein.

skin flap of the compound transfer. The flexor sheath is cleared out and the remaining volar plate is made thinner. The bone ends and the extensor mechanism are prepared. A separate approach (ideally horizontal) is performed in the first intermetacarpal space, with dissection of the radial artery and one superficial vein. The skin is undermined between the two incisions, providing a sufficient channel for the vascular bundle. The length of missing bone and vessels needed is measured and the dissection of the foot is completed. The phalanges of the toe are usually trimmed in a step fashion to allow intramedullary penetration at the recipient site. Then the vein and the artery are divided. When length permits, the dorsalis pedis artery and the proximal plantar arch are harvested so that the latter can be intercalated as a T-shaped graft (Fig. 30-7).

The compound joint is then transferred to the recipient finger and the bone secured. We have used different types of osteosynthesis (intramedullary screw, K-wire, bone peg, and wiring), and there has been no specific correlation with the final range of motion depending on the type of fixation. Most frequently, we have used a buried intramedullary pin and an oblique K-wire. Care has to be taken not to make the intercalated segment too long (it is preferable that it be too short). Then the remnant of flexor sheath of the toe is sutured to the rim of the recipient sheath to prevent bowstringing. The extensor mechanism is sutured with overlapping, with the joint in full extension. The extensor hallucis longus is secured to the medial tendon on the dorsum of the first phalanx and the extensor brevis to the intrinsic tendon. The bundle is then passed through the subcutaneous tunnel, avoiding any twisting, and the skin flap is carefully trimmed, inserted, and sutured. The vessels are then sutured end-to-side or end-to-end (T-shaped) for the artery and end-to-end for the sole vein (Fig. 30-6F). The tourniquet is then removed and the donor site is closed after hemostasis. Intermetatarsal ligament reconstruction is performed and the skin closed with drainage tubes.

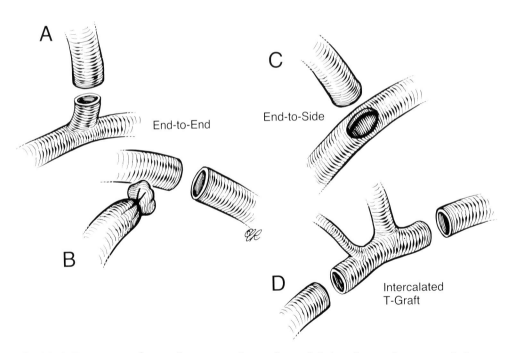

Fig. 30-7. Four types of arterial suture can be performed. (**A**) End-to-end suture with the princeps pollicis artery. (**B**) End-to-end suture with the radial artery. (**C**) End-to-side suture with the radial artery. (**D**) The dorsalis pedis artery in continuity with the plantar arch is intercalated as a T-shaped graft (in this case, two feeding arteries have been harvested from the foot).

Our policy of second ray amputation is based on problems encountered following donor site grafting (nonunion and delayed walking). On the other hand, a study by a foot surgeon based on 20 cases of second toe amputation[86] has demonstrated that when the metatarsal was left in place, there was a consistent tendency to hallux valgus deformity. This decreased after ray amputation except when the angle between the first and second metatarsals was greater than 20 degrees. In such cases, reconstruction of the second toe has to be considered.

The last steps are assessment of viability of the flap at the recipient site after release of tourniquet and application of the dressing.

Moderate elevation is prescribed postoperatively, and visualization of the skin allows direct

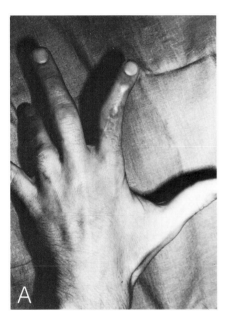
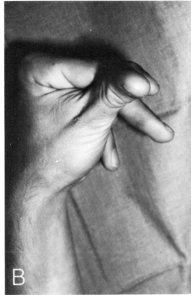
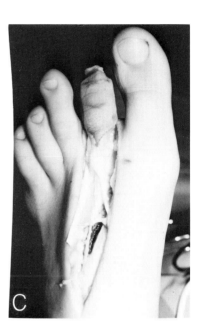

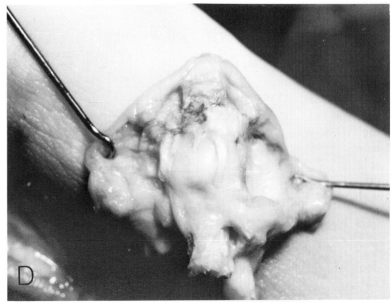

Fig. 30-8. An example of compound PIP joint transfer using the author's technique. (**A,B**) Multifinger involvement with a destroyed PIP joint of the second and fourth digits. (**C**) Preparation of a compound transfer of the PIP joint of the second toe. The first dorsal artery is visible proximally. (**D**) Plantar aspect of the transfer with intact volar plate. (*Figure continues.*)

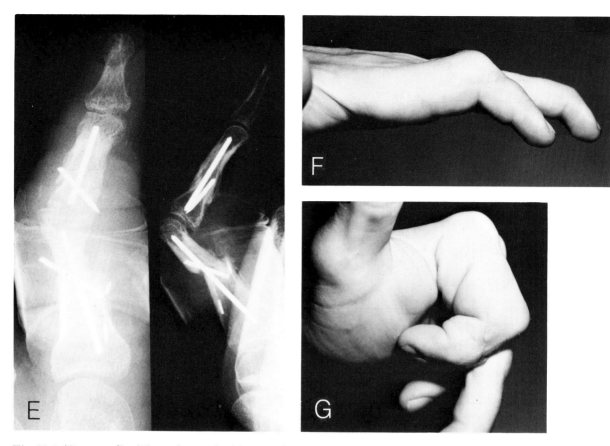

Fig. 30-8 *(Continued).* (**E**) A radiograph of the transferred joint in the PIP joint of the index finger. (**F,G**) Final range of motion 3 years after operation.

monitoring of the transfer. Low molecular Dextran is infused for 5 days with 1 g of aspirin daily. No antibiotics are given. The patient can be discharged from the hospital on the fifth day. A clinical trial of early mobilization with a dynamic dorsal splint did not correlate with the final range of motion; therefore, we routinely prescribe 3 weeks immobilization followed by active motion with dynamic extension splinting. Nightly passive flexion splinting is delayed until the fifth week. The pins are usually removed at 4 weeks. An illustrative case is shown in Figure 30-8.

OTHER TYPES OF RECONSTRUCTION

Four other techniques are worthy of mention: (1) double transfer for MPJ or PIPJ reconstruction; (2) TM joint reconstruction by MTPJ transfer; (3) joint transfer from a nonreplantable finger; and (4) "twisted two toes" for thumb reconstruction.

MP Joint Reconstruction

The MPJ can be reconstructed by using either the PIPJ or MTPJ of the toe. When two adjacent MPJ have to be reconstructed, it is possible to harvest both vascularized joints from the second toe (Fig. 30-9). The MTPJ is raised on the second plantar metatarsal artery and rotated 180 degrees on its axis. The PIPJ is raised on the first dorsal (or plantar) artery. This technique calls for a good extensor mechanism and good skin coverage.

Reconstruction of Adjacent PIP Joints

For reconstruction of an adjacent PIPJ, Tsai[115] has used the PIP joints of the second and third toes with partial syndactylization. To avoid this major cosmetic drawback, we prefer to harvest each joint on a separate pedicle (Fig. 30-10): a first plantar or

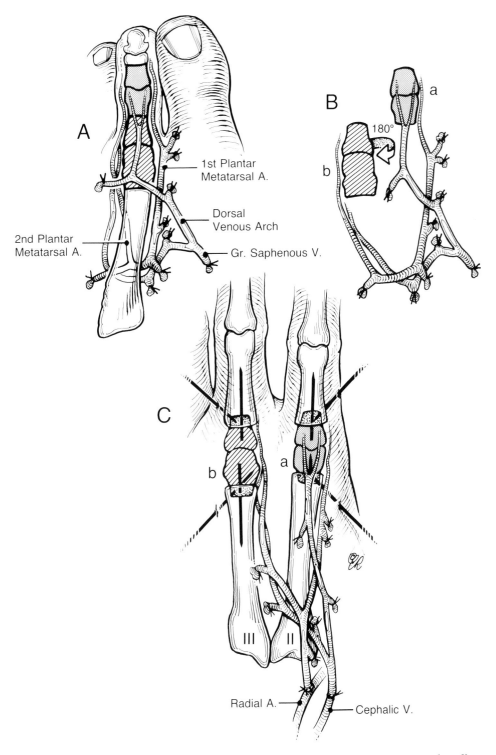

Fig. 30-9. The MTP joint and PIP joint of the second toe are lifted on separate bundles, allowing double MP joint reconstruction.

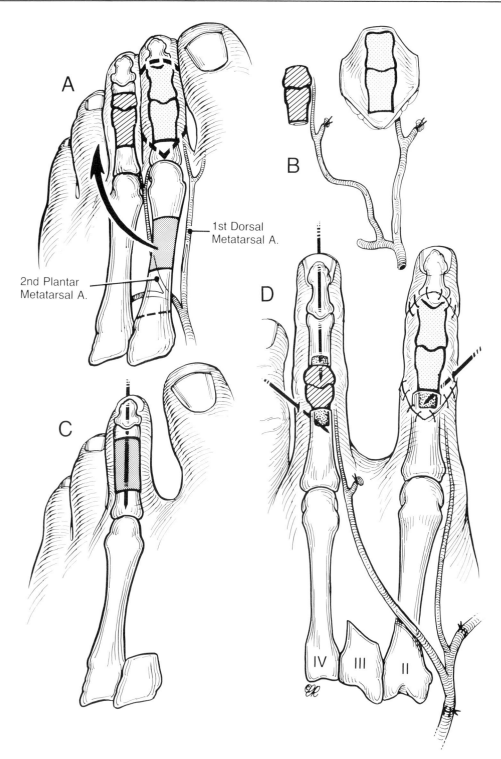

Fig. 30-10. The PIP joints of the second and third toes are harvested on separate bundles, which allows double PIP joint reconstruction.

dorsal metatarsal artery for the **PIPJ** of the second toe and the second plantar metatarsal artery for the third toe. In such cases, we amputate the second ray and use part of the second metatarsal for reconstruction of the third toe.

Trapeziometacarpal Joint Reconstruction

Reconstruction of the TMJ in certain cases of congenital thumb ray hypoplasia can be provided by an MTPJ transfer that provides bone stock, mobility, stability, and growth plates. The technique is not much different from that described above, ex-

cept that it is implanted on the carpus in hyperextension as described by Buck-Gramcko[3] in his pollicization technique. A skin flap can be transferred at the same time to improve the thenar eminence, thus facilitating an abductor digiti minimi opponensplasty.

Vascularized Joint Salvage from a Nonreplantable Finger

Occasionally, the ideal solution is to be able to harvest a compound VJT in an emergency setting from a nonreplantable finger. Either the PIPJ or the DIPJ can be used (Fig. 30-11). The technique is

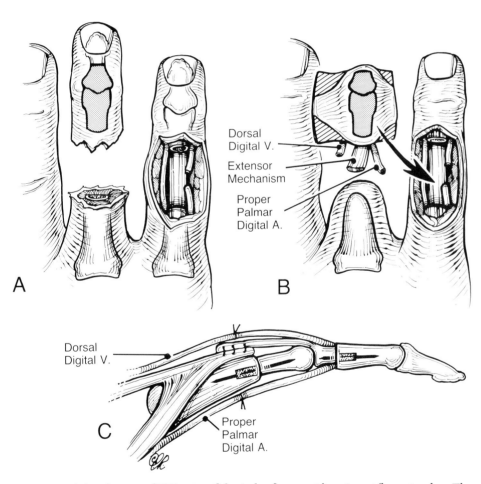

Fig. 30-11. (**A**) A destroyed PIP joint of the index finger with an intact flexor tendon. The third finger is not suitable for replantation, but the DIP joint is intact. (**B**) The third-finger DIP joint is harvested as a compound transfer for index finger PIP joint reconstruction. (**C**) The proper digital artery of the long finger is sutured to the recipient artery of the index finger.

very similar to the classic one except that the arterial anastomosis is usually performed in situ with a collateral digital artery. The proximal veins of the flap are sutured to the distal veins of the recipient finger. This technique can provide a quite normal range of motion (Fig. 30-12) and results can challenge those of VJT proposed recently.[116]

"Twisted Two Toes" (TTT) Technique

Finally, a VJT can be incorporated into a wraparound technique for thumb reconstruction in a so-called "twisted two toes" (TTT) technique.[31,36]

The skin and nail complex are taken from the ipsilateral big toe based on the first dorsal (or plantar) metatarsal artery. A piece of vascularized bone is incorporated into the flap to avoid bone resorption and to provide nail support. The PIP joint is lifted en bloc with the first and second phalanx on the second plantar (or, rarely, dorsal) metatarsal artery, the superficialis flexor, and the extensor mechanisms being harvested at the same time. Both arteries are taken in continuity with the dorsalis pedis artery, which is used for a T-shaped intercalated graft. The joint is buried into the big toe flap and the second phalanx is attached to the bone

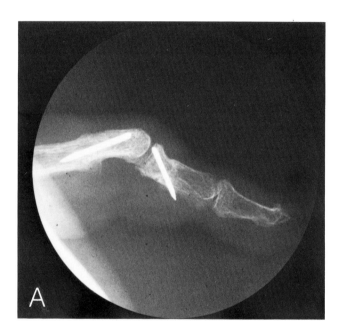

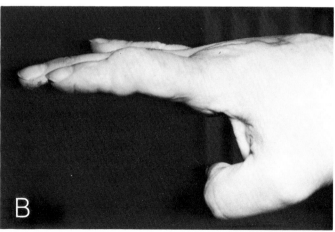

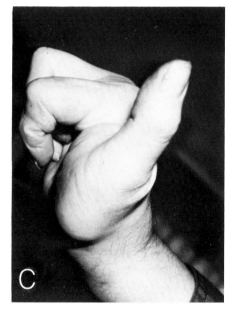

Fig. 30-12. (A) Radiograph of a transferred DIP joint at the PIP level. Final range of motion, showing (B) extension and (C) flexion.

of the big toe by a K-wire (Fig. 30-13). In this way, a two phalanx "custom-made" thumb is constructed and then may be transferred to the thumb stump in the standard manner. Either a graft or an ulnar-based flap, tailored from the stump, are used to cover the ulnar side of the filleted big toe skin. At the donor site, the proximal part of the second metatarsal bone is removed, the intermetatarsal ligament repaired and the filleted second toe skin is wrapped around the skeleton of the big toe with a Z-plasty.

Postoperative Complications

Thrombosis of the vessels is a classic complication of microvascular procedures that can be managed by careful monitoring of the skin flap incorporated into the transfer. In case of skin necrosis, mainly in very young patients, the transfer can be saved by moving a remote flap on to the "non"-vascularized joint. Infection, although not mentioned in the literature, should be managed with standard techniques.

Delayed bone healing does not seem to be a problem at the hand level, but has been mentioned frequently in the foot.[53,115,128] Stiffness of the VJT remains a major problem. We tried to improve joint mobility preoperatively in the foot by splinting at night, but without success. Even when early mobilization was employed, limitation of both active and passive extension as mentioned in total second toe transfers was found consistently after toe VJT.[30,31,34,36,37,53,115,128] There are several possible reasons for this: (1) pre-existing claw deformity of the donor toe; (2) deficient or insufficient tension on the extensor mechanism; (3) intercalated bony segment too long; and (4) bowstringing of the flexor tendons, increasing the lever arm as seen in digits with damaged pulleys.

As noted previously, some of these factors can be avoided by precise surgical technique. Despite constant efforts, our mean lack of extension has been 35 degrees with an active range of motion of 36 degrees, which is comparable to that reported in other series.[89,115,128.] At the MPJ level, motion is better, with a mean of 65 degrees, comparing favorably to other types of reconstruction.[34]

Indications

The potential advantages of vascularized joint transfers are several.

A useful range of motion in an acceptable arc can be obtained with good lateral stability providing strong opposition to the thumb in pinch.
Despite a rather short follow up period (10 years for our first case)[30] clinical *durability* has been found to corroborate experimental data with persistence of cartilage space.

Nevertheless, the two main advantages of this technique are the possibility of growth in young patients and the unique possibility of a compound transfer, providing not only joint but also bone stock, extensor mechanism, and skin, and as well allowing one-stage reconstruction.

However, several disadvantages must be emphasized as well: (1) the procedure is long, lasting 3½ hours on the average; (2) it must be performed under general anesthesia with hospitalization required (average 5.3 days); and (3) the danger of failure, as in other microsurgical procedures, exists.

In our opinion, at the PIPJ level, toe VJT falls short of its goal due to restricted range of motion. We think that it is not a definite answer to this problem, but remains useful, mainly in multiple PIP joint involvement, in young patients, and in complex losses (skin, bone, extensor tendon) with a normal flexor tendon.

At the MPJ level, indications are similar but in the case of double reconstruction, it seems better to reconstruct skin cover first. As for the PIPJ, the second and third rays are reconstructed most frequently. The MTJ joint transfer provides an acceptable solution to some cases of congenital thumb ray hypoplasia (second degree in Blauth's classification[1]). As we have already stressed, it improves the cosmetic aspect, allows growth and provides satisfactory stability and mobility (usually after muscle or tendon transfer). In thumb reconstruction, the "twisted two toes" technique is indicated in some amputations located close to the MPJ. It has several advantages over the classic "wraparound"[85] and total second toe transfer by providing: (1) a vascularized skeleton (avoiding resorption) with two

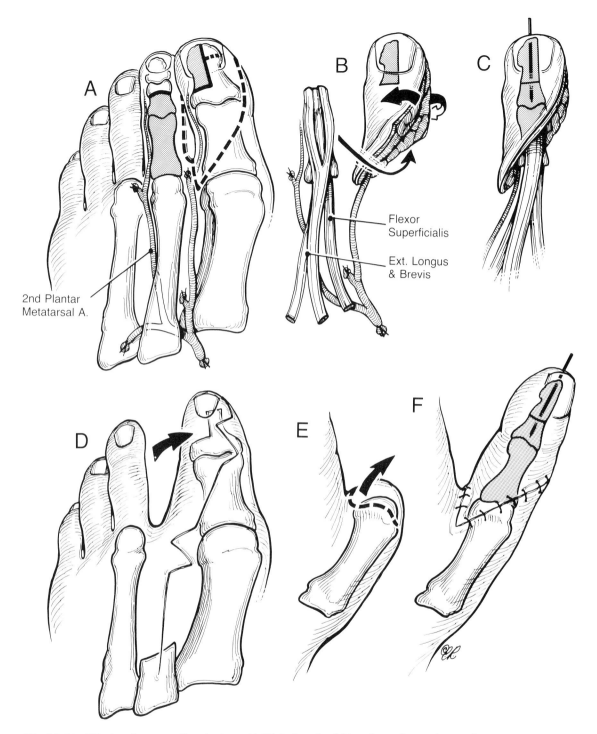

Fig. 30-13. "Twisted two toes" technique. **(A,B)** A sheath of skin, the nail complex, and a piece of bone are taken from the great toe; the **PIP** joint with extensor and flexor tendons is harvested from the second toe. **(C)** The bones of the first and second toes are joined by a K-wire and the skin wrapped around. **(D)** The filleted flap of the second toe covers the great toe defect. **(E,F)** A lateral flap is elevated from the thumb stump to cover the lateral aspect of the transfer.

Labels within figure:

2nd Plantar Metatarsal A.

Flexor Superficialis

Ext. Longus & Brevis

phalanges (matching the normal thumb); (2) one joint (plus a proximal hemi-joint when necessary) with extensor and flexor mechanism; (3) firm support for the nail; and (4) a growth plate in children.

Summary

Vascularized joint transfer may be indicated for PIPJ, MPJ, and TMJ reconstruction mainly in complex situations. This technique provides the unique advantage of a compound transfer of skin, bone, joint, tendons, and growth plate. Until vascularized homografts become clinically available, this is a worthwhile technique in limited complex situations.

REFERENCES

1. Blauth W, Schneider-Sickert F: Congenital Deformities of the Hand. An Atlas of their Surgical Treatment. pp. 136–153. Springer Verlag, Berlin, Heidelberg, New-York, 1980

2. Boyes JH: Bunnell's Surgery of the Hand. 4th Ed. pp. 318–320. JB Lippincott, Philadelphia, 1964

3. Buck Gramcko D: Pollicization of the index finger. Method and results in aplasia and hypoplasia of the thumb. J Bone Joint Surg 53A:1605–1617, 1971

4. Buncke HJ, Daniller AI, Schulz WP, Chase RA: The fate of autogenous whole joints transplanted by microvascular anastomoses. Plast Reconstr Surg 39:333–341, 1967

5. Bunnell S: Surgery of the Hand. Surgical Repair of Joints. pp. 300–304. JB Lippincott, Philadelphia, 1948

6. Burwell RG: Skeletal allografts for synovial joint reconstruction (Editorial). J Bone Joint Surgery 52B:10–13, 1970

7. Campbell CJ, Ishida H, Takahoashi H, Kelly F: The transplantation of articular cartilage. An experimental study in dogs. J Bone Joint Surg 45A:1579–1592, 1963

8. Campbell CJ: Homotransplantation of a half or whole joint. Clin Orthop 87:146–55, 1972

9. Carroll RE, Green DP: Reconstruction of hypoplastic digits using toe phalanges (Abstract). J Bone Joint Surg 57A:727, 1975

10. Colson P, Hovot R: Chirurgie réparatrice du pouce. Greffe articulaire. Lyon Chir 42:721–724, 1947

11. Colson P: Osteo articular transplants in the hand, tome II. pp. 678–684. Ed Tubiana, Masson, Paris, 1984

12. Comtet JJ, Bertrand HG, Moyen B: Free autogenous composite joint graft use in multiple finger injuries. Int J Microsurgery. 2:121–124, 1980

13. Cuthbert JB: The late treatment of dorsal injuries of the hand associated with loss of skin. Brit J Surg 33:66–71, 1945

14. Daniel G, Entin MA, Kahn DS: Autogenous transplantation in the dog of a metacarpophalangeal joint with preserved neurovascular bundle. Cand J Surg 14:253–259, 1971

15. Depalma AF, Sawyer B, Hoffman JD: Fate of osteochondral grafts. Clin Orthop 22:217–220, 1962

16. Depalma AF, Tsaltas TT, Mauler GG: Viability of osteochondral grafts as determined by uptake of S35. J Bone Joint Surg 45A:1565–1578, 1963

17. Dingman RO, Grabb WC: Reconstruction of both mandibular condyles with metatarsal bone grafts. Plast Reconstr Surg 34:441–451, 1964 Dingman RO: Follow-up clinic. Plast Reconstr Surg 47:594, 1971

18. Donski PK, Carwell GR, Sharzer LA: Growth in revascularized bone grafts in young puppies. Plast Reconstr Surg 64:239–243, 1979

19. Donski PK, O'Brien BMcC: Free microvascular epiphyseal transplantation. An experimental study in dogs. Br J Plast Surg 33:169–178, 1980

20. Ducuing J: Contribution Expérimentale à L'Étude des Greffes Articulaires Totales. Masson, Paris, 1912

21. Eades JW, Peacock EE: Autogenous transplantation of an interphalangeal joint and proximal phalangeal epiphysis. Case report and ten year follow-up. J Bone Joint Surg 48A:775–778, 1966

22. Entin MA, Alger JR, Baird RM: Experimental and clinical transplantation of autogenous whole joints. J Bone Joint Surg 44A:1518–1536, 1962

23. Entin MA, Daniel G, Kahn D: Transplantation of autogenous half-joints. Arch Surg 96:359–368, 1968

24. Erdelyi R: Experimental autotransplantation of small joints. Plast Reconstr Surg 31:129–139, 1963

25. Erdelyi R: Reconstruction of ankylosed finger joints by means of transplantation of joints from the foot. Plast Reconst Surg 31:140–150, 1963

26. Edwards EA: Anatomy of the small arteries of the foot and toes. Acta Anat 41:81–96, 1960

27. Ferlic DC, Clayton ML, Holloway M: Complications of silicone implant surgery in the metacarpophalangeal joint. J Bone Joint Surg 57A:991–994, 1975

28. Field PL, Hueston JT: Articular cartilage loss in long-standing immobilisation of interphalangeal joints. Brit J Plast Surg 23:186–191, 1970

29. Flatt AE: Studies in finger joint replacement. A review of the present position. Arch Surg 107:437–443, 1973

30. Foucher G, Merle M: Transfert articulaire au niveau d'un doigt en microchirurgie. Groupe d'avancement pour la microchirurgie. In lettre d'information du GAM n°7. 1976

31. Foucher G, Merle M, Maneaud M, Michon J: Microsurgical free partial toe transfer in hand reconstruction, a report of 12 cases. Plast Reconstr Surg 65:616–626, 1980

32. Foucher G, Denuit P, Braun FM, Merle M, Michon J: Le transfert total ou partiel du deuxième orteil dans la reconstruction digitale. A propos de 32 cas. Acta Orthop Belg 47:854–886, 1981

33. Foucher G, Van Genechten F, Merle M, Denuit P, Braun FM, Debry R, Sur H: Le transfert à partir d'orteils dans la chirurgie reconstructrice de la main. A propos de 71 cas. Ann Chir Main 3:124–138, 1984

34. Foucher G, Hoang Ph, Citron N, Merle M, Dury M: Joint reconstruction following trauma. Comparison of microsurgical transfer and conventional methods. A report of 61 cases. J Hand Surg 11B:388–393, 1986

35. Foucher G, Braun FM, Merle M, Michon J: Le transfert du deuxième orteil dans la chirurgie reconstructive des doigts longs. Revue de Chirurgie Orthopédique 67:235–240, 1981

36. Foucher G, Van Genechten F, Morrison WA: Composite tissue transfer to the hand from the foot. pp. 65–82. Jackson IT, Sommerlad BC (eds): In Recent Advances in Plastic Surgery. Churchill Livingstone, New York, 1985

37. Foucher G, Schuind F, Hoang P: Free vascularized joint transfers. Presented at the 1st meeting, American Society for Reconstructive Microsurgery, Las Vegas, 1985

38. Freeman BS: Reconstruction of thumb by toe transfer. Plast Reconstr Surg 17:393–398, 1956

39. Freeman BS: Growth studies of transplanted epiphysis. Plast Reconstr Surg 23:584–588, 1959

40. Freeman BS: Results of epiphyseal transplants by flap and by free graft. A brief survey. Plast Reconstr Surg 36:227–230, 1965 (Follow-up Clinic, 48:72, 1971)

41. Furnas DW: Growth and development in replanted forelimbs. Plast Reconstr Surg 46:445–453, 1970

42. Gibson T, Davis WB, Curran RC: The long-term survival of cartilage homografts in man. Brit J Plast Surg 11:177–187, 1958

43. Gilbert A: Composite tissue transfers from the foot: Anatomic basis and surgical technique. pp. 230–242. In Daniller AL, Strauch B (eds): Symposium on Microsurgery. CV Mosby, St Louis, 1976

44. Gill AB: Transplantation of entire bones with their joint surfaces. Ann Surg 61:658–660, 1915

45. Goebbel R: Ersatz von Fingergelenken durch Zehengelenke, München Med Wehnschi 60:1598–1601, 1913

46. Goldberg NH, Watson HK: Composite toe (phalanx and epiphysis) transfers in the reconstruction of the aphalangic hand. J Hand Surg 7:454-459, 1982

47. Goldberg VM, Porter BB, Lance EM: Transplantation of the canine knee joint on a vascular pedicle. J Bone Joint Surg 62:414–424, 1980

48. Goldberg VM, Heiple KG: Experimental hemijoint and whole-joint transplantation. A preliminary report. Clin Othop 174:43–53, 1983

49. Graham WC, Riordan DC: Reconstruction of a metacarpophalangeal joint with a metatarsal transplant. J Bone Joint Surg 30A:848–853, 1948

50. Graham WC: Transplantation of joints to replace diseased or damaged articulations in the hands. Am J Surg 88:136–141, 1954

51. Gregory CF: The current status of bone and joint transplants. Clin Orthop 87:165–166, 1972

52. Gross AE, McKee NH, Pritzker KPH, Langer F: Reconstruction of skeletal defects at the knee. A comprehensive osteochondral transplant program. Clin Orthop 174:96–106, 1983

53. Gu YD, Wu MM, Zheng YL, Yang DY, Li HR: Vascular variations and their treatment in toe transplantation. J Reconstr Microsurgery 1:227–232, 1985

54. Haas SL: Experimental transplantation of the ephiphysis with observations on the longitudinal growth of bone. JAMA 65:1965, 1915

55. Haas SL: Free transplantation of bones into the phalanges. Surg Gynecol Obstet 23:301–322, 1916

56. Haas SL: Further observations on the transplantation of the epiphyseal cartilage plate. Surg Gynecol Obstet 52:958–963, 1931

57. Harris WR, Martin R, Tile M: Transplantation of epiphyseal plates. An experimental study. J Bone and Joint Surg 47A:897–914, 1965

58. Herndon CH, Chase SW: Experimental studies in the transplantation of whole joints. J Bone Joint Surg 34A:564–578, 1952

59. Hoffman S, Siffert RS, Simon BE: Experimental and clinical experience in epiphyseal transplantation. Plast Reconstr Surg 50:58–65, 1972

60. Huang SL, Hou MZ, Yan CL: Reconstruction of the thumb by a free pedal neurovascular flap and composite phalanz-joint-tendon homograft: A preliminary report. J Reconstr Microsurg 1(4):299–303, 1985

61. Hurwitz PJ: Experimental transplantation of small joints by microvascular anastomoses. Plast Reconstr Surg 64:221–231, 1979

62. Imamaliev AS: Transplantation of hemijont in experiment. First report. Ortop Traum Protez 21:43–46, 1960

63. Imamaliev AS: Hemi-articular transplantation in experimental and clinical conditions. Ortop Traum Protez 23:9–15, 1962

64. Impallomeni G: Sul trapianto delle articolazioni. Arch Orthop 28:342, 1911

65. Johansson SH, Engkvist O: Small joint reconstruction by perichondreal arthroplasty. Clin Plast Surg 8:107–114, 1981

66. Judet H: Essai sur la greffe des tissus articulaires. CR Acad Sci Paris 146:193–196, 600–603, 1908

67. Judet H, Padovani JP: Transplantation d'articulation complète avec rétablissement circulatoire immédiat par anastomoses artérielle et veineuse. Mem Acad Chir 94:520–526, 1968

68. Judet H, Padovani JP: Transplantation d'articulation complète avec rétablissement circulatoire immédiat par anastomoses artérielle et veineuse chez le chien. Rev Chir Orthop 59:125–128, 1973

69. Kettelkamp DB, Alexander HH, Dolan J: A comparison of experimental arthroplasty and metacarpal head replacement. J Bone Joint Surg 50A:1564–1576, 1968

70. Kettelkamp DB, Ramsey P: Experimental and clinical autogenous distal metacarpal reconstruction. Clin Orthop 74:129–137, 1971

71. Kettelkamp DB: Experimental autologous joint transplantation. Clin Orthop 87:138–145, 1972

72. Kuo ET, Ji ZL, Zhao YC, Zhang ML: Reconstruction of metacarpophalangeal joint by free vascularised autogenous metatarsophalangeal joint transplant. J Reconstr Microsurg 1:65–74, 1984

73. Leung PC, Kok LC: Transplantation of the second toe. A preliminary report of sixteen cases. J Bone and Joint Surg 62A:990–996, 1980

74. Lexer E: Substitution of whole or half-joints from freshly amputated extremities by free plastic operation. Surg Gynecol Obstet 6:601, 1908

75. Lexer E: Joint transplantations and arthroplasty. Surg Gynecol Obstet 40:782–809, 1925

76. Lloyd GJ, McTavish DR, Soriano S, Wiley AM, Young MH: Fate of articular cartilage in joint transplantation. Can J Surg 16:306–320, 1973

77. Lopez A: Articular grafts. Med Exper 47:501–507, 1962

78. Lugnegard H: Autologous transplantation of a finger phalanx with articular surface. Report of a case. Acta Chir Scand 126:185–190, 1963

79. McKeever F: In discussion. Herndon and Chase. J Bone Joint Surg 34A:578–582, 1952

80. Mathes SJ, Buchannan R, Weeks PM: Microvascular joint transplantation with epiphyseal growth. J Hand Surg 5:586–589, 1980

81. May JW, Chait LA, Cohen BE, O'Brien BMc: Free neurovascular flap from the first web of the foot in hand reconstruction. J Hand Surg 2:387–393, 1977

82. May H: The regeneration of joint transplants and intracapsular fragments. Ann Surg 116:297–303, 1942

83. Menon J: Reconstruction of the metacarpophalangeal joint with autogenous metatarsal. J Hand Surg 8:443–446, 1983

84. Mooney V, Ferguson AB: The influence of immobilisation and motion on the formation of fibro-cartilage after joint resection in the rabbit. J Bone Joint Surg 48A:6–10, 1966

85. Morrison WA, O'Brien BMc, Macleod AM: Thumb reconstruction with a free neurovascular wrap-around flap from the big toe. J Hand Surg 5:575–583, 1980

86. Moyen B: Paper at the 8th International Meeting of Microsurgery. Panel on toe transfer. May 1982 (Unpublished)

87. Nettelblad H, Randolph MA, Weiland AJ: Free microvascular epiphyseal-plate transplantation. An experimental study in dogs. J Bone Joint Surg 66A:1421 and 1430, 1986

88. O'Brien BMc: Microvascular free small joint transfer. pp. 248–249. Microvascular Reconstructive Surgery. Churchill Livingstone, New York, 1977

89. O'Brien BMc, Gould JS, Morrison WA, Russel RC, Macleod AM, Pribaz JJ: Free vascularized small joint transfer to the hand. J Hand Surg 9(5):634–641, 1984

90. Pap K, Kronpecher S: Arthroplasty of the knee. Experimental and clinical experiences. J Bone Joint Surg 43A:523–530, 1961

91. Parrish FF: Treatment of bone tumours by total excision and replacement with massive autogenous and homologous grafts. J Bone Joint Surg 48A:968–972, 1966

92. Peacock EE: Reconstructive surgery of hands with injured metacarpophalangeal joints. J Bone Joint Surg 38A:291–302, 1956

93. Porter BB, Lance EL: Limb and joint transplantation. A review of research and clinical experience. Clin Orthop 104:249–274, 1974

94. Planas J: Free transplantation of the finger joints. Rev Espan Cir Plast 1:21–26, 1968

95. Pritzker KPH, Gross AE, Langer F, Luk SC, Houpt JB: Articular cartilage transplantation. Human Pathology. 8:635–651, 1977

96. Rank BK: Long term results of epiphyseal transplants in congenital deformities of the hand. Plast Reconstr Surg 61:321–329, 1978

97. Reeves B: Orthotopic transplantation of vascularised whole knee joints in dogs. Lancet 1:500-502, 1969

98. Reeves B: Studies of vascularized homotransplants of the knee joint. J Bone Joint Surg 50B:226–227, 1968

99. Rinaldi E: Metacarpal loss treated by metatarsal substitution. Ital J Orthop Trauma 2:335–340, 1976

100. Ring PA: Transplantation of epiphyseal cartilage: An experimental study. J Bone Joint Surg 37B:642–647, 1955

101. Roffe JL, Latil F, Chamant M, Huguet JF, Bureau H: Intérêt chirurgical de l'étude radio-anatomique de la vascularisation artérielle de l'avant-pied. Ann Chir Main 1:84–87, 1982

102. Rutishauser E, Taillard W: L'ischémie articulaire en pathologie humaine et expérimentale. La notion de pannus vasculaire. Rev Chir Orthop 52:197–223, 1966

103. Sarrafian SK, Topouzian LK: Anatomy and physiology of the extensor apparatus of the toes. J Bone Joint Surg 51A:669–679, 1969

104. Schreiber A, Walker N, Nishikawa M: Autologe Gelenkentransplantationen mit mikrochirurgischer gefassplastik. Helv Chir Acta 43:151–155, 1976

105. Schreiber A, Walker N, Nishikawa M, Yargarsil MG: Transplantation d'articulation avec la technique de microchirurgie vasculaire. Acta Orthop Belg 45:403–411, 1979

106. Seligman GM, George E, Yablon I, Nutik G, Cruess RL: Transplantation of whole knee joints in the dog. Clin Orthop 87:332–344, 1972

107. Slome D, Reeves B: Experimental homotransplantation of the knee joint. Lancet 2:205–206, 1966

108. Snowdy HA, Omer GE, Sherman FC: Longitudinal growth of a free toe phalanx transplant to a finger. J Hand Surg 5:71–73, 1980

109. Smith PJ, Jones BM: Free vascularized transfer of a metatarsophalangeal joint to the hand. A technical modification. J Hand Surg 10B:109–112, 1985

110. Straub GF: Anatomical survival, growth and physiological function of an epiphyseal bone transplant. Surg Gynecol Obstet 48:687–690, 1929

111. Swanson AB: Arthroplasty in traumatic arthritis of the joints of the hand. Orthop Clin North Am 1:285–298, 1970

112. Tietze A: Ersatz des Resezierten Unteren Radiusendes durch eine Grosszehenphalange. Chir Kongre Verhandl 1:77–81, 1902

113. Tomita Y, Tsai TM, Steyers C, Ogden L, Juiter JB, Kutz JE: The role of the epiphyseal and metaphyseal circulations on longitudinal growth in the dog: An experimental study. J Hand Surg 11A:375–382, 1986

114. Tsai TM, Odgen L, Jaeger SH, Okubo K: Experimental vascularized total joint autografts. A primate study. J Hand Surg 7:140–146, 1982

115. Tsai TM, Jupiter JB, Kutz JE, Kleinert HE: Vascularized autogenous whole joint transfer in the hand: A clinical study. J. Hand Surg 7:335–342, 1982

116. Tsai TM, Singer R, Elliott E, Klein H: Immediate free vascularized joint transfer from second toe to index finger proximal interphalangeal joint. A case report. J Hand Surg 10B:85–89, 1985

117. Vercauteren ME, Van Vynckt C: A free total toe phalanx transplant to a finger. A case report. J Hand Surg 8:336–339, 1983

118. Volkov M: Allotransplantation of joints. J Bone Joint Surg 52B:49–53, 1970

119. Watanabe M, Katsumi M, Yoshizu T, Tajima T: Experimental study of autogenous toe-joint transplantation: Anatomic study of vascular pattern of toe joints as a base of vascularised autogenous joint transplantation. Orthop Surg (Tokyo) 29:1317–1320, 1978

120. Watanabe M, Katsumi M, Yoshizu T, Tajima T: Experimental study and clinical application of free toe-joint transplantation with vascular pedicle. Orthop Surg (Tokyo) 31:1411–1416, 1980

121. Whitesides ES: Normal growth in a transplanted epiphysis. Case report with 13 year follow up. J Bone Joint Surg 59A:546–547, 1977

122. Wilson JN: Epiphyseal transplantation. A clinical study. J Bone and Joint Surg 48A:245–256, 1966

123. Wilson JN, Smith CF: Transplantation of whole autogenous joints in the hand. J Bone Joint Surg 48A:1651–1654, 1966

124. Worsing RA, Engber WD, Lange TA: Reactive synovitis from particulate Silastic. J Bone Joint Surg 64A:581–585, 1982

125. Wray RC, Mathes SM, Young VL, Weeks PM: Free vascularized whole joint transplants with ununited epiphyses. Plast Reconstr Surg 67:519–525, 1981

126. Wray RC, Young VL: Drug treatment and flap survival. Plast Reconstr Surg 73:939–942, 1984

127. Yablon IG, Brandt KD, Delellis R, Covall D: Destruction of joint homografts. An experimental study. Arthritis Rheum 20:1526–1537, 1977

128. Yoshizu T, Watanabe M, Tajima T: Etude expérimentale et applications cliniques des transferts libres d'articulation d'orteil avec anastomoses vasculaires. pp. 539–551. In Chirurgie de la Main. Tome II, ed. Tubiana, Masson, Paris, 1984

129. Zaleske DJ, Ehrlich MG, Piliero C, May JW, Mankin HJ: Growth plate behavior in whole joint replantation in the rabbit. J Bone Joint Surg 64A:249–258, 1982

130. Zaleske DJ: Revascularized joint transplants. pp. 377–385. In Friedlender, Mankin, Sell (eds): Osteochondreal Allografts. Little Brown, Boston, 1983

131. Zrubecky: Freie Verpflanzung von zehengelenken in der Handchirurgie. 2:67–71, 1970

Microneurovascular Great-Toe–to–Hand Transfer for Thumb Reconstruction

31

James W. May, Jr.
Rodney J. Rohrich

The thumb is essential for normal hand function. Without a thumb the functional capacity of the normal hand is reduced by 40 to 50 percent.[6] In the severely mutilated hand, the thumb assumes far greater importance and in such cases a mobile sensate thumb greatly improves prehensile function and may convert a useless extremity into a satisfactory assisting hand.[5] The great-toe–to–hand free tissue transfer can provide functional thumb reconstruction in carefully selected patients with thumb amputation or absence.

Numerous reconstructive procedures have evolved to reconstruct a congenitally absent or traumatically amputated thumb.[6,7,9–14,17,18,26–28] With the advent of microvascular technique, it became possible to transfer distant tissues in a single stage, thereby leading Buncke to perform the first great-toe–to–hand transfer in a primate in 1964.[3] Cobett successfully performed the procedure in the human in 1968.[8] At present, the great-toe–to–hand microvascular transfer for thumb reconstruction has proven not only to be functional, but also a safe and reliable method of thumb reconstruction.[15,20] This method of thumb reconstruction maximizes the free tissue transfer concept by providing multiple component tissues in a single reconstructive procedure. It avoids local tissue sacrifice from an already injured extremity and furthermore, it can provide a dexterous and remarkably aesthetic thumb.[19,22]

Great-toe–to–hand free tissue transfer is a technically demanding procedure for even the most experienced surgeon. A thorough understanding of the anatomy of the donor and recipient site is fundamental in the successful performance of this procedure.[20] This chapter outlines our current approach to the selection of an appropriate patient for this procedure, and presents the pertinent anatomy and procedural detail needed for the great-toe–to–hand transfer for thumb reconstruction. Attention to detail and adherence to these principles has allowed this procedure to be safe, reliable, and functional.

INDICATIONS

Free great-toe–to–hand transfer is our preferred method of thumb reconstruction in those instances in which the thumb has been lost near the

MP joint and adjacent injured digits are not available for pollicization. Pollicization remains our treatment of choice for the care of the patient with a congenitally absent thumb in a hand with four normal fingers.[1,30,32]

Toe-to-thumb transfer is also our choice for thumb reconstruction when the badly damaged hand may be deficient in remaining digits. The great toe is always preferred, as we believe that this makes a far better thumb than any other toe.[22] The donor site after great toe transfer may be worse aesthetically than after the second toe transfer, but this single disadvantage is worth the multiple advantages in the hand that great toe transfer provides. This procedure is preferred over pollicization of a normal index finger for replacement of the amputated thumb because great toe transfer adds a digit that looks and feels more like a normal thumb than does an index finger and does not borrow tissue from an already injured hand. Furthermore, a great toe transfer is functionally more powerful than a pollicization procedure when normal thenar muscles remain in the hand.[25] The primary goal in great-toe–to–hand transfer is to attain a maximally functional and aesthetic thumb.

ANATOMIC CONSIDERATIONS

Skin Incision and Flap Design

The proper foot incision allows for ample tissue to be left in the foot, including thick plantar skin for adequate wound closure. This involves the use of a racket-type incision, with a linear dorsal component beginning proximally and dorsally in the area of the palpable dorsalis pedis artery (Fig. 31-1). The incision extends distally to join a circular incision at the great toe plantar flexion crease. The flap over the thumb stump should be radial and palmar to allow sufficient length to cover the medial and plantar surface of the great toe transfer. A skin graft or a previously placed groin flap can be used to cover the dorsal and/or first web region.

Vasculature

Angiography of both donor and recipient vessels is necessary when planning a toe-to-thumb transfer. Both studies can be performed at the same time via a transfemoral approach. In a previously injured hand it is essential to identify the vessels in the recipient area that are most useful, and not to devascularize this region of an already compromised hand. We have often found the best recipient vessel to be the dorsal radial artery in the anatomic snuffbox area. In the foot, biplaner angiography is used to delineate the dominant vasculature in the first web space.

The dorsal foot dissection is technically straightforward and provides less foot morbidity than volar

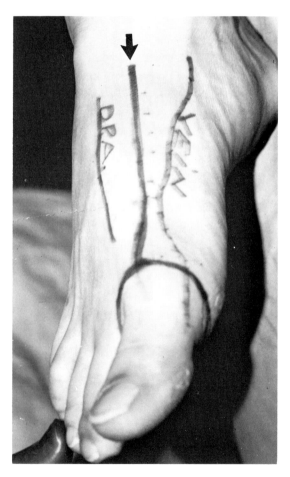

Fig. 31-1. The dorsal foot incision *(arrow)* is located midway between the dorsalis pedis artery *(DPA)* and the greater saphenous vein.

dissections. In a previous study,[21] the first dorsal metatarsal artery (FDMA) was found to reliably supply the first web space by giving rise to small dorsal digital vessels just distal to the transverse metatarsal ligament. The FDMA vessel continues distally as the distal communicating artery and ultimately joins the large plantar digital vessels to the great and second toe. Seventy-eight percent of the 50 cadaveric dissections in this study showed the first dorsal metatarsal artery (FDMA) emerging from the dorsalis pedis artery (DPA) in a relatively superficial plane (dorsal to the midmetatarsals), with the mean length of the FDMA vessel being 7 cm to the web space skin. In 22 percent, however, the origin was more deeply situated in the first metatarsal space. If more than 7 cm of arterial vascular length is required, the proximal dorsalis pedis artery is carried with the transferred toe. This is usually the case, and allows the large dorsalis pedis artery to be the donor artery. By use of the first dorsal metatarsal artery or the large dorsalis pedis artery, adequate vessel caliber is attained to facilitate a safe and reliable anastomosis, in most cases. The dorsal arterial system has been used in all but 2 of the 37 great-toe–to–thumb transfers performed at the Massachusetts General Hospital.

The venous anatomy of the foot and recipient area is assessed preoperatively by the use of a venous tourniquet. Typically, a distal cephalic vein in the hand becomes the recipient vessel. In the foot, the transverse venous arch, including the proximal saphenous vein, serves as the donor vessel. This arch gives rise to two or more dorsal veins on either side of the great toe. Great care must be taken to preserve the superficial venous plexus to the dorsal skin of the foot to prevent flap necrosis while ascertaining the largest venous arch to the great toe. These veins, in continuity with the saphenous vein, are preserved along with the intervening soft tissue, which not only provides coverage for tendons, but also provides a suitable bed for skin grafting in the hand when needed after the toe is transferred to the hand.

Bone

The ipsilateral great toe is preferable for transfer, as most great toes angulate laterally 10 to 15 degrees; this allows the reconstructed thumb to form a better pinch with the adjacent fingers. The general principle of making the reconstructed part slightly shorter and therefore less conspicuous than its normal counterpart should be followed. The length of the great toe measured from the metatarsophalangeal (MTP) joint distally is slightly greater than that of the thumb in the same individual. If the level of the thumb amputation is proximal to the midmetacarpal level, the toe MP joint should be taken with the transfer, with appropriate shortening to allow the overall length of the reconstructed thumb to be slightly less than that of the normal thumb. It is imperative to note that the great toe MP joint is primarily an extension joint while that of the thumb is primarily a flexion joint (Fig. 31-2). Therefore, the toe metatarsal osteotomy should be angulated approximately 60 degrees in a dorsal to plantar direction so that upon transfer the MP joint of the toe can be placed in a 60 degree hyperextended position, thus converting it into a flexion joint (Fig. 31-3). This maneuver provides joint stability and full flexion. In doing so the volar plate should be anchored in such a way as to provide an additional restraint against MP hyperextension in the new thumb position. With the MP joint reconstructed as described, 30 to 60 degrees of active motion can be expected following the transfer. The angled osteotomy can be positioned so that the volar extent enters the joint, while the volar plate is divided distal to the sesamoid bones along the proximal volar plate (Fig. 31-4). Leaving the sesamoids with the great toe metatarsal adds 5 to 10 mm of height to the soft tissues beneath the metatarsal head and helps prevent descent of the metatarsal head in the foot. It also maintains a desirable pushoff surface in the foot.

Tendon

Tendon reconstruction of the transferred toe is dependent upon recipient tissue availability (Fig. 31-5). Accurate length measurements are made for each tendon required in the recipient hand prior to transection of the great toe tendons, to allow for adequate tendon reconstruction. The extensor hallucis longus (EHL) and extensor hallucis brevis (EHB) are divided over the midmetatarsal and repaired to the extensor pollicis longus (EPL) and extensor pollicis brevis (EPB), respectively, in the

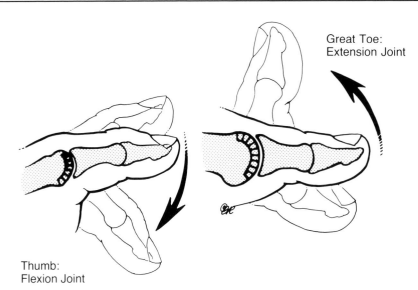

Great Toe:
Extension Joint

Thumb:
Flexion Joint

Fig. 31-2. The thumb metacarpophalangeal joint is primarily a flexion joint, while the great toe metatarsophalangeal joint is primarily an extension joint.

snuffbox area, distal to the dorsal retinaculum. The flexor hallucis longus (FHL) is divided in the midfoot (which usually requires a second transverse incision) and is joined to the flexor pollicis longus (FPL) proximal to the wrist. If the FPL is not available or lacks adequate excursion (less than 2 cm), the FHL may be joined to a superficialis flexor tendon with adequate excursion from an adjacent digit. If functional thenar muscles and the thumb adductor pollicis are present they are joined into

the thumb extensor mechanism just proximal to the MP joint. If there is insufficient length for them to be joined, a slip of the EHL can be split from proximal to distal and turned medially and laterally from the radial and ulnar sides and connected to the abductor pollicis brevis (APB) and the adductor pollicis (AP), respectively. In the absence of thenar musculature, the extensor hallucis brevis (EHB) tendon can be left long for future use as an opposition transfer. Similarly, an adductor transfer can be

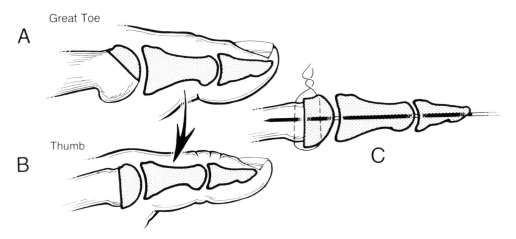

Great Toe

A

Thumb

B

C

Fig. 31-3. (A,B) The great toe metatarsal osteotomy is angulated approximately 60 degrees, so that after transfer the toe MP joint is converted to a flexion joint in the hand. (C) A longitudinal K-wire is used to fix the toe into the thumb metacarpal. Interosseous compression wire fixation is used at the osteotomy site.

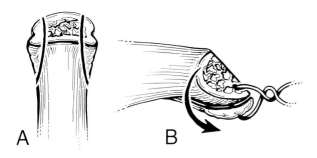

Fig. 31-4. Narrowing of the distal end of the first metatarsal with the sesamoids fixed in the plantar position.

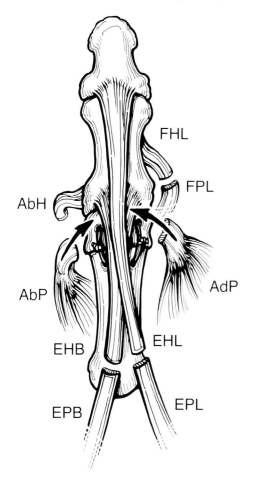

Fig. 31-5. Right toe transferred to a right thumb with approximate donor and recipient tendons. *(AbH,* abductor hallucis; *FHL,* flexor hallucis longus; *FPL,* flexor pollicis longus; *EHL,* extensor hallucis longus; *EHB,* extensor hallucis brevis; *EPL,* extensor pollicis longus; *EPB,* extensor pollicis brevis; *AbP,* abductor pollicis brevis; *AdP,* adductor pollicis.) (The FPL to FHL juncture is made proximal to the wrist, but is shown here diagrammatically.)

performed at a later date. When the tension of each tendon repair is adjusted, the interphalangeal joint of the toe should be placed in full extension, as there is a tendency for the development of a flexion contracture of the interphalangeal joint following the transfer. The thumb CM joint and the new MP joint from the toe should be in a neutral position.

Nerve

Like the thumb, the great toe has both a dorsal and a plantar nerve supply. The deep peroneal nerve (DPN) is identified beneath the EHB tendon in the foot, from which point it proceeds distally to supply the first web space. The nerve can be sutured to a branch of the superficial radial nerve in the hand, thus providing sensation to the dorsolateral area of the transferred toe.

In the toe, the plantar digital nerves are identified distal to the MP joint and dissected proximally through a short plantar foot incision. The common digital nerve can be dissected and split longitudinally to preserve plantar sensation to the second toe. Both nerves are divided in the soft tissues proximal to the metatarsal head in an area of the foot where neuroma formation should cause no symptoms. The thumb digital nerve stumps must be carefully checked for residual scar with the microscope prior to cutting of the toe nerves, to allow adequate length for tension-free neurorrhaphies to the thumb digital nerves. In the young patient, one can expect the ultimate two-point discrimination in the transferred toe to be in the range of the original two-point discrimination in the toe donor site following careful nerve repair. In 50 normal patients, two-point discrimination in the lateral pulp of the normal great toe was found to be an average of 11 mm.[20]

OPERATIVE TECHNIQUE

Patient Preparation

The donor and recipient areas of the patient are given a thorough preparation with surgical soap the evening before surgery. Shaving is performed by the surgeon in the operating room. One gram of cephazolin is given intravenously in the operating room. The patient is placed on an air mattress and all pressure points are well padded. Following induction of general anesthesia, a Foley catheter is inserted, and upper and lower extremity tourniquets are positioned. Routine antiseptic preparation is performed on the donor and recipient sites, including a hip donor area in the event that skin grafting is necessary. An Esmarch bandage is not routinely used in the leg, as it is desirable to have some blood remaining in the arteries and veins to assist in vascular identification.

Foot Dissection

Under 2.5 power loupe magnification, a racket-shaped skin incision is made as shown in Figure 31-1, and the medial and lateral dorsal foot flaps are raised for exposure. Hemostasis is achieved with bipolar electrocoagulation. The continuation of the saphenous vein is identified in a deep subareolar plane and the dorsal foot flaps are kept as thick as possible to prevent flap necrosis. Division of the EHB tendon allows identification of the FDMA and DPN. They are exposed as far proximally as the DPA to provide adequate arterial length and size. The DPA and FDMA anatomy must be correlated with the lateral view of the foot arteriogram. This is the most critical part of the foot dissection. The continuation of the DPA as it passes to the plantar side of the foot is ligated only after the take-off of the FDMA is seen and the FDMA is traced into the great toe. On the plantar surface, the FHL is identified along with the plantar digital nerves and arteries on either side. The first plantar metatarsal (FPM) artery also supplies the first and second toes. The FDMA crosses over the transverse metatarsal ligament before joining the FPMA. By dissection into the web space, the FPMA is divided (preserving adequate length for use as a back-up system), as are vessels to the second toe. The DPN is split and the fibers to the great toe are divided with adequate proximal length. On the volar surface, the digital nerves are divided. Adequate length is preserved, and those fibers to the second toe that have been split off are spared. The FHL is divided through a separate incision in the midfoot, from which the FHL is pulled into the distal wound. At this point the tourniquet is released and adequate circulation is confirmed. The great toe is perfused for 20 minutes prior to completion of the dissection and transfer of the great toe to the hand.

Hand Dissection

Shortly after the toe dissection is begun, the hand is prepared by a separate surgical team. A radially based palmar thumb skin flap is raised, and the dorsal incision extends into the anatomic snuffbox, where the cephalic vein, superficial radial nerve, dorsal dominant branch of the radial artery, and extensor tendons are identified. The tendon repairs will be done distal to the extensor retinaculum and Lister's tubercle. On the volar surface of the wrist, a transverse incision is made that allows identification of the FPL tendon and repair of the FHL proximal to the carpal tunnel. The thumb metacarpal or phalanx is cut squarely at a right angle to its long axis with the power saw after appropriate measurements of length have been made. If no carpometacarpal joint exists, the trapezium is freshened to allow osteosynthesis between the toe metatarsal and the trapezium. In many cases a groin flap will have been done prior to the toe transfer if there is inadequate soft tissue coverage. A bone graft can be done at the time of the groin flap to lengthen the bony skeleton in anticipation of the toe transfer in selected cases.

Microvascular Free Tissue Transfer

As the toe is dissected, vessels, nerves, and tendons are folded distally over the toe and wrapped in protective gauze for cooling with iced saline. Following amputation, the toe is joined to the thumb stump by two vertically placed #26-gauge interosseous compression wires and a longitudinally placed K-wire, which helps hold the digit in proper extension. Extensor tendon repairs are performed with an overlapped side-to-side technique. The flexor tendons are joined by weave tenorrhaphy, and the abductor and adductor tendons are repaired to the extensor mechanism. The vascular repairs are then completed in an end-to-end or end-to-side fashion as vessel caliber and position permit, using standard microvascular techniques. Following removal of vessel clamps, capillary filling of the thumb ensues, although this may take several minutes to become apparent. Flow should be confirmed by vessel patency tests. Subsequently, the superficial radial nerve and DPN are joined dorsally, and the digital nerve repairs are completed volarly. Vessel patency is again assessed. Skin closure is then undertaken, with drains used as deemed necessary by the surgeon. If a skin graft is required, a thick split-thickness or full-thickness skin graft is placed dorsally over the area of the confluence of the dorsal veins that were intentionally preserved during the toe dissection. Surface differential thermocouple probes are placed on the new thumb and a control digit before volar and dorsal supporting plaster splints are fashioned.[23] This method of monitoring tissue perfusion is used as an adjunct to clinical judgement.

The great toe donor site is closed by removal of the metatarsal condyles to reduce bony prominence. The remaining volar plate and sesamoids are sutured into the distal metatarsal through two drill holes (see Fig. 31-4). The wounds are closed over a suction catheter. A well-padded posterior plaster splint is applied to the lower leg and foot.

Illustrative Case

A 57-year-old, left-hand dominant male was referred to the Massachusetts General Hospital one year after amputation of his left thumb at the proximal MP level following an unsuccessful attempt at replantation (Fig. 31-6). The patient had found the stump of his thumb to be functionally too short and aesthetically unpleasing. Thus a left great-toe–to–thumb transfer was suggested after discussing other reconstructive options with the patient. Preoperative gait analysis performed by Dr. Sheldon Simon at the Boston Children's Hospital showed normal gait, with the exception that no significant weight bearing of the great toe metatarsal head was seen. Preoperative angiography of the left foot revealed normal arterial anatomy, showing a dominant superficial circulatory pattern[21] with a large first dorsal metatarsal artery (Fig. 31-7A). Simultaneous angiography of the hand revealed a patent radial artery supplying the remaining thumb stump (Fig. 31-7B).

On 11 August 1981 a left microvascular great-

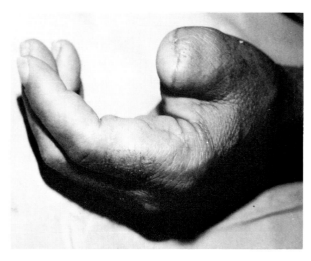

Fig. 31-6. Left thumb amputation stump at the proximal MP level.

toe to left-thumb reconstruction was performed. After appropriate longitudinal incisions were made on the dorsum of the foot, the DPA and FDMA were identified, along with the greater saphenous vein and the DPN. On the volar surface the FHL, digital nerves, and vascular pedicles were identified. After making the appropriate measurements of the tendons and neurovascular bundles to guarantee adequate length in the hand, the tendons and nerves were divided and the plantar digital vessels were ligated. The tourniquet was deflated prior to vessel division and transfer.

Simultaneously, in the hand a second operative team proceeded with the hand dissection. A dorsal incision permitted the raising of a flap and exposure of the dorsal radial nerve, superficial radial artery, and cephalic vein. On the palmar side, two volar thumb digital neuromas were identified. The EPL and EPB tendons were identified, and the FPL tendon was located through a separate transverse incision in the wrist. The thumb proximal phalanx was freshened transversely with an oscillating power saw.

The DPA and saphenous vein were then divided. The great toe was brought to the hand (Fig. 31-8) and bony fixation was achieved with two interosseous compression wires and a longitudinal K-wire. The appropriate tendons were sutured to allow for full thumb extension. The operating microscope

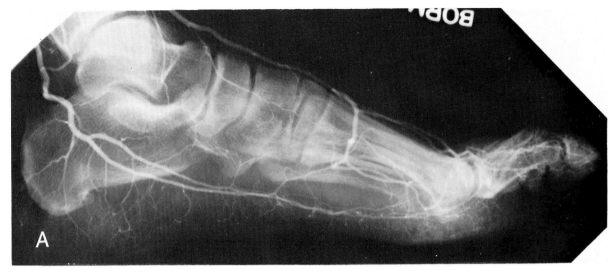

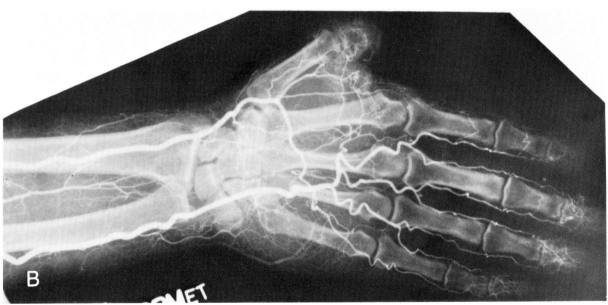

Fig. 31-7. (**A**) Lateral view angiogram of the left foot revealed the first dorsal metatarsal artery in a superficial location. (**B**) Left hand angiogram revealed patent radial and ulnar arteries supplying the hand.

was brought into the field and the arterial and venous anastomoses were performed with interrupted 10–0 nylon followed by neurorrhaphies, dorsally and volarly. Release of the microvascular clamps revealed prompt capillary filling and good venous return. A full-thickness skin graft was taken from the right groin and sutured into the first web space defect (Fig. 31-9). The incisions in the hand were closed, followed by placement of two thermocouple probes on the great toe and adjacent index finger to monitor the free tissue transfer postoperatively.

The toe metatarsal was narrowed, the volar plate capsuloplasty was performed as previously described (see Fig. 31-4), and the skin was approximated over a suction catheter. A bulky supportive

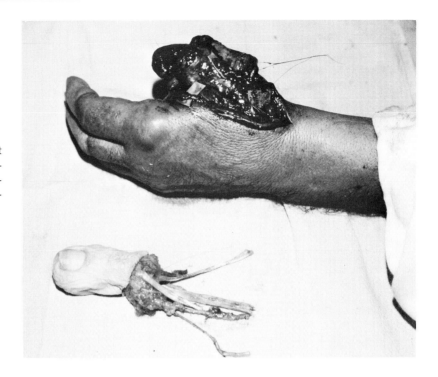

Fig. 31-8. The detached left great toe is shown adjacent to the dissected left hand prior to bony fixation, tendon, vessel, and nerve repair.

plaster dressing was applied to the hand and the foot and both were elevated on two pillows.

Postoperative Management

The splinted hand is elevated on pillows, with the thumb monitored hourly both clinically and with the use of skin temperature probes by a skilled nursing staff familiar with microvascular reconstructive procedures. The patient is kept at bed rest for 7 days while intravenous (IV) cephazolin and low molecular weight Dextran are given, in addition to daily aspirin (1 g). On the seventh day after surgery the original dressing is changed and the hand is immobilized for an additional week. Gentle, active range of motion exercises are then

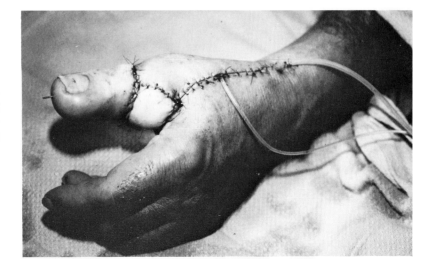

Fig. 31-9. Completion of left great-toe–to–thumb transfer, showing drains and skin graft prior to placement of thermocouple skin probes and dressing.

initiated at 2 weeks. Passive exercises are begun after approximately 6 weeks. The original foot dressing and drains are removed after the seventh day and replaced with a snug-fitting elastic dressing. The patient is allowed full weight bearing at 3 weeks.

Complications

Most complications occur in the immediate postoperative period and relate to the microvascular repairs. Venous occlusion is characterized by a cyanotic or purplish color of the transferred toe, with a concomitant drop in measured temperature. In addition, when the toe is pierced with a pin-prick, dark, de-oxygenated blood can be seen. Arterial occlusion is also accompanied by a temperature drop in conjunction with decreased tissue turgor, pallor, absent or sluggish capillary refill, and little, if any, bleeding upon pricking with a pin. If either situation occurs, the patient should be returned promptly to the operating room for exploration. Revisions of the vessel anastomoses with vein grafts taken from the foot may be required. In the 37 toe-to-hand procedures we have performed, a single loss of the transferred digit has been encountered.

Hand Rehabilitation Program

The hand rehabilitation program following a great-toe–to–thumb transfer is important to maximize the ultimate functional result.[31] The specific goals of therapy are to:

1. Prevent first web space contracture due to skin and adductor tightness;
2. Regain maximum range of motion in all joints of the affected upper extremity in addition to the toe-to-thumb transfer;
3. Facilitate sensibility of the transferred thumb;
4. Maximize strength, coordination, and endurance of the reconstructed toe-to-thumb.

Rehabilitation begins immediately after initial toe-to-thumb transfer, in that the affected extremity is elevated during the early postoperative course to decrease the amount of edema. At 2

weeks, gentle active mobilization of the thumb is begun with no isolated interphalangeal joint motion or abduction allowed until 6 weeks after surgery. A long opponens thermoplastic splint holds the thumb in palmar abduction at the wrist and 15 degrees of flexion to minimize tension at the vessel, nerve, and tendon anastomotic sites. The patient must observe all sensory precautions. Forceful activities are avoided. Compressive wrappings of the thumb using Coban reduce edema and light lanolin massage may help reduce scar tissue.

Postoperatively, passive mobilization of the thumb begins at 6 weeks and gradually more demanding activities are introduced. A sensory retraining program is designed and varies according to the patient's recovery process. As sensation returns over the first 6 months, the patient learns to reassociate the new sensation with thumb function. At 8 weeks after surgery, the long opponens splint is discontinued and three new splints are fabricated. A dynamic splint with elastic band traction flexes and extends the interphalangeal joint and promotes optimal gliding of the flexor pollicis longus tendon. Another splint extends and abducts the MP joint. These two are worn alternately throughout the day between active exercise sessions. The third splint, a web spacer, is regularly adjusted to counteract the inevitable first web space tightening, and this is worn at night. By 16 weeks following transfer, the patient can perform heavier and more strenuous tasks. Sensation will gradually improve throughout the next 6 to 12 months, and home or job related activities should be simulated in the therapy program. The splints may be discarded when mobilization and strength are sufficient, and therapy is discontinued when improvement plateaus.

Long-Term Follow-Up

Four and a half years following great-toe–to–thumb reconstruction, the patient whose case was illustrated demonstrates an aesthetically pleasing (Fig. 31-10) and functional thumb (Fig. 31-11). Key pinch measures 18 pounds and grip strength is 60 pounds. Two-point thumb pulp discrimination is 11 mm. Postoperative gait analysis was unchanged from preoperative. The donor site poses

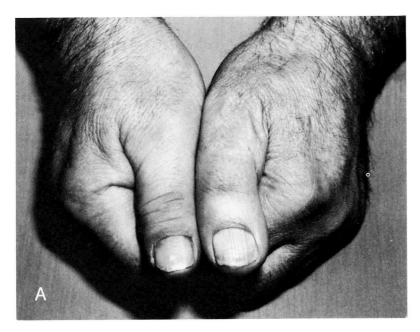

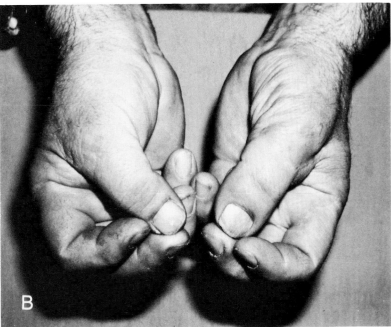

Fig. 31-10. (A,B) Aesthetic appearance of the left great-toe–to–thumb reconstruction five years postoperatively.

no problems and gait analysis on ambulation is unaffected (Fig. 31-12). The patient underwent a volar thumb pulp plasty reduction $3\frac{1}{2}$ years postoperatively to improve the aesthetic appearance of the reconstructed thumb.

Secondary Procedures

In most patients, the new thumb circumference atrophies 10 to 15 percent within the first 3 years. If the volar pulp remains too full, an ellipse of volar

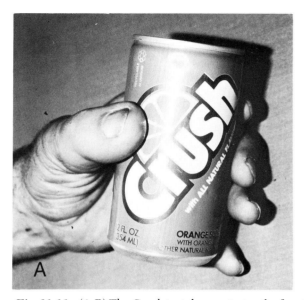
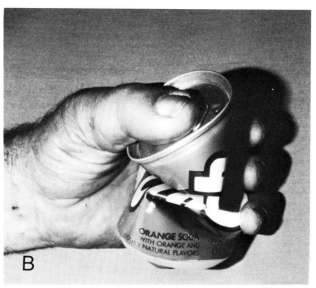

Fig. 31-11. (A,B) The Crush test demonstrates the functional capability of the great-toe–to–thumb reconstruction.

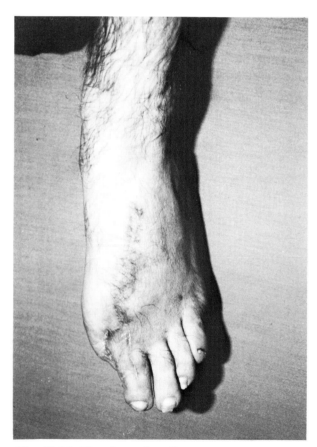

Fig. 31-12. The donor foot five years postoperatively poses no functional gait problems.

skin and fat can be removed from the pulp in a brief outpatient procedure under local anesthesia.

Secondary tendon transfers can be performed 6 months postoperatively after maximizing the hand rehabilitation program and delineating any residual functional deficits the patient may have prior to returning to work. Dependent upon the individual patient needs and functional result the following procedures can be performed:

1. Opponensplasty (FDS or EIP to FHB);
2. Adductorplasty (ECRB or BR plus tendon graft to proximal phalanx);
3. Tenolysis (extensor or flexor);
4. Tendon adjustment (extensor or flexor).

A web space and/or adductor contracture can be released with a thick split-thickness skin graft or local flap 6 months postoperatively if the contracture interferes with thumb function.[1,33]

An MP rotational wedge osteotomy or arthrodesis may be considered to maximize thumb positioning after tendon transfer and the hand rehabilitation program is completed.

One year following great-toe–to–thumb transfer, exploration of digital and superficial radial nerves can be considered with neurolysis and/or nerve grafting if sensory return has not allowed restoration of protective sensation.[24]

RE-EMPHASIS OF IMPORTANT POINTS

Great-toe–to–thumb transfers can provide a mobile and sensate thumb that greatly improves hand function as well as aesthetic appearance. This method of thumb reconstruction maximizes the free tissue transfer concept by providing multiple component tissues in a single reconstructive procedure and avoids local tissue sacrifice from an already injured extremity.

A good understanding of the normal anatomy of the thumb and great toe is essential so that modifications of the anatomy can be made when constructing a functional aesthetic thumb from the toe. This is a technically demanding procedure for even the most experienced surgeon. Therefore, careful preoperative assessment and angiography are important. Several points must be considered to optimize both the aesthetic and functional results.

1. A team approach is preferable, with one team removing the toe and the other preparing the recipient site. Both teams must have experience in complex hand reconstruction and microsurgery, and the two teams must communicate with each other.
2. The normal toe is aproximately 5 mm longer than the normal thumb in the adult; therefore, this length discrepancy plus the location of the growth epiphyses in a child must be considered if ultimate length is to be optimal.[22]
3. The normal great toe deviates laterally at the interphalangeal and metatarsophalangeal joints. This deviation will be optimal if the ipsilateral great toe is used in reconstruction, as ultimately the pulp will be more easily opposable and in contact with the remaining digits of the hand.
4. Skin incisions in the hand should be planned to allow volar and radial coverage over the flexor hallucis longus tendon and digital nerve repairs. If a cuff of soft tissue is taken with the extensor tendons and neurovascular structure of the toe, these tissues will support a thick skin graft in the hand when dorsal flap tissues are insufficient. Thick skin grafts are better tolerated in the hand than on the foot, and they frequently look better in the hand than bulky flap tissue. This method avoids depriving the foot donor site of specialized innervated thick plantar and dorsal skin.
5. Joint imbalance after toe transfer is avoided by reconstructing the metacarpophalangeal joint to avoid hyperextension and secondary interphalangeal joint flexion deformity.
6. Tendon imbalance and adhesion should be avoided. If the intrinsic muscles of the thumb are intact, the tendon of the abductor pollicis brevis and the adductor should be repaired to the extensor hallucis longus (EHL) to assist in interphalangeal joint extension. To complete the balance, the extensor pollicis longus (EPL) tendon should be repaired to the extensor hallucis longus (EHL). The extensor hallucis brevis (EHB) should be repaired to the extensor pollicis brevis (EPB) to help in metacarpophalangeal joint extension.
7. If adequate motors are lacking to assist the reconstructed thumb, one may include a primary adductor or abductor or opponens transfer at the time of the toe-to-thumb transfer. It is better to do only one tendon transfer at the initial procedure, as the splinting position may obviate an optimal result if more than one transfer is performed.
8. The sesamoids of the great toe are left in the foot to help postoperative initiation of push-off in normal gait. In a long-term follow-up of pre- and postoperative gait analysis of patients undergoing great-toe–to–thumb transfer we have found no major objective disturbance of foot function and gait following a great toe transfer.[16]
9. The institution of a specific, regimented hand rehabilitation program is critical in maximizing joint motion and tendon gliding, as well as in decreasing hand edema and enhancing thumb sensory re-education.
10. Secondary thumb soft-tissue tailoring can be done after the initial successful toe transfer. This approach is safer than complex tailoring at the time of initial toe transfer.

CONCLUSION

Great-toe–to–hand transfer for thumb reconstruction in selected cases may offer the patient an optimal aesthetic and functional reconstructive result. The elective amputation of the great toe provides no major objective disturbance in foot function and gait and therefore should not discourage this method of thumb reconstruction.[16] A thumb reconstruction that is aesthetically pleasing to the patient will encourage the patient to use the thumb more normally and effectively. Based upon these two major reconstructive goals (function and aesthetic appearance), the great-toe–to–thumb transfer has been found to be an ideal method of thumb reconstruction in carefully selected patients.

ACKNOWLEDGMENTS

The authors would like to thank the residents and fellows on the Plastic and Hand Surgical Service at the Massachusetts General Hospital who have made this successful series of thumb reconstructions possible. We are also indebted to Ms. Jeanne Spindler for her skills in manuscript preparation.

REFERENCES

1. Brown PW: Adduction-flexion contracture of the thumb. Correction with dorsal rotation flap and release of contracture. Clin Orthop 88:161–168, 1972
2. Buck-Gramcko D: Pollicization of the index finger; method and results in aplasia and hypoplasia of the thumb. J Bone Joint Surg 53A:1605–1617, 1971
3. Buncke HJ, Buncke CM, Schulz WP: Immediate Nicoladoni procedure in the Rhesus monkey, or hallux-to-hand transplantation, utilising microminature vascular anastomoses. Br J Plast Surg 19:332, 1966
4. Buncke HJ, McLean DH, George PT, Creech BJ, Chater NL, Commons GW: Thumb replacement: Great toe transplantation by microvascular anastomosis. Br J Plast Surg 26:194, 1973
5. Bunnell S: Physiological reconstruction of a thumb after total loss. Surg Gynecol Obstet 52:245, 1931
6. Campbell-Reid DA: Reconstruction of the thumb. J Bone Joint Surg 42B:444–465, 1960
7. Chase RA: An alternate to pollicization in subtotal thumb reconstruction. Plast Reconstr Surg 44:421, 1969
8. Cobett JR: Free digital transfer: Report of a case of transfer of a great toe to replace an amputated thumb. J Bone Joint Surg 51B:677–679, 1969
9. Flynn JE, Burden CN: Reconstruction of the thumb. Arch Surg 85:56, 1962
10. Gillies H, Reid DAC: Autograft of the amputated digit. Br J Plast Surg 7:338, 1955
11. Gosset J: La pollicisation de l'index. J Chir (Paris) 65:403, 1949
12. Gueullette R: Étude critique des procedes de restauration du ponce. J Chir (Paris), 36:1, 1930
13. Guermonprez F: Notes sur Quelques Resections et Restaurations du Ponce. P Asselin, Paris, 1887
14. Huguier PC: Remplacement du pouce par son metacarpien, par l'agrandissement du premier espace interosseux. Arch Gen Med (Paris) 1:78, 1874
15. Lister GD, Kalisman M, Tsai T: Reconstruction of the hand with free microneurovascular toe-to-hand transfer: Experience with 54 toe transfers. Plast Reconstr Surg 71:372, 1983
16. Lipton HA, May JW Jr, Simon R: Preoperative and postoperative gait analyses of patients undergoing great toe-to-hand transfer. J Hand Surg, 12A:66–69, 1987
17. Littler JW: The neurovascular pedicle method of digital transposition for reconstruction of the thumb. Plast Reconstr Surg 12:303, 1953
18. Matev IB: Gradual elongation of the first metacarpal as a method of thumb reconstruction. Communication at the Anglo-Scandinavian Meeting of Hand Surgery, Lausanne. In Stoeh HG, Bolton H (eds): The Second Hand Club. The British Society for Surgery of the Hand, London, 1975
19. May JW Jr: Aesthetic and functional thumb reconstruction: Great toe to hand transfer. Clinics Plast Surg 8:357, 1981
20. May JW Jr, Bartlett SP: Great toe to hand free tissue transfer for thumb reconstruction. Hand Clinics 1:271, 1985
21. May JW Jr, Chait LA, Cohen BE, Bernand McC, O'Brien MS: Free neurovascular flap from the first web of the foot in hand reconstruction. J Hand Surg 2:387–393, 1977

22. May JW Jr, Daniel RK: Great toe to hand free tissue transfer. Clin Orthop 133:140–153, 1978

23. May JW Jr, Lukash FN, Gallico GG III, Stirrat CR: Removable thermocouple probe microvascular patency monitor: An experimental and clinical study. Plast Reconstr Surg 72:366, 1983

24. Moberg E: Aspects of sensation in reconstructive surgery of the upper extremity. J Bone Joint Surg 46A:817–825, 1964

25. Michon J, Merle M, Bouchor Y, Foucher G: Functional comparison between pollicization and toe-to-hand transfer for thumb reconstruction. J Reconstr Microsurg 1:103, 1984

26. Nicoladoni C: Daumenplastic und organischer ersatz der fingerspitze (anticheiroplastic und daktyloplastik). Arch Clin Chri 61:606, 1900

27. Nicoladoni C: Daumenplastik. Wein Klin Wocehnschr 10:663, 1897

28. Noesske K: Uber den plastischen ersatz von ganz oder teilweise verlorene fingern, isbesondere des daumens, und uber hand teller plastik. Munch Med Worchenschr 56:1403, 1909

29. O'Brien B, McC, MacLeod AM, Sykes PJ, Donahoe S: Hallux-to-hand transfer. Hand 7:2, 128–133, 1975

30. Peacock EE Jr: Reconstruction of the thumb. In Flynn, JE (ed): Hand Surgery. Williams & Wilkins, Baltimore, 1966

31. Robbins F, Reece T: Hand rehabilitation after great toe transfer for thumb reconstruction. Arch Phys Med Rehabil 66:109, 1985

32. Tanzer RC, Littler JW: Reconstruction of the thumb by transposition of adjacent digit. Plast Reconstr Surg 3:533, 1948

33. Woolf RM, Broadbent TR: The four-flap Z-plasty. Plast Reconstr Surg 49:48, 1972

Other Microvascular Reconstruction of the Thumb

32

James R. Urbaniak

Microsurgical procedures for restoring thumb function are becoming increasingly more common, and in some institutions they have become more conventional than the standard staged procedures. The best method, when possible, of replacing an amputated thumb is replantation of the severed digit. In many microsurgical centers toe-to-hand free tissue transfers for thumb reconstruction are being performed on a routine basis. These procedures best duplicate the function and appearance of the absent thumb.

The advantages of transferring a toe or partial toe to the hand by microvascular techniques include the following: (1) usually a one stage procedure; (2) cosmetically and functionally duplicates the thumb; (3) hospitalization is usually short; and (4) sensory function is generally good. The disadvantages of these free transfers are: (1) sacrifice of a toe or part of a toe; (2) the procedure may fail (with loss of toe as well as thumb); (3) a preoperative arteriogram is recommended; and (4) the operation is lengthy and requires microvascular expertise.

Because of the relative reliability and excellent functional and cosmetic results that can be achieved by using a vascularized toe or partial toe, I prefer these methods over the established methods of restoring the amputated thumb. Certainly many of the favored conventional methods described in Chapters 56 and 57 continue to be useful and valuable in specific patients on whom microvascular procedures are ill advised.

May and Rohrich describe in detail in Chapter 31 the method of transferring the great toe (hallux) to the hand for thumb reconstruction. In this chapter, alternative methods to restore thumb function using vascularized tissue transfers from the foot will be presented. Comparisons of and specific indications for the different types of toe-to-hand transfers will be discussed.

VASCULAR ANATOMY

An accurate knowledge of the vascular anatomy of the donor foot and recipient hand is essential prior to these elective procedures. Palpation of the pedal pulses and Doppler evaluation are helpful, but preoperative biplane arteriography is strongly recommended prior to the toe-to-hand tissue transfers.[5,21] Preoperative detection of alterations in the vascular tree secondary to atypical anatomic variations or trauma is vital to determine the feasibility of selecting the appropriate tissue transfer, to choose the optimal surgical approach, and to avoid or diminish surgical difficulties. Since these procedures are technically demanding, the prudent surgeon will be prepared with this anatomic information.

The foot, similar to the hand, has two connected arterial arches: the dorsal arch arises from the dorsalis pedis artery and the plantar arch from the medial and lateral branches of the posterior tibial artery (Fig. 32-1). The dorsal arch is usually less dominant but is easier to dissect. The main arterial supply of the great and second toes is by the *first metatarsal artery*, which is an extension of the dor-

salis pedis artery. Because of the relatively large caliber of the dorsalis pedis artery, most tissue transfers using donor tissue from the great or second toe are usually successful; additionally, the dissection is relatively easy because of its superficial position.

The first metatarsal artery has been described as being dorsal to the metatarsal in 80 percent of dissected feet by May[13] and Gilbert.[4] If this pattern is present, the donor tissue dissection is usually rapid and simple. However, I have found that in about 50 percent of our own surgical dissections in this area, the first metatarsal artery is plantar to the first me-

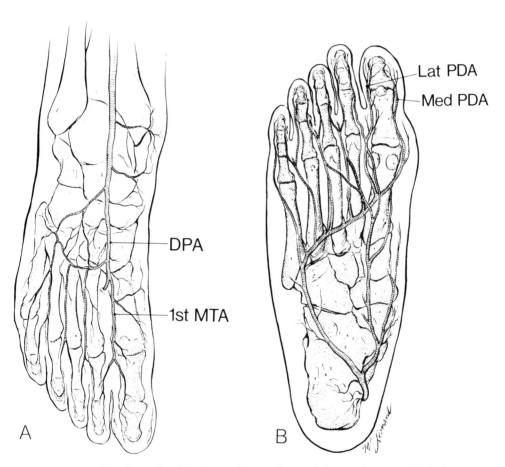

Fig. 32-1. Major blood supply of the first and second toes. **(A)** Dorsal view and **(B)** plantar view. The dorsalis pedis artery *(DPA)* or its extension, the first metatarsal artery *(1st MTA)*, is the primary artery in first or second toe transfers. The plantar digital artery *(PDA)* may be used if the first metatarsal artery is deficient. (Reproduced with permission from Urbaniak JR: Elective microsurgery for orthopaedic reconstruction. Part II. Thumb reconstruction by microsurgery. In AAOS Instructional Course Lectures. Vol. 33. CV Mosby, St Louis, 1984.)

tatarsal[10,21] (Buncke HJ: Personal communication, 1983). Accurate preoperative awareness of the vascular anatomy of the first metatarsal artery or blood supply to the first and second toes simplifies the dissection of the donor tissue. Actually, I believe that it is no more difficult to approach the *common plantar digital artery* of the first web space through a longitudinal plantar incision than it is to dissect the dorsalis pedis artery dorsally. If the preoperative study of the vascular anatomy is thorough and clearly understood, basing the donor tissue on the plantar vessel is often easier and quicker. The disadvantage is that the plantar vessel is usually smaller in diameter and shorter in length.

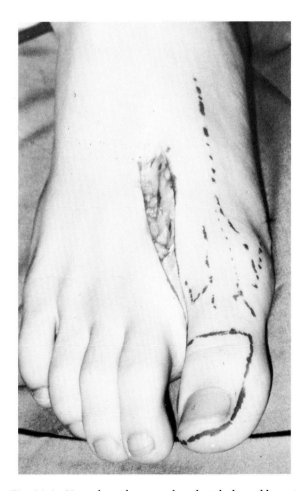

Fig. 32-2. Veins have been outlined with dotted lines in preparation for a wraparound graft. Prior to tourniquet elevation and skin incision, the foot was depressed to demonstrate the superficial veins.

Therefore, a supplemental vein graft for additional length may theoretically be required, although I cannot recall a case in which this was necessary.

There is no difficulty in locating two or three large dorsal veins draining the great and second toes. These veins are best identified preoperatively by depressing the foot, warming the forefoot with a moist cloth, or using a venous tourniquet. Since the more medial veins are the largest, I recommend selecting them. It is useful to trace selected veins with a marking pencil (Fig. 32-2).

The deep peroneal nerve accompanies the first metatarsal artery and supplies the skin of the first web space. This nerve is dissected as an important structure of the donor tissue. Additional nerves and other significant anatomy will be described in the specific surgical techniques.

SELECTION OF PROCEDURE

The surgeon who elects to reconstruct a thumb by a vascularized toe transfer must be knowledgeable about the standard alternative methods of thumb restoration[18,19] and must deem the free tissue transfer to be the most reasonable method of management. Several different microvascular reconstructive procedures for vascularized toe transfers are available.[1,20] The goals of the patient must be considered when deciding the type of technique to be used. In general, the aim in thumb reconstruction is to duplicate the structure and function of the absent thumb. Motion and stability are necessary for a strong pinch and grip. Sensitive pulp tissue and good skin texture are essential for prehension and fine manipulation. The single-staged free toe transfers may fulfill all of these goals.

The surgeon and patient must initially determine if thumb reconstruction is necessary. In most individuals, if 1 or 2 cm of proximal phalanx with good glabrous skin is present, adequate function exits. This type of thumb can be cosmetically improved by the wraparound procedure, but only minimal functional gain is likely to be obtained. The length of available thumb remaining, the patient's occupation, expected thumb performance and appearance, and the patient's choice of donor tissue to be sacrificed all must be considered when selecting the method.

I have found it useful to present the options to patients by showing them clinical photographs or drawings of the various methods in order for them to appreciate the amount of toe to be lost and the anticipated final appearance of the thumb.

In most patients with congenital deficiency or absence of the thumb, I favor index pollicization for thumb reconstruction. In the hand with a congenitally absent thumb and only three fingers, pollicization is usually not indicated, and some type of toe transfer may be reasonable. In most instances of traumatic amputation near the MP joint, I prefer a toe transfer over pollicization. These techniques avoid the additional loss of digits from an already insufficient hand. The major disadvantage of toe transfer is that if the procedure fails, the patient with the absent thumb also loses part or all of a toe. I advise the patient and family that there is a 10 percent possibility that the procedure may fail.

Essentially four methods of free tissue transfers are available for thumb reconstruction: (1) great toe transfer, (2) wraparound procedure, (3) second toe transfer, and (4) intercalary augmentation. The first method is described in Chapter 31 and the latter three methods will be described in this chapter.

The major *contraindications* against toe-to-hand free tissue transfers are patients with (1) diabetes mellitus; (2) peripheral vascular disease; (3) previous damage to the donor toe (although the contralateral toe may be used); and (4) an inadequate vascular tree of the donor or recipient sites as determined by arteriography.

PREOPERATIVE MANAGEMENT

After the decision to perform a vascularized toe-to-hand transfer for thumb reconstruction has been made, the patient preparation is similar for all of the procedures. A model or mold of the thumb size and shape is fashioned from a rubber glove. This pattern aids in designing the skin incision and de-termining the amount of tissue that will be transferred.

A preoperative arteriogram of the donor and recipient sites should always be obtained[5] to assist in determining whether or not a vascularized tissue transfer is even advisable. This study also influences the choice of incisions, planning for vein grafts, and choosing arteries to be dissected. Since most of these procedures will require a minimum of 5 hours of surgery, adequate operating time and assistance (two teams) must be scheduled.

A gram of cephalosporin antibiotic is administered to the patient on call to the operating room. A Foley catheter is inserted to monitor the urinary output, which should approximate 100 ml an hour to ensure adequate patient hydration. The operating room temperature must be warm, and the patient kept well hydrated to diminish peripheral vasospasm.

The operating table is well padded and the patient's hand and foot are properly positioned to permit two teams to operate simultaneously and comfortably. Tourniquets are used on the arm and the thigh, but an Esmarch wrap is not applied, to permit better identification of the vessels.

WRAPAROUND PROCEDURE

Foot Dissection

This procedure was introduced by Morrison in 1980.[15] Basically, the great toe flap is patterned to deglove the toe, except for a peninsular portion of skin with its neurovascular pedicle on the medial border and tip of the great toe, which is retained on the toe. The dimensions of the skin flap are determined by measuring the circumference of the normal opposite thumb (or one of a similar-sized individual). The retained medial skin flap on the toe should be at least 10 mm in width (Fig. 32-3). The tip of the retained medial skin peninsula is tapered and extends to the lateral edge of the toenail plate. It is important to retain as much skin as possible on the toe for protection and appearance. The length

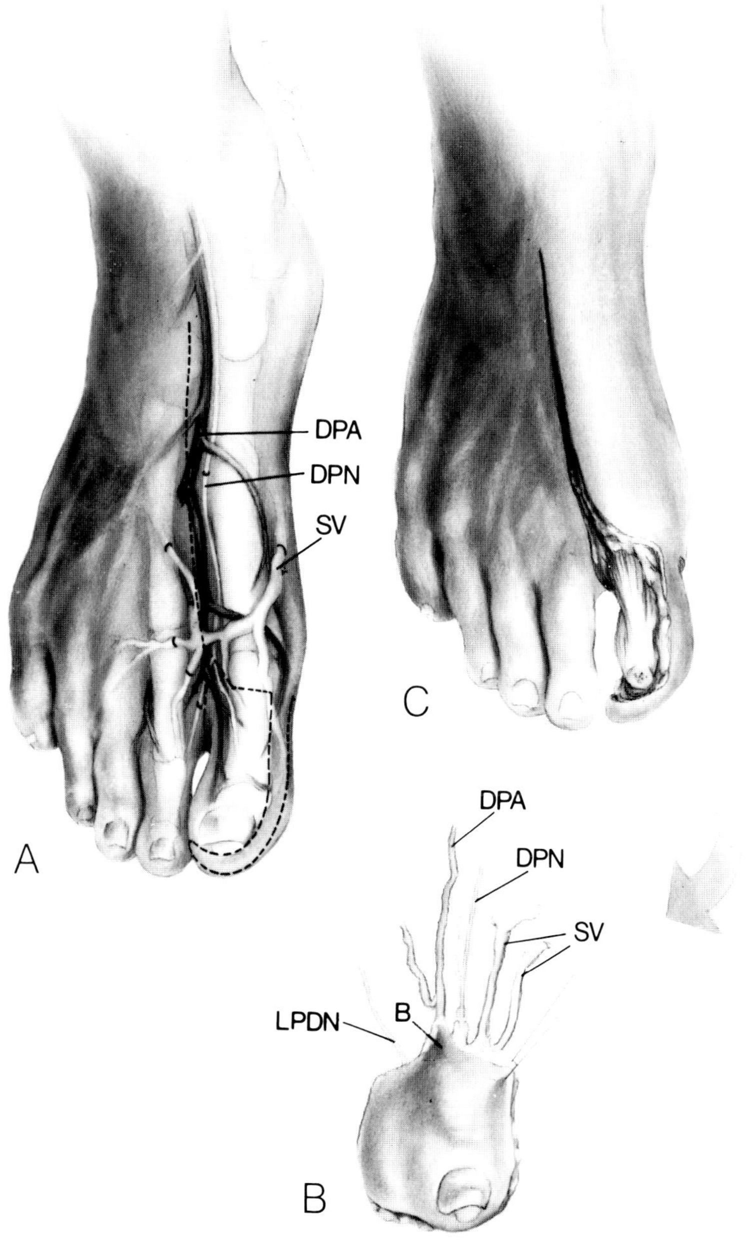

Fig. 32-3. Wraparound procedure. **(A)** The medial aspect of the great toe with its neurovascular bundle remains on the foot, as indicated in the dashed lines for skin incisions. The dorsalis pedis artery *(DPA)*, deep peroneal nerve *(DPN)*, and major branches of the saphenous veins *(SV)* are transected proximally. **(B)** The flap with long neurovascular pedicles is freed from the toe *(LPDN,* lateral plantar digital nerve). The triangular projection of skin is from the first web space. **(C)** The distal 7–10 mm of the distal phalanx are removed to allow the medial skin flap to be advanced for closure. *(Figure continues.)*

of the donor flap is determined by the length of the reconstructed thumb (or coverage of the bone graft). In normal hands, the end of the thumb usually falls approximately 5 mm short of reaching the PIP joint of the index finger. A shorter thumb is more desirable than one that is longer than normal. It is preferable to preserve the first web space skin

on the foot if possible to allow better healing of the foot.

Using loupe magnification, the foot dissection begins with a longitudinal incision between the first and second metatarsals to locate the dorsalis pedis artery (Fig. 32-3). The artery is carefully dissected distally to locate the first dorsal metatarsal

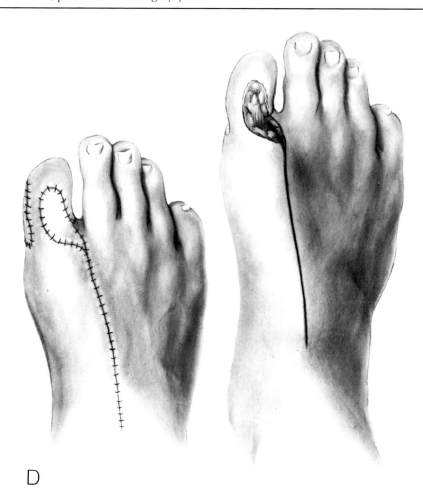

D

Fig. 32-3 *(Continued).* **(D)** A split-thickness graft covers the retained fatty tissue and paratenon of the flexor and extensor tendons.

artery. The application of papavarine (1:20) and minimal trauma to the vessel will diminish unwanted vasospasm. If the preoperative arteriogram shows the first metatarsal artery to be plantar or that the dominant vessel to the great toe is the plantar digital vessel, then the lateral plantar digital vessel is located in the first web space (similar to the approach for a Morton's neuroma) and dissected proximally through a longitudinal plantar incision. All arterial feeders to the donor flap are carefully preserved and the branches to the second toe are severed. The small branches of the arteries and veins may be occluded with mini silver hemoclips or bipolar cautery.

The deep peroneal nerve is located adjacent to the dorsalis pedis artery and included with the toe flap. It is transected proximally at the determined length. The previously outlined dorsal veins are dissected with the donor skin flap. An effort is made to harvest a vascular pedicle with as much length as possible. A vein graft may be used if the plantar artery serves as the main feeder to the flap, but this is seldom if ever necessary.

The elevation of the toe flap is begun after the artery, veins, and nerves are isolated. The skin is opened on the outline of the toe flap. A triangular projection of skin on the proximal lateral border (first web space) of the flap is designed to allow closure of the hand incisions without constriction over the vascular pedicle (Fig. 32-3). When making the transverse incision, the surgeon must *avoid transecting the subcutaneous veins* that drain the toe flap. The medial neurovascular bundle is located, so it can be retained with the medial flap on the toe. The lateral plantar neurovascular bundle is located in order to retain it with the medial flap on the toe.

The lateral plantar neurovascular bundle is dissected and tagged if it was not previously isolated.

The dorsal toe flap is separated from the bone by subperiosteal peeling of the nail plate to avoid damage to the germinal matrix of the nail (Fig. 32-3). I suggest including the distal 7 to 10 mm of the distal phalanx with the flap to optimize toe closure and minimize bone resorption and shrinkage in the thumb. The paratenon on the extensor hallucis longus is preserved to permit the coverage by a split-thickness graft.

The plantar portion of the flap is elevated, with an effort made to retain some subcutaneous fat on the toe. This dissection is meticulous since the vascular supply to the skin flap must not be damaged. The dissection begins distally and proceeds to the medial neurovascular bundle and the first metatarsal artery. The lateral digital artery is severed unless it has been selected as the donor artery. If so, it is isolated and transected more proximally through a longitudinal plantar incision. The lateral digital nerve is divided from the common digital nerve in the first web space. The entire toe flap is now free except for the dorsal vascular pedicle (Fig. 32-3). The tourniquet is released to observe the flap for distal perfusion, which may require longer than 20 minutes because of vasospasm. The early application of local papaverine solution (i.e., prior to the pedicle dissection) plus warming the foot has diminished the local vasospasm in our experience.

Hand Dissection

As the foot is dissected, a second team is operating on the hand that is to receive the donor tissue. A radial triangular flap is designed in the skin incision on the thumb stump (Fig. 32-4A). This flap is interposed between the proximal edges of the donor skin flap to permit a loose closure. A zigzag skin incision extends to the anatomic snuffbox to dissect the following: (1) dorsal radial artery and first metacarpal artery (princeps pollicis); (2) one or two dorsal veins (usually the cephalic vein); and (3) a terminal branch of the superficial radial nerve (Fig. 32-4). A palmar incision parallel to the thenar crease is necessary to isolate the ulnar and radial digital nerves in the thumb stump.

Accurate measurements to determine the length of the vessels and nerves needed in the transfer are important. These determinations will usually obviate the need for vascular or nerve grafts, which are seldom necessary in this procedure. However, if there is any problem with tension, then grafts must be harvested. The vein grafts should be obtained from the volar forearm before the vascular pedicle of the toe is severed. The vein grafts are stored in Ringer's lactate solution containing papaverine.[2]

The remnant of the proximal phalanx is exposed by subperiosteal dissection. The end is squared with a power saw in such a way that as much length as possible is preserved. A full-thickness (tri-cortical) bone graft is obtained from the iliac crest. The size is determined by measurement of the normal or opposite thumb. The size of the bone will usually have to be fashioned to a smaller size than estimated in order to receive the toe flap. It is not necessary to fashion the bone to simulate the thumb phalanx, as some resorption and remodeling will occur. Slight flexion can be achieved by directing the cephalic cortical surface of the graft dorsalward (Fig. 32-4). Stabilization of the bone graft to the proximal phalangeal skeletal surface is achieved by two intramedullary or crossed K-wires. Preparation of the hand usually requires less time than dissection of the toe flap.

Transfer of the Toe Flap to the Hand

After the bone peg is properly secured and its appropriate length rechecked, the toe flap is ready to be detached from the foot if perfusion is evident. The donor veins and artery are severed at the appropriate lengths (Fig. 32-5C). The toe flap is wrapped around the bone graft and the distal and radial skin edges are sutured with 4–0 nylon.

The bone fragment harvested with the toe flap must be fixed to the major bone peg. This may be achieved by one of two methods: (1) the proximal end of the bone fragment is pre-drilled to correspond with the two protruding K-wires from the fixed bone on the proximal phalanx, and the fragment is then positioned with the flap onto the K-wires; or (2) two K-wires are first inserted longitudinally through the major bone graft. The bone graft is then connected to the fragment of bone

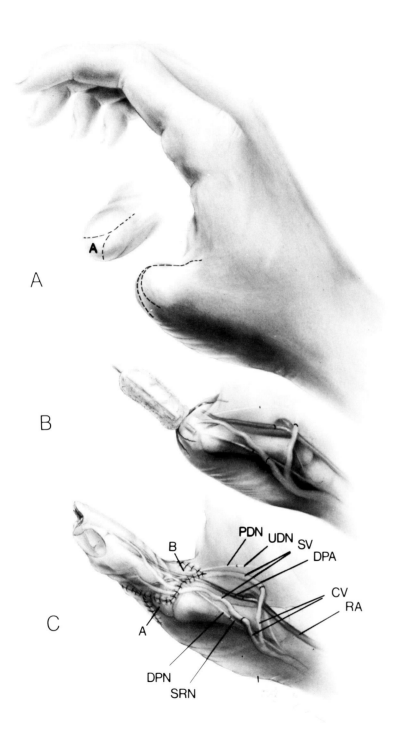

Fig. 32-4. Wraparound procedure—Hand preparation and toe transfer. (A) The radial triangular flap incision on the thumb stump is designed to prevent constriction at the juncture site of the skin closure. (B) An iliac crest bone graft (cortical side is dorsal) is fixed to the remaining proximal phalanx with one or two intramedullary K-wires. (C) The flap is wrapped around the bone graft. The following structures are connected: dorsalis pedis artery *(DPA)* to first metacarpal artery (branch of radial artery) *(RA)*; saphenous vein *(SV)* to cephalic vein *(CV)*; plantar digital nerve *(PDN)* to ulnar digital nerve *(UDN)*; deep peroneal nerve to superficial radial nerve *(SRN)*.

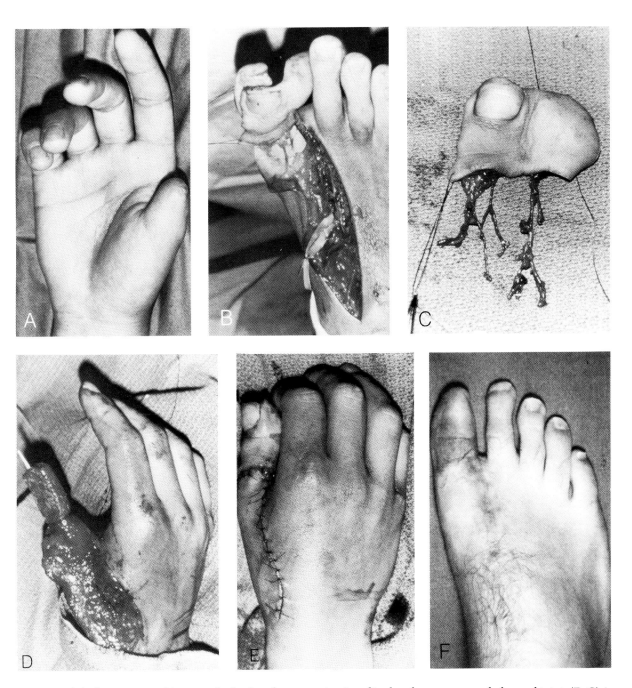

Fig. 32-5. (A) This 22-year-old patient had a thumb amputation just distal to the metacarpophalangeal joint. (**B, C**) A skin flap has been dissected with a neurovascular pedicle. (**D**) An iliac crest bone graft is pinned to the proximal phalanx. (**E**) The completed transfer is shown. (**F**) The appearance of the toe of the donor foot. (Reproduced with permission from Urbaniak JR: Elective microsurgery for orthopaedic reconstruction. Part II. Thumb reconstruction by microsurgery. In AAOS Instructional Course Lectures. Vol. 33. CV Mosby, St Louis, 1984.)

attached to the toe flap by retrograde drilling of the wires through the proximal end of the fragment. The joined toe flap with the distal fragment and bone peg is attached to the proximal phalanx with advancement of the K-wires. I prefer the second method, since this permits distal extraction of the longitudinal pins when bony union occurs (usually at 2 or 3 months). However, this method requires more caution to protect the neurovascular structures of the toe flap from being injured by the advancing K-wires.

The operating microscope is positioned for repair of the neurovascular structures. I have found it easier to repair the nerves first because the exposure is better prior to the vascular connections. The ulnar digital nerve of the thumb is connected to the lateral plantar digital nerve and the radial digital nerve to the donor deep peroneal nerve with 9-0 nylon. An alternative method is to suture the superficial radial nerve to the deep peroneal nerve or the dorsal medial nerve of the flap.

The dorsalis pedis artery (or lateral plantar digi-

tal artery) is anastomosed to the first metacarpal artery or to the radial artery in the dorsal wrist area. The choice of a more distal end-to-end anastomosis or more proximal end-to-side anastomosis depends on which one is easier with regard to vessel size orientation and facilitation of vessel positioning. The largest vein of the toe flap is usually connected to the cephalic vein at the dorsal wrist level. A second vein anastomosis is recommended if an additional vein is present in the transfer, and it usually is. Again, the anastomosis may be end-to-end or end-to-side depending on the vessel size discrepancy and ease of the connection. The vascular anastomoses are performed usually with 9-0 nylon. After the microclips are removed from the anastomosis site, good distal perfusion should occur within a few minutes. After continuous perfusion is assured, meticulous hemostasis is obtained and the skin edges are closed without tension (Fig. 32-6). Skin grafts are used if direct skin closure would cause even the slightest tension.

There are at least three sources of error that can

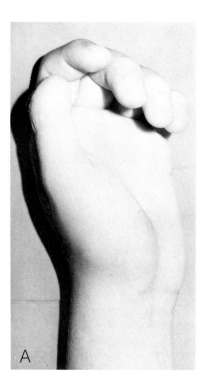
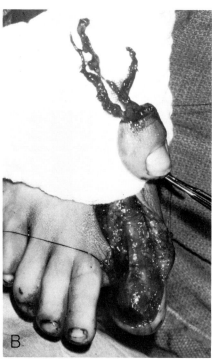
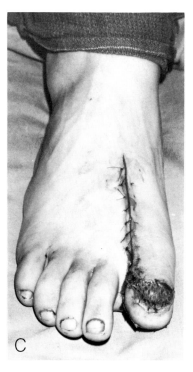

Fig. 32-6. **(A)** A 13-year-old patient with loss of the thumb through the distal portion of the proximal phalanx. **(B)** The harvested toe flap with its neurovascular pedicles of appropriate length. **(C)** Closure of the foot with a split-thickness graft over the fatty tissue and paratenon of the flexor and extensor tendons. *(Figure continues.)*

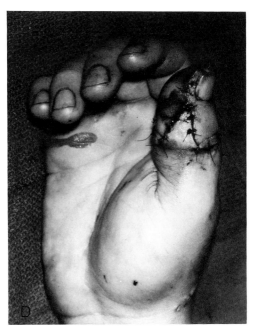 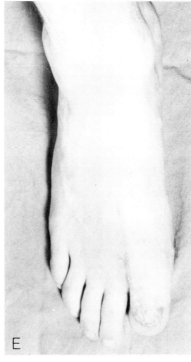 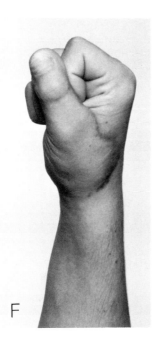

Fig. 32-6 *(Continued).* **(D)** Immediate postoperative appearance of the wraparound procedure. Note the triangular flap on the thumb stump illustrated in Figure 32-4A. **(E)** Appearance of the foot 2 months after surgery. **(F)** The hand 3 months after surgery.

result in vascular obstruction and failure: (1) twisting of the vascular pedicle when passing it beneath a skin bridge; (2) constriction of the pedicle by tight skin closure; and (3) kinking of the pedicle because of excessive length, since a long pedicle is harvested with this method. With proper execution, all of these errors can be avoided. I no longer pass the vascular pedicle beneath a skin bridge but choose to open the skin. The designed triangular projection of skin on the donor flap, the planned incision on the stump, and/or the use of split-thickness or full-thickness skin grafts for closure eliminate constriction.

A bulky dressing with a volar-radial splint incorporating the elbow is applied. The pulp of the thumb is exposed for monitoring of the circulation.

Closure of the Foot

If the surgeon has preserved paratenon over the extensor hallucis longus and flexor hallucis longus tendons and some pulp fat has been retained on the plantar toe skeleton, a cosmetic closure is possible with a split-thickness graft (Fig. 32-6C and E). Since the distal phalanx of the great toe has been shortened, the retained medial skin may be advanced around the tip of the bone to cover all or most of the lateral border of the great toe. The remaining fatty tissue on the plantar and dorsal surfaces is spread to cover the exposed bone and tendons. A small split-thickness graft completes the closure.

SECOND TOE TRANSFER FOR THUMB RECONSTRUCTION

The second toe may be selected for reconstruction of a missing thumb.[6-8,11,14,16,22-24] Personally I do not use the second toe for thumb reconstruction, because I consider the esthetic results to be considerably inferior to the great toe transfer or the wraparound method. As a result, the clinical application of the second toe as a transfer is seldom recommended for thumb reconstruction; however, it is occasionally used to restore length or restore the pulp and/or nail bed and plate of other digits.[3,20] (See Chapter 27 for a more detailed discussion of the use of the second toe as a free flap.)

The second toe transfer is favored by some reconstructive microsurgeons, especially in Oriental societies where the inhabitants are reluctant to sacrifice the great toe because of cultural beliefs and the necessity of the great toe for foot apparel (thongs). There is certainly less donor site morbidity from using the second toe instead of the hallux and therefore the second toe may be chosen as the donor if the patient has a strong aversion to losing the great toe or part of it.

Second Toe Dissection

The surgical technique for second toe transplantation is similar to the hallux transfer (see Chapter 31), except that the dissection remains medial to the first metatarsal artery, so that the dorsal digital artery to the great toe can be divided while vessels to the second toe are kept intact (Fig. 32-7). The skin incision is determined by the level of toe that is chosen for the transfer. If transfer is at the metatarsophalangeal joint or distal to it, no additional skin flap is needed. If the metatarsophalangeal joint is included in the transfer, extra skin must be obtained from the dorsum of the foot to cover the medial side of the metatarsophalangeal joint (Fig. 32-7D). The size of the skin flap on the foot should be restricted to the amount that allows primary closure of the donor site. Split-thickness skin is usually necessary to complete the coverage of the hand, especially for more proximal reconstructions.

In the process of making circumferential (transverse) incisions, care must be taken to avoid cutting the neurovascular structures to be transferred, especially the veins, which are vulnerable because of their superficial position. The sequence of harvesting the donor structure of the foot is as follows: veins (usually two), dorsalis pedis artery, branch of the deep peroneal nerve (optional), extensor tendon, osteotomy (second metatarsal or more dis-

tally), and first metatarsal artery. On the plantar surface both digital nerves are harvested prior to severing the flexor tendons. As in the wraparound procedure, the vascular dissection is influenced by the anatomic variations identified in study of the preoperative arteriogram.

The length of the tendons, nerves, and vessels must be measured before these structures are severed to ensure sufficient length for the connections at the recipient sites (usually wrist for vessels and tendons and thenar area for nerves). The level of bone transection is determined by the level of the thumb amputation. If the reconstruction will occur proximal to the MP joint, an oblique osteotomy of the metatarsal neck is performed at a 60-degree angle, with the dorsal cut proximal and the plantar cut distal. This oblique cut allows the new MP joint of the thumb to be prepositioned in hyperextension to prevent a recurvatum-type deformity that would result from the inherent hyperextension of the toe MTP joint[12] (see Fig. 31-2 on page 1298). After the structures have all been isolated, the vascular pedicle is left intact and the tourniquet is released. Perfusion of the donor tissue should occur within a few minutes. If not, the tissue should be covered with a warm, moist cloth, and papavarine (1:20) should be applied to the vascular pedicle.

Hand Dissection and Preparation

The preparation of the hand for receiving the second toe transfer is similar to that of the great toe transfer described in Chapter 31, and differs from that of the wraparound in only two steps: (1) no bone graft is necessary, and (2) the flexor pollicis longus and extensor pollicis longus tendons need to be located.

Once the structures are all isolated, the tourniquet is released to be certain that there is good flow through the donor artery and for obtaining hemostasis.

Toe-to-Hand Transfer

Bone fixation is obtained by crossed K-wires, which are cut adjacent to the bone to prevent teth-

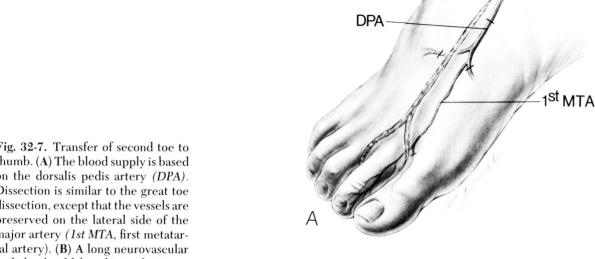

Fig. 32-7. Transfer of second toe to thumb. (A) The blood supply is based on the dorsalis pedis artery *(DPA)*. Dissection is similar to the great toe dissection, except that the vessels are preserved on the lateral side of the major artery *(1st MTA, first metatarsal artery)*. (B) A long neurovascular pedicle should be obtained. Direct closure of the foot incision is possible. The artery, vein, and digital nerves are isolated for transfer. *(Figure continues.)*

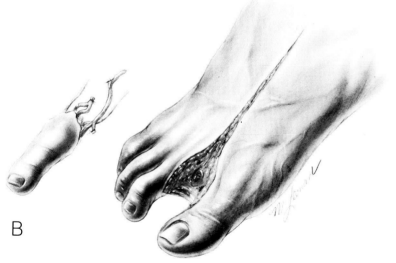

ering of the vessels. Leung prefers to use only an intramedullary bone peg for osteosynthesis.[8] The flexor pollicis longus is attached to the flexor digitorum longus at the wrist level if possible. The digital nerves are repaired next. The palmar wounds may then be closed.

The extensor pollicis longus is attached to the extensor digitorum longus, and the dorsal sensory nerves may be approximated if they have been harvested. The vascular anastomoses are performed in a fashion similar to the wraparound procedure.

The skin edges are loosely approximated and a split-thickness skin graft is frequently necessary for coverage. A commonly seen deformity of the sec-

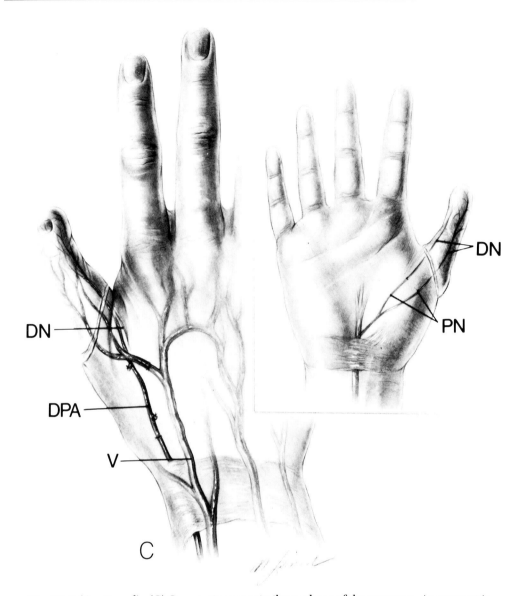

Fig. 32-7 *(Continued).* **(C)** Connections are similar to those of the great toe. An attempt is made to do the microvascular anastomoses at wrist level where vessel size is larger. Tendon connections are also at or proximal to the wrist to achieve maximal excursion. *(Figure continues.)*

ond toe transfer is a flexed position of the PIP joint and hyperextension at the metatarsophalangeal joint. Temporary insertion of a K-wire across the PIP joint for 6 weeks will obviate the flexion deformity. The oblique osteotomy of the metatarsal described in the dissection section eliminates the hyperextension deformity.

INTERCALARY AUGMENTATION

Vascularized composite tissue from the second toe for thumb reconstruction may include phalanges, epiphyseal plates, and joints to restore thumb length and provide growth or articular surfaces.

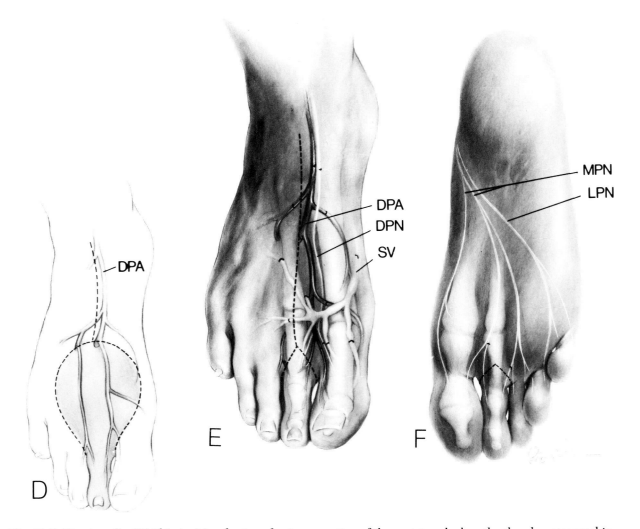

Fig. 32-7 *(Continued).* **(D)** Skin incision for transferring a portion of the metatarsal when the thumb metacarpal is absent. **(E, F)** Skin incisions for a transfer distal to the metatarsophalangeal joint. (A–C Reproduced with permission from Urbaniak JR: Elective microsurgery for orthopaedic reconstruction. Part II. Thumb reconstruction by microsurgery. In AAOS Instructional Course Lectures. Vol. 33. CV Mosby, St Louis, 1984.)

Intercalary augmentation of a hypoplastic thumb in a 4-year-old girl is presented as an example (Fig. 32-8). In this patient, the proximal phalanx with a medial skin island and neurovascular pedicle based on the dorsalis pedis artery was transferred to the thumb. The involved vessels at this age are approximately 1 to 1.5 mm in diameter and adequate for safe microvascular reconstruction.

The foot dissection for transfer of a composite tissue graft of the second toe is similar to that of the second toe transfer. The first metatarsal artery is dissected in a fashion that preserves the branches supplying the medial skin and proximal phalanx of the second toe. A sufficient skin island is harvested for skin coverage in the thumb-index web space and for monitoring the patency of the anastomoses. The digital nerve may be included in the tissue transfer if indicated. Growth of the transferred

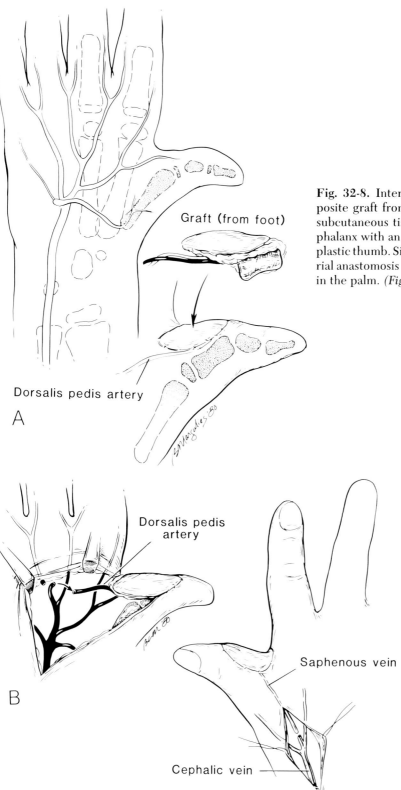

Graft (from foot)

Dorsalis pedis artery

A

Dorsalis pedis artery

Saphenous vein

Cephalic vein

B

Fig. 32-8. Intercalary augmentation. **(A,B)** A composite graft from the second toe, consisting of skin, subcutaneous tissue, vascular pedicle, and proximal phalanx with an epiphysis was transferred to a hypoplastic thumb. Since the radial artery was absent, arterial anastomosis was made to a common digital artery in the palm. *(Figure continues.)*

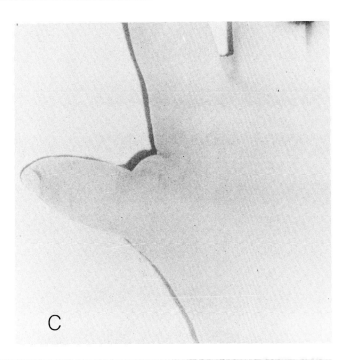

Fig. 32-8 *(Continued).* **(C)** Preoperative hypoplastic thumb in 2-year-old girl. **(D)** Outline of the skin incision for obtaining vascularized composite tissue, based on the dorsalis pedis artery. **(E)** The reconstructed thumb is longer, has an increased thumb-index web space, and a growing epiphysis. (Reproduced with permission from Urbaniak JR: Elective microsurgery for orthopaedic reconstruction. Part II. Thumb reconstruction by microsurgery. In AAOS Instructional Course Lectures. Vol. 33. CV Mosby, St Louis, 1984.)

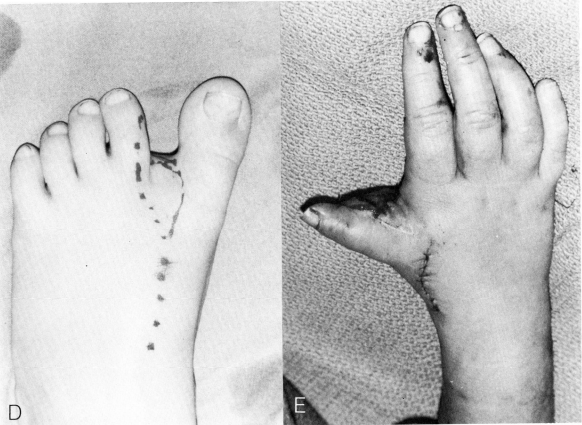

phalanx should continue because of the continued growth potential of the vascularized physis that is included in the transfer.

In a similar manner, the vascularized PIP joint of the second toe may be transferred to replace a damaged MP or interphalangeal joint of the thumb. Such a transfer is rarely indicated for thumb reconstruction, and seldom suggested for improving other digits[3] (see Chapter 30).

The toe defect can usually be directly closed without grafting. A small bone graft may be used to replace the donor proximal phalanx. Use of a K-wire from the tip of the toe into the metatarsal head for several weeks will diminish the toe deformity.

POSTOPERATIVE CARE

The postoperative care is similar for all toe or partial toe transfers to the hand. Small suction drainage tubes are used but care is taken not to place them near the anastomoses. A loose bulky dressing with volar splints that incorporate the elbow is applied. The splints are not placed on the dorsal surface of the hand, to allow close inspection of the major incisions if there is an early postoperative complication. A portion of the skin surface, usually the digital pulp, is left exposed for visible monitoring. The extremity is elevated to improve venous drainage.

As in replantation surgery, the most reliable method of monitoring is clinical observation of color, capillary refill, and pulp turgor. I generally rely on temperature monitoring in these types of transfers, since it is dependable, inexpensive, and uncomplicated.[17] The surface temperature should remain over 30°C.

The patient's room temperature is maintained at a constant warm level (74° to 76°F). No smoking is allowed, and the patient is kept well hydrated and normotensive.

Aspirin (300 mg/day), Persantine (50 mg twice a day), and Dextran 40 (500 cc/day) are administered for 7 days. Heparin is seldom used in elective microvascular surgery.

A smaller protective splint is applied 7 to 10 days postoperatively, and active protective motion is initiated at 3 weeks. Patients who have had the wraparound procedure require minimal hand therapy, as no additional joint motion is involved. In the other transfers flexor and extensor outriggers are used for rehabilitating the transferred digits. A normal gait pattern is to be expected after healing of the donor site of the foot.

FUNCTIONAL RESULTS AND COMPARISONS

Essentially all of the toe-to-hand transfers provide adequate sensibility (approximately 15 mm of two-point discrimination), pinch, length, and stability (see Table 32-1). Of course, the sensibility is not as good as with index pollicization, which should be normal.

Table 32-1. Comparison of Three Methods of Vascularized Toe Transfers for Thumb Reconstruction[a]

	Great Toe	Second Toe	Wraparound
Duplicates thumb			
Esthetically	++	+	+++
In size	++	0	+++
Preserves toe	0	0	++
Motion			
IP	+++	++	0
MP	++	++	0
Stability	+++	++	+++
Sensibility	+++	+++	+++
Pinch and grasp	+++	++	++
Reconstruct thumb on hand with 2 or more fingers absent	+++	++	0
Maintains bone stock	+++	+++	+
Donor vessel size			
Caliber	++	++	++
Length	+++	++	+++
Viability potential	+++	++	++
Ease of dissection	++	++	+
Growth potential	++	++	0

[a] Key: 0 = none; + = fair, ++ = good, +++ = excellent

A definite advantage of the wraparound procedure over the complete toe transfers is that it preserves the toe skeleton of the foot, thus providing a nearly normal appearing and functional foot (Figs. 32-5 and 32-6). Pinch and grip strength is strongest with the great toe transfer. Pinch strength of 30 to 50 percent of the normal side can be expected with the wraparound method.

A major disadvantage of the wraparound procedure is the loss of motion at the interphalangeal joint. If this procedure is used for reconstruction proximal to the MP joint, then loss of motion exists at both the MP and IP joints. This method should not be used in children under 10 or 11 years of age because of the failure of the bone to grow. Some surgeons have reported a problem of bone resorption with this technique.[9] This is an additional reason for transferring a small portion of the distal toe phalanx with the flap. Functional use of the thumb by the patient increases the stress concentration on the bone graft and minimizes the occurrence of resorption. Only two of our patients have experienced some resorption of the bone peg. The wraparound procedure is technically more difficult than a toe transfer and the chances of failure are greater. Three of our first eighteen wraparound transfers partially or totally necrosed; we have not experienced a failure with the hallux transfer.

REFERENCES

1. Buncke HJ, Buncke CB, Schultz WP: Immediate Nicoladoni procedure in the rhesus monkey or hallux-to-hand transplantation, utilizing microminiature vascular anastomoses. Br J Plast Surg 19:332–337, 1966

2. Catinella FP, Cunningham JN Jr, Baumann FG, et al: An ultrastructural comparison of endothelial preservatinn in vein grafts prepared by various techniques. J Clin Surg 6:393–402, 1982

3. Coleman DA, Urbaniak JR: Osteocutaneous flaps for thumb and digit reconstruction. Hand Clinics 1:717–728, Nov 1985

4. Gilbert A: Composite tissue transfers from the foot: Anatomic basis and surgical technique. pp. 230–242. In Danhiller AI, Strauch B (eds): Symposium on Microsurgery. CV Mosby, St Louis, 1976

5. Koman LA, Pospisil RF, Nunley JA, Urbaniak, JR: Value of contrast arteriography in composite tissue transfer. Clin Orthop 172:195–206, 1983

6. Leung PC: The "throbbing sign"—an indication of early venous congestion in replantation surgery. J Hand Surg 4:409–411, 1979

7. Leung PC: Thumb reconstruction using second-toe transfer. Hand 15:15–21, 1983

8. Leung PC: Thumb reconstruction using second-toe transfer. Hand Clinics. 1:285–295, May 1985

9. Leung PC, Ma FY: Digital reconstruction using the toe flap: Report of 10 cases. J Hand Surg 7:366–370, 1982

10. Leung PC, Wong WL: The vessels of the first metatarsal web space—an operative and radiographic study. J Bone Joint Surg 65A:235–238, 1983

11. Lister GD, Kalisman M, Tsai T: Reconstruction of the hand with free microneurovascular toe-to-hand transfer: Experience with 54 toe transfers. Plast Reconstr Surg 71:372–384, 1983

12. May JW Jr: Aesthetic and functional thumb reconstruction: Great toe to hand transfer. Clin Plast Surg 8: 357–362, 1981

13. May JW, Chait LA, Cohen BE, O'Brien BM: Free neurovascular flap from the first web of the foot and in hand reconstruction. J Hand Surg 2:387–393, 1977

14. Michon J, Merle M, Bouchon Y, Foucher G: Functional Comparison between Pollicization and Toe-to-Hand Transfer for Thumb Reconstruction. J Reconstr Microsurg 1:103–112, 1984

15. Morrison WA, O'Brien BM, MacLeod AM: Thumb reconstruction with a free neurovascular wraparound flap from the big toe. J Hand Surg 5:575–583, 1980

16. O'Brien, BM, MacLeod AM, Sykes PJ, Browing FSC, Threlfall GN: Microvascular second toe transfer for digital reconstruction. J Hand Surg 3:123–133, 1978

17. Stirrat CR, Seaber AV, Urbaniak JR, Bright DS: Temperature monitoring in digital replantation. J Hand Surg 3:342–347, 1978

18. Strickland JW: Restoration of thumb function following partial or total amputation. pp. 379–406. In Hunter JM, Schneider LH, Mackin EJ, Bell JA (eds): Rehabilitation of the Hand. CV Mosby, St Louis, 1978

19. Strickland JW: Thumb reconstruction. pp. 1563–1618. In Green DP (ed): Operative Hand Surgery. 1st Ed., Vol. 2. Churchill Livingstone, New York, 1982

20. Urbaniak JR: Elective Microsurgery for Orthopaedic Reconstruction. Part II. Thumb Reconstruction by Microsurgery. pp. 425–446. AAOS Instructional Course Lectures. Vol. 33. CV Mosby, St Louis, 1984

21. Urbaniak JR: Wrap-around procedure for thumb reconstruction. Hand Clinics 1:259–269, May 1985

22. Wang W: Keys to successful second toe-to-hand transfer. A review of 30 cases. J Hand Surg 8:902–906, 1983

23. Yang D, Yudong G: Thumb reconstruction utilizing second toe transplantation by microvascular anastomosis. Report of 78 cases. Chinese Med J (Engl) 92:295–301, 1979

24. Yoshimura M: Toe to hand transfer. Plast Reconstr Surg 66:74–83, 1980

The Perionychium

33

Elvin G. Zook

Fingernails are used for scratching, in defense and, more obviously, by humans to pick up small objects. However, the nail also protects the fingertip, contributes to tactile sensation,[33,36,49,59] and plays an important role in regulation of the peripheral circulation.[49] An abnormal nail is both a cosmetic and a functional problem, in that it catches on objects, particularly cloth, causing finger pain and damage to the object. Although nail injuries are among the most common of those of the hand,[37] until recently they have received little attention in the standard textbooks on hand surgery.[11,24,44]

ANATOMY

The perionychium consists of the paronychium and the nail bed[41] and has been described by many authors.[8,36,42,49,53,60,65,66,71] The nail anatomy is shown in diagrammatic form in Figure 33-1. The proximal nail fits into a depression called the *nail fold*. The skin over the dorsum of the nail fold is the *nail wall*. The thin membrane extending from the nail wall onto the dorsum of the nail is the *eponychium*. The *lunula* is the curved, white opacity in the nail found just distal to the eponychium and is roughly at the junction of the intermediate (germinal) and ventral (sterile) matrixes.

The nail fold is divided into the dorsal roof and the ventral floor by the nail. The *nail bed (matrix)* is all the soft tissue immediately beneath the nail that participates in nail generation and migration. The mass of keratin between the distal nail and the nail bed is the *hyponychium*. This is very resistant to infection, as shown by the fact that bacterial contamination in the area is heavy, yet infections are uncommon.

The embryology of the nail bed has been described by several authors.[36,41,42]

The nail is made up of material from three areas of the nail bed. Lewis[41] attributed production of the vast majority of the nail volume to the ventral floor *(germinal matrix)* of the nail fold. He also suggested that the tissue produced by the dorsal roof and the ventral nail bed *(sterile matrix)* are nail (Fig. 33-2). This is in spite of the fact that the contributions to the nail are produced in two different ways. Zaias[65] stated that only the portion produced by the ventral floor (germinal matrix) is true nail (Fig. 33-3). There is little doubt that some material is added to the undersurface of the nail by the "sterile matrix" as it progresses distally, since the distal nail is thicker than the proximal portion[8] and

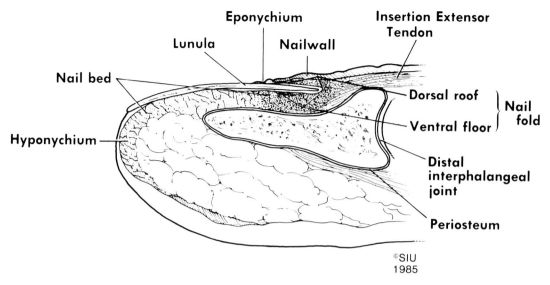

Fig. 33-1. The anatomy of the nail bed is shown in sagittal section.

a subungual hematoma that starts proximally beneath the nail becomes incorporated into the nail as it grows distally.[60] This argument, however, is primarily theoretical and has little effect on the practical care of the nail bed.

The arterial blood supplied to the nail bed comes from two terminal branches of the volar digital artery (Fig. 33-4). They communicate in the nail bed to form blood sinuses that are surrounded by muscle fibers and help to regulate the blood pressure and blood supply to the extremities.[49]

The venous drainage of the perionychium coalesces in the proximal portion of the nail bed and the skin proximal to the nail fold, and the veins then course in a random fashion over the dorsum of the finger.[45,66] Lymphatic vessels are more numerous in the nail bed, particularly in the area of the hyponychium, than in any other dermal area.[68]

The nerve supply to the perionychium comes from the dorsal branch of the volar digital nerve. Varying patterns of branching[64,66] have been reported.

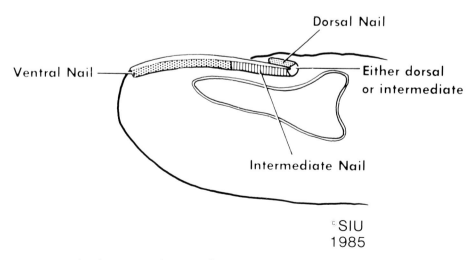

Fig. 33-2. The three areas that contribute to nail production are shown.

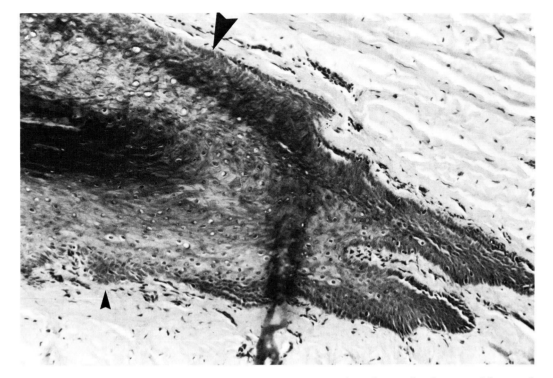

Fig. 33-3. The small arrow denotes intermediate nail production by the ventral floor and the large arrow shows the nail production of the dorsal roof, which contributes the shine of the nail.

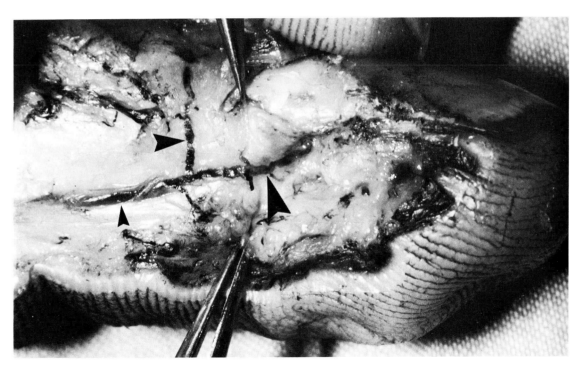

Fig. 33-4. The small arrow shows the common volar digital artery, the intermediate arrow the dorsal branch to the nail fold, and the large arrow the artery that progresses along the paronychium giving branches to the nail bed. The terminal branch to the pad of the finger is not shown. (Zook EG, Van Beek AL, Russell RC, Beatty ME: Anatomy and physiology of the perionychium. J Hand Surg 5:528–536, 1980.)

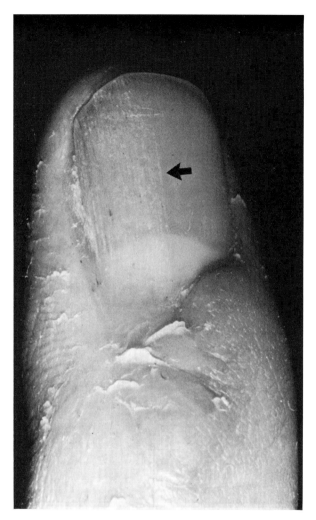

Fig. 33-5. A nail that has sustained avulsion of the nail-producing tissue of the dorsal roof from one side of the nail fold has lost its normal shine. (Zook EG: The perionychium: Anatomy, physiology, and care of injuries. Clin Plas Surg 8:21–31, 1981. Reprinted with permission from WB Saunders Co., Philadelphia.)

Physiology

Complete longitudinal nail growth takes approximately 70 to 160 days,[36,49] at a rate of approximately 0.1 mm a day,[3] 25 mm a week,[31] or $1\frac{1}{2}$ inches a year.[17] Baden[3] described a 21-day delay in distal growth of the nail after injury, during which time it thickens proximal to the injury site. Nail generation continues to be greater than normal for the next 50 days and then is less for 30 subsequent days. This accounts for the bulge in the surface of a regrowing nail. Nail growth, therefore, is not physiologically normal for 100 days following injury. Nail growth is slower in children younger than 3 years and then is progressively faster until approximately age 30. After 30 it gradually slows as the individual ages. Fingernails grow more rapidly than do toenails by a ratio of 4 to 1, and grow progressively faster on the longer fingers.[49]

The nail progresses distally because of the confinement of the nail fold. As the matrix cells enlarge they are flattened by the pressure of newly forming cells beneath them. As this pressure is exerted, restriction of the nail fold results in a distal vector. Kligman[40] has shown that a germinal matrix graft placed on the forearm will grow upward in a vertical cylinder.

The material produced by the roof of the nail fold is responsible for the shiny surface of the nail. If the dorsal roof is removed, the nail surface will be dull in appearance[66] (Fig. 33-5). Hashimoto[29] has shown in monkeys that a smooth nail bed is essential for regrowth of a normal nail. Scar does not produce any type of nail, so if the nail bed is not accurately approximated, primary healing with minimal scar cannot result and deformity may occur.

If the scar is on the dorsal roof, a dull streak will appear; if it is in the intermediate nail (germinal matrix), a split or absent nail will occur; and if it is in the ventral nail (sterile matrix), a split or nonadherence of the nail beyond the scar will occur.

TREATMENT OF ACUTE INJURIES

Twenty years ago Ashbell et al[2] classified nail bed injuries, but made no mention of subungual hematomas, although blood beneath the nail comes from disruption of the nail bed blood vessels. I will use a simplified classification of simple lacerations, stellate lacerations, severe crush, and avulsions.[70]

Late reconstruction of the nail bed is unpredictable and frequently little, if any, improvement, is obtained. It is therefore preferable to treat the injury early and properly to prevent deformity. "There's never time to do it right, but there is always time to do it over" (Meskimen's Law of Bureaucracies)[43] is an adage that should *not* be applied to the treatment of nail bed injuries.

Epidemiology of the Injury

Nail deformities can occur secondary to anything that causes injury or deformation of the nail bed. This may include infection, self-mutilation, tumor, and trauma. Doors are the most common source of injury, followed by smashing between two objects, saws, and lawn mowers. The age group most commonly injured is the older child and young adult. The digits of the left and right hand are injured with equal frequency. The long finger, being the longest and most exposed, is the most frequently injured, with the ring, index, small, and thumb following in that order. Injuries to the nail bed alone are six times less common than injuries that involve the paronychium and tip. The most common type of injury is the simple laceration, followed by stellate laceration, crush, and avulsion in decreasing frequency. The middle and distal third of the nail bed are the most frequent site of injury and 50 percent of injuries involve fracture of the distal phalanx and/or tuft.[70]

Injuries of the nail bed most commonly result from localized trauma to the nail that causes compression of the nail bed between the bent or broken nail and the bone (Fig. 33-6A). This causes a straight or stellate, tearing laceration of the nail bed. When the nail is compressed between a larger object and the bone, an exploding type of injury results in stellate lacerations or multiple fragments of nail bed (severe crush and/or avulsion; Fig. 33-6B). It is rare to have a truly sharp laceration of the nail bed, for commonly when a sharp object strikes the nail hard enough to perforate it, it goes through and amputates the tip.[70]

Subungual Hematoma

The nail bed is a highly vascular structure. A compression laceration of the nail bed secondary to a blow causes bleeding. If the nail is not broken or

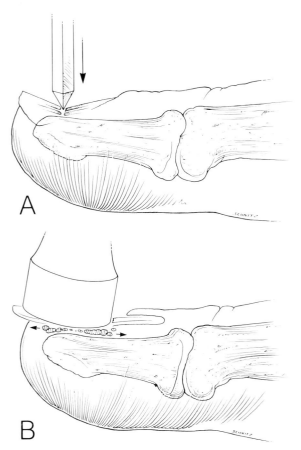

Fig. 33-6. (A) A relatively sharp object compressing the nail between the nail and bone causes a splitting laceration. (B) A wider area of compression of the nail bed between the nail and the bone causes an exploding-type injury that results in multiple fragments.

the edge dislodged, the pressure of the hematoma beneath the nail will frequently cause severe throbbing pain, and evacuation of the hematoma is indicated. If more than 25 percent of the visible portion of the nail is undermined by hematoma, it is best to remove the nail, inspect the nail bed, and repair the injury.[67-69] It is essential to surgically scrub the finger prior to perforation of the nail to prevent contamination of the subungual area and the subsequent risk of infection and potential osteomyelitis. I prefer a Betadine soap scrub for five minutes followed by Betadine solution application.

Use of a drill, needle,[46] or paper clip heated in an alcohol lamp or Bunsen burner until red hot, have

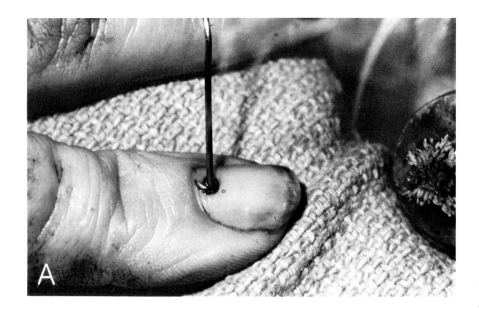

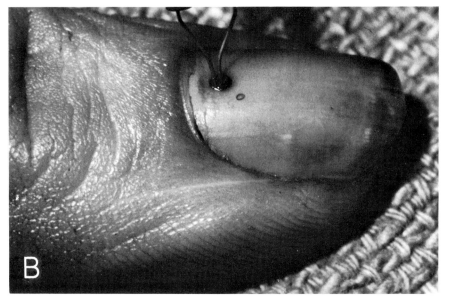

Fig. 33-7. (**A**) The time-honored method of burning a hole through the nail is with a heated paper clip. (**B**) The author's preferred method of burning a hole through the nail is with an ophthalmic battery-powered cautery.

been advocated (Fig. 33-7A). I prefer the battery-powered microcautery unit, available in most emergency rooms (Fig. 33-7B). The heated tip passes through the nail, is cooled by the hematoma and does not injure the nail bed. The hole burned in the nail must be large enough to allow prolonged drainage. Some methods create a small hole that decompresses the hematoma immediately, but the hematoma reforms when clot seals the hole.

Simple Lacerations

Simple laceration is the most common injury. Warning signs of significant injury to the nail bed other than the obvious are subungual hematoma involving over 25 percent of the visible nail and/or avulsion of the nail from the nail fold or paronychium (see Fig. 33-13A). A surgical prep and finger tourniquet are necessary to allow an adequate view of the nail bed. The nail is removed by gentle opening and closing of iris scissors inserted beneath the free edge of the nail hyponychium and worked proximally. A small periosteal elevator may also be worked proximally from the hyponychium to free the nail. I find the Kutz periosteal elevator to be better than the Freer, since the former is smaller and does less damage to the nail bed. After the nail is removed it is cleaned by scraping the residual soft tissue from its undersurface and soaked in Betadine solution while the nail bed is being repaired.

The nail bed is explored with loupe magnification and the injury is evaluated to estimate the degree of crush and irregularity of the edges (Fig. 33-8A). Irregularities are trimmed, if it can be done without sacrificing so much tissue that tension on the repair occurs. If this is in doubt, it is usually advisable not to trim the edges. One millimeter of undermining of the nail bed from the periosteum will allow slight eversion of the wound edges and accurate wound approximation. Five–0 chromic catgut[63] and 6–0 plain catgut[2] have been advo-

cated for suture. I prefer 7–0 chromic on a micropoint spatula, double-arm, GS-9, ophthalmic needle (Ethicon). The curve of this needle allows easier passage through the nail bed that is adherent to the periosteum, and the double needle provides a spare in case one is bent or broken. After the nail bed is accurately approximated (Fig. 33-8B), a round hole is drilled or burned through the nail at a point not over the repair site, to allow drainage of serum or hematoma from the subungual area after the nail is reinserted into the nail fold. Schiller in 1967[54] described replacing the fingernail into the nail fold to keep the fold open and better approximate the edges of the repair (Fig. 33-8C). I hold the nail in place with a 5–0 monofilament nylon suture placed through the fingertip and the distal free border of the nail. The fingertip is then dressed with nonadherent gauze, a small dressing, and a splint that immobilizes the DIP joint and protects the tip. The dressing is changed in 5 to 7 days and the nail checked for subungual seroma or hematoma. If present, the hole is reopened or the nail

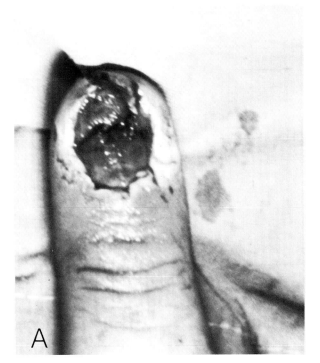

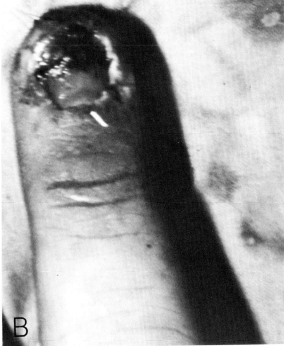

Fig. 33-8. **(A)** An injury in the simple laceration category. This laceration, although straight, is a crushing type of injury. **(B)** The nail bed has been sutured with 7–0 chromic sutures under magnification. *(Figure continues.)*

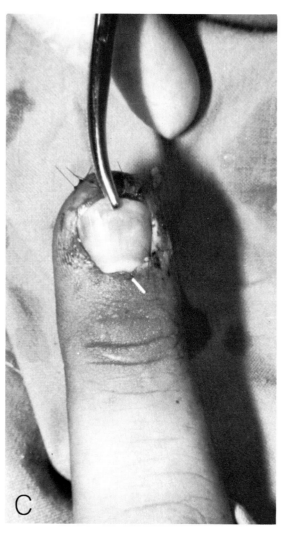

raised at the paronychium to permit drainage. The suture is removed from the tip at three weeks. The nail will frequently adhere to the nail bed for 1 to 3 months until pushed off by the new nail. Replacement of the nail creates a much less tender fingertip while a new nail is growing (Fig. 33-8D).

If the nail is unavailable or too badly damaged for a portion of it to be replaced, a nail-shaped sheet of 0.020-inch silicone may be used as a substitute. A 6–0 nylon suture is brought from the nail wall through the proximal portion of the nail fold, placed through the edge of the silicone sheet at each corner and returned through the nail fold onto the dorsum of the finger (Fig. 33-9). The silicone sheet approximates the edges of the repair and keeps the nail fold open. If a suture is not used proximally to hold the silicone sheet in the nail fold, the softness of the sheet may allow it to slip out; however, the use of more firm prosthetic materials does not allow the accurate conformation and smoothing of the nail bed desired.

A single thickness of nail-shaped adaptic or other nonadherent gauze may be placed in the nail fold if the nail is not available. It will adhere adequately to stay in place and will loosen after healing has occurred. I start t.i.d. soapy water soaks 7 days after injury to clean the wound.

If the nail is avulsed with a distal base, sutures should be placed through the proximal portion of the fold, into the free margin of the nail bed and

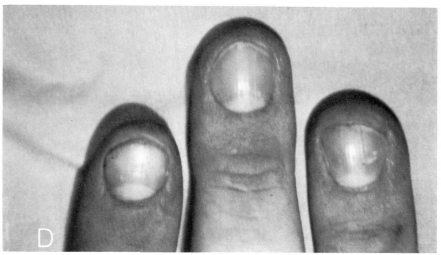

Fig. 33-8 *(Continued).* **(C)** The nail, after it has been cleaned and soaked in Betadine, is replaced into the nail fold. A hole will be drilled in the nail to allow drainage, although it is easier to do this before the nail is reinserted into the nail fold. **(D)** The nail 1 year postinjury. (Reproduced by permission from Zook EG: Fingernail injuries. In Strickland JW, Steichen JB (eds): Difficult Problems in Hand Surgery. CV Mosby, St Louis, 1982.)

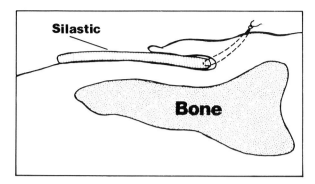

Fig. 33-9. A horizontal mattress suture through the nail wall is used to hold a silicone sheet into the nail fold.

brought back out through the dorsal roof of the nail fold, drawing the nail bed back into the nail fold (Fig. 33-10A and B). Accurate approximation in the nail fold may require an incision in the eponychium. The incision should be made perpendicular to the lateral curved portion of the eponychial fold and may be necessary on both sides (Fig. 33-11).

If the laceration involves the dorsal roof and the ventral fold, it is important that both be similarly repaired. The fine chromic catgut sutures approximating the nail bed should have the knots placed in the nail fold, not buried in the soft tissue of the nail wall or matrix. The nail wall (skin) is then approximated with 6–0 nonabsorbable sutures. It is especially important with this type of injury to place the nail, silicone sheet, or gauze in the nail fold to prevent adhesions (Fig. 33-12A and B).

Stellate Lacerations

The etiology of stellate lacerations is similar to simple lacerations, but is caused by a more widely distributed force that involves more of the nail surface. Accurate approximation of the stellate points is necessary (Fig. 33-13C); meticulous repair plus the use of the nail, silicone sheet, or nonadherent gauze as described previously will in most cases give a surprisingly good result (Fig. 33-13). The use of porcine xenografts[21] has been published showing good results. I have had no experience with this method.

Severe Crushing Injuries

Severe crushing injuries carry a poorer prognosis[70] than do the previously described injuries. In the severe crushing injury it is important that all fragments of the nail bed be returned to the nail bed and repaired as accurately as possible (Fig. 33-14A–C). Any fragments attached by tissue strands should be accurately replaced as free grafts. Any segments of nail bed attached to the detached nail should be removed with a small periosteal elevator and used as free grafts to complete

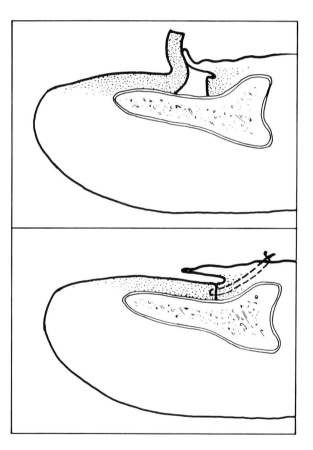

©SIU
1985

Fig. 33-10. (A) The nail bed has been torn in the proximal nail fold and stripped from the nail fold. (B) A horizontal mattress suture through the nail wall is used to replace the nail bed. The nail is then returned to the nail fold to mold the wound edges.

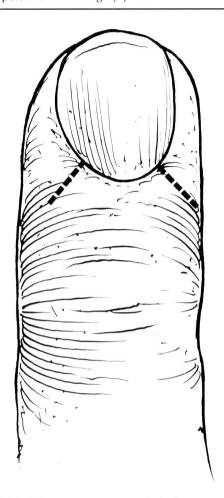

Fig. 33-11. When incisions are made in the eponychium, they should be made at 90-degree angles from the eponychium to prevent deformity.

the nail bed. Nail, silicone sheet, or adaptic is used to approximate the edges and maintain the nail fold open until healing results.

Lacerations Associated with Fractures of the Distal Phalanx

Approximately 50 percent of nail bed injuries have an accompanying fracture of the distal phalanx.[70] If the fracture is nondisplaced, the nail bed should be repaired and the nail replaced as a splint. The replaced nail, due to its close proximity to the periosteum, makes an excellent splint to maintain fracture reduction. Displaced fractures are accu-

rately reduced and fixed with a fine longitudinal K-wire if unstable.

If the patient is seen late with a displaced fracture that has not been reduced prior to a recent nail bed repair, the wound should be opened unless contraindicated by the presence of infection. The fracture should be accurately reduced, pinned if necessary to maintain reduction, and the nail bed re-repaired. If the dorsal cortex of the distal phalanx is left uneven it will cause a nail bed deformity.

Avulsions of the Nail Bed

Nail bed avulsion frequently leaves the fragment of nail bed attached to the undersurface of the avulsed nail. An attempt should be made to find the nail if it does not accompany the patient. Schiller[54] suggested that the nail to which the nail bed is attached is the optimum shape and tension to aid inosculation of the nail bed. It is therefore advisable to replace the nail as accurately as possible onto the avulsion site. One to two millimeters of nail may be freed and trimmed from the nail bed in the area to be sutured if the fragment is large (Fig. 33-15). This allows easier and more accurate placement of sutures.

Further injury to the nail bed might ensue if attempts are made to remove a fragment of nail bed from a small piece of nail, so the nail should be replaced accurately without disturbing the nail bed to optimally position the nail bed (Fig. 33-16).

Free Nail Bed Graft

All retrievable fragments of nail bed should be replaced as free grafts. A graft 1 cm in diameter will frequently live by inosculation and ingrowth of circulation from the periphery, even on the bare cortex of the distal phalanx. Iselin[32] recommended storing the avulsed fragment in mild antiseptic solution for 2 to 4 days prior to replacement to determine viability of the bed. Swanker in 1947 advocated allowing small areas of nail bed avulsion to heal by secondary intention while covered by tantalum sheet. This increases the amount of scarring, and I believe that it decreases the chances of adherence of the nail. He advocated the use of full-thickness nail bed grafts from an adjacent amputated finger or a 0.020-inch split-thickness nail bed graft

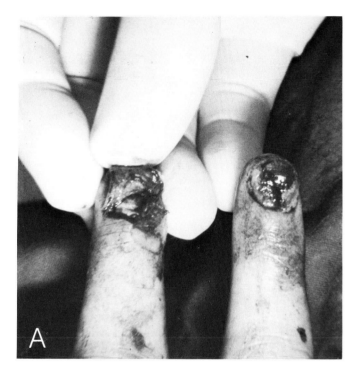
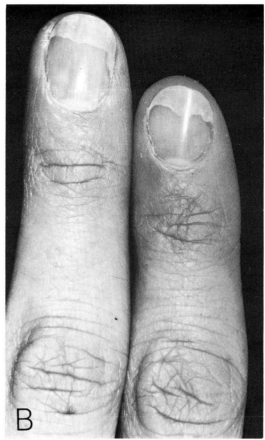

Fig. 33-12. (A) This through-and-through laceration of the nail fold was repaired as described in the text. (B) The nail 1 year postinjury. (Reproduced by permission from Zook EG: Fingernail injuries. In Strickland JW, Steichen JB (eds): Difficult Problems in Hand Surgery. CV Mosby, St Louis, 1982.)

from another finger to replace large avulsed segments.[61] Hoerner and Cohen,[31] Flatt,[22,23] and Hanrahan[28] advocate split-thickness skin grafts while Ashbell et al[2] and Claybaugh[18] advocate using reverse dermal grafts.

If an adjacent finger has been amputated or is so severely crushed that it is to be amputated, removal of a full-thickness nail bed graft or split-thickness nail bed graft is a good choice for coverage of avulsions. Saita et al[51] have shown excellent results using free full-thickness nail bed grafts from toes in the acute nail bed avulsion injury. These have the disadvantage of causing deformity of a toenail and contradict Iselin's[32] suggestion of delay.

Shepard[58] in 1983 demonstrated excellent results using split-thickness nail bed grafts from the adjacent nail bed of the injured finger or from a toe nail bed. It has been my experience that if there is inadequate undamaged area on the injured nail bed from which a split-thickness nail bed graft can be harvested, one must go to the large toe to acquire a large enough graft (Fig. 33-17A and B).

The toenail is removed from the great toe with a periosteal elevator under toe block anesthesia. A split-thickness nail bed graft (I suggest approximaty 0.014 inches thick, for no one knows the best thickness) of the toenail bed is removed with a surgical blade. It is better for the graft to be too thin than too thick. A surgical blade can be used with a back-and-forth sawing technique to tangentially remove a small fragment of nail bed (Fig. 33-17C and D). The curve of the nail bed makes it impossi-

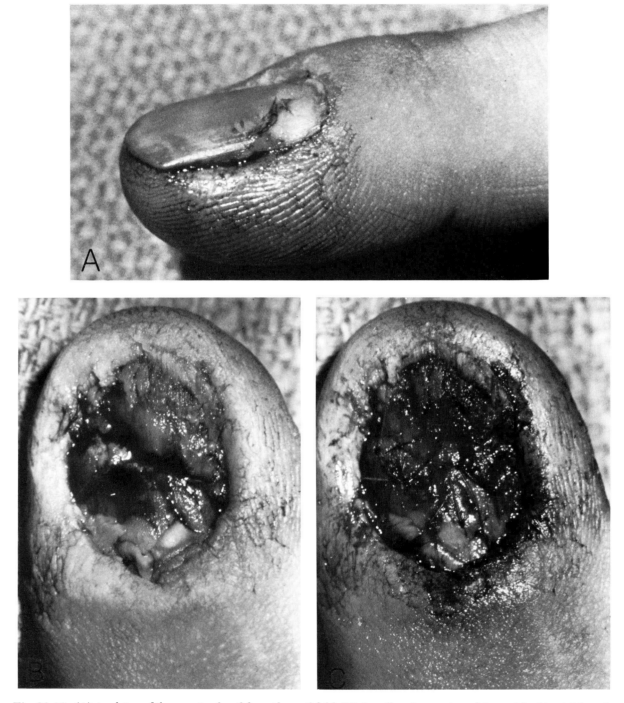

Fig. 33-13. (**A**) Avulsion of the proximal nail from the nail fold. (**B**) A stellate laceration of the nail bed is visible only after the nail has been removed. (**C**) The lacerations are approximated as accurately as possible with fine (7–0) chromic sutures and using magnification. *(Figure continues.)*

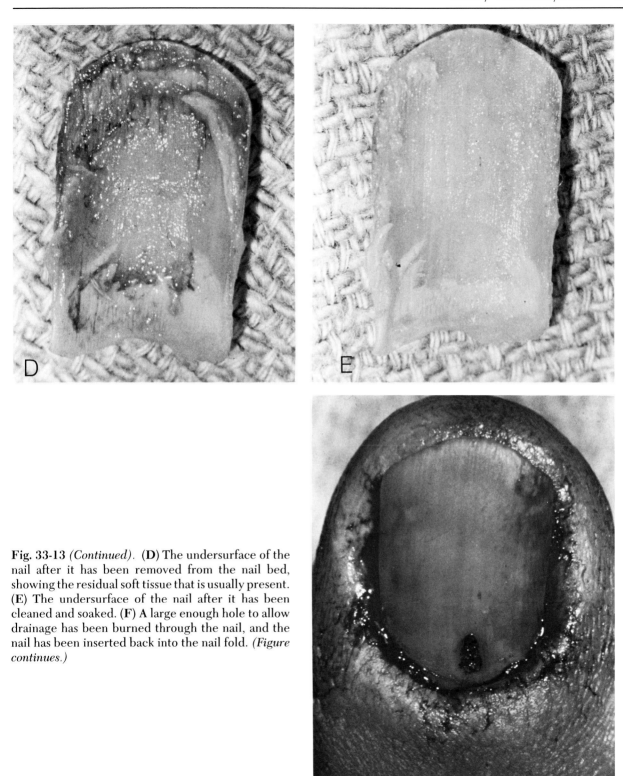

Fig. 33-13 *(Continued)*. **(D)** The undersurface of the nail after it has been removed from the nail bed, showing the residual soft tissue that is usually present. **(E)** The undersurface of the nail after it has been cleaned and soaked. **(F)** A large enough hole to allow drainage has been burned through the nail, and the nail has been inserted back into the nail fold. *(Figure continues.)*

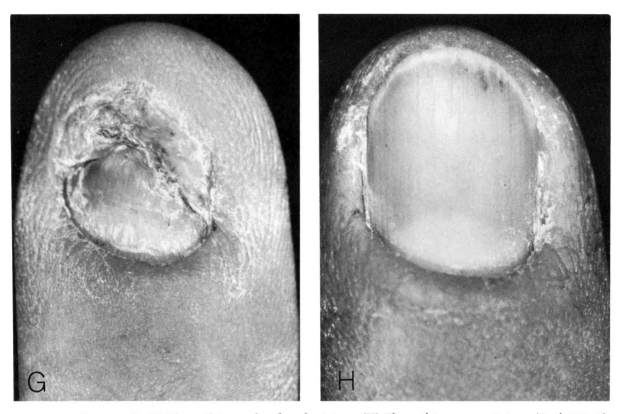

Fig. 33-13 *(Continued).* **(G)** The nail 2 months after the injury. **(H)** The nail 1 year postinjury. (Zook EG: The perionychium: Anatomy, physiology, and care of injuries. Clin Plas Surg 8:21–31, 1981. Reprinted with permission from WB Saunders Co., Philadelphia.)

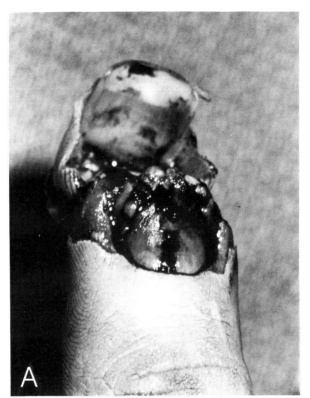

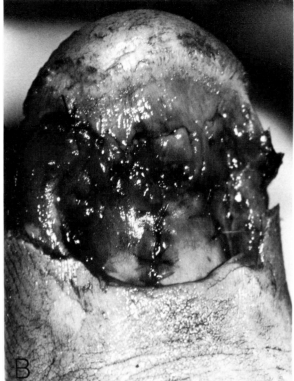

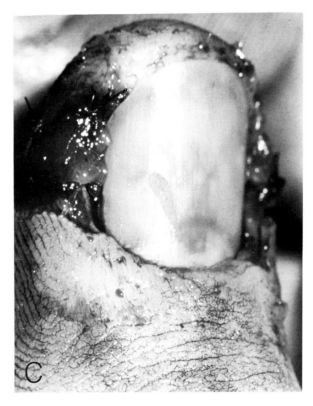

Fig. 33-14. (**A**) A severe crushing injury of the nail bed with avulsion of the nail and laceration of the tip. (**B**) The nail bed is approximated and sutured as accurately as possible. (**C**) The nail is replaced to maintain reduction of the fracture and to approximate the edges of the nail bed.

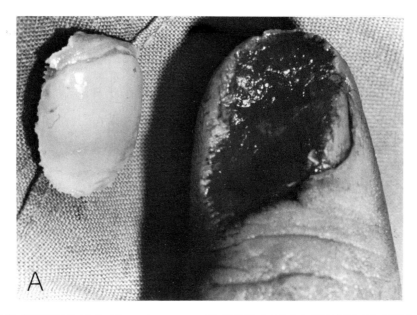

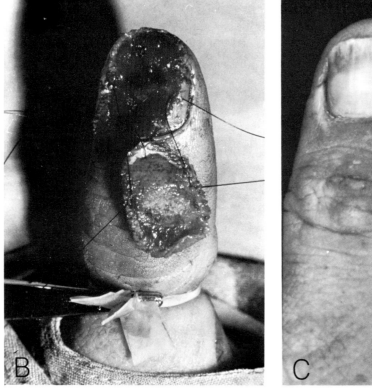

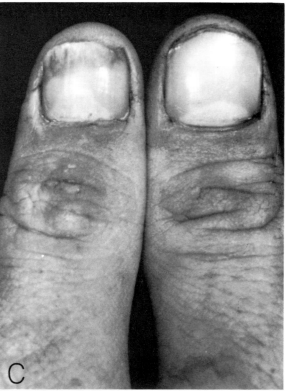

Fig. 33-15. (**A**) An avulsion of approximately 80 percent of the nail and nail bed. The nail bed is still attached to the nail. (**B**) The nail is dissected from the outer 2 mm of the nail bed to allow accurate suture placement, and the nail bed is replaced. (**C**) The repaired nail 1 year later with satisfactory growth, but some lack of complete adherence distally, compared with the normal side. (Reproduced by permission from Zook EG: Fingernail injuries. In Strickland JW, Steichen JB (eds): Difficult Problems in Hand Surgery. CV Mosby, St Louis, 1982.)

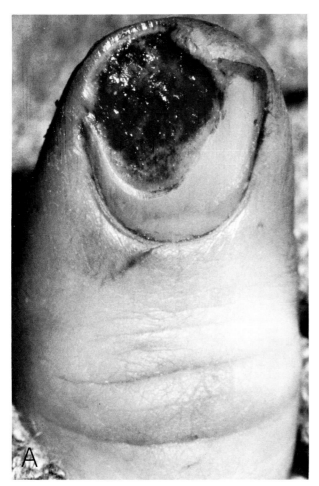

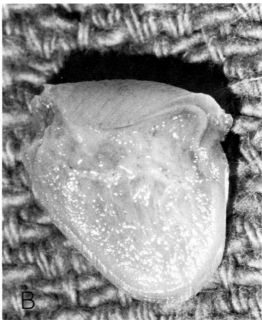

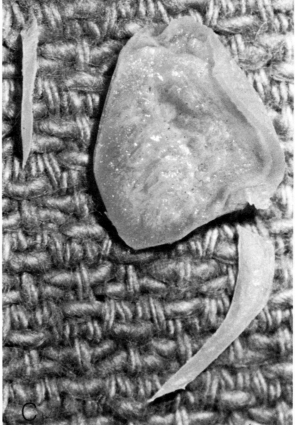

Fig. 33-16. (**A**) Avulsion of a small portion of the nail and nail bed. (**B**) The undersurface of the nail fragment with the attached nail bed is shown. (**C**) Only that portion of the nail that is overhanging the nail bed is removed. No attempt is made to dissect nail bed from the nail on small pieces. *(Figure continues.)*

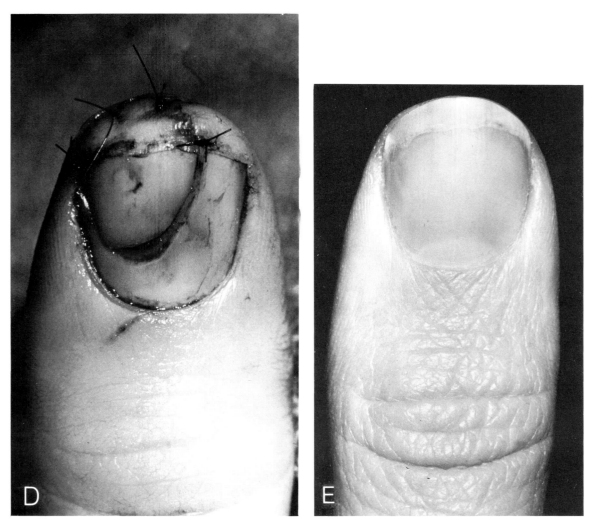

Fig. 33-16 *(Continued).* **(D)** The nail with attached nail bed is then accurately approximated and held in place with a few fine chromic sutures. **(E)** The nail 12 months postinjury.

Fig. 33-17. (A) A nail bed and fingertip injury with avulsion of approximately 25 percent of the nail bed. **(B)** The tip skin and nail bed surrounding the avulsion have been repaired. The white area at the distal left portion of the nail bed is bare cortical bone of the distal tuft. **(C)** The technique of harvesting a small, split-thickness nail bed graft. **(D)** The large toe after the nail has been removed and a split-thickness graft has been removed from the sterile matrix. The germinal matrix should not be included in a split-thickness graft. *(Figure continues.)*

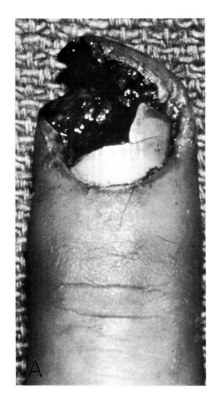
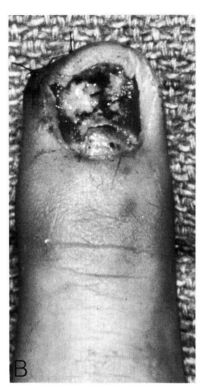
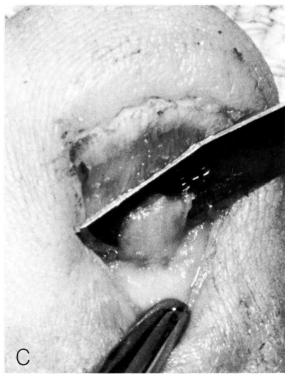
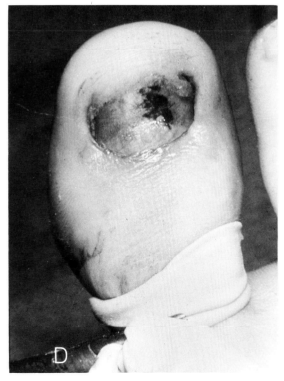

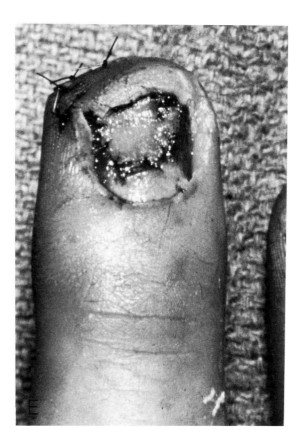
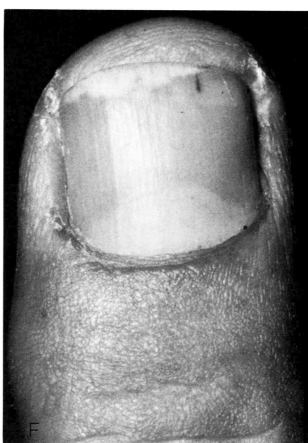

Fig. 33-17 *(Continued).* **(E)** The split graft of sterile matrix is sutured in place on the nail bed. **(F)** The fingernail 1 year later.

ble to obtain a large fragment with this technique. If a larger nail bed graft is needed, it is necessary to use the tip of the blade while picking up the edge of the graft being removed with fine forceps. The graft is sutured into the defect with fine chromic catgut sutures (Fig. 33-17E and F), and if the nail is available, it is replaced. The toenail is replaced into the nail fold after perforation and sutured distally as previously described.

A fragment of the tip is often avulsed with the nail bed in children. In such cases, I accurately approximate the edges of the nail bed and tip skin as a composite graft. Debridement should be minimal as the maximum possible inosculation effect is essential. The younger the child, the better the chances for "take" of a composite graft.

LATE RECONSTRUCTION OF THE NAIL BED

Reconstructive procedures of the nail bed are commonly not as successful as the surgeon or the patient would desire. These less than satisfactory results have discouraged attempts at reconstruction and hindered progress of knowledge. Every reconstructive problem of the nail bed is different and must be approached individually. Unfortunately, no one has reported a large series and knowledge is limited. A thorough knowledge of the anatomy and physiology of the nail bed of the fingers and toes is essential to devise a treatment plan and carry it out.

Reconstruction can be divided into problems involving the sterile and germinal matrix. They may also be divided into deformity categories such as nonadherence, split nails, absence of nail, and so on. Deformities may also involve the sterile and/or germinal matrix, and the treatment plan must take this into consideration.

Ridges

Nail ridges are caused by scar beneath the nail bed or an irregularly healed fracture. Since nail growth follows the shape of the nail bed, a nail ridge occurs. If an underlying ridge is transverse, the deformity can range from a transverse nail groove to distal nonadherence. If the ridge is longitudinal, a longitudinal nail ridge will result. Correction of the ridged nail requires surgical reduction of the scar and/or smoothing the irregularity of the bone to create a flat nail bed.[2,62]

Minor transverse ridges of the nail are frequently seen following hypoxic illnesses or use of the arm tourniquet for upper extremity surgical procedures, and these resolve as new nail grows out to replace the deformed area.

Split Nail

A split nail may be caused by a ridge or longitudinal scar in the germinal and/or sterile matrix. Since scar does not produce nail cells, there is a blank area between the regions of normal nail production and subsequent split. Carter in 1928[14] and 1930[15] and Seckel in 1986[55] have reported successful treatment of distal split nails. Seckel's technique, a piece of 0.20-inch silicone sheet between the nail and nail bed, seems to be the more reasonable approach to me.

If the scar involves the sterile matrix, it can be treated by resection of the scar and closure of the adjacent edges of matrix. However, in my experience, if the scar is wide enough to cause a split nail, it is frequently too wide to approximate the defect without significant tension and recurrence of the split. In such cases, I recommend resection of the scar of the nail bed and replacement with a split-thickness nail bed graft from an adjacent portion of the same nail or from a toenail.

If the split is due to scar in the germinal matrix with lack of nail production, the scar must be eliminated and replaced. The eponychium should be elevated with incisions at right angles from the corners (see Fig. 33-11). The nail is removed, and under magnification the scar identified and resected. Johnson[34] has advocated incisions in the lateral paronychial folds with advancement of the germinal matrix toward the center of the nail, but I have had little success with this technique. My preference is to use a toe germinal matrix graft similar in size and shape to the resected scar as a free composite graft (Fig. 33-18). This requires elimination of a toenail in most cases. I usually use the second toenail bed since this is more acceptable to most individuals, particularly women, than having significant deformity of the large toenail.

Nonadherence

When the scars of the sterile matrix are transverse or diagonal and wide, the non-nail producing scar may cause the nail to loosen and not re-adhere distal to the scar. Resection of the scar is essential, and my preference for replacement is a split-thickness sterile matrix graft from either an adjacent area of the nail bed or from a toenail bed (Fig. 33-19). If the majority of the sterile matrix is lost, a split- or full-thickness nail bed graft may be applied after the scar is excised. A satisfactory result can be obtained with this technique (Fig. 33-20).

Absence

Absence of a nail may be congenital or may result from avulsion, severe crush, infection, or burn, among other things, and is a disconcerting deformity to the patient and/or the family.

I find that the simplest treatment is to resect an area of skin in the shape of and slightly larger than a normal nail. A full- or split-thickness skin graft is applied, and after healing, it mimics to some degree the appearance of a nail. The graft may also be done along with reconstruction of a pouch, into which an artificial nail can be placed.[4,12] However, in my experience this type of reconstructed nail fold is only initially satisfactory; as time passes it becomes

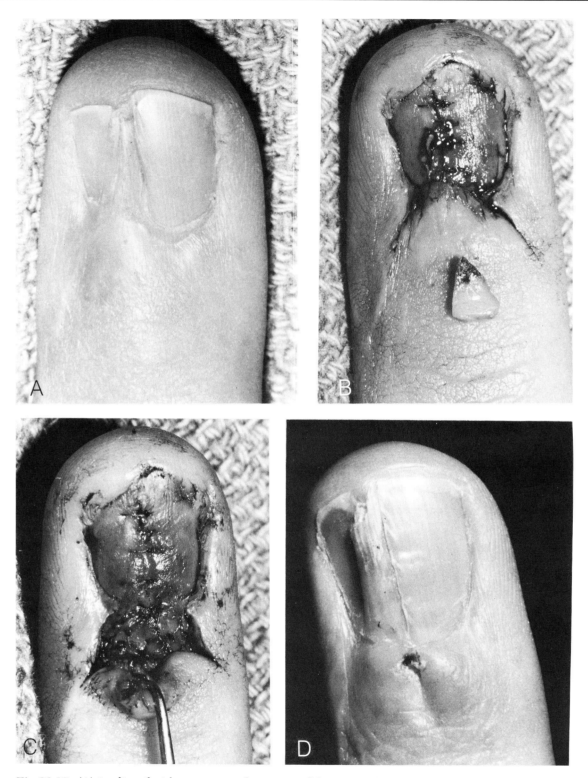

Fig. 33-18. **(A)** A split nail with a pterygium due to scar of the germinal matrix. **(B)** The scar of the germinal matrix has been removed and a fragment of germinal matrix from the second toe cut to shape to fit the defect. **(C)** The germinal matrix graft sutured in place. **(D)** Six months later nail can be seen growing from the germinal matrix graft.

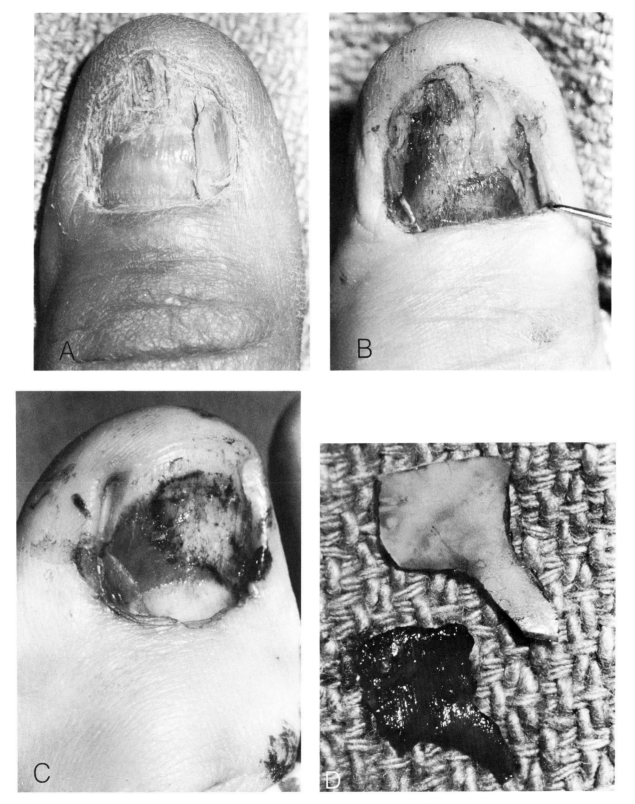

Fig. 33-19. (A) Preoperative view of a thumbnail in which the nail grows out and becomes nonadherent every 2 to 3 months following injury by a car door. (B) The nail remnant has been removed and scar can be seen in the nail bed on the right side.(C) The scar of the nail bed is marked for excision. (D) An exact template in the configuration of the scar is used to shape a split-thickness nail bed graft from sterile matrix of the toe. *(Figure continues.)*

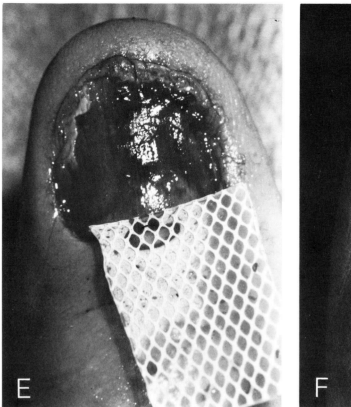
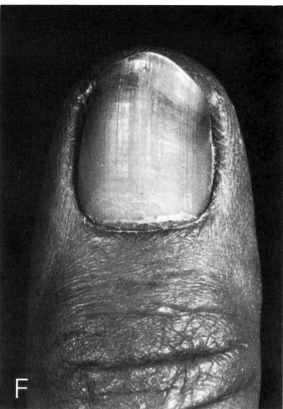

Fig. 33-19 *(Continued).* **(E)** The split-thickness nail bed graft has been sutured in place and a silicone sheet placed over it and into the nail fold. **(F)** The nail 11 months postoperative showing complete adherence of the nail.

obliterated and will not hold the edge of the prosthetic nail.

Composite Nail Bed Grafts

Good results with composite toenail grafts have been reported.[9,48,57] The reported cases are few, and composite nail bed grafts are unpredictable in adults, but in my experience give fairly good results in children. The younger the child, the better the results. I do not know the age at which the success rate falls significantly, but it is probably somewhere between 8 and 15 years. The chances of free composite toenail grafts in adults giving a satisfactory result are so poor that I do not believe that they warrant the loss of the toenail.[72] The nail bed frequently "takes" but no nail is produced, much to the patient's consternation.

In selecting a donor site for composite grafts, I prefer to use the second toe, since it is usually approximately the width of the fingernail. A toenail is, however, not as long as the finger nail, and a split-thickness sterile matrix graft from another toe needs to be placed distal to the germinal matrix graft to lengthen the attachment area (Fig. 33-21). The large toenail or a portion of it is necessary for thumbnail reconstruction with composite grafts.

Free Microvascular Grafts

Free microvascular transfer of the dorsal tip of the toe, including the nail bed, is the most reliable treatment to produce a growing nail in adults. However, this requires very skilled microvascular care, and also has some risk of failure and leaves significant scars on the foot, toe, and finger.

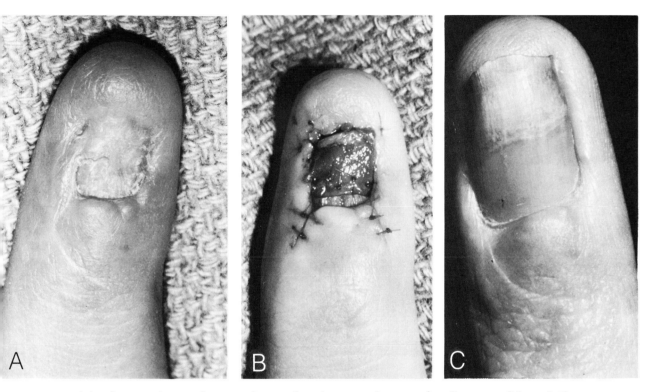

Fig. 33-20. (A) A finger with normal germinal matrix but absent sterile matrix for adherence of the nail. The patient had had repeated infections beneath the nail.(B) The scarred nail bed has been removed and a full-thickness sterile matrix graft from the second toe used to replace it. (C) One year later the nail adheres to the full-thickness toenail graft but does not adhere to the distal scar. (Zook EG: The perionychium: Anatomy, physiology, and care of injuries. Clin Plas Surg 8:21 – 31, 1981. Reprinted with permission from WB Saunders Co., Philadelphia.)

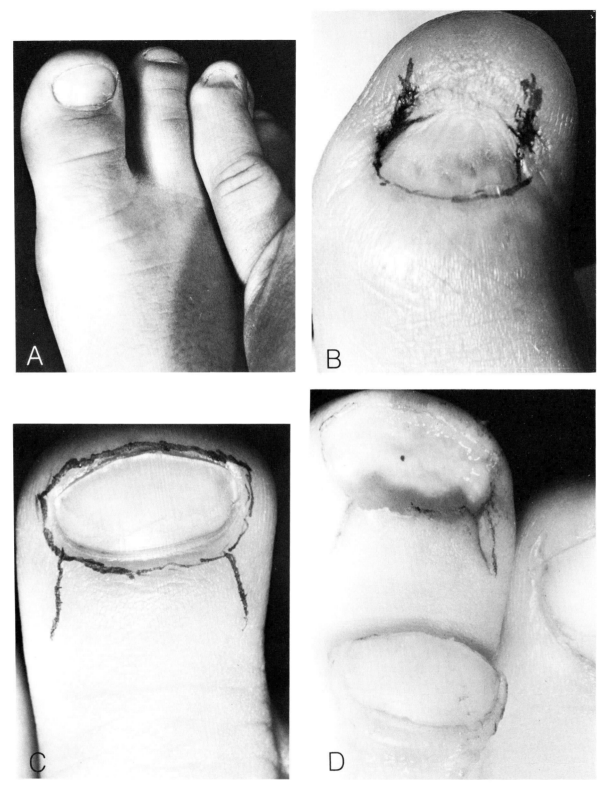

Fig. 33-21. **(A)** A 7-year-old child with post-traumatic absence of the index nail, showing the comparison in width of the fingernail and the second toe nail. **(B)** The nail bed is seen close-up at the time of the surgery. **(C)** The second toe is marked for removal of the composite nail and nail bed graft. **(D)** The composite graft excised. *(Figure continues.)*

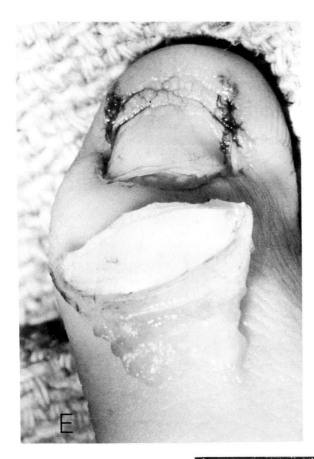

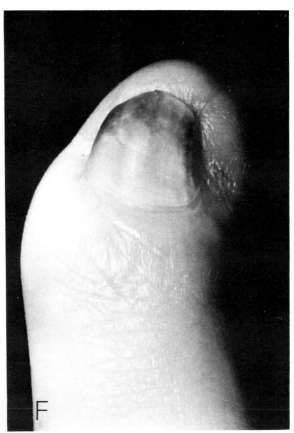

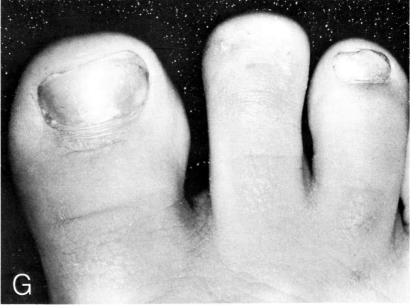

Fig. 33-21 *(Continued).* **(E)** The composite graft placed on the dorsum of the finger after the nail fold has been created. Note that the toenail does not have as much length as the normal fingernail. The sterile matrix was advanced distally to create a recipient site for the graft. **(F)** The nail 1 year postoperative. **(G)** Postoperative view of the second toe. A split-thickness skin graft was applied to the periosteum.

Pterygium and Eponychial Deformities

A pterygium of either the eponychium or hyponychium may occur secondary to trauma or ischemia. Pterygia of the hyponychial area may follow denervation injuries or ischemic injuries of the upper extremity. The pad of the finger becomes atrophic, and the hyponychial attachment to the nail becomes painful and tender. This is treated by removing the distal 5 mm of nail from the nail bed and hyponychial area. A strip of nail bed and hyponychium 3- to 4-mm wide is resected and re-

placed by a split-thickness skin graft. This causes nonadherence in the hyponychial area and usually provides relief of pain.

A persistent pterygium of the eponychium is treated by freeing the dorsal roof of the nail fold from the nail and inserting a small piece of silicone sheet with a horizontal mattress suture as shown in Figure 33-9. The undersurface of the nail fold epithelializes, releasing the adherence. If this is unsuccessful, a more radical approach is to separate the dorsal roof from the nail and place a thin split-thickness skin graft on the undersurface of the eponychium to prevent the adherence.

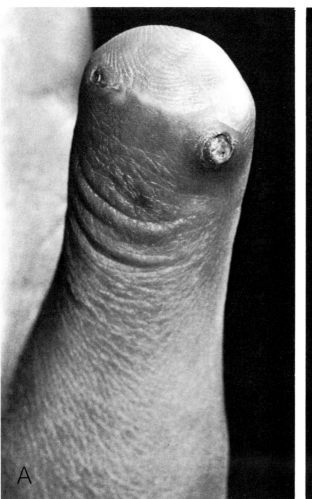
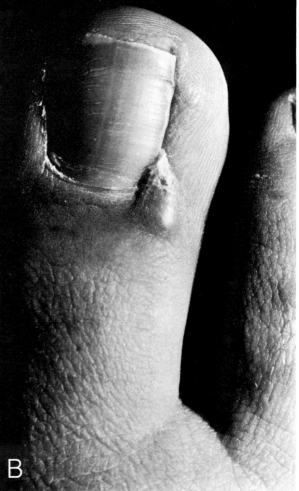

Fig. 33-22. (A) Nail cysts following amputation of the fingertip without complete removal of the nail bed. (B) A nail spike resulting from incomplete removal of nail bed after resection of an ingrown toenail.

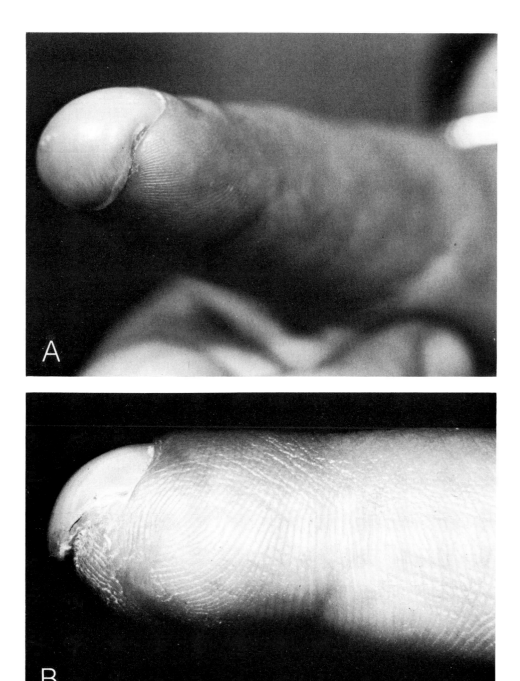

Fig. 33-23. (**A**) A hooked nail deformity due partially to some loss of bony support, but primarily because the nail bed was pulled over the tip to close the amputation. (**B**) Loss of bony support to hold the nail bed flat.

A notched eponychium may be reconstructed by a composite toe eponychial graft, the helical rim of the ear,[50] or rotation flaps.

Cornified Nail Bed

When the germinal matrix is removed to eliminate nail growth, the patient frequently has continued problems with keratinized material growing from the sterile matrix. To relieve this, the sterile matrix is excised and a split-thickness skin graft applied.

Nail Spikes and Cysts

Nail cysts most commonly occur following amputation of a fingertip and failure to remove all of the germinal matrix from the nail fold (Fig. 33-22A). Complete resection of the nail cyst and its wall is curative.

Nail spikes are also the result of incomplete removal of germinal matrix and are similar to nail cysts, except that they grow distally (Fig. 33-22B). It is a frequent occurrence following removal of the side of a nail and nail bed for ingrown toenail. The treatment is complete removal of the spike and the germinal matrix creating it.

Hooked Nail

The growing nail follows the nail matrix. The hooked nail is most commonly caused by either tight closure of a fingertip amputation (Fig. 33-23A) and/or loss of bony support for the nail bed (Fig. 33-23B). The nail bed should not be pulled over the distal phalanx to close a fingertip amputation, as this will almost surely cause a hooked nail. When the bone is absent, it must either be replaced or the nail bed trimmed back to the end of the bone so that the nail bed does not curve over the end and cause hooking.

When a hooked nail is present, a decision must be made whether to shorten the bone or attempt to add support to the nail bed. If the distal nail bed has been pulled over the end of the finger, a V-Y advancement flap, cross-finger flap, or full-thickness skin graft can be used to replace the soft tissue of the tip, allowing replacement of the nail bed onto the dorsum of the bone. This usually improves the hook, although complete correction is uncommon.

Correction of the hooked nail with maintenance of nail length requires replacement of the distal phalanx or tuft with a bone graft. This may require additional tip soft tissue prior to or at the time of bone graft. Initially, bone grafts support the nail bed satisfactorily, but, as with most bone grafts that do not have bone opposition on both ends, in time they tend to resorb and loose the correction.

INFECTION

Perionychial infections of the subungual area are the most common infection in the hand. These are most frequently chronic fungal infections, although superimposed bacterial infections may occur[64] and are usually treated medically by dermatologists.[5,6,64] The medical treatment may require surgical removal of the nail to reach the subungual infection on occasion. After removal of an isolated nail, I have the patient apply 4 percent Mycolog with Vioform ointment twice a day to the nail bed until the nail has completely regrown. Griseofulvin or other systemic antifungal agents may also be used, if indicated.

Bacterial infections of the nail most commonly involve the paronychium. The dermal and epidermal layers of the paronychium are arranged in an overlapping fashion, much like the shingles of a house. When one of these layers is pulled up, an open wound (hangnail) is created. *Staphylococcus aureus* most frequently cause the infection. If the infection involves the paronychium but is above the nail, it can be drained by lifting the paronychium away from the nail, followed by soaks to encourage adequate drainage.

If the infection process and purulence has progressed beneath the edge of the nail (Fig. 33-24A), a portion of the nail must be removed to permit adequate drainage. The nail is dissected from the underlying nail bed and the overlying proximal eponychium with fine scissors or a periosteal elevator (Fig. 33-24B). The nail is then split longitudi-

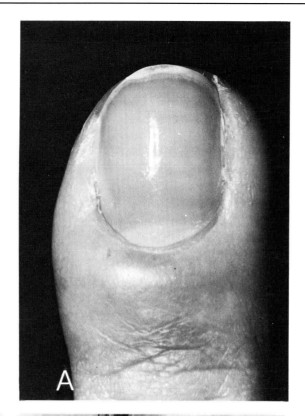

Fig. 33-24. (**A**) A paronychia of the left parony-chium, with pus extending beneath the nail. (**B**) A fine pair of iris scissors is used to elevate the side of the nail from the nail bed and the epo-nychium from the dorsum of the nail. (**C**) The loosened fragment of nail is then split longitudi-nally and removed from the nail fold. *(Figure continues.)*

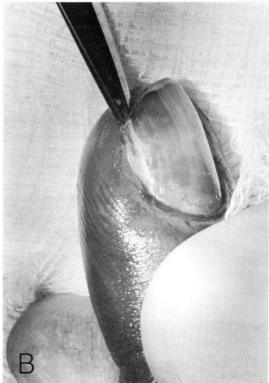

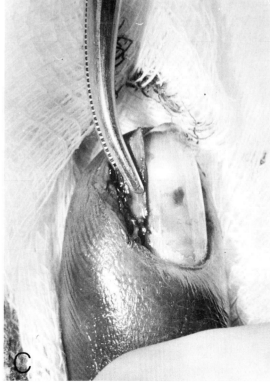

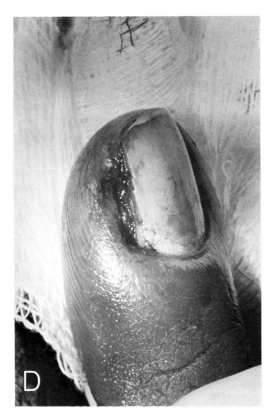
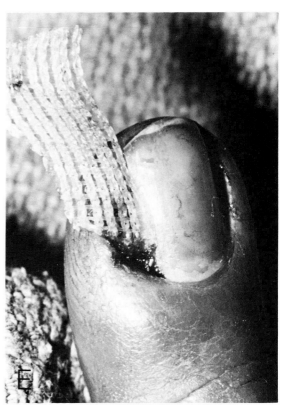

Fig. 33-24 *(Continued)*. **(D)** Adequate drainage of the paronychia after partial removal of the nail. **(E)** A small wick of gauze is used to promote drainage.

nally and the undermined portion removed to allow drainage (Fig. 33-24C–E). Adequate open drainage is maintained with soapy water soaks 3 to 4 times a day. Antibiotics are indicated if there is tissue cellulitis.

If the abscess dissects beneath the dorsal roof of the nail fold or beneath the nail in the nail fold, the proximal portion of the nail must be removed. The distal portion of the nail may be left in place to decrease discomfort.

In neither of these instances should incisions be made in the eponychium to drain the infection, in my opinion. The incision will frequently not heal primarily in the face of infection, and a notch or square corner in the eponychium may result. I have never seen a paronychia or a runaround that could not be adequately drained without incision in the eponychium.

Chronic paronychia usually occur between the nail and the dorsal roof of the nail fold. They are chronic in nature and are tender, erythematous, and swollen (Fig. 33-25A). The infection is most commonly caused by mixed gram negative organisms with an occasional fungus. The treatment is an arc-shaped excision of the dorsal roof of the nail fold that is allowed to heal secondarily, as described by Keyser and Eaton[38] (Fig. 33-25B and C). I have found this treatment to be generally successful (Fig. 33-25D).

Pyogenic granulomas manifest themselves as a rapidly growing lesion with a round red elevated area similar to granulation tissue growing through the nail (Fig. 33-26). They are usually the result of perforations of the nail by trauma or iatrogenic causes. The treatment is repeated silver nitrate cauterization or hyfurcation, but some nail deformity usually results. The differential diagnosis is squamous cell carcinoma or amelanotic melanoma.

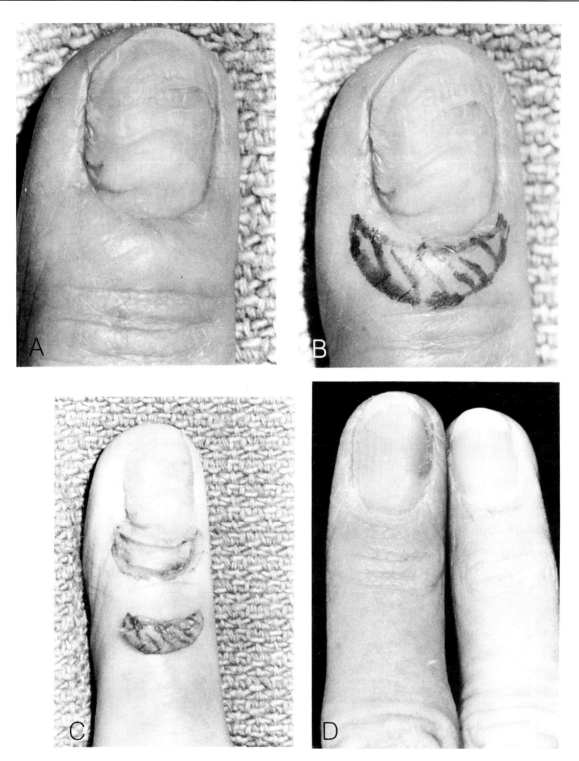

Fig. 33-25. (A) A chronic paronychia that has been present for 2 years. (B) The area on the dorsal roof is marked for excision. (C) The dorsal roof of the nail fold has been removed down to the nail. (D) The appearance 1 year postinjury with no further infection.

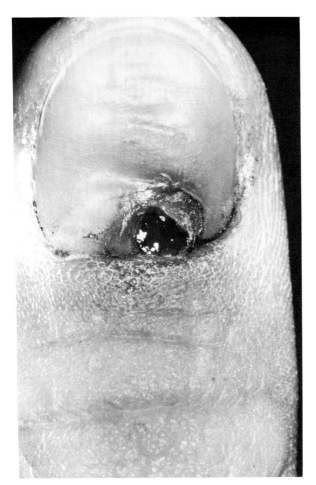

the nail bed might leave a nail deformity and so he recommended a watch and wait policy for at least the thumb and index finger. Clark and Fleegler (personal communication, 1985) now believe that the danger of malignant degeneration at puberty is significant, and they recommend nail bed biopsy prior to that time. If atypical cells are present, they recommend removal of the involved portion of the nail bed.

Bands of pigmentation may develop after trauma, particularly in black people with darkly pigmented skin. Areas of adult onset subungual pigment formation must be followed closely. If there is any question, a biopsy should be carried out. The most common differential diagnosis is subungual hematoma, even if no injury is known. In

Fig. 33-26. A pyogenic granuloma growing through the nail following perforation of the nail with cuticle scissors.

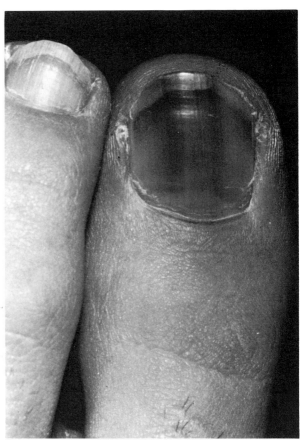

Fig. 33-27. A pigmented nevus of the large toenail present since birth that was biopsied at puberty and showed atypical melanocytes. The entire nail bed was excised.

BENIGN TUMORS

Subungual Nevi

Nevi of the nail bed are not uncommon. The nail produced by the nail bed involved by a pigmented nevus will be pigmented. Roughening of the nail surface usually does not occur, but elevation and ridging of the nail may (Fig. 33-27). A nevus is frequently present at birth or is noticed shortly thereafter and as years pass they may become lighter or darker in color. Samman[52] in 1938 remarked that if a dark streak was present at birth or shortly thereafter, removal of the nail and biopsy of

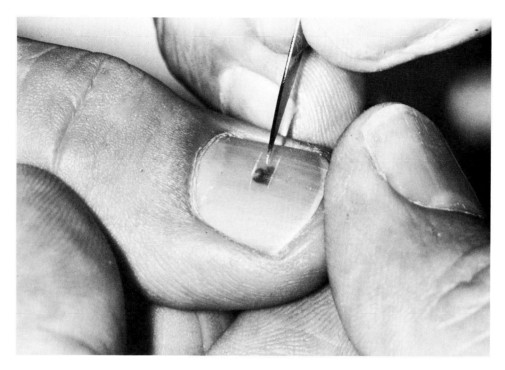

Fig. 33-28. Marking the nail over a pigmented area to measure change in relation with growth (see text).

this case, I make a cut into the surface of the nail at the proximal and distal borders of the pigmented area (Fig. 33-28). If the pigmentation is a hematoma, it will progress toward the free edge of the nail with the scratches. If the pigment is a foreign body, nevus, or melanoma in the nail bed, the scratches will progress distally away from the area of pigmentation enough in 3 weeks to make a determination.

Viral Warts (Verruca Vulgaris)

Viral warts, although not a common occurrence in the perionychium, are a significant cosmetic problem. Treatment with subsequent nail deformity and disfigurement has been frequent. Halpren and Lane[27] recommended treatment with monochloroacetic acid and 40 percent salicylic acid plaster as well as the use of 3 percent formalin. Removal of the nail may be necessary to allow treatment of the underlying warts. I have had some success with cauterizing perionychial warts with the CO_2 laser. One should err on the side of treat-

ing too superficially rather than too deeply, and therefore multiple applications of the laser may be necessary. For some unexplained reason, spontaneous remission of warts after application of the CO_2 laser to other warts may occur. Unfortunately, many patients seen by the hand surgeon have been treated unsuccessfully by other methods, creating sufficient scar tissue to make a return of the nail to normal after eradication of the wart impossible.

Ganglions (Mucous Cysts)

Ganglions are the most common tumors that deform the nail bed. They have been called clear cysts, mucous cysts, and other names.[45,65]

Kleinert[39] reported a communication between these cysts and the DIP joint in the area of an arthritic spur.

When the cystic expansion of the ganglion is between the floor of the nail fold and the periosteum, the upward pressure on the nail bed causes a ridge in the nail, a curve of the entire nail, or a ragged nail (Fig. 33-29). If the cyst is in the dorsal roof of the

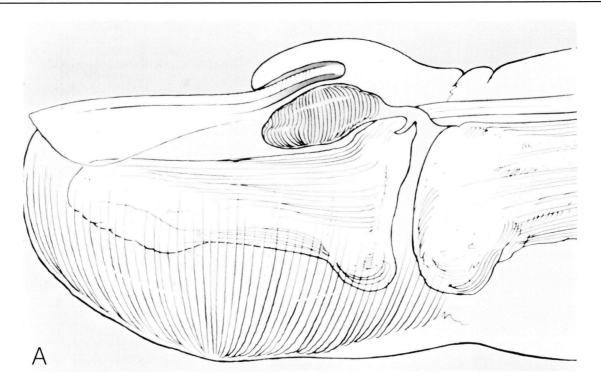

A

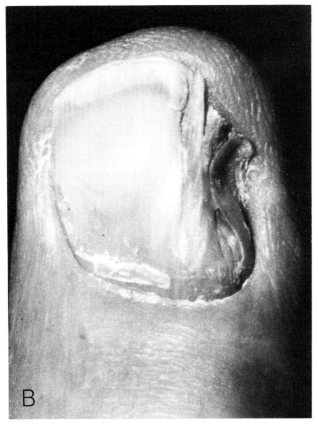

B

Fig. 33-29. (**A**) Dissection of a ganglion between the periosteum of the distal phalanx and the nail bed. (**B**) The typical deformity when the ganglion is located as shown in (**A**).

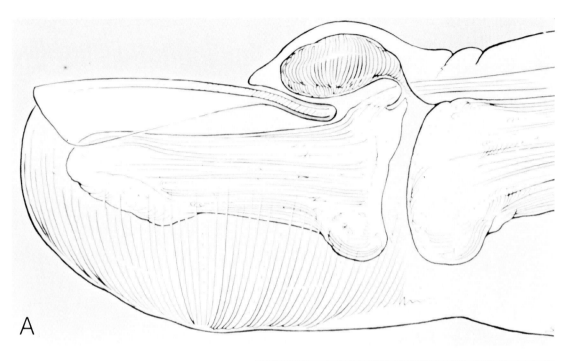

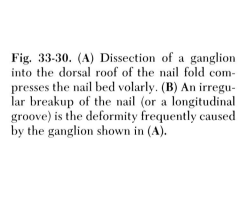

Fig. 33-30. (A) Dissection of a ganglion into the dorsal roof of the nail fold compresses the nail bed volarly. (B) An irregular breakup of the nail (or a longitudinal groove) is the deformity frequently caused by the ganglion shown in (A).

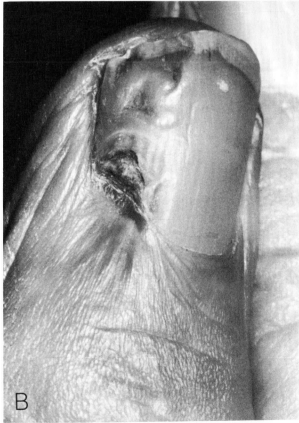

nail fold the pressure is downward on the nail, and a groove, thinning, or roughening may occur (Fig. 33-30).

Zaias[65] recommends intracystic steroid injections. Even if injection were to eliminate the cyst, the nail deformity maintains the nail bed in the deformed position, with the result that the cavity where the cyst was fills with scar tissue and at least to some degree perpetuates the deformity.

If there is a nail deformity, I believe that the best treatment is removal of the nail followed by resection of the ganglion through an incision over the DIP joint. Even if the skin over the ganglion is very thin, the ganglion can usually be resected without perforation of the skin. If the skin is perforated, it is draped over the defect and will rapidly heal. After the cyst is removed, I place a piece of 0.020-inch silicone sheet into the nail fold to flatten the nail bed back into its normal position. The joint osteophytes should be removed to prevent recurrence.

Ganglions occasionally rupture and drain through the nail fold or the overlying skin. If infection occurs, permanent nail deformity and limitation of joint motion may result. If the ganglion ruptures, the appropriate treatment is with antibiotics until the skin is closed, followed then by surgical removal before the ganglion reruptures. A draining ganglion should not be surgically resected while it is actively draining, since this may lead to subsequent joint infection and greater deformity.

Subungual Glomus Tumor

The glomus tumor first described in 1924 by Barre and Masson,[7] while greatly publicized, is rare. It is formed from the vasculo-musculo-neuro "glomus" elements of the nail bed that affect regulation of the blood flow.[16] Proliferation of this angiomatous tissue may cause pressure on the nerve plexuses and exquisite pain. The nail may be tender to pressure, and temperature changes (particularly cold) may cause pain. There may be a bluish discoloration beneath the nail in the area of the glomus. The entire nail bed should be carefully examined for multiple tumors after the nail is removed.

Treatment consists of removal of the nail, identification of the glomus tumor or tumors and surgical

excision. If the glomus is small and in the sterile matrix, the defect can be closed primarily. A split-thickness nail bed graft from another portion of the same nail or a toenail will be required for larger defects. A full-thickness sterile matrix graft from a toe can be used, but causes significant toenail deformity.

Resection will usually cause deformity if the glomus is in the germinal matrix. The defect may be closed primarily by using relaxing incisions in the lateral paronychial fold or by a free germinal matrix graft from a toe. In the nonscarred nail bed, relaxing incisions are much more successful than in post-traumatic deformities, such as the split nail discussed on page 1351.

Giant Cell Tumors (Nodular Synovitis)

Enlargement of this benign synovial tumor that arises distal to the DIP joint may cause pressure on the nail-forming elements, with resultant nail plate deformities. The treatment is complete resection of the tumor and removal of the nail plate to allow the nail bed to return to its original configuration.

MALIGNANT TUMORS

Basal Cell Carcinoma

Basal cell carcinoma is rare in the hand and even more so in the finger.[1,29] Complete resection of the tumor with frozen section examination of the margins to insure complete removal, is necessary even if the nail deformity is the result. Split-thickness skin graft coverage is usually necessary. Basal cell carcinomas most frequently occur after radiation exposure or other chronic problems of the nail bed, and some deformity of the nail is frequently present prior to resection. If the bone of the distal phalanx is involved, amputation at the DIP joint level is necessary.

Squamous Cell Carcinoma

Squamous cell carcinomas, although infrequent, are the most common malignant tumor of the perionychium and are commonly secondary to radiation exposure[1,13,56] (Fig. 33-31).

Squamous cell carcinomas are frequently misdiagnosed as paronychia, and the average length of time between appearance and treatment was 4 years in Carroll's series.[13] Squamous cell carcinomas are more common in males, and the thumb is the most frequently involved digit.[13] Dentists' hands are commonly involved due to their repeated radiation exposure.[56]

A perionychial squamous cell carcinoma with no bone involvement necessitates resection of the entire lesion with adequate margins, frequently re-

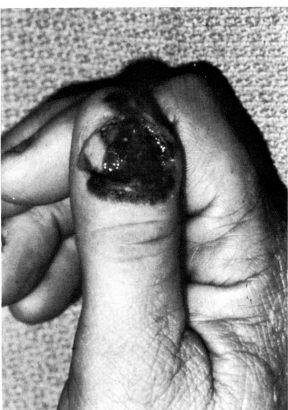

Fig. 33-32. A malginant melanoma of the nail bed.

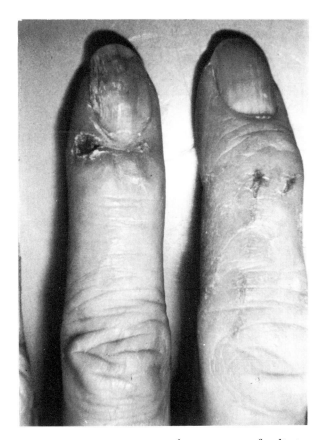

Fig. 33-31. A veterinarian with many years of radiation exposure to his fingers presented with a squamous cell carcinoma of the perionychium.

quiring a skin graft. If the carcinoma has a long existence, is large, or bony changes are present, amputation of the distal phalanx or even more proximally if necessary is indicated. Node dissection is indicated only if nodes do not disappear after amputation, since most nodal enlargements appear to be inflammatory.[20,56]

Subungual Melanoma

Melanomas of the hands and feet have a poorer prognosis than elsewhere on the body.[19] They are almost always pigmented with or without nail deformity (Fig. 33-32). Melanoma of the nail bed is frequently mimicked by other paronychial conditions, and the diagnosis may be delayed.[26] Pack and Orpeza[47] reported on subungual melanoma in 72 patients. Forty of these were of the fingernail and

32 were of the toenails. Almost two-thirds occurred in the thumb or large toe. Almost all of the patients had fair complexions, red or sandy hair, and blue or hazel eyes. Eighteen and one-half percent of the subungual melanomas occurred in blacks. Pigmented areas had been present beneath the nail for many years in 29 percent of their patients. Nodal involvement was present in 38.8 percent of the patients at the first visit, and at the time of resection, only 2 percent of patients did not have nodes containing melanoma.

The recommended treatment for stage I (local disease only) subungual melanoma is metacarpal or metatarsal ray amputation after the diagnosis is made.[26,47] Authors vary on the advisability of node dissection and timing of regional node dissection.[10,25] Pack and Orpeza[47] reported that patients with nonpalpable nodes but with microscopic evidence of tumor in resected nodes were found to have a cure rate twice that of individuals in whom node dissection was not done. They recommended amputation of the digit and node dissection when nodes are palpable. (See Chapter 60 for further discussion of melanomas.)

REFERENCES

1. Alport LI, Zak FG, Werthamer S: Subungual basal cell epithelioma. Arch Dermatol 106:595, 1972
2. Ashbell TS, Kleinert HK, Putcha S, Kutz JE: The deformed fingernail, a frequent result of failure to repair nail bed injuries. J Trauma 7:177–190, 1967
3. Baden HP: Regeneration of the nail. Arch Dermatol 91:619–620, 1965
4. Barfod B: Reconstruction of the nail fold. Hand 4:85–87, 1972
5. Baran R: Onychia and paronychia of mycotic, microbial and parasite origin. Chapter 6. In Pierre M (ed): The Nail. Churchill Livingstone, New York, 1981
6. Baran R, Zais N: The Nail In Health and Disease. SP Medical and Scientific Book, New York, 1980
7. Barre JA, Masson PV: Anatom-clinical study of certain painful subungual tumors (Tumors of the neuromyo-arterial glomus of the extremities). Bull Soc Frac de Dermat et Symph 31:148, 1924
8. Barron JN: The structure and function of the skin of the hand. Hand 2:93–96, 1970
9. Berson MI: Reconstruction of the index finger with nail transplantation. Surg 27:594–599, 1950
10. Booher RJ, Pack GT: Malignant melanoma of the feet and hands. Surg 42:1084, 1957
11. Boyes JH: Bunnell's Surgery of the Hand. 5th Ed., Philadelphia, JB Lippincott, 1970
12. Buncke HJ, Gonzalez RI: Fingernail reconstruction. J Plast Reconstr Surg 30:452–461, 1962
13. Carroll RE: Squamous cell carcinoma of the nail bed. J Hand Surg 1:92–97, 1976
14. Carter WW: Treatment for split fingernails. JAMA 90:1619–1620, 1928
15. Carter WW: Treatment of split fingernails. Med J Rec 131:599–600, 1930
16. Clark WE, Buxton LHD: Studies in nail growth. Br J Dermatol 52:21, 1938
17. Clark WE, LeGros, Buxton LHD: Studies in nail growth. Br J Dermatol 50:221–235, 1938
18. Clayburgh RH, Wood MB, Cooney WP: Nail bed repair and reconstruction by reverse dermal grafts. J Hand Surg 8:594–599, 1983
19. Day CL, Lew RA, Mihn MC, et al: A multi-variate analysis of prognotic factors for melanoma patients with lesions more than 3.65 millimeters in thickness. Ann Surg 195:44, 1982
20. Ellis VH: Squamous cell carcinoma of the nail bed. J Bone Joint Surg 30B:656–658, 1948
21. Ersek RA, Gadaria U, Denton DR: Nail bed avulsions treated with porcine xenografts. J Hand Surg 10A:152–153, 1985
22. Flatt AE: Nailbed injuries. Br J Plast Surg 8:38–43, 1955
23. Flatt AE: Minor hand injuries. J Bone Joint Surg 37B:117–125, 1955
24. Flynn IE: Hand Surgery. Williams & Wilkins, Baltimore, 1966
25. Fortner JG, Booher RJ, Pack GT: Results of groin dissection for malignant melanoma in 220 patients. Surg 55:485, 1964
26. Goldsmith HS: Melanoma: An overview. CA Cancer J. for Clinicians, 29:194–215, 1979
27. Halpern LK, Lane CW: Treatment of periungual warts. Missouri Medical, 50:765, 1953
28. Hanrahan EM: The split thickness skin graft as a cover following removal of a fingernail. Surg 20:398–400, 1946
29. Hashimoto H: Experimental study of histogenesis of the nail and its surrounding tissues. Niigato Med J 82:254, 1971
30. Hoffman S: Basal cell carcinoma of the nail bed. Arch Dermatol 108:828, 1973
31. Horner RL, Cohen BI: Injuries to the fingernail. Rocky Mt Med J 63:60–62, 1966
32. Iselin M: Avulsion injuries of the nail. Chapter 15. In

Pierre M (ed): The Nail. Churchill Livingstone, New York, 1981

33. Iselin M, Iselin F: Treatise on surgery of the hand. Medicales Flammarion, Paris, 1967

34. Johnson RK: Nailplasty. Plast Reconstr Surg 47:275–276, 1971

35. John HG: Primary skin cancer of the fingers stimulating chronic infection. Lancet 1:662, 1956

36. Jones FW: The Principles of Anatomy as Seen in the Hand. 2nd Ed., Bailliere, Tindall, and Cox, London, 1941

37. Kelsey JL, Pastides H, Kreiger N, Harris C, Chernow RA: Upper Extremity Disorders: A Survey of Their Frequency and Cost in the United States. CV Mosby, St Louis, 1980

38. Keyser JJ, Eaton RG: Surgical care of chronic paronychia by eponychial marsupialization. J Plast Reconstr Surg 58:66–70, 1976

39. Kleinert HE, Kutz JE, Fishman JH, McGraw LH: Etiology and treatment of the so-called mucous cyst of the finger. J Bone Joint Surg 54A:1455–1458, 1972

40. Kligman, AM: Why do nails grow out instead of up? Arch Dermatol 84:313–315, 1961

41. Lewis BL: Microscopic studies of fetal and mature nail and surrounding soft tissue. AMA Arch Dermatol 70:732–747, 1954

42. McCash, CR: Free nail grafting. Br J Plast Surg 8:19–33, 1956

43. Meskinen JK: The Official Rules. Ed. Dickson P, p.117 Delacorte Press, New York, 1978

44. Milford L: The Hand. CV Mosby, St Louis, 1971

45. Moss SH, Schwartz KS, von Drasek-Ascher G, Ogden LL, Wheeler CS, Lister GD: Digital venous anatomy. J Hand Surg 10A:473–482, 1985

46. Newmeyer WL, Kilgore ES: Common injuries of the fingernail and nail bed. Am Fam Physician 16:93–95, 1977

47. Pack GT, Orpeza R: Subungual melanoma. Surg Gynecol Obstet 124:751, 1967

48. Papavassiliou NP: Transplantation of the nail: A case report. Br J Plast Surg 22:274–280, 1969

49. Pardo-Castello V: Disease of the Nail. 3rd Ed. Charles C Thomas, Springfield, 1960

50. Rose EH: Nailplasty utilizing a free composite graft from the helical rim of the ear. J Plast Reconstr Surg 66:23–29, 1980

51. Saita H, Suzuki Y, Fujino K, Tajima T: Free nail bed graft for treatment of nail bed injuries of the hand. J Hand Surg 8:171–178, 1983

52. Samman PD: The Nails and Disease. 3rd Ed., Year Book Medical Publishers, Chicago, 1938

53. Sammon PD: The Nails in Disease. 2nd Ed., Charles C Thomas, Springfield, IL, 1972

54. Schiller C: Nail replacement in fingertip injuries. Plast Reconstr Surg 19:521–530, 1957

55. Seckel BR: Self advancing silicone rubber splint for repair of split nail deformity. J Hand Surg 11A:143–144, 1986

56. Shapiro L, Baraf CS: Subungual epidermoid carcinoma and keratoacanthoma. Cancer 25:141, 1970

57. Sheehan JE: Replacement of thumb nail. JAMA 92:1253–1255, 1929

58. Shepard GH: Treatment of nail bed avulsions with split thickness nail bed grafts. J Hand Surg 8:49–54, 1983

59. Shoemaker JV: Some notes on the nails. JAMA 15:427–428, 1890

60. Stone OJ, Mullins JF: The distal course of nail matrix hemorrhage. Arch Dermatol 88:186–187, 1963

61. Swanker WA: Reconstructive surgery of the injured nail. Am J Surg 74:341–345, 1947

62. Tajima T: Treatment of open crushing type of industrial injuries of the hand and forearm: Degloving, open circumferential, heat press and nail bed injuries. J Trauma, 14:995–1011, 1974

63. Weckesser EC: Treatment of Hand Injuries: Presentation and Restoration of Function. Year Book Medical Publishers, Chicago, 1974

64. Wilgis EFS, Maxwell GP: Distal digital nerve graft: Clinical and anatomical studies. J Hand Surg 4:439–443, 1979

65. Zaias N: The Nail. Spectrum Publishers, Jamaica, NY, 1980

66. Zook EG, Van Beek AL, Russell RC, Beatty ME: Anatomy and physiology of the perionychium: A review of the literature and anatomic study. J Hand Surg 5:528–536, 1980

67. Zook EG: The perionychium: Anatomy, physiology, and care of injuries. Clin Plas Surg 8:21–31, 1981

68. Zook EG: Injuries of the fingernail. In Green, DP (ed.): Operative Hand Surgery. New York, Churchill Livingstone, 1982

69. Zook EG: Fingernail injuries. In Strickland JW, Steichen JB (eds.): Difficult Problems in Hand Surgery. CV Mosby, St Louis, 1982

70. Zook EG, Guy RJ, Russell RC: A study of nail bed injuries: Causes, treatment and prognosis. J Hand Surg 9A:247–252, 1984

71. Zook EG: Nail bed injuries. Hand Clinics 1:701–716, November, 1985

72. Zook EG: Complications of the perionychium. Hand Clinics 2:407–427, May, 1986

Nerve Repair and Grafting 34

E. F. Shaw Wilgis

HISTORICAL REVIEW

The historical development of nerve repair and reconstruction came about during the past century. Although some ancient medical philosophers advised nerve repair, the concept of direct nerve repair was generally not accepted until after 1850.

From 1850 to 1900 vast discoveries were made in every phase of medical knowledge.[20] Nerve repair was attempted and regeneration was studied. Several authors postulated that a severed nerve should be repaired immediately. Paget in 1847 described an 11-year-old patient with a median nerve division and repair who made a complete recovery in 1 month. Marie Jean Pierre Flourens in 1828 reportedly transposed nerves of rooster wings, crossing the nerves of the extensor muscles to the flexors.[68]

In 1850, Augustus Waller presented his classic work that showed distal degeneration after nerve division. He worked with primitive equipment and first proposed the concept of Wallerian degeneration from his home laboratory. Waller's study on the glossopharyngeal and hypoglossal nerves of the frog showed not only distal degeneration, but also the orderly progress of regeneration down the preserved axis cylinder. He noted that the progress of regeneration was more rapid in the young, and that galvanic stimulation did not increase the speed of recovery.[7]

Many other investigators have contributed to the development of nerve repair. There was much duplication of information due to poor communication. However, in the development of knowledge, duplication enhances confirmation.

In the twentieth century the names of Tinel, Seddon, Woodhall, and Moberg were associated with major advances in nerve repair.

A positive consequence of past military conflicts has been the resulting expansion of medical knowledge. The medical demands for innumerable battle casualties and the available material for study have stimulated many discoveries. Fortunately, military physicians have used this opportunity to advance current knowledge of nerve repair and reconstruction. From his experiences during the Civil War, Weir Mitchell reported his observations on gunshot wounds and other injuries of the nerves. His article was first published in 1864 and included the first description of causalgia. Mitchell then expanded these studies and in 1872 published his classic, *Injuries of Nerves and Their Consequences.*

During World War I, Tinel in France and Hoffman in Germany studied the regeneration of repaired nerves, and in 1915 Tinel published his description of the regenerating nerve. He described pain as a sign of nerve irritation and tingling as a sign of regenerating axons. An interesting footnote of history is that after a great contribution in World War I, Tinel spent two years imprisoned during World War II for his work with the French underground.

However, other investigators were ready to carry on the tradition of Mitchell and Tinel. Sir Herbert Seddon, with the help of other British war surgeons, studied and reported on various traumatic lesions of the peripheral nervous system from the brachial plexus to the digital nerves.[71] The standards for all modern nerve repair and grafting procedures come from this work. Seddon continued his clinical work and research until his death in 1977.[64]

In the United States, Barnes Woodhall,[89] a great neurosurgeon, led American military surgeons in the area of peripheral nerve repair and reconstruction.[84] Both Woodhall and Seddon performed and studied bridge grafts, cable grafts, and primary and secondary repair. The principle of secondary nerve repair was advanced by these war studies and has remained a viable treatment alternative.

Sir Sidney Sunderland of Australia must be included in this historical account for his exhaustive study and detailed information on internal nerve anatomy. His work supports the modern concept of grouped fascicular repair and reconstruction.[76,77]

Erik Moberg, working in Göteborg, Sweden, and traveling extensively throughout the world, has detailed the evaluation of recovery of sensory function. He has demonstrated the importance of sensibility and its evaluation using two-point discrimination.[50,51]

Advances in nerve repair and grafting will continue to be made, and current investigators will be mentioned in future reviews as the quest for the perfect repair technique goes on.

ANATOMY AND TERMINOLOGY

Before repairing or grafting a damaged peripheral nerve, the detailed surgical anatomy of these structures must be appreciated. Some confusion exists concerning the types of repairs, due to a lack of conformity in the use of anatomic terminology. Sunderland has detailed the internal topography of all the peripheral nerves, and one must be familiar with his work before attempting to repair lacerated nerves.

In their passage from the spinal cord, motor, sensory, and sympathetic fibers contribute to the formation of the peripheral nerves. Spinal nerves from several segments in the spinal cord participate in plexus formations from which emerge the major peripheral nerves and the limbs. In these plexuses, the motor and sensory fibers from the spinal cord and the sympathetic fibers from the gangulated trunk are intermingled and rearranged. These fibers do not run independent courses as single units, but are collected into funiculi, or fascicles, that are bound together by connective tissue surrounded by blood vessels and lymphatics.[75,77] The cross-sectional anatomy is depicted in Figure 34-1.

Perineurium

A fascicle is a bundle of nerve fibers surrounded by a thin sheath of connective tissue, the perineurium. Each fascicle may contain motor, sensory, or sympathetic fibers in various numbers. The number and size of the fascicles may vary in any given nerve and along the course of the nerve.

There are three concentric zones or layers of the perineurium that have been identified, and these layers are responsible for the physiological action of this structure. The thickness of the perineurium can range from 1.3 to 100μ, and there is a relationship between the diameter of the fascicle and the thickness of the perineurial sheath. There are several functional considerations of the perineurium.

First, the perineurium serves to protect the nerve fibers within its boundaries. The perineurium also maintains an intrafascicular pressure, which is important in promoting the proximal to distal flow of the axoplasm. In areas where the perineurium is relatively thicker (i.e., over joints), such an arrangement affords greater protection to the nerve fibers during joint motion. The perineurium also serves to protect the nerve fiber from stretch injury, and the elastic properties and integrity of a nerve undergoing elongation are retained as long as the perineurium remains intact.[74] The perineu-

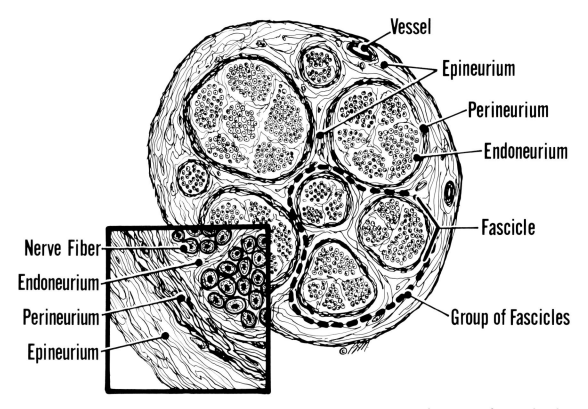

Fig. 34-1. Cross-sectional anatomy of a peripheral nerve.

rium acts as a diffusion barrier; this is particularly true of its intermesothelial lining, which blocks the passage of a wide range of macromolecular substances, from the epineurium to the contents of the fascicle and vice versa. The lining also restricts the movement of endoneurial fluid from the fascicle, thereby slowing the elimination of endoneurial edema. There is evidence that serum proteins may be transported across the barrier by the pinocytotic activity of the perineurial cells. Rupture of the perineurial sheath has serious consequences for the contained nerve fibers in that the fibers lose their conduction properties, whereas the removal of the epineurium, as in neurolysis, is not harmful. Finally, the perineurium is a barrier to the spread of infection.

Endoneurium

The endoneurium is the supporting connective tissue that fills the fascicle. This tissue provides the packing between individual nerve fibers. The only vessels found in the endoneurium are capillaries; there are no intrafascicular lymphatics. The endoneurium has a special relationship to the nerve fibers in which the collagen fibrils are closely packed around each nerve fiber to form the supporting wall of what is conveniently referred to as an *endoneurial tube*, which is occupied by a cylinder of tissue comprising the axon, Schwann's cell sheath, and the myelin.

The main functional consideration of the endoneurium is that it resists elongation under tension and thereby protects the delicate nerve fiber.

Epineurium

In studying the cross-sectional area of peripheral nerve trunks, Sunderland has concluded that the percentage of cross-sectional area of the nerve trunk devoted to fascicles varies irregularly along the nerve, from nerve to nerve, and from individual to individual.[73] However, individual nerves — median, ulnar, and radial — present regional differences and peculiarities in this regard. Approximately 25 to 75 percent of the cross-sectional area of a nerve trunk is composed of fascicular (nerve) tissue.[79] The remainder is connective tissue, either epineurium or perineurium. As a protective mechanism, nerves contain more connective tissue where they cross joints. The epineurium, therefore, can account for 25 to 75 percent of the cross-sectional area of a given peripheral nerve. In the diseased state, however, the epineurium may indeed be thickened. The epineurium, being collagen tissue, also responds to damage and will react with collagen deposition during the repair process. In doing peripheral nerve surgery, especially repair and grafting of peripheral nerves, one must keep in mind the fact that the epineurium comprises much of the cross-sectional area of the nerve, and recognize the inevitable response of the epineurium to injury. The epineurium is the areolar connective tissue that separates the fascicles and also binds them loosely together. This connective tissue structure is condensed at the surface of the nerve to form a definitive investing sheath. The sheath then delineates the nerve from surrounding structures to which it is loosely attached so that the nerve trunk enjoys considerable mobility in its bed. When a nerve is related to an artery, the epineurium is securely attached to the vessel, and there is an investing sheath around the neurovascular bundle.

The functional consideration of the epineurium is that the particular arrangement allows the nerve to lengthen without the fascicles being strained. The epineurium also protects the fascicles by providing the packing around it.

Finally, one must remember that the ultimate responsibility of the epineurium is to respond to injury with proliferation of collagen.

Fascicles (Funiculi)

A fascicle is a group of nerve fibers or axons surrounded by perineurial connective tissue. Each fascicle may contain motor, sensory, or sympathetic fibers in varying numbers; but as they approach the target organs, they become more pure in their arrangement of motor or sensory fibers. The fascicles coursing through the internal epineurium seem to arrange themselves in groups. This pseudoanatomic grouping plays an important role in modern nerve repair. These *groups of fascicles* remain constant over a long stretch of the nerves and may contain varying numbers of smaller fascicles; e.g., one large and several small, or several small, or one large fascicle. In the peripheral region near the target organ, the motor fascicles tend to group themselves into a definable bundle. Sunderland has studied this concept of fascicular grouping. Millesi has based his interfascicular nerve grafting procedure on this concept of groups of fascicles. Jabaley, Wallace, and Heckler,[30] and more recently, Chow,[12] have illustrated this anatomical concept in dissections of peripheral nerves. They point out that the anatomical grouping of fascicles can be traced for long distances throughout the course of the median and ulnar nerves in the wrist and forearm. Sunderland pointed out that there is cross-migration of nerve fibers from one fascicle to another and that fascicular plexuses form throughout the course of the nerve. This is particularly true of the proximal nerves, such as the musculocutaneous nerve. The majority of this cross-branching occurs within the fascicular group to which the fascicle belongs. When attempting nerve repair, particularly repair in which fascicular structures are matched, one should have a detailed knowledge of the cross-sectional appearance of the nerves, as depicted by Sunderland. The bundle of fascicles or bundle-group, representing a branching system of fascicles, may alter its position in the nerve trunk without scattering fascicles to other bundle groups, so that transverse sections taken centimeters apart will show the fascicular group in different positions in the nerve. Knowledge of the cross-sectional anatomy of each nerve at all levels in the extremity, prior to repair, is of paramount importance because one should constantly try to match fascicular groups. The true significance of fascicular plexuses and the internal cross-branching is not truly known, but is thought to be a product of mesenchymal condensations that occur during development, regardless of the destination and function of the fibers.

It is important to re-emphasize that most cross-branching occurs between fascicles of the same fascicular group, although there is some cross-branching between the fascicles of different fascicular groups. Thus, when considering nerve repair and grafting, the fascicular group concept should be kept in mind and the matching of fascicular groups in the proximal and distal ends is of paramount importance. If one maintains a knowledge of the cross-sectional anatomy, then the chances of matching fascicular groups between the proximal and distal stumps of the nerve are better, even when bridging a gap.

In summary, detailed knowledge of the anatomy of the nerve is important. The anatomy changes as the nerve courses from the shoulder to the fingertips. The basic structure of the fascicle branches in the fascicular plexuses and travels throughout the nerve in various locations. The fascicles seem to be grouped into bundles that course through the loose epineurial matrix to form the peripheral nerve as we know it. The anatomic and functional characteristics of the perineurium, which lines each fascicle, and the epineurium, which surrounds and binds together the fascicles and groups of fascicles, and finally invests the entire nerve as the organizing connective tissue element within the peripheral nerve trunk, are anatomic details that must be considered when faced with the repair of a peripheral nerve.

Longitudinal Excursion of Nerves

During limb movement, the peripheral nerve must accommodate to changes in the length of its bed. The longitudinal excursion of the nerve during motion has been recently studied in several ways. McLellan and Swash[45] recorded action potentials in the median nerve before and during active and passive motion of the limb. They found that active and passive movement had equal effects. The greatest excursion was produced by extension of the wrist and fingers and by flexion of the elbow. Extension of the wrist and fingers causes an excursion of 7.4 mm; flexion of the elbow, 4.3 mm. They estimated that hyperextension of the wrist caused the median nerve to have an excursion of 10 to 15 mm. They also found that displacement of the median nerve during flexion of the wrist and fingers was 2 to 4 times greater at the wrist than in the upper arm. Dellon, McKinnon, and Pestronk[18] postulated that the radial sensory nerve had a sig-

nificant excursion on radial and ulnar deviation of the wrist. Wilgis and Murphy,[87] using 15 fresh intact adult cadaver arms, dissected the entire peripheral nerve system and studied the longitudinal excusion of these nerves. They found that the brachial plexus had an average excursion of 15 mm when ranged in the frontal plane with the arm in full abduction as compared to full adduction in relation to the body. The median and ulnar nerves at the elbow moved an average of 7.3 and 9.8 mm respectively with full motion. The greatest excursion of the peripheral nerves occurred at the wrist proximal to the carpal tunnel. Here the median and ulnar nerves had 15.5 and 14.8 mm of longitudinal sliding, respectively, with the wrist ranged through a full arc of flexion and extension in the sagittal plane. These studies are consistent with the studies of McLellan and Swash.[45] In the palm and digits, the excursion was considerably less. In summarizing the amount of motion of the median nerve and the digital nerves at the wrist and fingers, one sees that the excursion of this component approaches 2 cm.

When considering the repair of a divided peripheral nerve, the surgeon must consider not only the internal elastic tension of the nerve, but also the necessities for longitudinal excursion during limb movement. For example, the normal retraction of the median nerve at the level of the wrist is 1.5 cm after a clean division. If one then adds the 1.5 cm of longitudinal excursion needed when taking the wrist from full flexion to full extension, the immediate demands for appropriate length of the nerve become apparent. In the acute situation, when the nerve can be brought together and approximated under normal tension, one would expect the normal amount of longitudinal excursion to occur once the local scarring factors had subsided. However, in the secondary situation, the conditions are different. The nerve has lost its normal elasticity because of injury and subsequent scarring. It therefore cannot be approximated under normal tension and maintain normal excursion without acute flexion of an adjacent joint. In other words, the length of the nerve substance has been shortened because of the injury. Because of this overall shortening, excursion cannot take place. If the nerve is sutured under tension with the wrist in acute flexion, there is no way the nerve can slide to its appropriate and normal distance when the adjacent joint is taken into the opposite mode of action from the position in which it was placed for the acute repair. The already existing gap between the two ends is effectively increased because of the excursion factor. For instance, if one approaches a secondary repair of the median nerve at the wrist, and the existing gap after resection of a neuroma is 2 cm, one must also consider that there is an additional 1.5 cm that must be present in order to accommodate the nerve's need for longitudinal excursion. This, then, makes a realistic gap of 3.5 cm, which may cause the surgeon to choose an alternative method of bridging the gap, such as nerve grafting. At the elbow, the excursion need can be met by transposing the ulnar nerve anteriorly, thereby reducing its need for longitudinal excursion and bridging the gap.

This aspect of nerve anatomy in its dynamic state must be understood and taken into account by the surgeon approaching repair of a peripheral nerve.

TIMING OF REPAIR

There are many factors that influence a decision regarding the time of repair of a damaged peripheral nerve. These factors include the metabolic and structural changes that occur in the central cell, as well as the proximal and distal nerve trunk, the muscle cell, and the sensory end organ. Other factors that must be considered are the condition of the patient, the condition of the wound, and associated injuries.

Metabolic Changes in the Nerve

Following acute transection of a peripheral nerve, the central nerve cell body progressively enlarges within 4 to 20 days. Enlargement persists as long as there is active regeneration; then the nerve slowly returns to normal size when conduction matures. This nerve cell body enlargement results from an increased metabolism, resulting in an increase in the total amount of protein in the cell body. These proteins in turn migrate through the cell's axon to the site of injury, where they are used

in axonal regeneration. Ducker, Kempe, and Hayes[19] have postulated that on the basis of these metabolic changes most nerve repairs should be carried out in the second to third week after injury, when the changes are at their peak activity. There have been no clinical studies to date to support this hypothesis. In the proximal nerve stump, there is a marked swelling within 1 hour of nerve division, from the point of severance proximally for a distance of approximately 1 cm. The cross-sectional area of the nerve increases approximately three times. This swelling consists of both intra- and extracellular edema, mostly a gel-like amorphous substance that contains a large quantity of acid mucopolysaccharides. It persists for 1 week or more and subsides slowly thereafter. Within 2 to 3 days after the nerve transection, there are signs of demarcation of the nerve stump or healing over of the open end of the neuron. After 7 days there is vigorous sprouting of the axon. In blast injuries the axonal sprouting may be 1, 2, or 3 cm proximal to the point of the actual severed end. In a clean section it is just a few millimeters proximal to the last intact node of Ranvier. The onset of this budding and regeneration occurs concomitantly with the anabolic hypertrophic phase of the cell body in the spinal cord or dorsal ganglion. Theoretically, it would be nice to have the distal stump prepared and ready for the maximum axonal regeneration to cross the anastomotic site.

The neuronal elements within the distal nerve trunk following division are separated from their trophic centers and die. The distal nerve trunk undergoes a series of changes that end in Wallerian degeneration. Wallerian degeneration is initiated because of neuronal death. After injury, digestive enzymes are present in the axonal segments. These axonal segments may isolate themselves in small units and can survive up to 2 weeks, but the majority of neuronal elements break down in 1 week. The surrounding myelin then fragments and is digested by Schwann's cells. By 3 weeks the majority of this cellular debris is phagocytosed by metabolically active Schwann's cells. By 6 weeks the natural debridement is complete. The fascicular anatomy persists and the endoneurial sheaths shrink and the tubes close. In time, the shrinkage becomes irreversible and minimizes the chances of regeneration. The mesenchymal elements are in part dependent on the nerve fibers to maintain anatomic and metabolic existence.

Muscle Cell Changes

The muscle cells are also metabolically dependent on the central nerve cell. After nerve injury, when the muscles no longer receive repeated stimuli, the cells shrink, endomysium and perimysium thicken, and the muscle spindles atrophy. These events begin in 3 to 4 months in animals and somewhat later in humans, and after 2 years the muscle fibers may fragment and disintegrate. These changes take place in the muscles progressively, in spite of extrinsic electrical stimulation or other physical modalities. The denervation atrophy of the muscle can only be halted by reinnervation, when stimuli from the nerve results in the improved metabolism of the muscle cell. The thickening of the muscle sheath hinders end plate formation, and because of the fibrous tissue formation around the end plate, the thickening interferes with the nerve regrowth and muscle contraction. Thus, the sooner a nerve establishes connection to the muscle cells, the more likely it is that the metabolism and anatomy of the muscle cell will be normal. If reinnervation is delayed for 1 year, function can at best be extremely poor. A delay of 18 to 24 months allows irreversible changes to take place in the muscle cells; any hope of motor return at that time is essentially nonexistent.[6]

Sensory End Organs

The sensory end organs, however, survive without nerve innervation. One study from World War II showed that there was no correlation from the time of injury to nerve repair in the ultimate sensory recovery.[53] We have had cases with varied delayed recovery of protective sensibility following nerve suture after more than 1 year of nerve division. However, the surgeon must realize that protective sensibility is the best result that can be achieved after a long delay. The quality of sensation is greatly dependent on the ability of the brain to decode the messages that are being received from the sensory end organs. These messages are altered because of the altered innervation. Young

people, because of natural central reorganization powers, can accomplish this change; older people may need sensory retraining.

Condition of the Patient

Another factor influencing the timing of repair is the condition of the patient. Nerve repair is an exacting operative undertaking, and ideal operating conditions, including a well patient, are mandatory. An intoxicated patient who can neither be adequately studied preoperatively nor reliably anesthetized is not a candidate for primary neurorrhaphy. A patient with serious systemic illness must also be approached with some caution.

Condition of the Wound

The condition of the wound is another factor that must be considered. Skin loss, vascular insufficiency and skeletal stability must be dealt with prior to nerve repair. In acutely injured patients, one must assure adequate skin coverage, have a viable extremity from a vascular standpoint, and have skeletal stability by either internal or external fixation prior to considering nerve repair. The nerve itself must not be damaged to the extent that the surgeon is unable to determine the degree of injury. Faced with a sharply cut nerve, the damaged ends can be seen and approximated; presented with a severely crushed or avulsed nerve, the damage may extend proximally and distally for quite some distance from the actual nerve division. In this case it is perhaps better to effect a secondary approach to the nerve.

Satisfactory secondary nerve repair can only be accomplished in a bed of healthy, well-vascularized tissue with a minimum of fibrosis and scar formation. It is preferable that the neurorrhaphy be surrounded by healthy muscle, fat, or a clean gliding surface rather than by scarred subcutaneous tissue. Adherence of a repaired nerve to moving tendons or to cutaneous scar may not only interfere with axonal regrowth but may stimulate abnormal collagen formation around the neuroma and lead to paresthesias and dysesthesia, which can present more of a problem to the patient than the lack of nerve function. Application of a muscle pedicle flap or local rotation flap may be helpful, or the nerve may have to be moved to a different location to avoid these problems.

Primary versus Secondary Nerve Repair

With due consideration given to all of the above factors, I believe that the earlier the nerve suture is done, the better are the chances of motor and sensory return. A primary neurorrhaphy is defined as the repair of a lacerated nerve performed soon after injury. A primary neurorrhaphy can be done immediately after injury or within 5 to 7 days. A secondary neurorrhaphy is one in which the repair is done after many of the metabolic and anatomic changes have taken place following the injury. Secondary neurorrhaphy always involves recutting the nerve and removing the neuroma. In short, the secondary neurorrhaphy creates another primary situation in more nearly ideal circumstances. It is agreed that secondary neurorrhaphy under favorable circumstances will give better results than a primary neurorrhaphy under unfavorable circumstances. However, it appears to me that a primary neurorrhaphy under favorable circumstances will give even better results.[24,25] I recommend performing primary neurorrhaphy when presented with the following conditions: (1) a clean, sharply incised nerve with no element of crush; (2) minimal contamination; (3) no associated injuries precluding skeletal stability, adequate circulation, or skin cover; (4) an appropriate operating staff with facilities for magnification[67]; and (5) a patient who is in suitable condition to undergo surgery. If primary neurorrhaphy is not done, then tying the ends together at the time of the initial wound care will minimize retraction of the ends and allow the nerve to assume its normal tension.

On the other hand, it is far better to delay nerve suture until these conditions can be met than to have an inadequate primary suture done. The reason for this is that once a suture is done, it will take many months before the surgeon can decide to re-explore the nerve suture site, determine whether to excise the neuroma, and then do a nerve graft or perform a neurolysis. Therefore, the initial decision must be undertaken with a great deal of thought. There is no room in nerve surgery for the concept "we will repair this and see how it does because we can always redo it." The first job must be the best job.

TYPES OF REPAIR AND TECHNIQUES

When choosing a method of nerve repair, the surgeon should be familiar with the many techniques available. Depending on the individual nerve lacerated and the level of injury in the extremity, there may be an indication for one of several repairs.

Primary Repair

If primary repair has been chosen, there are essentially four different techniques that can be employed: epineurial repair, fascicular repair, grouped fascicular repair, or a mixed repair, involving one or more of the above methods.

EPINEURIAL REPAIR

The technique of epineurial repair has been the traditional method. Any nerve repair can be enhanced with the use of magnification, either magnifying loupes or the operating microscope. I personally use magnification on every nerve repair. In performing the epineurial suture technique in the primary situation, the surgeon must first cut back the nerve ends until all visible signs of damage have been debrided. This then leaves the nerve with the fascicles mushrooming from the end, and the epineurium is slightly retracted. The goal of the epineurial repair is to establish continuity without tension and in the proper rotational alignment. The nerve should be inspected for longitudinal blood vessels in the epineurium that can be aligned. Also, the fascicular arrangement should be noted and matched with the two ends of the divided nerve. This then assures appropriate rotational alignment. The neurorrhaphy is carried out using nonabsorbable suture. I recommend 8-0 nylon in larger nerves and 10-0 nylon in small nerves, such as digi-

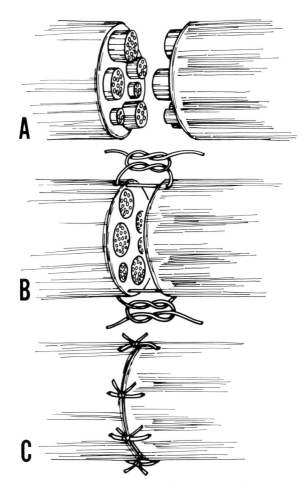

Fig. 34-2. Primary or secondary epineurial repair.

If the nerve cannot be brought together with an 8-0 nylon suture, I consider the tension to be excessive, and either further mobilization or a secondary procedure should be done. The nerve should be turned over and the posterior aspect sutured in a similar fashion. There should be no fascicles protruding between the suture lines.

FASCICULAR REPAIR

The technique of primary fascicular repair is depicted in Figure 34-3. I believe that fascicular sutures should be reserved for nerves with few fascicles, such as the digital nerve in the finger.[10] Other nerves, such as the ulnar nerve at the elbow, can be repaired with fascicular suture technique because, according to Sunderland,[76] the ulnar nerve in the region of the elbow has only three or four large fascicles, and these can be appropriately sutured. Therefore, I must reiterate that knowledge of the

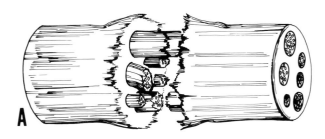

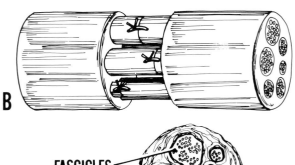

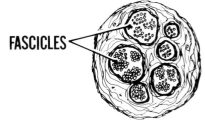

Fig. 34-3. Primary fascicular, or funicular, repair.

tal nerves. The nylon is passed through the epineurium proximally and distally and tied (Fig. 34-2). The surgeon must remember that the epineurium should not be closed so tightly that the fascicular ends become totally mismatched and malaligned. It is much better to have a small gap in the epineurium held together by a suture, with the fascicular ends in a more appropriate alignment. Therefore, the suture should not be tied tightly, and should be there only as a guiding suture, not as a retention suture. The second suture should be placed opposite the first suture, and then the epineurium should be closed by halving the distance on the anterior and posterior sides of the nerve. The number of sutures used should be as few as possible to adequately assure the approximation of the nerve.

anatomy throughout the course of the extremity is important. In my opinion, a nerve with many fascicles, such as the median nerve in the proximal forearm, should not be sutured with fascicular suture technique because the margin of error in being able to match up each fascicle to the proper fascicle on the distal end is too great.

In performing fascicular technique, the cut ends of the nerve are freshened back to noninjured tissue. The cross-sectional anatomy is then inspected proximally and distally and the fascicular pattern noted. The cut ends of the fascicles are then sutured together with interrupted sutures of 10-0 nylon, using the operating microscope. The suture is placed through the interfascicular epineurium and the perineurium of the individual fascicle.[2,82] Individual dissection of the fascicles tends to confuse the situation from an anatomic standpoint and, physiologically, will cause more scarring in the nerve juncture area. There is no tension allowed in the fascicular suture technique, and if the sutured ends cannot be held together with 10-0 nylon, perhaps another method should be used.

GROUPED FASCICULAR REPAIR

A potentially more accurate technique is the grouped fascicular repair. In this method, I employ the anatomic dissections of Sunderland[76] and Millesi's concepts[47,48] and group a number of fascicles together for matching. Again, the nerve ends must be matched by resecting damaged tissue, followed by a careful analysis of the anatomic cross-sectional appearance of the nerve. Fascicular groups should then be drawn out and dissected and the groups of fascicles joined by interfascicular epineurial suture. In the median nerve at the forearm level it is possible that five groups of fascicles will be found; in the ulnar nerve at the wrist, approximately four. In this technique the margin of error is reduced considerably in that axons remaining in the same groups of fascicles will cross the juncture and reinnervate the appropriate area. The interfascicular anatomic arrangement of the nerve is thus preserved better than with a fascicular repair.

FASCICULAR IDENTIFICATION

In performing any of the above types of repair, proper fascicular identification is mandatory. Several techniques have been proposed. Hakstian,[27] Jabaley,[30] and Gaul[21] have proposed using electrical stimulation to aid in the identification of the fascicular structure. Intraoperative nerve stimulation can be helpful in identifying specific motor and sensory bundles. For about 3 or 4 days after injury, stimulation of distal motor branches will generate a response in the appropriate muscle. Stimulation of the proximal stump will then allow precise matching of the motor fascicles and the appropriate groups of sensory fascicles. After these 3 or 4 days, distal motor branches can only be identified with certainty by directly dissecting them from the main nerve. Jabaley reports that in secondary repairs, experience with stimulation of the unanesthetized proximal nerve end in the awake patient has proven helpful.[30] The patient must be carefully coached and well prepared so that he can distinguish between motor and sensory stimulation. He can also identify specific sensory bundles and associate them with appropriate cutaneous territories. Identification of the motor fascicles in the distal stump can sometimes be done by direct stimulation and observing the appropriate muscle action. This motor response will be present in the acute situation and will last for 3 or 4 days. However, once Wallerian degeneration takes place, there will be no motor response in the distal stump. In the proximal stump, identification of the motor fascicles will elicit no sensory response from the patient. In other words, if a fascicle is stimulated and there is no sensory identification, this fascicle must be a motor fascicle by process of elimination. This is useful in the forearm, wrist, and hand. In the more proximal arm, localization becomes less precise and stimulation is of limited value. To perform this technique, the patient must be well prepared and coached in the preoperative state. The operation must be performed under a local anesthetic and the nerve ends very carefully and precisely stimulated to obtain the appropriate response from the patient.

A second aid in the proper identification of fascicles is the use of histochemical reactions and staining techniques. Gruber and Feilinger[26] reported histochemical differentiation between motor and sensory nerve fibers using acetylcholinesterase staining techniques. Carbonic anhydrase activity can be used for fascicular staining as well, as reported by Riley and Lang.[57] This histochemical method can be accomplished within 3 to 4 hours after receiving the tissue. The main objection to the staining techniques is that it takes some time for the staining effect to be useful to the surgeon. In the acetylcholinesterase stain, at least 12 hours is required, which makes the repair a two-stage procedure. The carbonic anhydrase stain takes 3 to 4 hours, which makes it possible to be accomplished in one operation if the neuroma is resected, the stain done, and other reconstructive work done before the nerve is sutured.

However, these staining techniques are in their infancy and are not readily clinically applicable at this time because of the delay between doing the stain and obtaining the information.

AUTHOR'S PREFERRED METHOD

I prefer to use a combination of the above types of repairs applied to a given area in the extremity. For instance, the ulnar nerve at the elbow is composed of approximately four fascicles. A fascicular repair would be the appropriate repair here. When faced with division of the ulnar nerve at the wrist, I would prefer to do a fascicular repair of the motor branch and then a grouped fascicular repair of the sensory branches, supported by an epineurial repair of the sensory component of the nerve. In the median nerve, I prefer to do a grouped fascicular repair of the fascicles to the motor branch and then a loose epineurial repair of the remainder of the sensory nerve (Fig. 34-4). I would like to emphasize that strict adherence to one type of repair or

another is not useful in peripheral nerve surgery. I believe that the surgeon should have all of the techniques in his armamentarium and use them in the appropriate situations. The anatomic arrangement of the nerve differs considerably throughout the extremity, and the surgeon must customize the nerve repair for the anatomic arrangement as he finds it. In my opinion, it is desirable to match, on a fascicular or grouped fascicular basis, motor nerves with motor nerves; and it is inappropriate to proceed with intricate interneural dissection as this causes more scarring that will ultimately detract from the results of nerve surgery.

Secondary Repair

There are several factors to be considered when faced with a secondary repair. First, the nerve ends have to be sectioned back to good nerve tissue. This then leaves a gap to be bridged. Because of the tension required to close the defect, I believe that there is very little chance for either grouped fascicular or fascicular repair in the secondary situation. The standard suture employed in secondary repair is the epineurial suture, which was popularized by Seddon and was used traditionally in the post–World War II era.[93,94] In freshening the nerve ends one must be sure to remove enough of the scar tissue so that appropriate axonal regeneration will occur. This can be done by either visually examining the cut ends of the nerve under magnification or even doing frozen sections to make sure that the epineurial thickening is not so severe that axonal regrowth will not occur.

Once the proximal and distal ends have been resected, a gap exists that may be from 1.5 to 5 cm. Usually a gap of 4 cm can be overcome by local mobilization of the nerve ends. The surgeon must remember that the price paid for extensive mobilization of nerve ends is destruction of the collateral blood supply of the nerve. Neviaser and others found that mobilization of the proximal nerve end was not as damaging as mobilization of the distal segment.[65,69] Nicholson and Seddon found that extensive mobilization of the median nerve of the forearm impaired recovery somewhat.[52] Zachary has demonstrated that the median nerve can be mobilized 7 to 9 cm, the ulnar nerve a similar distance, and, when anterior transposition is added, as much as 13 cm of ulnar nerve gap can be bridged.[94]

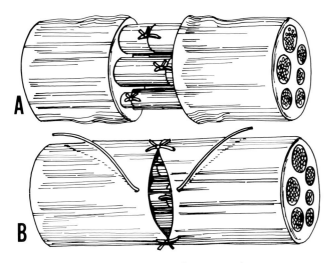

Fig. 34-4. Mixed fascicular and epineurial repair.

The radial nerve can be mobilized 8 cm. At the limits of mobilization, joints proximal and distal to the nerve suture can be flexed.

A third method of overcoming the gap is bone shortening, which I find to be radical and probably unjustified, except in the most rare circumstances. We must realize, then, that there is a limit to mobilization and closure of gaps. Highet and Holmes found that when large gaps had been closed, recovery did not take place. This was investigated experimentally, and it was found that the failure was due to extensive scarring of the nerve very similar to that in a traction injury.[28] Extensive stretching of a nerve had devascularized it. It seems logical, then, that an operation that is technically possible can be nonetheless undesirable and that there is a biological limit for the closure of large gaps that is stricter than the anatomic limit. It is my policy not to extensively mobilize nerves or flex joints to close gaps greater than 4 cm. In our experience nerve recovery has been better by using other techniques, such as interfascicular grafting, rather than by attempting heroic measures to overcome large gaps. The ultimate answer to this question, however, is not found in the literature. The case for primary or secondary repair with funicular suture can only be proved by controlled clinical trials. The type of injury must be uniform. The age range must be similar, and to date this clinical information is not available. However, based on our personal experience, I have adopted the policy that recovery following closure of gaps greater than 4 cm is not satisfactory and that other measures should be employed.

NERVE GRAFTING

In the previous section, I have recommended nerve grafting for gaps of 4 cm or more. Other authors, including Millesi, have recommended grafting for gaps of 2.5 cm or more.[46] Seddon recommended nerve grafting for "large gaps" of nerves.

There are three types of available nerve grafts:

heterograft, homograft, and autograft. Heterografts have not been successful. Homografts have enjoyed a limited success, mostly compromised by the immunologic response of the recipient patient. Preserved homografts have been used with some limited success. However, the ultimate fate of the homograft has proved to be an abundance of fibrous tissue, with limited results. Autologous nerve grafts, on the other hand, preserve the endoneurial structures and contain proliferated Schwann's cells that represent an excellent skeleton in which to receive the ingrowing axons.

Historical Review

It is interesting to reexamine the history of nerve grafting, which began in the Listerian era. In November 1866, Lister wrote a letter to his friend, Sir Hector Cameron, about a patient with a tumor of the sciatic nerve. He suggested that after removal of the tumor, it would be worthwhile to form a channel of catgut stitches between the two ends of the nerves so that new nerve tissue might grow down this channel to reinnervate the distal stump. In 1870, Philipeaux and Vulpian performed an experiment in which the lingual nerve was used to bridge a gap in the hypoglossal nerve. In a review of World War I surgery, British surgeons concluded that autogenous grafting was unsuccessful.[8] This effectively set back nerve grafting and retarded progress for approximately 20 years. In 1927 Bunnell published a paper on digital nerve grafting,[11] and in 1942 Sanders reviewed the history of nerve grafting, reported animal experimentation, and prompted a further attempt to use autografts in treatment of patients with large nerve gaps.[60] In 1947 and again in 1963, Seddon reported some measure of success in over 100 patients with nerve grafts.[61,63] The greater successes occurred in children and in the small nerves, such as the digital nerves. Seddon reached an important conclusion: the results of grafting nerve lesions in the digits were far better than secondary suture because the resection of the distal stump could be more generous. This then leads us to the rationale currently employed for nerve grafting.

Millesi, Meissl, and Berger made two important

contributions in their experimental work.[47,48] First, the ultimate result of the nerve repair was related to the amount of connective tissue proliferation at the suture site. Inasmuch as epineurium is the primary source of connective tissue at the site of injury to a nerve, they concluded that resection of the epineurium led to less connective tissue (i.e., scarring) at the suture site. Second, these authors concluded that tension at the suture site compromises nerve regeneration and ultimate recovery. This is again related to scar tissue. Tension increases scar tissue and prohibits axonal regeneration. Furthermore, the increased hypertrophied scar tissue due to the tension-ridden nerve juncture causes axonolysis and damage to the already regenerating nerve axons. Millesi, Meissl, and Berger[48] then compared nerve grafting using liberal resection of the damaged ends, epineurectomy, and suture without tension to standard nerve repair with epineurial suture under some tension. They concluded, in this experiment using rabbits, that nerve grafting was better than a suture under tension.

In a second series of experiments, Millesi[47] transected the sciatic nerves of rabbits, sutured the nerves under normal tension, and then grafted a 5-mm section under normal tension. He found no significant difference in the recovery of the two legs in these animals. He then concluded that under favorable conditions, with no tension, there was no difference between nerve suture and nerve grafting.

Repair Versus Grafting

If one could transform Millesi's experimental data into clinical practice, it might be concluded that a gap in a nerve of 4 cm or more cannot be closed without undue tension and therefore should be grafted. We see gaps of 4 cm in those cases in which nerve tissue has been lost or in secondary cases where the nerve ends have retracted and stuck to adjacent soft tissues. After resection of the neuroma and glioma, the gap is ultimately 4 cm or more and therefore will require a nerve graft. In making the decision to graft, the surgeon should use the operating microscope so he can examine the cut nerve endings and be absolutely certain that there is a minimum of fibrous tissue and normal fascicular grouping.

We have not seen the situation in which a primary nerve graft should be employed because of wound conditions. However, one might encounter a partially injured nerve in the brachial plexus, such as the lateral cord or a peripheral nerve in the forearm, where there is a significant gap in the injured portion and the normal portion is of normal length. In this unique situation, I could imagine using a primary nerve graft if the conditions are such that one would normally do a primary nerve suture, i.e., those conditions mentioned earlier on page 1380. Thus far in my practice I have not seen an instance where all of these criteria have been met, but I do think it is a theoretical possibility.

Therefore, most if not all nerve grafting will be carried out as a secondary procedure. The surgeon thus has an opportunity to explain to the patient the problem involved and discuss the source of the graft. The appropriate facilities include the operating microscope and a microsurgical team. The surgeon must also study and have a thorough knowledge of the neuroanatomy of the involved peripheral nerve. He must study the charts of Sunderland for the cross-sectional anatomy in the region to be surgically approached. In our experience it has been quite helpful to have Sunderland's charts in the operating room for evaluation after visualization of the cut ends of the nerve. I consider this no reflection on the surgeon's confidence, but rather an indication of his thoroughness. After the above, careful preparation, the operation should be customized to the individual patient and the individual nerve. Again, I should mention that children will ultimately do far better than adults, and patients over the age of 50 will have limited recovery even with an excellent nerve graft.

Types of Nerve Grafts

There are many types of grafts that can be employed, and a thorough knowledge of all of the types will enable the surgeon to chose the appropriate one for each situation. I prefer different types of grafts in various situations, depending on the size of the recipient nerve, the fascicular structure, and the location in the extremity.

TRUNK GRAFT

The trunk graft uses a whole segment of nerve interposed between the proximal and distal cut ends of the damaged nerve (Fig. 34-5). Trunk grafts have not enjoyed a high success rate because in the revascularization process the center of the trunk graft has become fibrotic and the regenerating axons have been limited in the distal nerve stump. However, Seddon stated that predegeneration may improve this situation. Wallerian degeneration involves intense metabolic activity, but if it has already taken place, as in the predegenerated graft, the metabolic requirements of the degenerated nerve are minimal. In large trunk grafts, such as might be employed for the radial nerve, I do recommend predegenerating the trunk graft, if at all possible. In such a situation the distal sensory branch of the radial nerve is, by definition, already degenerated and makes an ideal graft source. I usually use an already degenerated donor nerve as my graft source in these cases. In an unusual case, I have used a trunk graft from a damaged extremity, predegenerated it by local nerve division, and 4 weeks later taken the distal predegenerated nerve as a graft. This technique has only been used for trunk grafts, however.

In our experience, trunk grafts are used mainly in salvage situations where one is attempting to restore the median nerve and may use the already damaged distal ulnar nerve for reconstitution of the median nerve. In replacing one or two cords, we have had excellent results using the ulnar nerve as a trunk graft for brachial plexus lesions. One must be careful not to use a trunk graft for reconstruction when sacrificing the distal nerve precludes a more

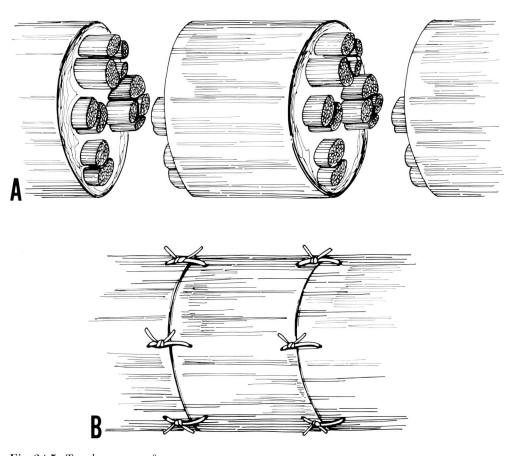

Fig. 34-5. Trunk nerve graft.

reasonable attempt at total reconstruction. However, in the isolated circumstance of a high median and ulnar nerve lesion, the surgeon may consider sacrificing the predegenerated distal ulnar nerve to graft the median nerve if he has decided to concentrate on the median supply to the hand. We have used this approach in hands with the ring and little fingers damaged beyond reconstruction, in which our reconstructive efforts are concentrated on the thumb and index and middle fingers.

CABLE GRAFT

The cable graft is mentioned primarily for historical interest, since other measures have essentially subplanted this technique. A cable was formed by uniting the strands of nerve graft into a unit and then suturing the unit in the gap to the proximal and distal stumps. This has limited success because of the low rate of precise anatomic continuity. However, it is encouraging to note that in Seddon's cases where a cable graft was used for the repair of partial lesions, there was only one failure out of 11 cases. There were also 45 successes out of 53 cases in his later group. He attributed this to many children being included in this group.[61,63]

PEDICLE NERVE GRAFT

A third type of graft, which has been employed in rare instances, is the pedicle graft described by Strange.[70,71] In this operation, which is of limited clinical use, the median and ulnar nerves were usually both divided. After transection through the healthy nerve ends, the proximal stumps of the median and ulnar nerves are united to form a U. The ulnar nerve is then transected proximally at an appropriate length so that it will bridge the gap in the median nerve. Doing this at the first stage allows the ulnar nerve to degenerate distally. The longitudinal blood vessels are disturbed as little as possible. The second stage leaves the anastomosis between the median and ulnar nerves intact, and the segment of ulnar nerve is swung down as a graft to the distal stump of the median nerve. This supposedly preserves the blood supply in the so-called pedicle fashion. However, the surgeon must mobilize the nerve stump to such an extent that I sincerely doubt there is significant blood supply to the grafted segment. This technique is rarely used in clinical practice for it involves two stages and sacrifice of the ulnar nerve.

INTERFASCICULAR NERVE GRAFT

In spite of the encouraging results reported by Seddon and others, nerve grafting in this country did not enjoy much popularity until the introduction of microneurosurgery and the interfascicular nerve grafting technique as described by Millesi[47] (Fig. 34-6). In using the anatomic principles of groups of fascicles, the interfascicular nerve graft (a better name perhaps is the grouped fascicular nerve graft) employs strands of grafted nerve between groups of fascicles appropriately dissected out and identified. For a successful grouped fascicular nerve graft the following conditions must be met: (1) the wound must be supple; (2) there must be an adequate vascularized bed in which the nerve graft has to lie; (3) the nerve ends must be adequately resected so that there is no scar tissue in the proximal stump; and (4) the nerve ends must be joined by a number of nerve grafts placed in the appropriate anatomic fashion without tension.

A wide exposure is used in this technique, with the tourniquet inflated. The dissection is done from the normal to abnormal tissue, attempting not to disturb the scar tissue in the pathologic site. The whole concept of the operation is to bridge normal nerve to normal nerve tissue. After the stumps are exposed, the operating microscope is employed, and the epineurium is inspected and incised just proximal to the neuroma and the dense scar. The investing epineurium is excised for a distance of approximately 1.5 cm, and then, using the anatomic structure and the operating microscope, one can appropriately map the groups of fascicles and separate these groups in the proximal nerve stump. Each fascicular group is transected at a different level so as not to make a circumferential scar. A similar procedure is done to the distal stump. The entire scarred neuroma and glioma need not be removed, but the nerve grafts must lie in an adequately vascularized bed.

After this dissection, which is tedious and time-consuming, the tourniquet is released and bleeders are electrocoagulated. The arm is then carefully wrapped in a slight compressive dressing while a

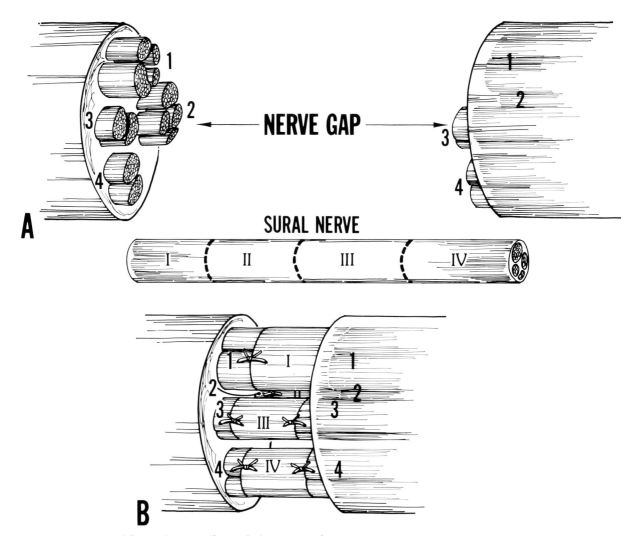

Fig. 34-6. Grouped fascicular (interfascicular) nerve graft.

search for the appropriate donor nerves is done. The sources of nerve graft are discussed in a separate section, but usually cutaneous nerves are used, the sural nerves being the appropriate first choice. After obtaining the donor nerve graft material, these wounds are closed and attention is then redirected to the upper extremity. A map is made of the proximal and distal nerve stumps, depicting the fascicular groups. These groups are then matched according to the maps that are drawn at the operating table, and the nerve graft is interposed between the fascicular groups. Mapping is relatively easy in small defects. However, in large defects (greater than 7 to 10 cm) there can be considerable varia-

tion in the fascicular anatomy between the two cut ends, and the best educated guess must be made, according to distribution of the fascicular groups and the different quadrants that might be united with those of the distal stump. Thus, fascicular grouping lessens the margin of error that would be encountered if "pure" fascicular grafting were undertaken. It is important to cut the donor nerve approximately 15 percent longer than the recipient defect to minimize the effective tension and to make the anastomosis easier. The epineurium must be retracted back from the ends so that it does not become interposed between the cut surfaces of the nerves and nerve grafts. The grafts are then placed between the corresponding fascicular groups. Exact, but loose approximation is used.

One or two 10-0 nylon sutures in each graft are usually sufficient to achieve this union. Hemostasis must be carefully maintained so as not to allow any hematoma between the cut ends of the nerve. Usually the graft on the farthest side from the operator is done first so that one does not disturb the existing grafts that are already in place. After completion of the entire grafting procedure, the wound is very carefully closed so as not to disrupt the grafts. The skin is closed and the limb is immobilized in the position in which the grafts were placed. Normally we prefer to have the wrist in neutral position and the elbow in slight flexion. Immobilization is maintained for 10 days, at which time the dressings are removed, the wound is inspected, sutures are removed (if ready), and motion can be begun. Motion, however, is restricted to very gentle motion for another 3 weeks.

The surgeon should expect an advancing Tinel's sign beginning 4 weeks postoperatively. The surgeon should carefully trace the Tinel's sign as it advances through the proximal and distal nerve sutures. In grafts of more than 10 cm, there is sometimes a retardation of axonal regrowth over the second suture line due to scarring, and, if the Tinel's sign does not advance appropriately over the second suture line, a resection of the more distal suture line should be done and primary nerve suture accomplished. I recommend resection of the distal suture site if the Tinel's sign, which had been advancing at the rate of 1 mm/day, ceases progression and is stationary for two return visits over a 2-month period. This is a rare occurrence, but it may salvage a satisfactory reconstruction out of one doomed to failure. Electrical testing is of little use until the Tinel's sign advances to a point where one would normally see motor reinnervation.

A review of Millesi's results with this technique shows that in young patients, below age 30, 60 percent achieved useful motor recovery with defects of 6 cm. Forty percent achieved excellent sensory recovery. The ulnar nerve results show 50 percent achieving excellent motor recovery and approximately 30 percent achieving excellent sensory recovery. These defects were in the range of 4 to 6 cm. In defects greater than 6 cm, the results tail off considerably, but there are isolated instances where very useful recovery was obtained from grouped fascicular nerve grafting in long defects. These defects were essentially irreparable by any other means.

FASCICULAR NERVE GRAFT

There are few indications for fascicular nerve grafts because the chances of matching corresponding fascicles decrease as the number of fascicles in the nerve increases. However, we have described fascicular nerve grafting in the distal digital nerve beyond the level of the DIP joint.[86] In this series, 11 patients were treated with 12 fascicular nerve grafts at the level of or beyond the terminal trifurcation of the digital nerve. These grafts all extended to a point beyond the DIP joint. All patients had improved sensibility. The technique is depicted in Figure 34-7. The small nerve graft is sutured to the proximal digital-nerve stump and then sutured distally into each individual fascicle of the trifurcated nerve. We have subsequently performed over 20 of these nerve grafts, and the donor site of choice at the present time is the terminal articular branch of the posterior interosseous nerve at the wrist (Fig. 34-8).

FREE VASCULARIZED NERVE GRAFT

There have been few reports of free vascularized nerve grafts. However, this concept can be applied in the case of long grafts in an unfavorable bed. Taylor and Ham[81] devised a technique in which the donor nerve, together with the arterial and venous supply, is transferred en toto to the graft site. In this case the neurovascular bundle of the superficial radial nerve and its associated radial artery and venae comitantes are used as the donor nerve. Bonney et al[1] reported on their experiences with vascularized nerve grafts to reconstruct the brachial plexus. They used the ulnar nerve vascularized by the ulnar artery or the ulnar collateral artery as a vascularized graft for the plexus. They have used this in 30 cases, and it was their impression that recovery in these patients is better than when conventional grafting is used. However, in no case was significant hand function restored through these grafts. Gilbert[22] used the sural nerve graft, vascularized by the sural artery in eight cases. Gilbert

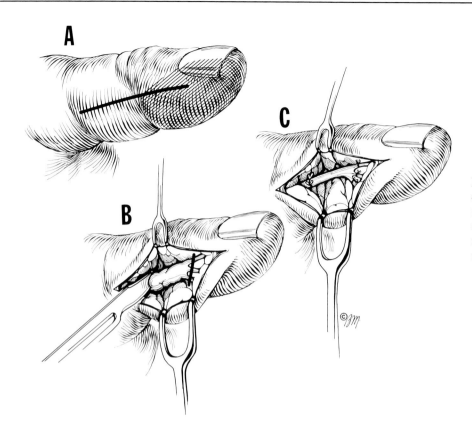

Fig. 34-7. Distal digital fascicular graft. (**A**) Incision line (shaded area indicates insensible region). (**B**) Resection of neuroma. (**C**) Graft to individual terminal fascicles.

states that the results in the vascularized nerve grafts are not better than those of classic interposition cutaneous grafts carried out in an excellent bed.

Rose,[58] however, used vascularized nerve grafts from the dorsum of the foot by the dorsalis pedis artery to restore sensibility in anesthetic scarred digits. He performed this in five cases with encouraging results. This emphasizes that this technique is only really acceptable in the situation where the bed is unacceptable for conventional grafting. The most promising situation would be one in which an already damaged or amputated limb could provide the surgeon with a major segment of nerve and its vascular supply to replace a large defect in another limb.

Source of Grafts

The source of the donor nerve should be chosen with great care.[80] The sural nerve in the posterior aspect of the lower leg represents the best source

of graft material in the majority of series (Fig. 34-9).

In positioning the patient for operation, the posterior aspect of the leg must be accessible to the surgeon. For short grafts where one sural nerve is being used, the semilateral position with support under the shoulder and hip contralateral to the operated hand will give access to the contralateral leg. If both sural nerves must be obtained, it is necessary to place the patient prone, obtain the grafts, and then turn the patient over to the usual position for the operative procedure on the hand. The surgeon, however, must be certain that a graft is feasible before removing the donor nerves. This may require repositioning during the operation.

The sural nerve can be found in the popliteal space just lateral to the lesser saphenous vein proximally, and it lies posterior to the lateral malleolus in the ankle. It may divide in the calf region. It is a little easier to identify the sural nerve distally and trace it proximally, using either a longitudinal or several transverse incisions. Up to 40 cm of graft

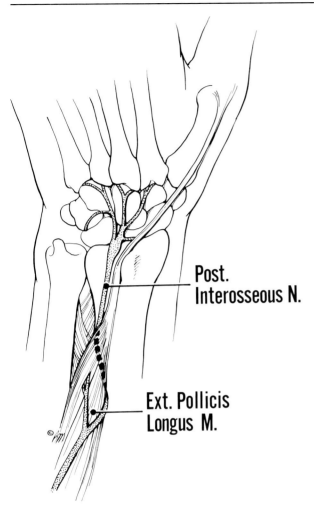

Fig. 34-8. Source of graft — terminal articular branches of posterior interosseous nerve (see text for details).

oblique incisions in the proximal forearm using the veins as landmarks.

The terminal branch of the posterior interosseous nerve (Fig. 34-8) has been used for the most distal digital nerve graft or as a single fascicular strand that can be used to replace one fascicle of the digital nerve. The use of this nerve is limited, but there is no deficit from taking the nerve as it is in articular branch, and, for this reason, it is the prime choice of donor graft for a very small nerve.[14]

The posterior interosseous nerve is found at the wrist level, lying on the interosseous membrane deep to the extensor tendons. As it branches distally, it usually lies just ulnar and deep to the extensor pollicis longus tendon and muscle. This nerve is obtained by a longitudinal dorsal wrist incision.

material can be obtained by this technique. The fasciculi are tightly packed in the interfascicular tissue, which is small in amount, thereby making this an excellent graft source. There are many other cutaneous nerves that can be used.

The medial and lateral antebrachial cutaneous nerves (Fig. 34-10), as well as the distal median and ulnar nerves, have been used for the grafting of digital nerves.[44] It should be noted, however, that these grafts have more interfascicular tissue than the sural nerve, and are thus theoretically a less desirable graft source. The antebrachial cutaneous nerves lie in the subcutaneous tissue adjacent to the basilic (medial) and cephalic (lateral) veins in the proximal forearm. They are obtained through

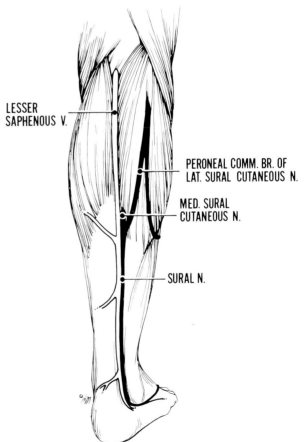

Fig. 34-9. Source of graft — sural nerve (see text for details).

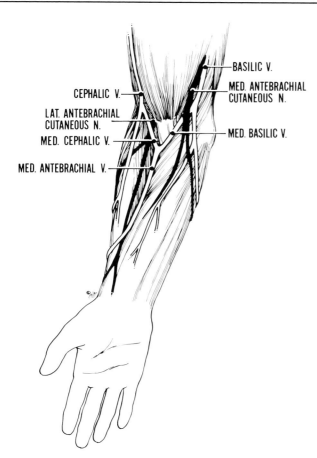

CEPHALIC V.

LAT. ANTEBRACHIAL
CUTANEOUS N.

MED. CEPHALIC V.

MED. ANTEBRACHIAL V.

BASILIC V.

MED. ANTEBRACHIAL
CUTANEOUS N.

MED. BASILIC V.

Fig. 34-10. Source of graft—medial and lateral antebrachial cutaneous nerves (see text for details).

After opening the extensor fascia, retraction of the extensor tendons reveals the nerve lying on the interosseous membrane. Care should be taken to preserve the extensor retinaculum.

Other cutaneous nerves, such as the lateral and posterior nerves of the thigh, can be used. The greatest amount of interfascicular tissue is found here, and there is considerable separation of the fascicles, limiting the use of these nerves as donors.

The superficial radial nerve is an excellent graft source in that the epineurial tissue is small in amount and the fascicles are tightly packed. However, the deficit from removing this is significant in the hand, especially in those hands with a concomitant median nerve injury; this nerve should never be taken for a graft in a patient with a median nerve deficit. The ideal use of the superficial radial nerve

is in the high radial nerve lesion that requires grafting. It is an excellent choice because the deficit is already present prior to excision of the superficial radial nerve, and this nerve is already predegenerated.

The dorsal branch of the ulnar nerve can similarly be used because one can obtain approximately 15 cm of nerve graft tissue. The deficit of numbness on the dorsum of the hand is not significant in the face of an intact median nerve, and this nerve can similarly be used for the same reasons as the superficial radial nerve to bridge small ulnar nerve defects in the forearm.

CHOICE OF TYPE OF NERVE GRAFT

The choice of the type of graft depends on the localization of the injury and the preference of the surgeon. In high injuries, we recommend interfascicular, or grouped fascicular, grafting and, in the most distal injuries, fascicular grafting. The donor graft must be chosen with care and the patient must be fully apprised of the deficit that will result from the choice of the donor graft. This is most important, and I have reported a prospective series of 28 nerve grafts in which the patients were questioned prior to and after the operation.[46] In a high percentage of cases, the patient did not fully understand the deficit that would result, and in a few cases, the deficit was greater than anticipated. A preoperative block of the graft source of the donor graft can be helpful to the surgeon in explaining the ultimate deficit that will occur.

In our opinion at the present time, autogenous grafting is preferable to any other type available.[42] One must be aware of the anatomic structures, the anatomic crossover, and the interfascicular anatomic pattern of the nerve before attempting to bridge a defect with a nerve graft. The nerve graft must be placed in a suitable bed so that vascularization will occur. The surgeon must be aware that tension at the suture line is undesirable and that the interval between injury and grafting should be as short as possible. If return of motor power is to be expected, grafting must be done before a 6-month interval after injury has elapsed. However, protective sensation can be restored after months or even years following injury.

Although there have been some reports on

wrapping the suture lines, there are no real clinical indications that this has been beneficial, and at the present time no part of the suture line nor the graft should be wrapped with a foreign material. However, taking all of these considerations into account, I prefer to use a grouped fascicular graft for defects of 4 cm in the median and ulnar nerve and for defects of smaller lengths in the digital nerves.

NEUROMA-IN-CONTINUITY

A neuroma-in-continuity of a major peripheral nerve in the upper extremity presents perhaps the greatest challenge to the managing surgeon. This is because such a lesion may initially be a partial one with sparing of a variable amount of important distal function; or when complete, may in some cases have the potential for spontaneous regeneration and restoration of function, while in other cases, no potential for recovery exists without resection and repair.

The main problem with a neuroma-in-continuity is its unpredictability. The biggest challenge to the treating physician is to utilize all of the available techniques, both surgical and nonsurgical, to arrive at a decision that would accurately predict either recovery without resection and repair or the need for such. It is important to realize that at least 60 percent of nerve injuries, even in civilian practice, do not transect the nerve, but leave it with some degree of continuity.[33] The location of a neuroma-in-continuity in relation to the extremity is another important consideration. A more proximal neuroma-in-continuity will present with a much more mixed distal lesion because of the fascicular arrangement of the proximal nerve; however, in the more distal part of the extremity, a clearer picture of the condition of the nerve may be elicited. Thus, partial lesions of the distal nerves are more likely to damage a fascicle destined for one or more specific distal sites; whereas proximal partial injuries are more likely to damage a cross section of fibers destined for many distal end organs.

Another crucial factor in managing a neuroma-in-continuity is the time element between injury and expected recovery. This is particularly true in the motor system because motor end plates as described earlier in this chapter begin to disintegrate after denervation and have no reinnervation potential after a period of 2 years. The reinnervation potential diminishes dramatically after 9 months. Therefore, it is critical to set time limits for decision making in watching the neuroma-in-continuity because it is very easy to be lulled into a sense of unwarranted optimism watching a portion of the nerve recover and not realizing that perhaps a more important portion of the nerve is *not* recovering. The neuroma-in-continuity can have all levels of axonal injury within the given nerve, including axonal disruption with no hope of regeneration and a physiologic impairment of conduction that has full potential for recovery. To reiterate, when managing a neuroma-in-continuity, the surgeon must take into account the elapsed time from injury and the proposed time of recovery when planning surgery. The total time must not exceed 2 years. This is particularly true in brachial plexus injuries, where recovery could approach 18 months.

Evaluation

The evaluation of a neuroma-in-continuity should include: (1) a precise knowledge of the wounding agent; (2) careful and frequent evaluation; (3) the use of Tinel's test; and (4) electrodiagnosis.

MECHANISM OF INJURY

A precise knowledge of the wounding agent is important, and careful examination should be done. Sharp injuries, while likely to lead to transection, sometimes leave the nerve in gross continuity and some of these can recover without resection and suture. Gunshot wounds and crush injuries or nerve contusions due to local open fractures are more likely to recover spontaneously.

CLINICAL EXAMINATION

The necessity for careful and frequent clinical evaluation is paramount to be sure that the nerve is regenerating. I would recommend evaluation at monthly intervals since more frequent evaluation will sometimes cloud the issue by presenting conflicting data. Many times a therapist performing periodic objective sensory and motor evaluation can aid the clinician in this.

TINEL'S TEST

Tinel's sign is another valuable tool that has been and is still used by many clinicians to signify regeneration. This is a valuable test but only as long as its limitations are kept in mind. Tinel's test is based on the irritability of fine regenerating fibers. Tapping over the course of the nerve where such fibers are present produces paresthesias or tingling in the distribution of the nerves; this signifies regeneration and is a positive sign.[49] Unfortunately such fibers may or may not subsequently increase enough in caliber or gain enough myelination to lead to useful function. A Tinel's sign that is obtained well distal to the injury site tells us that fine fibers have regenerated to that point; its continued progression down the distal course of the nerve would suggest further regeneration, although it does not guarantee functional recovery. A Tinel's sign that cannot be elicited below the injury site 3 to 4 months after injury or suture would mean that not even fine fibers have reached the point being tapped. Thus, the absence of a Tinel's sign distal to the injury becomes an important negative finding warranting the need for exploration.

ELECTRODIAGNOSIS

Another set of useful diagnostic tools utilizes electrodiagnosis. Electromyography (EMG) tests the innervation of muscles. Signs of denervation, such as fibrillations and denervation potentials, can be seen 2 to 4 weeks after serious injury, the length of interval depending on how far the lesion is from the muscle being tested. If muscles in the distribution of the injured nerve do not show denervational changes, one must make sure that the innervation is not coming from adjacent nerves. With re-input of axons into muscle and some motor end-plate reconstruction, the electromyographer finds an increase in insertional activity and a decrease in the number of fibrillations and denervation potentials. If signs of reinnervation in proximal muscles are seen by EMG, they should progress with time into more distal muscles and not remain relegated to

one muscle or one set of muscles. However, it should be cautioned that electromyographic evidence of regeneration does not guarantee subsequent useful clinical function because electromyography is a physiologic rather than a functional test. Nonetheless, electromyograms done in a careful and serial fashion can provide valuable information as long as the temporal and interpretive limitations of the test are understood.

Conduction studies are an additional electrodiagnostic aid. However, conduction studies done in the usual fashion are not helpful in the more serious and complete nerve injuries and are mostly used in mild or partial injuries. Nerve action potentials, postulated by Kline,[34–36] on the other hand, have been helpful. These are obtained in a noninvasive fashion by stimulating above and below the lesion and then amplifying the response and summing them up by computer. Nerve action potentials of early regeneration can sometimes be recorded. This technique works best for median, ulnar, and some radial nerve lesions, but can be used to stimulate and record from elements distal to the injury where the brachial plexus is involved. This test, along with the other electrical tests, must be used in conjunction with careful clinical observation. No decision should be made exclusively on the presence or absence of a positive noninvasive electrical test. A further electrical test, involving noninvasive evaluation of spinal cord or peripheral nerve–evoked responses, is a useful adjunct to more accurate preoperative delineation of brachial plexus injuries. This technique, popularized by Van Beek,[83] uses the fact that brachial plexus avulsion produces Wallerian degeneration in motor axons only. Some sensory axons are intact because the central cell location is outside the cord. Therefore, a nerve action potential will be transmitted by a sensory axon. Because avulsion has occurred, a spinal cord–evoked response should not be present. All of these electrical aids can be more useful in the operative setting where direct stimulus of the nerve and more accurate recording can be effected.

Surgical Management

If a decision is reached that the state of the neuroma-in-continuity of a given peripheral nerve will not allow sufficient and useful regeneration, then operative intervention becomes necessary. Many times this decision is precipitated by the time factor. The clinician will just not be able to make a total determination even from the clinical and non-invasive studies and will have to make a surgical decision because the available recovery time has elapsed from the time of injury. The patient should be apprised of the various possibilities that may arise at the time of exploration, including neurolysis or resection with either suture repair or nerve grafting of a portion of or the entire nerve.

At surgery, careful proximal and distal exposure of the suspected lesion-in-continuity is essential. Exposure should be generous, and dissection of the lesion itself delayed until both proximal and distal elements have been isolated and identified. Longitudinal blood supply to the nerve should be preserved, but most collaterals can be sacrificed so that a 360-degree exposure of the nerve itself can be obtained. If the neuroma is fusiform, a swelling of up to twice the normal diameter can be compatible with a lesion of the nerve in the Sunderland Grades I–III[76] (Table 34-1); whereas swelling larger than that favors a Sunderland IV or V lesion. Firmness or hardness suggests a heavy internal scar and total nerve division. In general, the internal architecture of the neuroma is almost always worse than it appears on inspection or palpation. A lateral neuroma suggests partial transection. The injection of saline or other physiologic solutions into lesions-in-continuity in an attempt to delineate fascicles has not proven beneficial because much of the scar preventing regeneration is intrafascicular rather than perineural. I do not advise injecting anything into the nerve to determine the advisability of resection.

After inspection and palpation of the lesion, the nerve can be stimulated both proximal and distal to the lesion to see if muscle function proximal and distal to the lesion can be observed. The standard nerve stimulators in most operating rooms are useful for this technique.[29]

INTRAOPERATIVE ELECTRODIAGNOSTIC STUDIES

Intraoperative electrodiagnostic techniques using either nerve action potentials or evoked responses are very helpful.[31,32] The surgeon faced with the need for this very sophisticated technique should either be familiar with the instrumentation and technique or have a working relationship with an electromyographer who can attend at the operative session. While there are some surgeons with particular research interest in this field, most clinical surgeons must maintain a relationship with an electromyographer. The equipment used is the standard, commercially available equipment for electrodiagnosis. A special probe for direct stimulation of the nerve can be modified from existing equipment or by using the probe from an existing nerve stimulator. The electromyographer can assist the surgeon with any modification necessary. In the operating room, there must be a dearth of background electrical activity. Most modern operating rooms are well grounded, but it is best to try the machine in the operating room prior to the clinical situation. Sometimes one operating room in a corner of an operating suite is more conducive to this method of diagnosis than one in the center of the operating suite due to the background electri-

---

Table 34-1. Sunderland's Grades of Nerve Injury[65]

Grade I
Interruption of axonal conduction at the site of injury.
Axonal continuity is preserved.
There may be segmental demyelinization without Wallerian degeneration.
This condition is totally reversible.

Grade II
The axon is severed and the axon fails to survive below the level of injury and for a variable, but short distance proximal to it.
The endoneurium is preserved.
Full recovery is expected.

Grade III
The axon is severed and disintegrated with Wallerian degeneration.
Endoneurial tube continuity is lost and disorganization of the internal structure of the fascicles occurs (this is the typical traction lesion).
Recovery is slower and is usually incomplete.

Grade IV
Total destruction of the internal architecture of the nerve with continuity of the nerve trunk preserved through the epineurium.
A neuroma forms in this injury.
Spontaneous recovery can occur, but rarely proceeds to a useful degree.
This fourth degree injury is an indication for surgical repair of the nerve.

Grade V
There is loss of continuity of the nerve trunk.
Surgical repair is mandatory for any useful recovery.

cal activity. The electromyographer can be scheduled to come into the operating room at the appointed time and does not necessarily need to be available during the whole procedure. As the equipment is fairly portable, it can be stored on a cart and be brought readily into the operating room. In our experience, the electromyographer's time is usually no longer than 30 minutes. Kline[33-37] has popularized intraoperative nerve action potential recordings across lesions-in-continuity. Those lesions with flat traces will require resection while those with evoked nerve action potentials need only neurolysis. Kline has been able to do partial repairs because only a portion of the element is regenerating and is responsible for the recorded nerve action potential. In a more distal neuroma-in-continuity, axons may regenerate through a lesion well into the distal stump, and yet be months away from a measurable distal input. For many years, Kline has recorded nerve action potentials across all of these injuries and has reported that this technique is a great aid in decision-making. Therefore, with the lesion exposed, both the stimulating and recording electrodes are placed proximally; if the stimulating and recording system is working correctly, a nerve action potential should be recorded from the proximal stump. In rare circumstances, stretch or lengthy contusions to the nerve extending above the lesion site will make recording of a healthy proximal nerve action potential difficult. Once the nerve action potential is recorded proximally, the recording electrode is moved distally beyond the lesion to see if a nerve action potential can be evoked through the area of injury. If a potential is recorded immediately distal to the neuroma-in-continuity, recording electrodes are moved further down the distal stump to see how far the potential, and presumably, the regenerating fibers of adequate size, have extended. If a nerve action potential cannot be recorded distal to the injury, voltage and amplification are gradually increased until it is difficult to visualize that portion of the trace following the stimulus artifact. Attention should be paid to electrode contact, and blood should be irrigated away from the region of the electrodes. It is generally best to elevate the nerve away from surrounding soft tissue by means of the electrodes, but if need be, the nerve can be stimulated and recorded by isolating short segments on either side of the lesion and placing the electrodes on them.[88]

Van Beek[83] used a technique in which cutaneous EEG electrodes are placed in the midfrontal area for reference, deltoid area for ground, C-4 posterior neck for recording spinal cord–evoked response, and Erb's point for recording peripheral nerve evoked response. The stimulating electrodes are positioned in the operative field and mechanically held. The wide separation of the intraoperative stimulator electrode and the cutaneously applied recording electrode permits separation between the stimulus artifact and the recording evoked response. The whole nerve, groups of fascicles, or fascicles can be stimulated and the recordings can be made using cutaneous recording electrodes placed at appropriate monitoring sites. In this technique, nerve dissection is minimized. Both measurements of a nerve's compound action potential from a near field by direct electrode application or measurement of a response from a far field taking advantage of volume conduction are possible with a computerized system. Van Beek[83] reported that electrically stimulating a nerve during the operation and then recording the evoked response has been useful in approximately 40 percent of his neuroma-in-continuity cases. In his experience the surgical management was altered because of the intraoperative findings.

One of the limitations of this particular technique is that there currently is a lack of definitive criteria to determine the appropriate surgical treatment. Any evoked response across the neuroma seems to mandate neurolysis, and the lack of a response, resection and repair. In Van Beek's[83] series he would not resect nerve segments producing greater than 40 μV evoked response across an injury using direct recording techniques. Using the cutaneous recording technique, normal amplitude ranges between 0.5 to 2.0 μV depending on the nerve and the recording site.

NEUROLYSIS VERSUS RESECTION

By using all of the available maneuvers including inspection, palpation, nerve stimulation, direct recording across the site, and distant recording through a cutaneous electrode, the surgeon can gather much useful information. The ultimate decision on whether to neurolyse or resect the neuroma-in-continuity must be made after distillation of all of the above information and not on one single determination. If a neuroma-in-continuity is large, appears very hard, and has no electrical activity across the area that can be determined, then resection is clearly the treatment of choice. If electrical activity can be discerned and even some muscle contraction noted, then neurolysis is clearly the choice. In the grey area between these two alternatives, all of the factors must be taken into the decision-making process.

Neurolysis

If neurolysis is considered, the nerve must be exposed and, with sufficient magnification, the epineurium carefully opened and resected. All scarred tissue should be removed. Internal dissection of the nerve, however, should be discouraged if there is any danger of fascicular interruption with the surgical technique. Sometimes groups of fascicles can be separated and intrafascicular scar removed. Once done, the local bed of a neurolysed nerve must be evaluated. The scar tissue that will form around the nerve postoperatively as a result of the surgical intervention will sometimes interfere with nerve regeneration. Therefore, if the local muscle bed is not adequate, the use of a local muscle as a bed for an injured nerve or to change the environment of the nerve will allow that nerve to recover with minimal scar tissue.[64,76] This is particularly true if the scarring between the fascia, subcutaneous tissue, and nerves can be eliminated. The nerve, once neurolysed, must regain its normal excursion in the local bed to maintain its ultimate function. In the brachial plaxus, a local muscle flap including the pectoral, sternocleidomastoid, and latissimus dorsi can be used to preserve an adequate bed and change the environment from a scarred bed to a more natural environment for the recovering nerve. In the upper arm and forearm, local muscles usually surround the nerve and can be utilized to improve the bed. The ulnar nerve at the elbow would normally be transposed in a submuscular position to improve its bed. Throughout the forearm, the large muscle groups also serve to protect the nerve.

Muscle Flaps for Nerve Coverage

At the level of the wrist, however, there are no muscles covering the nerves, but there are several muscle flaps that can be utilized. The pronator quadratus flap initially described by MacKinnon and Dellon[13] is created by mobilizing the pronator quadratus muscle from the volar aspect of the wrist to cover neuromas-in-continuity of the median or ulnar nerves proximal to the wrist crease. This muscle is a small, flat quadrilateral muscle extending across the volar aspect of the distal radius and ulna. The muscle is supplied by a branch of the volar interosseous artery and nerve, and acts as a pronator of the forearm. However, its removal causes patients to lose pronator ability only when the elbow is markedly flexed or if there is an absence or dysfunction of the pronator teres. The pronator quadratus can be detached from the radius and ulna and elevated to cover either the median or ulnar nerve. More distally, the abductor digiti minimi (ADM) muscle can provide a useful flap to cover neuromas-in-continuity of the ulnar or median nerve distal to the wrist crease and in the region of the carpal canal, as first described by Milward et al.[49] The ADM is a broad, fleshy muscle that arises at the pisiform and ends in a flat tendon inserting at the base of the proximal phalanx of the little finger. It is supplied by a branch of the ulnar nerve and a branch of the ulnar artery and can be mobilized on this neurovascular bundle to cover neuromas-in-continuity throughout the wrist and into the palm. The lumbrical muscle flap described by Wilgis[85] can be used by taking one of the lumbrical muscles on its neurovascular bundle, which arises from the common digital artery and nerve, detaching it from the profundus tendon and using it to cover neuromas-in-continuity of the common and proper digital nerves.

Summary of Surgical Management

When faced with a neuroma-in-continuity the surgeon must develop a time-based protocol for its management. Monthly examinations, with electrical studies interspersed, will aid in the diagnostic management. At critical points the surgeon must make a decision whether operative intervention is necessary. Once this decision is reached, and it frequently is triggered by the time factor — a limit of recovery time — then the surgeon must have a prescribed protocol for treatment during the operation consisting of exposure of the lesion, nerve stimulation, recording techniques, and a clear plan whether neurolysis alone or resection of the neuroma-in-continuity and grafting will be necessary. If resection must be employed, then it is rare that an end-to-end suture can be effected without severe nerve mobilization and flexion of the adjacent joints. One would then resort to nerve grafting techniques as described elsewhere in this chapter.

REHABILITATION OF PATIENTS WITH NERVE REPAIRS

No chapter on the reconstruction of nerve injuries can be complete without a section on rehabilitation and end evaluation of nerve surgery.[90] I think it should be stated at the outset that Onne and others have shown that the ultimate result of nerve suture and/or graft cannot be appropriately evaluated until a period of 3 or possible 5 years has elapsed.[54] Therefore, the reader should note that most of the series presented in the literature today have had inadequate follow-up.

In the proper evaluation of end results of nerve repair and grafting, the other intact nerves must be anesthetized so that any overlap in sensory or motor input can be eliminated. As an example, sensory contribution of the radial nerve overlaps the tips of the thumb and index finger, often giving false information following median nerve suture. The sensory branch of the radial nerve should be locally anesthetized to allow accurate recording of the median nerve recovery. It is also well known that the ulnar nerve may supply some of the thenar muscles, and therefore objective evaluation of the end results of median nerve recovery should be done with the ulnar nerve blocked. Currently, the most widely accepted method of evaluation of nerve repair is the system devised by Highet[28] (Table 34-2), although this method needs clarification and updating with respect to individual nerves.

The chart shown in Figure 34-11 outlines our recommended 1-year period of rehabilitation. Follow-up should then continue for several more years following nerve suture. Essentially, we can summarize the postoperative care by saying that in the first 3 weeks the repair or graft is protected by plaster splintage and limited motion. In the period between 3 weeks and 3 months, the range of motion gradually increases, taking care not to stretch the repair site. Nerve repairs can be subjected to traction injuries if the suture line is stretched beyond the tensile strength of the nerve. The patient should be examined carefully during this period of time so that secondary deformity is prevented. Prevention may involve the use of external splints, such as a thumb web splint in a median nerve injury or a lumbrical bar in an ulnar nerve injury to prevent hyperextension of the MP joints and resultant clawhand deformity with stiffness of the PIP joints in flexion. Once the joints are maintained in a supple position, in the period between 3

Table 34-2. Highet's Method of End Result Evaluation[64]

Motor Recovery	
M0	No contraction.
M1	Return of perceptible contraction in the proximal muscles.
M2	Return of perceptible contraction in both proximal and distal muscles.
M3	Return of function in both proximal and distal muscles of such a degree that all important muscles are sufficiently powerful to act against resistance.
M4	Return of function as in Stage 3; in addition, all synergistic and independent movements are possible.
M5	Complete recovery.
Sensory Recovery	
S0	Absence of sensibility in the autonomous area.
S1	Recovery of deep cutaneous pain sensibility within the autonomous area of the nerve.
S2	Return of some degree of superficial cutaneous pain and tactile sensibility within the autonomous area of the nerve.
S3	Return of superficial cutaneous pain and tactile sensibility throughout the autonomous area, with disappearance of any previous overresponse.
S3+	Return of sensibility as in Stage 3; in addition, there is some recovery of two-point discrimination within the autonomous area.
S4	Complete recovery.

Proximal muscles are defined as extrinsic, and distal as intrinsic muscles in the hand.

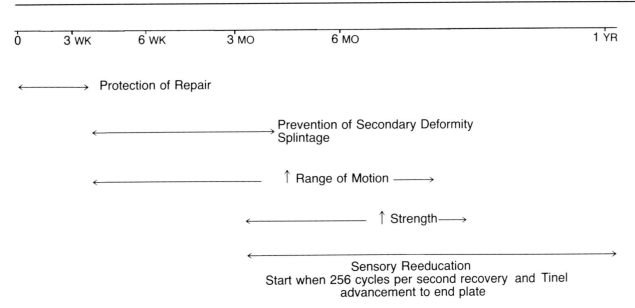

Fig. 34-11. Chart of postoperative rehabilitation of nerve injuries. The goal is to minimize recovery time and maximize functional recovery.

and 6 months, the strength of the hand is increased. During this time, the surgeon should be evaluating the nerve repair and studying Tinel's sign. If Tinel's sign does not advance significantly in the period between 3 and 6 months postoperatively, the surgeon must consider redoing the nerve repair or graft. The period of 6 months since the time of injury is critical, as explained earlier in this chapter, because metabolic changes occur both in the muscle and in the proximal nerve cell. Therefore, one must make a decision between 3 and 6 months whether the nerve regeneration is proceeding satisfactorily. If the nerve regeneration is proceeding satisfactorily and advancing Tinel's sign is present, sensory reeducation should be instituted.

Sensory Reeducation

Sensory reeducation was first reported by Dellon, Curtis, and Edgerton when they found near-normal sensation in four adults following nerve repair and intensive sensory retraining.[13–15] This was confirmed by Wynn-Parry and Salter in 1976.[91] Reid reviewed the testing of 150 adult patients with median nerve injury 1 to 5 years postinjury and found that these patients had very poor sensi-

bility.[56] Reeducation was then begun when 256 cycles per second with a tuning fork could be detected at the fingertips. He noticed an improvement in sensibility in all patients using two-point discrimination, point localization, and the Moberg pick-up test as clinical tests. The patients in this study maintained their improvement in two-point discrimination after many years. One woman with a primary repair of her median nerve was found to have two-point discrimination greater than 45 mm 6 months postoperatively. Following 6 weeks of sensory retraining, the two-point discrimination was 11 to 15 mm, and 7 years later the two-point discrimination was 7 mm over the thumb and index finger. This method of sensory retraining is the same spontaneous retraining that a child undergoes following nerve injury. Onne reported excellent recovery of two-point discrimination in children but poor recovery of two-point discrimination in adults.[54] Therefore, I believe that sensory retraining in adults is mandatory following nerve injury. Patients with hyperesthesia or pain cannot be retrained until desensitization is carried out with reduction in the hyperesthesia. After nerve repair one follows Tinel's sign, constant and moving touch, perception of vibration at 30 cycles per second and 256 cycles per second. When 256 cycles per second stimulus is perceived at the fingertips, sensory retraining should be introduced. The method of the training sessions is essentially repetitive use with constant objects. These sessions should last about 10 to 15 minutes, with maximum concentration on the patient's part. The items used are soft objects (such as an eraser of a pencil), various sizes of square, hexagonal, and round objects (such as metal nuts and washers), and the objects used in daily living (such as keys, coins, buttons, and safety pins). The patient must constantly feel these objects, practicing and testing himself repetitively. I emphasize again that this is a very natural process for the child, but in the adult we must encourage the retraining process. Following repair of a lacerated peripheral nerve, axons regenerate to reinnervate mechanical receptors in the skin. The regrowth is frequently disorderly. The number of nerve endings is not the same as prior to injury, and there is a reduction in the peripheral density of innervation. This altered profile must then be patterned in the brain so that the patient can again decode the information that is being produced by the mechanical receptors in the fingertips.

It is thought that the end-stage of nerve recovery is not reached until approximately 3 to 5 years post-injury. It is our hope that patients will be followed for this 5-year period and that suitable clinical information will be forthcoming. Unfortunately, there are very few reports of clinical series in the literature followed for this length of time. Only with this information will the clinician be able to determine the ultimate results of nerve repair and grafting.

FUTURE CONSIDERATIONS

In summary, many advances have been made in nerve repair and grafting over the last 130 years. However, we must be cognizant of the fact that the ultimate results of nerve repair and grafting are still unpredictable.[38,43,59,91] My opinion is that a major breakthrough in the understanding of nerve physiology and regenerative capacities is needed in order to make a significant step in assuring excellent results following nerve repair. With the advent of microsurgery, major steps have been made in the anatomic repair of nerves, from the standpoint of primary, secondary, and nerve grafting procedures. However, the ultimate results are still that children do better than adults and that repairs in adults, and sometimes even repairs in children, are unpredictable. The surgical world adopted microsurgery as the ultimate answer to neurosurgery, but evidence now indicates that there has not been significant difference in fascicular and perineurial repairs in clinical studies.[9,93] Exciting experimental work in pharmacologic suppression of neuroma formation is being done and may yield some useful techniques.[3,5] Recent experimental data indicate that there is more to nerve regeneration than axonal regrowth.[39,40]

Lundborg[41] has described an experimental model for nerve regeneration in which a well-organized nerve trunk regenerates without pre-existing structural guidance through a preformed tissue space. This stump regenerates in the presence of factors with strong neuronotrophic efforts on neurons in vitro. He interprets this process to suggest that the intrinsic regenerative potential of the nerve trunk can be expressed more effectively with appropriately permissive experimental conditions. He suggests that the secret of nerve regeneration is not only the needle, suture, and microscope, but also the need for ways to promote the full expression of the genetic program of the nerve cell under an optimal environment where potential neuronotrophic and neurite promoting factors are free to act.

It seems to me that we need to know more about the axoplasmic circulation and the actual conduction of the nerve through the repair site. If the ultimate answer is better anatomic fixation, then our present methods are inadequate. Central reprogramming of the imprint of the brain as advocated by the sensory education information has been helpful, and more study is needed in this field. We know that basically nerves are trying desperately to regenerate when injured, and all of our experimental efforts must be directed toward harnessing this regenerative energy and directing it into the proper channel so that normal neuroanatomy and physiology can be restored.

REFERENCES

1. Bonney G, Birch R, Jamieson A, Eames R: Experience with vascularized nerve grafts. Clin Plast Surg 11:137–142, 1984

2. Bora FW: Peripheral nerve repair in cats: The fascicular stitch. J Bone Joint Surg 49A:659–666. 1967

3. Bora FW: Improved axon regeneration after nerve injury by the pharmacological suppression of neuroma formation. Presented at the 35th Annual Meeting, American Society for Surgery of the Hand. Atlanta, 1980

4. Bora FW, Pleasure DE, Didizian NA: A study of nerve regeneration and neuroma formation after nerve suture by various techniques. J Hand Surg 1:138–143, 1976

5. Bora FW, Richardson S, Black J: The biomechanical responses to tension in a peripheral nerve. J Hand Surg 5:21–25, 1980

6. Bowden REM, Gutmann E: Denervation and reinnervation of human voluntary muscle. Brain 67:273, 1944

7. Boyes JA: On the Shoulders of Giants. JB Lippincott, Philadelphia, 1976

8. Brooks D: The place of nerve grafting in orthopaedic surgery. J Bone Joint Surg 37A:299–305, 1955

9. Brushart TM: A comparison of motoneuron pool organization after epineurial and perineurial repair of the rat sciatic nerve. Presented at the 35th Annual Meeting, American Society for Surgery of the Hand. Atlanta, 1980

10. Buncke HJ: Digital nerve repairs. Surg Clin North Am 52:1267, Oct 1972

11. Bunnell S: Surgery of nerves of the hand. Surg Gynecol Obstet 44:145, 1927

12. Chow JA, Van Beek AL, Meyer DL, Johnson MC: Surgical significance of the motor fascicular group of the ulnar nerve in the forearm. J Hand Surg 10A:867–872, 1985

13. Dellon AL, Mackinnon SE: The pronator quadratus muscle flap. J Hand Surg 9A:423–427, 1984

14. Dellon AL, Seif SS: Anatomic dissections relating the posterior interosseous nerve to the carpus, and the etiology of dorsal wrist ganglion pain. J Hand Surg 3:326, 1978

15. Dellon AL, Curtis RM, Edgerton MT: Reeducation of sensation in the hand following nerve injury. J Bone Joint Surg 53A:813, 1971

16. Dellon AL, Curtis RM, Edgerton MT: Evaluating recovery of sensation in the hand following nerve injury. The Johns Hopkins Med J 130:235, 1972

17. Dellon AL, Curtis RM, Edgerton MT: Reeducation of sensation in the hand after nerve injury and repair. J Plast Reconstr Surg 53:297, 1974

18. Dellon AL, Mackinnon S, Pestronk A: Implantation of sensory nerve into muscle: Preliminary clinical and experimental observations on neuroma formation. Ann Plast Surg 12:30, 1984

19. Ducker TB, Kempe LG, Hayes GJ: The metabolic background for peripheral nerve surgery. J Neurosurg 30:270, 1969

20. Garrison FH: An Introduction to the History of Medicine. 4th Ed. WB Saunders, Philadelphia, 1929

21. Gaul JS: Electrical fascicle identification as an adjunct to nerve repair. J Hand Surg 8:289–296, 1983

22. Gilbert A: Vascularized sural nerve graft. Clin Plast Surg 2:73–77, 1974

23. Gordon L, Buncke H, Jewett DL, Muldowney B, Buncke G: Predegenerated nerve autografts as compared with fresh nerve autografts in freshly cut and precut motor nerve defects in the rat. J Hand Surg 4:42–47, 1979

24. Grabb WC: Median and ulnar nerve suture. An experimental study comparing primary and secondary repair in monkeys. J Bone Joint Surg 50A:964–972, 1968

25. Grabb WC, Bement SL, Koepke GH, Green RA: Comparison of methods of peripheral nerve suture in monkeys. Plast Reconstr Surg 46:31, 1970

26. Gruber H, Freilinger G, Holle H, Mandl H: Identification of motor and sensory funiculi in cut nerves and their selective reunion. Br J Plast Surg 29:70, 1976

27. Hakstian RW: Funicular orientation by direct stimulation. An aid to peripheral nerve repair. J Bone Joint Surg 50A:1178, 1968

28. Highet WB, Holmes W: Traction injuries to the lateral popliteal nerve and traction injuries to peripheral nerves after suture. Br J Surg 30:212, 1943

29. Jabaley ME: Electrical nerve stimulation in the awake patient Bull Hosp Joint Dis Orthop Inst 44:248–259, 1984

30. Jabaley ME, Wallace WH, Heckler FR: Internal topography of major nerves of the forearm and hand: A current view. J Hand Surg 5:1–18, 1980

31. Jones SJ: Investigation of brachial plexus traction lesions by peripheral and spinal somatosensory evoked potentials. J Neurol Neurosurg Psychiatr 42:107, 1979

32. Jones SJ, Parry CB, Landi A: Diagnosis of brachial plexus traction lesions by sensory nerve action potentials and somatosensory evoked potentials. Injury 12(5):376, 1981

33. Kline DG: Early evaluation in peripheral nerve le-

sions in continuity with a note on nerve recording. Am Surg 34:77, 1968

34. Kline DG: Evaluation of the neuroma in continuity. Ch. 27. In Omer G, Spinner M (eds): Management of Peripheral Nerve Problems. WB Saunders, Philadelphia, 1980

35. Kline DG, Hackett ER: Value of electrophysiologic tests for peripheral nerve neuromas. J Surg Oncol 2:299, 1970

36. Kline DG, Nulsen FE: The neuroma in continuity: Its preoperative and operative management Surg Clin North Am 52:1189, 1972

37. Kline DG, Hackett ER, Happel LH: Surgery for lesions of the brachial plexus Arch Neurol 43:170, 1986

38. Larsen RD, Posch JL: Nerve injuries in the upper extremity. Arch Surg 77:469, 1958

39. Lundborg G: The intrinsic vascularization of human peripheral nerves: Structural and functional aspects. J Hand Surg 4:34–41, 1979

40. Lundborg G, Hansson H: Nerve regeneration through preformed pseudosynovial tubes. J Hand Surg 5:35–38, 1980

41. Lundborg G, Dahlin L, Danielsen N, Hansson H, Johannesson A, Longo FM, Varon S, Engin D: Nerve regeneration across an extended gap: A neurobiological view of nerve repair and the possible involvement of neuronotrophic factors. J Hand Surg 7:580–587, 1982

42. Marmor L: Regeneration of peripheral nerves by irradiated homografts. J Bone Joint Surg 46A:383–394, 1964

43. McEwan LE: Median and ulnar nerve injuries. Aust NZ J Surg 32:89, 1962

44. McFarlane RM, Mayer JR: Digital nerve grafts with the lateral antebrachial cutaneous nerve. J Hand Surg 1:169–173, 1976

45. McLellan DL, Swash M: Longitudinal sliding of the median nerve during movements of the upper limb. J Neurol Neuros Phys 39:566, 1976

46. Millesi H: Indication, technique and results of nerve grafting. Handchirurgie, suppl. 2, 1977

47. Millesi H, Meissl G, Berger A: The interfascicular nerve-grafting of the median and ulnar nerves. J Bone Joint Surg 54A:727–749, 1972

48. Millesi H, Meissl G, Berger A: Further experience with interfascicular grafting of the median, ulnar and radial nerves. J Bone Joint Surg 58A:209–218, 1976

49. Milward TM, Stott WG, Kleinert HE: The abductor digiti minimi muscle flap. Hand 9:82–85, 1977

50. Moberg E: Methods of examining sensibility of the hand. p. 236. In Flynn JE (ed): Hand Surgery. Williams & Wilkins, Baltimore, 1966

51. Moberg E: Nerve repair in hand surgery — An analysis. Surg Clin North Am 48:985, Oct 1968

52. Nicholson OR, Seddon HJ: Nerve repair in civilian practice. Results of treatment of median and ulnar nerve lesions. Br Med J 2:1065, 1957

53. Oester YT, Davis L: Recovery of sensory function. p. 241. In Woodhall B, Beebe GW (eds): Peripheral Nerve Regeneration. Washington, DC, US Government Printing Office, 1956

54. Onne L: Recovery of sensibility and sudomotor activity in the hand after nerve suture. Acta Chir Scand suppl. 300, 1962

55. Poppen NK, McCarroll HR, Doyle JR, Niebauer JJ: Recovery of sensibility after suture of digital nerves. J Hand Surg 4:212, 1979

56. Reid RL: Preliminary results of sensibility reeducation following repair of the median nerve. American Society for Surgery of the Hand Newsletter 15, 1977

57. Riley DA, Lang DH: Carbonic anhydrase activity of human peripheral nerves: A possible histochemical aid to nerve repair. J Hand Surg 9A:112–120, 1984

58. Rose EH, Kowalski TA: Restoration of sensibility to anesthetic scarred digits with free vascularized nerve grafts from the dorsum of the foot. J Hand Surg 10A:514–521, 1985

59. Sakellarides H: A follow up study of 172 peripheral nerve injuries in the upper extremity in civilians. J Bone Joint Surg 44A:140, 1962

60. Sanders FK: The repair of large gaps in the peripheral nerves. Brain 65:281, 1942

61. Seddon HJ: The use of autogenous grafts for the repair of large gaps in peripheral nerves. Br J Surg 35:151, 1947

62. Seddon HJ: War injuries of peripheral nerves. In wounds of the extremities. Br J Surg War Surgery Suppl. 2:325, 1948

63. Seddon HJ: Nerve grafting. J Bone Surg 45B:447, 1963

64. Seddon HJ: Surgical Disorders of the Peripheral Nerves. Williams & Wilkins, Baltimore, 1972

65. Seddon HJ, Holmes W: Ischaemic damage in the peripheral stump of a divided nerve. Br J Surg 32:389, 1945

66. Seddon HJ, Medawar PB, Smith H: Rate of regeneration of peripheral nerves in man. J Physiol (Lond.) 102:191, 1943

67. Smith JW: Microsurgery of peripheral nerves. Plast Reconstr Surg 33:317, 1964

68. Spinner M: Injuries to the Major Branches of Peripheral Nerves of the Forearm. 2nd Ed. WB Saunders, Philadelphia, 1978

69. Starkweather RJ, Neviaser RJ, Adams JP, Parsons DB: The effect of devascularization on the regenera-

tion of lacerated peripheral nerves: An experimental study. J Hand Surg 3:163, 1978

70. Strange FGStC: An operation for nerve pedicle grafting, preliminary communication. Br J Surg 34:423, 1947

71. Strange FGStC: Case report on pedicled nerve graft. Br J Surg 37:331, 1950

72. Sunderland S: The intraneural topography of the radial, median and ulnar nerves. Brain 68:243, 1945

73. Sunderland S: The adipose tissue of peripheral nerves. Brain 68:118, 1945

74. Sunderland S: The effect of rupture of the perineurium on the contained nerve fibres. Brain 69:149, 1946

75. Sunderland S: The connective tissues of peripheral nerves. Brain 88:841, 1965

76. Sunderland S: Nerves and Nerve Injuries. Williams & Wilkins, Baltimore, 1968

77. Sunderland S: Nerves and Nerve Injuries. 2nd Ed. Churchill Livingstone, Edinburgh, 1978

78. Sunderland S: The pros and cons of funicular nerve repair. Founder's Lecture, The American Society for Surgery of the Hand. J Hand Surg 4:201, 1979

79. Sunderland S, Bradley KC: The cross-sectional area of peripheral nerve trunks devoted to nerve fibres. Brain 72:428, 1949

80. Sunderland S, Ray LJ: The selection and use of autografts for bridging gaps in injured nerves. Brain 70:75, 1947

81. Taylor GI, Ham FJ: The free vascularized nerve graft. A further experimental and clinical application of microvascular techniques. Plast Reconstr Surg 57:413, 1976

82. Tupper J: Fascicular nerve repair. p. 215. AAOS Symposium on Microsurgery. CV Mosby, St Louis, 1979

83. Van Beek A, Hubble B, Kinkead L, Torros S, Suchy H: Clinical use of nerve stimulation and recording techniques. Plast Reconstr Surg 71:225, 1983

84. Walker EA: History of Neurological Surgery. Williams & Wilkins, Baltimore, 1951

85. Wilgis EFS: Local muscle flaps in the hand anatomy as related to reconstructive surgery. Bull Hosp Joint Dis 44:552, 1984

86. Wilgis EFS, Maxwell GP: Distal digital nerve grafts: Clinical and anatomical studies. J Hand Surg 4:439, 1979

87. Wilgis EFS, Murphy R: The significance of longitudinal excursion in peripheral nerves. Hand Clinics 2:761–766, 1987

88. Williams HB, Terzis JK: Single fascicular recordings: An intraoperative diagnostic tool for the management of peripheral nerve lesions. Plast Reconstr Surg 57:562, 1976

89. Woodhall B, Nulsen FE, White JC, Davis L: Neurosurgical implications. In Woodhall B Beebe GW (eds): Peripheral Nerve Regeneration. Washington, DC, US Government Printing Office, 1956

90. Wynn-Parry CB: Diagnosis and aftercare of peripheral-nerve lesions in the upper limb. Founder's Lecture, The American Society for Surgery of the Hand. J Bone Joint Surg 48A:607, 1966

91. Wynn-Parry CB, Salter M: Sensory re-education after median nerve lesions. Hand 8:250, 1976

92. Yahr MD, Beebe GW: Recovery of motor function. p. 71. In Woodhall B, Beebe GW (eds): Peripheral Nerve Regeneration. Washington, DC, US Government Printing Office, 1965

93. Young L, Weeks PM, Wray RC: A comparison of sensation after epineural and fascicular digital nerve repairs. Presented at the 35th Annual Meeting, American Society for Surgery of the Hand. Atlanta, 1980

94. Zachary RB: Results of nerve suture. In Seddon JH (ed): Peripheral Nerve Injuries. Her Majesty's Stationery Office, London, 1954

95. Zachary RB, Holmes W: Primary suture of nerves. Surg Gynecol Obstet 82:632, 1946

Neuromas

35

James H. Herndon

The painful neuroma is a critical problem in the injured hand. A simple hypersensitive neuroma in a finger amputation stump may impair function of the whole hand (Fig. 35-1). Many neuromas remain relatively asymptomatic, but 20 to 30 percent are problematic regardless of what technique of local treatment has been employed.[63]

Neuroma formation, that is, a nodule developing on the severed end of the proximal nerve stump, was first described by Odier in 1811.[64] Wood,[89] Virchow,[87] and Mitchell[58] added further reports of this lesion in the nineteenth century. The nodule forms as a result of injury to the Schwann's cell-endoneurial barrier that confines axons to their endoneurial tubes. Once this barrier is damaged, regenerating axons escape into the surrounding tissue in a disorganized fashion and are accompanied by proliferating fibroblasts, Schwann's cells, and blood vessels.[81]

Many nerve lesions are termed neuromas. In this chapter I discuss only those neuromas in the hand resulting from partial or complete severance of a nerve containing sensory fibers (solely or mixed with motor fibers). Only neuromas containing sensory fibers become painful. Other types of lesions such as Morton's neuroma, pacinian neuroma, acoustic neuroma, and gastric neuroma, and syndromes, such as multiple mucosal neuromas, are not discussed.

ANATOMY

Sunderland[81] has stressed the importance of Schwann's cell and the endoneurium in containing regenerating axons after injury. If this barrier is broken, regenerating axons grow out of the end of the severed nerve in an attempt to reenter their original endoneurial tubes distally to reach the end organs they originally innervated. If the barrier is not broken, regenerating axons remain contained in their original endoneurial tubes and grow distally until they reach their respective end organs.

After axonal continuity has been disrupted by crushing, cutting, or tearing, Wallerian degeneration occurs. After a period of recovery, regrowth of the axons occurs in the proximal portion of the damaged nerve. When these axons reach the end of the endoneurial tube, they escape into a disorga-

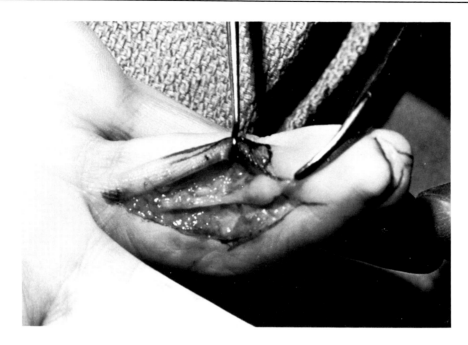

Fig. 35-1. A neuroma at the end of an amputation stump.

nized mass of connective tissue containing fibroblasts, Schwann's cells, macrophages, and capillaries. The axons grow out in many directions and branch irregularly, seeking to restore continuity of the nerve trunk. The growth and direction of the axons are influenced by the barrier of the fibro-

blasts and Schwann's cells. As a result, axons zigzag through the tissue in a totally disorganized fashion. They branch irregularly and form whorls, spirals, and convolutions (Fig. 35-2). Most are contained in the disorganized mass or nodule of connective tissue that becomes encapsulated. A few escape at-

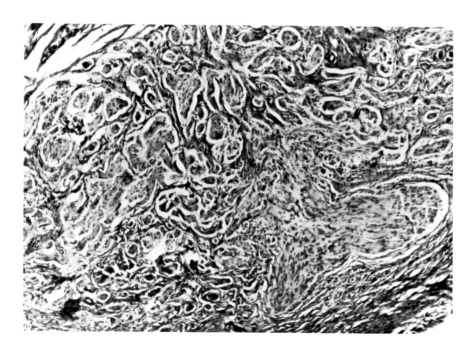

Fig. 35-2. Low-power photomicrograph of a neuroma, demonstrating disorganized tissue composed of axons, fibroblasts, Schwann's cells, and blood vessels.

tempting to reach the distal stump. This nodule at the stump end is called a *neuroma*. With time, progressive fibrosis converts an originally soft nodule into a firm, hard one.[48,78] Recently, myofibroblasts have been identified in neuromas. They increase in the scar tissue from 2 to 6 months after injury and then decrease as the collagen content of the scar increases. Within neuromas the matrix consists of glucosamine-glycosaminoglycan compared to minimal amounts of glycosaminoglycan in normal nerves.[1]

In the distal stump, the axons undergo degeneration as well, but since their cell bodies are proximal, they do not regenerate. There is a cellular response in the area of injury with some Schwann's cell and fibroblastic proliferation. However, the response is much less than that in the proximal stump, and without any regenerating axons the nodule that forms is small (always smaller than a neuroma) and is termed a *glioma*.

The size of a neuroma depends on the amount of proliferating connective tissue fibroblasts, Schwann's cells, vessels, and macrophages, but primarily on the number of axons and the extent of axonal ingrowth. Axonal growth is more active the closer the lesion is to the neuron. Therefore, neuromas tend to be larger in nerves injured proximally and smaller when injured peripherally. Also, increased size with more axonal growth is seen in nerves with large amounts of connective tissue and small, widely separated funiculi compared to nerves with large, closely packed funiculi. Petropoulos and Stefanko[69] have shown that in dogs the degree of anisomorphism is directly related to the size of the neuroma, that is, there was a marked disarray of all elements compared to smaller neuromas that were isomorphic or had a regular arrangement of all elements. Size and consistency of the neuroma are also affected by the presence of infection or foreign bodies and by repeated irritation such as pressure, friction, or repeated trauma.[7,9,17] Petropoulos and Stefanko have also shown that (in the dog) the blood supply to the nerve stump does not affect neuroma size, but in malnourished animals, the neuromas are always small and atrophic.[69] In addition to these known influences on size, consistency, and symptomatology, other unknown factors exist. For example, a patient with an amputated finger may have a painful neuroma develop in one digital nerve while the other digital nerve remains asymptomatic, even though both received identical primary treatment.

CLASSIFICATION OF NEUROMAS (TABLE 35-1)

Neuromas-in-Continuity

Neuromas-in-continuity are neuromas in a nerve that has not been completely severed. Sunderland described two types: those in which the perineurial sheath is intact and those in which there has been partial division of the nerve.

SPINDLE NEUROMAS

Spindle neuromas are swellings or enlargements in an intact nerve secondary to chronic irritation, friction, or pressure. Although they are called neuromas, they are not true neuromas. Histologically, the bulbous area contains increased connective tissue. With repeated continuous trauma, the fibrous tissue proliferates, constricting nerve fibers and interfering with their nutrition. Eventually the swelling becomes a large collagenized mass with fibrotic replacement of the nerve fibers and vessels.[81]

The only exception to this course of events was demonstrated by Spencer, in experiments in which he crushed nerves but kept the perineurium intact. He showed that regenerating axons in such circumstances did grow through the intact perineurium, forming a true neuroma-in-continuity.[78] I am not

Table 35-1. Classification of Neuromas

I. Neuromas-in-continuity
  A. Spindle neuromas. Lesions in which the perineurium is not broken
  B. Lateral neuromas. Lesions in which the perineurium of some funiculi is broken
  C. Neuromas following nerve repair
II. Neuromas in completely severed nerves
III. Amputation stump neuromas

(Modified from Sunderland S: Nerves and Nerve Injuries. 2nd Ed. Churchill Livingstone, Edinburgh, 1978.)

aware of any examples of this type of neuroma having been reported in humans.

Examples of this type of spindle neuroma are those occurring in Morton's metatarsalgia, the ulnar digital nerve of the thumb in bowler's thumb, the greater occipital nerve where it pierces the trapezius fascia, the lateral femoral cutaneous nerve where it passes beneath the inguinal ligament in meralgia paresthetica, the posterior interosseous nerve on the back of the wrist, the branch of the axillary nerve to the teres minor, and the lateral branch of the deep peroneal nerve where it crosses the tarsal navicular bone.[19,57,60,61,74]

LATERAL NEUROMAS

This type of neuroma occurs when part of the nerve with its perineurium has been injured, and is commonly seen by surgeons dealing with trauma. The size of the neuroma depends on how many funiculi have been damaged and the distance between the severed funiculi. Obviously, the more axons injured, the more will regenerate and therefore the larger the neuroma. Size also depends on the distance between the severed funiculi. For instance, if there is minimal retraction of the ends, the gap is rapidly bridged by proliferating Schwann's cells and fibroblasts, reestablishing the tubes to allow regenerating axons to find their way to their proper distal sheaths and end organs. If the funicular gap is large, this area is not bridged quickly by Schwann's cells and fibroblasts, allowing regenerating axons to escape from their sheaths and thus form a true neuroma on the side of an otherwise intact nerve.

The treatment of lateral neuromas-in-continuity, which can be exceedingly difficult, is discussed in Chapter 34.

NEUROMAS FOLLOWING NERVE REPAIR

Upon inspection of previously repaired severed nerves, the surgeon often finds a neuroma-in-continuity. This does not always happen, but it does occur frequently. Although not proven, funicular repair may decrease the incidence and size of this neuroma by providing end-to-end contact of fascicles, thus minimizing axonal escape. Sunderland

has shown that this type of neuroma is more common in severed nerves that contain small, widely separated funiculi, and/or in nerves where the injury has occurred at a level where the cut ends have dissimilar funicular patterns. An example of this would be where a segment of nerve has been excised or destroyed.

Neuromas in Completely Severed Nerves

This is the classic neuroma that surgeons encounter. It forms on the proximal stump of any severed peripheral nerve. Its formation and structure have been discussed earlier under the section on anatomy.

Amputation Stump Neuromas

The neuroma forming at the end of a severed nerve in an amputation stump is the same as the neuroma that forms on the end of a completely severed nerve. There are two important differences, however. In the amputation stump, if the nerve lies near the end of the stump and secondary healing occurs, it is subject to increased fibrosis. It is also subject to repeated trauma from pressure, friction, and concussion, which leads to increased size, edema, fibrosis, and increased sensitivity. In such cases, the neuroma may become so painful that the amputation stump or the whole part becomes useless.

To avoid this problem, the initial treating surgeon should transect the nerve in such a way as to allow it to retract into a bed of healthy soft tissues away from the working surface of the amputation stump. If the tissues are not satisfactory, the end of the nerve should be transferred to an area away from the working surface of the stump, usually dorsally, as is described in the section on relocation of the intact neuroma.

DIAGNOSIS

The diagnosis of a painful neuroma is usually easy to make. Direct tapping over the nerve elicits painful paresthesias. A palpable mass that is tender to touch may be present, and pressure on this mass recreates the patient's symptoms. The pain produced often has a peculiarly intense and unpleasant quality.

In some patients, especially in worker's compensation cases, it may be difficult to determine if the neuroma is indeed the major cause of the patient's pain. In such cases, Green (personal communication) uses differential diagnostic blocks, first with saline and then with lidocaine.

Rarely, one may be fooled by a mass over an intact nerve causing symptoms of a neuroma secondary to pressure on the nerve by the mass. I have had such a case recently of an inclusion cyst overlying one of the terminal branches of the digital nerve in the tip of the finger. The patient presented with classic history and physical findings of a neuroma.

TREATMENT

Sunderland states, "there is no procedure that is completely and consistently successful in preventing neuroma formation."[81] Because of this, the literature is extensive on the subject. Although many different techniques have been described, no universally successful method of treatment has been found. Guttmann and Medawar[40] showed that only destruction of the cell body would inhibit axonal regeneration completely. Any severed nerve will form a neuroma. Probably the best way to minimize neuroma formation is by a careful repair or grafting to allow the regenerating axons the best possible chance to extend into the distal empty funiculi. The debate on the optimal type of repair still persists in the literature, however. Bora, Pleasure, and Didizian[6] have measured the amount of collagen and myelin in the distal portion of severed nerves in rabbits. They found that there was more collagen near the neuroma in the immediate epineurial repair, but 60 percent of the normal myelin production was found in the distal nerve segment compared to 28.3 percent in the immediate perineurial group and less in the delayed groups. In other words, the epineurial repair resulted in more collagen about the periphery of the nerve repair site, whereas the perineurial repair resulted in more

internal scarring and therefore less axonal regrowth into the distal segment. I know of no studies comparing the neuroma formation in humans with each of these two types of repair, however. Clinically, Tupper and Booth have noted that a well-sealed epineurial repair of a severed nerve rarely results in a painful neuroma.[86]

Nonoperative techniques such as tapping, massage, ultrasound, and other modalities have been tried. I am not aware of any controlled studies to prove their effectiveness, and I therefore believe that operative treatment by repair or translocation to avoid or minimize neuroma formation provides the best likelihood of success. However, I do not believe, as some have suggested, that delay of operative treatment compromises the result.

Resection

Resection of an acutely severed nerve, allowing it to retract back into an area of uninjured soft tissue, is the most commonly preferred treatment of irreparable nerve injuries, especially in amputation stumps.[24] This technique is also used for treatment of a painful neuroma in an area of old injury. Tupper and Booth[86] reported a large series of 316 neuromas treated by simple excisional neurectomy. Injuries were divided into crush, jagged lacerations, and sharp lacerations. They reported that 65 percent of all of these injuries together had satisfactory or excellent results (36.5 percent excellent) from a single resection. Satisfactory or excellent results increased to 78 percent (45 percent excellent) following a second simple neurectomy.

Operative Technique

It is usually easier to first identify the nerve in an area of normal anatomy, isolate the neuroma, and then dissect the nerve free proximally. If it is a terminal branch, it may be helpful to dissect this branch from the main nerve under magnification to avoid any injury to the nerve. The proximal limits of the dissection should be an area of healthy soft tissue, free of scar, where the new nerve end will be well covered and protected. Gentle traction is then applied to the nerve (Fig. 35-3). Excessive traction is avoided to prevent intraneural axonal tears and possible additional neuroma formation. The nerve

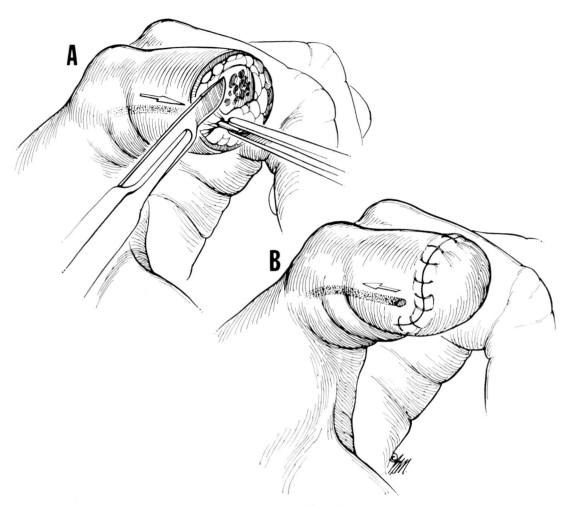

Fig. 35-3. Simple resection of a neuroma. (**A**) The end of the nerve is grasped, pulled gently into the wound, and severed sharply as far proximally as possible. (**B**) The transected nerve end retracts into the proximal normal soft tissues.

is then sectioned as far proximally as possible with a sharp knife, scissors, or razor blade, allowing it to retract into the bed of healthy soft tissue.

Crushing

Attempting to suppress axonal regrowth at the end of the severed nerve by crushing the end of the nerve was one of the earliest reported techniques, and it proved to be ineffective in preventing neuroma formation.[49] Stevenson combined the technique of crushing the nerve end with ligating the stump as well.[79]

Multiple Sectioning

Some surgeons believe that if a nerve is sectioned and then repaired at multiple levels proximal to the site of injury, many axons will not find their way back to the original injury site. If they do, the time course will have been sufficiently prolonged so that the end of the nerve will hopefully be covered over with scar, thereby impeding neuroma formation. As Sunderland points out, however, this method is not recommended, for it increases neuroma formation at multiple sites, and if the distal endoneurial tubes are closed, neuroma formation is not inhibited, but rather enhanced.[27,54]

Ligation

Ligation of the severed nerve to prevent neuroma formation is controversial. Sunderland believes that the method is of value in limiting neuroma formation.[81] Chavannaz[13] and Jegorow[59] have noted atrophy of the nerve distal to the ligature and reduced volume of the terminal neuroma. The rationale for ligation is to close the funiculi by the suture, thereby preventing axonal regrowth. The technique requires that the ligature be placed around the nerve 5 to 10 cm above the cut end and tied tightly enough to seal the funiculi, but not so tightly as to cut through them. I think this is where the problem arises, for it is probably impossible to secure a ligature around the nerve tightly enough to close the funiculi and not damage the perineurium, with resulting new sites for neuroma formation. Indeed, Petropoulos and Stefanko[68] found terminal neuromas above the ligation site and also reported a neuroma at the nerve end after ligature. The neuroma was smaller, but contained regenerating fibers. Below the ligation, the fibers were nonmedullated, and the authors thought that the nerve fibers had become smaller in order to penetrate the area of the ligature.[68] Other investigators have also found ligation unreliable, experimentally as well as clinically.[14,18,44,45] Ligation has been used in conjunction with other modalities, with mixed success. Such methods have included crushing, injecting the stump with gentian violet, covering the nerve with tannic acid powder and collodion, or the use of gentian violet, formaldehyde, or alcohol as chemical coagulants.[18,44,48,65,79]

Operative Technique

The nerve is dissected free proximally. An area somewhere between 5 and 10 cm above the severed end of the nerve is the site of the ligature. Nonabsorbable material is used. The suture is tied circumferentially around the nerve tightly enough to stop the bleeding, but not so tight as to cut through the nerve. Excess nerve distally may be resected for adequate stump closure (Fig. 35-4).

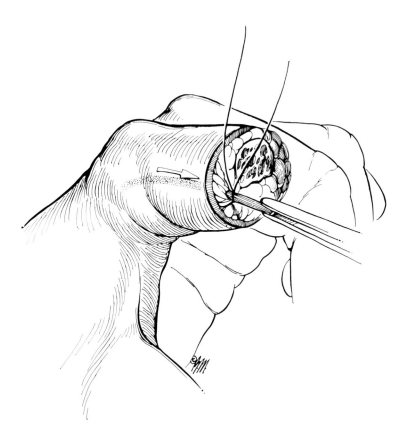

Fig. 35-4. Ligation of a neuroma. The severed nerve end is ligated proximally and the distal portion excised.

RADIOACTIVE LIGATURES

Perl and Whitlock[67] in rats and Gorman, Nold, and King[39] in horses used radioactive phosphate-impregnated chromic ligatures on severed nerves. In rats, axonal regeneration was inhibited by 88 percent. In horses, the neuromas were smaller, but the stumps were more sensitive. Limited use of an injection of a radioactive solution into nerve stumps in patients has produced some favorable results.[67] This is a concept that needs more investigation and may be an area to explore in the future.

Epineurial Closure

Three types of epineurial closure have been described. Chapple drew the epineurium over the end of the sectioned nerve, suturing it closed in an attempt to seal the endoneurial tubes.[12] Corner removed a wedge of the distal nerve in order to close the epineurium. Neuroma formation was not prevented.[16] A combination of crushing and ligation with transposition of the nerve end into muscle was reported by Munro and Mallory[62] Their results were better than those of Chapple or Corner.

Tupper and Booth[86] reported a third method—funiculectomy and epineurial ligation—in 45 neuromas in 28 patients. When this method was used as a primary procedure for a neuroma, 81 percent obtained excellent or satisfactory results (53.1 percent excellent). Three patients had to undergo a second funiculectomy and each showed nerve tissue growing past the ligature site. If a second funiculectomy was done, 87 percent of the patients obtained satisfactory or excellent results. In their hands, this method was better than a simple neurectomy, but they stated that the number of cases was too small to be conclusive.

Operative Technique

With the use of a microscope, the nerve is transected proximal to the neuroma. The epineurium is then carefully peeled back over the nerve trunk. Each funiculus is identified and individually sectioned 1 cm proximally. The empty epineurial tube is then doubly ligated with 6–0 nylon (Fig. 35-5). The nerve end is then placed in adjacent healthy tissue.

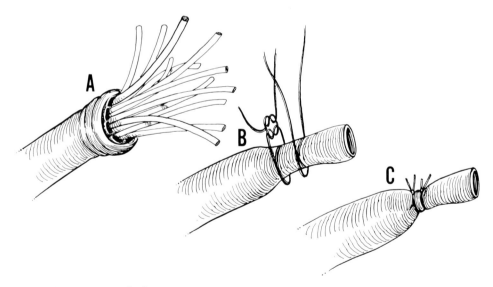

Fig. 35-5. Epineurial closure. (**A**) The epineurium is rolled proximally, exposing the fascicles, which are severed and allowed to retract. (**B**) The epineurium is then pulled distally, forming an empty tube. A double ligature is applied just distal to the severed ends of the fascicles. (**C**) The empty epineurial tube is sealed by the double ligature to prevent axonal outgrowth.

Transposition

In this technique the neuroma is usually excised (in contrast to relocation of the intact neuroma) and the distal portion of the proximal cut end of the nerve is turned back on itself.[13,15] The severed end is placed in an area devoid of scar, essentially similar to resection that allows the cut end to retract into healthy soft tissue. A neuroma still develops at the end of the nerve, but theoretically, there will be less irritation in the new healthy bed. If the nerve is twisted during the procedure, however, small terminal neuromas have been observed in the twisted area.[68] In such cases, the barrier provided by Schwann's cells and endoneurium is disrupted by stretching, and thus the nerve must be handled gently with this technique.

TRANSPOSITION WITH IMPLANTATION

Implantation of the nerve stump into surrounding tissue has been reported with good success. A requirement for success with this technique appears to be that the central stump of the cut nerve should be dissected out into its longitudinal funiculi, and each of these is implanted into the tissue.[68] The fact that surgeons have implanted the whole nerve stump into surrounding tissue with variable results has possibly led to the relative disfavor of this technique. Tissues used have been the nerve itself, muscle, bone, fascia, and blood vessels, but little is contained in the literature except for the use of the nerve, bone, and muscle. Even with these tissues, the reports are neither conclusive nor comparable.

Implantation into the Same Nerve (Neurocampsis)

Bardenheuer is credited with describing this technique.[68] The cut end of the nerve is implanted into the nerve trunk proximally through an opening made in the epineurium. Petropoulos and Stefanko found that with this technique in dogs a spiral-shaped neuroma was formed that was twice the size of the control neuromas. The neuroma formed was very hypertrophic with prolific regeneration of nerve components.[68] I found no studies in the literature using this technique in humans.

Implantation into Muscle

In dogs, Petropoulos and Stefanko dissected out the individual funiculi of the sectioned nerve and implanted each into neighboring muscle tissue.[68] They found no neuroma formation and observed only laminar formations that became lost in the muscle. Dellon et al also recently reported observations that suggest that a classic neuroma does not form when a transected nerve is implanted into muscle.[21]

In humans, I would suspect that even if this technique prevents neuroma formation, it may result in discomfort for the patient because of traction on the nerve end with movement and muscle contraction. Laborde et al abandoned this procedure because of an unacceptably high re-operative rate of 65 percent.[51]

Implantation into Bone

In this method, the nerve end is implanted within the medullary canal of bone.[15,29,77] Boldrey described a technique whereby a suture on the end of the nerve is drawn through a drill hole in bone, securing the amputated nerve stump in the medullary canal. Such a technique has two objectives: (1) to contain the nerve stump in a rigid compartment, thereby restricting neuroma size, and (2) by containing the nerve stump in bone, to protect the neuroma from direct trauma. However, with the nerve fixed in bone, tension on the nerve may result with movement of the extremity. Boldry reported successful use of his technique in one patient, but Munro and Mallory abandoned the procedure.[62] Mass et al recently presented 18 successful results in 20 attempts with this technique.[55] In 11 cases Goldstein and Sturim had excellent or satisfactory results in 10.[36] One additional patient required reoperation because of technical failure when one of two transposed nerves pulled out of the bone. They stressed some important technical details: adequate mobilization of the nerve; no tension on the nerve; avoidance of an excessively acute angle of the nerve as it enters the bone; and no implantation of the nerve just distal to a joint.

Implantation into Another Nerve

Cross union of the terminal ends of two severed nerves in proximity was reported by Langley and Anderson.[52] They demonstrated that axons will not grow into funiculi already containing axons. However, the axons will continue to grow and branch into the epineurial tissue about the funiculi, forming a neuroma-in-continuity. No reports have been found using a funicular repair in such cases. For this procedure to prevent neuroma formation, there must be an even match of funiculi in the two nerves, which is not a likely possibility.

Centrocentral Nerve Union. A new operative procedure, centrocentral nerve union with autogenous transplantation, was recently described by Gorkisch et al.[38] In this technique two nerves of central origin are sutured together with a simple epineurial repair just as described by Langely and Anderson.[52] In addition however, one of the nerves is severed more proximally, about 10 mm from the epineurial repair. This iatrogenic laceration is also repaired, thus creating an autograft segment. In their 30 patients, only one had complaints suggestive of a neuroma formation. Gonzalez-Darder et al were able to reduce the size of neuroma formation in rats using this technique.[37]

Two mechanisms have been suggested as the possible means by which this technique prevents neuroma formation: (1) the proximal axons are removed from the influence of their distal "targets"; and (2) confinement of the proliferative axons and eventual overlapping may increase the intraperineural pressure, which results in a reduction and eventual cessation of protein production and axoplasm flow.[72]

Relocation of Intact Neuroma

In 1967 Littler, realizing that all techniques for management of painful neuromas were subject to the same unknown factors that caused the symptoms in the initial neuroma, developed a new technique.[43] Every effort is made to keep the neuroma intact with its mature encapsulating scar, while transposing it en bloc to an adjacent area free of scar and not subjected to repeated trauma.

A subsequent evaluation of this technique[43] revealed that 82 percent of cases with amputation neuromas and 63 percent of cases with terminal branch neuromas had excellent results and were essentially symptom-free. In the nonamputee group, elimination of the iatrogenic lesions increased the excellent results to 86 percent. Fourteen of the 15 patients with amputations were worker's compensation cases and all but three returned to work. In 28 percent of the neuromas transferred, no sensitivity to percussion could be elicited, and in 73 percent, there was absent to mild sensitivity to direct percussion at the new location. No patient who initially had a successful transfer of the neuroma had recurrent symptoms after prolonged follow-up. Similar long term success with dorsal translocation has been reported by Laborde et al.[51]

Operative Technique

The neuroma with its fibrous capsule is carefully isolated. A proximal area that is free from scar and away from local trauma is selected, preferably deep to a muscle, in a web space, or between the shafts of adjacent metacarpals. A dorsal site is preferable to a palmar location that might lead to pressure on the neuroma with manual activity such as the gripping of tools.

The neuroma-in-continuity with its nerve is then carefully dissected proximally until the neuroma bulb can be transferred to its new location without tension on the nerve. A 5–0 catgut suture is then placed through the capsule (not the neuroma) and tied. Another knot is tied 3 to 4 mm away from the neuroma. The free ends of the suture are then tunneled subcutaneously and passed through the skin proximal to the location selected for the neuroma. This suture is drawn through the skin and tied, maintaining a 3- to 4-mm separation between the dermis and neuroma (Figs. 35-6 and 35-7). The nerve trunk is carefully examined to make certain that no tension or twisting exists along its path. A similar technique is used when the neuroma is buried in muscle. For neuromas in the finger stumps, I prefer to transfer the nerve end into the web space; for neuromas in the palm, the nerve ends are transferred to the dorsum of the hand between the metacarpals.

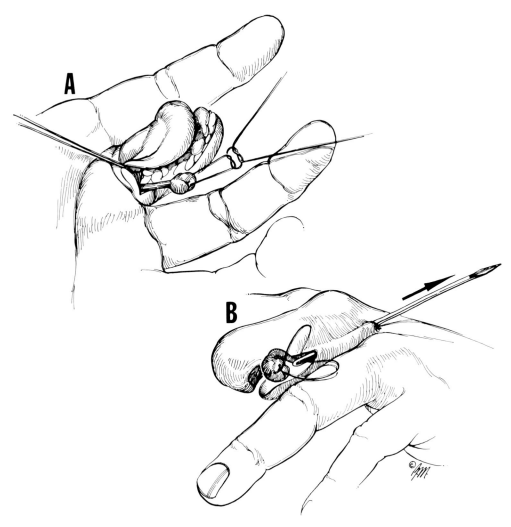

Fig. 35-6. Relocation of an intact neuroma. (**A**) After the neuroma is dissected free, a suture is placed in its capsule. A second knot is tied about 3 to 4 mm from the capsule. (**B**) A tunnel is bluntly dissected in the soft tissues. The neuroma is pulled through the tunnel into an area free from recurrent trauma. The suture is passed through the skin and tied, pulling the second knot up to the dermis.

Coagulation

In an effort to suppress regeneration of axons or to prevent their longitudinal growth by sealing the funicular ends with scar, many investigators have used various types of methods of coagulation of the nerve stump. These include hot water, heat (cauterization), freezing, electrocoagulation, application of chemical coagulants, and radioactive substances.[2,26,27,29,42,49,53,68]

PHYSICAL METHODS

Petropoulos and Stefanko studied the use of freezing, cauterization, and electrocoagulation in neuroma formation in dogs.[68] Neuromas did form, but they were smaller than controls. They were typical terminal neuromas of Schwann's type with little perineurial connective tissue proliferation. Others have reported similar findings with only temporary obstruction to regenerating axons.[27]

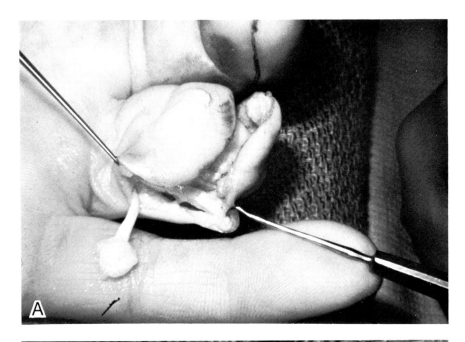

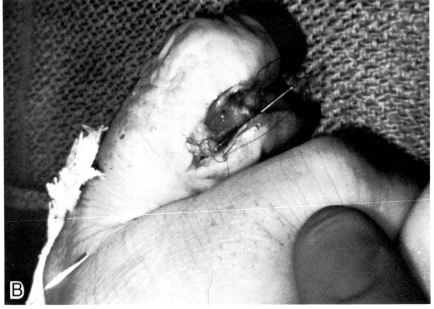

Fig. 35-7. Clinical photographs showing relocation of an intact neuroma. (**A**) The neuroma dissected free. (**B**) Transposition of the neuroma.

As Sunderland has pointed out, these methods are generally unsuccessful because it is almost impossible to suppress axonal growth.[81] Holmes and Young[46] and Duncan and Jarvis[23] have shown that in animals, axons have the capacity to regenerate for years. Clinically, this is true in humans as well.

In Italy, Maturo et al have been developing a technique of treating painful amputation neuromas with a CO_2 laser. Twenty-one of their 25 patients had total disappearance of their pain with CO_2 laser beam photocoagulation.[56]

CHEMICAL METHODS

Basically, these chemicals are all sclerosing agents. Sunderland has noted that no agent has been shown to effectively suppress all axonal regeneration.[81] These agents create scar tissue at the nerve gaps and may therefore possibly inhibit regrowth of axons into surrounding tissue. The list of agents tried is extensive, including procaine, alcohol, osmic acid, tannic acid, picric acid, chromic acid, hydrochloric acid and pepsin, formaldehyde, iodine, uranium nitrate, gentian violet, phenol, mercuric chloride solution, and nitrogen mustard.[3,4,18,27–30,32,33,40,47,48,65,69–71,73,80]

Sunderland, in his thorough review of the use of these agents, stated that "unfortunately the results of using these chemical agents have been disappointing and the concensus of opinion is that they have no real value in preventing the formation of neuromas."[81] Petropoulos and Stefanko showed that in animals 80 percent alcohol produced the greatest amount of necrosis of the nerve stump and formaldehyde the least.[69] Their best results were with the use of either local or systemic nitrogen mustard. Often no neuroma was present in these animals. If there was a neuroma, it was small and atrophic, with marked inhibition of Schwann's cell proliferation and minimal scar formation. Guttmann and Medwar in their studies found that formaldehyde and gentian violet were the most effective and alcohol the least effective in inhibiting neuroma formation.[40] Their series was small and the data were not conclusive.

The technique for using these agents locally is to free the distal end of the nerve from all soft tissues. A ligature may or may not be placed proximally (1 to 5 cm). The funiculi are then meticulously dissected apart, and the solution is carefully injected into every individual funiculus. Some investigators also then soak the distal nerve stump in the solution.

ANTI-INFLAMMATORY AGENTS (TRIAMCINOLONE)

Smith and Gomez injected triamcinolone acetonide into the painful neuroma and surrounding scar tissue in 22 patients.[75] They used either a needle or the Dermo-Jet, injecting the steroid at multiple sites in the deep dermal and subdermal levels. Their rationale was based on the observation that hypertrophic scars and keloids often become soft and flattened after intralesional injection of triamcinolone. Success was obtained in 19 of 34 neuromas so treated, but there was a 29 percent failure rate. This technique worked best in localized digital neuromas and was less successful for deeper neuromas in the palm and wrist.[66,75]

In the rat, some injured sensory fibers ending in an experimental neuroma of the sciatic nerve discharge spontaneously. Corticosteroids have been shown to produce a rapid and prolonged suppression of these discharges, suggesting a membrane action rather than an anti-inflammatory action.[20]

Capping the Nerve End

The divided end of the nerve has been ensheathed in numerous materials in an attempt to diminish neuroma formation. Materials reported include silicone, millipore, gold foil, tantalum, methylmethacrylate, polyethylene, silver, cellophane, Vitallium, glass caps, collodion, Lucite, tin, decalcified bone, fascia, vessel lumen, placental tissue, rubber and plastic femoral artery replacements, dried plasma, and arterial wall tissue.[5,18,25,27,31,34,35,71,76,82,83,85,88]

Petropoulos and Stefanko[69] showed that in dogs neither tantalum, silver, nor gold inhibited neuroma formation, and, in fact, the neuromas were larger than those in the controls. Other reports are inconclusive, with neuromas continuing to form about the material used. It is difficult to seal the funiculi completely. Poth and Bravo-Fernandez used similar materials plus cellophane, Vitallium, and glass with very unpredictable results.[71] Early success with tantalum was reported by White and Hamlin, but there have been no long-term results reported.[88] Sunderland noted that tantalum does evoke a severe delayed foreign body reaction.[81]

Methylmethacrylate was used by Edds but neuromas continued to form.[25] Collodion has been ineffective. Campbell and colleagues used millipore filters, without success, and it is no longer used.[10]

SILICONE CAPPING

Use of silicone rubber caps over the end of the severed nerve has been more effective than any of the other capping techniques.[5,31,82–84] Swanson, Boeve, and Lumsden reported a series of 18 patients with 38 neuromata.[83] Follow-up averaged 41 months. Fifteen patients had relief of their symptoms, one patient had recurrence of pain and was relieved by recapping, and two patients developed causalgia. Prior to its use in humans, Swanson and colleagues studied the technique in rabbits and demonstrated severed nerves with no neuroma formation. They have shown that several factors are important in inhibiting axonal growth and re-

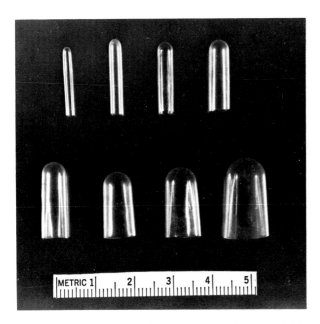

Fig. 35-8. Silicone caps (Swanson design) are available in several sizes. A cap only slightly larger than the diameter of the nerve should be used.

sultant neuroma formation: (1) the length-to-diameter ratio should be a minimum of 5 : 1, that is, the shorter the cap, the more likely a neuroma will form; and (2) the nerve cap should be only slightly larger than the nerve. It should not fit too loosely, allowing axons to grow back proximally between the cap and the epineurium.

Operative Technique

In Swanson's technique, the first step is to resect the neuroma. A silicone cap slightly larger than the nerve, but not too tight, is chosen (Fig. 35-8). It is trimmed to the appropriate length (5 to 10 times the nerve's diameter). Using a 5 – 0 nonabsorbable Bunnell-type suture, the cap is secured over the freshly amputated nerve stump (Fig. 35-9). Swanson and colleagues also recommend transfer of the nerve stump to healthy soft tissue if necessary.

Tupper and Booth reported a series of 32 neuromas in 17 patients in whom they used two types of silicone caps.[86] The first was a silicone rubber Ducker-Hayes tube that was passed over the end of the nerve. The proximal portion of the tube was sutured to the epineurium and the distal end was ligated beyond the end of the nerve. In two of these that were reexplored, the cap remained in place, but nerve fibers had grown through the loose proximal opening.

The second type was a Frackelton cap that was fit snugly over the nerve end. Both types of caps became dislodged in six patients. None of the Frackelton caps that were reexplored showed any evidence of funicular escape and neuroma formation. Only 25 percent of their results were excellent. This increased to 31 percent when a second capping was done. If compared to a third simple neurectomy, the results were no different. Tupper and Booth concluded that, in their hands, capping did not improve their results over simple excisional neurectomy.

Soft Tissue Coverage

Brown and Flynn reported four cases of patients with painful neuromas in the hand after multiple operations in whom resection of the scarred area and replacement with abdominal pedicle tissue gave relief of their symptoms.[8] Instead of transfer-

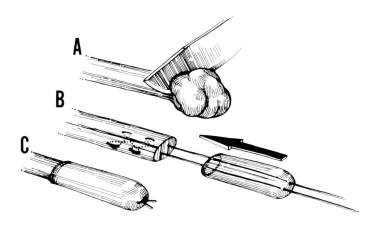

Fig. 35-9. Silicone capping. (A) The neuroma is excised. (B) A suture is passed through the nerve and the distal end of the silicone cap. (C) The silicone cap is pulled over the end of the nerve and secured by tying the suture.

ring the nerves to a healthy bed, they moved a healthy bed of tissue to the damaged area. This rather drastic approach represents a possible salvage procedure in patients with scarred tissues in whom other relatively easier methods of treatment have been tried without success.

Author's Preferred Method

The tremendous capacity for axons to regenerate and the many unknown influences resulting in symptomatic neuromas have led to the failure or unpredictability of many of the procedures described in this chapter. Sunderland concluded that silicone capping or ligation combined with the use of a chemical coagulant offers the best chances for success.[81] Petropoulos and Stefanko concluded from their studies that local or systemic nitrogen mustard provided the best results.[69] Swanson, Boeve, and Lumsden prefer silicone capping, and Tupper and Booth obtained better results with resection than with silicone capping.[83,86] Mass et al and Goldstein and Sturim reported good results with transfer of the neuroma into bone.[36,55] The unique concept of centrocentral nerve union described by Gorkisch et al is intriguing, and in selected cases may be potentially very useful.[38] Finally, the CO_2 laser may have a future role in the control of neuroma formation.[56] None of these studies is conclusive, however.

In the management of an amputated nerve end or an irreparable terminal branch laceration, I prefer simple resection, allowing the cut end of the nerve to retract into healthy soft tissues. If the bed is not adequate, I transfer the severed end to another location where local trauma will be minimal. For established neuromas, I prefer relocation of the intact neuroma as described on page 1414. If, however, the distal end of the nerve is present, I would attempt to minimize neuroma formation by resection of the neuroma and repair of the nerve. If too large a gap exists, grafts would be my next choice. Only if the distal portion of the severed nerve were absent or irreparable, would I recommend neuroma relocation. This applies to the commonly encountered neuromas of the superficial branch of radial nerve and the palmar cutaneous branch of median nerve. In case of amputation neuromas, I prefer relocation.

I believe that local nitrogen mustard, local radioactive materials, and silicone capping are all interesting possibilities, and more investigation and clinical use are necessary to find the best method, if one exists. At present, however, I prefer to leave the neuroma intact and transfer it to an area free from local trauma. This is an effective, proven method, even in the difficult, work-injured patient.

REFERENCES

1. Badalamente MA, Hurst LC, Ellstein J, McDevitt CA: The pathobiology of human neuromas: An electron microscopic and biochemical study. J Hand Surg 10B:49–53, 1985

2. Bate JT: Method of treating nerve ends in amputation stumps. Am J Surg 64:373–374, 1944

3. Benedikt M: Ueber neuralgien und neuralgische Affectionen und deren Behandlung. Klin Z Streitfragen 6:67, 1892

4. Beswerschenko AP: Traumatische Neurome. Entstehungsbedingungen der Neurome und Mittel zur ihren Verhutung. Experimentalle Untersuchungen Zentralbl Chir 56:455, 1929

5. Biddulph SL: The prevention and treatment of painful amputation neuroma. Proceedings of the South African Orthopaedic Association. J Bone Joint Surg 54B:379, 1972

6. Bora FW, Pleasure DE, Didizian NA: A study of nerve regeneration and neuroma formation after nerve suture by various techniques. J Hand Surg 1:138–143, 1976

7. Boyes JH: Bunnell's Surgery of the Hand. p. 426. 3rd Ed. JB Lippincott, Philadelphia, 1956

8. Brown H, Flynn JE: Abdominal pedicle flap for hand neuromas and entrapped nerves. J Bone Joint Surg 55A:575–579, 1973

9. Bunnell S, Boyes JH: Nerve grafts. Am J Surg 44:64–75, 1939

10. Campbell JB, Bassett CAL, Girado JM, Seymour RJ, Rossi JP: Application of mono-molecular filter tubes in bridging gaps in peripheral nerves and for prevention of neuroma formation. A preliminary report. J Neurosurg 13:635, 1956

11. Campbell JB, Bassett CAL, Husby J, Thulin CA, Feringa ER: Microfilter sheaths in peripheral nerve surgery, a laboratory report and preliminary clinical study. J Trauma 1:139–157, 1961

12. Chapple WA: Prevention of nerve bulbs in stumps. Br Med J 1:399, 1918

13. Chavannaz G: A propos de la technique de l'amputation de cuisse. La ligature du nerf grand sciatique. Bull Acad Med 123:123, 1940

14. Cieslak AK, Stout AP: Traumatic and amputation neuromas. Arch Surg 53:646–651, 1946

15. Contini V: Experimental study of amputation neuromas. Arch Ital Chir 56:569–575, 1939

16. Corner EM: The structure, forms and conditions of the ends of divided nerves: With a note on regeneration neuromata. Br J Surg 6:273–278, 1918

17. Davis L, Perret G, Hiller F: Experimental studies in peripheral nerve surgery. Effect of infection on regeneration and functional recovery. Surg Gynecol Obstet 81:302–308, 1945

18. DeCarvalho Pinto VA, Junqueira LCU: A comparative study of the methods for prevention of amputation neuroma. Surg Gynecol Obstet 99:492–496, 1954

19. Devor M, Wall PD: Type of sensory nerve fibre sprouting to form a neuroma. Nature 262:705–707, 1976

20. Devor M, Govrin-Lippmann R, Raber P: Corticosteroids suppress ectopic neural discharge originating in experimental neuromas. Pain 22:127–137, 1985

21. Dellon AL, MacKinnon SE, Pestronk A: Implantation of sensory nerve into muscle: Preliminary clinical and experimental observations on neuroma formation. Ann Plast Surg 12:30–40, 1984

22. Dobyns JH, O'Brien ET, Linscheid RL, Farrow GM: Bowler's thumb: Diagnosis and treatment. A review of seventeen cases. J Bone Joint Surg 54A:751–755, 1972

23. Duncan D, Jarvis WH: Observations on repeated regeneration of the facial nerve in cats. J Comp Neurol 79:315, 1943

24. Eaton RG: Painful neuromas. pp. 195–202. In Omer CE, Spinner M, (eds): Management of Peripheral Nerve Problems. WB Saunders, Philadelphia, 1980

25. Edds MV: Prevention of nerve regeneration and neuroma formation by caps of synthetic resin. J Neurosurg 2:507–509, 1945

26. Erlacher P: Untersuchung und Wiederherstellung der Leitung im peripheren Nerven durch thermische und chemische Mittel. Arch Orthop 23:287, 1924

27. Evans LH, Campbell JB, Pinner-Poole B, Jenny J: Prevention of painful neuromas in horses. J Am Vet Med Assoc 153:313, 1968

28. Fellinger K, Reimer E: Nitrogen Mustard in der Internen Klinik. Wien Klin Wochenschr 61:681–684, 1949

29. Fernandez J: Regeneracao nervosa apos diversos metodos cirgicos visando a prevencao do neuroma de amputacao. Archos Neuropsiquiat 18:341, 1960

30. Foerster O: Therapie der Schussverletzungen der peripheren Nerven. p. 1703. Berlin, 1929

31. Frackelton WH, Teasley JL, Tauras A: Neuromas in the hand treated by nerve transposition and silicone capping. Proceedings of the American Society for Surgery of the Hand. J Bone Joint Surg 53A:813, 1971

32. Fraenkel E: Ueber parenchymatose uberosmimsaure Injektion. Berl Klin Wochenschr 21:234, 1884

33. Frankenthal L: Histologische und experimentelle Untersuchungen über die Wirkungsweise der Injektionstherapie bei Neuralgien, augleich eine histologische Studie über die Nadelstichverletzungen der Nerven. Beitr Klin Chir 143:237, 1928

34. Garrity RW: The use of plastic and rubber tubing in

the management of irreparable nerve injuries. Surg Forum 6:517, 1955

35. Gluck T: Ueber Neuroplastik auf dem Wege der Transplantation. Arch Klin Chir 25:606, 1880

36. Goldstein SA, Sturim HS: Intraosseous nerve transposition for treatment of painful neuromas. J Hand Surg 10A:270–274, 1985

37. Gonzalez-Darder J, Baber J, Abell MJ, Mora A: Centrocentral anastomosis in the prevention and treatment of painful terminal neuroma. An Experimental Study in the Rat. J Neurosurg 63:754–758, 1985

38. Gorkisch K, Boese-Landgraf J, Vaubel E: Treatment and prevention of amputation neuromas in hand surgery. Plast Reconstr Surg 73:293–296, 1984

39. Gorman TN, Nold MM, King JM: Use of radioactivity in neurectomy of the horse. Cornell Vet 52:542, 1952

40. Guttmann L, Medawar PB: The chemical inhibition of fibre regeneration and neuroma formation in peripheral nerves. J Neurol Psychiatr 5:130, 1942

41. Hedri A: Zur Behandlung des Nervenquer-schnittes bei Amputationsstumpfen. Munch Med Wochenschr 67:1148, 1920

42. Hedri A: Ein einfaches Verfahren zur Verhutung der Trennungsneurome. Arch Klin Chir 117:842, 1921

43. Herndon JH, Eaton RG, Littler JW: Management of painful neuromas in the hand. J Bone Joint Surg 58A:369–373, 1976

44. Herrmann LG: Painful amputation stumps: Relation to treatment of large mixed nerves at time of amputation. Lyon Chir 52:476, 1956

45. Herrmann LG, Gibbs EW: Phantom limb pain: Its relation to treatment of large nerves at time of amputation. Am J Surg 67:168–180, 1945

46. Holmes W, Young JZ: Nerve regeneration after immediate and delayed suture. J Anat 77:63, 1942

47. Huber GC: Injection into Divided Nerve to Prevent Amputation Neuroma. p. 1125. Series Nos. 3 and 4, Medical Dept. of the United States Army in the World War, Vol. 1 (surgery). Government Printing Office, 1920

48. Huber GC, Lewis D: Amputation neuromas. Their development and prevention. Arch Surg 1:85–113, 1920

49. Kirk NT: Amputations: Monograph from Lewis Practice of Surgery, Vol 3. Harper & Row, Hagarstown, MD, 1943

50. Kreuger H: Ueber Nervenquetschung zur Verhutung schmerzhafter Neurome mach Amputation. Munch Med Wochenschr 63:368, 1916

51. Laborde KJ, Kalisman M, Tsai TM: Results of surgical treatment of painful neuromas of the hand. J Hand Surg 7:190–193, 1982

52. Langley JN, Anderson HK: The union of different kinds of nerve fibres. J Physiol 31:365, 1904

53. Lawen A: Ueber Nervenverisung bei Amputationen. Amputationsneuromen Angiospasmen, Erythromelalgie, seniler Gangren und Ulcus Cruris Varicosum. Beitr Klin Chir 133:405, 1925

54. Leriche R: La Chirurgie de la Douleur. Masson, Paris, 1949

55. Mass DP, Ciano MC, Tortosa R, Newmeyer WL, Kilgore ES Jr: Treatment of painful hand neuromas by their transfer into bone. Plast Reconstr Surg 74:182–185, 1984

56. Maturo L, Del Duce G, Gobbato GP: Painful amputation neuromas: treatment with CO_2 laser (unpublished data).

57. Minkow FV, Bassett FH: Bowler's thumb. Clin Orthop 83:115–117, 1972

58. Mitchell SW: Traumatic neuralgia. Section of median nerve. Am J Med Sci 67:2–16, July 1874

59. Molotkow S: Leczenje Ogienstreichlnch Ramneni Perifericzeskich. Nerwow, Leningrad, 1942

60. Morton TG: A peculiar and painful affection of the fourth metatarso-phalangeal articulation. Am J Med Sci 71:37, 1876

61. Mukherjee K, Bassett IB: Meralgia paraesthetica. Br Med J 2(648):55, 1969

62. Munro D, Mallory GK: Elimination of the so-called amputation neuromas of divided peripheral nerves. N Engl J Med 260:358, 1959

63. Nelson AW: The painful neuroma: The regenerating axon versus the epineural sheath. J Surg Res 23:215–221, 1977

64. Odier L: Manual de Medecine Pratique. p. 362. JJ Paschaud, Geneva, 1811

65. Padovani PL: Les douleurs des amputes. Sem Hop Paris 25:817, 1949

66. Pataky PE, Graham WP III, Munger BL: Terminal neuromas treated with triamcinolone acetonide. J Surg Res 14:36–45, 1973

67. Perl JI, Whitlock DG: Use of radioactive colloidal chromic phosphate for prevention of amputation neuroma. J Int Coll Surg 29:77, 1958

68. Petropoulos PC, Stefanko S: Experimental observations on the prevention of neuroma formation. J Surg Res 1:241–248, 1961

69. Petropoulos PC, Stefanko S: Experimental studies of posttraumatic neuromas under various physiologic conditions. J Surg Res 1:235–240, 1961

70. Polley TZ, Brixey AJ Jr: The clinical use of nitrogen mustard. Med Times 79:1–6, 1951

71. Poth EJ, Bravo-Fernandez E: Prevention of neu-

roma formation by encasement of the severed nerve ends in rigid tubes. Proc Soc Exp Biol Med 56:7–8, 1944

72. Seckel BR: Discussion of treatment and prevention of amputation neuromas in hand surgery. Plast Reconstr Surg 73:297–299, 1984

73. Sicard JA: Traitment des nevrites douloureuses de guerre (causalgie) par l'alcoolisation nerveuse locale. Press Med 24:241, 1916

74. Siegel IM: Bowling thumb neuroma. JAMA 192:263, 1965

75. Smith JR, Gomez NH: Local injection therapy of neuromata of the hand with triamcinolone acetonide. A preliminary study of twenty-two patients. J Bone Joint Surg 52A:71–83, 1970

76. Snow JW: Silastic overlay for troublesome neuromata. Am Soc Surg Hand 15:1980

77. Solerio B, Ferrero R: Fixation of nerve stump in bone canal. Minerva Chir 6:640–645, 1951

78. Spencer PS: The traumatic neuroma and proximal stump. Bull Hosp Joint Dis 35:85–102, 1974

79. Stevenson GH: Amputations with special reference to phantom limb sensation. Edinb Med J 57:44, 1950

80. Stookey BP: Surgical and Mechanical Treatment of Peripheral Nerves. WB Saunders, Philadelphia and London, 1922

81. Sunderland S: Nerves and Nerve Injuries, 2nd Ed. Churchill Livingstone, Edinburgh, 1978

82. Swanson AB, Boeve NR, Biddulph SL: Silicone-rubber capping of amputation neuromas. Investigational and clinical experience. Inter-Clin Inf Bull 11:1, 1972

83. Swanson AB, Boeve NR, Lumsden RM: The prevention and treatment of amputation neuromata by silicone capping. J Hand Surg 2:70–78, 1977

84. Synder CC, Knowles RP: Traumatic neuromas (Abstract). J Bone Joint Surg 47A:641, 1965

85. Tauras AP, Frackelton WH: Silicone capping of nerve stumps in the problem of painful neuromas. Surg Forum 18:504, 1967

86. Tupper JW, Booth DM: Treatment of painful neuromas of sensory nerves in the hand: A comparison of traditional and newer methods. J Hand Surg 1:144–151, 1976

87. Virchow R: Die Krankhaften Geschwulste, Vol. 3. A Hirschwald, Berlin, 1863

88. White JC, Hamlin H: New uses of tantalum in nerve suture, control of neuroma formation and prevention of regeneration after thoracic sympathectomy, illustration of technical procedures. J Neurosurg 2:402–413, 1945

89. Wood W: Observations on neuromas, with cases and histories of the disease. Trans Med—Chir Soc Edinb 3:68, 1828–1829

Entrapment and Compression Neuropathies 36

William W. Eversmann, Jr.

Entrapment neuropathies of the upper extremity occur in predictable areas, are generally evaluated in a similar manner, and probably have a common pathophysiology. Entrapment neuropathies are nerve injuries. Because the degree of nerve injury is unknown preoperatively or even at the time of surgical release, the prognosis following surgical exploration of an entrapment neuropathy is often uncertain until the patient's clinical response is observed. As a general rule, however, unless an entrapment neuropathy is severe or longstanding, the neuropathy will be relieved by release of the compression on the nerve.

PATHOPHYSIOLOGY

Since the success of surgical treatment is dependent on an understanding of the pathophysiology of nerve compression, a review of the current concepts of pathophysiology is important in understanding the operative procedures involved in the entrapment neuropathies. There is little doubt that ionic, mechanical, and vascular lesions are all involved in the pathophysiologic mechanism of entrapment neuropathies.[109] Which of these mechanisms is the initiating one in the neurologic disturbance of a compression neuropathy in any given patient is uncertain, and it immediately becomes apparent that a shroud of confusion can easily encompass the pathophysiologic mechanisms. In recent years, the vascular lesions seem to have become most understandable from the standpoint of the pathophysiologic mechanisms.[219] The vascular anatomy of nerves has been studied since the seventeenth century.[106,107] A segmental vascular supply to the nerve trunk is carried in a mesoneurium, which permits motion and allows changes of position and tension of the nerve with motion of the extremity.[106,107,159] The arcades in the mesoneurium vary with location. The median nerve at the wrist is supplied by the mesoneurium from the volar-ulnar side of the nerve proximal to the transverse carpal ligament, as well as by a mesoneurium from the superficial palmar arch distal to the transverse carpal ligament.[7] The nerve trunk is supplied by this mesoneurium in a regional pattern, the small vessels entering the epineurium of the nerve and immediately dividing into ascending and descending epineurial branches. The epineurial network of vessels forms an anastomotic network that further subdivides into a vascular plexus in the perineurium. The capillary bed within the nerve

1423

itself is contained within the fascicles of the nerve so that below the perineurial level of vascular plexus, small end arteries and capillary beds form the remainder of the vascular pattern within the nerve trunks.[106,107]

If there is obstruction of venous return from the nerve by a mechanism as simple as prolonged flexion of the wrist or as complex as a distal radius fracture, venous congestion within the nerve results. Because of this venous congestion within the epineurial and perineurial vascular plexus, there is a generalized slowing of the circulation, not only in the epineurial plexus but in the intrafascicular tissues as well. Anoxia of a nerve segment results, which leads to dilatation of the small vessels and capillaries within that segment of the nerve, and endoneurial edema of the tissue results.[336] The edema of the nerve segment increases the effect of the original compression, which may have initiated the venous obstruction. If this increased compression or the edema persists for a prolonged period of time, proliferation of fibroblasts within the nerve ensues. This proliferation of fibroblasts eventually leads to scarring within the nerve, further rendering segments of the nerve anoxic because of a barrier of fibroblasts that further inhibits circulation within the nerve and exchange of vital nutrients between the vascular system and the nerve fibers.

The axioplasmic transport system within an axon combines a system of transport filaments, microtubules, and neurofilaments to transport protein molecules synthesized in the endoplasmic reticulum of the cell body to a location in the axon where they will be chemically active, such as in the wall of the axon or at the terminal endings.[120] Accordingly, protein polypeptides, glycoproteins, glycolipids, catecholamines, and acetylcholinesterase are transported from the cell body along the axon to their active site using the segmental axonal mitochondria and oxidative phosphorylation to generate the high-energy phosphate necessary for the transport and maintenance of the cell. When a portion of the axon is rendered ischemic with as small a reduction in blood flow as 30 to 50 percent of normal, the reduction in oxidative phosphorylation and production of high-energy phosphate decreases the efficiency of the sodium pump, the axioplasmic transport system, and the integrity of the cell membrane, which will in turn eventually lead to a loss of conduction or transmission along the nerve fiber.[219]

According to studies of various authors, it seems likely then that the primary lesion of entrapment neuropathies is vascular compromise of a segment of the axon.[68,109,120,219,336] That segment of the axon rendered ischemic or relatively ischemic through either a change of position, local anatomy, or internal pressure will react not only through a series of vascular mechanisms but, by so doing, will alter its ionic relationship to its environment and further aggravate the normal internal pressure of the nerve trunk to a degree to account for increased vascular changes and a deterioration of normal function of the nerve trunk. In our studies of intraoperative motor conduction latencies associated with carpal tunnel syndrome we have suggested that the rapidity of our patients' recovery and restitution of a normal conduction velocity could only be explained by a vascular lesion.[219]

ENTRAPMENT NEUROPATHIES OF THE MEDIAN NERVE

Three distinct entrapment neuropathies of the median nerve have been described. They differ in clinical presentation, physical findings on examination, and surgical treatment. Although there are differentiating points on clinical presentation and examination, the many similarities that these entrapment neuropathies possess often confuse the surgeon, and, as a result, the presentation of any one will usually add at least one of the other two to the differential diagnosis.

Pronator Syndrome

The most proximal entrapment neuropathy of the median nerve, which has been widely studied, is the pronator syndrome.[148] The pronator syndrome presents with pain in the proximal volar surface of the distal arm and forearm, which generally increases with activity. There is reduced sensibility or at least sensory symptoms in the radial three and one-half digits. The wrist flexion test of Phalen is notably negative in this syndrome, and signs are not limited to the deep volar compartment of the forearm, specifically loss of active flexion of the DIP joint of the index finger or the interphalangeal joint of the thumb.

There are four sites of potential compression, all of which produce the signs and symptoms of pronator syndrome. The first of these is compression of the median nerve in the distal third of the humerus beneath a supracondylar process and the ligament of Struthers. The second potential site of compression occurs at the lacertus fibrosus, which courses across the median nerve at the level of the elbow joint. The third site of compression is within the pronator teres muscle, caused either by hypertrophy of the pronator teres muscle or by the aponeurotic fascia on the deep surface of the superficial head or the superficial surface of the deep head of the pronator teres. The final area of potential compression in the pronator syndrome occurs at the arch of the flexor digitorum superficialis muscle as the median nerve passes beneath that muscle to lie immediately deep to and within the muscle fascia of the flexor digitorum superficialis.

Functional testing of the muscles of the proximal forearm may give some indication of the site of compression in pronator syndrome. If symptoms are aggravated by flexion of the elbow against resistance between 120 and 135 degrees of flexion, the surgeon must be suspicious of a Struthers' ligament compression. Compression by the lacertus fibrosus will be manifest and aggravated by active flexion of the elbow with the forearm in pronation, and probably only occurs when the median nerve is superficial to and along the lateral edge of the flexor muscle mass where the lacertus fibrosus crosses from the bicipital tendon across the flexor muscle mass.[115,116,136,146,161,177] If the symptoms are increased by resistance to pronation of the forearm, usually combined with flexion of the wrist (to relax the flexor digitorum superficialis), the surgeon should be particularly careful to explore the median nerve as it passes through the pronator teres muscle.[109,137,143,167] If the symptoms of pronator syndrome are aggravated by resisted flexion of the superficialis muscle of the middle finger, the surgeon should be careful to inspect the superficialis arch at the time of exploration.

Electrodiagnostic studies should confirm the clinical diagnosis. In most cases these studies will localize the level of the lesion, will confirm whether the nerve injury is partial or complete, and in some patients may define a myopathic origin of upper extremity pain. The surgeon should always be aware that nerve conduction velocity determinations are subject to a multitude of variables, including the age of the patient, his temperature, vascular supply of the extremity, regenerating fibers within the nerve, obesity or edema in the extremity, as well as a myriad of technical problems associated with the determination itself. All these factors must be weighed by the surgeon in evaluating the results of electrodiagnostic studies. When the electrodiagnostic studies do not confirm the clinical impression of a pronator syndrome, but the clinical tests for this syndrome continue to implicate the pronator syndrome as the level of compression neuropathy, it is prudent to wait 4 to 6 weeks, at which time repeat electrodiagnostic studies, including nerve conduction velocity and electromyogram, should be repeated. If, on the other hand, the surgeon suspects a pronator syndrome but the clinical signs of this syndrome are absent or questionable, a more proximal lesion such as a vascular anomaly of the brachial plexus should be considered.

Operative Technique

The operative technique for the release of a pronator syndrome consists of a detailed exploration of the median nerve in the proximal forearm. Although some surgeons prefer to limit the exploration to the suspicious area of the nerve on diagnostic evaluation, operations of limited scope carry with them an inherent risk of failure to recognize more than a single compression, if in fact a single site of compression is isolated.

The exploration for pronator syndrome should begin with an incision at least 5 cm above the elbow joint over the medial neurovascular bundle, zigzagging across the elbow flexion crease to lie midway between the flexor and extensor muscle masses, extending to the midforearm.

A small hook-shaped process of bone, the supracondylar process, may be found 5 cm above the medial epicondyle, projecting anteromedially

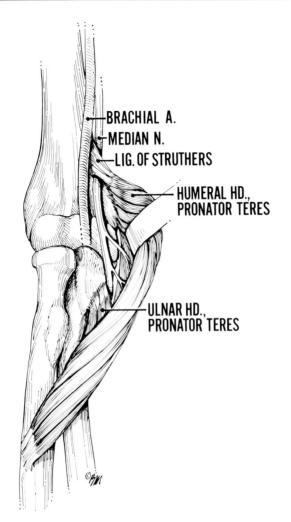

Fig. 36-1. The brachial artery may be superficial to the ligament of Struthers, which forms an accessory origin for the pronator teres.

from the surface of the humerus. This process may form an accessory origin for the pronator teres muscle (Fig. 36-1) through a ligament that was described by Struthers and bears his name.[115,116,177] If the median nerve is entrapped either beneath the supracondylar process or the ligament of Struthers, it is generally accompanied by the brachial artery and veins and lies on the medial aspect of the artery and veins. Following release of the ligament of Struthers, with or without resection of the supracondylar process, the median nerve must be traced distally to the second potential area of compression, the fascia of the lacertus fibrosus. Although thickening of the lacertus fibrosus can create a

compression neuropathy of the median nerve,[150] it probably only does so when the median nerve lies along the lateral edge and is uncovered by the flexor muscle mass and is, therefore, immediately beneath the lacertus fibrosus. This compression is probably only recognized with the forearm in pronation, which tightens the lacertus fibrosus over the neurovascular bundle and flexor muscle mass. The lacertus fibrosus should be divided routinely during surgery for pronator syndrome. The median nerve is then traced distally as it begins to dive into the pronator muscle.

It is important to recall Henry's admonition that the branches of the median nerve arise from the medial side as the nerve is followed in the proximal forearm.[39] The pronator teres muscle has two heads of origin: the humeral or superficial head arising from the medial epicondyle and the supracondylar ridge; and the ulnar or deep portion arising from the medial side of the coronoid process of the ulna, joining the superficial head at an acute angle. The median nerve enters the forearm between the two heads of the pronator teres.[42] Hypertrophy of the pronator teres muscle, reflections of the muscle fascia forming fibrous bands, and the sharp aponeurotic edge of the deep head of the pronator muscle have all been implicated in compression neuropathies of the median nerve at this level.[109,137,143, 167] The operation is continued by exploration of the median nerve as it enters the pronator teres muscle. After the entrance of the nerve into the muscle is inspected, the superficial head of the muscle can be elevated by dissecting the distal insertion of that head from a conjoined tendon with the deep head, which inserts at the midportion of the radius. The superficial head can be elevated, separated along the course of its fibers, and reflected ulnarly in order to explore the median nerve. Elevation of the superficial head of the pronator teres allows the surgeon to see the fourth and last potential compression site of the pronator syndrome, that is, the arch of the superficialis muscle. The flexor digitorum superficialis is the largest muscle of the superficial group in the proximal forearm. The muscle arises from the medial epicondyle of the humerus, joining with a common tendon origin from the ulnar collateral ligament of the elbow joint, and from the intermuscular septum between the ulnar collateral ligament and the remaining muscles of the superficial volar compartment.[36a] As the ulnar compartment of the superficialis joins the radial origin arising from the oblique fibers of the radius emanating from the radial tuberosity, a tendinous aponeurotic arch is formed, under which the median nerve passes. This aponeurotic arch of the superficialis origin constitutes the distal extent of the exploration for entrapment of the median nerve when the patient presents with symptoms and signs of pronator syndrome.

Author's Preferred Method. The author's preferred method of surgical exploration is to begin the exploration of the median nerve 5 cm proximal to the elbow and to trace it distally, taking care to explore all the individual branches to the superficial compartment of muscles. I often isolate a variety of fibrous bands that usually arise beneath the lacertus fibrosus or fascia of the pronator muscle, which will encircle some of the muscular branches of the median nerve as they arise from the medial side of the main trunk. Each of these potential sites of compression must be divided to ensure that a comprehensive release of the median nerve has been accomplished. Preoperative electrodiagnostic findings within the flexor carpi radialis, palmaris longus, flexor digitorum superficialis, or pronator teres do not isolate the area of compression at or above the lacertus fibrosus, since the separate fascial bands affecting individual muscular branches may lead the surgeon away from recognizing a compression neuropathy within the body of the pronator muscle or at the superficialis arch. Therefore, a complete exploration from the area of the ligament of Struthers through the arch of the superficialis is necessary to be considered an adequate release for the pronator syndrome.

Postoperative Management. Since during the closure of the operative wound the superficial head of the pronator teres is either sutured loosely to the tendinous insertion or allowed to lie on the deep head to seek its own level, postoperative care can usually be limited to a soft dressing. A posterior elbow splint may be used for support of the arm during the early postoperative period, positioning the elbow in 45 to 90 degrees flexion. The patient is permitted to begin flexion and extension exercises of the elbow by the fifth postoperative day. If, as a part of the surgical procedure, the entire pronator teres muscle has been detached from its insertion, which I believe is rarely necessary, the arm should be maintained in some degree of pronation, allowing only flexion and extension exercises of the elbow until tendinous healing of the reattached pronator teres is complete. This immobilization can be accomplished with a Muenster-type cast applied with the forearm in pronation so that some flexion and extension, but usually not full extension, of the elbow is permitted by the cast.

Anterior Interosseous Syndrome

A compression neuropathy of the anterior interosseous nerve is generally manifested by a vague pain in the proximal forearm that increases with exercise and is relieved with rest. On clinical examination, there is weakness or paralysis of the flexor digitorum profundus of the index finger, the flexor pollicis longus, and the pronator quadratus muscles. The patient will assume an unusual posture of pinch because of loss of function of the profundus to the index finger and the flexor pollicis longus, hyperextending the DIP joint of the index finger and the interphalangeal joint of the thumb.[171] This syndrome characteristically has no sensory symptoms or signs.[176] The diagnosis may be confirmed with electrodiagnostic studies of changes in the electrical pattern in the deep volar compartment muscles.[165] After the diagnosis of an anterior interosseous syndrome is made clinically and the involvement of the deep volar compartment is confirmed electrodiagnostically, surgical exploration of this branch of the median nerve is indicated.[171] If electrodiagnostic studies fail to confirm the diagnosis of anterior interosseous syndrome, the surgeon must consider a higher origin of nerve injury, such as pronator syndrome or vascular anomaly of the brachial plexus, as the cause of symptoms. If these possibilities are excluded, the surgeon should delay exploration of the forearm and the patient should be restudied electromyographically in 4 to 6 weeks.

Pertinent Anatomy

Although nearly a dozen variations of muscle-tendon units, blood vessels, or enlarged bursae or other tumors have been described as causative of anterior interosseous syndrome, the single common denominator in all these clinical cases has been that the anterior interosseous branch of the median nerve has been compressed in the area of the proximal forearm.[141,142,151,155,163,166,168,169,175, 178,180,182,200] Under ordinary circumstances, a detailed exploration of the median nerve, beginning above the anterior interosseous branch and extending into the deep volar compartment, will be sufficient to identify and isolate the area of compression and/or entrapment neuropathy of the anterior interosseous nerve.

Operative Technique

The operation for anterior interosseous syndrome begins as described above for the pronator syndrome, with an incision 5 cm above the elbow joint over the medial neurovascular bundle, zigzagging across the volar elbow crease and continuing to the midforearm between the flexor and extensor muscle masses (Fig. 36-2). The exploration of the median nerve begins proximal to the elbow joint by identifying the median nerve at the level of the elbow and tracing the nerve distally into the proximal forearm. After the median nerve is isolated medial to the brachial artery and veins, the surgeon can divide the lacertus fibrosus (Fig. 36-3) and trace the nerve distally as it enters the forearm at the level of the pronator teres. The surgeon must be careful to identify those small muscular branches that may have fascial reflections causing

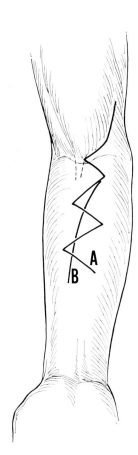

Fig. 36-2. The incision to explore the median and anterior interosseous nerves in the proximal forearm begins at least 5 cm above the elbow flexion crease. Although I prefer the zigzag incision *A*, which offers wider exposure, incision *B* is also adequate.

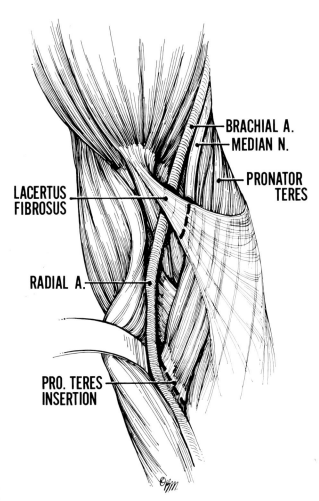

Fig. 36-3. The lacertus fibrosus may act as a compressive band across the flexor muscle mass in pronation; it should be divided with any exploration of the median nerve.

isolated compression neuropathies. At the proximal edge of the pronator teres muscle, the superficial head may again need to be elevated, as it was for the pronator syndrome, by detachment of its conjoined tendon insertion at the midportion of the radius and by separation of the muscle fibers of the superficial head from those of the deep head, to expose the median nerve (Fig. 36-4). It may also be necessary to divide the insertion of the deep head of the pronator teres to obtain a satisfactory view of the anterior interosseous nerve as it enters the deep volar compartment beneath the superficialis arch. In rare cases, reflection of the flexor digitorum superficialis muscle origin, as described by Henry in the subcutaneous transfer of the median

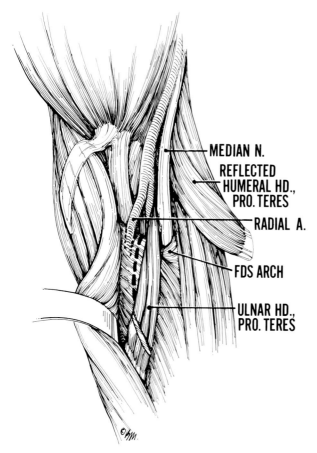

Fig. 36-4. Exposure of the median and anterior interosseous nerves by reflection of the humeral head (superficial head) of the pronator teres also exposes the arch of the superficialis.

nerve, may be necessary.[39] In those cases, separation of the origin of the superficialis from its radial border, as well as elevation of the muscle reflecting it ulnarly, will allow the surgeon to see the entire median nerve lying beneath the superficialis arch and within the fascia on the deep surface of the superficialis muscle (Fig. 36-5). This exploration deep to the superficialis muscle requires an extensive incision on the volar forearm, extending nearly to the junction of the middle and distal thirds. With this technique, however, the entire median nerve can be explored, and even transposed subcutaneously, placing the superficialis muscle beneath the median nerve but, of course, superficial to the anterior interosseous nerve and resuturing the pronator teres muscle to its insertion beneath the median nerve as well. The usual findings upon exploration of the anterior interosseous nerve are compression either by fascial bands on the deep head of the pronator teres or by the tendinous origin of the flexor superficialis as the nerve separates from the median nerve and comes to lie with a branch of the ulnar artery in the deep volar compartment. Thrombosed or aberrant vessels, as well as enlarged bursae, may also be seen. A variety of aberrant muscles and muscle-tendon units, such as an accessory head of the flexor pollicis longus (Gantzer's muscle[156]), the so-called palmaris profundus,[94] and the flexor carpi radialis brevis,[109] have all been identified as creating a compression neuropathy of the anterior interosseous nerve.

Postoperative Management. The postoperative management following exploration of the anterior interosseous nerve is simplified if the tourniquet is reduced and meticulous hemostasis of the wound is secured. Closure of the subcutaneous tissue and the skin can be accomplished in the usual manner. Most patients are comfortable in a soft dressing supported with a plaster splint for the elbow and wrist, with the wrist in neutral position, the forearm in 45 degrees pronation in order to reduce tension on the pronator teres muscle, particularly if it has been divided and repaired, and the elbow in 45 degrees flexion for comfort. It is important in the early postoperative period that the patient maintain adequate motion of his shoulder, and ordinarily by the end of the first week, flexion and extension of the elbow are begun, although prona-

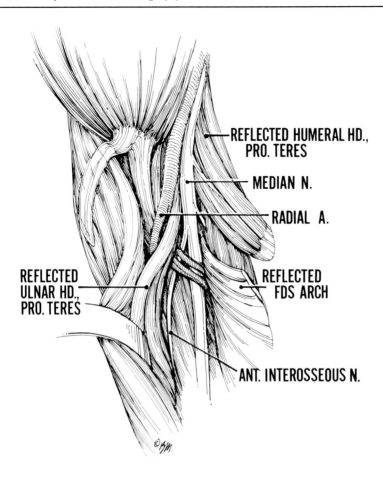

REFLECTED HUMERAL HD.,
PRO. TERES

MEDIAN N.

RADIAL A.

REFLECTED
ULNAR HD.,
PRO. TERES

REFLECTED
FDS ARCH

ANT. INTEROSSEOUS N.

Fig. 36-5. The radial origin of the superficialis muscle is elevated by subperiosteal dissection to expose the deep volar compartment and the anterior interosseous nerve.

tion and supination of the forearm are usually delayed to allow healing of the pronator teres tendon. Rupture of the repair of the pronator teres tendon has not been a problem, and if it should occur, I would not undertake a surgical repair.

Carpal Tunnel Syndrome

Carpal tunnel syndrome is the most common compression neuropathy in the upper extremity. Some authors have attributed the original description of carpal tunnel syndrome to Sir James Paget, who noted the clinical stigmata of the syndrome in 1863.[269] Marie et Foix in 1913 described the pathological changes of the median nerve.[283] Moersch coined the name of the syndrome in 1938, and Cannon and Love in 1946 described the first series of patients with median nerve compression.[203] In 1947, Brain, Wright, and Wilkerson[197] described

six patients who were treated surgically for bilateral carpal tunnel syndrome by surgical release of the transverse carpal ligament. In a series of articles beginning in 1950,[90,307,308,309,310,311,312] Phalen repeatedly directed the attention of the American medical community to the carpal tunnel syndrome. His contribution to both physicians and surgeons in the recognition and the treatment of carpal tunnel syndrome has been immeasurable.

A variety of symptoms[206,209,229,263,264,332,355] have been associated with carpal tunnel syndrome and a multitude of diseases[27,187,195,205,213,221,231,234,235,243, 255,260,261,267,269,273,274,285,286,288,295,303,313,315,319,320, 325,335,346,347,349,352] have presented with this syndrome as the presenting symptom complex. The usual symptoms of carpal tunnel syndrome are weakness or clumsiness in the hand, hypesthesia or paresthesias in the distribution of the median nerve, aggravation of the symptoms as the patient uses the hand (especially with grasping), awakening from sleep with numbness in the fingers, and pain in the wrist or distal forearm. Presenting symptoms of shoulder pain or upper arm pain are not uncommon,[206,209,229,264] and proximal migration of pain from the area of the wrist toward the proximal forearm and elbow are relatively common. Although most authors have felt in the past that this syndrome is seen more frequently in females than in males by a ratio of more than 2 to 1, recent reports indicate that the syndrome may be much more common in males than had previously been suggested. Except in selected populations, 50 percent of cases occur in patients between 40 and 60 years of age.[194] Distal lancinating paresthesias in the distribution of the median nerve with percussion of the median nerve at the wrist are suggestive of carpal tunnel syndrome,[334] and reproduction of symptoms with the wrist flexion test as described by Phalen[308] is generally diagnostic. Symptoms are often relieved by splinting the wrist in a neutral position, taking care that the splint does not lie over the median nerve on the volar surface of the forearm.

Decreased sensibility in the distribution of the median nerve and thenar atrophy are *advanced* signs of this entrapment neuropathy. Although electrodiagnostic studies are widely used to confirm the diagnosis of carpal tunnel syndrome (prolonged motor or sensory conduction latency across the carpal tunnel),[26,67,200,247,256,275,276,284,294,316,325,340,341] the diagnosis of this syndrome is at least 85 percent certain in the patient with a wrist flexion test that reproduces the symptoms, sensitivity to percussion of the median nerve at the wrist, and objective sensory findings limited to the median nerve distribution. The electromyogram is most useful in those patients in whom the surgeon wishes to differentiate the carpal tunnel syndrome from syndromes of the thoracic outlet and compression syndromes of the lower cervical roots.[294]

The conditions that have been associated with carpal tunnel syndrome include rheumatoid arthritis,[295,327] thyroid imbalance, particularly myxedema,[27,315] acromegaly,[320,354] multiple myeloma,[213] amyloidosis,[269] diabetes mellitus,[269,313] local trauma to the wrist,[183,190,222,257,293] alcoholism, hemophilia,[243,244,260] local tumors such as lipomata or ganglia,[178] hormonal changes associated with menopause,[269,319] pregnancy,[231,267,285] plen-

osteosis,[349] gout[234,303,347] and a variety of anatomic anomalies,[94,188,189,193,198,202,251,323] such as aberrant muscles, vascular tumors,[343] and even thrombosis of a persistent median artery[271,287] lying adjacent to the median nerve in the carpal tunnel. Although many anatomic variations have been reported as factors in the carpal tunnel syndrome, there has always been some question about whether such aberrant muscles as the palmaris profundus,[109] anomalous lumbrical muscles,[202,251,323] flexor superficialis muscles,[193,226] or palmaris longus[94,188,189,198] can be a factor in the carpal tunnel syndrome. On the other hand, an enlarged median artery can certainly be a factor in neuritic symptoms of the median nerve. Thrombosis of a persistent median artery[271,287] will precipitate the onset of an acute, extremely painful median neuritis that often requires early surgical care. Carpal tunnel syndrome has been reported in children,[329] presenting as atrophy of the index finger in a juvenile, as described by Lettin.[270] Some authors believe that 60 percent of patients with fractures of the distal radius have at some time during their fracture treatment symptoms of compression of the median nerve in the area of the carpal tunnel. Obviously, not all of these patients require surgical care.

The indication for operative intervention in the carpal tunnel is a failure to respond to conservative therapy. The conservative treatment for median neuritis consists of splinting of the wrist, injection with corticosteroid into the carpal tunnel, and oral nonsteroidal anti-inflammatory medications.

Splinting of the wrist in a neutral position will usually reduce and may even completely relieve the symptoms of carpal tunnel syndrome. In most cases, I apply a dorso-ulnar plaster splint across the wrist so that no portion of the splint lies over the median nerve on the volar aspect of the wrist. The patient wears the splint continuously day and night for the first 3 to 4 weeks, followed by nighttime splinting for an additional 4 weeks. If the patient's symptoms have been completely relieved with the use of the dorso-ulnar gutter splint, but the symptoms recur with removal of the splint after its use for several weeks, the patient is a candidate for operative intervention.

Once popular in the late 1950s and early 1960s[222a,230a,308,309] injection of corticosteroid into the carpal tunnel has regained popularity in the early 1980s.[227a,233,354a] The method of injection must be precise and consistent, and there is ample evidence that imprecise placement of the needle, or the use of a needle that is too large, can result in prolonged disability, even permanent injury, to the median nerve. Accordingly, it has been recommended by Wood[354a] that needle placement be practiced at the time of carpal tunnel operation, inserting the needle prior to skin incision and then visualizing the actual site of placement after the transverse carpal ligament has been sectioned. Green[233] has suggested the injection of a small amount of local anesthetic to insure correct placement of the needle prior to injection of corticosteroid. In the hands of most skilled surgeons, injection of the carpal tunnel is an effective, though usually transient, therapeutic modality, after which between 65 and 90 percent of patients can be expected to have some recurrence of symptoms that may require carpal tunnel surgical release.

In my opinion, corticosteroid injection into the carpal tunnel[254] is indicated when the entrapment of the median nerve can be predicted to be temporary, such as in pregnancy, or when the patient's activity can be sufficiently modified to anticipate a reduction in stress symptoms at the wrist. In patients with temporary carpal tunnel syndrome, particularly that associated with pregnancy, splinting and an injection of a cortisone preparation combined with a local anesthetic, with care taken to avoid the median nerve, have generally reduced symptoms sufficiently for the patient to complete the pregnancy. Following pregnancy the symptoms of carpal tunnel syndrome usually regress rapidly, certainly over the first 4 to 6 weeks postpartum. Nevertheless, many patients who exhibit signs and symptoms of carpal tunnel syndrome during pregnancy will have repeated and increasing symptoms during subsequent pregnancies, and will often eventually require surgical release of the transverse carpal ligament either between pregnancies or as they reach the menopausal years.

The repetitive or cumulative trauma syndromes associated with carpal tunnel syndrome that are commonly seen in the work place will normally respond to a combination of conservative treatment consisting of splinting, corticosteroid injection into the carpal tunnel, and change of job ac-

tivity. If the patient's treatment program does not include a permanent change of job activity, the combination of splinting and injection will provide the patient with only temporary relief of symptoms and the return to repetitive, stressful activity may very well be accompanied by increasing neuropathy of the median nerve.

Although nonsteroidal anti-inflammatory medications have been prescribed for patients with carpal tunnel syndrome, their effect in the treatment of this condition is uncertain. Presently, I do not use nonsteroidal anti-inflammatory medications as a routine part of conservative treatment of carpal tunnel syndrome.

Pertinent Anatomy

The volar radiocarpal ligament and the volar ligamentous extensions between the carpal bones form the floor of the carpal tunnel. The transverse carpal ligament is a thick fibrous band that arches over the concave surface of the carpal bones, attaching on the radial side to the tuberosity of the scaphoid and a portion of the trapezium and on the ulnar aspect to the pisiform and hook of the hamate. This ligament completes the tunnel through which the long flexor tendons and median nerve pass (Fig. 36-6). The median nerve ordinarily lies superficial, directly beneath the transverse carpal ligament. Of the many anatomic variations that can be associated with carpal tunnel syndrome none are more important to the surgeon than the variations of the motor branch of the median nerve, which must be protected during the surgical exposure and division of the transverse carpal ligament. Lanz[266] has classified the anatomic variations of the median nerve into four subgroups: (1) variations in the course of the thenar branch of the median nerve, (2) accessory variations of the thenar branch at the distal carpal tunnel, (3) high divisions of the median nerve, and (4) accessory branches proximal to the carpal tunnel. The normal position for the motor branch of the median nerve is the extra ligamentous recurrent course from the median nerve just distal to the transverse carpal ligament, supplying innervation to the thenar muscles (Fig. 36-7). This branching of the median nerve occurs in approximately one-half of cases. The next most common variation of the motor median nerve is the subliga-

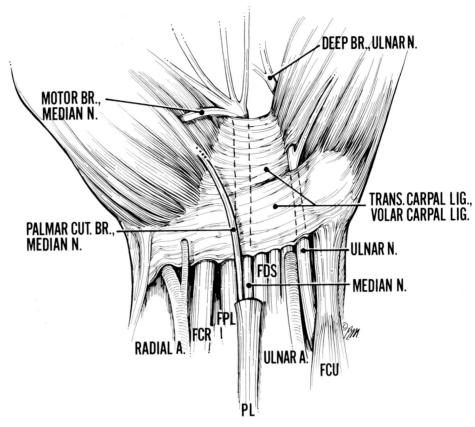

Fig. 36-6. The median nerve and the long flexor tendons traverse the carpal tunnel, lying beneath the transverse carpal ligament.

mentous branching in which the recurrent median branch divides from the median nerve beneath the transverse carpal ligament, lies close to the median nerve, and innervates the thenar muscles with a recurrent course distal to the transverse carpal ligament (Fig. 36-8). This subligamentous variation occurs in approximately one-third of cases. The third most common course for the motor branch of the median nerve is transligamentous. In this variation the motor branch of the median nerve divides from the common median nerve beneath the transverse carpal ligament and in its course to the thenar muscles pierces the transverse carpal ligament between 2 and 6 mm from its distal border (Fig. 36-9). This variation, according to Poisel as reported by Lanz,[266] occurs in approximately one out of five patients. The remaining variations in the course of the thenar branch of the median nerve are generally considered to be extremely rare and yet

variations have been reported by numerous authors[193,232,253,280,302,305] (Fig. 36-10).

The second group of variations seen with the motor branch of the median nerve consists of various accessory branches that innervate the thenar muscles. These multiple branches of the median nerve are considered to be rare, but they have been reported occurring distally and coursing parallel to the thenar muscles from the median nerve. High divisions of the median nerve in the carpal tunnel are classified in Lanz's Group 3[215,259] (Fig. 36-11). Although these high divisions may arise in the proximal or middle third of the forearm, they generally run parallel to the nerve and are divided from it by a persistent median artery[259] or an aberrant muscle.[323] The median nerve and the motor branch pass deep to the transverse carpal ligament and then divide into the usual multiple branches. In recognizing the possibility of a high division of the

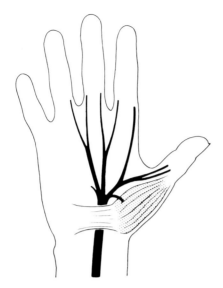

Fig. 36-7. The most common pattern of the motor branch of median nerve is extraligamentous and recurrent. (Lanz U: Anatomical variations of the median nerve in the carpal tunnel. J Hand Surg 2:44–53, 1977.)

median nerve, the careful surgeon will generally have little problem dealing with these variations. The fourth and final classification of anatomic variations of the median nerve at the carpal tunnel includes accessory branches of the median nerve

supplying the thenar muscles proximal to the transverse carpal ligament [272,302] (Fig. 36-12). These branches may course superficial to the transverse carpal ligament, arising from the common median nerve proximal to the carpal tunnel and then rejoining the main nerve distal to the ligament prior to again branching from it and supplying motor innervation to the thenar muscles. The transligamentous course of an accessory branch of the median nerve has been reported, as has an ulnar take-off of the accessory transligamentous branch proximal to the carpal tunnel.[266] In addition, I have observed multiple accessory branches of the median nerve passing either proximal and distal to the carpal ligament or transligamentous to supply innervation to the thenar muscles.

Operative Techniques

Although release of the transverse carpal ligament is the basic procedure for the treatment of carpal tunnel syndrome, the approaches to the release of that ligament may vary considerably in the hands of different surgeons. Keeping in mind the many variations that can occur in the motor branch of the median nerve, it seems prudent to design an incision through which the surgeon can protect the

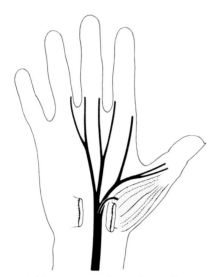

Fig. 36-8. Subligamentous branching of a recurrent median nerve. (Lanz U: Anatomical variations of the median nerve in the carpal tunnel. J Hand Surg 2:44–53, 1977.)

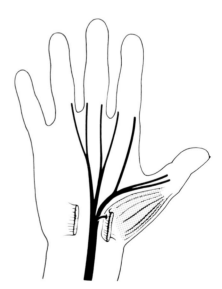

Fig. 36-9. Transligamentous course of the recurrent branch of the median nerve. (Lanz U: Anatomical variations of the median nerve in the carpal tunnel. J Hand Surg 2:44–53, 1977.)

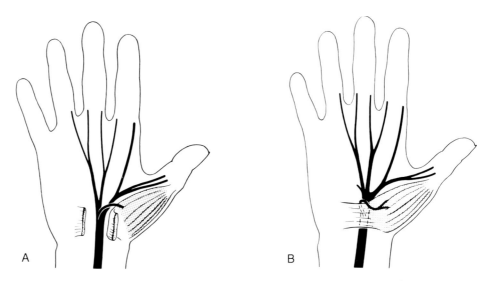

Fig. 36-10. Less common thenar branch variations incude (**A**) a branch from the ulnar border of the median nerve and (**B**) a branch lying on top of the transverse carpal ligament. (Lanz U: Anatomical variations of the median nerve in the carpal tunnel. J Hand Surg 2:44–53, 1977.)

branches, even the rare variations, and yet at the same time perform an adequate division of the carpal ligament. A small transverse incision at the base of the palm or in the proximal wrist crease does not allow adequate exploration of the carpal tunnel and endangers the branches of the median nerve, especially those branches that may communicate occasionally with the ulnar nerve at the distal border of the carpal tunnel[266,352] and those variations of the motor branch previously discussed. The surgeon is

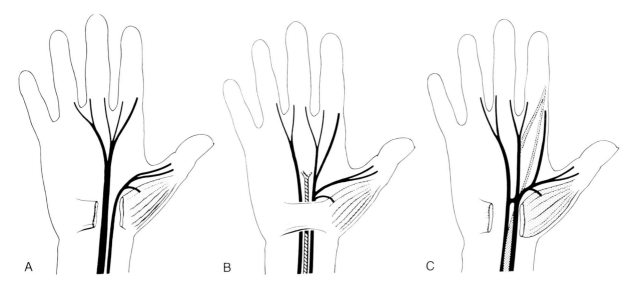

Fig. 36-11. Group III variations of the thenar branch include (**A**) high divisions of the median nerve that may be separated by (**B**) a persistent median artery or (**C**) an aberrant muscle. (Lanz U: Anatomical variations of the median nerve in the carpal tunnel. J Hand Surg 2:44–53, 1977.)

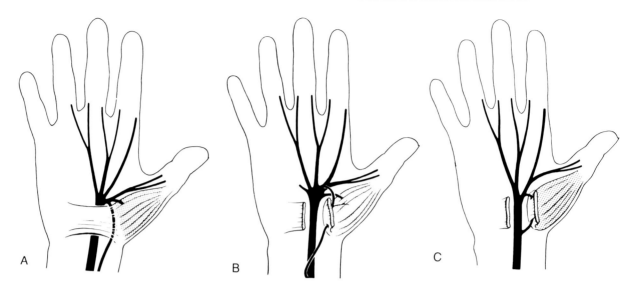

Fig. 36-12. Group IV variations of the thenar branch include those rare instances in which the thenar branch leaves the median nerve proximal to the carpal tunnel. (Lanz U: Anatomical variations of the median nerve in the carpal tunnel. J Hand Surg 2:44–53, 1977.)

also more likely to injure the palmar cutaneous branch of the median nerve with the transverse incision in the wrist crease.

A limited approach to the transverse carpal ligament parallel to longitudinal creases at the base of the palm may have some application in exploration of the transverse carpal ligament but will not identify those motor branches of the median nerve that divide proximal to the transverse carpal ligament and may jeopardize the more unusual variations that arise in the distal third of the forearm. Several authors[204,120] have pointed out the necessity of avoiding the palmar cutaneous branch of the median nerve in designing an incision to release the transverse carpal ligament. Taleisnik[338] has suggested that an incision over the palm of the hand lie ulnar to the axis of the ring finger at the base of the palm to avoid the medial branch of the palmar cutaneous nerve. Others have emphasized the use of a limited fasciotomy of the distal third of the forearm in the treatment of carpal tunnel syndrome to avoid a constricting band of forearm fascia across the median nerve as it rises from beneath the superficialis muscles or at the wrist flexion crease.

Author's Preferred Method. To accommodate the many anatomic variations and to ensure an adequate release of the median nerve, as well as per-

form an adequate division of the transverse carpal ligament, I have used an incision that begins distally at the distal border of the transverse carpal ligament and follows the longitudinal crease of the palm, crossing the base of the palm in a zigzag fashion ulnar to the long axis of the ring finger (Fig. 36-13). The incision continues above the proximal wrist crease for approximately 3 cm. Through the proximal portion of this incision, the superficial fascia of the forearm is isolated and divided longitudinally. The ulnar border of the median nerve is identified and a fasciotomy of the distal third of the forearm is performed. By remaining on the ulnar side of the median nerve, often using a hemostat to protect the deep structures, the transverse carpal ligament is divided. The dissection is done in layers, dividing the palmar fascia initially and then extending through the transverse carpal ligament throughout its course.

This exposure and technique allows maximum protection of the median nerve, as well as the tendons of the carpal canal. The transverse carpal ligament is sectioned under direct vision throughout its entire length and those structures on the ulnar side of the incision, that is, the ulnar neurovascular bundle and the superficial vascular arch of the palm, can be seen and protected. This approach at the base of the palm lies ulnar to the axis of the ring

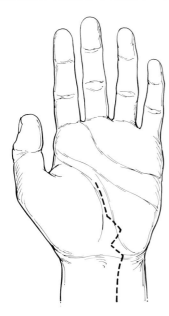

Fig. 36-13. The author's preferred carpal tunnel incision. At the base of the palm the incision is ulnar to the axis of the ring finger.

finger and is in close proximity to Guyon's canal, which may also be released at the time of carpal tunnel decompression if the surgeon feels that its release is indicated.[461] Following release of the transverse carpal ligament, exploration of the motor branch to identify a transligamentous course of the branch is necessary. If the motor branch of the median nerve passes distal to the transverse carpal ligament, assuming its usual recurrent course to the thenar muscles, no further dissection of the branch is necessary. If, however, a transligamentous course of the motor branch is identified, the branch should be freed from its transligamentous passage by further division of the transverse carpal ligament.[266,109] This procedure will eliminate any possibility of compression neuropathy or traction neuropathy at the transligamentous passage as a result of the division of the transverse carpal ligament. If no additional surgery of the median nerve is anticipated (see discussion of internal neurolysis that follows), the skin can be closed, taking care to approximate the skin of the palm anatomically.

Postoperative Management. The postoperative care consists of a period of wrist immobilization from 3 to 14 days, during which time the patient is encouraged to use the hand. Flexion and extension exercises of the fingers and flexion, extension, and rotational exercises of the thumb are encouraged. The usual postoperative course is punctuated with an almost immediate relief of pain and some improvement in the sensibility of the fingers if the patient does not have an axonotmetic or neurotmetic lesion of the median nerve. After the initial and usually dramatic improvement in sensibility, the patient experiences some slight decrease in improvement (about 1 week postoperatively). Improvement will again be realized after this transient partial relapse. The changes in the conduction velocity seem to parallel the patient's clinical response. It has been demonstrated at operation that an immediate improvement in conduction velocity can be anticipated in most cases of carpal tunnel release.[219] In the postoperative period, the conduction velocity, which was prolonged before surgery and returned to a normal range immediately following release of the ligament, rises to some intermediate value at approximately 1 week postoperatively, followed by a gradual return to its normal range within 8 to 12 weeks. Those patients who have a prolonged return of conduction velocity to normal must be anticipated to have a more profound neuropathy, possibly associated with other factors such as diabetes mellitus. Patients with an axonotmesis, of course, can be anticipated to have an advancing Tinel's sign and eventually regain nearly full return of function in the median nerve.

Following carpal tunnel release, swelling at the base of the palm superfical to the carpal tunnel can be expected to persist for 12 to 16 weeks following surgery. During this period of time and probably concurrent with the swelling, the patient may experience aching pain in the thenar or hypothenar eminences, which has been termed "pillar pain." Heavy activity and gripping will aggravate the pain, which may be accompanied by aching in the distal portion of the forearm or shooting sensations in the distal third of the forearm, which are usually only momentary in duration. Resolution of the swelling at the base of the palm is accompanied by relief of "pillar pain" and distal forearm symptoms.

The return of strength following carpal tunnel release is prolonged. By 6 weeks following surgical release of the deep transverse carpal ligament, patients will usually have only about 50 percent of their preoperative grip strength. As long as the patient is able to exercise and work effectively on increasing grip strength, which should be begun in the second or third postoperative week, by 8 to 10 weeks following carpal tunnel release 75 percent of grip strength will usually be regained. Maximum grip strength and, possibly more importantly, the endurance of grip strength often does not return until 6 months or even longer after surgical release of the carpal tunnel. Perhaps as many as 15 or 20 percent of patients who have had carpal tunnel release will never regain full strength after surgical release of the deep transverse carpal tunnel ligament. Whether this is due to some change in the carpal bone configuration with release of the deep transverse carpal ligament or to the loss of the pulley mechanism contributed to by the deep transverse carpal tunnel ligament is uncertain. It is probably premature to suggest that grip strength will not ultimately be restored unless the patient has been engaged in an active and vigorous rehabilitation program, has returned to his or her usual activities, and 1 year has elapsed since surgery.

As carpal tunnel syndrome becomes increasingly recognized in the work place as a repetitive trauma or cumulative trauma syndrome, it seems more and more certain that modification of the work environment by redistribution of work mechanics, modification of tools and handles to be more compatible with hand function, and the attention of biomechanical engineering designed to protect the worker will create a focus on the *prevention* of this syndrome rather than the repeated treatment of the syndrome by release of the deep transverse carpal ligament. An important part of the evaluation of industrial biomechanics will be the evaluation of the employee prior to his or her assuming a position in the work place, combined with a knowledge of the amount of stress applied to the worker's hands in a particular working environment. It should then be possible, through knowing the stress to which the worker is exposed in doing a specific job and that worker's capacity for stress, to provide a suitable match of the worker's abilities with the job requirement and thereby, hopefully, to reduce the incidence of cumulative trauma or stress-related carpal tunnel syndrome.

Internal Neurolysis

Internal neurolysis or endoneurolysis has been described as an adjunct to the treatment of carpal tunnel syndrome.[210,227] It is known that internal fibrosis of the peripheral nerve will constrict axons and mechanically reduce axoplasmic transport. Internal fibrosis can also reduce blood supply to the axons by producing an unfavorable interface between capillaries and the axon membrane. Internal fibrosis of a peripheral nerve may also act as a barrier to regeneration of axons, and constriction of regenerating axons may reduce recovery of the peripheral nerve. Therefore, I believe this procedure is indicated in those lesions of peripheral nerve in which either some degree of internal fibrosis or constriction by the epineurium can be anticipated to continue to prevent neurologic healing and recovery of periperal nerve function.

Although the indications for internal neurolysis differ among hand surgeons, my indications for internal neurolysis in conjunction with release of the carpal tunnel are: (1) atrophy of the thenar muscles; (2) *constant* loss of sensibility in the distribution of the median nerve; (3) deterioration of light touch or two-point discrimination sensibility; (4) severe causalgia confined to the distribution of the median nerve (usually associated with traumatic injuries of the distal radius or carpus); and (5) true neuroma-in-continuity of the median nerve at the time of operation.[210] The latter indication is not apparent until epineurotomy of the nerve is performed in an area of swelling of the median nerve, usually just proximal to the constriction of the transverse carpal ligament. With epineurotomy, the internal fibrosis of the nerve is visualized and internal neurolysis completed.

The risks of internal neurolysis are the destruction of the interfascicular plexus and further vascular damage due to interference of the capillary network within the peripheral nerve segment.[101] These risks have been studied in detail in a primate model by Dellon and MacKinnon,[278a] who have shown that with microsurgical technique the increase in scarring and anatomical disruption of the nerve segment is minimal with internal neurolysis. It is, however, true that the end result of any surgical procedure, including internal neurolysis, may be the formation of new scar within the peripheral nerve, and that this new scar may be as detrimental as any other fibrosis.

Because of the marked danger of destruction of the interfascicular plexus, internal neurolysis should be limited to those areas of peripheral nerves where the interfascicular plexus is minimal. Usually these are the more distal areas of the peripheral nerves, such as the median nerve at the wrist or distally, the ulnar nerve at the wrist or distally, and the radial nerve at the elbow and through the supinator muscle. The risks of internal neurolysis are increased in more proximal nerve segments such as the ulnar nerve at the elbow.

Internal neurolysis should not be confused with epineurotomy. The incising of the epineurium, considered by some authors to be a "fasciotomy" of a peripheral nerve, is a much simpler procedure and can be performed with appropriate care at any level of a peripheral nerve.

Also, the procedure of internal neurolysis should not be confused with epineurectomy or removal of the epineurium, which is used by some surgeons to decompress segments of peripheral nerves. Epineurectomy will routinely interfere with the blood supply to a segment of a peripheral nerve by excision of the subepineurial plexus of vessels, which lie on the undersurface of the excised epineurium. Although this procedure may have some place in the dissection of peripheral nerves with internal tumors, in my opinion it has no place in the treatment of entrapment neuropathy.

By relieving scar constriction within the nerve trunk, internal neurolysis effectively decompresses the constricted circulation and constricted fascicles within the segment of the peripheral nerve. In this procedure it is important *not* to breach the perineurium since dissection of the peripheral nerve at that level will injure the end artery circulation of the axon at the capillary level. One might compare the internal neurolysis procedure to that of epineurotomy so that if epineurotomy were a fasciotomy of the nerve trunk, internal neurolysis would be a fasciotomy of the fascicles.

The procedure of internal neurolysis must be performed with adequate magnification to allow the interfascicular plexus of nerves to be seen and to protect these vital communications between fascicles. Ordinarily this requires at least $3.5 \times$ magnification. I have found that, while learning the procedure, an operating microscope of at least $7 \times$ is necessary for the surgeon to perform the procedure and evaluate the dissection. After the procedure is learned, however, most surgeons can perform it using $3.5 \times$ loupe magnification. The internal neurolysis procedure is limited to the area of the median nerve that is severely affected and must conform to the indications for the procedure, which have been previously described. If, for example, the indication for the internal neurolysis is atrophy of the thenar muscles, the surgeon should begin the procedure by isolating the motor branch of the median nerve distally and tracing those fascicles contributing to the motor branch through the course of the carpal tunnel. Only those fascicles contributing to the motor branch will then undergo internal neurolysis. Similarly, if a patient has constant loss of sensibility in only the middle finger and intermittent loss of sensibility in the index finger and thumb, only those fascicles contributing to the middle finger need undergo internal neurolysis by tracing the fascicles from distal to proximal through the area of compression.

The procedure is begun by epineurotomy on the radial side of the median nerve at the wrist. The opening of the epineurium should be on the radial side of the median nerve since the segmental circulation of that nerve enters from the ulnar side proximal to the transverse carpal ligament and from the vessels of the superficial arch[106,107,336] distal to the transverse carpal ligament. If small vessels are seen within the nerve itself, the exposure through the epineurium should be to one side or the other of these epineurial vessels. The median nerve should *not* be elevated from its bed of areolar tissue and surrounding peritenon since microcirculation may enter the dorsal aspect of the nerve, and sacrifice of this circulation is contraindicated. Once the epineurium is opened, the fascicles are sighted and gently teased apart using small, sharp-pointed surgical scissors and microsurgical forceps. Separation of the fascicles is performed with care, preserving the interfascicular plexus of nerves. If no intrafascicular scarring is encountered at any point in the dissection, the dissection of the fascicles should be stopped. The wound is closed in the usual fashion for a carpal tunnel release by accurate anatomic approximation of the palmar skin. No deep closure is performed and no interposing tissue is drawn over the median nerve prior to skin closure. The postoperative care following internal neurolysis is the same as for carpal tunnel release. Although I generally splint the wrist in neutral position for ten days to two weeks following internal neurolysis, early, intermittent motion of the wrist in dorsiflexion and palmar flexion out of the splint several times a day may be desirable. The response to the surgery, except in cases of preoperative axonotmesis or neurotmesis of the median nerve, is identical to that seen with carpal tunnel release previously described. The initial response to surgical treatment, the diminution of that response at approximately 1 week postoperatively, and the gradual return of function within the distribution of the median nerve parallel the characteristic findings after simple carpal tunnel release. Based on a review of well over 500 cases of carpal tunnel syndrome, a 10 to 15 percent frequency for the use of the internal neurolysis procedure with carpal tunnel release seems to be constant in a general practice of hand surgery. This figure may be slightly higher if the hand surgeon has an exclusively referral practice, since many of the less severe compressions of the median nerve will be treated by other surgeons.

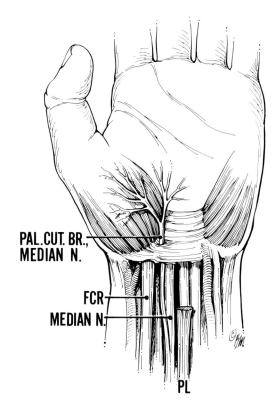

Fig. 36-14. The palmar cutaneous branch of the median nerve may be entrapped as it pierces either the volar carpal or transverse carpal ligament or at the antebrachial fascia.

Palmar Cutaneous Branch of Median Nerve

The palmar cutaneous branch of the median nerve arises from the median nerve in the distal third of the forearm, passes distally paralleling the median nerve, pierces either the antebrachial fascia, the volar carpal ligament or even the transverse carpal ligament at the wrist, and then divides into medial and lateral branches at the base of the palm (Fig. 36-14). As the palmar cutaneous branch courses superficial and ulnar to the flexor carpi radialis tendon, it enters a short tunnel in the volar carpal ligament or transverse carpal ligament at the end of which it divides into the medial and lateral branches.[42,338] The nerve eventually supplies sensibility to the thenar eminence and the proximal two-fifths of the palm on the radial side. Anatomic variations of the palmar cutaneous branch of the median nerve have included separation from the median nerve at any level in the distal third of the forearm, even at the proximal wrist crease, multiple branches from the median nerve arising at the same or separate levels, and total absence of the palmar cutaneous nerve, in which case a portion of the musculocutaneous nerve (lateral antebrachial cutaneous nerve) and/or the superficial radial nerve will supply sensibility on the radial side of the proximal palm.[42,109,120] Although most lesions of the palmar cutaneous branch of the median nerve are the result of lacerations or iatrogenic injury at the time of surgery,[204] compression neuropathy of the palmar cutaneous branch in its tunnel has been described by Stellbrink.[331] Release of the palmar cutaneous branch of the median nerve in its tunnel at the transverse carpal ligament relieved the patient of his hypesthesias over the thenar eminence.

ENTRAPMENT NEUROPATHIES OF THE ULNAR NERVE

Entrapment neuropathies of the ulnar nerve occur in two areas of the upper extremity. Because of differing clinical presentations, entrapment of the ulnar nerve at the elbow (cubital tunnel syndrome) will rarely be confused with entrapment of the ulnar nerve at the wrist in Guyon's canal (ulnar tunnel syndrome), unless the symptoms are minimal and the physical examination and electrodiagnostic studies are inconclusive.

Ulnar Nerve Entrapment at the Elbow (Cubital Tunnel Syndrome)

Entrapment syndromes of the ulnar nerve near the elbow joint generally present with pain of a lancinating or aching nature on the medial side of the proximal forearm.[386] This pain may migrate proximally or distally into either the arm or forearm. The pain is often accompanied by paresthesias, dysesthesias, or anesthesia in the ulnar one and one-half fingers—the sensory distribution of the ulnar nerve in the hand. Muscle wasting of the ulnar-innervated intrinsic muscles is not uncommon. The entrapment of the ulnar nerve may be localized by a positive percussion test over the ulnar nerve at the elbow, abnormal mobility of the ulnar nerve onto or over the medial epicondyle of the humerus,[366,367] or a positive elbow flexion test with increased numbness in the ulnar one and one-half fingers with full flexion of the elbow. Since electrodiagnostic studies[21,24,25,89,126,380] at the elbow are generally expressed as velocity in meters per second rather than as a latency in milliseconds, evaluation of reduced velocities of less than 25 percent are probably not significant and conduction velocities with a reduction across the elbow of greater than 33 percent are always significant.

(These percentages are based on our own unpublished studies.) Care must be taken that conduction velocities across the elbow of the ulnar nerve are recorded in a standard position because the flexed elbow position produces less segment-to-segment conduction velocity variation than those obtained with the elbow extended. Similar to other entrapment neuropathies, the use of conduction velocities as a sole indication for surgery is insufficient unless the patient has accompanying clinical findings, such as sensory symptoms and a positive percussion test over the ulnar nerve. The presence of intrinsic muscle wasting is a sign of prolonged compression neuropathy and ordinarily demands early operative intervention. The surgeon should be cautioned about muscle wasting of the intrinsic muscles of the hand in the geriatric patient since this may be a result of the normal aging process and may not be a manifestation of a compression neuropathy of the ulnar nerve. The presence of fibrillations within the ulnar intrinsic muscles of the hand in such a case is an important sign of neurologic injury.

Pertinent Anatomy

The ulnar nerve arises as the continuation and terminal branch of the medial cord of the brachial plexus after the medial cord contributes to the median nerve. At its origin, the ulnar nerve lies medial to the axillary and then the brachial artery as far as the middle third of the humerus. In the middle third of the arm, the ulnar nerve approaches the medial head of the triceps by piercing the medial intermuscular septum and runs along this head of the triceps muscle to the groove between the olecranon and the medial epicondyle of the humerus (Fig. 36-15). The cubital tunnel begins at the so-called ulnar groove just behind the medial epicondyle of the humerus. In the cubital tunnel the ulnar nerve is covered by multiple fascial layers and can be readily palpated coursing behind and beneath the medial epicondyle of the partially flexed elbow. Within the cubital tunnel the ulnar nerve comes to lie beneath the fascial arcade joining the two heads of the flexor carpi ulnaris, passing between these two heads and lying on the anterior or volar surface of the flexor digitorum profundus to the midportion of the forearm.

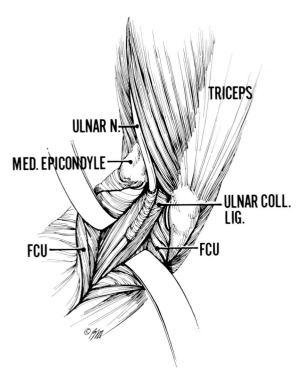

Fig. 36-15. The ulnar nerve lies on the medial head of the triceps muscle, entering the cubital tunnel behind the medial epicondyle and continuing distally beneath the arcade of fascia joining the heads of the flexor carpi ulnaris.

The anatomy of the cubital tunnel can be divided into three parts: the entrance of the tunnel just posterior to the medial epicondyle, the area of the fascial aponeurosis joining the two heads of the flexor carpi ulnaris, and the muscle bellies of the flexor carpi ulnaris itself. The elliptical, fibroosseous cubital tunnel is bordered laterally by the elbow joint, medially by the heads of the flexor carpi ulnaris origin, and anteriorly, at least at its origin, by the medial epicondyle. Within this canal the ulnar nerve passes from the extensor surface in the arm to the flexor surface in the forearm. Among the suggested causes of entrapment of the ulnar nerve at the elbow[405,406] are the arcade of Struthers[109,116,177]; the anconeus epitrochlearis[109]; the medial head of the triceps[409]; the aponeurosis of the flexor carpi ulnaris; osteophytes, ganglia or lipomata associated with the elbow joint[385,410]; subluxation of the ulnar nerve across the epicondyle[201,360,361,366]; or a combination of these causes,

particularly hypertrophy of the medial head of the triceps, which forces the ulnar nerve anteriorly around the medial epicondyle when the triceps contracts. This latter circumstance will produce an ulnar nerve that seems peculiarly subjected to trauma with flexion of the elbow.

Suggested surgical treatment of the cubital tunnel syndrome includes decompression of the ulnar nerve,[413,420] anterior transposition of the ulnar nerve,[361,364,371,393,395,398,407] medial epicondylectomy of the humerus,[370,378,387,389,400] and fascial repairs that prevent subluxation of the nerve. Since subluxation of the ulnar nerve occurs with flexion of the elbow and since fascial repair will create a band across the nerve to prevent its subluxation, it seems theoretically unsound to suggest an operation that might very well cause a compression with the repair. For this reason, although prevention of subluxation seems rational, these procedures have been abandoned and are not even discussed by most authors. The remaining procedures of decompression, transposition, and medial epicondylectomy deserve detailed discussion concerning their use for ulnar nerve entrapment at the elbow.

OPERATIVE TECHNIQUES

Decompression

The basic operation for ulnar nerve entrapment at the elbow when the compression is by the aponeurosis between the heads of the flexor carpi ulnaris, or the muscle itself, is decompression of the ulnar nerve. The advantages of this operation are (1) simplicity, since the aponeurosis is simply divided over the ulnar nerve; (2) safety, since the ulnar nerve is not disturbed and therefore not robbed of its intrinsic or extrinsic blood supply; and (3) predictability. With this localized compression we can anticipate that the patient will experience immediate relief of paresthesias and dysesthesias and increased sensibility in a short time, if the degree of injury is neurapratic rather than axonotmetic or neurotmetic, and recovery of the intrinsic muscles of the hand with neurapratic and axonotmetic nerve injuries. These results have not been duplicated with anterior transposition. The disadvantage of decompression is the inability to localize the site of compression. If the compression neuropathy is not limited to the aponeurosis or muscle of the flexor carpi ulnaris, the operation will not prove to be sufficient for the patient. The most useful localizing sign of compression is a positive percussion test over the ulnar nerve as the ulnar nerve lies between the superficial and deep heads of the flexor carpi ulnaris. This preoperative finding, combined with the finding at operation of an indentation of the nerve beneath the stout portion of the aponeurosis overlying the heads of the flexor carpi ulnaris (usually with a swelling of the nerve proximal to the site of the compression), is the most reliable indication that the site of compression of the ulnar nerve was indeed localized and can be relieved by decompression.

Decompression begins with an incision from a point midway between the tip of the olecranon and the medial epicondyle of the humerus, extending distally about 6 cm, parallel to the subcutaneous border of the ulna. This incision will normally not cross the small branches of the medial brachial or medial antebrachial cutaneous nerves, but they should be looked for and preserved if encountered. The dissection is deepened through the flexor aponeurosis over the ulnar nerve, taking care to isolate the ulnar nerve in the proximal end of the incision. The aponeurotic band (fibrous arcade of the flexor carpi ulnaris muscle) over the nerve is divided as the nerve is traced distally between the two heads of the muscle. Continuing the fasciotomy of the flexor carpi ulnaris is prudent; I believe that the ulnar nerve should be explored to at least the midportion of the proximal third of the forearm. The branches of the ulnar nerve to the two heads of the flexor carpi ulnaris and to the ulnar half of the profundus are identified, as is the occasional articular branch of the ulnar nerve to the elbow joint. The ulnar nerve is not disturbed in its bed, nor are the accompanying vessels dissected from the nerve. If the typical findings of compression are found within the cubital tunnel and if there is swelling of the nerve proximal to the compression, epineurotomy can be performed to relieve whatever compression may continue from the epineurium. Internal neurolysis of the ulnar nerve at the elbow is unwise, however, because of the rich interfascicular plexus of nerves, a portion of which may be injured with a complete internal neurolysis of the ulnar nerve. Following completion of the release, passive flexion and extension of the elbow should be done to be sure that decompression of the nerve is complete and that the nerve does not now subluxate from its bed, which may cause the patient further problems and necessitate reoperation. If, following the decompression, subluxation of the nerve does occur, anterior transposition or, preferably, medial epicondylectomy should be performed. A skin closure is the only closure necessary after decompression of the ulnar nerve. The postoperative care generally consists of a soft, supporting, well-padded dressing over the elbow; immediate active motion of the elbow in flexion and extension is encouraged.

Anterior Transposition of the Ulnar Nerve

Anterior transposition of the ulnar nerve may be indicated for several syndromes involving compression of the ulnar nerve at the elbow. These indications include: subluxation of the ulnar nerve onto or over the medial epicondyle with flexion of the elbow; persistent or progressive valgus deformity, usually secondary to fracture malunion; and a persistently positive elbow flexion test with severe neuritic signs with prolonged flexion of the elbow. It is well-known that transposition is used to gain length for repair of the ulnar nerve after laceration. Anterior transposition is also appropriate for those patients in whom a decompression procedure has failed. These patients have usually had a decompression of the ulnar nerve at least 6 and often 12 months or more prior to considering anterior transposition. Although there has been some early improvement following the procedures, the patient's clinical course has not continued to improve, and the symptoms seem now to be aggravated by use of the arm, particularly with repetitive flexion and extension of the elbow. The symptoms improve with careful immobilization of the elbow in a well-padded cast. In such a clinical presentation anterior transposition of the ulnar nerve must be considered.

Some surgeons have used the method of McGowan[398,416] to grade the degree of ulnar neuropathy. In McGowan's first stage (Grade I), the symptoms of ulnar neuropathy are subjective, consisting of minor hypesthesia and paresthesias, whereas in the intermediate stage (Grade II), weakness and wasting of the interossei are found in addition to the hypesthesia. In the final stage (Grade III), marked weakness and wasting of the interossei, adductor pollicis, and hypothenar muscles are combined with complete or partial anesthesia in the ulnar one and one-half fingers. Accordingly, anterior transposition for Grade III and decompression for Grade I and II neuropathy would be appropriate procedures. The degree to which the anterior transposition is performed can vary. The subcutaneous transposition, which gained popularity a few years ago, and the partial or complete submuscular transposition, in which the ulnar nerve is placed parallel to the median nerve as it enters the forearm, have gained wide acceptance as an indicated treatment for cubital tunnel syndrome. The advantage of anterior transposition is that any pathology, visualized or not, will be left behind as the nerve is transposed from the cubital tunnel to its new bed. Tension is removed from the nerve by transposition, and removal of tension may improve blood supply to the nerve. Most authors who transpose to beneath the flexor muscle mass believe that one of the advantages of submuscular transposition is the placement of the nerve in a well-vascularized muscular bed.[361,371,393,408] Learmonth has expanded this concept by showing that nerves usually run in intramuscular beds.[393] The consummate advantage of anterior transposition, according to those authors who favor this procedure, is that the results obtained are better with this procedure than with either decompression or medial epicondylectomy in indicated patients with cubital tunnel syndrome.[361,364,371,395,398,408]

The disadvantages of anterior transposition are that the surgery is more complex than either external decompression or medial epicondylectomy and that the extensive exposure of the ulnar nerve not only places the branches of the nerve at some risk (especially those to the flexor carpi ulnaris), but also increases the scar in the new bed to which the nerve is transposed. During the transposition the ulnar nerve may be dissociated from its blood supply, which accompanies it. Interference with the medial brachial and medial antebrachial cutaneous nerves is not uncommon during transposition and may produce annoying dysesthesias. Anterior transposition may also create a new site of compression[364,395,408] of the ulnar nerve if the arcade of

Struthers, medial intermuscular septum, and flexor muscle mass are not mobilized and/or repaired properly. Another disadvantage of anterior transposition is the more complex postoperative management, consisting of immobilization of the elbow, which may allow cicatrix formation around the ulnar nerve during this period. Finally, some surgeons who do not prefer anterior transposition have indicated that in their patients there seems to be less improvement of motor function of the intrinsic muscles of the hand than with decompression or medial epicondylectomy. To my knowledge, no controlled study to evaluate improvement of motor function in comparable patients treated by different techniques is available to evaluate this objection.

Subcutaneous Transposition. The skin incision for anterior transposition[393] of the ulnar nerve parallels the nerve, curving along the posterior margin of the medial epicondyle to lie 0.5 to 1 cm anterior to the nerve. This incision is desirable to prevent interference with the medial brachial and medial antebrachial cutaneous nerves, a neuroma of which may be distressing to the patient and confusing to the surgeon in the postoperative period. The ulnar nerve is most easily identified immediately behind the medial epicondyle of the humerus. The fascia is thin over the nerve and the nerve can be palpated easily. By lifting the fascia away from the nerve with fine forceps, exposure of the nerve can be safely achieved. Identification of the nerve behind the epicondyle is desirable since this is an unlikely site of compression by fascia and the area of entrapment can be preserved for detailed examination later during the operation. The ulnar nerve, extending from behind the medial epicondyle, is followed proximally for at least 8 cm. The ulnar nerve lies along the medial head of the triceps, and any encroachment of the muscle on the ulnar nerve[409] or the appearance of an anomalous muscle, such as the anconeus epitrochlearis,[109] can be identified and its importance in the compression neuropathy evaluated. After the ulnar nerve is traced distally from behind the medial epicondyle, the tight fascia bridging the heads of the flexor carpi ulnaris must be divided with care since this area (i.e., the cubital tunnel) is narrowed and is often the site of the nerve compression.

The exploration distally should be continued to

between the heads of the flexor carpi ulnaris, where the arcade and fascia of the flexor carpi ulnaris are divided into the proximal third of the forearm. Care must be taken to protect the muscular branches of the nerve. After the ulnar nerve is exposed from at least 8 cm above the medial epicondyle to between the heads of the flexor carpi ulnaris in the proximal forearm, the surgeon should elevate the nerve from its bed, taking care to include both the arteries and veins accompanying the ulnar nerve in the bulk of tissue to be transposed. After the neurovascular bundle is mobilized, it is transposed anteriorly beneath the elevated skin flap, if a subcutaneous transposition has been chosen (Fig. 36-16). During transposition care must be taken that a new site of constriction is not created proximally by the arcade of Struthers or by the medial intermuscular septum. The medial intermuscular septum can be excised to relieve the ulnar nerve. The third area of concern with subcutaneous transposition is beneath the fascial arcade between the two heads of the flexor carpi ulnaris. If a band has been created, excision of muscle fascia is indicated.[364,395,408,109]

Following subcutaneous transposition, a suture from the anterior skin flap to the medial epicondyle seems advisable to prevent a position change of the transposed ulnar nerve. The skin and subcutaneous tissues are approximated in the usual way.

Submuscular Transposition. If, after mobilization of the neurovascular bundle (Fig. 36-17), the surgeon intends to proceed with a submuscular or partial submuscular transposition, elevation of the flexor muscles from the medial epicondyle is performed. Since the anterior flap of skin and subcutaneous tissue has been reflected anteriorly and the location of the median nerve in the distal third of the brachium is certain, a large hemostat can be directed beneath the flexor muscle mass to elevate the superficial head of the flexor carpi ulnaris with the flexor carpi radialis, palmaris longus, pronator teres, and a portion of the flexor digitorum superficialis. If a partial submuscular transposition is to be performed, a portion of the pronator teres remains unelevated but the other muscles are elevated from their origin on the medial epicondyle. The division of these muscles from the medial epicondyle is performed using sharp dissection, and the muscle origin is reflected distally, preserving the innervation

of the superficial head of the flexor carpi ulnaris (Fig. 36-18). If an intermuscular fascial band is encountered between these muscles, it should be excised to allow an uninterrupted bed for the transposed ulnar nerve. Following the formal transposition of the ulnar nerve into the submuscular position, the surgeon must again reexplore the proximal segment of the ulnar nerve to be sure that a fascial band has not encroached upon the nerve. The arcade of Struthers and the medial intermuscular septum should be examined and excised if necessary. Repair of the flexor aponeurosis to the medial epicondyle is undertaken (Fig. 36-19) making sure that a fascial band across the nerve is not created by the repair of the muscles to the medial epicondyle. Rather than closing the fascia over the cubital tunnel, the fasciotomy of the proximal third of the forearm is allowed to remain open to accommodate additional swelling.

A technique of submuscular transposition by osteotomy of the medial epicondyle has been described,[397] in which the ulnar nerve is transposed through the osteotomy site of the epicondyle to a position lying beneath and within the flexor muscle mass similar to submuscular transposition. This technique seems to this author to be unnecessarily difficult, to not provide the surgeon with the needed exposure to insure that a secondary site of compression is not created, and therefore to offer little benefit to the previously described method of detachment of the flexor muscle origin and reattachment and repair of that origin after transposition of the ulnar nerve.

Postoperative Management. The postoperative management of the patient who has undergone anterior transposition of the ulnar nerve begins with the application of a bulky dressing over the operative site for several days; the dressing should be of sufficient size to provide support and padding for the extremity and the transposed ulnar nerve. A supporting plaster splint across the elbow may be added as long as care is taken that there is *no* pressure over the operative incision or over the transposed nerve that could interfere with the viability of the skin or the recovery of the ulnar nerve. With submuscular transposition, because of the elevation of the flexor origin, it may be advisable to immobilize the elbow and wrist for a few weeks to allow healing of the repaired flexor muscle origin.

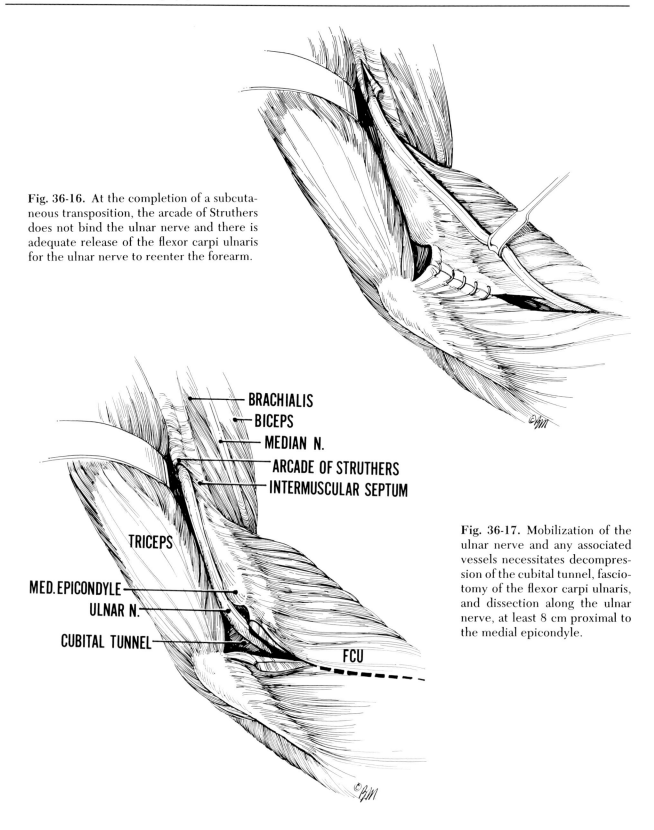

Fig. 36-16. At the completion of a subcutaneous transposition, the arcade of Struthers does not bind the ulnar nerve and there is adequate release of the flexor carpi ulnaris for the ulnar nerve to reenter the forearm.

BRACHIALIS
BICEPS
MEDIAN N.
ARCADE OF STRUTHERS
INTERMUSCULAR SEPTUM
TRICEPS
MED. EPICONDYLE
ULNAR N.
CUBITAL TUNNEL
FCU

Fig. 36-17. Mobilization of the ulnar nerve and any associated vessels necessitates decompression of the cubital tunnel, fasciotomy of the flexor carpi ulnaris, and dissection along the ulnar nerve, at least 8 cm proximal to the medial epicondyle.

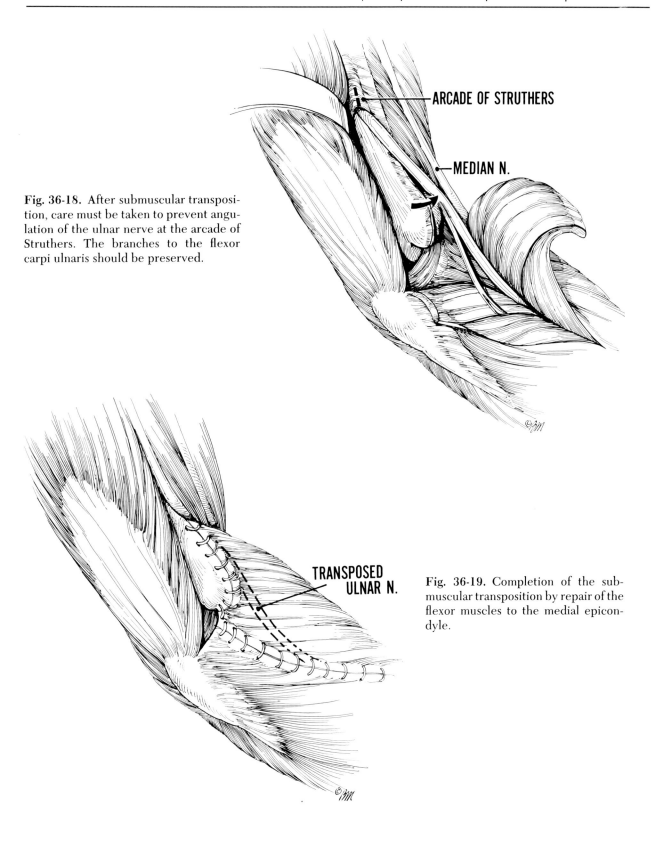

Fig. 36-18. After submuscular transposition, care must be taken to prevent angulation of the ulnar nerve at the arcade of Struthers. The branches to the flexor carpi ulnaris should be preserved.

ARCADE OF STRUTHERS

MEDIAN N.

TRANSPOSED ULNAR N.

Fig. 36-19. Completion of the submuscular transposition by repair of the flexor muscles to the medial epicondyle.

Following immobilization, gentle exercises are begun, with flexion and extension of both wrist and elbow. These exercises are generally accompanied by some sensation in the distribution of the ulnar nerve, but the exercises can be continued as long as the discomfort is tolerated by the patient.

Medial Epicondylectomy

Nearly 40 years ago, King and Morgan[389] published their experience with medial epicondylectomy for the treatment of traumatic ulnar neuritis. Their concept was that removal of the medial epicondyle, as one would remove an offending tumor or encroaching foreign body on a nerve, would permit that nerve to find its own optimal position. Though attractive in its simplicity, the concept has not been widely accepted by surgeons, although there have been several favorable studies reported.[370,378,387] The advantage of the procedure is that the nerve is not disturbed during the course of the removal of the medial epicondyle of the humerus. Consequently there is minimal exposure of the nerve, no damage to the proximal muscular branches, and no interference with the blood supply to the nerve. The tension on the nerve as it passes behind the medial epicondyle is removed, and the nerve, by necessity, slides forward and seeks its own position following removal of the restricting epicondyle. The motion possible in the early postoperative period allows the patient to return to his usual activities in the shortest possible time. The disadvantage of this procedure includes the loss of the protecting prominence of the medial epicondyle, which may subject the ulnar nerve to repeated direct external trauma. The failure to identify the site of compression of the ulnar nerve is a criticism of this procedure. Since the nerve is not explored during the course of the procedure, one cannot identify a compressive lesion and the danger of partial or no correction of a compression is a potential disadvantage. However, removal of the epicondyle probably decompresses the nerve at all points implicated in the cubital tunnel syndrome as long as the flexor carpi ulnaris is opened concomitantly. Subluxation of the ulnar nerve following medial epicondylectomy can potentially create a band at the medial intermuscular septum proximally or at the fascia of the flexor carpi ulnaris

distally as the nerve seeks its new position. Finally, the detachment of the flexor muscle mass arising from the medial epicondyle, even with provision for their reattachment, and the possibility of injury to the elbow joint if the medial collateral ligaments are detached may be greater disadvantages than other authors have indicated. The indications for this procedure[370,378,387,389,400] have been the occurrence of an ulnar neuropathy at the elbow caused by valgus deformity, nerve displacing callus, and irritating ununited medial epicondyle. Occupational trauma, arthritis of the elbow joint, adhesions, foreign bodies, tumors, blood vessel aberrations, shortening of the nerve after anastomosis for laceration in the forearm, as well as a group of unknown causes account for the rest of the patients in the series reported.[389,400]

A skin incision approximately 8 cm long is made parallel to the ulnar nerve and 1 cm behind the prominence of the medial epicondyle. The center of the incision is at the posterior aspect of the medial epicondyle. The incision is carried to the deep fascia, with care taken to protect any small branches of the medial antebrachial or medial brachial cutaneous nerves that lie over the distal portion of the incision and generally supply the skin over the olecranon prominence below the medial epicondyle. The epicondyle is exposed by sharp, subperiosteal dissection reflecting off the common flexor-pronator origin (Fig. 36-20). The ulnar nerve lies immediately behind the medial epicondyle and should be identified either by palpation or, preferably, under direct vision since its exposure will ease the ability of the surgeon to protect the nerve during excision of the medial epicondyle. Descriptions of the operation[370,378,389,410] note that there is no need to expose the ulnar nerve or its branches or to disturb its natural bed, since these techniques will result in unwanted scar formation about the nerve. In practice, however, it is safer to expose the nerve, carefully protecting all of the branches, natural bed, and blood supply. After the medial epicondyle and adjacent supracondylar ridge are fully exposed, the entire medial epicondyle and the ridge, or at least a portion of the ridge, are removed using either ronguers, osteotome, or bone saw. A natural guide for the proper plane of the osteotomy is the medial border of the trochlea (Fig. 36-21). By removing the distal portion of the

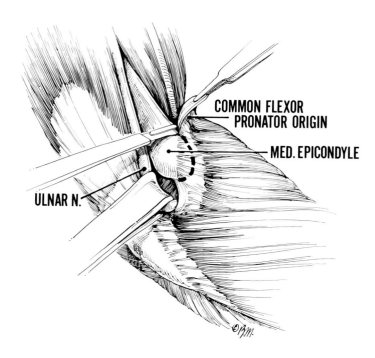

COMMON FLEXOR PRONATOR ORIGIN

MED. EPICONDYLE

ULNAR N.

Fig. 36-20. Medial epicondylectomy is begun by protecting the ulnar nerve and elevating the common flexor pronator origin from the medial epicondyle.

Fig. 36-21. The guide for the proper plane of the osteotomy for the medial epicondyle is the medial border of the trochlea. The sharp posterior edge of the osteotomy must be smoothed and rounded.

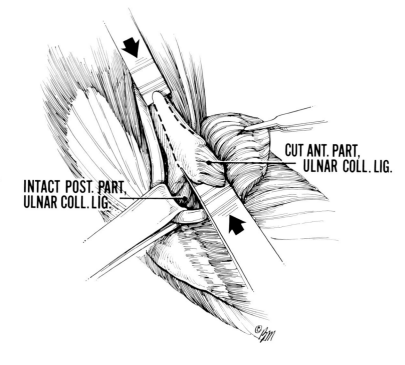

CUT ANT. PART, ULNAR COLL. LIG.

INTACT POST. PART, ULNAR COLL. LIG.

supracondylar ridge, the surgeon will release the intermuscular septum and remove the septum as a possible cause of complications in the postoperative period. The sharp bony edges must be smoothed off posteriorly, but one must not remove so much bone as to enter the elbow joint. If the elbow joint is entered, some elbow stiffness in either flexion or extension in the postoperative period is likely to result. Care should also be taken to leave the collateral ligaments intact. Before periosteal closure of the bone surface is done, bone wax may be pressed into the cancellous bone to reduce bleeding. The periosteum that was elevated is closed over the bone surface to reattach the origins of the flexor muscle mass (Fig. 36-22). The skin and subcutaneous tissues are closed in the usual fashion, once again being careful to protect any small branches of the medial brachial or medial antebrachial cutaneous nerves.

Only a soft dressing is required postoperatively, and range of motion exercises of the elbow can be begun within a few days after the operation. Except for the extremes of extension of the elbow, range of motion of the elbow is regained rapidly and even the extremes of extension should be regained within several months.

Author's Preferred Method. Careful preoperative evaluation of the patient with an ulnar entrapment neuropathy at the elbow determines, in my opinion, the selection of the procedure for relief of the neuropathy. If the patient has percussion sensitivity over the ulnar nerve distal to the medial epicondyle in the cubital tunnel, a decompression procedure will be used to relieve the neuritis present at the site of percussion sensitivity. Normally, the decompression will continue between the two heads of the flexor carpi ulnaris. If however, at the time of operation, no site of compression can be localized within the cubital tunnel from its entrance behind the medial epicondyle and extending distally between the heads of the flexor carpi ulnaris, I now recommend that the operation be continued by performing a medial epicondylectomy and decompression of the ulnar nerve. Decompression of the ulnar nerve combined with medial epicondylectomy has been most effective with my patients in relieving ulnar neuropathy at the elbow. The decompression continues distally between the heads of the flexor carpi ulnaris and proximally for approximately 10 cm proximal to the medial epicondyle. Such a decompression combined with medial epicondylectomy, as has been outlined pre-

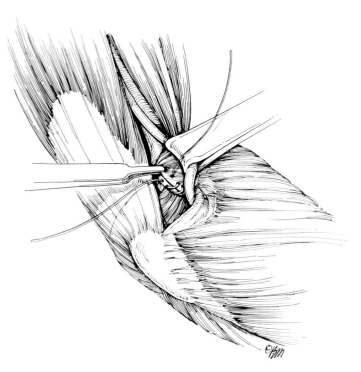

Fig. 36-22. Repair of the flexor-pronator origin to the humerus. After repair of the muscles, the ulnar nerve is allowed to seek its own position, and the arcade of the flexor carpi ulnaris must be opened sufficiently to prevent impingement on the nerve (not shown in the drawing).

viously, satisfies many of the criticisms of the medial epicondylectomy procedure. Specifically, the nerve is explored during this procedure, and the medial intermuscular septum is relieved proximally, as is the flexor carpi ulnaris distally. By carrying the exploration of the ulnar nerve 10 cm proximal to the medial epicondyle, the arcade of Struthers, should one exist, can also be decompressed, preventing a secondary neuropathy at the arcade of Struthers. The main criticism of the medial epicondylectomy procedure that remains unanswered with this surgical approach is the loss of the protecting prominence of the medial epicondyle. In a few of my patients — and I would emphasize that this has been less than 10 percent — this has been a minor problem, but has not contributed to increased neuropathy of the ulnar nerve and has not required any secondary treatment, either surgical or orthotic.

Some surgeons have suggested that medial epicondylectomy may weaken flexor-pronator muscle power, but the incidence and severity of this has not been well documented. If measurements are made in the early postoperative period, relative weakness may represent continuing ulnar neuropathy, and long-term follow-up studies are needed to resolve this question.

If the patient exhibits subluxation or dislocation of the ulnar nerve, a static or progressive valgus deformity of the elbow, or a positive elbow flexion test reproducing symptoms within 30 seconds of full flexion of the elbow preoperatively, I have found it advisable to proceed with medial epicondylectomy and ulnar nerve decompression as the primary surgical procedure for the relief of ulnar nerve neuropathy. During the course of the operation, I have explored the ulnar nerve from 10 cm proximal to the medial epicondyle to 7 to 8 cm distal to the medial epicondyle, carefully maintaining the tissue contiguous to the ulnar nerve, particularly the vascular structures associated with the nerve.

I now prefer medial epicondylectomy decompression over anterior transposition of the ulnar nerve because of the reduced morbidity following operation, improved postoperative results, and earlier return of patients to work.

In the postoperative period, I prefer a soft dressing of sufficient size to support the elbow for the first 4 to 5 days. After the first dressing change, the patient begins range of motion exercises in a light dressing with enough gauze pads to provide some protection of the operative area for an additional week to 10 days. I have not found it necessary to immobilize the flexor muscle repair nor to reattach that repair in a secondary operation in any patient in the last several years.

Symptoms in the early postoperative period of ulnar neuritis are usually associated with wrinkles in or a poorly applied dressing causing direct pressure over the ulnar nerve and the operative site. A simple change in dressing will relieve these symptoms. I have seen one patient who reformed bone at the medial epicondyle in the postoperative period and again became symptomatic approximately 6 months after medial epicondylectomy. Re-excision of the newly formed bone was sufficient to relieve the recurrent symptoms of ulnar neuritis. At the time of re-excision, the ulnar nerve was noted to snap over the new bone exostosis with flexion and extension of the elbow, much as an ulnar nerve might snap over a medial epicondyle as it subluxated from the ulnar groove.

The diagnosis of ulnar neuropathy at the elbow requires two essential determinations by the examining physician and surgeon. The examiner must make the diagnosis of ulnar nerve neuropathy and he must localize that neuropathy to the elbow. In my experience an electrodiagnostic study is extremely helpful in these determinations. The presence of an ulnar neuropathy can be determined by an efficient and complete electrodiagnostic study, usually an electromyogram. An electromyogram that includes studies of the flexor carpi ulnaris, flexor digitorum profundus of the ulnar two fingers, the abductor digiti quinti, the first dorsal interosseous, and the third palmar interosseous generally provides the useful information necessary to confirm an ulnar nerve neuropathy. I would emphasize that the use of the third palmar interosseous is extremely helpful and seems to be a muscle that is affected very early by the neuropathic process at the elbow. The finding of fibrillations or positive sharp waves in the third palmar interosseous or other ulnarly innervated muscles will confirm the diagnosis of neuropathy in the ulnar nerve.

Localization of the neuropathic process to the area of the elbow may be more difficult electrodiagnostically, and the delay of treatment until the conduction velocity is reduced significantly (30 percent or greater) may lead to an irreversible neuropathic process. I would emphasize that the conduction delay across the elbow in the ulnar nerve is a late sign of cubital tunnel syndrome and may not appear until irreversible damage has been done to the ulnar nerve. As a consequence, the appearance of a conduction delay across the elbow may be a valuable prognostic sign in the evaluation of cubital tunnel syndrome since it may often herald an irreversible lesion. In my experience, the appearance of a significant conduction delay in the ulnar nerve across the elbow has been associated in the postoperative period with a prolonged recovery of ulnar nerve function, if ulnar nerve function recovers at all.

Ulnar Nerve Entrapment in Guyon's Canal (at the Wrist)

Entrapment neuropathy of the ulnar nerve at the wrist may present with a variety of signs and symptoms[427,437,445,453,459,460,463,466,467,470,475] depending on whether the ulnar nerve itself or the superficial or deep branch of the nerve is compressed. An isolated sensory neuropathy or an isolated or even partial motor neuropathy of the deep branch of the ulnar nerve only heralds the anatomic site of compression. The presence of a combined motor and sensory neuropathy of the ulnar nerve indicates that the location of the entrapment[463] is at or proximal to the wrist or in Guyon's canal before the division of the nerve into superficial and deep branches. If there is involvement of the dorsal sensory branch of the ulnar nerve with concomitant involvement of motor and sensory fibers of the ulnar nerve, the site of compression must be at or proximal to the origin of the dorsal branch of the ulnar nerve in the distal third of the forearm. In such cases, the most likely site of compression is in the cubital tunnel.

The confirmed presence of entrapment neuropathy in the region of the wrist, especially if it is progressive, is sufficient indication for operative intervention, except in those few patients where an occupational neuritis with repeated blunt trauma to the hypothenar eminence of the palm might suggest that discontinuance of the blunt trauma would allow resolution of the neuropathic symptoms.[354,428,440,471,475]

Preoperative examination for an ulnar entrapment neuropathy of the wrist includes Allen's test for confirmation of ulnar collateral circulation to the superficial or deep palmar arches. Thrombosis or aneurysm of the ulnar artery or one of its branches can be a cause of ulnar neuropathy, which may be predicted if Allen's test reveals slowed circulation from the ulnar artery (see Chapter 63).

Pertinent Anatomy

Three years following his graduation from medical school, Felix Guyon, in 1861,[434] published a description of the canal at the base of the hypothenar eminence that bears his name. He later concentrated on the urinary tract and became renowned for his operations on the prostate gland.

Joined by the ulnar artery in the midportion of the forearm, the ulnar nerve lying deep to the flexor carpi ulnaris muscle gives off a large dorsal branch in the distal third of the forearm, which passes to the dorsum of the wrist between the flexor carpi ulnaris and the ulna. This dorsal branch eventually divides into two dorsal digital nerves that supply sensation of the ulnar one and one-half fingers. The ulnar nerve continues to the base of the palm and enters Guyon's canal (Fig. 36-23), which is a triangular canal. The roof is formed by the volar carpal ligament, which is blended with the tendinous insertion of the flexor carpi ulnaris into the pisiform bone, and the distal extension of the flexor carpi ulnaris, the pisohamate ligament. The lateral wall is formed by the hook of the hamate and the insertion of the transverse carpal ligament. The medial wall is formed by the fibrous attachments to the pisohamate ligament and the pisiform bone itself.[426,463] The ulnar nerve and artery traverse Guyon's canal. Within the canal, the ulnar nerve bifurcates into the superficial and deep branches; the superficial branch passes distally to the fat pad in the canal; the deep branch, along with a larger branch of the ulnar artery, passes distally and deeply between the origins of the abductor digiti quinti and flexor digiti quinti brevis muscles to supply the deeper interosseous muscles of the hand. There are no tendons or tendon sheaths tra-

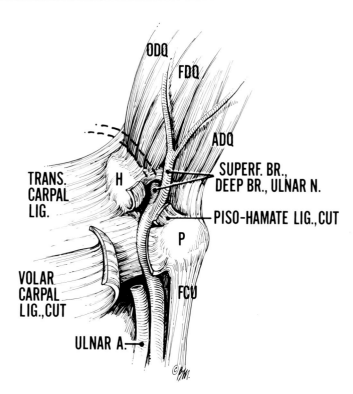

Fig. 36-23. The canal of Guyon with the ulnar nerve traversing from forearm to hand (*H*, hook of hamate; *P*, pisiform).

versing Guyon's canal as there are in the carpal tunnel, and the roof of this canal is relatively loose and fibrous rather than rigid and unyielding as is the transverse carpal ligament over the carpal tunnel.

Unlike the carpal tunnel syndrome, in which a majority of patients seem to have an ill-defined onset of the compression neuropathy, compression of the ulnar nerve in Guyon's canal is often associated with an occupational cause, predisposing the nerve to repeated blunt trauma,[421,422,428,471,474] an occult tumorous condition,[432,437,439,442,443,450,452,453,457,462,463,469] particularly a ganglion or lipoma in the region of the ulnar nerve and Guyon's canal, or fractures of the hamate or triangular bone[456,472,475] or ring and little metacarpal bases.[432] Some cases have been attributed to anatomic variations in Guyon's canal. These reports have been concerned with accessory or anomalous muscles[459,460,466,470] traversing Guyon's canal, arising from the deep fascia of the forearm and passing obliquely through the canal to blend with fibers of the abductor digiti minimi. Anatomic variations in the arrangement of the branches of the ulnar nerve[95,425,428,429,444,447] in the region of the pisiform bone have been described but rarely are the cause of motor or sensory signs. The palmar cutaneous branch of the ulnar nerve,[216] which may arise as far proximally as the middle portion of the forearm, accompanies the ulnar nerve and artery to the hand, perforating the volar carpal ligament and terminating in the skin and at the base of the palm. It may also communicate with the palmar branch of the median nerve. Although recent work has called attention to the presence of this nerve,[216] if the incision to decompress Guyon's canal is not carried ulnarly over the hypothenar eminence, injury to the palmar cutaneous branch of the ulnar nerve will most likely be avoided.

Operative Technique

An incision on the radial border of the flexor carpi ulnaris, beginning several centimeters above the proximal wrist crease and extending in a zigzag fashion across the crease along a line to the ring finger, will provide exposure of Guyon's canal and the ulnar nerve and artery. The ulnar nerve should be isolated above the wrist and traced distally through Guyon's canal by reflecting ulnarly the flexor carpi ulnaris, pisiform bone, and pisohamate ligament. The branches of the ulnar nerve to the hypothenar muscles and the palmaris brevis muscle, as well as the superficial and deep branches of the ulnar nerve, can be identified and preserved with this incision. Just as the palmar cutaneous branch of the median nerve is not exposed during carpal tunnel release, so also is the palmar cutaneous branch of the ulnar nerve not exposed during release of Guyon's canal. Although neuromata of the palmar cutaneous branch of the ulnar nerve have been mentioned as a possible cause of continuing symptoms in the hypothenar eminence,[216] I have not found this to be a problem using the incision described. Since this incision lies near the incision used for carpal tunnel release, when release of Guyon's canal is combined with release of the transverse carpal ligament, a single incision, that for the carpal tunnel, is used. In exploring Guyon's canal at the time of carpal tunnel decompression, the surgeon must be careful to release the band at the proximal wrist flexion crease that may create a new site of compression across the ulnar nerve if neglected.

Postoperative complications peculiar to the release of Guyon's canal are few. Neuroma of the palmar cutaneous branch of the ulnar nerve has been suggested[216] but I have not identified this as a cause of continuing pain at the base of the palm. Failure to release Guyon's canal into the distal third of the forearm can be associated with a continuing entrapment neuropathy in the proximal wrist crease.

COMPRESSION NEUROPATHIES OF THE RADIAL NERVE

Compression neuropathies of the radial nerve occur in predictable areas along the course of the nerve. The lateral intermuscular septum where the radial nerve passes from the posterior to the anterior compartment of the arm is a more common site for compression neuropathy than is generally reported.[499,501] Recorded cases of compression neuropathy relieved surgically[501] at the lateral intermuscular septum are sparse except in those cases associated with major trauma to the arm, particularly in fractures of the humerus.[83,153,487,507,511]

Displaced fractures of the humerus associated with radial nerve palsy are often related to the entrapment of radial nerve at the lateral intermuscular septum of the humerus, and decompression of the nerve at the intermuscular septum with or without internal stabilization of the fractured humerus may be beneficial to the recovery of radial nerve function. The radial nerve seems to be in jeopardy also at the lateral intermuscular septum during open reduction and interal fixation of a fractured humerus, particularly when a plate and screws are applied from the anterolateral approach to the humerus. During the internal fixation of the humeral fracture from the anterolateral approach, the radial nerve should be isolated, protected, and relieved from its entrapment at the lateral intermuscular septum so that undue tension and neuropathy are not created by the placing of a plate for fixation.

The radial tunnel syndrome,[498,515] a compression neuropathy of the radial nerve from the radial head to the supinator muscle, is the most common entrapment neuropathy of the radial nerve. A patient with this syndrome presents with aching pain in the extensor-supinator muscle mass in the proximal forearm that commonly radiates to the distal arm and distal forearm. If the fascicles of the superficial radial nerve are involved in the entrapment, radiation to the dorsal radial aspect of the hand and dysesthesias and paresthesias in the superficial radial distribution can be found. Two-point discrimination testing of the superficial radial nerve has not been helpful in my patients.

Most authors agree that there are four potential sites of compression within the radial tunnel.[274,514] The first is by fibrous bands lying anterior to the radial head at the entrance to the radial tunnel. The second site occurs at a fan-shaped leash of vessels (the radial recurrent vessels, the so-called leash of Henry), lying across the radial nerve and supplying the brachioradialis and extensor carpi radialis longus muscles. The third potential site of compression occurs at the tendinous margin of the extensor carpi radialis brevis. The fourth and most frequent site is at the arcade of Frohse, which forms a ligamentous band over the deep radial nerve as it enters the supinator muscle.

In my patients, I have observed that the tendinous margin of the extensor carpi radialis brevis and the arcade of Froshe may overlap, forming a scissorlike effect on the deep branch of the radial nerve that may combine to cause the radial tunnel syndrome. I believe that what we actually test with the flexor-pronator test is the combined tightening of the supinator muscle with pronation of the forearm and tightening of the ECRB with wrist flexion. At the operating table it is important therefore to recognize this potential combined cause of compression of the radial nerve, and to treat both aspects by not only dividing the arcade of Froshe but also by excision of a portion of the tendinous margin of the extensor carpi radialis brevis. Recently, a fifth cause of radial tunnel syndrome has been described.[522] As the deep branch of the radial nerve passes through the supinator muscle and exits along its distal lateral border, a fascial arcade is often present, lining the superficial head of the supinator muscle just above the existing deep branch of the radial nerve. Because this site has been described as a cause of radial tunnel syndrome, some surgeons now release the entire superficial head of the supinator muscle in order to preclude overlooking this area as a cause of continuing compression of the deep branch of the radial nerve.

In some cases the site of compression can be suspected by the physical findings on examination. If the symptoms of radial compression are reproduced by full flexion of the elbow with the forearm in supination and the wrist in neutral position, the fibrous bands anterior to the radial neck must be suspect. If the symptoms are reproduced with passive pronation of the forearm (elbow at 45 to 90 degrees flexion, wrist in full flexion), particularly if relieved with wrist extension alone, compression by the extensor carpi radialis brevis is likely. When the symptoms are reproduced by isometric active supination from the fully pronated position, compression at the arcade of Frohse is likely.

Electrodiagnostic studies of the radial nerve are helpful if signs of denervation are present on electromyogram. Conduction velocity of the radial nerve across the radial tunnel has not been helpful in my experience.

Since the onset and distribution of pain are similar in the radial tunnel compression and in tennis elbow, these syndromes must be differentiated. Usually the point of maximal tenderness in tennis elbow is over the lateral epicondylar ridge, lateral epicondyle, or radial head, whereas in radial tunnel compression the maximal tenderness is over the supinator muscle, four fingerbreadths distal to the lateral epicondyle. The widely acclaimed, but much less useful, middle finger test (extension of the middle finger against resistance, with the wrist in neutral and the elbow in 45 to 90 degrees) often produces diffuse pain over the extensor muscle mass, which, if localized to the area of maximal tenderness, may be helpful. In the absence of positive findings with the functional tests for radial tunnel syndrome (see above), I have used diagnostic local anesthetic blocks with Xylocaine to differentiate these syndromes. When the instillation of 0.5 to 1 cc of 1 percent Xylocaine four fingerbreadths distal to the lateral epicondyle relieves pain and is accompanied by a deep radial palsy, and a complementary injection more proximal in the region of the lateral epicondyle (usually given on a day after the patient has recovered from the first) does not relieve the patient's symptoms, I have made the diagnosis of radial tunnel compression.

The most distal compression of the radial nerve involves only the superficial (sensory) branch and occurs in the distal third of the forearm. This syndrome, described by Wartenberg[527] in 1932, as "cheiralgia paresthetica," was so named because of its similarity, in Wartenberg's opinion, to meralgia paresthetica of the lateral femoral cutaneous nerve.

Pertinent Anatomy

The radial nerve is a continuation of the posterior cord following separation of the axillary nerve at the inferior border of the glenohumeral joint. It crosses the posterior aspect of the humerus, accompanied by the profunda brachii artery, and reaches the lateral side of the posterior aspect of the arm where it pierces the lateral intermuscular septum at the junction of the middle and distal thirds of the humerus (Fig. 36-24). In the anterior compartment, the radial nerve lies between the brachialis and brachioradialis muscles. At the radial head the nerve enters the radial tunnel and then

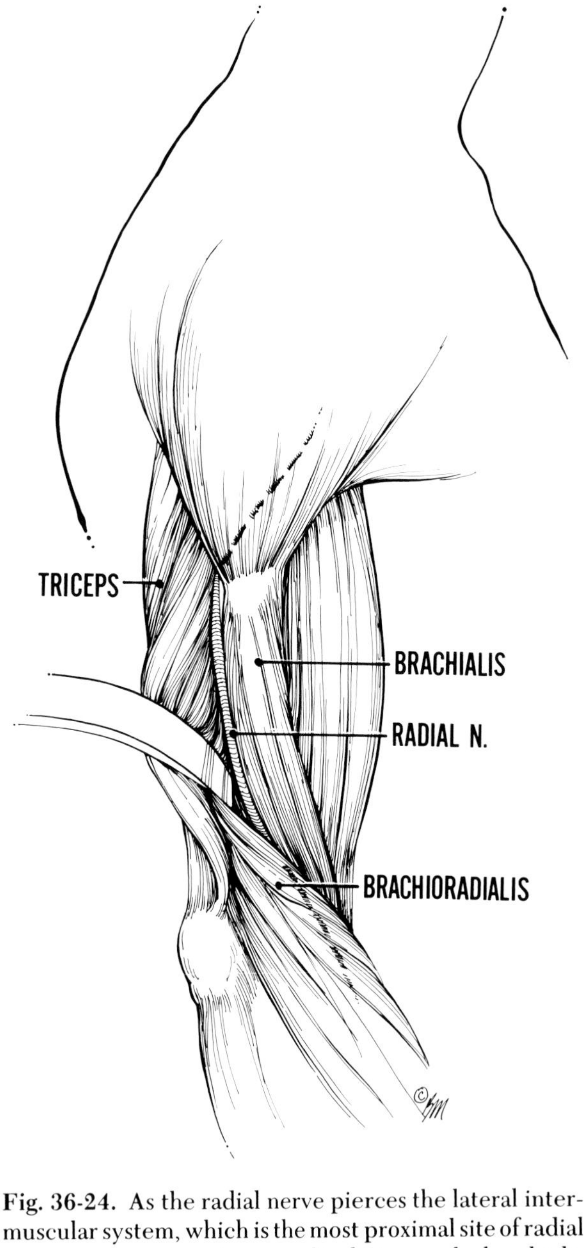

Fig. 36-24. As the radial nerve pierces the lateral intermuscular system, which is the most proximal site of radial nerve compression, the nerve lies between the brachialis and brachioradialis muscles.

divides into superficial and deep branches. The superficial branch lies beneath the muscle and tendon of the brachioradialis to the distal third of the forearm, where it exits dorsally to supply sensibility on the dorsal radial aspect of the hand. It is well-known that sensibility to the dorsoradial aspect of the hand may be overlapped by branches of the musculocutaneous nerve and ulnar nerve in a significant percentage of patients.

The deep branch of the radial nerve within the radial tunnel passes to the dorsal lateral aspect of the forearm, around the lateral side of the radius, and between the superficial and deep heads of the supinator muscle, exiting from this muscle at its distal border as multiple muscular branches to the ulnar wrist extensor, the extensor muscles of the fingers, and the extensor and abductor longus muscles of the thumb.

Radial Tunnel Syndrome

Operative Techniques

The basic indication for operation is the persistence of a compression neuropathy that has been documented to be progressive, unrelieved by conservative treatment, and localized by physical examination or electrodiagnostic studies.[252] If a peripheral compression neuropathy is neurapratic and associated with muscular effort, immobilization of the extremity should lead to rather prompt improvement of the neuropathy. If with restitution of muscular effort the neuropathy reappears, surgical decompression of the peripheral nerve is indicated. The basic operation for neuropathies of the radial nerve secondary to entrapment above the level of the radial tunnel is exploration of the radial nerve along its course. Exploration may be carried out either with an incision parallel to the course of the radial nerve or a series of longitudinal incisions, the first lying on the posterior lateral aspect of the distal brachium where the radial nerve can be observed piercing the intermuscular septum, and the second anterior to the lateral intermuscular septum. The longitudinal incisions are preferred to a single incision overlying the course of the radial nerve because the separation of the muscular bundles to expose the nerve is more easily performed through the longitudinal incisions.

Posterior Muscle-Splitting Approach to the Radial Tunnel. Exposure of the radial nerve within the radial tunnel can be accomplished by using either of two surgical approaches. If the compression neu-

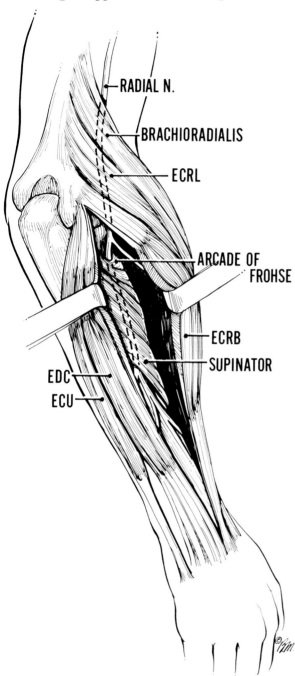

RADIAL N.

BRACHIORADIALIS

ECRL

ARCADE OF FROHSE

ECRB

SUPINATOR

EDC

ECU

Fig. 36-25. The posterior muscle-splitting approach to the radial tunnel and the arcade of Frohse.

ropathy in the radial tunnel is located at the arcade of Frohse, excellent exposure can be provided by a direct approach through the extensor muscles. The muscle bundles are separated distally and the incision is extended proximally, developing the plane between the superficial and deep muscles on the extensor surface to expose the radial nerve as it enters the supinator muscle at the arcade of Frohse (Fig. 36-25). An incision beginning 2 cm from the lateral epicondyle of the humerus and extending distally 7 cm will provide adequate exposure. To develop the interval between the extensor muscles, the dissection is begun in the superficial layer distally, developing the incision from distal to proximal and exposing the supinator muscle and, more proximally, the radial nerve. Exploration of the radial nerve, supinator muscle, arcade of Frohse, and their relationship to each other can be undertaken without difficulty. The advantage of this approach is the limited dissection and, thus, limited morbidity of the patient in the postoperative period. If the compression neuropathy can be localized preoperatively to the arcade of Froshe or to the fascial arcade as the deep branch of the radial nerve exits from the supinator muscle, adequate exposure for the release is possible through this incision. The disadvantage of this approach is the limited anatomic exposure that can be developed through this incision. Inability to localize the lesion to the arcade of Frohse is a contraindication to the use of this limited anatomic approach. The postoperative management after using this approach to the supinator muscle is to splint the wrist for support for the early postoperative period, allowing full flexion/extension and pronation/supination by the fourth postoperative day.

Anterolateral Approach to the Radial Tunnel. Since the radial tunnel syndrome[498,515] has been associated with four compressive anatomic lesions, an understanding of these potential lesions (see page 1454) is germane to a discussion of the more generalized approach to decompression of the radial tunnel. In those patients where the entrapment neuropathy of the radial nerve cannot be isolated preoperatively to the arcade of Frohse, a more generalized approach to the radial tunnel will be necessary to identify the site of compression, explore the radial nerve, and release the compressive le-

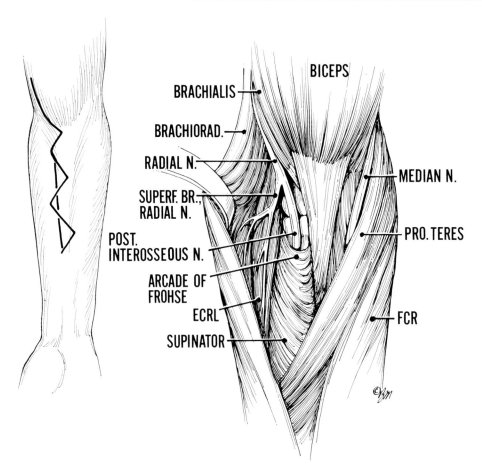

Fig. 36-26. The anterolateral approach to the radial nerve provides the best exposure of the radial tunnel when the compressive lesion cannot be localized to the arcade of Frohse. Although I prefer the zigzag incision for wider exposure, the linear incision is usually adequate.

sion. Consequently, an anterolateral approach to the radial nerve is advised in these patients (Fig. 36-26). The incision is begun laterally 5 cm above the flexor crease of the elbow and continues across that flexor crease along the ulnar border of the mobile wad. The incision is deepened and the flaps are elevated to the level of the deep fascia of the arm and forearm. The radial nerve is located between the brachioradialis and brachialis muscles, just above the flexor crease of the elbow. It is advisable to trace the radial nerve from this point distally since the first potential lesion, that of the fibrous band lying anterior to the radial head, will be lost if the exploration is begun further distally. The radial recurrent vessels forming a fanlike vascular arcade anteriorly across the radial nerve must be ligated and divided to continue the operation. Since the dissection is generally done with the forearm in supination, it is hard to visualize the potential for compression of the sharp tendinous margin of the extensor carpi radialis brevis unless the surgeon, during the operation, passively pronates the forearm and volarly flexes the wrist. If, during this maneuver, the border of the extensor carpi radialis brevis conforms to an indentation of the radial nerve or if this tendinous margin is otherwise suspected as the cause of the entrapment neuropathy, the fibrous margin should be excised. Finally, the exploration is continued to the arcade of Frohse, where the deep branch dives into the substance of the supinator muscle beneath the arcade. The arcade should be divided with care so that the branch of the radial nerve to the superficial head of the muscle is not also transected during division of the arcade. I have found it desirable to completely divide the superficial head of the supinator muscle as it lies across the deep radial nerve, since the fascial surface on the deep side of this superficial head continues across the nerve for some distance and cannot be adequately explored, except by cutting the superficial head. Complete muscle division also allows exploration of the nerve to the point where the nerve arborizes and leaves the distal margin of the supinator muscle. It seems prudent to free the nerve at the distal margin completely, as well as the proximal arcade, since there can be a fibrous band at the distal margin of the supinator. This exploration can be completed with the forearm in marked pronation and retraction of the superficial layer of extensor muscles laterally to expose the distal border of the supinator.

Postoperative Management. Following completion of the exploration of the radial nerve throughout its course in the radial tunnel, the wound is closed with subcutaneous and skin sutures in the usual fashion. Although I usually provide the patient with a supportive splint for the elbow and forearm, I prefer to begin early motion in pronation and supination of the forearm and flexion and extension of the elbow within 1 week postoperatively. Between therapy sessions, the patient should continue to use the supportive splint for 1 or 2 more weeks, depending on his progress following operation.

The postoperative recovery after radial tunnel decompression is generally prolonged when compared to the more common compressive neuropathies of the upper extremity. Accordingly, the patient can anticipate an early and definite improvement in symptoms with relief of the dysesthetic pain in the distribution of the radial nerve. Ultimate recovery of the radial nerve, however, seems to be prolonged over a 3- to 4-month period, during which time neurologic recovery of the neuropathy is anticipated.

Author's Preferred Method. Because of its more general applicability to entrapment neuropathies within the radial tunnel, the generalized (antero-

lateral) approach to the decompression of the tunnel is to be preferred. The ability of the surgeon to evaluate the entire nerve from above the elbow to the distal end of the supinator muscle cannot be overemphasized. Although the incision is less cosmetic than the more limited approach, the completeness of this exploration for neuropathies within the radial tunnel far outweighs the cosmetic disadvantage.

Radial Nerve Compression at the Wrist (Wartenberg's Syndrome)

Wartenberg[527] described an isolated neuritis of the superficial radial nerve (cheiralgia paraesthetica), which still bears his name. The syndrome was described in five patients and was associated with persistent pain on the dorsal radial surface of the distal third of the forearm radiating to the dorsum of the hand, thumb, and index and middle fingers. The location of pain may involve all or part of the distribution of the superficial radial nerve. On examination, there is sensitivity to percussion over the radial nerve within several centimeters of the radial styloid along the dorsal edge of the brachioradialis muscle. The percussion sensitivity radiates to the area of pain and is often associated with numbness. The indication for operative correction is the failure of conservative treatment to relieve the isolated neuritis of the superficial radial nerve.

Isolated neuritis of the superficial radial nerve has been associated with a number of seemingly unrelated causes. Although hemorrhage in the proximal forearm, extrinsic or intrinsic tumors of the radial nerve, and thrombosis of the recurrent radial vessels have been implicated in neuritic syndromes of the superficial radial nerve, injury to the branches of the superficial radial nerve in the distal third of the forearm or dorsum of the wrist are most often iatrogenic or traumatic.[204] The wearing of jewelry, such as elastic watchbands or elastic or tight-fitting bracelets, will produce a neuritis of this nerve, which can be easily relieved with removal of the watchband or bracelet. Anomalies of the muscles along the course of the superficial radial nerve can produce neuritic symptoms associated with numbness and sensitivity to percussion. Some of these muscle anomalies result in tight fascial bands across the nerve, creating an entrapment neuropathy. In those patients in whom the removal of jewelry does not relieve the neuritic symptoms, and immobilization either does not relieve the neuritic symptoms or following reinstitution of active motion the neuritic symptoms promptly reappear, surgical exploration of the superficial radial nerve is indicated.

Dellon and Mackinnon[485a,486a] have recently reviewed a series of 51 patients with complaints related to entrapment of the superficial radial nerve. Surgical exploration was carried out in 35 hands, and among this group, 49 percent of the patients rated their pain relief as good, but only 37 percent felt that the relief was excellent. It would thus appear, that, as with other affections of the superficial radial nerve, such as iatrogenic and industrial trauma, many of these patients will continue to have persistent dysesthesias, especially aggravated by motion of the wrist.

Pertinent Anatomy

The superficial branch of the radial nerve arises as the distal sensory branch approximately 4 cm distal to the lateral epicondyle of the humerus. The nerve passes distally along the lateral border of the forearm beneath the brachioradialis muscle. During much of its course in the forearm it is accompanied by the radial artery and concomitant vein. At the junction of the middle and distal thirds of the forearm, the superficial radial nerve begins to pass dorsally from beneath the cover of the brachioradialis tendon. The nerve pierces the deep fascia of the distal forearm, divides into two or more branches, and supplies the sensory innervation on the dorsum of the radial side of the hand to the tip of the thumb and to the PIP joints of the index, middle, and possibly the radial half of the ring fingers. An important volar branch innervates a small area at the base of the thumb on the volar aspect of the thenar eminence.

Several important variations of the superficial radial nerve should be noted. The superficial branch of the radial nerve may supply the entire dorsum of hand, encroaching on the area usually supplied by the ulnar nerve on the dorsum of the ring and little fingers, as well as on the index and middle fingers. Another variation of the superficial radial nerve is its passage superficial rather than deep to the brachioradialis muscle along its course from the proximal third of the forearm to the wrist. The musculocutaneous nerve may innervate the area usually supplied by the superficial radial nerve in varying degrees, even to replace the entire distribution of the superficial radial nerve on the dorsal radial aspect of the hand.

Operative Technique

To accommodate the many variations that have been outlined in the anatomic course of distribution of the superficial radial nerve, the operation should begin on the volar edge of the brachioradialis with an incision extending from the midportion of the lateral surface of the forearm, curving in a serpentine or lazy-S pattern to the dorsoradial aspect of the wrist just distal to the carpometacarpal joints. Through this incision, and by elevating the brachioradialis muscle in the proximal aspect of the incision, the superficial radial nerve can be identified beneath the muscle several centimeters more proximally. The nerve is then traced distally beneath the brachioradialis muscle and can be identified as it begins to pass dorsally and radially in the distal third of the forearm. The distal subcutaneous dissection beneath the incision is then carefully deepened to identify the brachioradialis tendon and the superficial radial nerve passing dorsal from it in the distal third of the forearm. When entrapped by either the tendinous margin of the brachioradialis, the margin of the extensor carpi radialis longus, or a bridge of superficial fascia of the forearm between these muscles, the entrapment can be relieved by excision of the tendon margin or adjacent fascia. The nerve must be carefully dissected and identified throughout its course to ensure relief of the entrapment. Except when the nerve has been injured and is entrapped in cicatrix or has been partially or completely transected at a previous surgical procedure, I have not identified an entrapment distal to the carpometacarpal joints of the fingers and thumb.

Postoperatively, the skin is closed in a single layer, taking care not to place the sutures so deep as to incarcerate the superficial nerve in the suture line. I prefer to mobilize the wrist as soon as possible to prevent fixed cicatrix formation about the nerve.

THORACIC OUTLET SYNDROME

Thoracic outlet syndrome may present with a variety of vague and confusing symptoms, including pain in the shoulder or supraclavicular fossa, radiating down the extremity in a radicular pattern and often involving the medial border of the arm and forearm. The symptoms are often vague, ill-defined and inconsistent, but may be provoked by a particular activity, such as working overhead, reaching down and behind repetitively, or lying in a particular position (e.g., with the hands overhead, behind the head, or on the side), allowing the symptomatic shoulder to fall away on the upward side.

The common denominator of thoracic outlet syndrome is a vascular and/or neurologic symptom complex related to the subclavian artery and/or the lower trunk of the brachial plexus. Occasionally the middle trunk of the plexus is also involved, thereby involving the seventh cervical root, in addition to the eighth cervical and first thoracic roots. In those cases with middle trunk involvement, the lower trunk is also involved. The vascular lesion may be caused by mechanical compression of the subclavian artery with resultant irritation and spasm of the artery. It may also be neurologic in origin, in which case an endoneuritis of the lower trunk of the brachial plexus creates an irritative lesion of the sympathetic fibers and resultant physiologic susceptibility rather than mechanical compression of the subclavian artery.[120] In either mechanical or neurologic vascular lesions, the subclavian artery is compressed or narrowed, resulting in reduced blood flow to the upper extremity, incipient reduction of the venous outflow if the concomitant subclavian vein is also involved, and relative ischemia of the upper extremity, which may be most marked during provocative muscular tests of the upper limb. The neurologic component of the thoracic outlet syndrome involves a compression neuropathy of the lower trunk of the brachial plexus as it arises from the lower cervical and first thoracic roots, passing superiorly and laterally across the first rib to pass between the scalenus medius muscle posteriorly and the scalenus anterior muscle anteriorly.[1,8,9,60,71,110,132,134] A number of anatomic variations that affect the passage of the neurovascular structures across the first rib may be involved in the neurovascular compression syndrome, including the slope of the first rib,[1] the site of attachment of the anterior scalenus muscles,[8] the size or cross-sectional area of the cleft between the scalenus muscles,[8,132] and variations in the attachment of the scalenus minimus muscle.[110] A common insertion of the anterior and medius scalenus muscles will elevate the vessel and nerve in the passage of the neurovascular structures through the scalene cleft.[120,132] Also, a crescent-type insertion of the anterior scalenus will have a tendency to push the artery and nerve posteriorly and superiorly, making them more susceptible to compression by a sharp tendinous margin of the scalenus medius.[8] A thickening or a prominent suprapleural membrane, also known as Sibson's fascia, may translocate the nerve more posteriorly making it more susceptible to compression, again by the margin of the scalenus medius.[8]

As with other entrapment syndromes of the upper extremity, thoracic outlet syndrome represents a series of anatomic variations, many of which have specific diagnostic maneuvers to confirm their presence. In Adson's test[1] the patient inhales deeply, holds his breath, elevates his chin, and turns it toward the affected side. If this series of maneuvers reduces or obliterates the radial pulse and/or reproduces the symptoms of the patient's complaint, the scalene muscles, particularly the scalenus anterior, may be the offending agent.

Malalignment of the shoulder, such as from sagging with increasing age, fatigue, ill health, or even poor posture, may narrow the costoclavicular space into which the neurovascular structures pass following the crossing of the scalene cleft. Narrowing of the costoclavicular space and resultant compression in the thoracic outlet may also occur with abnormal cervical ribs,[9,35] fracture calluses of the first rib or clavicle,[31,43] or abnormal posturing of the pectoral girdle, as in the brace syndrome.[60,134] The so-called costoclavicular maneuver, in which the shoulders are drawn downward and backward after which the patient takes a deep breath (with the head and neck in neutral), calls attention to compression in the costoclavicular space in this maneuver reproduces symptoms or obliterates the radial pulse. Many people will have reduced radial pulse with this test, and this in itself, without reproducing symptoms, has no clinical significance.

Wright's hyperabduction syndrome[134] is another

form of thoracic outlet entrapment, in which neurovascular symptoms in the upper extremities accompany repetitive or long-standing hyperabduction positioning of the pectoral girdle. The posturing assumed by a patient is one in which the arms are above or behind the head with elbows flexed. Wright indicated that two potential sites of entrapment might exist, the first being at the tendon of the pectoralis minor, and the second behind the clavicle, between it and the first rib. Once again, to make the diagnosis of Wright's hyperabduction syndrome, symptoms must be reproduced by this maneuver.

The neurologic signs and symptoms of thoracic outlet syndrome include fullness in the supraclavicular fossa, muscle wasting, atrophy, and weakness. Clumsiness of the hand, particularly apparent in activities of daily living and manipulation of fine objects of the hand, can be seen secondary to weakness or partial paralysis of the intrinsic muscles of the hand or the flexor pollicis longus or flexor digitorum profundus muscles.[66,132] A variety of sensory complaints can be associated with this syndrome. Many of these sensory complaints may be aggravated by cold weather, particularly with vascular involvement, or by carrying objects in the hand or on the shoulder, particularly if those objects displace or reposition the shoulder while being carried. The symptoms are usually increased after a long or tiring day, can be worse at night, and, if the patient sleeps on his side, affect the upper shoulder rather than the shoulder on which the patient sleeps. The shoulder on which the patient sleeps is usually relieved of thoracic outlet symptoms because of the compression of the shoulder and a widening of the costoclavicular space and scalene cleft while in this position. Similarly, elevation of the shoulder relieves the symptoms, and the patient may notice relief as he rests on a table or bar with his shoulders elevated but relaxed while leaning on the elbows. Several authors have noted (but have not explained), that vasomotor changes usually affect the radial side of the hand, specifically the thumb and index finger, rather than the ulnar side of the hand and palm. The vascular signs and symptoms of thoracic outlet syndrome include venous congestion of the upper limb and a bruit or thrill in the supraclavicular fossa, usually more marked with activity of the hand at either eye level or above the head. The symptoms of mild ischemia, particularly during work, may be described by the patient as a tiring or early fatiguing of the hands or arms, and, when dependent, the hand may be congested or bluish in color, possibly turning ischemic or white with elevation, particularly when the elevation is associated by exercise or cold.

Operative Treatment

Operative treatment for thoracic outlet syndrome may vary, depending on the success of localizing the origin of the compression. Although scalenotomies,[8] particularly of the scalenus anterior, have been popular in the past, the relatively frequent failure of this procedure in the treatment of thoracic outlet syndrome has led to the theory that the costoclavicular compression may be the principle mechanism. The correction of this compression syndrome by resection of the first rib has evolved. First rib resection is to be preferred to claviculectomy because decompression of the lower trunk of the brachial plexus as it crosses the first rib with the subclavian vessels is ensured by rib resection. The complications of claviculectomy, particularly those of traction neuritis of the entire brachial plexus, have mitigated against the use of this procedure.

Even though first rib resection is the treatment of choice in thoracic outlet syndrome, the method of removal is disputed. The transaxillary approach[96] has largely replaced the subclavicular, anterior extrapleural, and posterior thoracoplasty approaches, all of which have been used in the past. It should be emphasized that, with resection of the first rib, the attachments of the scalenus muscles are removed and that any cervical rib should be resected at the same operation. This operation results in a thorough removal of the bony structures that may be involved in the compression syndrome at the thoracic outlet, effectively removing the attachment of all of the scalenus muscles (medius, anterior, and minimus) and relieving any incarceration of the neurovascular structures within the scalene cleft at the first rib. As always, the value of this surgical procedure is only as good as the diagnostic procedures, which localize the compression neuropathy, and the skill of the surgeon will be weighed by the preoperative evaluation rather than the intraoperative treatment.

The details of operative procedures for thoracic outlet syndrome are not included in this text as they usually fall outside the purview of most hand surgeons.

REFERENCES

General

1. Adson AW: Surgical treatment for symptoms produced by cervical ribs and the scalenus anterior muscle. Surg Gynecol Obstet 85:687, 1947
2. Backhouse KM: Innervation of the hand. Hand 7:107–114, 1975
3. Barber KW Jr, Bianco AJ Jr, Soule EH, MacCarty CS: Benign extraneural soft tissue tumors of the extremities causing compression of nerves. J Bone Joint Surg 44A:98–104, 1962
4. Bateman JE: Trauma to Nerve in Limbs. WB Saunders, Philadelphia, 1962
5. Behse F, Buchthal F, Carlsen F, Knappeis GG: Hereditary neuropathy with liability to pressure palsies: Electrophysiological and histopathological aspect. Brain 95:777–794, 1972
6. Belsole RJ, Lister GD, Kleinert HE: Polyarteritis: A cause of nerve palsy in the extremity. J Hand Surg 3:320–325, 1978
7. Blunt MJ: The vascular anatomy of the median nerve in the forearm and hand. J Anat 93:15, 1959
8. Bonney G: The scalenus medius band. A contribution to the study of the thoracic outlet syndrome. J Bone Joint Surg 47B:268–272, 1965
9. Brannon EW: Cervical rib syndrome. An analysis of nineteen cases and twenty-four operations. J Bone Joint Surg 45A:977–998, 1963
10. Brooks DM: Nerve compression by simple ganglia. J Bone Joint Surg 34B:391–400, 1952
11. Brooks DM: Nerve compression syndromes (Editorial). J Bone Joint Surg 45B:445–446, 1963
12. Brown BA: Internal neurolysis in traumatic peripheral nerve lesions in continuity. Surg Clin North Am 52:1167–1175, 1972
13. Chalmers J: Unusual causes of peripheral nerve compression. Hand 10:168–175, 1978
14. Clein LJ: Suprascapular entrapment neuropathy. Neurosurgery 43:337, 1975
15. Cliffton EE: Unusual innervation of the intrinsic muscles of the hand by median and ulnar nerve. Surgery 23:12, 1948
16. Craig WS, Clark JMP: Of peripheral nerve palsies in the newly born. J Obstet Gynecol Br Commonw 65:229–237, 1958
17. Cruz-Martinez A, Barrio M, Perez-Conde MC, Ferrer MT: Electrophysiological aspects of sensory conduction velocity in healthy adults. Ratio between the amplitude of sensory evoked potentials at the wrist on stimulating different fingers in both hands. J Neurol Neurosurg Psychiatry 41:1097–1101, 1978
18. Daube JR: Nerve conduction studies in the thoracic outlet syndrome. Neurology 25:347, 1975
19. Denny-Brown D, Brenner C: Paralysis of nerve induced by direct pressure and by tourniquet. Arch Neurol Psychiatry 51:1–26, 1944
20. Earl CJ, Fullerton PM, Wakefield GS, Schutta HS: Hereditary neuropathy with liability to pressure palsies. A clinical and electrophysiological study of four families. Q J Med 33:481–498, 1964
21. Eisen A: Early diagnosis of ulnar nerve palsy: An electrophysiological study. Neurology 24:256, 1974
22. Eisen A, Schomer D, Melmed C: The application of F-wave measurements in the differentiation of proximal and distal upper limb entrapments. Neurology 27:662–668, 1977
23. Eversmann WW: Compression and entrapment neuropathies of the upper extremity. J Hand Surg 8:759–766, 1983
24. Felsenthal G: Median and ulnar distal motor and sensory latencies in the same normal subject. Arch Phys Med Rehab 58:297, 1977
25. Felsenthal G: Median and ulnar evoked muscle and sensory action potentials. Am J Phys Med 57:167, 1978
26. Felsenthal G: Comparison of evoked potentials in the same hand in normal subjects and in patients with carpal tunnel syndrome. Am J Phys Med 57:228–232, 1978
27. Fincham RW, Cape CA: Neuropathy in myxedema. A study of sensory nerve conduction in the upper extremities. Arch Neurol 19:464, 1968
28. Froshe F, Frankel M: Die Muskeln des menschlichen Armes. pp. 164–175. In Bardeleben's Handbuch der Anatomie des Menschlichen. Fisher, Jena, 1908
29. Furnas DW: Muscle tendon variations in the flexor compartment of the wrist. Plast Reconstr Surg 36:320–324, 1965
30. Gage MP: Scalenus anterior syndrome. Am J Surg 73:252, 1947

31. Gelberman RH, Verdeck WH, Brodhead WT: Supraclavicular nerve entrapment syndrome. J Bone Joint Surg 57A:119, 1975

32. Gilliatt RW: Disorders of peripheral nerve. JR Coll Phys London 1:50, 1966

33. Gilliatt RW, Melville ID, Velate AS, Willison RG: A study of normal nerve action potentials using an averaging technique (barrier grid storage tube). J Neurol Neurosurg Psychiatry 28:191, 1965

34. Gilliatt RW, Ochoa J, Rudge P, Neary D: The cause of nerve damage in acute compression. Trans Am Neurol Assoc 99:71–74, 1974

35. Gilliatt RW, Willison RG, Dietz V, Williams IR: Peripheral nerve conduction in patients with a cervical rib and band. Ann Neurol 4:124, 1978

36. Gilliatt RW, Wilson TG: Ischaemic sensory loss in patients with peripheral nerve lesions. J Neurol Neurosurg Psychiatry 17:104, 1954

36a. Goss CM: Anatomy of the Human Body by Henry Gray. 27th Ed., Lea & Febiger, Philadelphia, 1959

37. Gruber W: Ueber die Verbindung des Nervus medianus mit dem Nervus ulnaris am Unterarme des Menschen under Sängethiete. Arch Anat Physiol 37:501–522, 1870

38. Hakstian RW: Funicular orientation by direct stimulation. J Bone Joint Surg 50A:1178–1186, 1968

39. Henry AK: Extensile Exposure. 2nd Ed., Williams & Wilkins, Baltimore, 1970

40. Herbison GJ, Staas WE: Electrical testing: Neuromuscular physiology and clinical application. In Littler JW, Cramer LM, Smith JW (eds): Symposium on Reconstructive Hand Surgery. CV Mosby, St Louis, 1974

41. Hodes R, Larrabee MG, German W: The human electromyogram in response to nerve stimulation and conduction velocity of motor axons. Arch Neurol Psychiatry 60:340–365, 1948

42. Hollinshead WH: Anatomy for surgeons. The Back and Limbs, Vol. 3. 2nd Ed., Hoeber, New York, 1969

43. Howard FM, Shafer SJ: Injuries to the clavicle with neurovascular complications. A study of fourteen cases. J Bone Joint Surg 47A:1335–1346, 1965

44. Howe JF, Loeser JD, Calvin WH: Mechanosensitivity of dorsal root ganglia and chronically injured axons: A physiological basis for the radicular pain of nerve root compression. Pain 3:25, 1977

45. Hunt JR: The thenar and hypothenar types of neural atrophy of the hand. Am J Med Sci 141:224–241, 1911

46. Hunt JR: Thenar and hypothenar types of neural atrophy of the hand. Br Med J 2:642, 1930

47. Jabaley ME, Wallace WH, Heckler FR: Internal topography of major nerves of the forearm and hand. A current review. J Hand Surg 5:1–18, 1980

48. Johnson EW, Olsen KJ: Clinical value of motor nerve conduction velocity determination. JAMA 172:2030–2035, 1960

49. Kaplan EB: Functional and Surgical Anatomy of the Hand. 2nd Ed., JB Lippincott, Philadelphia, 1965

50. Karpati G, Carpenter S, Eisen AA, Feindel W: Familial multiple peripheral nerve entrapments— An unusual manifestation of a peripheral neuropathy. Trans Am Neurol Assoc 98:267–269, 1973

51. Karpati G, Carpenter S, Eisen AA, Wolfe LS, Feindel W: Multiple peripheral nerve entrapments. Arch Neurol 31:418, 1974

52. Kelso JS, Wallace S, Stelmach G, Weitz G: Sensory and motor impairment in the nerve compression block. Q J Exp Psychol 27:123, 1975

53. Kimura J, Murphy MJ, Varda DI: Electrophysiological study of anomalous innervation of intrinsic hand muscles. Arch Neurol 33:842–844, 1976

54. Kline DG, Hackett ER, May PR: Evaluation of nerve injuries by evoked potentials and electromyography. J Neurosurg 31:128–136, 1969

55. Kline DG, Nulsen FE: The neuroma in continuity. Surg Clin North Am 52:1189–1209, 1972

56. Kopell HP, Thompson WAL: Peripheral Entrapment Neuropathies. Williams & Wilkins, Baltimore, 1963

57. Kuczynski K: Functional micro-anatomy of the peripheral nerve trunks. Hand 6:1–10, 1974

58. Kudrjavcev T: Neurologic complications of thyroid dysfunction. Adv Neurol 19:619, 1978

59. Lahey MD, Aulicino PL: Anomalous muscles associated with compression neuropathies. Orth Rev 15:19–28, 1986

60. Lain TM: The military brace syndrome: A report of sixteen cases of Erb's palsy occurring in military cadets. J Bone Joint Surg 51A:557–560, 1969

61. Leonard MH: Immediate improvement of sensation on relief of extraneural compression. J Bone Joint Surg 51A:1282–1284, 1969

62. Levine J, Spinner M: Neurolysis in elderly patients. Clin Orthop 80:13–16, 1971

63. Linell EA: The distribution of nerves in the upper limb with reference to variabilities and their clinical significance. J Anat 55:79–112, 1921

64. Lister GD: The Hand Diagnosis and Indications. Churchill Livingstone, Edinburgh, 1977

65. Littler JW: Principles of reconstructive surgery of the hand. In Converse JM (ed): Reconstructive Plastic Surgery. WB Saunders, Philadelphia, 1964

66. London GW: Normal ulnar nerve conduction velocity across the thoracic outlet: Comparison of two measuring techniques. J Neurol Neurosurg Psychiatry 38:756–760, 1975

67. Ludin HP, Lutschg J, Valsangiacomo F: Comparison of orthodromic and antidromic sensory nerve conduction. 1. Normals and patients with carpal tunnel syndrome. EEG EMG 8:173, 1977

68. Lundborg G: Ischemic nerve injury. Experimental studies on intraneural microvascular pathophysiology and nerve function in a limb subjected to temporary circulatory arrest. Scand J Plast Reconstr Surg (suppl.) 6:1–113, 1970

69. Lundborg G, Gelberman RH, Minteer-Convery M, Lee YF, Hargens AR: Median nerve compression in the carpal tunnel — Functional response to experimentally induced controlled pressure. J Hand Surg 7:252–259, 1982

70. Marinacci AA: Some unusual causes of pressure neuropathies. Bull Los Angeles Neurol Soc 25:223–231, 1960

71. McIntyre DI: Subcoracoid neurovascular entrapment. Clin Orthop 108:27–30, 1975

72. McRae DL: The significance of abnormalities of the cervical spine. Am J Roentgenol 84:3, 1960

73. Miller R: Observations upon the arrangement of the axillary artery and brachial plexus. Am J Anat 64:143–163, 1939

74. Moldaver J: Tourniquet paralysis syndrome. Arch Surg 68:136, 1954

75. Morrison JT: A palmaris longus muscle with a reversed belly, forming an accessory flexor muscle of the little finger. J Anat Phys 50:324, 1916

76. Murai Y, Anderson I: Studies of sensory conductions: Comparison of latencies of orthodromic and antidromic sensory potentials. J Neurol Neurosurg Psychiatry 38:1187, 1975

77. Nakano KK: The entrapment neuropathies of rheumatoid arthritis. Orthop Clin North Am 6:837, 1975

78. Neary D, Eames RA: The pathology of ulnar nerve compression in man. Neuropathol Appl Neurobiol 1:69–88, 1975

79. Neary D, Ochoa J, Gilliatt RW: Subclinical entrapment neuropathy in man. J Neurol Sci 24:283–298, 1976

80. Nicolle FV, Woolhouse FM: Nerve compression syndromes of the upper limb. J Trauma 5:313–319, 1965

81. Ochoa J: Schwann cell and myelin changes caused by some toxic agents and trauma. Proc R Soc Med 67:131–133, 1974

82. Ochoa J, Fowler TJ, Gilliatt RW: Anatomical changes in peripheral nerves compressed by pneumatic tourniquet. J Anat 113:433–455, 1972

83. Omer GE: Injuries to nerves of the extremity. J Bone Joint Surg 56A:1615–1624, 1974

84. Omer GE, Spinner M: Peripheral nerve testing and suture techniques. pp. 122–143. In AAOS Instructional Course Lectures, Vol. 24. CV Mosby, St Louis, 1975

85. Paget J: Lectures on Surgical Pathology. 1st Ed., Lindsay & Bakiston, Philadelphia, 1854

86. Pandya NJ: Surgical decompression of nerves in leprosy. An attempt at prevention of deformities. A clinical, electrophysiologic, histopathologic and surgical study. Int J Lepr 46:47, 1978

87. Parks BJ: Postoperative peripheral neuropathies. Surgery 74:348, 1973

88. Parsonage MJ, Turner JWA: Neuralgic amyotrophy. The shoulder-girdle syndrome. Lancet 1:973, 1948

89. Payan J: Electrophysiological localization of ulnar nerve lesions. J Neurol Neurosurg Psychiatry 32:208, 1969

90. Phalen GS, Kendrick JI, Rodriguez JM: Lipomas of the upper extremity. Am J Surg 121:298–306, 1971

91. Rainer WG, Mayer J, Sadler TR Jr, Dirks D: Effect of graded compression on nerve conduction velocity. Arch Surg 107:719, 1973

92. Rank RK, Wakefield AR, Hueston JT: Surgery of Repair as Applied to Hand Injuries. 3rd Ed., Williams & Wilkins, Baltimore, 1968

93. Rask MR: Suprascapular nerve entrapment: A report of two cases treated with suprascapular notch resection. Clin Orthop 123:73–75, 1977

94. Reimann AF, Daseler EH, Anson BJ, Beaton LE: The palmaris longus muscle and tendon. A study of 1600 extremities. Anat Rec 89:495–505, 1944

95. Riche P: Le nerf cubital et las muscles de l'eminence thenar. Bul Mem Soc Anat Paris 5:251–252, 1897

96. Roos D: Transaxillary approach for first rib resection to relieve thoracic outlet syndrome. Ann Surg 163:354, 1966

97. Rowntree T: Anomalous innervation of the hand muscles. J Bone Joint Surg 51B:505–510, 1949

98. Rudge P, Ochoa J, Gilliatt RW: Acute peripheral nerve compression in the baboon. J Neurol Sci 23:403–420, 1974

99. Rydevik B, Lundborg G: Permeability of intraneural microvessels and perineurium following acute, graded experimental nerve compression. Scand J Plast Reconstr Surg 11:179, 1977

100. Rydevik B, Lundborg G Bagge U: Effects of graded

compression on intraneural blood flow. J Hand Surg 6:3–12, 1981

101. Rydevik B, Lundborg G, Nordborg C: Intraneural tissue reactions induced by internal neurolysis. Scand J Plast Reconstr Surg 10:3–8, 1976

102. Seddon HJ: Three types of nerve injury. Brain 66:237–287, 1943

103. Seddon HJ: Surgical Disorders of the Peripheral Nerve. 2nd Ed., Churchill Livingstone, Edinburgh, 1975

104. Simpson JA: Fact and fallacy in measurement of conduction velocity in motor nerves. J Neurol Neurosurg Psychiatry 27:381–385, 1964

105. Smith GE: An account of some rare nerve and muscle anomalies with remarks on their significance. J Anat Physiol 29:84, 1895

106. Smith JW: Factors influencing nerve repair. I. Blood supply to peripheral nerves. Arch Surg 93:335–341, 1966

107. Smith JW: Factors influencing nerve repair. II. Collateral circulation of the peripheral nerves. Arch Surg 93:433–436, 1966

108. Spencer PS, Weinberg HJ, Raine CS, Prineas JW: The perineurial window—A new model of focal demyelination and remyelination. Brain Res 96:323–329, 1975

109. Spinner M: Injuries to the Major Branches of Peripheral Nerves of the Forearm. 2nd Ed., WB Saunders, Philadelphia, 1978

110. Spinner M: Cryptogenic infraclavicular brachial plexus neuritis (Preliminary report). Bull Hosp Joint Dis 37:98, 1976

111. Spinner M, Freundlich BD: An important variation of the palmaris longus. Bull Hosp Joint Dis 28:126, 1967

112. Spinner M, Spencer PS: Nerve compression lesions of the upper extremity. A clinical and experimental review. Clin Orthop 104:46–67, 1974

113. Strain RE, Olson WH: Selective damage of large diameter peripheral nerve fibers by compression. An application of Laplace's law. Exp Neurol 47:68, 1975

114. Straus WL Jr: The phylogeny of the human forearm extensors. Hum Biol 13:23, 203, 1941

115. Struthers J: On a peculiarity of the humerus and humeral artery. Monthly J Med Sci 8:264–267, 1848

116. Struthers J: On some points in the abnormal anatomy of the arm. Br Foreign Medico-Chirurgical Rev 12:523–533, 1854

117. Sunderland S: The intraneural topography of the radial, median and ulnar nerves. Brain 68:243–299, 1945

118. Sunderland S: The innervation of the flexor digitorum profundus and lumbrical muscles. Anat Rec 93:317–321, 1945

119. Sunderland S: Traumatic injuries of peripheral nerves. I. Simple compression injuries of the radial nerve. Brain 68:56–72, 1945

120. Sunderland S: Nerves and Nerve Injuries. Williams & Wilkins, Baltimore, 1968

121. Thomas JE, Lambert EH: Ulnar nerve conduction velocity and H reflex in infants and children. J Appl Physiol 15:1–9, 1960

122. Thomas PK, Sears TA, Gilliatt RW: The range of conduction velocity in normal motor nerve fibers to the small muscles of the hand and foot. J Neurol Neurosurg Psychiatry 22:175–181, 1959

123. Trojaborg W: Prolonged conduction block with axonal degeneration. J Neurol Neurosurg Psychiatry 40:50–57, 1977

124. Turner JWA, Parsonage MJ: Neuralgic amyotrophy (paralytic brachial neuritis.) Lancet 2:209, 1957

125. Upton ARM, McComas AJ: The double crush nerve entrapment syndromes. Lancet 2:359, 1973

126. Wagman IH, Lesse H: Maximum conduction velocities of motor fibers of ulnar nerve in human subject of various ages and sizes. J Neurophysiol 15:235, 1952

127. Watson-Jones R: Primary nerve lesions in injuries of the elbow and wrist. J Bone Joint Surg 12:121, 1930

128. Weir MS: Injuries of Nerves and Their Consequences. JB Lippincott, Philadelphia, 1872

129. White WL, Hanna DC: Troublesome lipomata of the upper extremity. J Bone Joint Surg 44A:1353–1359, 1962

130. Wilbourn AJ, Lambert EH: The forearm median-to-ulnar nerve communication; electrodiagnostic aspects. Neurology 26:368, 1976

131. Williams HB, Terzis JK: Single fascicular recordings: An intraoperative diagnostic tool for the management of peripheral nerve lesions. Plast Reconstr Surg 57:562–569, 1976

132. Williams HT, Carpenter NH: Surgical treatment of the thoracic outlet compression syndrome. Arch Surg 113:850, 1978

133. Wortis H, Stein MH, Jolliffee N: Fiber dissociation in peripheral neuropathy. Arch Intern Med 69:222, 1942

134. Wright IS: The neurovascular syndrome produced by hyperabduction of the arms. Am Heart J 29:1, 1945

Pronator Syndrome

135. Agnew DH: Bursal tumor producing loss of power of forearm. Am J Med Sci 46:404–405, 1863

136. Barnard LB, McCoy SM: The supracondyloid process of the humerus. J Bone Joint Surg 28:845–850, 1946

137. Beaton LE, Anson BJ: The relation of the median nerve to the pronator teres muscle. Anat Rec 75:23–26, 1939

138. Bell GE Jr, Goldner JL: Compression neuropathy of the median nerve. South Med J 49:966–972, 1956

139. Bucher TPJ: Anterior interosseous nerve syndrome. J Bone Joint Surg 54B:555, 1972

140. Buchthal F, Rosenfalck A, Trojaborg W: Electrophysiological findings in entrapment of the median nerve at wrist and elbow. J Neurol Neurosurg Psychiatry 37:340, 1974

141. Farber JS, Bryan RS: The anterior interosseous nerve syndrome. J Bone Joint Surg 50A:521–523, 1968

142. Fearn CBd'A, Goodfellow JW: Anterior interosseous nerve palsy. J Bone Joint Surg 47B:91–93, 1965

143. Ferner H: Ein Abnormaler verlauf des Nervus medianus vor dem M. pronator teres. Anat Anz 84:151–156, 1937

144. Finelli PF: Anterior interosseous nerve syndrome following cutdown catheterization. Ann Neurol 1:205–206, 1977

145. Gardner-Thorpe C: Anterior interosseous nerve palsy: Spontaneous recovery in two patients. J Neurol Neurosurg Psychiatry 37:1146–1150, 1974

146. Kessel L, Rang M: Supracondylar spur of the humerus. J Bone Joint Surg 48B:765–769, 1966

147. Kiloh LG, Nevin S: Isolated neuritis of the anterior interosseous nerve. Br Med J 1:850–851, 1952

148. Kopell HP, Thompson WAL: Pronator syndrome. N Engl J Med 259:713–715, 1958

149. Krag C: Isolated paralysis of the flexor pollicis longus muscle. An unusual variation of the anterior interosseous nerve syndrome. Case report. Scand J Plast Reconstr Surg 8:250–252, 1974

150. Laha RK, Lunsford D, Dujovny M: Lacertus fibrousus compression of the median nerve. Case report. J Neurosurg 48:838, 1978

151. Lake PA: Anterior interosseous nerve syndrome. J Neurosurg 41:306–309, 1974

152. Leffert RD, Dorfman HD: Antecubital cyst in rheumatoid arthritis. Surgical findings. J Bone Joint Surg 54A:1555–1557, 1972

153. Lipscomb PR, Burleson RJ: Vascular and neural complications in supracondylar fractures of the humerus in children. J Bone Joint Surg 37A:487–492, 1955

154. Macon WL, Futrell JW: Median-nerve neuropathy after percutaneous puncture of the brachial artery in patients receiving anticoagulants. N Engl J Med 288:1396, 1973

155. Maeda K, Miura T, Komada T, Chiba A: Anterior interosseous nerve paralysis. Report of 13 cases and review of Japanese literatures. Hand 9:165–171, 1977

156. Mangani U: Flexor pollicis longus muscle. Its morphology and clinical significance. J Bone Joint Surg 42A:467–470, 1960

157. Mannerfelt L: Median nerve entrapment after dislocation of the elbow. Report of a case. J Bone Joint Surg 50B:152–155, 1968

158. Matev I: A radiological sign of entrapment of the median nerve in the elbow joint after posterior dislocation. J Bone Joint Surg 58B:353–355, 1976

159. McLellan DL, Swash M: Longitudinal sliding of the median nerve during movements of the upper limb. J Neurol Neurosurg Psychiatry 39:566, 1976

160. Mills RH, Mukherjee K, Bassett IB: Anterior interosseous nerve palsy. Br Med J 2:555, 1969

161. Mittal RL, Gupta BR: Median and ulnar nerve palsy: An unusual presentation of the supracondylar process. Report of a case. J Bone Joint Surg 60A:557–558, 1978

162. Morris HH, Peters BH: Pronator syndrome: Clinical and electrophysiological features in seven cases. J Neurol Neurosurg Psychiatry 39:461–464, 1976

163. Nakano KK, Lundergan C, Okihiro MM: Anterior interosseous nerve syndromes. Diagnostic methods and alternative treatments. Arch Neurol 34:477–480, 1977

164. Neundorf B, Kroger M: The anterior interosseous nerve syndrome. J Neurol 213:341, 1976

165. O'Brien MD, Upton ARM: Anterior interosseous nerve syndrome. A case report with neurophysiological investigation. J Neurol Neurosurg Psychiatry 35:531–536, 1972

166. Schmidt H, Eiken O: The anterior interosseous nerve syndrome. Scand J Plast Reconstr Surg 5:53–56, 1971

167. Seyffarth H: Primary myoses in the M. pronator teres as cause of lesion of the N. medianus (the pronator syndrome). Acta Psychiatr Neurol (suppl.) 74:251–254, 1951

168. Sharrard WJW: Anterior interosseous neuritis. Report of a case. J Bone Joint Surg 50B:804–805, 1968

169. Smith BH, Herbst BA: Anterior interosseous nerve palsy. Arch Neurol 30:330–331, 1974

170. Solnitzky O: Pronator syndrome: Compression neuropathy of the median nerve at level of prona-

tor teres muscle. Georgetown Med Bull 13:232–238, 1960

171. Spinner M: The functional attitude of the hand afflicted with an anterior interosseous nerve paralysis. Bull Hosp Joint Dis 30:21, 1969

172. Spinner M: The anterior interosseous-nerve syndrome. With special attention to its variation. J Bone Joint Surg 52A:84–94, 1970

173. Spinner M, Schreiber SN: The anterior interosseous-nerve paralysis as a complication of supracondylar fractures in children. J Bone Joint Surg 51A:1584–1590, 1969

174. Steiger RN, Larrick RB, Meyer TL: Median-nerve entrapment following elbow dislocation in children. J Bone Joint Surg 51A:381–385, 1969

175. Stern MB, Rosner LJ, Blinderman EE: Kiloh-Nevin syndrome. Clin Orthop 53:95–98, 1967

176. Stern PJ, Kutz JE: An unusual variant of the anterior interosseous nerve syndrome. J Hand Surg 5:32–34, 1980

177. Struthers J: Anatomical and Physiological Observations. Part I. Sutherland & Knox, Edinburgh, 1854

178. Thomas DF: Kiloh-Nevin syndrome. J Bone Joint Surg 44B:962, 1962

179. Thomsen PB: Processus supracondyloidea humeri with concomitant compression of the median nerve and the ulnar nerve. Acta Orthop Scand 48:391–393, 1977

180. Vichare NA: Spontaneous paralysis of the anterior interosseous nerve. J Bone Joint Surg 50B:806–808, 1968

181. Warren JD: Anterior interosseous nerve palsy as a complication of forearm fractures. J Bone Joint Surg 45B:511–512, 1963

182. Weins E, Lau SCK: The anterior interosseous nerve syndrome. Can J Surg 21:354, 1978

Carpal Tunnel Syndrome

183. Abbott LC, Saunders JB: Injuries of the median nerve in fractures of the lower end of the radius. Surg Gynecol Obstet 57:507, 1933

184. Aiache AE: An early sign of carpal tunnel syndrome. Plast Reconstr Surg 61:130, 1978

185. Amadio PC: Pyridoxine as an adjunct in the treatment of carpal tunnel syndrome. J Hand Surg 10A:237–241, 1985

186. Ariyan S, Watson HK: The palmar approach for the visualization and release of the carpal tunnel. An analysis of 429 cases. Plast Reconstr Surg 60:539–547, 1977

187. Arnold AG: The carpal tunnel syndrome in congestive cardiac failure. Postgrad Med J 53:623, 1977

188. Ashby BS: Hypertrophy of the palmaris longus muscle. J Bone Joint Surg 46B:230–232, 1964

189. Backhouse KM, Churchill-Davidson D: Anomalous palmaris longus muscle producing carpal tunnel-like compression. Hand 7:22, 1975

190. Bacorn RW, Kurtze JF: Colles fracture: A study of two thousand cases from the New York State Workmen's Compensation Board. J Bone Joint Surg 35A:643–658, 1953

191. Barfred T, Höjlund AP, Bertheussen K: Median artery in carpal tunnel syndrome. J Hand Surg 10A:864–867, 1985

192. Barfred T, Ipsen T: Congenital carpal tunnel syndrome. J Hand Surg 10A:246–248, 1985

193. Baruch A, Hass A: Anomaly of the median nerve (letter). J Hand Surg 2:331–332, 1977

194. Bendler EM, Greenspun B, Yu J, Erdman WJ: The bilaterality of carpal tunnel syndrome. Arch Phys Med Rehabil 58:362–364, 1977

195. Blodgett RC Jr, Lipscomb PR, Hill RW: Incidence of hematologic disease in patients with carpal tunnel syndrome. JAMA 182:814, 1962

196. Borgman MF: Carpal tunnel syndrome. Nurse Pract 3:21, 1978

197. Brain WR, Wright AD, Wilkerson M: Spontaneous compression of both median nerves in the carpal tunnel. Six cases treated surgically. Lancet 1:277, 1947

198. Brones MF, Wilgis EFS: Anatomical variations of the palmaris longus, causing carpal tunnel syndrome: Case reports. Plast Reconstr Surg 62:798–800, 1978

199. Brown EZ Jr, Snyder CC: Carpal tunnel syndrome caused by hand injuries. Plast Reconstr Surg 56:41–43, 1975

200. Buchthal F, Rosenfalck A: Sensory conduction from digit to palm and from palm to wrist in the carpal tunnel syndrome. J Neurol Neurosurg Psychiatry 34:243–252, 1971

201. Buchthal F, Rosenfalck A, Trojaborg W: Electrophysiological findings in entrapment of the median nerve at wrist and elbow. J Neurol Neurosurg Psychiatry 37:340, 1974

202. Butler B, Bigley EC: Aberrant index (first) lumbrical tendinous origin associated with carpal tunnel syndrome. A case report. J Bone Joint Surg 53A:160–162, 1971

203. Cannon BW, Love JB: Tardy median palsy: Median neuritis: Median thenar neuritis amenable to surgery. Surgery 20:210, 1946

204. Carroll RE, Green DP: The significance of the palmar cutaneous nerve at the wrist. Clin Orthop 83:24, 1972

205. Champion D: Gouty tenosynovitis and the carpal tunnel syndrome. Med J Aust 1:1030, 1969

206. Cherington M: Proximal pain in the carpal tunnel syndrome. Arch Surg 108:69, 1974

207. Crow RS: Treatment of the carpal-tunnel syndrome. Br Med J 1:1611–1615, 1960

208. Crymble B: Brachial neuralgia and carpal tunnel syndrome. Br Med J 3:470–471, 1968

209. Cseuz KA, Thomas JE, Lambert EH, Love JG, Lipscomb PR: Long-term results of operation for carpal tunnel syndrome. Mayo Clin Proc 41:232–241, 1966

210. Curtis RM, Eversmann WW: Internal neurolysis as an adjunct to the treatment of the carpal-tunnel syndrome. J Bone Joint Surg 55A:733–740, 1973

211. Das SK, Brown HG: In search of complications in carpal tunnel decompression. Hand 8:243–249, 1976

212. DeLuca FN, Cowen NJ: Median-nerve compression complicating a tendon graft prosthesis. J Bone Joint Surg 57A:553, 1975

213. Doll DC, Weiss RB: Unusual presentations of multiple myeloma. Postgrad Med 61:116–121, 1977

214. Eboh N, Wilson DH: Surgery of the carpal tunnel. Technical note. J Neurosurg 49:316–318, 1978

215. Eiken O, Carstram N, Eddeland A: Anomalous distal branching of the median nerve. Scand J Plast Reconstr Surg 5:149–152, 1971

216. Engber WD, Cmeiner JG: Palmar cutaneous branch of the ulnar nerve. J Hand Surg 5:26–29, 1980

217. Engel J, Zinneman H, Tsur H, Farin I: Carpal tunnel syndrome due to carpal osteophyte. Hand 10:283–284, 1978

218. Entin MA: Carpal tunnel syndrome and its variants. Surg Clin North Am 48:1097–1112, 1968

219. Eversmann WW Jr, Ritsick JA: Intraoperative changes in motor nerve conduction latency in carpal tunnel syndrome. J Hand Surg 3:77–81, 1978

220. Fissette J, Onkelinx A, Fandi N: Carpal and Guyon tunnel syndrome in burns at the wrist. J Hand Surg 6:13–15, 1981

221. Folkers K, Ellis J, Watanabe T, Saji S, Kaji M: Biochemical evidence for a deficiency of vitamin B6 in the carpal tunnel syndrome based on a crossover clinical study. Proc Natl Acad Sci USA 75:3410–3412, 1978

222. Folmar RC, Nelson CL, Phalen GS: Ruptures of the flexor tendons in hands of non-rheumatoid patients. J Bone Joint Surg 54:579–584, 1972

222a. Foster JB: Hydrocortisone and the carpal tunnel syndrome. Lancet 1:454–456, 1960

223. Freshwater MF, Arons MS: The effect of various adjuncts on the surgical treatment of carpal tunnel syndrome secondary to chronic tenosynovitis. Plast Reconstr Surg 61:93–96, 1978

224. Fullerton PM: The effect of ischaemia on nerve conduction in the carpal tunnel syndrome. J Neurol Neurosurg Psychiatry 26:385, 1963

225. Gainer JV Jr, Nugent GR: Carpal tunnel syndrome: Report of 430 operations. South Med J 70:325–328, 1977

226. Gardner RC: Confirmed case and diagnosis of pseudocarpal-tunnel (sublimis) syndrome. N Engl J Med 282:858, 1970

227. Gassmann N, Segmuller G, Stanisic M: Carpal tunnel syndrome. Indication, technique and results following epineural and interfascicular neurolysis. Handchirurgie 9:137, 1977

227a. Gelberman RH, Aronson D, Weisman MH: Carpal tunnel syndrome. Results of a prospective trial of steroid injection and splinting. J Bone Joint Surg 62A:1181–1184, 1980

228. Gilliatt RW, Wilson TG: A pneumatic tourniquet test in the carpal-tunnel syndrome. Lancet 2:595, 1953

229. Golding DN: Brachial neuralgia and the carpal tunnel syndrome. Br Med J 3:803, 1968

230. Goodman HV, Gilliatt RW: The effect of treatment on median nerve conduction in patients with the carpal-tunnel syndrome. Ann Phys Med 6:136, 1961

230a. Goodman HV, Foster JB: Effect of local corticosteroid injection on median nerve conduction in carpal tunnel syndrome. Ann Phys Med 6:287–294, 1962

231. Gould JS, Wissinger HA: Carpal tunnel syndrome in pregnancy. South Med J 71:144–145, 1978

232. Graham WP, III: Variations of the motor branch of the median nerve at the wrist. Plast Reconstr Surg 51:90–93, 1973

233. Green DP: Diagnostic and therapeutic value of carpal tunnel injection. J Hand Surg 9A:850–854, 1984

234. Green EJ, Dilworth JH, Levitin PM: Tophaceous gout. An unusual cause of bilateral carpal tunnel syndrome. JAMA 237:2747–2748, 1977

235. Grokoest AW, Demartini FE: Systemic disease and the carpal tunnel syndrome. JAMA 155:635, 1954

236. Grundberg AB: Carpal decompression in spite of normal electromyography. J Hand Surg 8:348–349, 1983

237. Gutmann L: Median-ulnar nerve communications and carpal tunnel syndrome. J Neurol Neurosurg Psychiatry 40:982–986, 1977

238. Guyon MA, Honet JC: Carpal tunnel syndrome or trigger finger associated with neck injury in auto-

mobile accidents. Arch Phys Med Rehabil 58:325–327, 1977

239. Harding AE, LeFanu J: Carpal tunnel syndrome related to antebrachial Cimino-Brescia fistula. J Neurol Neurosurg Psychiatry 40:511–513, 1977

240. Harris CM, Tanner E, Goldstein MN, Pettee DS: The surgical treatment of the carpal-tunnel syndrome correlated with preoperative nerve-conduction studies. J Bone Joint Surg 61A:93, 1979

241. Harrison MJ: Lack of evidence of generalized sensory neuropathy in patients with carpal tunnel syndrome. J Neurol Neurosurg Psychiatry 41:957–959, 1978

242. Hart VL, Gaynor V: Roentgenographic study of the carpal canal. J Bone Joint Surg 23:382–383, 1941

243. Hartwell SW Jr, Kurtay M: Carpal tunnel compression caused by hematoma associated with anticoagulant therapy. Report of a case. Cleve Clin Q 33:127, 1966

244. Hayden JW: Median neuropathy in the carpal tunnel caused by spontaneous intraneural hemorrhage. J Bone Joint Surg 46A:1242–1244, 1964

245. Helm PA, Johnson ER, Carlton AM: Peripheral neurological problems in the acute burn patient. Burn 3:123, 1977

246. Holtmann B, Anderson CB: Carpal tunnel syndrome following vascular shunts for hemodialysis. Arch Surg 112:65, 1977

247. Hongell A, Mattsson HS: Neurographic studies before, after, and during operation for median nerve compression in the carpal tunnel syndrome. Scand J Plast Reconstr Surg 5:103, 1971

248. Hunt CM, Abbott K, Robert WH: The median nerve and carpal tunnel syndrome historical features anatomical basis and clinical experiences. Bull Los Angeles Neurol Soc 25:211, 1960

249. Hunt JR: The neural atrophy of the muscles of the hand without sensory disturbances. A further study of compression neuritis of the thenar branch of the median nerve and the deep palmar branch of the ulnar nerve. Rev Neurol Psychiatry 12:137, 1914

250. Hunt WE, Luckey WT: The carpal tunnel syndrome. Diagnosis and treatment. J Neurosurg 21:178–181, 1964

251. Jabaley ME: Personal observations on the role of the lumbrical muscles in carpal tunnel syndrome. J Hand Surg 3:82–84, 1978

252. Jackson DW, Harkins PD: An aberrant muscle belly of the abductor digiti quinti associated with median nerve paresthesias. Bull Hosp Joint Dis 33:111–115, 1972

253. Johnson RK, Shrewbury MM: Anatomical course of thenar branch of the median nerve — usually in a separate tunnel through the transverse carpal ligament. J Bone Joint Surg 52A:269–273, 1970

254. Jones KG: Carpal tunnel syndrome. J Arkansas Med Soc 75:58, 1978

255. Kaplan H, Clayton M: Carpal tunnel syndrome secondary to *Mycobacterium kansasii* infection. JAMA 208:1186, 1969

256. Kemble F: Electrodiagnosis of the carpal tunnel syndrome. J Neurol Neurosurg Psychiatry 31:23, 1968

257. Kendall D: Non-penetrating injuries of the median nerve at the wrist. Brain 73:84, 1950

258. Kenzora JE: Dialysis carpal tunnel syndrome. Orthopedics 1:195, 1978

259. Kessler I: Unusual distribution of the median nerve at the wrist. A case report. Clin Orthop 67:124–126, 1969

260. Khunadorn N, Schlagenhauff RE, Tourbaf K, Papademetriou T: Carpal tunnel syndrome in hemophilia. NY State J Med 77:1314–1315, 1977

261. Klofkorn RW, Steigerwald JC: Carpal tunnel syndrome as the initial manifestation of tuberculosis. Am J Med 60:583, 1976

262. Koenigsberger MR, Moessinger AC: Iatrogenic carpal tunnel syndrome in the newborn infant. J Pediatr 91: 443–445, 1977

263. Kremer M, Gilliatt RW, Golding JSR, Wilson TG: Acroparesthesiae in the carpal-tunnel syndrome. Lancet 2:590, 1953

264. Kummel BM, Zazanis GA: Shoulder pain as the presenting complaint in carpal tunnel syndrome. Clin Orthop 92:227–230, 1973

265. Langloh ND, Linscheid RL: Recurrent and unrelieved carpal tunnel syndrome. Clin Orthop 83:41–47, 1972

266. Lanz U: Anatomical variations of the median nerve in the carpal tunnel. J Hand Surg 2:44–53, 1977

267. Layton KB: Acroparesthesia in pregnancy and the carpal tunnel syndrome. Obstet Gynecol 65:823, 1958

268. Lazaro L III: Carpal-tunnel syndrome from an insect sting. J Bone Joint Surg 54A:1095–1096, 1972

269. Leach RE, Odom JA: Systemic causes of the carpal tunnel syndrome. Postgrad Med 44:127–131, 1968

270. Lettin AWF: Carpal tunnel syndrome in childhood. J Bone Joint Surg 47B:556–559, 1965

271. Levy M, Pauker M: Carpal tunnel syndrome due to thrombosed persisting median artery. A case report. Hand 10:65–68, 1978

272. Linburg RM, Albright JA: An anomalous branch of the median nerve. A case report. J Bone Joint Surg 52A:182–183, 1970

273. Linscheid RL, Peterson LFA, Juergens JL: Carpal tunnel syndrome associated with vasospasm. J Bone Joint Surg 49A:1141–1146, 1967

274. Lipscomb PR: Tenosynovitis of the hand and the wrist: Carpal tunnel syndrome, de Quervain's disease, trigger digit. Clin Orthop 13:164–181, 1959

275. Loong SC, Seah SC: Comparison of median and ulnar sensory nerve action potentials in the diagnosis of the carpal tunnel syndrome. J Neurol Neurosurg Psychiatry 34:750, 1971

276. Loong SC: The carpal tunnel syndrome: A clinical and electrophysiological study of 250 patients. Proc Aust Assoc Neurol 14:51, 1977

277. Love JG: Median neuritis; carpal tunnel syndrome; diagnosis and treatment. NC Med J 16:463, 1955

278. Mainland D: An uncommon abnormality of the flexor digitorum sublimus muscle. J Anat 62:86–89, 1927

278a. Mackinnon SE, Dellon AL: An experimental study of treatment methods of chronic nerve compression. Proceedings of the American Society for Surgery of the Hand. J Hand Surg 11A:759, 1986

279. Mangani U: Carpal-tunnel syndrome. Proceedings of the American Society for Surgery of the Hand. J Bone Joint Surg 44A:1036, 1962

280. Mannerfelt L, Hybbinette CH: Important anomaly of the thenar branch of the median nerve. Bull Hosp Joint Dis 33:15–21, 1972

281. Mannerfelt L, Normal O: Attritional ruptures of flexor tendons in rheumatoid arthritis caused by bony spurs in the carpal tunnel. J Bone Joint Surg 51B:270–277, 1969

282. Manske PR: Fracture of the hook of the hamate presenting as carpal tunnel syndrome. Hand 10:181, 1978

283. Marie et Foix P: Atrophie isolé de l'éminence thènar d'origine nevritiqué. Role du ligament annulaire antér ieur de carpe dans la pathogènie de la lèsion. Rev Neurol 26:647, 1913

284. Marinacci AA: Comparative value of measurement of nerve conduction velocity and electromyography in diagnosis of carpal tunnel syndrome. Arch Phys Med Rehabil 45:548, 1964

285. Massey EW: Carpal tunnel syndrome in pregnancy. Obstet Gynecol Surg 33:145, 1978

286. Massey EW, O'Brian JT, Georges LB: Carpal tunnel syndrome secondary to carpopedal spasm. Ann Intern Med 88:804–805, 1978

287. Maxwell JA, Keyes JJ, Ketchem LD: Acute carpal tunnel syndrome secondary to thrombosis of a persistent median artery. J Neurosurg 38:774, 1973

288. Mayers LB: Carpal tunnel syndrome secondary to tuberculosis. Arch Neurol 10:426, 1964

289. MacDonald RI, Lichtman DM, Hanlon JJ, Wilson JN: Complications of surgical release for carpal tunnel syndrome. J Hand Surg 3:70–76, 1978

290. MacDougal B, Weeks PM, Wray RC Jr: Median nerve compression and trigger finger in the mucopolysaccharidoses and related diseases. Plast Reconstr Surg 59:260–263, 1977

291. McClain EJ, Wissinger HA: The acute carpal tunnel syndrome: Nine case reports. J Trauma 16:75–78, 1976

292. McCormack RM: Carpal-tunnel syndrome. Surg Clin North Am 40:517, 1960

293. Meadoff N: Median nerve injuries in fractures in the region of the wrist. Calif Med 70:252–256, 1949

294. Melvin JL, Schuckmann JA, Lanese RR: Diagnostic specificity of motor and sensory nerve conduction variables in the carpal tunnel syndrome. Arch Phys Med Rehabil 54:69, 1973

295. Michaelis LS: Stenosis of carpal tunnel, compression of median nerve, and flexor tendon sheaths, combines with rheumatoid arthritis elsewhere. Proc R Soc Med 43:414, 1950

296. Moffat JH: Traumatic neuritis of the deep palmar branch of the ulnar nerve. Can Med Assoc J 91:230–231, 1964

297. Muller LH: Anatomical abnormalities of the wrist joint causing neurological symptoms in the hand. J Bone Joint Surg 45B:431, 1963

298. Newman PH: Median nerve compression in the carpal tunnel. Postgrad Med J 24:264, 1948

299. Nissen KI: Etiology of carpal tunnel compression of the median nerve. Proceedings of the Joint Meeting of the Orthopaedic Associations of the English-Speaking World. J Bone Joint Surg 34B:514, 1952

300. Nissenbaum M, Kleinert HE: Treatment considerations in carpal tunnel syndrome with co-existing Dupuytren's disease. J Hand Surg 5:544–547, 1980

301. Ocker K, Seitz HD: A rare anatomical condition causing carpal tunnel syndrome. Handchirurgie 9:25, 1977

302. Ogden JA: An unusual branch of the median nerve. J Bone Joint Surg 54A:1779–1781, 1972

303. O'Hara LJ, Levin M: Carpal tunnel syndrome and gout. Arch Intern Med 120:180, 1967

304. Paine KWE: The carpal-tunnel syndrome. Can J Surg 6:446, 1963

305. Papathanassiou BT: A variant of the motor branch of the median nerve in the hand. J Bone Joint Surg 50B:156–157, 1968

306. Patrick J: Carpal-tunnel syndrome. Br Med J 1:1377, 1965

307. Phalen GS: Spontaneous compression of the me-

dian nerve at the wrist. JAMA 145:1128, 1951

308. Phalen GS: The carpal-tunnel syndrome: Seventeen years' experience in diagnosis and treatment of six hundred fifty-four hands. J Bone Joint Surg 48A:211–228, 1966

309. Phalen GS: Reflections on 21 years' experience with the carpal tunnel syndrome. JAMA 212:1365–1367, 1970

310. Phalen GS: The carpal tunnel syndrome. Clinical evaluation of 598 hands. Clin Orthop 83:29–40, 1972

311. Phalen GS, Gardner WJ, LaLonde AA: Neuropathy of the median nerve due to compression beneath the transverse carpal ligament. J Bone Joint Surg 32A:109–112, 1950

312. Phalen GS, Kendrick JI: Compression neuropathy of median nerve in carpal tunnel. JAMA 164:524, 1957

313. Phillips RS: Carpal tunnel syndrome as manifestation of systemic disease. Ann Rheum Dis 26:59, 1967

314. Posch JL, Marcotte DR: Carpal tunnel syndrome. An analysis of 1201 cases. Orthop Rev 5:25, 1976

315. Purnell DC, Daly DD, Lipscomb PR: Carpal-tunnel syndrome associated with myxedema. Arch Int Med 108:751, 1961

316. Richier HP, Thoden U: Early electroneurographic diagnosis of carpal tunnel syndrome. EEG EMG 8:187, 1977

317. Rietz KA, Onne L: Analysis of sixty-five operated cases of carpal-tunnel syndrome. Acta Chir Scand 133:443, 1967

318. Robbins H: Anatomical study of the medial nerve in the carpal tunnel and etiologies of the carpal tunnel syndrome. J Bone Joint Surg 45A:953–966, 1963

319. Sabour MS, Fadel HE: The carpal tunnel syndrome—A new complication ascribed to the "Pill." Am J Obstet Gynecol 107:1265, 1970

320. Schiller F, Kolb FO: Carpal tunnel syndrome in acromegaly. Neurology 4:371, 1954

321. Schmitt O, Temme C: Carpal tunnel syndrome in developing pseudarthrosis following isolated fracture of os capitatum. Arch Orthop Trauma Surg 93:25, 1978

322. Schorn D, Hoskinson J, Dickson RA: Bone density and the carpal tunnel syndrome. Hand 10:184–186, 1978

323. Schultz RJ, Endler PM, Huddleston HD: Anomalous median nerve and an anomalous muscle belly of the first lumbrical associated with carpal-tunnel syndrome. J Bone Joint Surg 55A:1744–1746, 1973

324. Silver MA, Gelberman RH, Gellman H, Rhoades CE: Carpal tunnel syndrome: Associated abnormalities in ulnar nerve function and the effect of carpal tunnel release on these abnormalities. J Hand Surg 10A:710–713, 1985

325. Simpson JA: Electrical signs in the diagnosis of carpal tunnel and related syndromes. J Neurol Neurosurg Psychiatry 19:275, 1956

326. Smith EM, Sonstegard DA, Anderson WH Jr: Carpal tunnel syndrome: Contribution of flexor tendons. Arch Phys Med Rehabil 58:379–385, 1977

327. Smukler NM, Patterson JR, Lorenz H, Weiner L: The incidence of the carpal tunnel syndrome in patients with rheumatoid arthritis. Arthritis Rheum 6:298, 1963

328. Spindler HA, Dellon AL: Nerve conduction studies and sensibility testing in carpal tunnel syndrome. J Hand Surg 7:260–263, 1982

329. Starreveld E, Ashenhurst EM: Bilateral carpal tunnel syndrome in childhood. Neurology 25:234, 1975

330. Stein AH Jr: The relation of median nerve compression to Sudeck's syndrome. Surg Gynecol Obstet 115:713–720, 1962

331. Stellbrink G: Compression of the palmar branch of the median nerve by atypical palmaris longus muscle. Handchirurgie 4:155–157, 1972

332. Stephens J, Welch K: Acroparesthesia, a symptom of median nerve compression at the wrist. Arch Surg 73:849, 1956

333. Sterling AP, Eshraghi A, Anderson WV, Habermann ET: Acute carpal tunnel syndrome secondary to a foreign body in the median nerve. Bull Hosp Joint Dis 33:130–134, 1972

334. Stewart JD, Eisen A: Tinel's sign and the carpal tunnel syndrome. Br Med J 2:1125–1126, 1978

335. Stratton CW, Phelps DB, Reller LB: Tuberculoid tenosynovitis and carpal tunnel syndrome caused by mycrobacterium szulgai. Am J Med 65:349–351, 1978

336. Sunderland S: The nerve lesion in the carpal tunnel syndrome. J Neurol Neurosurg Psychiatry 39:615–626, 1976

337. Sutro CJ: Carpal tunnel syndrome caused by calcification in the deep or volar radio-carpal ligament. Bull Hosp Joint Dis, 30:23, 1969

338. Taleisnik J: The palmar cutaneous branch of the median nerve and the approach to the carpal tunnel. An anatomical study. J Bone Joint Surg 55A:1212–1217, 1973

339. Tanzer RC: The carpal-tunnel syndrome. A clinical

and anatomical study. J Bone Joint Surg 41A:626–634, 1959

340. Thomas JE, Lambert EH, Cseuz KA: Electrodiagnostic aspects of the carpal tunnel syndrome. Arch Neurol 16:635, 1967

341. Thomas PK: Motor nerve conduction in the carpal tunnel syndrome. Neurology 10:1045, 1960

342. Thomas PK, Fullerton PM: Nerve fibre size in the carpal tunnel syndrome. J Neurol Neurosurg Psychiatry 26:520, 1964

343. Tomkins DG: Median neuropathy in the carpal tunnel caused by tumor-like conditions. J Bone Joint Surg 49A:737–740, 1957

344. Vichare NA: Anomalous muscle belly of the flexor digitorum superficialis. J Bone Joint Surg 52B:757–759, 1970

345. Wainapel SF: Carpal tunnel syndrome (letter). Arch Phys Med Rehabil 59:43, 1978

346. Wallace TJ, Cook AW: Carpal tunnel syndrome in pregnancy. Am J Obstet Gynecol 73:1333, 1957

347. Ward LE, Bicker WH, Corbin KB: Median neuritis (carpal tunnel syndrome) caused by gouty tophi. JAMA 167:844, 1958

348. Warren DJ, Otieno LS: Carpal tunnel syndrome in patients on intermittent haemodialysis. Postgrad Med J 51:450, 1975

349. Watson-Jones R: Léri's pleonosteosis, carpal tunnel compression of the median nerve and Morton's metatarsalgia. J Bone Joint Surg 31B:560–571, 1949

350. Werschkul JD: Anomalous course of the recurrent motor branch of the median nerve in a patient with carpal tunnel syndrome. J Neurosurg 47:113–114, 1977

351. Wesser DR, Calostypis F, Hoffman S: The evolutionary significance of an aberrant flexor superficialis muscle in the human palm. J Bone Joint Surg 51A:396–398, 1969

352. Wilson JN: Profiles of the carpal canal. J Bone Joint Surg 36A:127–132, 1954

353. Winkelman NZ, Spinner M: A variant high sensory branch of the median nerve to the third web space. Bull Hosp Joint Dis 34:161–166, 1973

354. Woltman HW: Neuritis associated with acromegaly. Arch Neurol Psychiatry 45:680, 1941

354a. Wood MR: Hydrocortisone injections for carpal tunnel syndrome. Hand 12:62–64, 1980

355. Yamaguchi DM, Lipscomb PR, Soule EH: Carpal-tunnel syndrome. Minn Med 48:22, 1965

356. Zachary RB: Thenar palsy due to compression of the median nerve in the carpal tunnel. Surg Gynecol Obstet 81:213, 1945

Cubital Tunnel Syndrome

357. Adson AW: The surgical treatment of progressive ulnar paralysis. Coll Paper Mayo Clin 10:944, 1918

358. Adson AW: Progressive ulnar paralysis. Minn Med 1:455, 1918

359. Apfelberg DB, Larson SJ: Dynamic anatomy of the ulnar nerve at the elbow. Plast Recontr Surg 51:76–81, 1973

360. Arkin AM: Habitual luxation of the ulnar nerve. J Mt Sinai Hosp 7:208, 1940

361. Broudy AS, Leffert RD, Smith RJ: Technical problems with ulnar nerve transposition at the elbow: Findings and results of reoperation. J Hand Surg 3:85–89, 1978

362. Bryan RS, Lipscomb PR, Svien HJ: Tardy paralysis of the ulnar nerve due to a cyst of the elbow: Report of case. Proc Staff Meeting Mayo Clin 31:473, 1956

363. Burman MA, Sutro CJ: Recurrent luxation of the ulnar nerve by congenital posterior position of the medial epicondyle of the humerus. J Bone Joint Surg 21:958, 1939

364. Campbell JB, Post KD, Morantz RA: A technique for relief of motor and sensory deficits occurring after anterior ulnar transposition. J Neurosurg 40:405–409, 1974

365. Carr JA: Spontaneous ulnar nerve paresis. Br Med J 2:1415, 1957

366. Childress HM: Recurrent ulnar-nerve dislocation at the elbow. J Bone Joint Surg 38A:978–984, 1956

367. Childress HM: Recurrent ulnar-nerve dislocation at the elbow. Clin Orthop 108:168, 1975

368. Clark CB: Compression of the ulnar nerve. Orthop Rev 6:33–38, 1977

369. Clark CB: Cubital tunnel syndrome. JAMA 241:801–802, 1979

370. Craven PR, Green DP: Cubital tunnel syndrome. Treatment by medial epicondylectomy. J Bone Joint Surg 62A:986–989, 1980

371. Curtis BF: Traumatic ulnar neuritis: Transplantation of the nerve. J Nerv Ment Dis 25:480, 1898

372. Ekerot L: Postanesthetic ulnar neuropathy at the elbow. Scand J Plast Reconstr Surg 11:225–229, 1977

373. Farquhar-Buzzard E: Some varieties of traumatic and toxic ulnar neuritis. Lancet 1:317, 1922

374. Feindel W, Stratford J: The role of the cubital tunnel in tardy ulnar palsy. Can J Surg 1:287–300, 1958

375. Feindel W, Stratford J: Cubital tunnel compression

in tardy ulnar palsy. Can Med Assoc J 78:351–353, 1958

376. Foster RJ, Edshage S: Factors related to the outcome of surgically managed compressive neuropathy at the elbow level. J Hand Surg 6:181–192, 1981

377. Fragiadakis EG, Lamb DW: An unusual cause of ulnar nerve compression. Hand 2:14–16, 1970

378. Froimson AI, Zahrawi F: Treatment of compression neuropathy of the ulnar nerve at the elbow by epicondylectomy and neurolysis. J Hand Surg 5:391–395, 1980

379. Gay JR, Love JG: Diagnosis and treatment of tardy paralysis of the ulnar nerve. Based on a study of 100 cases. J Bone Joint Surg 29:1087–1097, 1947

380. Gilliatt RW, Thomas PK: Changes in nerve conduction with ulnar nerve lesions at the elbow. J Neurol Neurosurg Psychiatry 23:312–320, 1960

381. Gurdjian ES: Traumatic ulnar neuritis due to strapping of the elbow and the forearm to the operating table. JAMA 96:944, 1931

382. Hagstrom P: Ulnar nerve compression at the elbow. Results of surgery in 85 cases. Scand J Plast Reconstr Surg 11:59–62, 1977

383. Hirasawa Y, Sawamaura H, Sakakida K: Entrapment neuropathy due to bilateral epitrochleoanconeus muscles: A case report. J Hand Surg 4:181–184, 1979

384. Ho KC, Marmor L: Entrapment of the ulnar nerve at the elbow. Am J Surg 121:355, 1971

385. Hunt JR: Tardy or late paralysis of the ulnar nerve. A form of chronic progressive neuritis developing many years after fracture dislocation of the elbow joint. JAMA 66:11–15, 1916

386. James GGH: Nerve lesions about the elbow. J Bone Joint Surg 38B:589, 1956

387. Jones RE, Gauntt C: Median epicondylectomy for ulnar nerve compression syndrome at the elbow. Clin Orthop 139:174–178, 1979

388. Kincaid JC, Phillips LH, Daube JR: The evaluation of suspected ulnar neuropathy at the elbow. Arch Neurol 43:44–47, 1986

389. King T, Morgan FP: The treatment of traumatic ulnar neuritis. Mobilization of the ulnar nerve at the elbow by removal of the medial epicondyle and adjacent bone. Aust NZ J Surg 20:33–45, 1950

390. King T, Morgan FP: Late results of removing the medial humeral epicondyle for traumatic ulnar neuritis. J Bone Joint Surg (Br) 41B:51–55, 1959

391. Kumar K: Surgical management of leprous ulnar neuritis. Clin Orthop 163:235–242, 1982

392. Kurlan R, Baker P, Miller C, Shoulson E: Severe compression neuropathy following sudden onset of Parkinsonian immobility. Arch Neurol 42:720, 1985

393. Learmonth JR: A technique for transplanting the ulnar nerve. Surg Gynecol Obstet 75:792–793, 1942

394. Leffert RD: Anterior submuscular transposition of the ulnar nerves by the Learmonth technique. J Hand Surg 7:147–155, 1982

395. Lluch AL: Ulnar nerve entrapment after anterior transposition at elbow. NY State J Med 1:75–76, 1975

396. Magee RB, Phalen GS: Tardy ulnar palsy. Am J Surg 78:470, 1949

397. Mass DP, Silverberg B: Cubital tunnel syndrome: Anterior transposition with epicondylar osteotomy. Orthopedics 9:711–715, 1986

398. McGowan AJ: The results of transposition of the ulnar nerve for traumatic ulnar neuritis. J Bone Joint Surg 32B:293–301, 1950

399. Murakami Y, Komiyama Y: Hypoplasia of the trochlea and the medial epicondyle of the humerus associated with ulnar neuropathy. J Bone Joint Surg 60B:225–227, 1978

400. Neblett C, Ehni G: Medial epicondylectomy for ulnar palsy. J Neurosurg 32:55–62, 1970

401. Osborne G: The surgical treatment of tardy ulnar neuritis. J Bone Joint Surg 39B:782, 1957

402. Osborne GV: Ulnar neuritis. Postgrad Med J 35:392, 1959

403. Osborne GV: Compression neuritis of the ulnar nerve at the elbow. Hand 2:10–16, 1970

404. Panas J: Sur une cause peu connue de paralysie du nerf cubital. Arch Generales che Med 2:5, 1878

405. Pechan J, Julis I: The pressure measurement in the ulnar nerve. A contribution to the pathophysiology of the cubital tunnel syndrome. J Biomech 8:75, 1975

406. Platt H: The pathogenesis and treatment of traumatic neuritis of the ulnar nerve in the postcondylar groove. Br J Surg 13:409–431, 1926

407. Reis ND: Anomalous triceps tendon as a cause for snapping elbow and ulnar neuritis: A case report. J Hand Surg 5:361–362, 1980

408. Richards RL: Traumatic ulnar neuritis. The results of anterior transposition of the ulnar nerve. Edinburgh Med J 52:14–21, 1945

409. Rolfsen L: Snapping triceps tendon with ulnar neuritis. Acta Orthop Scand 41:74–76, 1970

410. Sherren J: Remarks on chronic neuritis of the ulnar nerve due to deformity in the region of the elbow joint. Edinburgh Med J 23:500, 1908

411. Skillern PG Jr: Surgical lesions of the ulnar nerve at the elbow. Surg Clin North Am 2:251, 1922

412. Spinner M, Kaplan EB: The relationship of the ulnar nerve to the medial intermuscular septum in the arm and its clinical significance. Hand 8:239–242, 1976

413. Thomsen PB: Compression neuritis of the ulnar nerve treated with simple decompression. Acta Orthop Scand 48:164–167, 1977

414. Vanderpool DW, Chalmers J, Lamb DW, Whiston TB: Peripheral compression lesions of the ulnar nerve. J Bone Joint Surg 50B:792–803, 1968

415. Wadsworth TG: The cubital tunnel and the external compression syndrome. Anesth Analg 53:303–308, 1974

416. Wadsworth TG: The external compression syndrome of the ulnar nerve at the cubital tunnel. Clin Orthop 124:189–204, 1977

417. Wadsworth TG, Williams JR: Cubital tunnel external compression syndrome. Br Med J 1:662, 1973

418. Wadsworth TG, Williams RM: The cubital tunnel external compression syndrome. Nurs Times 73:1357–1359, 1977

419. Wartenberg R: A sign of ulnar nerve palsy. JAMA 112:1688, 1939

420. Wilson DH, Krout R: Surgery of ulnar neuropathy at the elbow: 16 cases treated by decompression without transportation. Technical note. J Neurosurg 38:780–785, 1973

Ulnar Tunnel Syndrome (at the Wrist)

421. Bakke JL, Wolff HG: Occupational pressure neuritis of the deep palmar branch of the ulnar nerve. Arch Neurol Psychiatry 60:549–553, 1948

422. Blunden R: Neuritis of deep branch of the ulnar nerve. J Bone Joint Surg 40B:354, 1958

423. Brooks DM: Traumatic ulnar neuritis (Editorial). J Bone Joint Surg 32B:291–292, 1950

424. Comtet JJ, Quicot L, Moyen B: Compression of the deep palmar branch of the ulnar nerve by the arch of the adductor pollicis. Hand 10:176–180, 1978

425. Denman EE: An unusual branch of the ulnar nerve in the hand. Hand 9:92–97, 1977

426. Denman EE: The anatomy of the space of Guyon. Hand 10:69–76, 1978

427. Dupont C, Cloutier GE, Prevost Y, Dion MA: Ulnar-tunnel syndrome at the wrist. A report of four cases of ulnar-nerve compression at the wrist. J Bone Joint Surg 47A:757–761, 1965

428. Eckman PB, Perlstein G, Altrocchi PH: Ulnar neuropathy in bicycle riders. Arch Neurol 32:130–131, 1975

429. Fenning JB: Deep ulnar-nerve paralysis resulting from an anatomical abnormality. A case report. J Bone Joint Surg 47A:1381–1385, 1965

430. Fissette J, Onkelinx A, Fandi N: Carpal and Guyon tunnel syndrome in burns at the wrist. J Hand Surg 6:13–15, 1981

431. Freundlich BD, Spinner M: Nerve compression syndrome in derangements of the proximal and distal radioulnar joints. Bull Hosp Joint Dis 19:38–47, 1968

432. Gore DR: Carpometacarpal dislocation producing compression of the deep branch of the ulnar nerve. J Bone Joint Surg 53A:1387–1390, 1971

433. Greene MH, Hadied AM: Bipartate hamulus with ulnar tunnel syndrome—Case report and literature review. J Hand Surg 6:605–609, 1981

434. Guyon F: Note sur une disposition anatomique proper á la face antérieure de la région du poignet et non encores décrite par la docteur. Bull Soc Anat Paris, 2nd series 36:184–186, 1861

435. Harrelson JM, Newman M: Hypertrophy of the flexor carpi ulnaris as a cause of ulnar-nerve compression in the distal part of the forearm. Case report. J Bone Joint Surg 57A:554–555, 1975

436. Harris W: Occupational pressure neuritis of the deep palmar branch of the ulnar nerve. Br Med J 1:98, 1929

437. Hayes CW: Ulnar tunnel syndrome from giant cell tumor of tendon sheath: A case report. J Hand Surg 3:187–188, 1978

438. Hayes JR, Mulholland RC, O'Connor BT: Compression of the deep palmar branch of the ulnar nerve. J Bone Joint Surg 51B:469–472, 1969

439. Howard FM: Ulnar nerve palsy in wrist fractures. J Bone Joint Surg 43A:1197–1201, 1961

440. Hunt JR: Occupation neuritis of the deep palmar branch of the ulnar nerve. A well defined clinical type of professional palsy of the hand. J Nerv Ment Dis 35:673–689, 1908

441. Hunt JR: The neural atrophy of the muscles of the hand without sensory disturbances. A further study of compression neuritis of the thenar branch of the median nerve and the deep palmar branch of the ulnar nerve. Rev Neurol Psychiatry 12:137, 1914

442. Jeffery AK: Compression of the deep palmar branch of the ulnar nerve by an anomalous muscle. J Bone Joint Surg 53B:718–723, 1971

443. Kalisman M, Laborde K, Wolff TW: Ulnar nerve compression secondary to ulnar artery false aneurysm at the Guyon's canal. J Hand Surg 7:137–139, 1982

444. Kaplan EB: Variation of the ulnar nerve at the wrist. Bull Hosp Joint Dis 24:85–88, 1963

445. Kleinert HE, Hayes JR: The ulnar tunnel syndrome. Plast Reconstr Surg 47:21–24, 1971

446. Lamb D: Ulnar nerve compression lesions at the wrist and hand. Hand 2:17–18, 1970

447. Lassa R, Shrewbury MM: A variation in the path of the deep motor branch of the ulnar nerve at the wrist. J Bone Joint Surg 57:990–991, 1975

448. Lipscomb PR: Duplication of hypothenar muscles simulating soft-tissue tumor of the hand. J Bone Joint Surg 42A:1058–1061, 1960

449. Magee KR: Neuritis of the deep palmar branch of ulnar nerve. Arch Neurol Psychiatry 73:200–202, 1955

450. Mallet BL, Zilkha KJ: Compression of the ulnar nerve at the wrist by a ganglion. Lancet 1:890, 1955

451. Mannerfelt L: Studies on the hand in ulnar nerve paralysis. A clinical-experimental investigation in normal and anomalous innervation. Acta Orthop Scand (suppl.) 87:1966

452. McDowell CL, Henceroth WD: Compression of the ulnar nerve in the hand by a ganglion. Report of a case. J Bone Joint Surg 59A:980, 1977

453. McFarland GB, Hoffer MM: Paralysis of the intrinsic muscles of the hand secondary to lipoma in Guyon's canal. J Bone Joint Surg 53A:375–376, 1971

454. McFarlane RM, Mayer JR, Hugill JV: Further observations on the anatomy of the ulnar nerve at the wrist. Hand 8:115–117, 1976

455. Muller LH: Anatomical abnormalities of the wrist joint causing neurological symptoms in the hand. J Bone Joint Surg 45B:431, 1963

456. Poppi M, Padovani R, Martinelli P, Pozzati E: Fractures of the distal radius with ulnar nerve palsy. J Trauma 18:278–279, 1978

457. Richmond DA: Carpal ganglion with ulnar nerve compression. J Bone Joint Surg 45B:513–515, 1963

458. Russell WR, Whitty CWM: Traumatic neuritis of the deep palmar branch of the ulnar nerve. Lancet 1:828–829, 1947

459. Salgebac S: Ulnar tunnel syndrome caused by anomalous muscles. Case report. Scand J Plast Reconstr Surg 11:255–258, 1977

460. Schjelderup H: Aberrant muscle in the hand causing ulnar nerve compression. J Bone Joint Surg 46B:361, 1964

461. Sedal L, McLeod JG, Walsh JC: Ulnar nerve lesions associated with carpal tunnel syndrome. J Neurol Neurosurg Psychiatry 36:118, 1973

462. Seddon HJ: Carpal ganglion as a cause of paralysis of the deep branch of the ulnar nerve. J Bone Joint Surg 34B:386–390, 1952

463. Shea JD, McClain EJ: Ulnar nerve compression syndromes at and below the wrist. J Bone Joint Surg 51A:1095–1103, 1969

464. Smith RJ: Ulnar nerve compression secondary to ulnar artery false aneurysm at Guyon's canal (letter to the editor). J Hand Surg 7:631–632, 1982

465. Stein AH Jr, Morgan HC: Compression of the ulnar nerve at the level of the wrist. Am Prac 13:195–198, 1962

466. Swanson AB, Biddulph SL, Baughman FA, DeGroot G: Ulnar nerve compression due to an anomalous muscle in the canal of Guyon. Clin Orthop 83:64–69, 1972

467. Taylor AR: Ulnar nerve compression at the wrist in rheumatoid arthritis. J Bone Joint Surg 56B:142–143, 1974

468. Tonkin MA, Lister GD: The palmar brevis profundus. An anomalous muscle associated with ulnar nerve compression at the wrist. J Hand Surg 10A:862–864, 1985

469. Toshima Y, Kimata Y: A case of ganglion causing paralysis of intrinsic muscles innervated by the ulnar nerve. J Bone Joint Surg 43A:153, 1961

470. Turner MS, Caird DM: Anomalous muscles and ulnar nerve compression at the wrist. Hand 9:140–142, 1977

471. Uriburu IJF, Morchio FJ, Marin JC: Compression syndrome of the deep branch of the ulnar nerve. (Piso-hamate hiatus syndrome). J Bone Joint Surg 58A:145–147, 1976

472. Vance RM, Gelberman RH: Acute ulnar neuropathy with fractures at the wrist. J Bone Joint Surg 60A:962–965, 1978

473. Vanderpool DW, Chalmers J, Lamb DW, Whiston TB: Peripheral compression lesions of the ulnar nerve. J Bone Joint Surg 50B:792–803, 1968

474. Worster-Drought C: Pressure neuritis of the deep palmar branch of the ulnar nerve. Br Med J 1:247, 1929

475. Zoega H: Fracture of the lower end of the radius with ulnar nerve palsy. J Bone Joint Surg 48B:514–516, 1966

Radial Nerve Compression Syndromes

476. Austin R: Tardy palsy of the radial nerve from a Monteggia fracture. Injury 7:202–204, 1976

477. Barton NJ: Radial nerve lesions. Hand 5:200–208, 1973

478. Blakemore ME: Posterior interosseous nerve paralysis caused by a lipoma. J R Coll Surg Edinb 24:113, 1979

479. Bowen TL, Stone KH: Posterior interosseous nerve

paralysis caused by a ganglion at the elbow. J Bone Joint Surg 48B:774–776, 1966

480. Bryan FS, Miller LS, Panijayanond P: Spontaneous paralysis of the posterior interosseous nerve: A case report and review of the literature. Clin Orthop 80:9–12, 1971

481. Campbell CS, Wulf RF: Lipoma producing a lesion of the deep branch of the radial nerve. J Neurosurg 11:310–311, 1954

482. Capener N: Tennis elbow and posterior interosseous nerve. Br Med J 2:130, 1960

483. Capener N: Posterior interosseous nerve lesions. Proceedings of the Second Hand Club. J Bone Joint Surg 46B:361, 1964

484. Capener N: The vulnerability of the posterior interosseous nerve of the forearm. A case report and anatomical study. J Bone Joint Surg 48B:770–773, 1966

485. Davies F, Laird M: The supinator muscle and the deep radial (posterior interosseous) nerve. Anat Rec 101:243–250, 1948

485a. Dellon AL, Mackinnon SE: Radial sensory nerve entrapment in the forearm. J Hand Surg 11A:199–205, 1986

486. Dharapak C, Nimberg GA: Posterior interosseous nerve compression. Report of a case caused by traumatic aneurysm. Clin Orthop 101:225–228, 1974

486a. Ehrlich W, Dellon AL, Mackinnon SE: Cheiralgia paresthetica (entrapment of the radial sensory nerve). J Hand Surg 11A:196–199, 1986

487. Garcia A, Maeck BH: Radial nerve injuries in fractures of the shaft of the humerus. Am J Surg 99:625, 1960

488. Gassel MM, Diamantopoulos E: Pattern of conduction times in the distribution of the radial nerve. Neurology 14:222–231, 1964

489. Goldman S, Honet JC, Sobel R, Goldstein AS: Posterior interosseous-nerve palsy in the absence of trauma. Arch Neurol 21:435–441, 1969

490. Hagert CG: Lundborg G, Hansen T: Entrapment of the posterior interosseous nerve. Scand J Plast Reconstr Surg 11:205, 1977

491. Hobhouse N, Heald CB: A case of posterior interosseous paralysis. Br Med J 1:841, 1936

492. Hustead A, Mulder D, MacCarty C: Nontreatment progressive paralysis of the deep radial (posterior interosseous) nerve. Arch Neurol Psychiatry 79:269, 1958

493. Jebsen RH: Motor conduction velocity of distal radial nerve. Arch Phys Med Rehabil 47:12–16, 1966

494. Kruse F Jr: Paralysis of the dorsal interosseous nerve not due to direct trauma. A case showing spontaneous recovery. Neurology 8:307–308, 1958

495. Learmonth JR: A variation in the distribution of the radial branch of the musculo-spiral nerve. J Anat 53:371–372, 1919

496. Lichter RL, Jacobsen T: Tardy palsy of the posterior interosseous nerve with a Monteggia fracture. J Bone Joint Surg 57A:124–125, 1975

497. Linscheid RL: Injuries to radial nerve at wrist. Arch Surg 91:942–946, 1965

498. Lister GD, Belsole RB, Kleinert HE: The radial tunnel syndrome. J Hand Surg 4:52–59, 1979

499. Lotem M, Fried A, Levy M, Solzi P, Najenson T, Nathan H: Radial palsy following muscular effort. A nerve compression syndrome possibly related to a fibrous arch of the lateral head of the triceps. J Bone Joint Surg 53B:500–506, 1971

500. Lubahn JD, Lister GD: Familial radial nerve entrapment syndrome: A case report and literature review. J Hand Surg 8:297–298, 1983

501. Manske PR: Compression of the radial nerve by the triceps muscle. Case report. J Bone Joint Surg 59A:835–836, 1977

502. Marmor L, Lawrence JF, Dubois EL: Posterior interosseous nerve paralysis due to rheumatoid arthritis. J Bone Joint Surg 49A:381–383, 1967

503. Marshall SC, Murray WR: Deep radial nerve palsy associated with rheumatoid arthritis. Clin Orthop 103:157–162, 1974

504. Mayer JH, Mayfield FH: Surgery of the posterior interosseous branch of the radial nerve. Surg Gynecol Obstet 84:979–982, 1947

505. Millender LH, Nalebuff EA, Holdsworth DE: Posterior interosseous nerve syndrome secondary to rheumatoid synovitis. J Bone Joint Surg 55A:753–757, 1973

506. Moon N, Marmor L: Parosteal lipoma of the proximal part of the radius. J Bone Joint Surg 46A:608–614, 1964

507. Morris AH: Irreducible Monteggia lesion with radial-nerve entrapment. J Bone Joint Surg 56A:1744–1746, 1974

508. Moss SH, Switzer HE: Radial tunnel syndrome: A spectrum of clinical presentations. J Hand Surg 8:414–420, 1983

509. Mulholland RC: Non-traumatic progressive paralysis of the posterior interosseous nerve. J Bone Joint Surg 48B:781–785, 1966

510. Nielsen HO: Posterior interosseous nerve paralysis caused by fibrous band compressioin at the supinator muscle. A report of four cases. Acta Orthop Scand 47:304–307, 1976

511. Packer JW, Foster RR, Garcia A, Grantham SA: The humeral fracture with radial nerve palsy: Is

exploration warranted? Clin Orthop 88:34–38, 1972

512. Popelka S, Vianio K: Entrapment of the posterior interosseous branch of the radial nerve in rheumatoid arthritis. Acta Orthop Scand 45:370–372, 1974

513. Richmond DA: Lipoma causing a posterior interosseous nerve lesion. J Bone Joint Surg 35B:83, 1953

514. Riordan DC: Radial nerve paralysis. Orthop Clin North Am 5:283, 1974

515. Roles NC, Maudsley RH: Radial tunnel syndrome. Resistant tennis elbow as a nerve entrapment. J Bone Joint Surg 54B:499–508, 1972

516. Salsbury CR: The nerve to the extensor carpi radialis brevis. Br J Surg 26:95–97, 1938

517. Schnitker MT: A technique for transplant of the musculospiral nerve in open reduction of fractures of the mid-shaft of the humerus. J Neurosurg 6:113–117, 1949

518. Sharrard WJW: Posterior interosseous neuritis. J Bone Joint Surg 48B:777–780, 1966

519. Silverstein A: Progressive paralysis of the dorsal interosseous nerve. Report of a case. Arch Neurol Phychiatry 38:885, 1937

520. Spinner M: The arcade of Frohse and its relationship to posterior interosseous nerve paralysis. J Bone Joint Surg 50B:809–812, 1968

521. Spinner M, Freundlich BD, Teicher J: Posterior interosseous nerve palsy as a complication of Monteggia fractures in children. Clin Orthop 58:141, 1968

522. Sponseller PD, Engber WD: Double-entrapment radial tunnel syndrome. J Hand Surg 8:420–423, 1983

523. Stein F, Grabias SL, Deffer PA: Nerve injuries complicating Monteggia lesions. J Bone Joint Surg 53A:1432–1436, 1971

524. Strachan JCH, Ellis BW: Vulnerability of the posterior interosseous nerve during radial head resection. J Bone Joint Surg 53B:320–323, 1971

525. Van Rossum J, Buruma OJS, Kamphuisen HAC, Onvlee GJ: Tennis elbow—A radial tunnel syndrome? J Bone Joint Surg 60B:197–198, 1978

526. Wadsworth TG: Injuries of the capitular (lateral humeral condylar) epiphysis. Clin Orthop 85:127–142, 1972

527. Wartenberg R: Cheiralgia Paraesthetic (Isolierte Neuritis des Ramus superficialis nervi radialis). Z Ges Neurol Psychiatr 141:145–155, 1932

528. Weinberger LM: Non-traumatic paralysis of the dorsal interosseous nerve. Surg Gynecol Obstet 69:358–363, 1939

529. Werner CO: Lateral elbow pain and posterior interosseous nerve entrapment. Acta Orthop Scand (suppl.) 174:1979

530. Whitely WH, Alpers BJ: Posterior interosseous palsy with spontaneous neuroma formation. Arch Neurol 1:226–229, 1959

531. Wilhelm A: Radialis kompressions syndrome. Hand Chir 8:113, 1976

532. Woltman HW, Learmonth JR: Progressive paralysis of the nervus interosseous dorsalis. Brain 57:25–31, 1934

533. Wu KT, Jordan FR, Eckert C: Lipoma, a cause of paralysis of deep radial (posterior interosseous) nerve. Report of a case and review of the literature. Surg 75:790–795, 1974

Radial Nerve Palsy

37

David P. Green

Loss of radial nerve function in the hand is a significant disability. The patient cannot extend the fingers and thumb and therefore has great difficulty in grasping objects. Perhaps more importantly, the loss of active wrist extension robs the patient of the ability to stabilize the wrist, further impairing grasp and especially power grip. The tendon transfers to restore function in radial nerve palsy are among the best and most predictable transfers in the upper extremity, but as Riordan[44] has pointed out, "in muscle tendon surgery there is very little hope that errors in technique can be overcome by local adaptation. The success or failure of an operation depends upon the technical competence of the operator and his painstaking after-care." Riordan[45] has also noted that "there is usually only one chance to obtain good restoration of function in such a paralyzed hand."

ANATOMY

Trauma to the upper extremity is such that most injuries of the radial nerve occur distal to the branches to the triceps in the upper arm. For this reason, transfers to restore triceps function are not included in this chapter.

It is imperative that the surgeon make the important distinction between complete radial nerve palsy (excluding the triceps) and posterior interosseous palsy. The radial nerve innervates the BR and ECRL° before it divides into its two terminal branches, the posterior interosseous (motor) and superficial (sensory) branches. Clinically, I believe it is extremely difficult, if not impossible, to determine the integrity of the ECRB in the presence of an intact ECRL, and the presence of the ECRB is variable in posterior interosseous nerve palsy. Usually the ECRB is absent in such cases, although it may be intact. Spinner[50] has noted that the ECRB receives its innervation in the majority of limbs (58 percent) from the superficial radial nerve rather than from the posterior interosseous nerve. In any case, patients with posterior interosseous nerve palsy will have at least one strong radial wrist extensor intact, resulting in radial deviation of the wrist with dorsiflexion, which may be rather marked in some patients (Fig. 37-1). This clinical finding may have significant implications in the

---

° For simplicity, the abbreviations used throughout this chapter are listed in Table 37-1.

1479

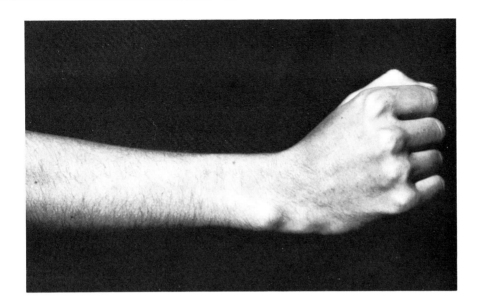

Fig. 37-1. In a patient with posterior interosseous nerve palsy the ECRL is intact, resulting in radial deviation of the wrist in dorsiflexion.

choice of appropriate tendon transfers, as discussed later in the chapter.

As it emerges from the supinator about 8 cm distal to the elbow joint, the posterior interosseous nerve splays out into multiple branches, which Spinner[50] has likened to the cauda equina. The difficulty in repairing an untidy laceration of the nerve at this level will often have an important influence on the timing of tendon transfers.

The surgeon who plans to perform transfers for radial nerve palsy must have a profound three-dimensional understanding of the anatomy of the flexor and extensor muscles of the forearm. This is a complex area of anatomy that is difficult to master, and continual review is mandatory. I find that the best sources for augmenting my knowledge of forearm anatomy are actual dissections in the laboratory, Henry's classic book,[22] and the superb atlas of anatomy by McMinn and Hutchings.[80]

Table 37-1. Abbreviations Used in This Chapter

PT	Pronator teres
FCU	Flexor carpi ulnaris
FCR	Flexor carpi radialis
PL	Palmaris longus
FDP	Flexor digitorum profundus
FDS	Flexor digitorum sublimis (superficialis)
FPL	Flexor pollicis longus
BR	Brachioradialis
ECRL	Extensor carpi radialis longus
ECRB	Extensor carpi radialis brevis
ECU	Extensor carpi ulnaris
APL	Abductor pollicis brevis
EPB	Extensor pollicis brevis
EPL	Extensor pollicis longus
EDC	Extensor digitorum communis
EIP	Extensor indicis proprius
EDM	Extensor digiti minimi
II	Index finger
III	Long finger
IV	Ring finger
V	Small finger

REQUIREMENTS IN THE PATIENT WITH RADIAL NERVE PALSY

The patient with irreparable radial nerve palsy needs to be provided with: (1) wrist extension, (2) finger (MP joint) extension, and (3) a combination of thumb extension and abduction. The motors available for transfer in a patient with an isolated radial nerve palsy are all the extrinsic muscles innervated by the median and ulnar nerves. This multitude of available motors provides the surgeon with a rather mind-boggling and almost limitless number of possible combinations of transfers. Indeed, almost every conceivable combination has been tried, and a careful historical review of transfers for radial nerve palsy (see page 1485) will save us from some of the errors of the past.

Unless the patient has a painful neuroma, the sensory part of the radial nerve can usually be ignored. Loss of sensibility on the radial side of the dorsum of the hand is perhaps bothersome but rarely a disability. The patient with a complete radial nerve palsy occasionally will have no demonstrable sensory deficit, because in some patients the superficial branch of radial nerve is absent and its function is preempted by the lateral antebrachial cutaneous nerve.[29,50]

NONOPERATIVE TREATMENT

By far the most important aspects of nonoperative management in the patient with radial nerve palsy are maintenance of full passive range of motion in all joints of the wrist and hand and prevention of contractures, including that of the thumb-index web. In most patients, the constant supervision of a therapist is not required, but the patient himself must be taught very soon after the original nerve injury how to carry out an appropriate exercise program to keep the joints supple. It is the patient's responsibility to do his exercises, and the role of the therapist at this point is to teach the

patient and to monitor his course to be certain that the exercise program is carried out correctly.

Many types of splints have been described for patients with radial nerve palsy.[4,39,54,55] Most of these incorporate some type of dynamic outriggers to extend the fingers and thumb with elastic traction, while allowing full mobility for active flexion. Not all patients with radial nerve palsy need this much elaborate splinting, and each patient's individual needs should dictate the type of splinting used; the same orthosis should not be prescribed for every patient. For example, a telephone operator who wishes to continue working could probably do so with the somewhat cumbersome dynamic splint shown in Figure 37-2. However, an insurance salesman who is more concerned about appearance might be content with only a small, inconspicuous volar cockup wrist splint. In some patients, merely stabilizing the wrist in dorsiflexion will impart remarkably good temporary function. Burkhalter[16] has observed that grip strength may be increased three to five times by simply stabilizing the wrist with a splint.

Early Transfers ("Internal Splint")

It is perhaps a contradiction in terms to discuss early tendon transfer under nonoperative treatment, but my point is to stress that the concept of

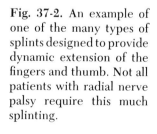
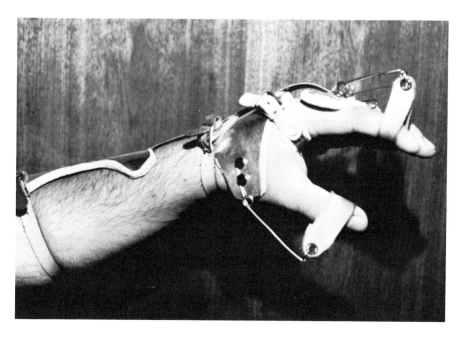

Fig. 37-2. An example of one of the many types of splints designed to provide dynamic extension of the fingers and thumb. Not all patients with radial nerve palsy require this much splinting.

early transfers is to provide a temporary "internal splint," and it should not be construed as definitive treatment of the radial nerve palsy.

Burkhalter[16] has claimed that the greatest functional loss in the patient with a radial nerve injury is weakness of power grip. Consequently, he has been perhaps the strongest advocate of an early PT to ECRB transfer to eliminate the need for an external splint and, at the same time, to restore a significant amount of power grip to the patient's hand. In advocating early tendon transfer, Burkhalter has been careful to emphasize what he calls three indications and three important principles. The *indications* are: (1) the transfer works as a substitute during regrowth of the nerve to eliminate the need for splintage, (2) the transfer works as a helper following reinnervation by aiding the power of a normal muscle to the reinnervated muscles, and (3) the transfer acts as a substitute in cases where the results of nerve repair are statistically poor or in cases where the nerve is irreparable. The important *principles* are: (1) the transfer should not significantly decrease the remaining function in the hand, (2) the transfer should not create a deformity if significant return occurs following nerve repair, and (3) the transfer should be a phasic one or capable of phase conversion.

Burkhalter believes that the PT to ECRB transfer fulfills all of these indications and principles, and he therefore suggests that the operation be done at the time of radial nerve repair or as soon as possible thereafter. The tendon juncture is done end-to-side, and the continuity of ECRB is not disrupted so that it may regain its own function if reinnervation should occur.

I have no personal experience with the use of this transfer as an internal splint, but its use is also supported by Omer[35] and Brand.[12]

OPERATIVE TREATMENT

Principles of Tendon Transfers

The application of certain fundamental principles is essential for successful transfer of muscle-tendon units. These important concepts were es-tablished by such masters as Mayer,[28] Steindler,[52] and Bunnell[10] and have been reemphasized by Littler,[26] Boyes,[7] Curtis,[18] White,[59] and Brand.[12] They have in fact been repeated so often that their significance may sometimes be obscured by their familiarity, but they remain essential elements in successful tendon transfers.

CORRECTION OF CONTRACTURE

From the outset in the management of any patient with a peripheral nerve palsy, it is imperative that all joints be kept supple since soft tissue contracture is far easier to prevent than to correct. The essential principle here, of course, is that maximum passive motion of all joints must be present before a tendon transfer is performed, because no tendon transfer can move a stiff joint, and it is impossible for a joint to have more active motion postoperatively than it had passively preoperatively.

ADEQUATE STRENGTH

The tendon chosen as a donor for transfer must be sufficiently strong to perform its new function in its altered position. An appreciation of the relative strengths of the forearm muscles is important to the surgeon in selecting an appropriate motor (Table 37-2). Perhaps even more important than the normal strength of a given motor is its current condition, and, in general, a muscle should not be used for transfer unless it can be graded as being at least good (Steindler said 85 percent of normal). If at all possible, I try to avoid using a muscle that has been reinnervated, that is, one that was paralyzed and now has returned function. Omer[34,36] has noted that a muscle will usually lose one grade of strength (on Highet's clinical scale) following transfer.

Table 37-2. Work Capacity of Forearm Muscles (Boyes[9])

Donor Muscles (Mkg)		Recipient Muscles (Mkg)	
BR	1.9	EPL	0.1
PT	1.2	APL	0.1
FCR	0.8	EPB	0.1
FCU	2.0	EDC	1.7
PL	0.1	EIP	0.5
FDS	4.8	ECRL	1.1
FDP	4.5	ECRB	0.9
FPL	1.2	ECU	1.1

AMPLITUDE OF MOTION

The surgeon must also have some appreciation of the amplitude of tendon excursion for each muscle. Although more precise values of these have been determined,[11,58,60] Boyes[9] has suggested the use of the following values for practical purposes.

Wrist flexors and extensors — 33 mm
Finger extensors and EPL — 50 mm
Finger flexors — 70 mm

These numbers have practical significance, since it is obviously impossible for a wrist flexor with an excursion of 33 mm to substitute fully for a finger extensor with an amplitude of 50 mm. Although the *true* amplitude of the tendon cannot be increased, two things can be done to augment its *effective* amplitude. First, a muscle can be converted from monoarticular to biarticular or multiarticular, thereby effectively utilizing the natural tenodesis effect. For example, when the FCU is transferred to the EDC, it is converted to a multiarticular muscle and the *effective* amplitude of the tendon is increased significantly by active volar flexion of the wrist, thereby allowing the transferred wrist flexor to extend the fingers fully (Fig. 37-3). The second factor that can increase amplitude is extensive dis-section of the muscle from its surrounding fascial attachments. This is particularly true of the brachioradialis.

STRAIGHT LINE OF PULL

The pioneers of tendon transfer surgery repeatedly emphasized that the most efficient transfer is one that passes in a direct line from its own origin to the insertion of the tendon being substituted. Although this is not always possible (e.g., in an opponensplasty), it is a desirable goal to seek and is particulary important in the FCU to EDC transfer, which is described later in this chapter.

ONE TENDON – ONE FUNCTION

It is obvious that a single tendon cannot be expected to do two diametrically opposing actions simultaneously, for example, flex and extend the same joint. It is perhaps not quite so obvious that the effectiveness of a tendon transfer is reduced when it is expected to produce two dissimilar functions even when they are not direct opposites. If a muscle is inserted into two tendons having separate functions, the force and amplitude of the donor tendon will be dissipated and less effective than it would be if it motored only a single tendon.[48]

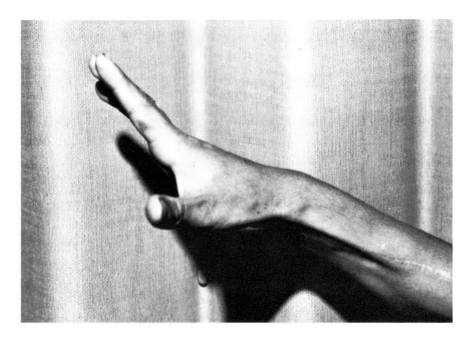

Fig. 37-3. A wrist flexor transferred to the finger extensors does not have sufficient amplitude of excursion to simultaneously extend the wrist and fingers. In this patient following FCU to EDC transfer, note that he uses the tenodesis effect created by active volar flexion of the wrist to enhance the effective excursion of the tendon and thereby achieve excellent active extension of the fingers (compare with Fig. 37-11).

SYNERGISM

There is debate among hand surgeons as to the importance of synergistic motion in the hand, that is, finger flexors acting in concert with wrist extensors and finger extensors with wrist flexors. Littler[26] has been a major advocate of the use of synergistic muscles for transfer whenever possible, and I personally believe it is easier to retrain muscle function after synergistic muscle transfers. A possible exception to this rule is the use of the superficialis (sublimis) tendons, which have more independent cortical control than other muscles in the hand, although I still find it more difficult to retrain the superficialis than synergistic transfers.

EXPENDABLE DONOR

Removal of a tendon for transfer must not result in unacceptable loss of function; there must be sufficient muscle remaining to substitute for the donor muscle. The classic example of this is the necessity of retaining one strong wrist flexor (PL is not adequate) in any combination of transfers for radial nerve palsy (see page 1485).

TISSUE EQUILIBRIUM

The timing of tendon transfers is somewhat controversial, but all authors agree that no transfer should be done until the local tissues are in optimal condition. Steindler's classic expression, "tissue equilibrium" (quoted by Boyes[7]) is a good term; it implies that soft tissue induration is gone, there is no reaction in the wounds, the joints are supple, and the scars are as soft as they are likely to become. To perform tendon transfers or any elective operation before tissue equilibrium has been reached is to invite disaster. If scar tissue remains after maximum recovery has been achieved, the surgeon must consider providing new skin coverage with flaps prior to transfer or else devise transfers that will avoid the scarred areas. Tendon transfers work best when passed between the subcutaneous fat and deep fascial layer; they are not likely to work at all in a pathway of scar. When performing tendon transfers, the surgeon should think in terms of trying to minimize scar formation, and skin incisions should be planned so as to place

tendon junctures beneath flaps rather than directly beneath incisions.[34]

Timing of Tendon Transfers

The appropriate time to perform transfers for radial nerve palsy is a somewhat controversial subject. As noted previously, several authors[12,16,35] advocate only a limited transfer (PT to ECRB) almost immediately after injury to act as an internal splint and also to supplement any return in the reinnervated extensor muscles. Brown[15] suggests that it is advisable to proceed with the full component of tendon transfers early when there is a questionable or poor prognosis from the nerve repair. For example, if there is a nerve gap of greater than 4 cm or if there is a large wound or extensive scarring or skin loss over the nerve, he recommends ignoring the nerve and proceeding directly to the tendon transfers. I basically agree with Brown; if the chances of nerve regeneration are poor, there is no point in waiting before doing the transfers. However, if a good repair of the nerve has been accomplished, it is my practice to wait a sufficient period of time before considering transfer. In my opinion, "sufficient time" is determined by using Seddon's[49] figures for nerve regeneration, i.e., approximately 1 mm per day. This means that it may take as long as 5 or 6 months before one sees return in the most proximal muscles (BR and ECRL) following nerve repair in the middle third of the arm. The remaining muscles should return in orderly progression at the same rate of 1 mm per day (Table 37-3).

To my knowledge, there is little if any popular support for the concept offered by Bevin[5] of never repairing the radial nerve and proceeding directly to tendon transfers. Although he demonstrated im-

Table 37-3. Distances (cm) from the Distal End of Supinator to the Point of Innervation (Spinner[50])

ECU	1.25
EDC	1.25–1.8
EDM	1.8
APL	5.6
EPB	6.5
EIP	6.8
EPL	7.5

pressive differences in disability times (8 weeks after tendon transfers, $7\frac{1}{2}$ months after nerve repair), I believe that most surgeons would agree that the results of radial nerve repair are sufficiently good to warrant routine repair in all cases except perhaps in those identified above by Brown as having a poor prognosis.

There does not appear to be any *upper* time limit as to how long a delay before transfers are done can be tolerated following nerve injury. Brodman[13] reported successful transfers 24 years after radial nerve injury, despite what he described as "gelatinous degeneration" (i.e., translucent appearance) of the paralyzed tendons at the time of operation.

Historical Review

As with the management of peripheral nerve injuries per se, the development of operative procedures for treatment of irreparable radial nerve palsy mainly evolved during the two world wars. Most of the important articles contributing to our knowledge of transfers for radial nerve palsy are to be found in the immediate post-war years. The tragedies of the wars enabled a few individuals to accumulate a lifetime of experience in a very short period of time. For example, Scuderi[48] reported 45 patients with radial nerve palsy in whom he performed transfers during a $12\frac{1}{2}$ month period.

Sir Robert Jones is credited with being the major innovator of radial nerve transfers, and all the articles in the post–World War I era acknowledge his fundamental contributions. However, the "classic" Jones transfer has been quoted and misquoted so many times in articles and texts that it is worthwhile to review his original articles[23,24] to see exactly what he did advocate. Part of the confusion arises from the fact that Jones did describe at least two slightly different combinations of transfers, as outlined in Table 37-4.

Although the Jones transfers came to be one of the more popular operations for radial nerve palsy, they were by no means universally accepted. Virtually every conceivable combination of transfers for radial nerve palsy has been reported, and the reader interested in this fascinating aspect of medical history is referred to Boyes' superb article,[8]

Table 37-4. Jones Transfers

1916[23]
PT to ECRL and ECRB
FCU to EDC III–V
FCR to EIP, EDC II, and EPL
1921[24]
PT to ECRL and ECRB
FCU to EDC III–V
FCR to EIP, EDC II, EPL, EPB, and APL

which outlines the multitude of procedures described between 1897 and 1959. For the purpose of this discussion, it is important to mention only some of the more important highlights in the development of transfers for radial nerve palsy.

The only part of the classic Jones transfer that has become universally accepted is the use of the PT to provide active wrist extension; however, even this acceptance came relatively recently. Saikku[47] pointed out that at the onset of World War II there were two schools of thought regarding the best method of restoring wrist dorsiflexion in the patient with radial nerve palsy. The British and Americans tended to favor Jones' transfer of the PT to the radial wrist extensors, while the Germans were influenced by the recommendation of Perthes, who advocated a tenodesis or arthrodesis to maintain a dorsiflexed attitude of the wrist. Saikku reviewed a large series comparing the two methods and concluded that the Jones transfer was superior, noting a high failure rate with tenodesis due to loosening. A few authors have favored wrist arthrodesis,[37,52] but most believe that it is important to maintain wrist motion in a patient with radial nerve palsy.[4,7,9,26,41,43,47,61]

The only current controversy regarding the pronator transfer centers around whether to insert the PT into both radial wrist extensors or only into the ECRB to minimize radial deviation[14,26,31,33,35] (see page 1491).

Major disagreement arises concerning the optimal method of restoring finger extension and thumb extension and abduction. It is clear that Jones advocated transferring both strong wrist flexors (FCU and FCR), a practice apparently not questioned by most of his contemporaries. Although Starr[51] in 1922 was the first to transfer the PL and leave one of the strong wrist flexors intact, his article leads the reader to wonder if he fully appreciated the significance of his contribution. Indeed, it was not until 1946 that Zachary[62] documented and convincingly illustrated the concept that it is desirable to leave one wrist flexor intact. He also showed that the PL is *not* adequate to provide satisfactory wrist flexion if both the FCU and FCR are transferred. Zachary's other contribution was the creation of a standard method of assessing results, which has been modified and used by numerous other authors since 1946.

In 1949, Scuderi[48] refined the PL to rerouted EPL transfer, emphasizing the important principle that function is better when the transfer is done into only one tendon (note in Table 37-4 that by 1921 Jones was suturing the FCR into four tendons with separate functions).

The results of these and other studies gradually evolved into what has been referred to by some as the "standard" set of tendon transfers for radial nerve palsy:

> PT to ECRB
> FCU to EDC II-V
> PL to rerouted EPL

However, the best combination of transfers is still not totally agreed upon. In 1960, Boyes[8] offered a reasonable alternative to the standard set of transfers that seems to have withstood the test of time.[17] Boyes reasoned that the FCU is a more important wrist flexor to preserve than the FCR, because the normal axis of wrist motion is from dorso-radial to volar-ulnar. I have also heard Paul Brand state in a lecture that the FCU is an "astonishingly important" muscle and that its function should be retained. Another reason for suggesting this new operation was to provide simultaneous wrist dorsi-flexion and finger extension. Because the amplitude of the wrist flexors is only about 33 mm and that of the finger extensors is 50 mm, full active extension of the fingers with an FCU or FCR transfer can be achieved only by simultaneous volar flexion of the wrist, relying upon the teno-desis effect of the transfer (Fig. 37-3). Boyes thus concluded that, because of their greater excursion (70 mm), the superficialis (sublimis) tendons would be ideal motors for finger extensors. Yet another reason for his new combination of transfers was to provide more independent control of the

Table 37-5. The Best Combinations of Tendon Transfers for Radial Nerve Palsy

Standard (FCU) transfer
PT to ECRB
FCU to EDC
PL to rerouted EPL
Superficialis transfer (Boyes[8,17])
PT to ECRL and ECRB
FDS III to EDC
FDS IV to EIP and EPL
FCR to APL and EPB
FCR transfer (Starr,[51] Brand,[12] Tsuge[57])
PT to ECRB
FCR to EDC
PL to rerouted EPL

thumb and index finger. The combination of transfers he described is as follows:

> PT to ECRL and ECRB
> FCR to EPB and APL
> FDS III to EDC (via interosseous membrane)
> FDS IV to EPL and EIP (via interosseous membrane)

Operative Techniques

Although there is almost an infinite number of possible combinations of transfers for radial nerve palsy, I believe it is safe to say that there are three sets of transfers that are currently considered to be the most reasonable alternatives (Table 37-5). Probably the most popular group is what I refer to as the "standard" (FCU) transfer, although Boyes' combination that utilizes the superficialis tendons for finger extension is another good combination. The third combination is that first proposed by Starr[51] in 1922 and more recently described in detail by Brand[12], which utilizes the FCR instead of the FCU. The operative techniques for these three procedures are described in detail below.

It is of course obvious that in a patient with posterior interosseous palsy the PT transfer is not necessary to restore wrist extension.

STANDARD (FCU) TRANSFER

Incision #1 (Fig. 37-4) is directed longitudinally over the FCU in the distal half of the forearm. Its distal end is J-shaped, with the transverse extension

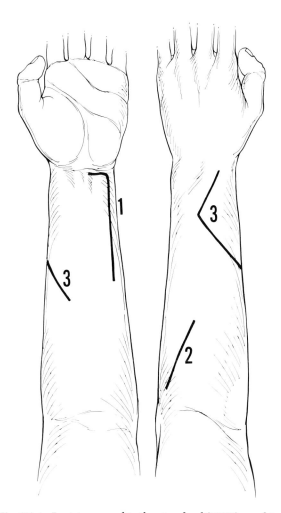

Fig. 37-4. Incisions used in the standard (FCU) combination of transfers (see text).

being long enough to reach the PL tendon. The FCU tendon is transected just proximal to the pisiform and freed up as far proximally as the incision will allow. Separation of this muscle from its particularly dense fascial attachments is facilitated by a special tendon stripper designed by Carroll (Fig. 37-5); however, if this tendon stripper is not available, the dissection of FCU can be done under direct vision by extending incision #1 more proximally. The muscle belly of the FCU is very long, extending usually to within a few centimeters of the insertion of the tendon. I prefer to excise rather generously that part of the muscle belly that is attached to the distal half of the tendon, as this will later facilitate the transfer and cause a less bulky appearance of the muscle in its new position around the ulnar border of the forearm.

Incision #2 begins 2 inches below the medial epicondyle and angles across the dorsum of the proximal forearm, aimed directly toward Lister's tubercle. The deep fascia overlying the FCU muscle belly is excised and the remainder of the fascial attachments to the muscle are incised. It is imperative that the FCU be completely freed up so that the entire muscle belly and tendon can be displaced into the proximal wound to redirect the muscle. The limiting factor in the dissection is the innervation of the FCU, which enters the muscle in its proximal 2 inches, and the dissection must not extend this far proximally.

Incision #3 begins on the volar-radial aspect of the midforearm, passes dorsally around the radial border of the forearm in the region of the insertion of the PT, and then angles back on the dorsum of the distal forearm toward Lister's tubercle. The tendon of the PT is identified in the volar aspect of the wound and followed to its insertion on the

Fig. 37-5. This instrument designed by Carroll facilitates division of the extensive fascial attachments of the muscle belly of FCU.

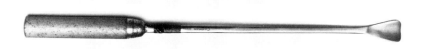

radius. It is important to free up the insertion with an intact long strip of periosteum in order to ensure that the length will be sufficient for a strong tendon juncture later (Fig. 37-6). The PT muscle and tendon are then passed subcutaneously around the radial border of the forearm, superficial to the BR and ECRL, to be inserted into the ECRB just distal to its musculotendinous junction.

A tendon passer or large Kelly clamp is then passed from the dorsal wound (incision #3) subcutaneously around the ulnar border of the forearm,

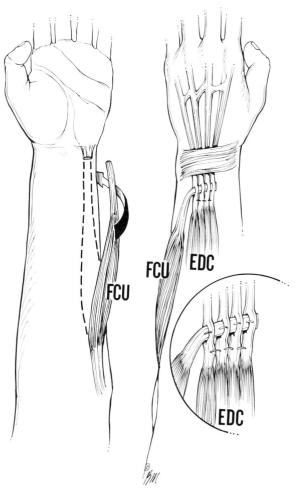

Fig. 37-7. FCU to EDC transfer. The FCU must be freed up extensively to create a direct line of pull from its origin to the new insertion into the EDC tendons just proximal to the dorsal retinaculum. End-to-side juncture is shown here. Moberg and Nachemson[32] have suggested that 4 to 5 cm of the paralyzed EDC tendons be resected proximal to the juncture, allowing an end-to-end suture and a more direct line of pull.

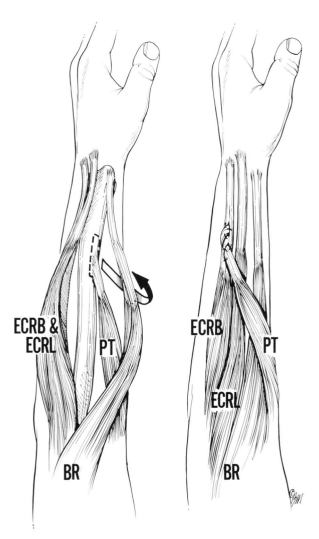

Fig. 37-6. PT to ECRB transfer. It is important to take a strip of periosteum in continuity with the PT insertion to ensure adequate length for the transfer.

and the tendon of the FCU is pulled into the dorsal wound (Fig. 37-7). At this point, if there is still excessive bulk of muscle overlying the ulnar border, the FCU muscle belly can be trimmed a bit more. It is imperative that the line of pull of the FCU be as straight as possible from the medial epicondyle to the EDC tendon just proximal to the dorsal retinaculum. If the previous dissection has not freed up all the fascial attachments of FCU, it will be impossible to achieve this important direct pull.

The EPL muscle is then identified in the dorsal wound; it is divided at its musculotendinous junction and rerouted out of Lister's canal toward the volar aspect of the wrist across the anatomic snuffbox (Fig. 37-8). The PL tendon is transected at the wrist, and the muscle-tendon unit is freed up proximally enough to allow a straight line of pull between the PL and the rerouted EPL tendon. The PL tendon is delivered into the dorsal wound in the region of the snuffbox.

A variation in technique recommended by Moberg and Nachemson[32] is to open the dorsal retinaculum to prevent ischemic necrosis of the tendons secondary to postoperative edema. I am not aware of this being a common problem, and I would be concerned about possible bowstringing if the retinaculum were completely cut (which is not mentioned by the authors). Consequently I have not used this modification.

At this point, I prefer to release the tourniquet, establish hemostasis, and close incisions #1 and #2 before doing the final tendon junctures.

Setting the proper tension in the transfers is a somewhat tricky task but is very critical to the outcome of the operation. It is difficult to describe precisely how to adjust tension in tendon transfers, and a certain amount of experience is essential in being able to "feel" the proper tension. In general, however, one should probably err on the side of suturing extensor tendon transfers too tightly rather than too loosely. The tendons must be tight enough to provide full extension of the wrist, fingers, and thumb, yet not so tight as to limit flexion of the digits. I usually suture the PT to ECRB (not including the ECRL) just distal to the musculotendinous junction. The long tongue of periosteum at the end of the PT tendon is woven through the tendon of the ECRB and secured with multiple 4–0 nonabsorbable sutures. (Omer[34] prefers larger [2–0 or 3–0] material). The tension is set with the PT in maximum tension and the wrist in moderate (45 degrees) dorsiflexion.

The FCU transfer is then sutured. I generally use the technique described by Omer[33] (and depicted in Fig. 37-7), weaving the FCU tendon through the EDC tendons at a 45-degree angle just proximal to the dorsal retinaculum. Moberg and Nachemson[32] have suggested that better results can be achieved if 4 to 5 cm of inactivated EDC muscle-tendon is resected just proximal to the intended site of suture. Although I have not used this technique, it would provide a more direct line of pull since the tendon juncture would be end-to-end rather than end-to-side.[20]

Most authors do not include the EDM in the transfer for fear of creating excessive tension in the small finger. I determine whether to include it by pulling on the EDC tendons with an Allis clamp (proximal to the intended site of juncture); if the small finger extends adequately, the EDM is not

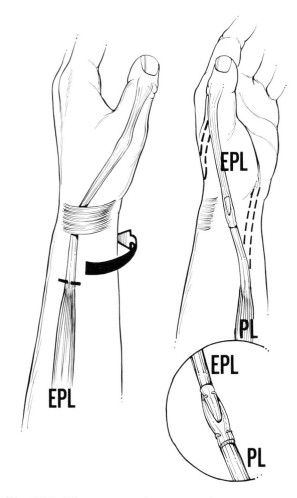

Fig. 37-8. PL to rerouted EPL transfer. By rerouting EPL out of the dorsal retinaculum, the transfer creates a combination of abduction and extension force on the thumb.

included, but if there is an extensor lag in the small finger (signifying an inadequate slip of EDC to the small finger), I include the EDM among the recipient tendons. It is important to suture the FCU tendon into each EDC slip separately and to adjust the tension in the EDC tendons individually so that all four MP joints extend synchronously and evenly. I prefer 4–0 nonabsorable suture, and the tension I use is with the wrist and MP joints in neutral (0 degrees) and the FCU under maximum tension. A good assistant is very helpful at this point to aid in holding the tension while the tendons are sutured.

Retraction on the distal end of incision #3 will allow the third and final juncture (PL to rerouted EPL) to be made in the region of the anatomic snuffbox superficial to the dorsal retinaculum. The direction of the tendons is essentially in line with the first metacarpal (Fig. 37-9). My preferred tension is with the wrist in neutral and with maximum tension on both the EPL and PL tendons.

The tension must be tested by passively moving the wrist to demonstrate the synergistic action of the new transfer; with the wrist in dorsiflexion, it should be possible to easily flex the fingers completely into the palm, and, with the wrist in volar flexion, the MP joints should pull into full extension but not hyperextension.

Incision #3 is then closed while an assistant stabilizes the position of the wrist and hand to protect the transfers. I prefer to close all three wounds with subcuticular sutures to avoid unattractive cross-hatches in the scars.

Postoperative Management

In the operating room, a long arm splint is applied, which immobilizes the forearm in 15 to 30 degrees pronation, the wrist in approximately 45 degrees dorsiflexion, the MP joints in slight (10 to 15 degrees) flexion, and the thumb in maximum extension and abduction. The PIP joints of the fingers are left free. Since limited elbow motion will not cause undue tension on the suture lines, a single sugar tong splint is a satisfactory alternative to the long arm splint. The splint and sutures are removed at 10 to 14 days, and a Munster-type long arm cast is applied in the same position as noted above. The cast is removed at 4 weeks postoperatively, and removable short arm splints to hold the wrist, fingers, and thumb in extension are made, which the patient wears for an additional 2 weeks, removing them only for exercise.

A planned exercise program, begun at 4 weeks, under the guidance of an experienced hand thera-

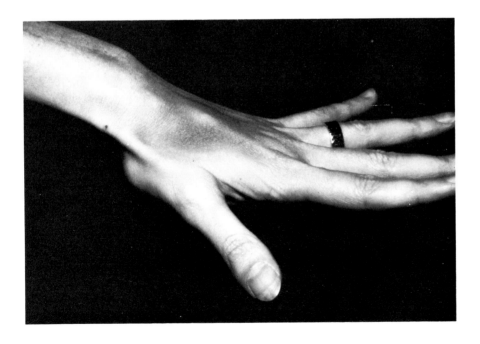

Fig. 37-9. PL to rerouted EPL transfer. Note that the line of pull is essentially in line with the thumb metacarpal.

pist is very beneficial to achieve the optimal results from this procedure. Following these transfers, I find it particularly useful to instruct the patient in synergistic movements. A well-motivated patient should have good control of function by 3 months, although many patients take as long as 6 months to reach maximum recovery.

Potential Problems

Excessive Radial Deviation. Removing the FCU (an important wrist flexor and the only remaining ulnar deviator) from the wrist in a patient with radial nerve palsy may contribute to radial deviation of the hand. This is likely to be further aggravated if the PT is inserted into the ECRL, which Youm et al[60] have shown to be mainly a radial deviator rather than an extensor of the wrist. Even if the transfer is into the more centrally located ECRB, there may be some radial deviation because the ECRB, although more centrally located than the ECRL, still imparts some radial deviation.[12] Also, significant intercommunication between the ECRL and ECRB has been identified by Albright and Linburg.[2] The problem is particularly severe in patients with *posterior interosseous nerve palsy* who have a normally functioning, strong ECRL; in my experience, removing the FCU in these patients can seriously aggravate the radial deviation problem.

Several solutions to the problem have been suggested and are listed below.

Avoidance. If the patient has significant radial deviation preoperatively (e.g., the patient with posterior interosseous nerve palsy), I will not do the FCU transfer. In such cases, I prefer to use Boyes' superficialis transfers.

Alter the Insertion. In some patients I have altered the insertion of the radial wrist extensors at the time of PT transfer. The simplest way to do this is to resect the distal 2 to 3 cm of the ECRL tendon and suture the tendon more proximally into the adjacent ECRB, thereby eliminating any possibility of pull through the ECRL insertion. A more radical approach is to shift the distal end of the ECRB into the tendon of the ECU[57] or to include the transposed ECU tendon in the PT to ECRB transfer as suggested by Said.[46]

Absence of the PL. Absence of the PL compromises the standard set of transfers since it obviously eliminates the important PL to rerouted EPL transfer. In this situation, several authors suggest simply including the EPL into the FCU to EDC transfer, although this significantly limits the abduction component of the transfer's effect on the thumb. Bevin[5] has suggested including all of the thumb extrinsics (EPL, EPB, and APL) in the FCU to EDC transfer, but this seriously violates the one tendon–one function principle. Milford[31] advocates the use of the BR, which is of course possible only in posterior interosseous nerve palsy and not in complete radial nerve palsy. If the BR is used as a transfer, extensive freeing up of the muscle belly is necessary to augment its excursion, and Beasley[4] has commented that the BR is more difficult to re-educate in the rehabilitation program. Tsuge[57] and Goldner[21] have substituted the FDS III or IV for an absent PL.

Not being totally satisfied with any of the above alternatives, I will generally do Boyes' superficialis transfers when the PL is absent.

Bowstringing of the EPL. Tsuge[57] has noted a relatively minor problem of bowstringing of the rerouted EPL tendon across the radial aspect of the wrist. He reported that this may be prevented by hooking the EPL around the insertion of the APL at the time of the tendon transfer. I have no experience with this modification.

SUPERFICIALIS TRANSFER (BOYES[8,17])

Through a long incision on the volar side of the radial aspect of the midforearm, the tendons of PT, ECRL, and ECRB are exposed. The insertion of the PT is removed with a 2- to 3-cm strip of periosteum, and this tendinous portion is interwoven through the ECRB just distal to the musculotendinous junctions. In the original descriptions of this transfer,[8,17] PT was sutured to both ECRL and ECRB, but for the reasons noted above, I use only ECRB.

The superficialis (sublimis) tendons of the long and ring fingers are exposed through a transverse incision in the distal palm or through separate transverse incisions at the base of each finger. The tendons are divided proximal to the chiasma, freed up, and delivered into the forearm wound. At a level just proximal to the pronator quadratus, two

1×2 cm openings are excised from the interosseous membrane, one on each side of the anterior interosseous artery. Care is taken to protect both the anterior and posterior interosseous vessels. Numerous authors,[1,4] including Boyes,[10] have recommended that the muscle bellies of the transferred muscles be passed through the interosseous space to minimize adhesions. This may necessitate a larger opening in the interosseous membrane than that recommended by Chuinard and colleagues.[17] Others[56] prefer to route the superficialis tendons around the radial and ulnar borders of the forearm, respectively, in an effort to avoid tendon adherence.

A J-shaped incision is then made on the dorsum of the distal forearm; the transverse limb runs from the radial styloid to the ulnar styloid, and the longitudinal limb extends proximally along the ulna. The flexor tendons are passed to the dorsum through the openings in the interosseous membrane, with FDS III routed to the radial side of the profundus mass, between FDP and FPL, and FDS IV to the ulnar side of the profundus muscle mass. Care must be taken to avoid kinking the median nerve as the muscles are passed into the opening. O'Brien (O'Brien ET: personal communication) has noted kinking of the nerve by a band of fascia on the superficialis muscle belly. FDS IV is interwoven into the tendons of EIP and EPL, and FDS III into EDC. The EDM is not included and the recipient tendons are not divided proximal to the tendon juncture. The suture lines are placed proximal to the dorsal retinaculum, which may be narrowed if there is danger of impingement by the tendon junctures.

Through a transverse incision at the base of the thumb, the FCR tendon is divided and freed up sufficiently to allow it to be turned dorsally and passed through the substance of the APL and EPB tendons, where it is sutured in place. Milford[31] and Omer[36] have stressed the importance of deflating the tourniquet prior to wound closure because of possible damage to the interosseous vessels.

Postoperative Management

Postoperative splints similar to those described on page 1490 are applied and worn for 4 weeks, at which time the sutures are removed and a Thomas splint is worn day and night for the next 2 weeks, except during exercise periods. All external support is then discontinued at 6 weeks postoperatively. The exercise program should emphasize specific control of the superficialis muscles in order to try to take advantage of the greater excursion of these tendons. It should *not* use the tenodesis techniques that are useful after the synergistic (FCU and FCR) transfers.

FCR TRANSFER (STARR,[51] BRAND,[12] TSUGE[57])

The PT to ECRB transfer, when required, is performed as described previously with the other transfers.

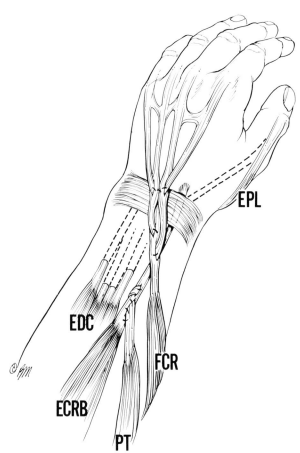

Fig. 37-10. FCR to EDC transfer. Brand[12] suggests that the EDC tendons be transected and transposed superficial to the dorsal retinaculum to create a straight-line end-to-end juncture with the FCR. (Redrawn from Brand PW: Tendon transfers in the forearm. In Flynn JE (ed): Hand Surgery. 2nd Ed. © 1975, The Williams & Wilkins Co, Baltimore.)

The FCR tendon is exposed through two transverse or a single longitudinal incision on the volar-radial aspect of the forearm. The tendon is divided at the wrist and freed up to the middle of the forearm so that it can be redirected around the radial border of the forearm in a straight line to the center of the wrist dorsally via a subcutaneous tunnel. A separate dorsal incision exposes the distal 3 inches of the forearm and the wrist. The juncture between the FCR and EDC can be made by leaving the EDC in continuity (similar to the FCU transfer depicted in Fig. 37-6), but Brand recommends that the EDC tendons be divided so that a formal end-to-end suture can be done between the FCR and EDC, as shown in Figure 37-10. To avoid the problem of multiple exposed raw tendon ends, Brand suggests burying each cut tendon end. The finger extensor tendons are all tested for extension of the MP joint, and "four good tendons are chosen."[12] These are divided at their musculotendinous junctions, withdrawn distally, superficial to the intact dorsal retinaculum, and redirected to a point over the distal radius where they can meet the FCR tendon in a straight line. They are then retested for effective pull-through at the MP joints in case the change of direction has placed some cross connection under tension. Brand leaves the two best tendons long to join the FCR, suturing the other two to their neighbors more distally. The tendon juncture is done as shown in Figure 37-10, passing the two slips of the EDC into slits in the FCR and burying their ends in a second slit. With the tendons left long, care is taken to ensure appropriate tension on each of the four tendons before making the final cut of the tendons and burying their ends. I would recommend suturing the tendons with the wrist and MP joints in neutral and the FCR tendon under maximum tension. Tsuge[57] has modified the FCR transfer by passing it through the interosseous membrane to obtain a straighter line of pull.

The PL to rerouted EPL transfer is performed as described on page 1490. If the PL is absent, the EPL is joined with the EDC to the FCR transfer.[12] Postoperative management is the same as that described on page 1490.

AUTHOR'S PREFERRED METHOD

I believe it is important for the hand surgeon to be well versed in a least two of the aforementioned transfers, for it is preferable to choose an operation for the individual patient rather than to try to adapt all patients to a single procedure.

In general, I prefer to use the standard (FCU) set

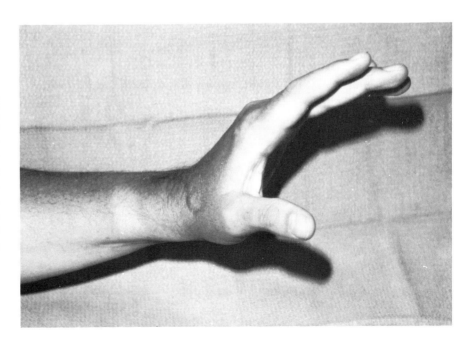

Fig. 37-11. Simultaneous extension of the fingers and wrist is not possible after transfer of a wrist flexor (FCR or FCU) to the finger extensors because of limited tendon excursion. It is possible to achieve this, however, with the Boyes superficialis transfer, as shown in this patient (compare with Fig. 37-3).

of transfers except in patients with posterior interosseous nerve palsy. In those patients, I believe that the resulting radial deviation is unacceptable, and I prefer to use Boyes' superficialis transfer. I agree with Boyes and colleagues that the only way to achieve simultaneous active extension of the wrist and fingers is with the superficialis transfer, although in my experience this goal is more likely to be achieved in children than in adults (Fig. 37-11).

Except for the FCU transfer in patients with posterior interosseous nerve palsy, I have been pleased with the results of both sets of transfers. I have had less experience with the FCR transfer, but its principles are sound, the credentials of its proponents are solid, and there may be some merit in preserving the important FCU as a wrist flexor.

RADIAL NERVE PALSY ASSOCIATED WITH FRACTURES OF THE HUMERUS

Few topics generate more heated or emotional discussion in a fracture conference than radial nerve palsy associated with fractures of the humerus. The literature dealing with this topic over the past 30 years serves only to add to the controversy, for one can find at least one article to support virtually any plan of management. It is therefore important to review this entire spectrum of contradictory articles and consider each in its proper context and perspective. An attempt has been made to do that in this section.

The reported incidence of radial nerve palsy associated with humeral fractures has varied from 1.8 to 16 percent,[68-70] although some of these studies were selected or referred series and probably do not reflect an accurate incidence. Using data from a consecutive series of humeral shaft fractures in a major trauma center,[71] the actual incidence is probably less than 10 percent.

There are basically three ways in which radial nerve palsy seen with a humeral shaft fracture can be managed; a discussion of each follows.

Early Exploration of the Nerve

Several authors[64,69,77] have advocated that all radial nerve injuries associated with humeral shaft fractures should be treated with early exploration. They cite the following theoretical advantages to support this position.

1. The status of the nerve (i.e., is it intact, contused, entrapped in the fracture site, impaled on a fragment, or divided?) can be ascertained at the time of injury, thereby facilitating decisions regarding nerve repair or tendon transfers.
2. Stabilization of the fracture by internal fixation protects the radial nerve from further damage.
3. Early operation is technically easier and safer.

Several aspects of these arguments require closer scrutiny. The first question has to do with how many of these patients have a "surgically correctable" lesion. Sim[77] stated that "remediable lesions were encountered too frequently to ignore early exploration," but Kettlekamp et al[67] came to exactly the opposite conclusion after having found *no* surgically correctable lesions in any of the 16 radial nerves that they explored.

In a paper published in 1963 that has since been frequently quoted, Holstein and Lewis[66] described a fracture of the distal humerus in which the radial nerve is in particular jeopardy. The proximal spike of this spiral fracture breaks through the lateral cortex of the humerus at or near the point where the nerve is most closely apposed to the bone as it passes through the lateral intermuscular septum from the posterior to the anterior compartment of the arm. Their findings in seven patients with this particular lesion led Holstein and Lewis to the conclusion that early operative intervention was indicated in all such patients. However, a more recent and larger collection of Holstein-Lewis fractures with radial nerve palsy reported by Szalay and Rockwood[79] concluded that early operative treatment is not necessary. Of their 15 patients with this combination of injuries, all 11 who were treated without exploration had complete nerve recovery, and in the 4 patients in whom exploration was carried out, the nerve was found to be in continuity and all had full recovery of nerve function.

Another point regarding early exploration deals

with those patients who develop "secondary" radial nerve paralysis in conjunction with a fractured humerus; that is, where the nerve is intact when the patient is first seen and subsequently goes out, usually following fracture reduction. In several articles,[63,64,76] this situation is given as an absolute indication for immediate nerve exploration, although Shah and Bhatti[75] offered convincing evidence that even secondary radial nerve paralysis can be treated nonoperatively with good expectations for full recovery in most cases.

Finally, the source of the clinical material for each of these studies must be examined. Those who most strongly advocate early exploration based their conclusions on series of patients treated in referral centers (The New York Orthopaedic Hospital[64,69] and the Mayo Clinic[77]), where the percentage of complicated problems and failures from other treatment facilities is unusually high. Sim[63] in fact acknowledged that his series from the Mayo Clinic was difficult to evaluate because most of the patients were referred. Conversely, in those studies drawn from major trauma centers where consecutive series of patients with humeral shaft fractures complicated by radial nerve palsy were evaluated, the authors[71,75,79] all agree that nonoperative management of the radial nerve palsy is the treatment of choice.

Exploration at 6 to 8 Weeks if no Return

Shaw and Sakellarides[76] reviewed a series of patients from the Massachusetts General Hospital in 1967 and concluded that the nerve should be explored at 7 to 8 weeks if there is no evidence of return of function. They offered the following reasons for this decision.

1. All patients in their series showed some signs of recovery of nerve function within the first 2 months.
2. An unnecessary operation will be avoided in most patients, in whom spontaneous nerve recovery will occur.
3. There is no interference with fracture healing.
4. The waiting period allows the neuroma to become well delineated and hence to be adequately resected, but is short enough to minimize nerve retraction.

Goldner and Kelley[65] advocated a similar position, but considered the absence of an advancing Tinel's sign to be an important added indication for exploration at 6 to 8 weeks. However, they went on to say that "a longer waiting period could not be criticized, because some of the patients in this group recovered completely without sign of motor recovery for 20 weeks."

Nerve Exploration if no Return After a Longer Waiting Period

Since it is well documented that the *initial* signs of motor recovery may not appear until 4 or 5 months after a radial nerve palsy associated with a fractured humerus, a third option is available. This plan of management is based upon the work of Seddon[72-74] regarding nerve regeneration and is best summarized in the abstract by Szalay and Rockwood.[79] Assuming that a nerve regenerates at the rate of approximately 1 mm a day and adding 30 days as Seddon has suggested,[72] the maximum length of time that *may be required* for motor recovery to *first* manifest itself can easily be calculated by measuring the distance on the x-ray from the fracture site to the point of innervation of the brachioradialis muscle (approximately 2 cm above the lateral epicondyle[74]). In most midshaft humerus fracures, this distance is approximately 90 to 120 mm (Fig. 37-12). Thus, if there is no evidence of return of function in the brachioradialis or radial wrist extensors by the calculated time interval (usually 4 to 5 months), exploration is indicated. The major advantages of this plan of management are: (1) unnecessary operative intervention is avoided in the large majority of patients; (2) most of these patients will regain full recovery of the radial nerve without surgical treatment; and (3) the humerus fracture will usually be healed.

A question that must be raised of course is whether or not the delay in nerve repair for those very few patients in whom neurorrhaphy becomes necessary is excessive and will lessen the chances for good functional recovery. According to Sunderland,[78] a delay of 12 months or even longer is

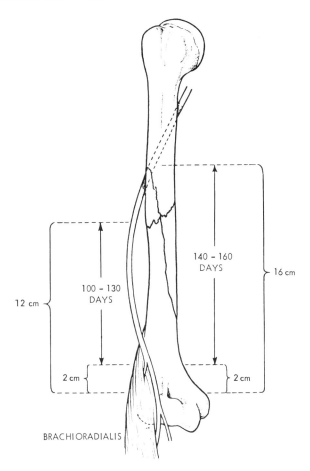

140 - 160
DAYS

16 cm

100 - 130
DAYS

12 cm

2 cm

2 cm

BRACHIORADIALIS

Fig. 37-12. Calculation of the time that must elapse before signs of recovery can be expected after fractures of the shaft of the humerus causing a degenerative lesion of the radial nerve. The information on the left is for a transverse fracture; on the right, for an oblique fracture. (Seddon HJ: Surgical Disorders of the Peripheral Nerves. 2nd Ed. p. 246. Churchill Livingstone, Edinburgh, 1975.)

not likely to jeopardize functional motor return following nerve repair, and Seddon[72,74] has reported that prognosis for good recovery worsens only after a 12-month delay.

Author's Preferred Method

It has long been my policy to treat most patients with radial nerve palsy associated with humeral shaft fractures nonoperatively, considering exploration of the nerve only after a *realistic* waiting time as outlined in the third option described above and illustrated in Fig. 37-12.

There are, however, certain specific indications for early operative treatment of humeral shaft fractures, which in my opinion, include the following: (1) open fractures; (2) fractures in which satisfactory alignment cannot be achieved by closed reduction techniques; and (3) fractures with associated vascular injuries. In all such cases, I believe that it is imperative to expose and make visible the radial nerve at the time of operative intervention.

Based upon studies previously cited, I do not consider a secondary nerve radial nerve palsy (i.e., occurring after fracture manipulation), to be *in itself* an absolute indication for early nerve exploration. Rather, I would still rely upon the three indications noted above for early nerve exploration.

Following these indications, it must be acknowledged that there will be a very few patients in whom spontaneous return of function will not occur, but my experience is similar to that of others who have shown that these patients will be so few that routine exploration of all radial nerve injuries is not justified.

Finally, although I favor the third option for management, I find less objection to early exploration than to exploration at 6 to 8 weeks. There may be some valid arguments for early exploration, but in my opinion there is no sound rationale for exploring the nerve at 6 to 8 weeks. If the decision has been made to await spontaneous return of function, I believe that it is only reasonable to wait an *appropriate* period of time.

REFERENCES

1. Adams J, Wood VE: Tendon transfers for irreparable nerve damage in the hand. Orthop Clin North Am 12:403–432, April 1981
2. Albright JA, Linburg RM: Common variations of the radial wrist extensors. J Hand Surg 3:134–138, 1978
3. Altman H, Trott RH: Muscle transplantation for paralysis of the radial nerve. J Bone Joint Surg 28:440–446, 1946
4. Beasley RW: Tendon transfers for radial nerve palsy. Orthop Clin North Am 1:439–445, Nov 1970
5. Bevin AG: Early tendon transfer for radial nerve transection. Hand 8:134–136, 1976

6. Billington RW: Tendon transplantation for musculo-spiral (radial) nerve injury. J Bone Joint Surg 4:538–547, 1922

7. Boyes JH: Tendon transfers in the hand. In Medicine in Japan in 1959 (Proceedings of the 15th General Assembly of the Japan Medical Congress), 5:958–969, 1959

8. Boyes JH: Tendon transfers for radial palsy. Bull Hosp Joint Dis 21:97–105, 1960

9. Boyes JH: Selection of a donor muscle for tendon transfer. Bull Hosp Joint Dis 23:1–4, 1962

10. Boyes JH: Bunnell's Surgery of the Hand. 4th Ed. JB Lippincott, Philadelphia, 1964

11. Brand PW: Biomechanics of tendon transfer. Orthop Clin North Am 5:205–230, 1974

12. Brand PW: Tendon transfers in the forearm. In Flynn JE (ed): Hand Surgery. 2nd Ed. Williams & Wilkins, Baltimore, 1975

13. Brodman HR: Tendon transfer for old radial nerve paralysis. Arch Surg 76:24–27, 1958

14. Brooks D: Peripheral nerve injuries: Reconstructive techniques. pp. 20–25. In Rob E, Smith R (eds): Operative Surgery, Vol. 8. Butterworths, London, 1969

15. Brown PW: The time factor in surgery of upper-extremity peripheral nerve injury. Clin Orthop 68:14–21, Jan–Feb 1970

16. Burkhalter WE: Early tendon transfer in upper extremity peripheral nerve injury. Clin Orthop 104:68–79, Oct 1974

17. Chuinard RG, Boyes JH, Stark HH, Ashworth CR: Tendon transfers for radial nerve palsy: Use of superficialis tendons for digital extension. J Hand Surg 3:560–570, 1978

18. Curtis RM: Fundamental principles of tendon transfer. Orthop Clin North Am 5:231–242, 1974

19. Dunn N: Treatment of lesion of the musculo-spiral nerve in military surgery. Am J Orthop Surg 16:258–265, 1918

20. Entin MA: Restoration of function of paralyzed hand. Surg Clin North Am 44:1049–1059, 1964

21. Goldner JL, Kelley JM: Radial nerve injuries. South Med J 51:873–883, 1958

22. Henry AK: Extensile Exposure. 2nd Ed. Williams & Wilkins, Baltimore, 1957

23. Jones R: On suture of nerves, and alternative methods of treatment by transplantation of tendon. Br Med J 1:641–643, 1916

24. Jones R: On suture of nerves, and alternative methods of treatment by transplantation of tendon. Br Med J 1:679–682, 1916

25. Jones R: Tendon transplantation in cases of musculospiral injuries not amenable to suture. Am J Surg 35:333–335, 1921

26. Littler JW: Restoration of power and stability in the partially paralyzed hand. pp. 3266–3280. In Converse JM (ed): Reconstructive Plastic Surgery. 2nd Ed. WB Saunders, Philadelphia, 1977

27. Luckey CA, McPherson SR: Tendinous reconstruction of the hand following irreparable injury to the peripheral nerves and brachial plexus. J Bone Joint Surg 29:560–581, 1947

28. Mayer L: The physiological method of tendon transplantation. Surg Gynecol Obstet 22:182–197, 1916

29. MacKinnon SE, Dellon AL: The overlap pattern of the antebrachial cutaneous nerve and the superficial branch of the radial nerve. J Hand Surg 10A:522–526, 1985

30. McMinn RMH, Hutchings RT: Color Atlas of Human Anatomy. Chicago, Year Book Medical, 1977

31. Milford LW: Radial nerve palsy. pp. 297-300. In Edmonson AS, Crenshaw AH (eds): Campbell's Operative Orthopaedics, Vol. 1. 6th Ed. CV Mosby, St Louis, 1980

32. Moberg E, Nachemson A: Tendon transfers for defective long extensors of the wrist and fingers. Acta Chir Scand 133:31–34, 1967

33. Omer GE: Evaluation and reconstruction of the forearm and hand after acute traumatic peripheral nerve injuries. J Bone Joint Surg 50A:1454–1478, 1968

34. Omer GE: The technique and timing of tendon transfers. Orthop Clin North Am 5:243–252, 1974

35. Omer GE: Tendon transfers for reconstruction of the forearm and hand following peripheral nerve injuries. In Omer GE, Spinner M (eds): Management of Peripheral Nerve Problems. WB Saunders, Philadelphia, 1980

36. Omer GE: Reconstructive procedures for extremities with peripheral nerve defects. Clin Orthop 163:80–91, 1982

37. Parker D: Radial nerve paralysis treated by tendon transplant and arthrodesis of the wrist. J Bone Joint Surg 45B:626, 1963

38. Parkes AR: Some useful tendon transplants. J Bone Joint Surg 41B:217, 1959

39. Penner DA: Dorsal splint for radial palsy. Am J Occup Ther 26:46–47, 1972

40. Pulvertaft RG: Techniques in hand surgery. J Bone Joint Surg 42A:907, 1960

41. Riordan DC: Surgery of the paralytic hand. pp. 79-90. AAOS Instructional Course Lectures, Vol. 16. CV Mosby, St Louis, 1959

42. Riordan DC: Tendon transfers for nerve paralysis of the hand and wrist. Curr Prac Orthop Surg 2:17–40, 1964

43. Riordan DC: Tendon transfers for median, ulnar or radial nerve palsy. J Bone Joint Surg 50B:441, 1968

44. Riordan DC: Radial nerve paralysis. Orthop Clin North Am 5:283–287, 1974

45. Riordan DC: Tendon transfers in hand surgery. J Hand Surg 8(2):748–753, 1983

46. Said GZ: A modified tendon transference for radial nerve paralysis. J Bone Joint Surg 56B:320–322, 1974

47. Saikku LA: Tendon transplantation for radial paralysis. Factors influencing the results of tendon transplantation. Acta Chir Scand 96:suppl. 132:7–100, 1947

48. Scuderi C: Tendon transplants for irreparable radial nerve paralysis. Surg Gynecol Obstet 88:643–651, 1949

49. Seddon H: Surgical Disorders of the Peripheral Nerves. 2nd Ed. p. 31. Churchill Livingstone, Edinburgh, 1975

50. Spinner M: The radial nerve. pp. 28–65. In Injuries to the Major Branches of Peripheral Nerves of the Forearm. WB Saunders, Philadelphia, 1972

51. Starr CL: Army experiences with tendon transference. J Bone Joint Surg 4:3–21, 1922

52. Steindler A: Operative treatment of paralytic conditions of the upper extremity. J Orthop Surg 1:608–624, 1919

53. Stiles HJ: Operative treatment of nerve injuries. Am J Orthop Surg 16:351–363, 1918

54. Thomas FB: A splint for radial (musculospiral) nerve palsy. J Bone Joint Surg 26:602–605, 1944

55. Thomas FB: An improved splint for radial (musculospiral) nerve paralysis. J Bone Joint Surg 33B:272–273, 1951

56. Thomsen M, Rasmussen KB: Tendon transfers for defective long extensors of the wrist and fingers. Scand J Plast Reconstr Surg 3:71–78, 1969

57. Tsuge K, Adachi N: Tendon transfer for extensor palsy of forearm. Hiroshima J Med Sci 18:219–232, 1969

58. Wehbe MA, Hunter JM: Flexor tendon gliding in the hand. Part I. In vivo excursions. J Hand Surg 10A:570–574, 1985

59. White WL: Restoration of function and balance of the wrist and hand by tendon transfers. Surg Clin North Am 40: 427–459, 1960

60. Youm H, Thambyrajah K, Flatt AE: Tendon excursion of wrist movers. J Hand Surg 9A:202–209, 1984

61. Young HH, Lowe GH: Tendon transfer operation for irreparable paralysis of the radial nerve. Surg Gynecol Obstet 84:1100–1104, 1947

62. Zachary RB: Tendon transplantation for radial paralysis. Br J Surg 23:350–364, 1946

Radial Nerve Palsy Associated with Fractures of the Humerus

63. Duncan DM, Johnson KA, Monkman GR: Fracture of the humerus and radial nerve palsy. Minn Med 57:659–662, 1974

64. Garcia A, Maeck BH: Radial nerve injuries in fractures of the shaft of the humerus. Am J Surg 99:625–627, 1960

65. Goldner JL, Kelley JM: Radial nerve injuries. South Med J 51:873–883, 1958

66. Holstein A, Lewis GB: Fractures of the humerus with radial-nerve paralysis. J Bone Joint Surg 45A:1382–1388, 1963

67. Kettelkamp DB, Alexander H: Clinical review of radial nerve injury. J Trauma 7:424–431, 1967

68. Klenerman L: Fractures of the shaft of the humerous. J Bone Joint Surg 48B:105–111, 1966

69. Packer JW, Foster RR, Garcia A, Grantham SA: The humeral fracture with radial nerve palsy: Is exploration warranted? Clin Orthop 88:34–38, 1972

70. Pennsylvania Orthopaedic Society: Fresh midshaft fractures of the humerus in adults: Evaluation of treatment in Pennsylvania during 1952-1956, made by Scientific Research Committee, Pennsylvania Orthopaedic Society. Penn Med J 62:848–850, 1959

71. Pollock FH, Drake D, Bovill EG, Day L, Trafton PG: Treatment of radial neuropathy associated with fractures of the humerus. J Bone Joint Surg 63A:239–243, 1981

72. Seddon HJ: Nerve lesions complicating certain closed bone injuries. JAMA 135:691–694, 1947

73. Seddon HJ: The practical value of nerve repair (President's Address). Proc Roy Soc Med 42:427–436, 1949

74. Seddon HJ: Surgical Disorders of the Peripheral Nerves. 2nd Ed. p. 242–249. Churchill Livingstone, Edinburgh, 1975

75. Shah JJ, Bhatti NA: Radial nerve paralysis associated with fractures of the humerus. Clin Orthop 172:171–176, 1983

76. Shaw JL, Sakellarides H: Radial-nerve paralysis associated with fractures of the humerus. A review of the forty-five cases. J Bone Joint Surg 49A:899–902, 1967

77. Sim FH, Kelly PJ, Henderson ED: Radial-nerve palsy complicating fractures of the humeral shaft (Abstract). J Bone Joint Surg 53A:1023–1024, 1971

78. Sunderland S: Nerves and Nerve Injuries. 2nd Ed. pp. 508-509. Churchill Livingstone, Edinburgh, 1978

79. Szalay EA, Rockwood CA Jr: The Holstein-Lewis fracture revisited. Orthop Trans 7:516, 1983

Median Nerve Palsy

38

William E. Burkhalter

INTRINSIC REPLACEMENT IN MEDIAN NERVE PARALYSIS (RESTORATION OF OPPOSITION)

Median nerve paralysis most frequently is caused by penetrating or perforating wounds of the forearm or wrist area, and less commonly may be secondary to a fracture of the contiguous skeleton along the course of the nerve. In rare instances, the wound may involve only the median nerve. More frequently, however, there is damage to the flexor tendons in lower injuries and damage to the brachial artery in proximal injuries. The motor deficit involves primarily loss of opposition of the thumb in injuries at the level of the wrist or distal forearm, or loss of opposition of the thumb and severe weakness of the extrinsic flexors of the hand in the more proximal injuries. Because of variations of innervation involving primarily the flexor pollicis brevis, unsatisfactory positioning of the thumb following complete median nerve laceration may occur in only 60 to 70 percent of the patients. In other words, 30 to 40 percent of the people with complete median nerve lacerations will not require an opponensplasty regardless of the quality of return following neurorrhaphy.[3,49]

Restoration of opposition of the thumb by tendon transfer is the most commonly employed tendon transfer in the hand. Restoration of opposition (i.e., the development of true pulp-to-pulp pinch between the thumb and index finger or the thumb and index and long fingers) is required only in those patients in whom satisfactory sensibility is likely to be achieved. These patients, then, require precision pinch activities, and true opposition is likely to be required. In patients with limited motor units or poor sensibility, pulp-to-side transfer (i.e., restoration of short flexor action) is functionally as important as restoration of true opposition.

Early articles on restoration of opposition of the thumb all dealt with the completely intrinsic-minus thumb. Methods of restoration in these cases were aimed at bringing about short flexor action rather than true opposition of the thumb, as pointed out by Bunnell.[34,35,39,46,50,55] Opposition is a composite of two motions: (1) rotation of the thumb into pronation so that the pulp surfaces of the thumb and index finger face one another, and (2) abduction or lifting of the thumb away from the palm of the hand (palmar abduction). This combination of the two motions is true opposition. In order to render the thumb maximally functional, not only must the thumb be positioned in true opposition, but it must have, in addition, short flexor action so that it can be brought against the fingers with reasonable

1499

power through the MP and carpometacarpal joints of the thumb. So-called adductor transfers for power pinch are really not necessary because the adductor pollicis functions as a supinator of the thumb and is a direct antagonist to the pronatory effects that are being restored. A reasonable compromise is a short flexorplasty rather than an adductorplasty (Curtis RM: personal communication). In order to have a maximally functional thumb, the patient should be able to put the thumb into opposition, but also should have short flexor action so that the thumb can be brought against the fingers with power.[58] Without satisfactory function of the short flexor muscles or a short flexor substitute, the extensor pollicis longus becomes the only satisfactory substitute for adductor action. This muscle, through its secondary actions, brings the thumb out of opposition into the supinated position, in addition to bringing about adduction of the first metacarpal.[36] Littler has pointed out that the extensor pollicis longus is the direct antagonist of opposition of the thumb, and although satisfactory opposition may be achieved by any type of opposition transfer, collapse of this opposed position will occur if the extensor pollicis longus is used to substitute for the short flexor adductor group of muscles.[31]

The literature on opposition transfer and the reasons for its failure are most interesting. As pointed out initially by Mayer, the most absolute reason for failure is contracture of the first web space, either the adduction type or the adduction-supination type[37] (Fig. 38-1). In both of these situations, the thumb cannot really be placed into the fully opposed position passively at the time of transfer. To perform an opponensplasty in the face of a web space contracture indicates either failure to appreciate the problem or to understand what a supination contracture is in terms of rotational deformity in the thumb.[25] If there is a persisting supination contracture, regardless of the motor or pulley used, the operation will bring about only short flexor action without true opposition.[8,18,22,38] If true opposition is to be obtained, the thumb needs to be brought away from the fingers, in addition to being rotated on its long axis into pronation.

Another cause of failure in opposition transfer is inaccurate evaluation of the strength of the individual motor to be used for transfer. If a patient has an isolated laceration of the median nerve, the radial and ulnar innervated musculature should certainly be graded normal or near normal, and we assume that such will be the case. However, in certain disease states or in spotty lesions associated with brachial plexus injury, the motor in question may not have normal strength and, in fact, may not provide sufficient power to position the thumb.[18] Much of our experience in determining individual muscle strength and the basic principles of tendon transfer came from a disease that we no longer see much of — poliomyelitis.

Another area of some concern is the use of reinnervated muscles in an opposition transfer. We are all partial to the use of the flexor digitorum superficialis of the ring finger as the motor for an opponensplasty. In an undamaged state, this muscle tendon unit is an excellent functional transfer and has certainly withstood the test of time.[19,27,30] However, in proximal nerve injury with reinnervation of extrinsic flexors, its use to achieve satisfactory opposition through a transfer should be discouraged. Reinnervated flexor digitorum superficialis muscles lack the strength and certainly the control to bring about satisfactory opposition of the thumb.[3] In summary, then, the two major causes for failure of opposition transfer are the persistence of a contracture, either adduction or adduction-supination, and the use of an inadequate motor for transfer.[1,2]

When choosing a specific type of opposition transfer for an individual patient, I think it is mandatory for the hand surgeon to consider what the situation is that requires the opposition transfer. Is this an isolated peripheral nerve injury or is there associated damage to muscle tendon units and to bone? Is there more than one nerve damaged? What is the level of injury? Has there been direct injury to the soft tissues and perhaps the bone of the thumb itself, in addition to its extrinsics or intrinsics? No single opposition transfer will work for all cases requiring opponensplasty because of the wide variety in patient requirements and associated deficits. In addition to having motors of adequate strength with satisfactory amplitude, a reasonable bed, and tissue equilibrium, the transfer should be expected to do only one other thing and that is to bring about opposition of the thumb. One of the precepts of Steindler[54] and Mayer[37] not often

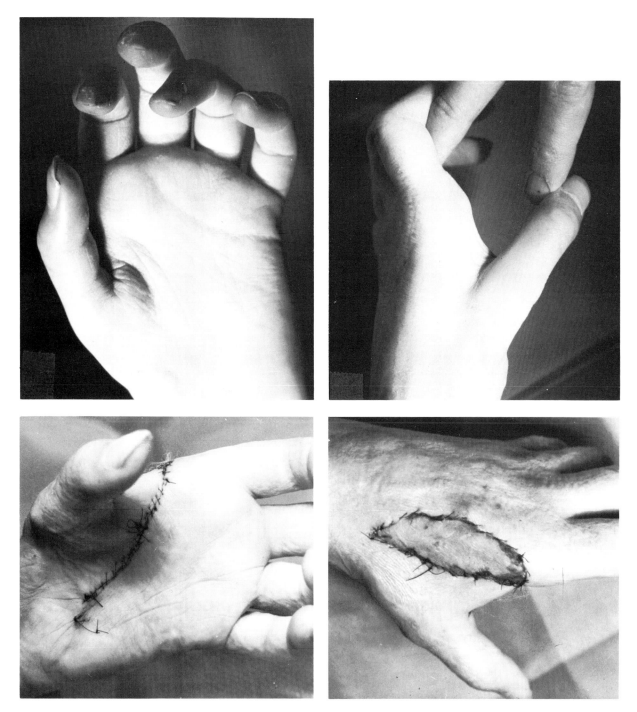

Fig. 38-1. Direct injury to the thenar area, in addition to median nerve laceration, resulted in a significant contracture of the thumb web space, which required release prior to opponensplasty. Position of the thumb was maintained by a threaded Steinmann pin, and a dorsal rotation flap with skin graft allowed good release of the first web space. In certain severe situations, osteotomy of the first metacarpal or excision of the trapezium may be indicated to satisfactorily position the thumb prior to opposition transfer.

considered is that the deficit created by the transfer should be acceptable to the patient. The use of the abductor digiti minimi for opposition transfer in a high median nerve injury will bring about satisfactory position of the thumb. However, the removal of this muscle tendon unit from the ulnar side of the hand will further compromise the already weakened strength on the flexor side, and I think this would be unacceptable to the patient.

Royle-Thompson Opponensplasty

The most frequently used motor for opponensplasty of the thumb is the flexor digitorum superficialis of either the ring or long finger. The so-called Royle-Thompson opposition transfer uses the motor from the ring finger as described by Royle.[50] Royle, however, used no pulley for the transfer; instead, he passed the motor up the sheath of the flexor pollicis longus and attached the split superficialis tendon to the superficial head of the flexor pollicis brevis and the opponens pollicis, respectively. Thompson's modification of this procedure was to use a pulley and a more superficial location of the transfer. The pulley for this procedure is the distal end of the transverse carpal ligament and the ulnar border of the palmar fascia.[57] The route of the transferred digitorum superficialis is subcutaneous across the palm to the area of the thumb MP joint. A dual attachment is made: one through a drill hole in the neck of the first metacarpal, while the other slip of the superficialis is drawn over the MP joint and sutured into the hood mechanism over the proximal phalanx. Three incisions are required for this procedure.

Some thought needs to be given to the removal of the superficialis tendon from the ring finger. Both a persistent flexion contracture of the PIP joint and swan-neck deformity have been reported in as many as 8 percent of the cases in which the superficialis was removed from a finger for a transfer.[26] A volar zigzag or transverse incision is used to cut the dual attachments of the flexor digitorum superficialis in the finger. The distal tags should be long enough so that the volar plate may be reinforced with a few nonabsorbable sutures to these tags. To remove the flexor digitorum superficialis from its insertion into the middle phalanx is to invite a swan-neck deformity. An additional palmar incision will probably be required so that the distal union of the superficialis can be longitudinally opened completely and the flexor digitorum superficialis freed from its loop about the flexor digitorum profundus. The perforation of the flexor digitorum superficialis by the profundus occurs beneath the fibrous (A2) pulley of the proximal phalanx, and it is best to operate distally and proximally to this, leaving the pulley intact.[24,28] This is the usual or classic description of removal of the flexor digitorum superficialis.

An easier method than to operate in the finger is to remove the tendon through an incision in the distal palm only. When using the flexor digitorum superficialis for an opposition transfer, there is adequate tendon length without going into the finger. Generally an incision at the base of the finger will allow opening the flexor tendon sheath between the MP (A1) pulley and the wide proximal phalangeal (A2) pulley. The superficialis begins to divide here and is still located superficial to the profundus. If the superficialis is divided here, the problem with the decussation is avoided and the volar area of the PIP joint is not violated.[41]

At this point another incision is made immediately distal to the carpal tunnel, toward the ulnar side, so that the palmar fascia can be retracted radially. The flexor digitorum superficialis to the ring finger is identified at the distal level of the carpal tunnel. An incision is then made over the dorsum of the MP joint of the thumb and a subcutaneous tunnel is created between the incision in the wrist and the area of the thumb MP joint. The flexor digitorum superficialis is delivered from the finger into the palmar incision and passed subcutaneously across the palm of the hand to the incision on the dorsum of the thumb MP joint. If done in the classic fashion, a drill hole is created through the neck of the first metacarpal and one slip of the superficialis is pulled through this, exiting on the ulnar aspect of the thumb (Fig. 38-2). The second slip of the superficialis is passed superficially over the extensor hood of the MP joint, under the ulnar lateral band of the extensor mechanism of the thumb, and out through a small transverse incision immediately dorsal to the lateral band. The two ends are then sutured together. Prior to this, the tourniquet

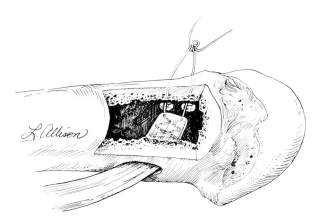

Fig. 38-2. Method of bony attachment of a tendon using internal sutures rather than external pull-out techniques. The opposite cortex from the area of entrance of the tendon is used to anchor the stitch. This, however, does require an incision on the side opposite to the tendon entrance for exposure of the cortex and tying of the suture.

should be released and hemostasis obtained. Before suturing the attachment of the transfer, all wounds should be closed, with the exception of the one in the area of the thumb MP joint.

The correct tension is always a major consideration in opposition transfer. In this particular transfer, it is not terribly important because of the enormous amplitude of the flexor digitorum superficialis. However, the tension should be adjusted primarily with the distal attachment in this case. If the reverse is done, no power will be transferred to the extensor pollicis longus or to the proximal phalanx of the thumb, and the transfer will act only on the first metacarpal. Tension is adjusted so that the thumb is in full opposition with the wrist in neutral position. This method of attachment makes the thumb MP joint extremely stable, with some abduction of the joint and some increase in power to the extensor pollicis longus. This transfer courses in line with the fibers of the flexor pollicis brevis superficial head and thus reproduces the action of this muscle. It does not give as wide abduction to the thumb as some other methods, but it is an extremely useful transfer for the completely intrinsic-minus thumb (combined median and ulnar palsy) and in situations with limited motors available for transfer.[23,48]

Classic Bunnell Opponensplasty

With this information as a background, other possible opposition transfers can be considered. In 1938 Bunnell established what have become the standard requirements for restoration of true opposition of the thumb. His precepts were that the transfer should come from the area of the pisiform to the thumb MP joint subcutaneously. The transfer should have a fixed pulley in the area of the pisiform, the transfer essentially being in line with the fibers of the abductor pollicis brevis. Bunnell's method of attachment distally was through a drill hole on the dorsal ulnar aspect of the proximal phalanx. The transfer thus passed distal to the axis of motion of the MP joint and thereby acted as an MP joint flexor in addition to being a rotator-abductor.[10] This flexion may not be desirable in an operation in which the main function is to position the thumb for use where true short flexor action is already available from other muscles within the hand.

The operative technique of Bunnell is as follows. The method of removal of the superficialis from the ring finger is as described on page 1502. At this point, a word should be said regarding the removal of the flexor digitorum superficialis of the long finger. Removal of this muscle has been done to restore opposition to the thumb, but I believe that this creates too much deficit on the flexor side of the hand. The superficialis to the long finger is an extremely powerful muscle with individual control. I believe that its removal creates an almost unacceptable deficit for the patient in terms of power grip. I suggest that other transfers be used rather than using the superficialis to the long finger. Once the ring finger superficialis is removed, another incision is made proximal to the wrist over the ulnar artery and nerve area. In this fashion the flexor digitorum superficialis to the ring finger can be readily found proximally and the tendon of the flexor carpi ulnaris identified. Three to four centimeters of flexor carpi ulnaris tendon are exposed proximal to the pisiform, and approximately one-half of the flexor carpi ulnaris tendon is divided at this proximal level; that is, a 3- to 4-cm strip of tendon is separated from the remaining portion of the intact flexor carpi ulnaris longitudinally, leaving it attached distally to the pisiform. An incision is then made on the dorsum of the thumb and a subcutaneous tunnel created across the palm from the thumb to the area of the pisiform. The flexor digitorum superficialis of the ring is then delivered into the wrist incision and passed subcutaneously from the pisiform to the thumb incision. The distally based slip of the flexor carpi ulnaris is then sutured to the area of the pisiform to create a fixed loop through which the flexor digitorum superficialis can easily pass passively. Care should be taken not to make this loop too tight, making free motion of the flexor superficialis impossible. It seems much easier to simply loop the flexor digitorum superficialis around the flexor carpi ulnaris prior to its subcutaneaous passage across the palm. However, the flexor carpi ulnaris soon becomes ineffective as a pulley, and the transfer then becomes incapable of positioning the thumb.[25] This occurs secondary to proximal migration of the point of direction change of the flexor digitorum superficialis (Fig. 38-3B). Other fixed pulleys in this area that might be used with the flexor digitorum superficialis transfer are the canal of Guyon, immediately radial to the flexor carpi ulnaris,[4] and a window created in the transverse carpal ligament.[53] Also, the slip of flexor carpi ulnaris that was developed to create the pulley loop may instead be sutured to the tendon of the extensor carpi ulnaris close to its attachment to the fifth metacarpal rather than to the pisiform.[51] All of these techniques are valuable and can be selected on the basis of individual preference and local conditions.

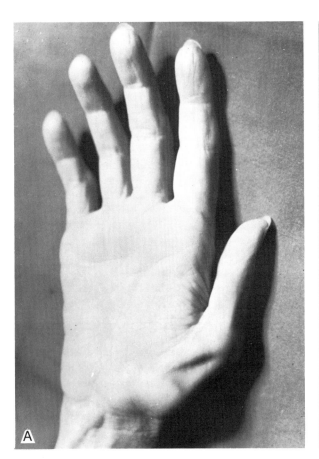
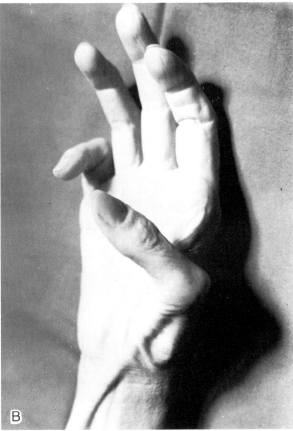

Fig. 38-3. A classic Bunnell transfer using the superficialis motor. However, there was no fixed pulley in the area of the pisiform and the transfer was too volar, acting more as a flexor of the MP joint than as a real abductor. Satisfactory opposition needs a fixed pulley at or near the area of the pisiform.

The method of attachment distally in the classic Bunnell transfer is through a drill hole in the proximal phalanx on its dorsal ulnar aspect. The tendon is passed subcutaneously across the palm, over the dorsum of the MP joint, but distal to the axis of motion of the joint. A drill hole is created from the dorsal ulnar aspect of the proximal phalanx to the midaxial line radially. This drill hole should be large enough to accommodate at least one slip of the flexor digitorum superficialis. Once the tendon is passed through the drill hole, it may be sutured upon itself, anchored to the periosteum on the radial aspect of the proximal phalanx, or held with a pull-out suture over a dental roll. Tension here is critical. At the completion of the operation, the thumb should rest in full opposition, with the wrist in neutral position.

Methods of Distal Attachment

Prior to discussing other transfers, the methods of distal attachment should be examined in some detail (Fig. 38-4). Both the Bunnell and Royle-Thompson operations use bony attachments. This is probably not necessary and complicates the procedure of opposition transfer unnecessarily. Littler feels that if the function of the abductor pollicis brevis can be duplicated by the opposition transfer, satsifactory function will result. Because of this, the transferred tendon is simply interwoven into the tendon of the abductor pollicis brevis muscle.[31] The Riordan attachment uses interweaving of the transfer into the abductor pollicis brevis tendon, but continuing distally into the hood of the thumb MP joint and to the extensor pollicis longus tendon over the proximal phalanx.[48] This course markedly increases the power of extension of the interphalangeal joint of the thumb. Without a functional flexor pollicis longus, a hyperextension deformity of the interphalangeal joint will likely result with this method of attachment. Brand's method of distal attachment interweaves one slip of the superficialis through the tendon of the abductor pollicis brevis and continues on to the extensor pollicis longus, similiar to Riordan's technique. The other slip, however, comes across the extensor mechanism subcutaneously and is attached to the area of the adductor pollicis. This method brings about considerable stability of the MP joint and is especially indicated in a combined median and ulnar nerve palsy.[4,44]

Phalen and Miller Opponensplasty (Extensor Carpi Ulnaris)

Other methods of distal attachment include the extensor pollicis brevis attachment.[29,45] Bunnell mentioned tenotomy of this muscle tendon unit and the use of the normal attachment of the extensor pollicis brevis as a method of attaching an opposition transfer to the thumb.[10] Using this technique, the extensor pollicis brevis is divided through a short incision at its musculotendinous junction proximal to the first dorsal compartment. An incision in the area of the MP joint is then used to expose the tendon immediately proximal to the MP joint, and the tendon is pulled distally and delivered into the wound. A subcutaneous tunnel is created from its attachment to the proximal phalanx toward the pisiform. Through another incision, the extensor carpi ulnaris is exposed immediately proximal to its attachment into the fifth metacarpal, cut, and freed proximally so that a subcutaneous passage can be made around the ulnar border of the wrist. Depending on the length of the extensor pollicis brevis tendon, the juncture will probably be in the area of the pisiform. This can be a difficult place in which to obtain a gliding tendon junction, but it does emphasize the subcutaneous border of the forearm as the pulley for tendon transfer, bringing about opposition of the thumb.[21] This border is used as a pulley for other transfers, notably the extensor indicis proprius and the extensor digiti minimi opponensplasties. In addition to being an awkward location for a tendon juncture, another problem may develop. The extensor pollicis brevis may slide volarly to the ulnar side of the MP joint so that it no longer acts as an extensor of the joint, acting as a flexor instead. This dorsal instability has been reported to be alleviated by looping the extensor pollicis brevis tendon around the tendon of the extensor pollicis longus prior to its attachment to the motor unit. This seems to provide better stability for the MP joint and prevent the flexion deformity.[28]

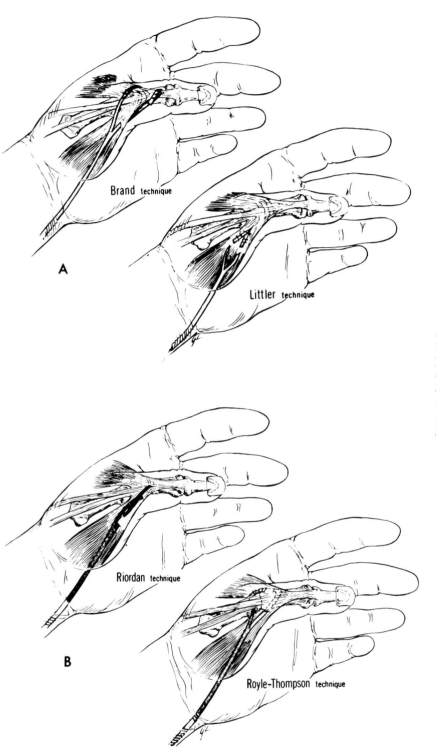

Fig. 38-4. Techniques of distal attachment as described by Brand, Littler, Riordan, and Royle-Thompson. (Curtis RM: Opposition of the thumb. Orthop Clin North Am 5:305–321, 1974. Reprinted with permission from WB Saunders Co, Philadelphia.)

Another combination of motor and distal attachment is the use of the extensor carpi radialis longus as a motor prolonged by the extensor pollicis longus tendon passed around the ulnar border of the wrist.[28] In my opinion, both the extensor carpi ulnaris–extensor pollicis brevis and extensor carpi radialis longus–extensor pollicis longus combination transfers are wasteful of motors that perform useful functions and also place undesirable forces on the MP joint of the thumb. It seems that the distal attachment techniques of Littler, Brand, and Riordan all reproduce the function of the abductor pollicis brevis, which is, after all, what the surgeon is trying to restore.

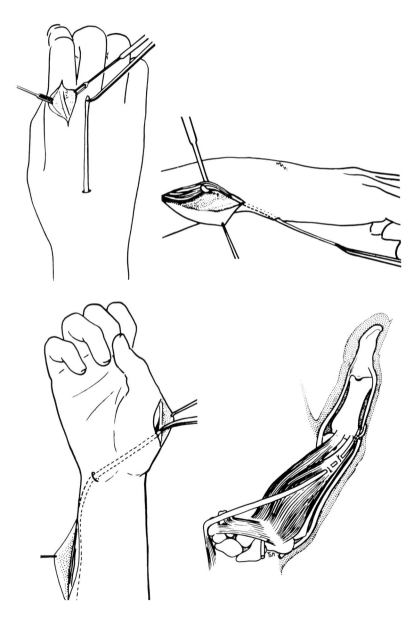

Fig. 38-5. The extensor indicis proprius tendon is removed with a small portion of extensor hood. The hood should be carefully repaired in order to avoid lag of the index finger in extension. An additional incision is usually required on the dorsum of the hand immediately distal to the retinaculum at the wrist. The extensor indicis proprius and extensor digitorum communis to the index finger may be joined in this area. A large incision on the dorsoulnar aspect of the wrist exposes the muscle belly of the extensor indicis proprius and allows the muscle to be placed on the ulnar aspect of the wrist. The tendon is passed subcutaneously around the ulnar aspect of the wrist, exiting in the area of the pisiform. Another subcutaneous passage is made across the palm to the area of the thumb joint. Riordan's technique of distal attachment is used if there is a functioning flexor pollicis longus. (Burkhalter WE, Christensen RC, Brown PW: Extensor indicis proprius opponensplasty. J Bone Joint Surg 55A:725–731, 1973.)

Proprius Extensor Tendon Opponensplasties

Recently both proprius tendon transfers have become popular because of the frequency of damage to muscle tendon units in the distal volar forearm. Both the extensor indicis proprius[11,15] (Fig.

38-5) and the extensor digiti minimi[52,56] (Fig. 38-6) have been described for restoration of opposition. These motors are both available in volar wrist injuries and combined median and ulnar nerve palsies, either high or low, and require only a single muscle tendon unit without a tendon graft. They do not significantly reduce remaining hand function and

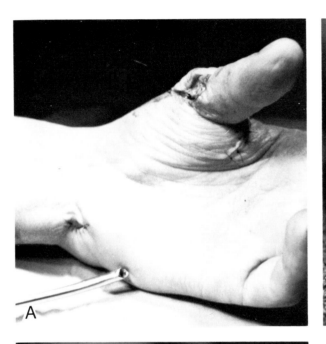

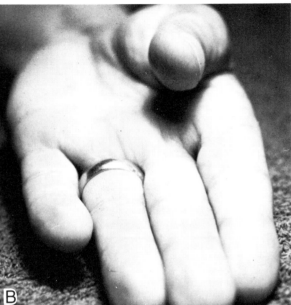

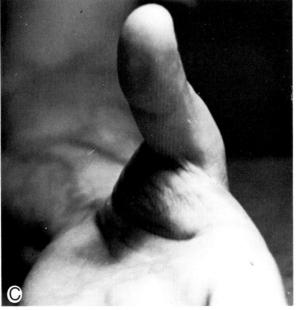

Fig. 38-6. Extensor digiti minimi transfer for opposition of the thumb. Note position at the time of surgery (**A**) and postoperative active abduction and rotation of the thumb (**B,C**) even with an immobile wrist.

the techniques of both are very similar. Short incisions are made over the MP joint of either the index or small finger. In the small finger, the presence of an extensor digitorum communis slip from the ring finger should be verified prior to removal of the extensor digiti minimi. Another short incision is made over the base of the fifth metacarpal, and a more extensive exposure is required over the distal forearm along its ulnar aspect. The extensor digiti minimi is brought into the more proximal incision, and a subcutaneous tunnel is created around the ulnar border of the forearm across the palm to the

area of the thumb MP joint. The method of attachment, as described by Schneider, uses Riordan's technique. As noted previously, the pulley for this transfer is the ulnar aspect of the forearm.[52]

In using the extensor indicis proprius, the tendon is removed along with a small portion of extensor hood. The removal of a portion of the extensor hood allows lengthening of the extensor indicis proprius tendon. The hood excision should taper from the tendon distally into the hood mechanism. This defect in the hood is carefully repaired with interrupted nonabsorbable sutures, an important

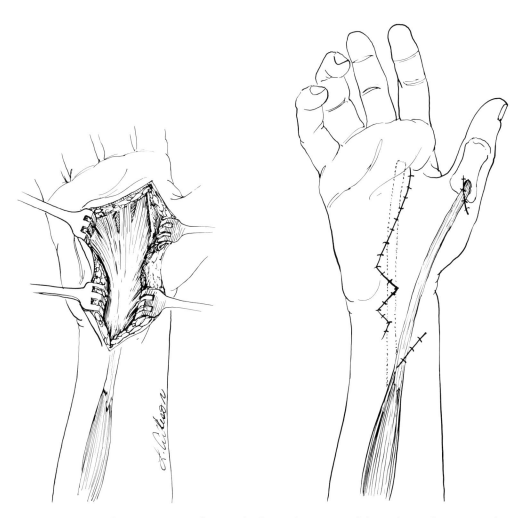

Fig. 38-7. The Camitz transfer in which an elongation of the palmaris longus via the palmar fascia is attached to the area of the abductor pollicis brevis. The subcutaneous tunnel for this transfer runs in a direct line from the wrist to the thumb.

step in preventing subsequent extensor lag by maintaining normal tension within the hood mechanism.[9]

An additional incision over the dorsum of the hand to separate the extensor indicis from the index communis is frequently required. A larger dorsal ulnar incision is made in the distal forearm. This is used to displace the tendon into the forearm on its ulnar aspect. An additional incision is usually made in the area of the pisiform as well as an incision in the area of the thumb MP joint. The tendon is then passed through the ulnar aspect of the wrist across to the MP joint. The attachment is made by Riordan's method, and the pulley again is the ulnar aspect of the forearm.[13]

All of the previously discussed opposition transfers require pulleys, whereas the following one does not.

Palmaris Longus Opponensplasty (Camitz)

A beautifully simple yet effective operation that brings about abduction of the thumb away from the fingers (palmar abduction) is transfer of the palmaris longus to the tendon of the abductor pollicis brevis. The palmaris longus will obviously not reach into the area of the MP joint of the thumb. The muscle tendon unit is prolonged by a strip of palmar fascia as originally described by Camitz[14] (Fig. 38-7). The area of the volar surface of the distal forearm, wrist, and palm are opened as for a generous carpal tunnel release. The palmaris longus tendon is exposed in the wrist, and the palmar skin flaps are elevated to expose the distal palmaris longus in continuity with the palmar fascia. A strip of palmar fascia in continuity with the palmaris longus is then removed. A subcutaneous tunnel is created from the volar surface of the distal forearm to the tendon of the abductor pollicis brevis. The palmar fascia is then pulled into the short incision in the area of the thumb MP joint and sutured into position. The tendon should pull in a straight line from the muscle belly to the thumb MP joint. This transfer does not bring about much in the way of rotation or pronation as the standard transfer, but does result in good palmar abduction of the thumb. The transfer loss is certainly accept-

able and the function is reasonable. The transfer has its greatest application in severe carpal tunnel syndromes with thenar paralysis and atrophy (Fig. 38-8). The procedure can be carried out simultaneously with carpal tunnel release.[6,33] Because of the proximity of the palmaris longus to the median nerve, its use in traumatic median nerve injuries at the wrist or distal forearm is limited. Similarly, the palmaris longus is denervated in the more proximal nerve injuries.

Hypothenar Muscle Opponensplasty (Huber)

Restoration of opposition of the thumb by transfer of an ulnar innervated intrinsic muscle was first described by Huber[24] and later by Nicolaysen,[40] and popularized by Littler and Cooley[32] (Fig. 38-9). The abductor digiti minimi muscle transfer is predicated on the fact that this muscle can survive and function on a thin neurovascular pedicle with almost its entire origin, and certainly its entire insertion, detached. The distal tendon is exposed by a midaxial incision over the proximal phalanx of the small finger ulnarly. The incision continues radially at the level of the distal palmar crease and then immediately radial to the hypothenar bulk. Proximally, the incision curves again ulnarly so as to cross the distal wrist crease. A separate incision is made over the thumb MP joint and a large subcutaneous tunnel created between the thumb area and that area immediately proximal to the pisiform. The flaps are raised and the ulnar digital nerve is carefully identified, elevated, and protected during this operation. The ulnar nerve and artery at the wrist are defined and traced distally until the branches can be seen entering the musculature of the abductor digiti minimi. Only after the neurovascular bundle has been isolated is the attachment of this muscle to the pisiform divided. At this point the muscle is held by its neurovascular pedicle and its attachment to the flexor carpi ulnaris (Fig. 38-10). The muscle is rotated 180 degrees on its long axis, much as one would close a book, and pulled through the subcutaneous tunnel into the thumb area. The distal tendon is then attached to the abductor pollicis brevis tendon only.

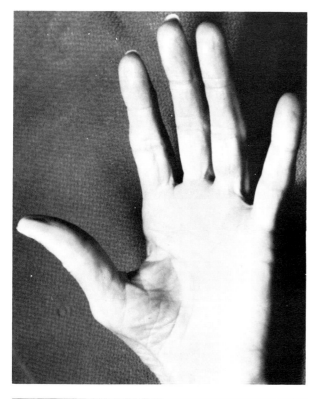

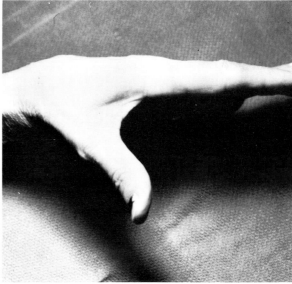

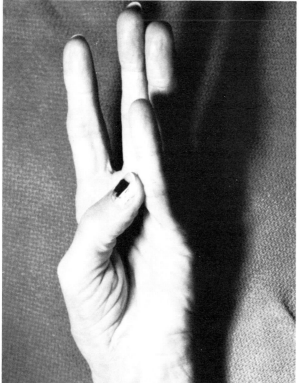

Fig. 38-8. A patient with a scapholunate dissociation and long-standing median nerve compression with thenar atrophy, treated at the time of carpal tunnel release by Camitz transfer. There was excellent improvement in abduction of the thumb, but note that there is not good active pronation of the thumb.

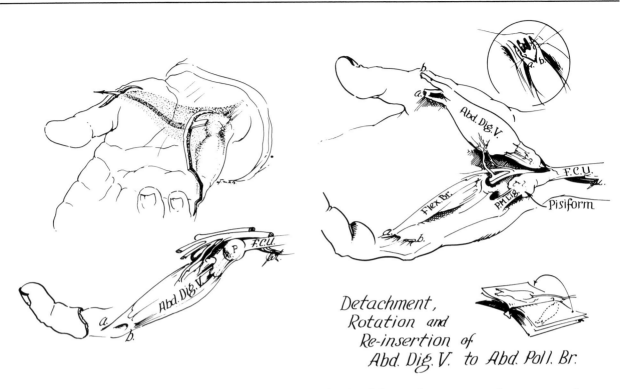

Fig. 38-9. Two incisions are required to expose and transfer the abductor digiti minimi. The neurovascular structures enter the muscle on its deep and radial aspect. The muscle is freed from its fascial attachments to the other hypothenar muscles and from its origin on the pisiform. The origin proximally is the flexor carpi ulnaris tendon. The muscle tendon unit is rotated 180 degrees on its long axis and passed between the palmar skin and palmar fascia to the area of the thumb MP joint. The distal attachment is into the tendon of the abductor pollicis brevis muscle. (Littler JW, Cooley SGE: Opposition of the thumb and its restoration by abductor digiti quinti transfer. J Bone Joint Surg 45A:1389–1396, 1963.)

In a more recent report,[59] the abductor digiti quinti is not detached from the pisiform and neurovascular structures are not exposed proximally. This limits mobility of this muscle unit proximally and moves the new origin more distally so that it acts more as a short flexor than as a true opponensplasty.

Other Opponensplasties

Another intrinsic opposition replacement, not done frequently in this country, is transfer of the adductor pollicis to the tendon of the superficial head of the flexor pollicis brevis. DeVecchi[17] described this procedure. Orticochea,[43] likewise, described the use of an innervated portion of the flexor pollicis brevis to bring about opposition to the thumb. The adductor pollicis transfer requires an extensive palmar incision, extending from the adductor attachment to the thumb into the palm in the area of the third metacarpal and then proximally toward the thumb. The carpal tunnel should be opened for exposure and protection of the median nerve and its branches. The adductor is released from the thumb, freed from the deep head of the flexor pollicis brevis, brought out from beneath the flexor tendons to the index finger, and passed over the tendons of the index finger, as well as the common neurovascular bundle to the adjacent sides of the index and long fingers. The transfer is then placed superficial to the flexor policis longus and attached to the flexor pollicis brevis superficial head only. This transfer restores function of the flexor pollicis brevis and gives some rotation to the thumb but does not bring about true opposition.[47]

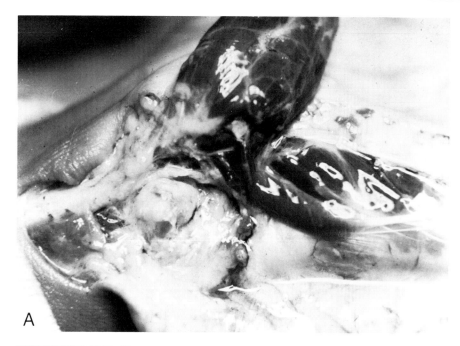

Fig. 38-10. Abductor digiti minimi opponensplasty. (**A**) Freeing of the abductor digiti minimi from the pisiform, leaving as its only remaining attachment the flexor carpi ulnaris, as well as the neurovascular bundle to its base. Satisfactory restoration of function has been achieved (**B,C**); note that the direction of pull is really from the area of the pisiform in this particular case. *(Figure continues.)*

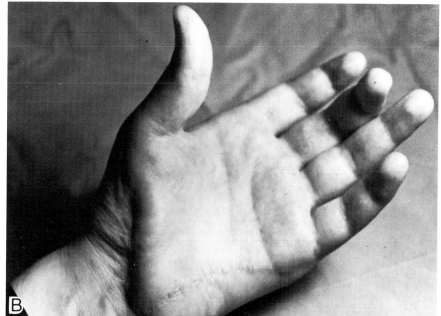

Importance of Flexor Pollicis Brevis Power

Opposition of the thumb requires only minimal power to position the thumb for function. To make the thumb maximally functional, however, short flexor action is required in addition to opposition. In most isolated median nerve injuries, the adductor pollicis and at least a portion of the flexor pollicis brevis are functional in addition to the normal extrinsic motors. If short flexor action is present, the thumb may be brought against the fingers with

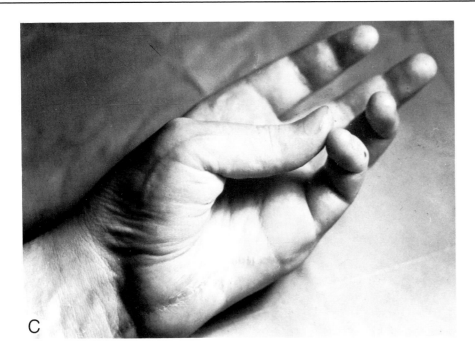

Fig. 38-10 *(Continued).*

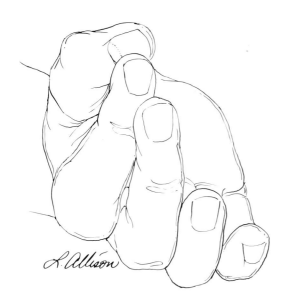

Fig. 38-11. With hyperflexion of the interphalangeal joint, a moment for supination of the thumb occurs if the index finger contacts the thumb with power. Brand calls this the crank-handle effect.

power. Two different motions are required: opposition of the thumb to position the thumb for action, and then short flexor action for power, either prehension or power grip. If both opposition and short flexor action are absent, both functions need to be restored. This will require two transfers or a single transfer to restore short flexor action only, which is a compromise between the two. If a strictly opposition transfer is performed in the absence of short flexor action, two things may occur. As the fingers close against the thumb and power is exerted, the thumb may collapse into supination. The fingers have a supinatory effect on the thumb, and as the thumb attempts to approach the fingers, the opposition transfer relaxes. The pronatory effect of the transfer is lost and collapse occurs. At the same time, because there is no carpometacarpal or **MP** joint flexor available (short flexor action), the thumb approaches the fingers by the action of the flexor pollicis longus. With this muscle active, the terminal joint flexes initially. As the index finger or index and long fingers contact the flexed interphalangeal joint of the thumb, a crank action is created on the thumb by the fingers, forcing it into supination (Fig. 38-11). In addition to this and in the absence of short flexor action, the only substitute for the abductor pollicis complex is the extensor pollicis longus.[36] The functions of this muscle are supination of the thumb and adduction of the metacarpal and proximal phalanx, and these tend to increase the thumb collapse deformity. Certain opposition transfers provide short flexor power. The Royle-Thompson operation does this by its angle of approach to the thumb, and Bunnell's bony attachment procedure does so by creating MP joint flexion in addition to true opposition.

True opposition transfers with soft tissue distal attachment bring about short flexor action through another method. Those distal attachments that insert into the extensor pollicis longus over the proximal phalanx increase extensor power to the thumb interphalangeal joint. This semiactive tenodesis effect limits passive interphalangeal joint motion of the thumb postoperatively and at the time of surgery, and persists long-term if the opposition motor has satisfactory strength. This limitation of passive interphalangeal joint motion means that when the flexor pollicis longus contracts, all of its excursion is not used up by interphalangeal joint flexion. The remaining excursion is thus available to provide MP and even carpometacarpal flexion. In such a case, short flexor action is achieved by limiting passive flexion of the interphalangeal joint of the thumb.[16] An arthrodesis of the thumb interphalangeal joint would give similar results. In the completely intrinsic-minus thumb in which satisfactory opposition has been obtained, improved function may be achieved by an arthrodesis of the MP joint. This added stability is valuable, but more importantly, the thumb can be hyperpronated so that the pulp of the thumb actually contacts the index finger or the index and long fingers straight on. The fingers then lose their supinatory effect on the thumb. This loss of the supination effect of the thumb can also be appreciated if the MP joint is not arthrodesed in full extension. If the MP joint maintains much flexion, another crank-handle effect for the fingers is created one joint proximally (Fig. 38-12). The fingers working against the thumb with a flexed MP joint force the thumb into supination because of the length of the moment arm. This moment arm actually consists of the entire length of the distal and proximal phalanges of the thumb. Arthrodesis of the thumb in full extension decreases the supinatory or the rotational defect on the thumb by the fingers (Fig. 38-13).

Thumb Extrinsic Opponensplasties

The use of thumb extrinsic muscles that contribute to deformities of the thumb to restore opposition is an attractive concept. To utilize a deforming force and alter its attachment or its muscle-tendon unit approach to the thumb is a concept that stems from the days of poliomyelitis. The two muscle-tendon units that are deforming forces on the thumb with intrinsic muscle paralysis are the flexor pollicis longus and the extensor pollicis longus. Both of these muscles, however, become deforming forces only in the presence of a complete or nearly complete intrinsic-minus thumb. With the absence of short flexor action to the thumb, secondary to injury or disease, overactivity of these two extrinsic muscles occurs. In disease states with progressive paralysis, dual motor tendon transfers to the thumb to provide both opposition and short flexor action is a luxury that cannot be afforded. Obviously, in order to render the thumb maximally functional, one tendon transfer coupled with a joint fusion in the thumb will probably be necessary. Also, in a severely involved hand, true opposition may not be necessary or desirable. Attaining short flexor action alone may render the thumb maximally functional.

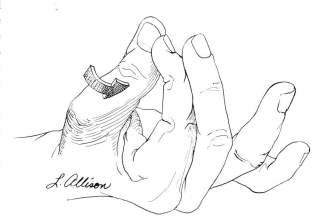

Fig. 38-12. With a flexed thumb MP joint, the index finger exerts a powerful supinatory effect on the thumb. The moment arm is the entire length of the distal and proximal phalanges of the thumb. This is the same crank-handle effect as seen in Figure 38-11, but with an even longer moment arm.

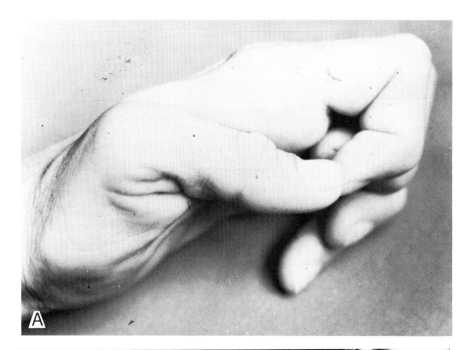

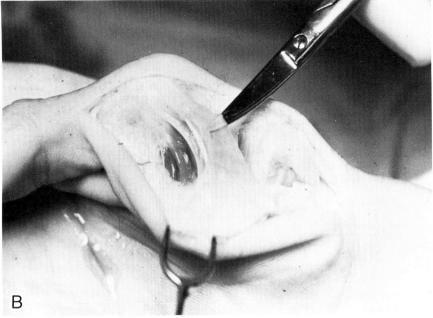

Fig. 38-13. (A,B) A completely intrinsic-minus thumb, in which only a single motor was used to reconstruct thumb function. *(Figure continues.)*

FLEXOR POLLICIS LONGUS OPPONENSPLASTY

One has only to observe the function of the intrinsic-minus thumb to notice the hyperflexed interphalangeal joint and the overactive extensor pollicis longus tendon (Fig. 38-14A,B). Such patients seem to be using both of these extrinsic motors in order to make up for the absence of intrinsic muscles. The hyperflexed interphalangeal joint impairs the pulp of the thumb from properly meeting the index finger in either pulp or key

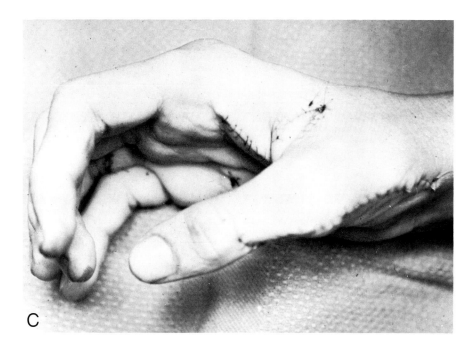

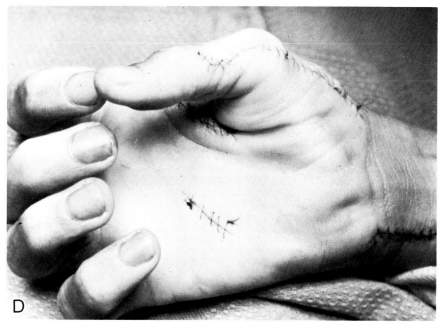

Fig. 38-13 (Continued). In spite of adequate release (C), this patient needed either an arthrodesis of the MP joint in full extension or a second transfer for a short flexor-adductor replacement. As the patient attempts to pinch with the thumb against the index finger (D), notice the tremendous crank-handle action that would be exerted on the thumb by the flexing index.

pinch. The fingers tend to strike the nail or the dorsum of the thumb. The flexor pollicis longus has previously been used for an opponensplasty, but classically the routing has been through either the carpal tunnel or its own tendon sheath. Utilizing the flexor pollicis longus tendon with the Thompson pulley or around the ulnar aspect of the flexor carpi ulnaris must be credited to Mangus and Snow.[35] Utilizing the ulnar border of the palmar fascia as a pulley to the rerouted flexor pollicis longus provides short flexor function. Distal attachment of the transferred tendon into the tendon of

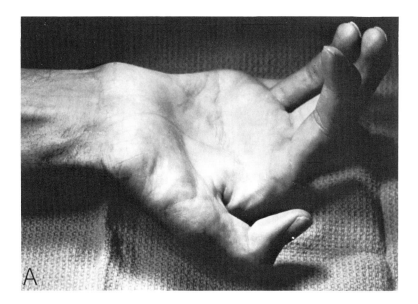

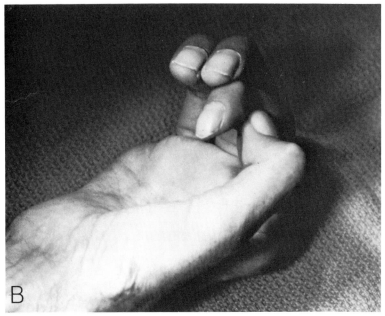

Fig. 38-14. Flexor pollicis longus opponensplasty. This 25-year-old man presented for improvement of hand function with a brachial plexus injury and the equivalent of an intrinsic-minus thumb. In this situation, the extrinsics of the thumb were creating a deformity (**A,B**) and transfer of the flexor pollicis longus with arthrodesis of the interphalangeal joint of the thumb restored much of the activity of the short flexor of the thumb as well as the extensor pollicis longus function. *(Figure continues.)*

the abductor pollicis brevis plus arthrodesis of the interphalangeal joint completes the opponensplasty. The flexor pollicis longus now becomes the superficial head of the flexor pollicis brevis. Arthrodesis of the interphalangeal joint in zero degrees allows the pulp of the thumb to meet the fingers correctly. Overactivity of the extensor pollicis longus in this situation tends to disappear. The patient seems to immediately sense without any

formal retraining that he now has a functional short flexor muscle and does not need to use the extensor pollicis longus as a secondary adductor (Fig. 38-14C,D,E). He instead now uses the extensor pollicis longus to clear the thumb away from the fingers and the "new flexor pollicis brevis" in prehension activity. Thus, an overactive thumb extrinsic muscle that had contributed to the deformity has now been rerouted to improve function. In cer-

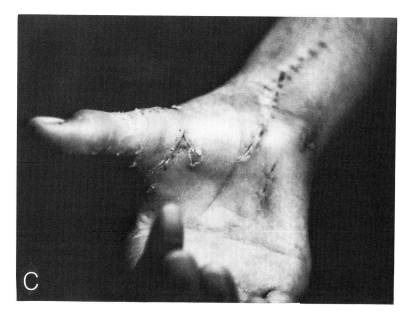

Fig. 38-14 *(Continued)*. Immediately upon removal of the cast, the patient's improved thumb function is apparent (**C–E**). The extensor pollicis longus now functions not as an adductor, but as an extensor, and the flexor pollicis longus now functions as a short flexor replacement. The pulley for the flexor pollicis longus was in the area of the pisiform, and the distal attachment was the tendon of the abductor pollicis brevis.

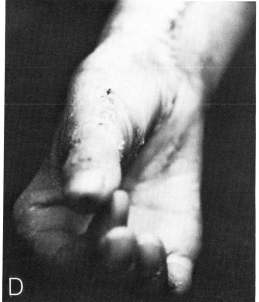

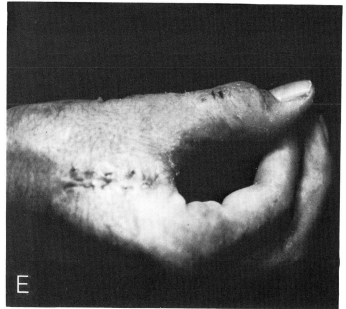

tain long-standing situations, the interphalangeal joint flexion deformity may become fixed. Even in this situation, with adequate excursion and power in the flexor pollicis longus, a satisfactory short flexor can be obtained.

In the case of peripheral nerve disease or spastic paralysis, the flexor pollicis longus may be too weak to utilize as a tendon transfer to improve thumb function. However, a flexion contracture of the interphalangeal joint of the thumb may occur even with a weak flexor pollicis longus. The overactive extensor pollicis longus and the tenodesis action of the flexor pollicis longus with extension and supination of the thumb from the extensor pollicis longus may produce the interphalangeal joint flexion contracture. With a weak flexor pollicis longus and a flexion contracture of the interphalangeal joint of the thumb, only one motor, the extensor pollicis longus, can be causing the deformity. The intrinsic muscles are weak or inactive. The flexor pollicis longus is weak, creating the deformity only by tenodesis. The only functioning motors are the extensor pollicis longus, extensor pollicis brevis, and abductor pollicis longus. All of these are supinators of the thumb. The extensor pollicis longus is also an adductor. Before considering an intermetacarpal bone block to control the thumb, some thought should be given to maintaining thumb mobility by using the only remaining long extrinsic motor, the extensor pollicis longus as described on page 1521. The extensor pollicis longus should, however, only be utilized as an opponensplasty if the patient has active control of this muscle-tendon unit. Using a transferred extensor pollicis longus that is spastic without voluntary control as an opponensplasty will result in a thumb that is always in the way of the fingers. Without voluntary control of the extensor pollicis longus, the abductor pollicis longus by itself cannot clear the thumb from the plane of the fingers during digital flexion.

Operative Technique of Flexor Pollicis Longus Opponensplasty

The distal attachment of the flexor pollicis longus is exposed through a volar zigzag incision, and the tendon is divided at its attachment to the terminal phalanx of the thumb. If there is adherence of the tendon throughout the radial bursa at all, additional, more proximal incisions are required, most commonly at the level of the A1 pulley. At this point, a Y-type incision is made over the dorsum of the interphalangeal joint of the thumb, flaps are developed radially and ulnarly, and the extensor pollicis longus tendon is divided at the level of the joint. The tendon is retracted proximally, the collateral ligaments are incised, and the joint surfaces are exposed. Using rongeurs and a burr, an arthrodesis of the interphalangeal joint is performed using any method of technique and any method of fixation deemed appropriate (see Chapter 4). I prefer to use some type of rigid fixation, either tension band wiring or a screw, because active motion will be begun within 3 or 4 weeks, and good osseous stability is required to allow unrestricted motion of

the thumb. I believe that the position of arthrodesis in this situation should be full extension regardless of the method of fixation.

An incision is then made on the radial volar aspect of the wrist, the muscle belly of the flexor pollicis longus is identified in the distal forearm, and the tendon delivered into the proximal wound. Usually the indications for a flexor pollicis longus opponensplasty suggest that there are no functioning ulnar or median intrinsic muscles to the thumb, and this is the reason for the overactivity of the flexor pollicis longus. In a completely intrinsic-minus thumb the only functioning extrinsic muscles (extensor pollicis longus, extensor pollicis brevis, and abductor pollicis longus) are all basically supinators of the thumb. If the flexor pollicis longus is to be used as an opponensplasty, it should have some pronatory effect, not just short flexor action; otherwise the thumb will not rotate enough after the transfer. The pulleys available with this method of opponensplasty are all of those that have been mentioned, including the fixed pulley at the level of the pisiform using a turned back strip of flexor carpi ulnaris; a loop of the tendon around the flexor carpi ulnaris; a window in the carpal tunnel; or the Thompson pulley (i.e., the ulnar border of the palmar fascia at the distal level of the carpal tunnel). The first three pulleys basically provide far more opposition than short flexor action, and in the completely intrinsic-minus thumb are probably not indicated. I believe that the Thompson pulley, which gives more short flexor action but some pronation action is a far better pulley to use in the completely intrinsic-minus thumb.

An incision for the pulley is then made at the ulnar border of the palmar fascia in line with the ulnar aspect of the ring finger. The flexor tendons can be seen coming from beneath the transverse carpal ligament in the most proximal extent of this incision. A Carroll tendon passer is then passed from distal to proximal, emerging in the proximal incision on the volar radial aspect of the wrist. The flexor pollicis longus tendon is then passed through the depth of the carpal tunnel and brought superficially into the palmar incision. The actual route of the tendon of the flexor pollicis longus should be between the tendons of the flexor digitorum superficialis and those of the flexor digitorum profundus. An incision is then made in the area of the metacarpophalangeal joint on the dorsoradial aspect of the thumb. It is very important in this type of opponensplasty not to attach the transferred tendon into the tendon of the abductor pollicis brevis. This basically is an abductor of the metacarpophalangeal joint, and such an insertion will only pull the metacarpophalangeal joint into a palmar position with abduction. The goal in this tendon transfer, in addition to providing some pronation and abduction, is to stabilize the metacarpophalangeal joint of the thumb in some flexion. This is the only way to achieve power of the thumb against the fingers. If the transfer is inserted into the abductor pollicis brevis tendon, the thumb will not oppose the fingers with nearly as much power as it will if it is sutured into a more volar position, actually attached to the superficial head of the flexor pollicis brevis. In this way, as the patient uses the single long flexor of the thumb to bring about useful thumb function, he will actually have flexion of the metacarpophalangeal joint with a stable distal joint rather than abduction, which he really does not need. Thus, the reason that the method of distal attachment is slightly different than in other opponensplasties is that what we are really trying to reproduce is short flexor action.

Again using a tunnelling forcep or a Carroll tendon passer, the tendon of the flexor pollicis longus is passed subcutaneously from the palmar incision to the thumb incision. There is so much excursion in the flexor pollicis longus that setting the tension in this transfer is even easier than in the flexor digitorum superficialis opponensplasty. As in other opponensplasties, the thumb should rest in almost the fully opposed position, not to the same extent that it does in the short excursion extensor proprius transfers, but high enough so that the patient has reasonable tension on the muscle-tendon unit when it tries to bring power to either side of the fingers or to the pulp of the fingers. In the patient with this type of severely involved hand, pulp-to-pulp pinch is not as important as pulp of the thumb to side of the index or long fingers.

After release of the tourniquet and hemostasis is established, simple wound closure is accomplished. The wrist is maintained in 30 to 40 degrees volar flexion, with the thumb in full opposition for about 3 to 4 weeks. Following this, rehabilitation is begun with active wrist dorsiflexion, which acts to bring the thumb into full opposition. This is followed by exercises to increase power of the transfer.

The desired end result is basically a single axis thumb, which has lost a lot of the rotation movement that it had with normal intrinsic muscles. This provides a thumb that is able to clear the fingers and still oppose the fingertips as well as the sides of the finger with considerable power. Results of this transfer in my experience have been very good, and there is practically no relearning required with this opponensplasty. I believe that there are distinct advantages to using this transfer in the completely intrinsic-minus thumb, which we have previously missed because we have felt that opposition is more important than short flexor action.

EXTENSOR POLLICIS LONGUS OPPONENSPLASTY

The extensor pollicis longus has been emphasized throughout this discussion as being a direct antagonist to opposition of the thumb. In certain cases in which improvement is not likely to occur following nerve injury, in those cases in which an extended period of time has gone by since the nerve injury, or in those patients who have a paralysis problem based on a progressive disease, some thought should be given to using the extensor pollicis longus as an opposition transfer. With an intrinsic-minus thumb from a median and ulnar nerve paralysis, only supinators and adductors of the thumb are present and true opposition of the thumb frequently cannot be achieved against these powerful muscles. I have performed a small number of cases of extensor pollicis longus opponensplasty, taking a muscle that is a deforming force in the intrinsic palsied thumb and converting it into a positive force. For this opponensplasty, patients have been selected who are not likely to improve or who are actually likely to get worse because of the associated disease.[47]

Operative Technique of Extensor Pollicis Longus Opponensplasty

The technique of the extensor pollicis longus opponensplasty is as follows (Fig. 38-15). The central portion of the extensor pollicis longus over the

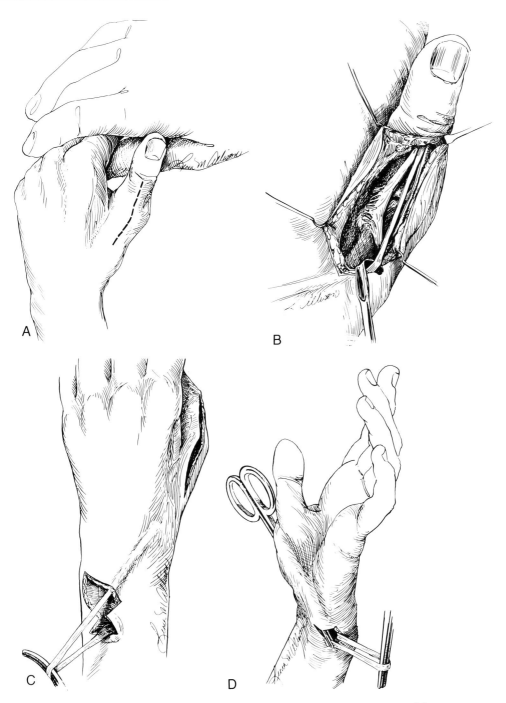

Fig. 38-15. Extensor pollicis longus opponensplasty. The middle portion of the extensor pollicis longus is exposed over the proximal phalanx of the thumb (**A**) and removed in continuity with the main extensor pollicis longus tendon proximal to the MP joint (**B**). This allows satisfactory length of the transfer. Following the freeing up of this and its transfer around the ulnar border of the wrist (**C,D**), an arthrodesis of the thumb MP joint is performed (**E**). *(Figure continues.)*

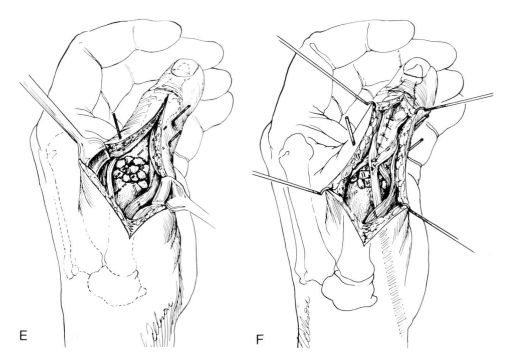

E   F

Fig. 38-15 *(Continued)*. The two lateral bands or the two most lateral portions of the extensor pollicis longus are sutured together and then the transfer is actually sutured into them (**F**). In addition to arthrodesis of the MP joint, the interphalangeal joint of the thumb should be pinned in extension in order to prevent inadvertent flexion during the healing of this transfer. (Riley WV, Mann RJ, Burkhalter WE: Extensor pollicis longus opponensplasty. J Hand Surg 5:217–220, 1980.)

proximal phalanx of the thumb is removed in continuity with the extensor pollicis longus tendon over the MP joint through the hood into the middle of the metacarpal area of the thumb. The width of the tendon over the proximal phalanx is approximately one-third of the tendon width that would normally be present. This tendon is then freed from the hood system. A small incision may be necessary over the dorsum of the hand to free it from some adhesions in the area of the third compartment, and a more generous incision is then made on the ulnar aspect of the distal forearm where the muscle belly is identified. The extensor pollicis longus tendon is then pulled into the more ulnar incision proximally. A subcutaneous tunnel is created along the ulnar border of the forearm. A small incision is usually made in the area of the pisiform. The muscle belly is transposed onto the ulnar aspect of the forearm subcutaneously; the tendon is brought out in the area of the pisiform and transferred directly

across the palm to the area of the MP joint. All of the patients in whom this operation has been done have had a concomitant arthrodesis of the MP joint of the thumb in full extension and hyperpronation. The elongated extensor pollicis longus tendon (i.e., elongated by the intrinsic portion of the tendon) is then interwoven between the two lateral bands that are brought together in the midline and the entire hood is repaired, using this interweaving technique of the transferred extensor pollicis longus and the lateral bands. The interphalangeal joint of the thumb is pinned in full extension at this time. It is most important to make sure that the fixation of the MP joint arthrodesis is secure because active use of this transfer is ideally started within about 4 weeks, at which time the arthrodesis is really not going to be solid. After 4 weeks of immobilization, the patient should be taught to differentiate function of the extensor pollicis longus from function of the abductor pollicis longus. It is

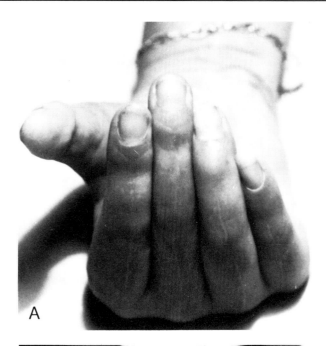

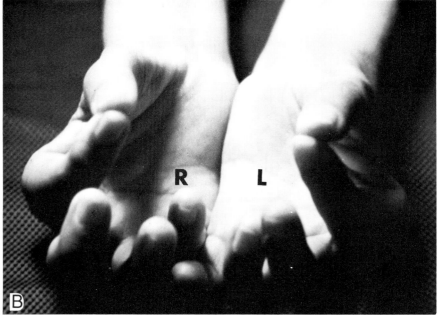

Fig. 38-16. This patient with Charcot-Marie-Tooth disease has undergone arthrodesis of the thumb MP joint as well as an extensor pollicis longus opponensplasty. Note the use of the abductor pollicis longus to move the thumb (**B**) so that power grip is possible as the fingers really clear the thumb. In addition, notice that in the left hand the MP joint has been arthrodesed in hyperpronation whereas in the right it has been done in almost neutral rotation. The crank-handle effect is much less obvious in the left thumb, suggesting that hyperpronation, as well as full extension, is the preferred position of arthrodesis of the thumb MP joint in a patient with combined median and ulnar palsy.

most important at the time the transfer is being performed that it is possible for the fingers to actually clear the opposed thumb with the wrist in neutral. No thumb extensor muscle remains, and there is only abductor pollicis longus function available to bring the thumb away so the fingers can close in power grip (Fig. 38-16). The patient is able to clear the thumb for the fingers during power grip activities using this abductor pollicis longus. Our results with this transfer have been most pleasing, and we continue to use it in situations in which the patient is not likely to have any evidence of improvement and has limited motors, or in which the patient's condition is likely to deteriorate, such as in syringomyelia or Charcot-Marie-Tooth disease.[47]

Postoperative Management of Opponensplasty

In general, the postoperative management of opponensplasties is related to whether or not the transfer crosses the wrist joint; if it crosses the wrist joint volarly, the wrist needs to be supported in some way. In most opponensplasties it has been our practice to leave the patient in a bulky dressing for several days postoperatively and then after this period of time to position the thumb in full opposition for approximately 4 weeks. If the transfer is one of the proprius transfers in which the excursion of the muscle tendon unit is relatively short, it is important that the wrist be placed at about 30 to 35 degrees volar flexion with the thumb in full opposition. If the transferred motor is the superficialis or some other type of transfer that has a considerable range of excursion, merely positioning the thumb in full opposition and the wrist in neutral is generally adequate. If the method of attachment distally involves the extensor pollicis longus over the middle phalanx or the abductor pollicis brevis tendon rather than some type of bony attachment, immobilization of the thumb interphalangeal joint in full extension will probably be required. If not, additional excessive tension will probably be placed on the suture line distally and might result in some attenuation of this attachment. Since at the present time most attachments of the opponensplasty distally use either Riordan's or Brand's method of attachment, certainly interphalangeal joint immobilization should be an integral part of the postoperative management. Since this is a tendon-to-tendon suture, 4 weeks of immobilization is generally adequate. After 4 weeks of immobilization, patients generally regain control very rapidly. Following cast removal in these patients, the emphasis early on should be on rehabilitation to regain wrist motion.

Those transfers that use an ulnar innervated intrinsic muscle (e.g., the abductor digiti minimi to replace a median innervated intrinsic muscle) do not need to be placed in any particular position as far as wrist flexion is concerned, but the thumb should be placed in full opposition.

In most patients, splinting is not required once mobility of the thumb and wrist is started. However, in certain disease states, primarily high median and ulnar nerve palsies or in patients with diseases such as Charcot-Marie-Tooth or leprosy, the extensors are so strong and the lack of sensibility may be so profound as to have the patient attenuate his own transfer prior to getting control over the muscle and strengthening of the tendon suture through collagen maturation. In such cases it is important to protect the transfer from overstretching by normal muscles working against the opponensplasty. It has generally been our impression that in such patients who have considerable loss of sensibility in the hand either from disease or injury, prolonged protection of the opponensplasty will be required for up to about 3 months. However, in patients who are less disabled than this and have only an isolated high or low median nerve injury, attenuation of the transfer has not been a major problem and generally these patients do not require immobilizaton past 4 weeks.

Authors Preferred Method of Opponensplasty

There are many different conditions associated with loss of opposition of the thumb, and there is probably no single opposition transfer that is applicable to all cases in which the thumb is nonfunctional secondary to loss of the abductor pollicis brevis function. Historically, the opposition transfer came about as a substitute primarily in diseased states such as poliomyelitis, in which the thumb usually had complete intrinsic paralysis. However, in present day situations it seems as if more problems with reduced thumb function occur following trauma with or without local injury in the area of the wrist. In these variable circumstances, a single choice of opponensplasty would obviously not be optimal in all cases.

The flexor digitorum superficialis opponensplasty using a fixed pulley in the area of the pisiform, with various methods of attachment in the area of the MP joint of the thumb, has been the standard opponensplasty for years. This is applicable in a low median nerve permanent paralysis without associated tendon injury, and should give excellent thumb function. However, in this type of patient, the intrinsic muscles that bring about short flexor action and adduction of the thumb are functioning, and therefore great strength of opposition is not required. Because of this I generally prefer to use a proprius tendon transfer opponensplasty, either the extensor digiti minimi or the extensor indicis proprius. These muscles with adequate strength and positioning capability allow the use of a muscle that in my opinion is more expendable than the strong flexor digitorum superficialis to the ring finger. There is a significant complication rate associated with superficialis removal from the finger,[26,41] and because of this I prefer to use one of the proprius tendons as my primary opponensplasty. Since my experience has been greatest with extensor indicis proprius, I prefer this opponensplasty as my operative procedure in the thumb without tendon injury and with normally functioning, ulnar-innervated intrinsic musculature.

In the case of a high median nerve paralysis or a low median nerve paralysis associated with tendon injury at the level of the wrist, a proprius tendon transfer would be my first choice. In the case of a low injury at the level of the wrist with a median nerve repair, however, often no opponens transfer is indicated. These patients generally regain some function of the abductor pollicis brevis within 6 months and, usually in the case of sharp lacerations, have reasonably good return of function within one year. In these low injuries, contractures can usually be prevented by a short opponens splint, and therefore no internal splint needs to be created by an operative procedure.

My experience with the extensor indicis proprius transfer has been good. The functional defect is acceptable and failures are few. Strength seems to be adequate with ulnar nerve muscles intact, and I continue to be amazed with how well the patients do postoperatively as far as regaining motion with minimal to no rehabilitation.

I think the method of distal attachment should be to the abductor pollicis brevis tendon only. In a high median nerve injury, suturing the distal attachment to the extensor pollicis longus has not been necessary and may result in excessive interphalangeal joint hyperextension, because in pa-

tients with a high injury there is no functioning flexor pollicis longus. Therefore, in the patient with an isolated high median nerve injury, I would not use this method of distal attachment, as advocated by Brand or Riordon, unless at the same time I had done some type of transfer to the flexor pollicis longus.

In the patient with a low injury to the median nerve that had required a nerve graft to regain continuity of the nerve, I would again think in terms of the extensor indicis proprius opponensplasty. With deficits involving the ulnar nerve musculature as well, the method of attachment should be to the extensor pollicis longus as well as to the abductor pollics brevis, as advocated by Riordon and Brand. I believe that this brings about greater rotation of the thumb and limits the interphalangeal joint motion by increasing the tension of the extensor pollicis longus. This high tension then limits passive interphalangeal joint motion so that the excursion of the flexor pollicis longus can provide more proximal control in the MP and carpometacarpal joints of the thumb, rather than just at the interphalangeal joint.

EXTRINSIC REPLACEMENT IN MEDIAN NERVE PARALYSIS

In high median nerve paralysis there is lack of function of the forearm wrist pronator-flexor group with the exception of the flexor carpi ulnaris. Absent muscles include all of the flexor digitorum superficialis, the two radial profundi, and the flexor pollicis longus. Although the radial half of the flexor digitorum profundus is classically denervated, flexion of the long finger is usually complete although considerable weakness of this digit is present. In the index finger only intrinsic flexion is present and overuse of the intrinsic flexors might bring about intrinsic-plus deformity of the index finger, with loss of passive DIP and PIP flexion. Likewise, the interphalangeal joint of the thumb may develop considerable stiffness secondary to the unopposed action of the extensor pollicis longus and the intrinsic interphalangeal joint extensors. In considering extrinsic replacement, the functions that need to be replaced must be determined. Basically what is desired is flexor power in the index and long fingers, range of motion in the index finger, and range of motion and power in the interphalangeal joint of the thumb. It is certainly desirable to have full finger flexion, but some power is also needed if there is to be minimal likelihood of extrinsic return following nerve graft or nerve repair. The only functions that actually need to be replaced are flexors to the index finger and thumb, or to the thumb and index, and long fingers

if more power is required. What are the available muscle-tendon units available for transfer? There are really only two or perhaps three. In a high median palsy the brachioradialis and the extensor carpi radialis longus are available and perhaps the extensor carpi ulnaris, if it is not being used for an opposition transfer.[45] Frequently, however, the removal of the extensor carpi ulnaris for transfer brings about a radial deviation deformity of the wrist. Therefore, in general, I think removing this muscle for functions other than an opposition transfer should be discouraged. An alternative to

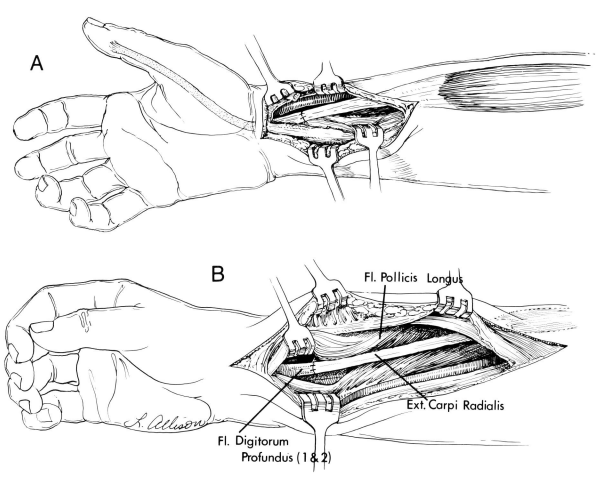

Fig. 38-17. Extrinsic replacement using the brachioradialis to the flexor pollicis longus (**A**) and the extensor carpi radialis longus to the profundi of the index and long fingers (**B**). In both situations the transfers as shown here are end-to-end. If there is felt to be any chance for extrinsic return following grafting, the transfer should be end-to-side. The end-to-end technique shown here would be used in the patient in whom there is no chance of extrinsic return.

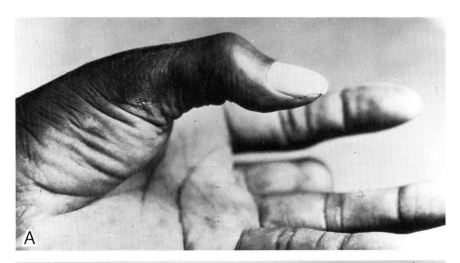

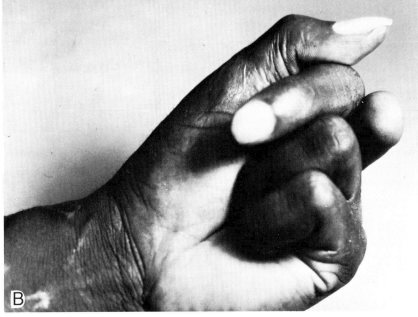

Fig. 38-18. A patient with high median nerve injury in whom the brachioradialis has been transferred to the flexor pollicis longus and the extensor carpi radialis longus to the index finger profundus tendon. There is good power in the flexor pollicis longus, but limited range with the wrist held still. Note the absence of flexion contracture of the index finger and thumb (**C**).

direct transfer for restoration of extrinsic function is side-to-side suture of the functioning flexor digitorum profundi of the ring and small fingers, which are ulnarly innervated, to the denervated portions on the radial side. This adds range of motion to the index finger and perhaps prevents stiffness but does nothing to the extreme weakness on the radial side, which involves both the index and long fingers. Two motors are available for transfer to the flexor pollicis longus: the extensor carpi radialis longus and brachioradialis. The use of these motors provides independent flexion in the interphalangeal joints of the thumb and index finger.

The use of the extensor carpi radialis longus to the flexor digitorum profundus of the index and long fingers is reserved for those patients who need radial side power and are unlikely to obtain significant reinnervation following neurorrhaphy (Fig. 38-17). In order to perform a tendon transfer of new motors to the index finger, or to the index and long fingers and thumb, there must be full range of motion of the wrist or an indifferent result will occur. Similarly, use of the brachioradialis to the flexor pollicis longus requires a full range of wrist motion. The reason for this is explained as follows. The suture line tension between the brachiora-

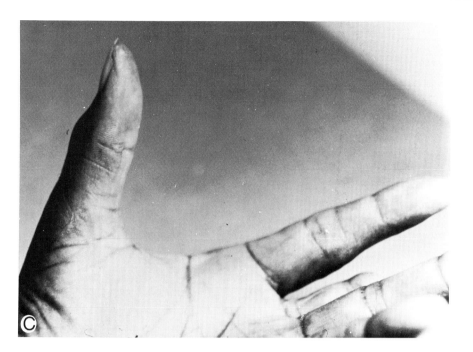

Fig. 38-18 *(Continued)*.

dialis and the flexor pollicis longus or the extensor carpi radialis longus and the profundus to the index and long fingers is most critical. There is significant disparity in excursion between the flexor digitorum profundus to the index and long fingers (about 50 mm) and the extensor carpi radialis longus (about 30 mm). Therefore, if excessive tension is placed on the transfer, either to the thumb or the index and long fingers, flexion contractures will result. Flexion contractures of the digits on the radial side of the hand reduce hand function considerably because precision activities, which are usually performed by the radial side of the hand, are performed with the interphalangeal joints of both the thumb and fingers in nearly full extension. The tension on this transfer should then be adjusted by the use of a dynamic tenodesis approach (i.e., with synergistic wrist motion). Full volar flexion of the wrist will bring about nearly complete extension of the fingers, and full dorsiflexion of the wrist will allow complete flexion of the fingers. This tenodesis action should be used to adjust the tension of the tendon transfer. Tension for the transfer should be adjusted so that with the wrist at about 30 degrees volar flexion the fingers come into nearly full extension. With the wrist in 30 to 45 degrees dorsiflexion the fingers should close passively so that the power of the transfer can exert its

force with the fingers partially flexed, i.e., the 30 mm of excursion of the extensor carpi radialis longus begins to act when the fingers are almost completely flexed passively by wrist dorsiflexion.

Use of the brachioradialis poses the same problem in terms of excursion, but it must be remembered that the brachioradialis tendon must be freed extensively up to the proximal third of the forearm, well past its musculotendinous junction, in order to develop 30 mm of excursion. Only with this dissection, freeing the tendon widely from the investing fascia of the forearm, is it possible to get 30 mm of excursion in this muscle. The tension then can be adjusted in essentially the same fashion described above for adjusting the tension in the fingers. With the wrist in about 30 degrees volar flexion it should be possible to passively extend all three joints of the thumb completely. This will result in lack of full flexion of the interphalangeal joint by the transfer, but it will essentially stabilize the tip of the thumb and give additional power of flexion to the thumb. As noted previously, most precision pinch activities are performed with the thumb interphalangeal joint in full extension. Therefore, a flexion contracture of this joint at this point can be extremely disabling[11] (Fig. 38-18). If these extrinsic tendon replacements are performed following a nerve repair or nerve graft, the method of attachment should be end-to-side rather than end-to-end. This is true even if considerable time has elapsed since the nerve surgery and all hope of nerve regeneration has been given up. Extremely late recovery is occasionally seen, and because of this, all suture lines should be end-to-side. This type of anastomosis, of course, allows any subsequent return of power in the reinnervated muscle to augment the transfer.

TIMING AND SELECTION OF TRANSFERS

Timing

I believe that the selection and timing of transfers performed for both intrinsic and extrinsic paralysis in high median nerve lesions needs some clarification. If a tendon is considered following a neurorrhaphy in the case of a high median nerve laceration, one should expect considerable return in extrinsic flexors. Consequently, probably no tendon transfer is indicated to restore function in the extrinsic flexors of the forearm. On the other hand, if a nerve repair has been performed several months before and no evidence of return has occurred, one should think of doing a transfer that would give additional power rather than just range of motion to the index and long fingers. I think that for all practical purposes, extrinsic replacement for high median nerve palsy is indicated only when nerve grafting is performed. In this case transfers should be performed end-to-side to take advantage of muscle power that may return following the nerve graft. If one elects not to perform extrinsic replacements, maintenance of mobility of the interphalangeal joints of the thumb and index finger will be necessary until recovery occurs. As stated before, because of the difference in amplitude of the muscles transferred, it is most important that the wrist have full range of motion prior to performing any of these short excursion motor transfers.

Regarding further transfers in the upper extremity, I believe that tendon transfers in the upper extremity should be performed as soon after injury and nerve repair as possible to improve overall hand function. Much has been said about the timing of transfers.[7,11,4] Transfers should be performed when it is obvious that no further return is going to occur, but this may be as long as several years following neurorrhaphy or grafting. Although there is some controversy regarding this point, I believe that transfers should be performed soon after repair of the nerve. In patients with median nerve palsy, sensory loss may be the most important single deterrent to satisfactory hand function. Even in the presence of sensory loss, however, some function of the hand is possible. Certainly a mobile, opposable thumb that can reach the normal sensible areas of the hand is much more useful than one that cannot be used and cannot even reach the areas of normal sensibility. The functional deficit associated especially with a high median lesion is so profound that I believe all attempts should be made to improve motor function early. Whether this includes just thumb opposition transfer or opposition and extrinsic transfer is frequently dependent on the individual patient, i.e., his requirements for return to work, motivation, need for splintage, and associated injury. I believe that a transfer can work as a substitute during regrowth of the nerve, while at the same time prevent contractures and eliminate the requirement for external splintage. External splintage may severely limit the patient's ability to use the palsied hand, and therefore I believe that the use of an internal splint, that is, the early transfer, is of considerable benefit in the rehabilitation of these patients.[12] If the patient ultimately regains only partial function in the muscles involved, the transfer may act at the same time as a helper. In such cases, the reinnervated muscles may then function with near-normal power. If essentially no return occurs from the neurorrhaphy or nerve graft, the transfer may then act as a permanent substitute. As previously noted, those patients who have significant power in the superficial portion of the flexor pollicis brevis may have a thumb that is maximally functional and will not require an opposition transfer. In my opinion, however, those patients who need an opposition transfer should have it performed soon after neurorrhaphy or grafting.

When asked what muscle substitutes for the abductor pollicis brevis, most physicians quickly respond with the flexor pollicis brevis. This is true, but if the superficial head of this muscle is paralyzed, what works as the substitute? Functional examination of patients with a median nerve palsy reveals that because they are really unable to bring the thumb into opposition, they either substitute by pronation of the forearm or internal rotation and abduction of the shoulder. In picking up an article from a table, the thumb is positioned so that the abductor pollicis longus can really open the hand. Therefore, although the thumb index web is open, it is done so not in pronation but in supination, because the abductor pollicis longus, extensor pollicis brevis, and extensor pollicis longus are all supinators. To compensate for this supination effect of the substitute musculature, the forearm pronates (Fig. 38-19). Because of lack of good sensibility in the median nerve distribution, the patient has a pattern of use that for all practical purposes is not useful to him. He cannot see the palm of his hand. The real reason for doing an opposition transfer early on after a median nerve paralysis is so that the patient can position his thumb in opposition with the wrist in either supination, neutral, or pronation. Almost all patients will preferentially select either supination or midrotation of the forearm to use the hand, because in these positions the palmar surface of the hand is exposed to the eyes and the patient can then use his eyes to make up for the lack of sensibility in the hand. If, in fact, the patient must use the hand in pronation because of his inability to position the thumb, his eyes are no longer an effective aid in hand use. I would therefore suggest that when thinking of the timing for opponensplasty, the surgeon watch the thumb position when the patient tries to perform activities, such as picking up a glass or change, and note if, in fact, the patient is using his hand in forearm pronation. If so, this patient probably does need an early tendon transfer to restore maximal function in the thumb and hand. If he is able to use the hand to pick up articles and transfer objects from hand to hand with the injured hand in a position other than full pronation, then he is probably not a candidate for early tendon transfer. This is probably because he has an innervated portion of the flexor pollicis brevis, which renders his hand fairly functional.

Selection of Motors

If the decision is made to perform an early tendon transfer to restore opposition of the thumb in a *high* median nerve palsy, what transfer should be used? Obviously, in this case the proprius tendons are the most readily available. These tendons position the thumb well, do not create significant functional deficit by their removal from the hand, and do not require a tendon graft for lengthening. The use of a paralyzed superficialis motored by a functional flexor carpi ulnaris as mentioned by Irwin[25] and Goldner[19] brings about strong opposition of the thumb. This has at least some theoretic objections in that the only remaining wrist flexor is eliminated. Moreover, strong opposition of the thumb is not required as long as there are functioning intrinsic muscles that are capable of acting as a short flexor or short flexor substitute.

To summarize, I would suggest that in a high median nerve injury, the surgeon should think of doing an opposition transfer if pronation of the forearm is a substitute motion used by the patient and that probably one of the proprius tendons is more appropriate for early tendon transfer than anything else. If a neurorrhaphy is possible, I do not think any extrinsic replacement should be used early in the management of the patient. Significant extrinsic power will generally return following a high median nerve neurorrhaphy, and this really does not create a problem. On the other hand, if the patient has required a nerve graft, especially if done late or under unfavorable conditions (e.g., long graft or a poor bed), the anticipated return of function is not likely to be satisfactory. In this patient one may consider doing the extrinsic flexor replacement as previously described, i.e., brachioradialis to flexor pollicis longus and extensor carpi radialis longus to the index and long profundus tendons. All of these transfers, both intrinsic and extrinsic replacements, can be performed at the same time. Since in the postoperative period the wrist is going to be in volar flexion, the thumb can easily be placed in full opposition to release the tension on the brachioradialis transfer to the flexor pollicis longus, as well as reducing the tension on the proprius tendon transfer. This will reduce the tension on the extensor carpi radialis longus transfer to the flexor digitorum profundi.

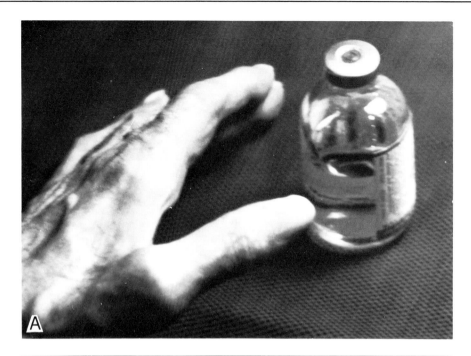

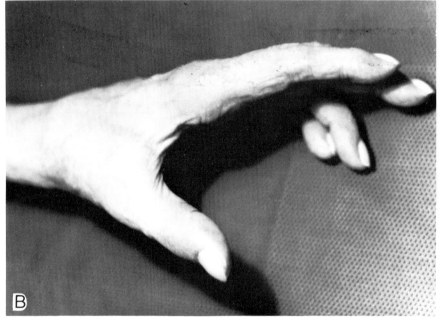

Fig. 38-19. A patient with a brachial plexus injury is shown attempting to pick up a bottle with the hand in full pronation (**A**). This is a substitute maneuver for an absent abductor pollis brevis or flexor pollicis brevis. Following opponensplasty (**B**), with the patient's forearm in neutral rotation, it is possible to position the hand for grasp. The patient can see the palmar surface of the hand.

SUMMARY

All of the significant functional deficits in median nerve injury cannot be restored by tendon transfer. Lack of normal sensibility on the radial aspect of the hand is a real deterrent to hand function. Opposition transfers are many and varied; almost every motor has been used, many pulleys are available, and distal methods of attachment are likewise innumerable. The major reasons for failure to achieve satisfactory opposition of the thumb with a transfer are persistence of a contracture within the thumb (recognized or unrecognized) and the selection of a poor motor. Early opposition transfer (i.e., very soon after neurorrhaphy) should be carried out in those patients who have a pronation attitude of the forearm as a substitute for the nonfunctioning abductor pollicis brevis. Extrinsic replacement probably should be required early only in those patients that have had a nerve graft in less than optimum situations or in those patients in whom, for one reason or another, neurorrhaphy of the median nerve is not considered.

REFERENCES

1. Beasley RW: Principles of tendon transfer. Orthop Clin North Am 1:433, 1970
2. Bohr HH: Tendon transposition in paralysis of opposition of the thumb. Acta Chir Scand 105:45, 1953
3. Boswick JA, Stromberg WB: Isolated injury to the median nerve above the elbow. A review of thirteen cases. J Bone Joint Surg, 49A:653, 1967
4. Brand PW: The hand in leprosy. p. 279. In Pulverlaft RG (ed): Clinical Surgery of the Hand. Butterworth's, London, 1966
5. Brand PW: Tendon transfer for median and ulnar nerve paralysis. Orthop Clin North Am 1:447, 1970
6. Braun RM: Palmaris longus tendon transfer for augmentation of the thenar musculature in low median palsy. J Hand Surg 3:488–491, 1978
7. Brown PW: The time factor in surgery of upper extremity peripheral nerve injury. Clin Orthop 68:14–21, 1970
8. Brown PW: Adduction-flexion contracture of the thumb. Correction with dorsal rotation flap and release of contracture. Clin Orthop 88:161, 1972.
9. Browne EZ, Teague MA, and Snyder CC: Prevention of extensor lag after indicis proprius tendon transfer. J Hand Surg, 4:168–172, 1979
10. Bunnell S: Opposition of the thumb. J Bone Joint Surg 20:269–284, 1938
11. Burkhalter WE: Tendon transfer in median nerve paralysis. Orthop Clin North Am 5:271, 1974
12. Burkhalter WE: Early tendon transfer in upper extremity peripheral nerve injury. Clin Orthop 104:68–79, 1974
13. Burkhalter WE, Christensen RC, Brown PW: Exten-
sor indicis proprius opponensplasty. J Bone Joint Surg 55A:725–732, 1973
14. Camitz H: Über die be Handlung der Oppositionslähmung. Acta Chir Scand 65:77, 1929
15. Chouhy-Aguirre S, Caplan S: Sobre secuelas de lesion alta e irreparable di nervio meidano y cubital y su tratamiento. Prensa Med Argentina 43:2341–2346, 1956
16. Curtis RM: Opposition of the thumb. Orthop Clin North Am 5:305–321, 1974
17. DeVeechi J: Oposición del pulgar fisiopatologia una nerva operaction transplante del aductor. Bol Soc Cir Uruguay 32:423, 1961
18. Goldner JL, Clippinger FW: Excision of the greater multangular bone as an adjunct to mobilization of the thumb. J Bone Joint Surg 41A:609–625, 1959
19. Goldner JL, Irwin CE: An analysis of paralytic thumb deformities. J Bone Joint Surg 32A:627–639, 1950
20. Groves RJ, Goldner JL: Restoration of strong opposition afer median nerve or brachial plexus paralysis. J Bone Joint Surg 57:112–115, 1975
21. Henderson ED: Transfer of wrist extensor and brachioradialis to restore opposition of the thumb. J Bone Joint Surg 44A:513–522, 1962
22. Herrick RT, Lister GD: Control of first web space contracture. Including a review of the literaure and a tabulation of opponensplasty techniques. Hand, 9:253–264, 1977
23. Hill NA: Restoration of opposition for the paralyzed thumb. Clin Orthop 61:234–249, 1968
24. Huber E: Hilfsoperation bei median Uslähmung. Dtsch Arch Klin Med 136:271, 1921
25. Irwin CE: Transplant to the thumb to restore function of opposition. End results. South Med J 35:257, 1942
26. Jacobs B, Thompson TC: Opposition of the thumb and its restoration. J Bone Joint Surg 42A:1015–1026, 1960
27. Jensen EG: Restoration of opposition of the thumb. Hand, 10:161–167, 1978
28. Kaplan I, Dinner M, Chait L: Use of extensor pollicis longus tendon as a distal extension for an opponens transfer. Plast Reconstr Surg 57:186–189, 1976
29. Kessler I: Transfer of extensor carpi ulnaris to tendon of extensor pollicis brevis for opponensplasty. J Bone Joint Surg 51A:1303–1308, 1969
30. Kirklin JW, Thomas CG: Opponens transplant. An analysis of the method employed and results obtained in 75 cases. Surg Gynecol Obstet 86:213, 1948
31. Littler, JW: Tendon transfers and arthrodesis in combined median and ulnar nerve paralysis. J Bone Joint Surg 31A:225–234, 1949

32. Littler JW, Cooley SGE: Opposition of the thumb and its restoration by abductor digiti quint transfer. J Bone Joint Surg 45A:1389–1396, 1963

33. Littler JW, Li CS: Primary restoration of thumb opposition with median nerve decompression. Plast Reconstr Surg 39:74–75, 1967

34. Makin M: Translocation of the flexor pollicis longus tendon to restore oppostion. J Bone Joint Surg 49B:458–461, 1967

35. Mangus DJ: Flexor pollicis longus tendon transfer for restoration of opposition of the thumb. Plast Reconstr Surg 52:155, 1973

36. Mannerfelt L: Structures of the hand in ulnar nerve paralysis. A clinical experimental investigation in normal and anomalies of innervation. Acta Orthop Scand suppl 87: 1966

37. Mayer L: Operative reconstruction of the paralyzed upper extremity. J Bone Joint Surg 21:377, 1939

38. Mutz SB: Thumb web contracture. Hand 4:236–246, 1972

39. Ney KW: A tendon transplant for intrinsic hand muscle paralysis. Surg Gynecol Obstet 33:342, 1921

40. Nicolaysen J: Transplantation des m. Abductor dig. V. Die Fenlender Oppositions Fehigkeit des Daumens. Dtsch Z Chir 168:133, 1922

41. North ER, Littler JW: Transferring the flexor superficialis tendon: Technical considerations in the prevention of proximal interphalangeal joint disabiity. J Hand Surg 5:498–501, 1980

42. Omer GE: The technique and timing of tendon transfers. Orthop Clin North Am 5:243, 1974

43. Orticochea M: Use of the deep bundle of the flexor pollicis brevis to restore opposition of the thumb. Plast Reconstr Surg 47:220, 1971

44. Palande DD: Opponensplasty in intrinsic muscle paralysis of the thumb in leprosy. J Bone Joint Surg 57A:489–493, 1975

45. Phalen GS, Miller RC: Transfer of wrist extensor muscles to restore or reinforce flexion power of the fingers and opposition of the thumb. J Bone Joint Surg 29:993–997, 1947

46. Ramselaar JM: Tendon Transfers to Restore Opposition of the Thumb. HE Stenfert Kroese NV, Leiden, Holland, 1970

47. Riley WB, Mann RJ, Burkhalter WE: Extensor pollicis longus opponensplasty. J Hand Surg 5:217–220, 1980

48. Riordan DC: Tendon transfers for nerve paralysis of the hand and wrist. Curr Pract Orthop Surg 2:17, 1964

49. Rowntree T: Anomalous innervation of the hand muscles. J Bone Joint Surg 31B:505–510, 1949

50. Royle ND: An operation for paralysis of the intrinsic muscles of the thumb. JAMA 111:612, 1938

51. Sakellarides HT: Modified pulley for opponens tendon transfer. J Bone Joint Surg 52:178–179, 1970.

52. Schneider LH: Opponensplasty using the extensor digiti minimi. J Bone Joint Surg 51A:1297–1302, 1969

53. Snow JW, Fink GH: Use of transverse carpal ligament window for the pulley in tendon transfers for median nerve palsy. Plast Reconstr Surg 48:238, 1971

54. Steindler A: Orthopaedic operations on the hand. JAMA 71: 1288, 1918

55. Steindler A: Flexorplasty of the thumb in thenar palsy. Surg Gynecol Obstet 50:1005, 1930

56. Taylor TR: Reconstruction of the hand; a new technique in tenoplasty. Surg Gynecol Obstet 32:237–248, 1921

57. Thompson TC: A modified operation for opponens paralysis. J Bone Joint Surg 24:632–640, 1942

58. Tubiana R, Valentin P: Opposition of the thumb. Surg Clin North Am 48:967, 1968

59. Wissinger HA, Singsen EG: Abductor digiti quinti opponensplasty. J Bone Joint Surg 59A:895–898, 1977

Ulnar Nerve Palsy

39

George E. Omer, Jr.

Ulnar nerve palsy results in an awkward hand with significant sensibility loss and profound weakness.

CLINICAL PICTURE

There are ten motor and sensory functions lost in ulnar nerve palsy, and it is imperative for the surgeon to understand these deficits before embarking on a reconstructive program.

Motor Loss

1. Loss of flexion of the proximal phalanges of the fingers, due to paralysis of the interossei and other intrinsic muscles. If extrinsic muscle function is intact, the ring and little fingers will claw (*Duchenne's sign*, 1867),[23,38] with hyperextension of the proximal phalanges and flexion of the middle and distal phalanges. However, if hyperextension is passively prevented by dorsal pressure, the extensor digitorum communis can extend the middle and distal phalanges (*Bouvier's maneuver*, 1851).[66] An

unconscious effort to extend the fingers by tenodesing the extensor tendon with palmar flexion of the wrist only increases the deformity (*André-Thomas sign*, 1917).[38]

2. Loss of integration of MP and interphalangeal joint flexion, due to paralysis of the lumbrical muscles to the ring and little fingers.[26] Normal finger flexion is initiated at the MP joint, and then all three finger joints flex simultaneously. In intrinsic paralysis, the MP joint does not flex until interphalangeal joint flexion has been completed. The fingers curl into the palm, and objects are pushed away instead of grasped.

3. Loss of lateral or key pinch of the thumb, due to paralysis of the adductor pollicis, which normally acts as a first metacarpal adductor, a flexor of the thumb MP joint, and an extensor of the thumb interphalangeal joint. Ulnar nerve palsy is obvious when the MP joint of the thumb is hyperextended to 10 to 15 degrees with key pinch or gross grip (*Jeanne's sign*, 1915).[13,55]

4. Flattened metacarpal arch (palmar arch) and loss of hypothenar elevation (*Masse's sign*, 1916),[38] due to paralysis of opponens digiti quinti and the decreased range of flexion of the little finger MP joint. These four lost functions are responsible for the inefficient power grip associated with low (distal) ulnar nerve palsy.

Power grip is even weaker in a high (proximal) ulnar nerve palsy.

5. Loss of extrinsic power to the ulnar innervated portion of the flexor digitorum profundus, with inability to flex the distal phalanges of the ring and little fingers (*Pollock's sign*, 1919).[38]

6. Partial loss of wrist flexion, due to paralysis of the flexor carpi ulnaris. The position of the wrist is significant in power grip, since it is held in neutral.[3] In a precision grip, the wrist is dorsiflexed until the thumb lies in line with the radius.

7. Precision grip is impaired in ulnar nerve palsy: loss of active lateral mobility with the fingers in extension, due to paralysis of the interossei and hypothenar muscles.[56,57] There is an inability to adduct the extended little finger to the extended ring finger (*Wartenberg's sign,* 1930)[2,38] due to the activity of the extensor digiti minimi, which is unopposed by the paralyzed third palmar interosseous.

8. Loss of distal stability and rotation for a tip pinch between the thumb and index finger (*Froment's sign,* 1915)[13,55] (*Bunnell's "O" sign,* 1956),[3,17,38] due to paralysis of the first dorsal and second palmar interossei and the adductor pollicis. The thumb interphalangeal joint may flex 80 to 90 degrees as the flexor pollicis longus attempts to hold the object. The impairment for power grip is greater than the loss of power for precise grip.[3]

Sensory Loss

9. Sensibility function is lost in ulnar nerve palsy over the volar side of the little finger and the ulnar aspect of the volar side of the ring finger.

10. In the high (proximal) ulnar nerve palsy, there is sensibility loss over the dorso-ulnar aspect of the palm and the dorsal side of the little finger.

Anomalous Innervation Patterns

These ten major functional deficiencies are found in the patient with the usual innervation pattern for the ulnar nerve. A careful examination of the extremity may demonstrate anomalous innervation patterns: the ulnar nerve always contains axons from the anterior divisions of C8 and T1, but often also contains axons from the anterior division of C7 root. In 5 to 10 percent of upper extremities, the motor axons to the flexor carpi ulnaris arise from the C7 root rather than from the C8 and T1 roots.[33] Therefore, it is not uncommon to observe a functioning flexor carpi ulnaris with a complete C8 and T1 lesion.

There are several potential anomalous neural patterns of the ulnar nerve in the forearm. The Martin (1763)-Gruber (1870) communication[33,38] occurs adjacent to the ulnar artery in the proximal forearm and is between the median nerve, or its anterior interosseous branch, and the ulnar nerve. There is a 15 percent occurrence of this anomaly, which carries motor axons from the median nerve to the ulnar nerve and on to many of the intrinsic muscles of the hand. There is a second potential communication in the distal forearm between the ulnar nerve and the median nerve that is far less frequent than the Martin-Gruber connection. There is also a communication within the flexor digitorum profundus between the ulnar nerve and the anterior interosseous branch of the median nerve, resulting in potential variations in the innervation of this muscle. The innervation of the flexor digitorum profundus may vary from all ulnar to all median to completely dual supply.

Riche (1897) and Cannieu (1897) described a potential connection between the motor branch of the ulnar nerve and the recurrent branch of the median nerve in the hand.[33] These anomalous neural patterns occasionally permit a hand to present without deformity even though a complete ulnar nerve palsy is present. For example, the median nerve may innervate all of the lumbricals, and there would be no clawing of the digits. The third lumbrical has dual innervation in 50 percent of upper extremities,[33] and in such a hand, a complete low (distal) ulnar nerve palsy would result in clawing in only the little finger. The first dorsal interosseous is innervated completely or partially by the median nerve in 10 percent of hands and by the radial nerve in 1 percent of hands.[33]

The dorsal cutaneous sensory branch of the ulnar nerve perforates the fascia 6 to 8 cm proximal to the wrist and supplies the dorso-ulnar surface of the hand and the little finger. However, this area can be supplied by the superficial branch of the radial nerve, which will lead to confusion concerning the level of the ulnar nerve lesion.

Diagnostic errors can be avoided with careful voluntary muscle testing, precise evaluation of sensibility and sudomotor activity, anesthetic blocks of intact nerves, and electrodiagnostic studies that include conduction times across segments of the ulnar nerve.

After complete evaluation of the patient, all possible surgical solutions should be considered. Nerve suture is the basic approach to a nerve palsy, but tendon transfers or joint arthrodeses may be acceptable alternate procedures. Each patient has special problems and reconstruction must be individualized.

TIMING OF TENDON TRANSFERS

Patient evaluation is a major factor in the clinical decision for tendon transfers. The patient must be able to understand what is to be done and be ready to accept the postoperative discipline. The surgeon should determine whether the patient desires an increased functional performance or cosmetic improvement.

Homeostasis of the involved extremity must be established before elective tendon surgery.[44] There should be stable skeletal alignment with near-normal passive motion of joints. Soft tissues should be free of scar contractures and have adequate circulation. Chronic wounds are contraindications to elective surgery. The functional performance expected after tendon transfer should be possible to effect by passive movement before surgery.

An important aspect of initial treatment is the appropriate use of individual splints, which should be fabricated for each patient and changed whenever indicated.[41,42] Problems in splinting the ulnar nerve palsy are the maintenance of the transverse palmar arch, and adequate lumbrical and thenar stops to maintain the functional position. External splints are sometimes awkward and often interfere with sensory function.

INTERNAL SPLINTS (EARLY TENDON TRANSFERS)

The objectives of selected early tendon transfers are to stimulate sensory reeducation and to improve the coordination of the residual muscle-tendon units during the interval between the injury and nerve regeneration secondary to suture. The transferred muscle-tendon units can temporarily substitute for the palsied motors until they are reinnervated, or the transferred muscle-tendon units may become the permanent replacement if the injured nerve does not recover.[18,19,47] A complete reconstructive program with multiple tendon transfers is not indicated for internal splinting; instead, the surgeon should use as few tendon transfers as required to maintain dynamic positions for functional coordination and sensory reeducation.

Low Ulnar Nerve Palsy Technique (Omer[4–43,46,48])

An isolated tendon transfer cannot restore all of the power requirements in a low ulnar nerve palsy, but a single flexor digitorum superficialis tendon can improve the integration of MP and interphalangeal joint flexion, key pinch for the thumb, and the flattened metacarpal arch. Arthrodesis of the MP joint of the thumb will improve distal stability for tip pinch. The flexor digitorum superficialis tendon of either the ring or long finger is suitable, but the ring finger superficialis is preferable if the ulnar-innervated portion of the flexor digitorum profundus is not paralyzed (Fig. 39-1).

The ring superficialis tendon is exposed through a finger volar zigzag incision that extends into the palm, and short longitudinal incisions are made over the abductor tubercle of the thumb and the dorsal side of the ring and little fingers at the level of the PIP joint. The radial slip of insertion of the superficialis tendon is released proximal to the PIP joint and tenodesed to prevent hyperextension of the joint after completion of the transfer. The ulnar slip of the superficialis tendon is released at its terminal insertion. The flexor sheath should be retained, especially the proximal A1 and A2 pulleys. The flexor digitorum superficialis is first split longi-

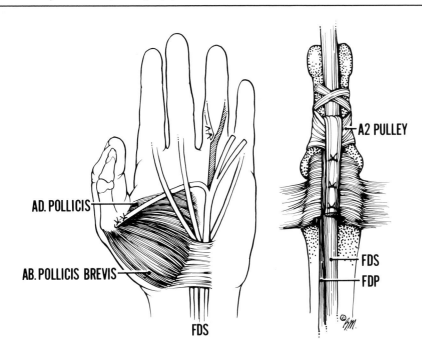

AD. POLLICIS

AB. POLLICIS BREVIS

FDS

A2 PULLEY

FDS

FDP

Fig. 39-1. Transfer of the flexor digitorum superficialis *(FDS)* as an "internal splint" for low ulnar nerve palsy. The radial half of the tendon passes volar to the adductor pollicis muscle and dorsal to the flexor digitorum profundus *(FDP)* tendons into the insertion of the abductor pollicis brevis. The ulnar half of the tendon is split into two slips that are directed distally and volar to the deep transverse metacarpal ligament and through the A2 annular pulley of the flexor sheath. The result is improved thumb-index pinch, and active flexion returns to the MP joint.

tudinally well into the palm, and the ulnar half of the tendon is split again into two slips. The two slips of the ulnar half of the tendon are directed volar to the deep transverse metacarpal ligament and then dorsally, to be sutured at the insertion of the central slip of the dorsal apparatus on the middle phalanx of the ring and little fingers. It is important that the dorsal apparatus is not injured because the slips are not inserted into the lateral bands of the dorsal apparatus. If preoperative testing reveals that the interphalangeal joints cannot be actively extended when the MP joint is stabilized in flexion, this is the insertion that should be performed. Traction on the transferred tendon slips should flex the MP joint and extend the PIP joint.

A different insertion for the two slips is preferred when increased power for grip is desirable. A longitudinal zigzag incision should be made on the volar side of the little finger, in addition to the incision on the volar side of the ring finger. The proximal edges of the flexor sheaths are exposed, and the superficialis slips are passed distally through the flexor sheaths and around the distal edge of the A2 pulley and sutured into place.[22] This insertion does not extend the PIP joint, and is similar to dynamic transfers for proximal phalanx flexion.[10,11,66]

The radial half of the superficialis tendon is directed transversely over the volar surface of the adductor pollicis but dorsal to the flexor tendons and neurovascular structures, and is sutured into the insertion of the abductor pollicis brevis. The pulley for this transfer is the distal edge of the palmar fascia inserted into the third metacarpal.[24] Traction on the transferred tendon half should adduct and pronate the first metacarpal.

The resting tension of the transferred tendon is adjusted at the insertion points while the wrist is in neutral flexion-extension and the hand is supinated into a palm-up position. The MP joints of the clawed fingers are placed in 45 degrees flexion, and the PIP joints in 0 degrees extension (10 degrees flexion if tenodesed). The first metacarpal is adducted so that it is parallel with the plane of the second metacarpal. This intrinsic-plus position is maintained in plaster immobilization for 4 weeks before active extension is allowed.

Distal stability for tip pinch between the thumb and index finger is improved by arthrodesis of the MP joint of the thumb and is indicated when the patient develops a positive Jeanne's sign following transfer of the flexor digitorum superficialis. The joint is approached through a longitudinal incision on the dorsal side of the thumb. The dorsal appa-

Table 39-1. Internal Splints for Low (Distal) Ulnar Nerve Palsy Using One Primary Tendon (Flexor Digitorum Superficialis)

Needed Function	Internal Splint Transfer	Supplemental Motors
Thumb adduction—key pinch	One-half flexor digitorum superficialis[43,45,47,48]	
Metacarpal (palmar) transverse arch	One-half flexor digitorum superficialis split tendon to ring and little fingers[35]	
Proximal phalanx power flexion—ring and little fingers	Flexor sheath insertion[11,66] or	
Integration of MP and interphalangeal motion—ring and little fingers	Central slip insertion[47,49] across PIP joint	
Thumb-index tip pinch	Arthrodesis of thumb MP joint[41,42]	Abductor pollicis longus slip to first dorsal interosseous[40] or Extensor pollicis brevis to first dorsal interosseous[15]
Adduction of little finger		Extensor digiti minimi[2]
Volar sensibility—ring and little fingers		

ratus is split between the extensor pollicis longus and brevis tendons. Synovium is excised, and the distal end of the first metacarpal and the proximal end of the proximal phalanx are denuded of soft tissue. The joint surfaces are cut back with a power saw to produce a chevron-shaped mortise, with the point of the chevron directed proximally. The apex

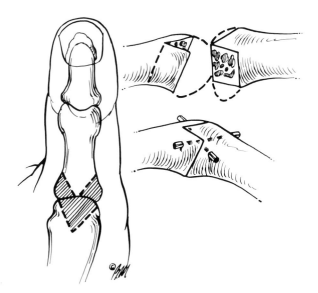

Fig. 39-2. Chevron-shaped mortise for arthrodesis of the MP or PIP joints. The proximal bone cut determines the amount of flexion. Crossed K-wires are used for fixation.

of the phalangeal half of the chevron mortise is made perpendicular to the long axis of the phalanx, while that of the metacarpal portion of the chevron is inclined palmarward to obtain the desired angle of flexion for the arthrodesed joint (Fig. 39-2). The desired flexion is 10 to 15 degrees, and the mortise is then stabilized with buried, crossed K-wires. The wires may be removed after bony healing.

This transfer of a single flexor digitorum superficialis tendon and arthrodesis of the thumb MP joint will improve four of the six lost motor functions in a low (distal) ulnar nerve palsy (Table 39-1). However, these internal splints do not provide adequate strength for power grip, which is the major problem in ulnar nerve palsy. These procedures are indicated during the period of nerve regeneration and are not a definitive reconstructive program.

PROXIMAL PHALANX FLEXION

Any surgical procedure that prevents MP joint hyperextension will control the claw deformity initiated by the extrinsic muscles. Brand believes that ulnar nerve palsy will result in a claw deformity in all four fingers,[9] although this may be apparent in the index and middle fingers only during power pinch.

Static Block Techniques (Howard,[17] Zancolli,[65] Mikhail[39,54])

Mikhail inserted a bone block on the dorsum of the metacarpal head to prevent hyperextension of the proximal phalanx and reported on six patients followed up to 4 years. Howard suggested a bone slab from the dorsal side of the metacarpal, which was directed distalward as a bone block. Arthrode-

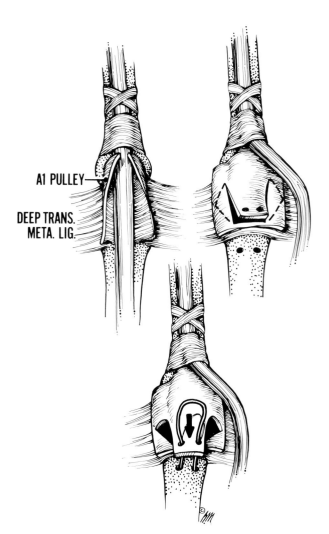

Fig. 39-3. Capsulodesis of the MP joint to control claw deformity. The excised triangles extend into the deep transverse metacarpal ligament and allow the flap to advance to a straight line. The flap is anchored to the metacarpal.

sis has been suggested,[17] but this limits flexion of the fingers into the palm.

Zancolli[65] approaches each MP joint through a volar longitudinal incision. A short flap with a distal base is cut from the volar plate and drawn proximally and sutured into the metacarpal neck with the joint in 20 degrees flexion. It is necessary to open the proximal pulley of the flexor sheath. The result is a pulley advancement with a mild flexion contracture of the MP joint.

Zancolli's procedure has had several modifications (Fig. 39-3). A transverse incision in the distal palmar crease and cutting a triangle into the deep transverse metacarpal ligament on each side of the volar plate flap have provided a better view and a more secure fixation of the flap.[41,42] The excision of a 1.5-cm wide ellipse of palmar skin has been recommended to prevent stretching of the volar plate flap.[12] The advanced volar plate has been inserted into the metacarpal neck and immobilized for a minimum of 6 weeks.[34] Long-term follow-up studies of patients with normally relaxed joint capsules have demonstrated recurrence of clawing.[12]

Bunnell[16,17] performed a flexor pulley advancement as an isolated procedure. Each side of the proximal pulley is split 1.5 to 2.5 cm to the middle of the proximal phalanx. The flexor tendons will then "bowstring," which increases the moment across the MP joint and the power of flexion. The procedure is not effective if there is damage to the extrinsic extensors or the dorsal apparatus of the finger. Fingers often develop ulnar drift when the pulley advancement is carried distal to the A2 pulley.

Tenodesis Techniques (Riordan,[52,54] Fowler,[53,54] Parkes[49])

Riordan uses a dorsal approach to expose the extensor carpi radialis longus and the extensor carpi ulnaris tendons. Each tendon is cut one-half through at the junction of the middle and distal thirds of the muscle. The freed half tendon is stripped distally but left attached to its insertion on a metacarpal. Each half tendon is then split once longitudinally to obtain a total of four slips. Each slip is routed through the interosseous space and

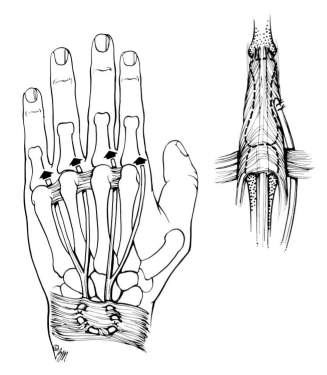

Fig. 39-4. Dorsal tenodesis to control claw deformity. The free graft is looped through the extensor retinaculum (dorsal carpal ligament); the slips pass volar to the deep transverse metacarpal ligament and into the lateral bands of the dorsal apparatus.

passed to the radial side of each finger; the slip passes volar to the deep transverse metacarpal ligament and is inserted into the lateral band of the dorsal apparatus. Only the extensor carpi ulnaris tendon is necessary in ulnar nerve palsy involving the ring and little fingers.

Fowler[53,54] developed a semiactive tenodesis by using wrist flexion to increase tension on the tendon grafts (Fig. 39-4). A long tendon graft, such as the plantaris, is obtained. One end of the tendon graft is sutured into the radial lateral band of the dorsal apparatus of the ring finger, then passed volar to the deep transverse metacarpal ligament on the radial side of the finger and proximally through a small hole in the dorsal carpal ligament. The route is then reversed so that the other end of the graft is sutured into the radial lateral band of the dorsal apparatus of the little finger. Tsuge fixes the proximal (high) point of the tenodesis through drill holes in the distal radius to be sure that the

movements of the wrist act dynamically upon the free tendon graft.[61] In a combined ulnar-median palsy, each end of the tendon can be split into two slips, or another tendon graft can be used for all four fingers. Both Riordan's and Fowler's tenodeses are sutured with the wrist in 30 degrees dorsiflexion and the MP joints in 80 degrees flexion with the interphalangeal joints in full (zero degrees) extension.

Kessler (personal communication, April 1980) has used the extensor retinaculum for the proximal point of a tenodesis, with the distal free tendon slips sutured around the A1 pulley similar to Zancolli's "lasso" procedure.[66] The tendon slips are directed from dorsal to volar through the intermetacarpal spaces and sutured with the MP joint in flexion. Extension is blocked for 3 weeks, but active flexion is continued.

Parkes[49] has devised a more distal tenodesis by placing a free tendon graft between the radial lateral band of the dorsal apparatus of the finger and the flexor retinaculum (deep transverse metacarpal ligament) in the palm (Fig. 39-5). The grafts function independently on each treated finger.

Dynamic Techniques (Brooks,[10,11] Burkhalter,[20] Zancolli[58,66])

The best available method to increase power for gross grip is to add an extra muscle-tendon unit to the power train for flexion of the proximal phalanx.

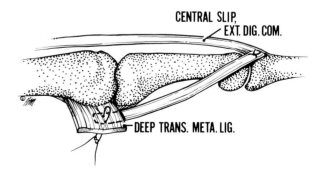

Fig. 39-5. Volar tenodesis to control claw deformity. A free graft passes from the central slip insertion at the PIP joint through the lumbrical canal to the deep transverse metacarpal ligament. The tension for each finger is adjusted individually.

Gross grip power is improved by transferring a wrist extensor or the brachioradialis to flex the MP joint (Fig. 39-6). The flexor digitorum superficialis will not increase gross grip power.

Burkhalter and Strait[20] use a free tendon graft, palmaris longus or plantaris, to prolong the extensor carpi radialis longus tendon. The free graft is split into two slips, which are passed through the intermetacarpal spaces between the long and ring fingers and the ring and little fingers. Each tendon

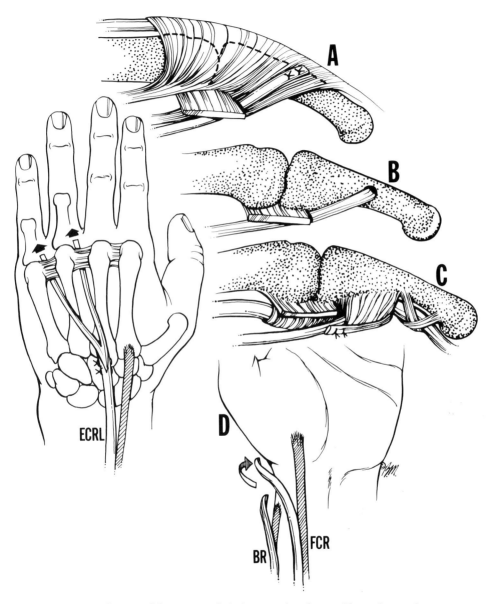

Fig. 39-6. Power flexion of the proximal phalanx can be obtained by utilizing the extensor carpi radialis longus *(ECRL)*, with a free graft, so that tendon slips pass volar to the deep transverse metacarpal ligament. The insertion can be either into (**A**) the lateral bands of the dorsal apparatus, (**B**) the bone of the proximal phalanx, or (**C**) the A2 pulley of the flexor sheath. (**D**) The brachioradialis *(BR)* or the flexor carpi radialis *(FCR)* may be used in place of the extensor carpi radialis longus as the motor.

slip is passed volar to the deep transverse metacarpal ligament and is attached to the radial aspect of the proximal phalanx of the ring and little fingers. A transverse drill hole is made, into which the tendon slip is inserted and held with a pull-out wire technique. It is important to remove all intermetacarpal fascia to minimize adhesions of the tendons. If the finger extensor tendons or the dorsal apparatus are injured, insertion into the extensor apparatus is not indicated, because finger extension is not assisted by the transfer.

Postoperative immobilization is continued for 4 weeks, with the wrist maintained in 45 degrees dorsiflexion and the MP joints in 60 degrees flexion. The extensor carpi radialis longus contracts during finger flexion and is easily retrained. The same procedure may utilize the brachioradialis as the motor muscle.

Brooks[10,11] has described using the flexor carpi radialis or extensor carpi radialis longus prolonged with toe extensor grafts through the carpal canal and attached to the A2 pulley of the flexor sheath. Each graft slip is sutured with the wrist held in maximum palmar flexion and the MP joints in neutral position.

Zancolli[58,66] performs the "lasso" procedure through a transverse incision at the level of the distal palmar crease. The proximal pulleys (A1) of the flexor sheaths are exposed, and the flexor digitorum superficialis tendon to be used is sectioned in the finger. Each superficialis tendon slip is passed volarward through the flexor sheath at the distal edge of the vaginal ligament (A1 pulley) and is looped and sutured to itself (I use the proximal edge of the A2 pulley [see Fig. 39-7B]). The tendon loop is sutured with the finger in neutral position, but with enough tension on the superficialis to complete its passive excursion.

Active (dynamic) flexion of the proximal phalanx does not provide active flexion of the two distal

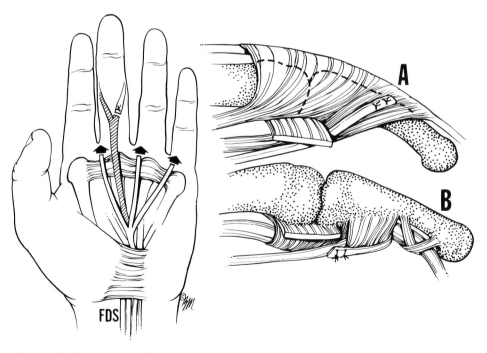

Fig. 39-7. Transfer of a flexor digitorum superficialis *(FDS)* to control claw deformity. The tendon is divided into two to four slips, which are passed through the lumbrical canals and volar to the deep transverse metacarpal ligament. Each slip may be inserted (**A**) into the lateral band of the dorsal apparatus or (**B**) into the A2 pulley of the flexor sheath. One-half of the distal tendon of the donor superficialis tendon is tenodesed across the PIP joint to prevent hyperextension deformity. This transfer does not add power to finger flexion.

phalanges. In a high (proximal) ulnar nerve palsy, active flexion must be restored to the distal phalanx. Also, active flexion of the proximal phalanx will not ensure extension of the DIP joints if they are stiff or the extrinsic tendons are ineffective. Long-standing ulnar nerve palsy may result in fixed PIP joint flexion contractures of the ring and little fingers. If the interphalangeal joint is painful and stiff, an arthrodesis should be considered.[35,63]

INTEGRATION OF FINGER FLEXION

The loss of simultaneous MP flexion with interphalangeal extension and flexion prevents the rhythm necessary to hold large and small objects. Most of the tendon transfers designed to improve the asynchronous motion of the finger joints found in ulnar nerve palsy attempt to duplicate the lumbrical muscles, and therefore pass volar to the deep transverse metacarpal ligament and insert into the lateral band of the dorsal apparatus.[27,37]

Superficialis Techniques (Stiles,[60] Stiles-Bunnell,[16] Riordan[52,53])

Bunnell's modification of Stiles's procedure transferred many tendon slips designed to provide both ulnar and radial deviation to each finger. Riordan's[52–54] modification is the standard technique: The flexor digitorum superficialis of the long finger is split into four slips, and one slip is passed through the lumbrical canal of each finger to be inserted into the radial lateral band of the dorsal apparatus (Fig. 39-7). The slip is sutured with the wrist in 30 degrees palmar flexion, the MP joints in 80 to 90 degrees flexion, and the interphalangeal joints in full extension. A variation in technique is to insert the index slip into the ulnar lateral band of the dorsal apparatus. This procedure should not be used in high (proximal) ulnar nerve palsy unless the index or long superficialis is used as the transfer. The superficialis is out of phase relative to interphalangeal joint motion. Brand's[6] long-

term follow-up studies have shown a high incidence of swan-neck deformity, and a Brooks' insertion[10,11] into the A2 pulley of the flexor sheath may be preferable. The procedure has better long-term results when the tendon slips are sutured under less tension, with the wrist in neutral flexion-extension, the MP joints in 45 to 55 degrees flexion, and the interphalangeal joints neutral. The operation is not indicated in patients with wrist flexion contracture. It is, however, indicated in those patients whose chief complaint is awkwardness of grip due to lack of synchronous motion of the finger joints.

Clinical studies suggest that a finger with intrinsic paralysis cannot give up the flexion activity of the flexor digitorum superficialis. Furthermore, when the superficialis is absent for flexion, it may be too powerful to be used as an extensor. However, if the patient cannot actively extend the interphalangeal joints when the MP joints are stabilized, the superficialis transfer should insert on the central slip at the base of the middle phalanx.[45] If the patient can actively extend the fingers when the proximal phalanx is stabilized, the superficialis transfer should insert into the A2 pulley of the flexor sheath.

COMBINED PROXIMAL PHALANX POWER FLEXION AND INTEGRATION OF FINGER FLEXION

Wrist Level Motors (Fowler,[25,27,54] Riordan,[52,53] Brand[5,7])

Brand has used two techniques that involve wrist extensors. The dorsal approach[5] is motored by the extensor carpi radialis brevis prolonged by plantaris tendon free grafts (Fig. 39-8). The tendon slips are passed superficial to the dorsal carpal ligament, through the intermetacarpal spaces, and then through the lumbrical canal volar to the deep transverse metacarpal ligament and attached to the radial lateral bands of the long, ring, and little

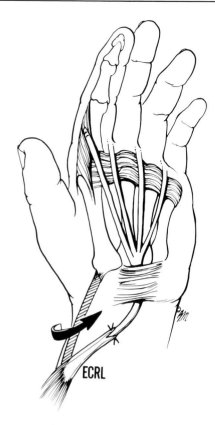

Fig. 39-8. Transfer of the extensor carpi radialis longus *(ECRL)* to control claw deformity. The extensor carpi radialis longus is passed around the radial side of the forearm and extended by a free graft, in two to four slips, through the carpal tunnel and volar to the deep transverse metacarpal ligament, into the lateral band of the dorsal apparatus. This transfer adds power to finger flexion.

fingers and the ulnar lateral band of the index finger. Brand noted that a stronger pinch can be obtained by stabilizing the index finger in adduction at the MP joint,[64] and thus a four-tailed (slips) graft could be used in an ulnar nerve palsy.

Brand has modified the dorsal approach by detaching the extensor carpi radialis longus at its insertion and passing it deep to the brachioradialis to the volar side of the forearm 7.5 cm proximal to the wrist.[7] The plantaris or palmaris tendons are used for the free grafts. The lateral bands are identified through dorsoradial incisions over the proximal phalanx (except the index finger, which has the ulnar lateral band exposed). The tendon slips are directed through the carpal tunnel volar to the deep transverse metacarpal ligaments and into the lateral bands. The tendons are sutured with the wrist dorsiflexed 45 degrees, the MP joints flexed 70 degrees, and the interphalangeal joints in neutral extension. Potential problems with this procedure are flexion deformity of the wrist secondary to removing a strong wrist extensor and possible carpal tunnel syndrome secondary to increased tissue in the carpal canal.

The original Fowler's technique[25,54] used the extensor indicis proprius tendon and the extensor digiti quinti tendons as direct transfers to the lateral bands of the dorsal apparatus. This technique required excessive tension, and an intrinsic-plus deformity was common. In addition, extension of the little finger was lost if the extensor digiti quinti was the only effective extensor of the little finger. Riordan modified the procedure by transferring the extensor indicis proprius to the ulnar side of the hand and dividing the tendon into two slips that are passed volar to the deep transverse metacarpal ligaments and into the radial lateral bands of the ring and little fingers. The technique is easier than one using free tendon grafts. If the median nerve is also involved, a free tendon graft can provide tendon slips for the long and index fingers.

Patients with ulnar nerve palsy often develop wrist palmar flexion deformity in an attempt to extend the clawed fingers. Riordan transfers the flexor carpi radialis, elongated with a brachioradialis, plantaris, or palmaris free graft. The flexor carpi radialis is passed to the dorsal side of the forearm, and the free tendon slips are passed through the intermetacarpal spaces, then volar to the deep transverse metacarpal ligaments, and into the radial lateral bands of the involved fingers. The flexor carpi radialis is in phase for interphalangeal extension, and minimal rehabilitation is necessary.

The wrist motor procedures use free grafts. The incidence of absence of the plantaris is about 8 percent, whereas the palmaris longus is absent in approximately 11 to 14 percent. There seems to be no relationship between the absence of the palmaris longus and that of the plantaris. When the plantaris is absent, it is usually absent bilaterally, but when the palmaris longus is absent, its absence is bilateral in 60 percent of cases.[48]

KEY PINCH AND FLAT METACARPAL ARCH

Biomechanical studies have shown the residual strength for pinching grip and palmar adduction of the thumb to be diminished as much as 75 to 85 percent in patients with ulnar nerve palsy. Most tendon transfers provide improved stability and pinch but only in the range of 25 to 50 percent of normal strength.[13,29,38]

Thumb Adduction Techniques (Bunnell,[17] Littler,[13,24,26,27] Boyes,[4] Goldner[28,29])

Bunnell's "tendon loop" utilizes the extensor digitorum communis to the index finger. The tendon is detached from the index dorsal apparatus and withdrawn to the dorsal carpal ligament. The tendon is elongated by a free tendon graft from the palmaris longus or plantaris, then passed subcutaneously around the ulnar border of the hand and across the palm deep to the flexor tendons, to be inserted into bone on the ulnar side of the base of the proximal phalanx of the thumb at the adductor tubercle. The communis tendon is selected because its muscle is stronger than the extensor indicis proprius. The dorsal apparatus (extensor hood) should be carefully closed to prevent extensor lag of the index finger.[14]

In contrast, the extensor indicis proprius has been used as the motor.[13] The tendon is passed volarward between the third and fourth metacarpals and then passed across the transverse muscle belly of the adductor pollicis. The tendon is sutured to the adductor pollicis insertion. Brand[8,24] recommends inserting the transfer into the abductor pollicis brevis tendon as a more functional placement of the insertion. Tension is achieved by holding the wrist in zero flexion-extension and the first and second metacarpals parallel to each other in both the lateral and anteroposterior planes. A pull of 2 to 3 kg is exerted on the tendon in this position before sutures are placed.

Boyes has advocated the brachioradialis as the donor muscle because its amplitude of motion is sufficient to allow action whether the wrist is flexed or extended (Fig. 39-9). He also illustrated the ex-

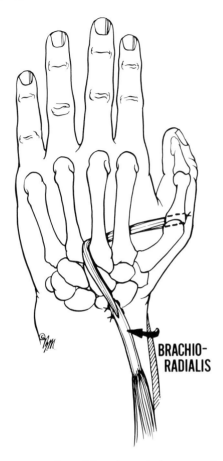

Fig. 39-9. Transfer of brachioradialis, extended with free tendon graft, through the interspace between the third and fourth metacarpals, to insert on the abductor tubercle of the thumb. This transfer will add power to key pinch.

tensor carpi ulnaris as the donor muscle.[4] The wrist extensors must be elongated with free grafts. Solonen and Bakalim[59] have used the extensor carpi radialis longus in a similar transfer.

Littler recommends a long or ring flexor digitorum superficialis transfer in those patients with hyperextension deformity of the MP joint of the thumb (Fig. 39-10). The superficialis is detached in the finger, the decussation is split, and withdrawn into the palm. Brown[13] cautions to leave enough distal tendon to prevent hyperextension (recurvatum) of the PIP joint. The superficialis tendon is tunneled across the volar surface of the adductor pollicis and sutured to the adductor pollicis tendon at its insertion. Edgerton and Brand[24] recommend

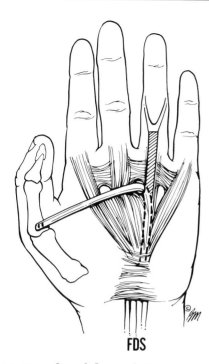

FDS

Fig. 39-10. Transfer of flexor digitorum superficialis *(FDS)*, through a fascial pulley, to the abductor tubercle of the thumb. This transfer will add power to key pinch, but will further weaken power grasp.

an abductor tubercle insertion for improved key pinch. The pulley for this procedure, and the procedure that I use,[43,45] is the vertical septum of the palmar fascia as described by Edgerton and Brand.[24] The thumb and wrist are immobilized for 4 weeks, and then active motion is allowed. Hamlin and Littler[32] reported their results for superficialis transfer and recorded a return of pinch power to 70 percent of the uninvolved hand.

Goldner[28,29] uses the long finger flexor digitorum superficialis that approaches the thumb on the dorsal surface of the hand. The superficialis is withdrawn to the volar side of the wrist. A hole 2 × 3 cm is made in the ulnar side of the pronator quadratus muscle, and the tendon is passed through the interosseous membrane proximal to the wrist joint. The superficialis is passed subcutaneously around the distal end of the extensor carpi ulnaris, which acts as a pulley. The superficialis is then directed under the extensor digitorum communis and other extensor tendons in a line parallel to the extensor pollicis longus. The tendon is su-

tured into a drill hole on the ulnar aspect of the thumb at the level of the adductor tendon insertion. Immobilization is continued for 3 weeks and maintains the wrist in 30 degrees palmar flexion, the MP joints in 45 degrees flexion, and the interphalangeal joints in 10 degrees flexion, while the thumb is held about 1 cm away from the index finger.

Metacarpal Arch Restoration (Bunnell,[4,17] Littler,[35] Ranney[50])

It is often emphasized that the wrist must be stable before an operation is performed to reconstruct the hand; therefore, a procedure to improve finger activity must first consider the stability of the transverse metacarpal arch. Instability (flattening) of the transverse metacarpal arch may contribute to recurrent clawing following lumbrical replacement procedures.[51]

Bunnell's "tendon-T" operation[4,17] gives adduction to the thumb and the little finger, while cupping the hand to restore the metacarpal arch. A free tendon graft spans the hand, dorsal to the flexor tendons, from the base of the proximal phalanx of the thumb to the neck of the metacarpal of the little finger. A flexor digitorum superficialis tendon is detached from its origin and is attached by a loop to the center of the free tendon, forming a T. On contraction of the superficialis, the T is made into a Y, and the metacarpal arch is restored.

Littler[35] transfers a flexor digitorum superficialis but does not use the free tendon graft across the palm. One slip of the superficialis is sutured to the adductor tubercle, the other slip to a bony insertion in the base of the proximal phalanx of the little finger.

Ranney[50] depresses the metacarpal arch with a volar transfer of the extensor digiti minimi to the neck of the fifth metacarpal. The extensor digiti minimi is step-cut at its insertion, leaving a strip to be sutured to the extensor digitorum communis. The muscle-tendon unit is withdrawn to the wrist and passed through the forearm between the abductor pollicis longus and the flexor carpi radialis. The extensor digiti minimi tendon then passes subcutaneously in a diagonal course to be sutured to the periosteum of the neck of the fifth metacarpal.

Ahern (personal communication, 1969) has produced an effect similar to that from Ranney's procedure by looping the flexor digitorum superficialis of the little finger around the deep transverse metacarpal ligament between the fourth and fifth metacarpals.

TIP PINCH

Index Abduction Techniques (Bunnell,[4,17] Graham and Riordan,[31] Bruner,[15] Neviaser, Wilson, and Gardner[40])

The flexion strength of the flexor pollicis longus often displaces the opposing index finger to an adducted position, which is particularly noted in pulp-to-pulp pinch. A tendon transfer to abduct and flex the index finger is essential to the reconstruction of tip pinch.

Bunnell[4,17] reported the transfer of the extensor indicis proprius to the tendon of the first dorsal interosseous. The tendon is divided from the index dorsal apparatus and withdrawn at the wrist through a short transverse incision and passed distally around the radial border of the second metacarpal to insert into the first dorsal interosseous tendon volar to the axis of the motion of the MP joint. The dorsal apparatus should be carefully closed to prevent extension lag of the index finger.[14] The transfer must be sutured under considerable tension (2 to 3 kg) for an adequate performance.[13] Success is demonstrated by stability during pulp-to-pulp pinching, in that there will be slight flexion of the index MP joint and no adduction of the index. Clippinger and Goldner[21,30] believe that this transfer is not a satisfactory procedure, perhaps secondary to a short moment arm and a narrow angle of approach. Solonen and Bakalin[59] improved the approach angle by rerouting the extensor indicis proprius from the wrist around the "dynamic pulley," consisting of the extensor tendons of the thumb.

Graham and Riordan[31] passed a flexor digitorum superficialis, usually from the ring finger, either to bone on the radial side of the proximal phalanx or to

the tendon of the first dorsal interosseous. The superficialis is withdrawn at the wrist and directed subcutaneously around the radial aspect of the forearm, over the anatomic snuffbox and the first dorsal interosseous space to the radial aspect of the index finger. Postoperative immobilization includes holding the index finger in abduction and extension with the wrist slightly flexed. At the end of 3 weeks, active motion is permitted.

Bruner[15] has transferred the extensor pollicis brevis (Fig. 39-11), but Graham and Riordan[31] stated that this tendon is lacking in strength. Burkhalter and Eversmann have prolonged the brachioradialis with a free tendon graft and inserted the tendon into the proximal phalanx of the index finger. Eyler and Coonrad[21] described a split insertion for a flexor digitorum superficialis transfer, with one-half of the superficialis through the lumbrical canal and the other half subcutaneously toward the dorsal surface.

Neviaser, Wilson, and Gardner[40] recommend the transfer of a slip of the abductor pollicis longus

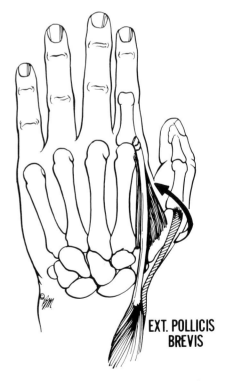

EXT. POLLICIS BREVIS

Fig. 39-11. Transfer of the extensor pollicis brevis to the insertion of the first dorsal interosseous to improve index abduction.

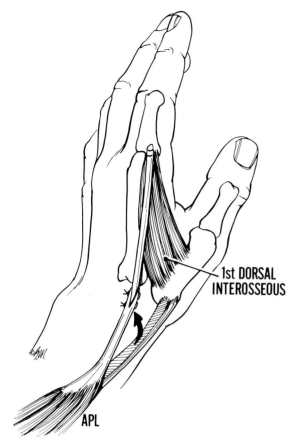

Fig. 39-12. Extension of a slip of the abductor pollicis longus *(APL)*, with a free graft, into the tendon of the first dorsal interosseous. The brachioradialis may be used as an alternative motor.

elongated with a free tendon graft — palmaris longus or plantaris — into the tendon of the first dorsal interosseous (Fig. 39-12). The abductor pollicis longus is exposed distal to the first dorsal compartment, and the insertion of its slips are inspected. Only the slip that inserts on the first metacarpal is essential; if there are additional slips, one may be used for the first dorsal interosseous transfer.

Arthrodesis of Thumb Joints (Omer,[41,48] Brand,[9] Brown,[13] Tubiana[62])

Brown notes that splinting the ulnar palsied thumb usually increases pinch strength by 1 to 2 kg. The position for arthrodesis of the interpha-

langeal joint of the thumb is 20 to 30 degrees flexion. Some patients have objected to the loss of motion and have considered this a greater problem than the ineffective tip pinch. Brown reserves this procedure for patients in whom the interphalangeal joint is noticeably unstable. Tubiana[62] prefers interphalangeal joint arthrodesis to fusion of the MP joint.

I[41,48] recommend arthrodesis of the MP joint when there is instability in the longitudinal arch of the thumb (Fig. 39-2). Brand[9] places the joint in 15 degrees flexion, 5 degrees abduction, and 15 degrees extra pronation. Barden[1] has reported normal active motion of the interphalangeal joint following arthrodesis of the MP joint of the thumb, with correction of Froment's sign.

LITTLE FINGER ABDUCTION

Blacker, Lister, and Kleinert[2] found that the extensor digiti minimi had the potential to abduct the little finger through its indirect insertion into the abductor tubercle on the proximal phalanx. The balancing force is provided by the third palmar interosseous, which is inactive in ulnar nerve palsy. The problem is corrected with a transfer of the ulnar half of the tendon of the extensor digiti minimi (Fig. 39-13). The ulnar half of the tendon is detached from the dorsal apparatus and dissected proximally to the distal edge of the dorsal carpal ligament (extensor retinaculum). A palmar incision is made that extends obliquely from the distal palmar crease to the proximal digital crease, which will expose the deep transverse metacarpal ligament and the flexor sheath of the little finger. The ulnar half of the extensor digiti minimi is passed between the fourth and fifth metacarpals into the palmar wound. If the little finger is clawed as well as abducted, the tendon slip is inserted into a radially based flap of the flexor tendon sheath just distal to the proximal A1 pulley (Brooks' insertion).[10,11] If the little finger is not clawed, the tendon slip is passed beneath the deep transverse metacarpal ligament and sutured into the phalangeal attachment of the radial collateral ligament of

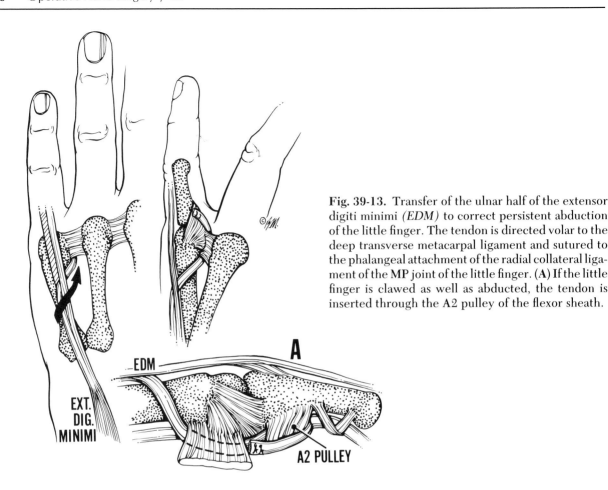

Fig. 39-13. Transfer of the ulnar half of the extensor digiti minimi *(EDM)* to correct persistent abduction of the little finger. The tendon is directed volar to the deep transverse metacarpal ligament and sutured to the phalangeal attachment of the radial collateral ligament of the MP joint of the little finger. **(A)** If the little finger is clawed as well as abducted, the tendon is inserted through the A2 pulley of the flexor sheath.

the MP joint of the little finger. The tendon is sutured with the wrist in neutral flexion-extension and the MP joint in 20 degrees flexion. The ring and little fingers are splinted for 4 weeks with the wrist extended and the MP joint flexed. The interphalangeal joints are left free, and motion is encouraged to prevent adhesions of the flexor tendons.

Goldner[29] detaches the entire extensor digiti minimi and withdraws the tendon to the level of the dorsal carpal ligament (extensor retinaculum). The tendon is passed under the extensor carpi radialis longus as a pulley and is inserted from the dorsal surface into the oblique fibers of the dorsal apparatus of the little finger or directly into bone. One must be certain that there is a functional slip of the extensor digitorum communis to the little finger prior to removing the entire extensor digiti minimi.

FINGER AND WRIST FLEXION

Brand does not consider the loss of flexor carpi ulnaris and the ulnar half of the flexor digitorum profundus to be a functional problem, and he states that tendon transfers should not be considered unless there is also median or radial nerve loss[8] (see Chapter 40). If there is marked weakness of the ring and little fingers in isolated ulnar nerve paralysis, the profundus tendons of the ring and little fingers are attached to the profundus tendon of the long finger in the forearm. The index profundus should be left free. Bunnell[17] believed it inadvisable to join the profundus of the long finger, because the more the long flexors are working, the more marked will be the clawhand deformity.

My own experience leaves me less pessimistic,

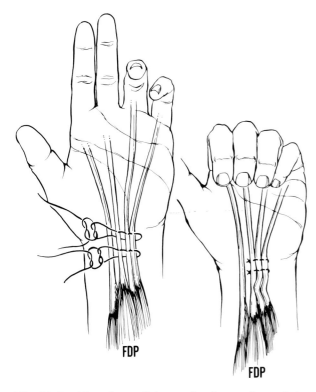

Fig. 39-14. Tenodesis of the profundus tendons of the ring and little fingers to the active flexor digitorum profundus *(FDP)* of the long finger to increase power for gross grip. A double line of sutures is important to prevent "whip-sawing" of the tendons during power grip.

and I believe that side-to-side tenodesis of the profundus tendons of the ring and little fingers to the profundus of the long finger in the forearm will increase the power for gross grip (Fig. 39-14). These patients should also have an intrinsic transfer and a procedure to restore the metacarpal arch. If the total series of procedures is impracticable, the surgeon should consider tenodesis of the flexor digitorum profundus across the DIP joints of the ring and little fingers. It would be equally useful to transfer the tendon of the flexor carpi radialis to the insertion of the flexor carpi ulnaris in a patient who wished to perform activities requiring strong wrist flexion. Ulnar deviation is as important for wrist flexion as radial deviation is for wrist extension.

AUTHOR'S PREFERRED METHODS

Ulnar nerve palsy results in a hand with so many functional problems that there is no "standard" accepted program that is suitable for reconstruction in all patients. Available tendon assets must be invested wisely. For example, the ubiquitous flexor digitorum superficialis has been overused for proximal phalanx flexion, as a substitute for the lumbri-

Table 39-2. Author's Preferred Reconstructive Program for Low (Distal) Ulnar Nerve Palsy

Needed Function	Preferred Transfer	Alternate Transfers
Thumb adduction — key pinch	Brachioradialis with free graft between third and fourth metacarpals and to abductor tubercle of thumb[4]	Flexor digitorum superficialis to abductor tubercle of thumb with palmar fascia[8,35,36] and flexor tendons as pulleys
Metacarpal (palmar) transverse arch Adduction for little finger	Extensor digiti minimi transfer volar to deep transverse metacarpal ligament[2] (extensor digitorum communis to little finger must be effective)	Flexor digitorum superficialis to little finger transferred volar to deep transverse metacarpal ligament between fourth and fifth metacarpals (Ahern, 1969) or Should be combined as single transfer with thumb adduction transfer[43,45,48]
Proximal phalanx power flexion and integration of MP and interphalangeal motion (clawed fingers)	Extensor carpi radialis longus to all four fingers using four-tailed free graft and flexor sheath insertion[5–7,9,11,20,66]	Flexor carpi radialis (if wrist flexion contracture) with four-tailed free graft and flexor sheath insertion[30,52,53,65]
Thumb-index tip pinch	Abductor pollicis longus slip to first dorsal interosseous tendon[40] and arthrodesis of MP joint of thumb[41,42]	Extensor pollicis brevis to first dorsal interosseous[15] (if thumb MP has been fused)
Volar sensibility — ring and little fingers	Free nerve graft (donor: sural nerve)	Free neurovascular cutaneous island flap on long nerve pedicle

Table 39-3. Author's Preferred Reconstructive Program for High (Proximal) Ulnar Nerve Palsy

Needed Function	Preferred Transfer	Alternate Transfers
Thumb adduction—key pinch	Brachioradialis with free graft between third and fourth metacarpals and to abductor tubercle of thumb[4]	Flexor digitorum superficialis to abductor tubercle of thumb[8,35,36] (long finger is only candidate)
Metacarpal (palmar) transverse arch Adduction for little finger	Extensor digiti minimi transfer volar to deep transverse metacarpal ligament[2] (extensor digitorum communis to little finger must be effective)	Long flexor digitorum superficialis as split transfer—to little finger and as thumb adductor[43,45,48]
Proximal phalanx power flexion and integration of MP and interphalangeal motion (clawed fingers)	Extensor carpi radialis longus to all four fingers through four-tailed graft and flexor sheath insertion[5–7,9,11,20,66]	Flexor carpi radialis (if wrist flexion contracture) with four-tailed graft and flexor sheath insertion[20,52,53,66]
Thumb-index tip pinch	Abductor pollicis longus slip to first dorsal interosseous tendon[40] and arthrodesis of thumb MP joint[41,42]	Extensor pollicis brevis to first dorsal interosseous[15] (if thumb MP has been fused)
Distal finger flexion—ring and little fingers	Flexor digitorum profundus (long) tenodesed to flexor digitorum profundus (ring and little)	Tenodesis, DIP joints, ring and little fingers
Wrist flexion—ulnar aspect	Flexor carpi radialis to insertion of flexor carpi ulnaris	Palmaris longus to insertion of flexor carpi ulnaris
Volar sensibility—ring and little fingers Dorsal sensibility—little finger ray	None available	Free neurovascular cutaneous island flap on very long nerve pedicles

cals, as a thumb adductor, to restore the metacarpal arch, as an index abductor—yet it provides the only flexor power in the ring and little fingers in a high (proximal) ulnar nerve palsy!

When a precise neurorrhaphy has been performed on a low (distal) ulnar nerve laceration, the prognosis for reinnervation of palsied muscles has improved during the past decade. In these patients, selected tendon transfers may be performed early as internal splints to support partial function while awaiting the potential nerve recovery (Table 39-1).

Patients with a severe extremity injury, a nerve graft, or a high (proximal) ulnar nerve lesion are all candidates for a complete reconstruction program. The author's preferred transfers, as well as alternative methods, are listed in Tables 39-2 and 39-3. The potential for functional motor action is better than recovery of sensibility in the high (proximal) ulnar nerve palsy.

REFERENCES

1. Barden GA: American Society for Surgery of the Hand, Correspondence Club Newsletter 47, 1978
2. Blacker GJ, Lister GD, Kleinert HE: The abducted little finger in low ulnar nerve palsy. J Hand Surg 1:190–196, 1976
3. Bowden Ruth EM, Napier JR: The assessment of hand functional after peripheral nerve injuries. J Bone Joint Surg 43B:481–492, 1961
4. Boyes JH: Bunnell's Surgery of the Hand. p. 514. 4th Ed. JB Lippincott, Philadelphia, 1964
5. Brand PW: Hand reconstruction in leprosy. p. 117. In British Surgical Practice. Surgical Progress 1954. Butterworth, London, 1954
6. Brand PW: Paralytic claw hand. J Bone Joint Surg 40B:618–632, 1958
7. Brand PW: Tendon grafting. Illustrated by a new operation for intrinsic paralysis of the fingers. J Bone Joint Surg 43B:444–453, 1961
8. Brand PW: Tendon transfers in the forearm. p. 331. In Flynn JE (ed): Hand Surgery. Williams & Wilkins, Baltimore, 1966
9. Brand PW: Tendon transfers for median and ulnar nerve paralysis. Orthop Clin North Am 1:447–454, 1970
10. Brooks AL: Tendon transfer for intrinsic minus fingers. American Society for Surgery of the Hand, Correspondence Club Newsletter, Nov. 24, 1969
11. Brooks AL, Jones DS: A new intrinsic tendon transfer for the paralytic hand. J Bone Joint Surg 57A:730, 1975
12. Brown PW: Zancolli capsulorrhaphy for ulnar claw hand. J Bone Joint Surg 52A:868, 1970
13. Brown PW: Reconstruction for pinch in ulnar intrinsic palsy. Orthop Clin North Am 5:323–342, 1974
14. Browne EZ Jr, Teague MA, Snyder CC: Prevention

of extensor lag after indicis proprius tendon transfer. J Hand Surg 4:168–172, 1979

15. Bruner JM: Tendon transfer to restore abduction of the index finger using the extensor pollicis brevis. Plast Reconstr Surg 3:197–201, 1948

16. Bunnell S: Surgery of the intrinsic muscles of the hand other than those producing opposition of the thumb. J Bone Joint Surg 24:1–31, 1942

17. Bunnell S: Surgery of the Hand. JB Lippincott, Philadelphia, 1944

18. Burkhalter WE: Early tendon transfer in upper extremity peripheral nerve injury. Proceedings of American Society for Surgery of the Hand. J Bone Joint Surg 53A:816–817, 1971

19. Burkhalter WE: Early tendon transfers in upper extremity peripheral nerve injury. Clin Orthop 104:68–79, 1974

20. Burkhalter WE, Strait JL: Metacarpophalangeal flexor replacement for intrinsic paralysis. J Bone Joint Surg 55A:1667–1676, 1973

21. Clippinger FW, Goldner JL: Tendon transfers as substitutes for paralyzed first dorsal and volar interosseous muscles. Proceedings of American Society for Surgery of the Hand. J Bone Joint Surg 47A:633, 1965

22. Doyle JA, Blythe W: The finger flexor tendon sheath and pulleys: Anatomy and reconstruction. pp. 81–87. In Hunter JM, Schneider LH (eds): AAOS Symposium on Tendon Surgery in the Hand. CV Mosby, St Louis, 1975

23. Duchenne GB: Physiology of Motion Demonstrated by Electrical Stimulation and Clinical Observation. p. 141. (Translated and edited by Kaplan EB.) WB Saunders, Philadelphia, 1959

24. Edgerton MT, Brand PW: Restoration of abduction and adduction to the unstable thumb in median and ulnar paralysis. Plast Reconstr Surg 36:150–164, 1965

25. Enna CD, Riordan DC: The Fowler procedure for correction of the paralytic claw hand. Plast Reconstr Surg 52:352–360, 1973

26. Flatt AE: Kinesiology of the hand. pp. 266–281. AAOS Instructional Course Lectures, Vol. 18. CV Mosby, St Louis, 1961

27. Fowler SB: Extensor apparatus of the digits. J Bone Joint Surg 31B:447, 1949

28. Goldner JL: Replacement of the function of the paralyzed adductor pollicis with the flexor digitorum sublimis—a ten year review. Proceedings of American Society for Surgery of the Hand. J Bone Joint Surg 49A:583, 1967

29. Goldner JL: Tendon transfers for irreparable peripheral nerve injuries of the upper extremities. Orthop Clin North Am 5:343–375, 1974

30. Goldner JL, Irwin CE: An analysis of paralytic thumb deformities. J Bone Joint Surg 32A:627–639, 1950

31. Graham WC, Riordan DC: Sublimis transplant to restore abductor of index finger. Plast Reconstr Surg 2:459–462, 1947

32. Hamlin C, Littler JW: Restoration of power pinch. Orthop Trans 3:319, 1979

33. Kaplan EB, Spinner M: Normal and anomalous innervation patterns in the upper extremity. pp. 75–99. In Omer GE, Spinner M (eds): Management of Peripheral Nerve Problems. WB Saunders, Philadelphia, 1980

34. Leddy JP, Stark HH, Ashworth CR, Boyes JH: Capsulodesis and pulley advancement for the correction of claw finger deformity. J Bone Joint Surg 54A:1465–1471, 1972

35. Littler JW: Tendon transfers and arthrodesis in combined median and ulnar nerve palsies. J Bone Joint Surg 31A:225–234, 1949

36. Littler JW: Restoration of power and stability in the partially paralyzed hand. p. 1675. In Converse JM (ed): Reconstructive Plastic Surgery, Vol. IV. WB Saunders, Philadelphia, 1964

37. Long C: Intrinsic-extrinsic muscle control of the fingers. Electromyographic studies. J Bone Joint Surg 50A:973–984, 1968

38. Mannerfelt L: Studies on the hand in ulnar nerve paralysis. A clinic-experimental investigation in normal and anomalous innervation. Acta Orthop Scand suppl 87, 1966

39. Mikhail IK: Bone block operation for clawhand. Surg Gynecol Obstet 118:1077–1079, 1964

40. Neviaser RJ, Wilson JN, Gardner MM: Abductor pollicis longus transfer for replacement of first dorsal interosseous. J Hand Surg 5:53–57, 1980

41. Omer GE Jr: Evaluation and reconstruction of the forearm and hand after acute traumatic peripheral nerve injuries. J Bone Joint Surg 50A:1454–1478, 1968

42. Omer GE Jr: Evaluation and reconstruction of the forearm and hand after acute traumatic peripheral nerve injuries. pp. 93–119. AAOS Instructional Course Lectures, Vol. 18J-1. CV Mosby, St Louis, 1973

43. Omer GE Jr: Restoring power grip in ulner palsy. Proceedings of American Society for Surgery of the Hand. J Bone Joint Surg 53A:814, 1971

44. Omer GE Jr: The technique and timing of tendon transfers. Orthop Clin North Am 5:243–252, 1974

45. Omer GE Jr: Tendon transfers in combined nerve lesions. Orthop Clin North Am 5:377–387, 1974

46. Omer GE Jr: Complications of treatment of peripheral nerve injuries. pp. 765–801. In Epps CH (ed):

Complications in Orthopaedic Surgery. JB Lippincott, Philadelphia, 1978

47. Omer GE Jr: Tendon transfers as early internal splints following peripheral nerve injury in the upper extremity. pp. 292–296. In Hunter JM, Schneider LH, Mackin EJ, Bell JA (eds): Rehabilitation of the Hand. CV Mosby, St Louis, 1978

48. Omer GE Jr: Tendon transfers for reconstruction of the forearm and hand following peripheral nerve injuries. pp. 817–846. In Omer GE, Spinner M (eds): Management of Peripheral Nerve Problems. WB Saunders, Philadelphia, 1980

49. Parkes A: Paralytic claw fingers—a graft tenodesis operation. Hand 5:192–199, 1973

50. Ranney DA: Reconstruction of the transverse metacarpal arch in ulnar palsy by transfer of the extensor digiti minimi. Plast Reconstr Surg 52:406–412, 1973

51. Ranney DA: The mechanism of arch reversal in the surgically corrected claw hand. Hand 6:266–272, 1974

52. Riordan DC: Tendon transplantations in median-nerve and ulnar-nerve paralysis. J Bone Joint Surg 35A:312–320, 1953

53. Riordan DC: Surgery of the paralytic hand. pp. 79–90. AAOS Instructional Course Lectures, Vol. 16. CV Mosby, St Louis, 1959

54. Riordan DC: Tendon transfers for nerve paralysis of the hand and wrist. Curr Pract Orthop Surg 2:17–40, 1964

55. Roullet J: Froment's sign. pp. 37–43. In Michon J, Moberg E (eds): Traumatic Nerve Lesions of the Upper Limb, Group d'Etude de la Main monograph #2. Churchill Livingstone, Edinburgh, 1975

56. Smith RJ: Balance and kinetics of the fingers under normal and pathological conditions. Clin Orthop 104:92–111, 1974

57. Smith RJ: Intrinsic muscles of the fingers: Function, dysfunction, and surgical reconstruction. pp. 200–220. AAOS Instructional Course Lectures, Vol. 24. CV Mosby, St Louis, 1975

58. Smith RJ: Surgical treatment of the clawhand. pp. 181–203. In Hunter JM, Schneider LH (eds): AAOS Symposium on Tendon Surgery in the Hand. CV Mosby, St Louis, 1975

59. Solonen KA, Bakalim GE: Restoration of pinch grip in traumatic ulnar palsy. Hand 8:39, 1976

60. Stiles HJ, Forrester-Brown MF: Treatment of injuries of the peripheral spinal nerves. p. 166. H Frowde and Hodder, Stoughton, 1922

61. Tsuge K: Tendon transfers in median and ulnar nerve paralysis. Hiroshima J Med Sci 16:29–48, 1967

62. Tubiana R: Palliative treatment of paralytic deformities of the thumb. Orthop Clin North Am 4:1141–1160, 1973

63. Tubiana R, Malek R: Paralysis of the intrinsic muscles of the fingers. Surg Clin North Am 48:1139–1148, 1968

64. White WL: Restoration of function and balance of the wrist and hand by tendon transfers. Surg Clin North Am 40:427–459, 1960

65. Zancolli EA: Claw-hand caused by paralysis of the intrinsic muscles. A simple surgical procedure for its correction. J Bone Joint Surg 39A:1076–1080, 1957

66. Zancolli EA: Structural and Dynamic Bases of Hand Surgery. 2nd Ed. pp. 168,174. JB Lippincott, Philadelphia, 1978

Combined Nerve Palsies 40

George E. Omer, Jr.

When multiple nerves are injured in a single extremity, the functional loss is severe. Circulation is usually impaired, which results in ischemic pain and increased fibrosis. The skeleton may be unstable, with loss of normal joint stability and motion. Muscle-tendon units are often lacerated and sometimes avulsed, increasing the neuromotor impairment, and the resulting scar complicates the technical transfer of remaining intact tendons. Unhealed or chronic wounds are contraindications to elective surgery. As joints stiffen and muscles atrophy, the maintenance of a mobile hand without deforming contracture demands persistent therapy and meticulous splinting. Reconstructive procedures should not be undertaken until normal joint motion has been established and skeletal alignment is stable.[40]

In addition to the physical condition of the involved extremity, successful tendon transfers depend on the etiology and prognosis of the motor imbalance. The etiology of the motor imbalance is important in predicting the further involvement of additional muscle-tendon units with progressive functional impairment. The extent of muscle imbalance is usually static after traumatic injury, but is often unstable in upper motor neuron problems, such as a series of cerebrovascular accidents. The prognosis for progressive muscle imbalance may be a contraindication for elective surgery. A major problem in multiple nerve palsy is sensory loss coupled with a loss of position sense and other normal feedback mechanisms. Spinal reflex arcs coordinate with the ventral horn motor neurons to produce a pattern of motor function. For each muscle there is an optimal tension at which force and motion are efficient.[35,22] In addition, one must consider the potential for excursion of each muscle in a new position.[9] Muscles with only temporary loss of function, such as a neurapraxia lesion, do not regain normal strength for elective transfer procedures.[33] Sensibility loss is more profound in combined nerve palsies, and motor return rarely passes two major joints distal to the injury.[39]

The motion expected after tendon transfer cannot exceed the passive movement present preoperatively. However, the longer one waits for nerve recovery, the more difficult it is to prevent deformity. Combined nerve palsies are further complicated by the fewer number of motor tendons that are available to stabilize residual function[29] or to provide additional function while awaiting potential nerve recovery following neurorrhaphy.[19,44] Therefore, it is difficult to utilize muscle-tendon units as internal splints to enhance patterns of motion in combined nerve palsies.

Tendon tranfers in combined nerve palsies are

more complicated than those in isolated nerve palsy because of complex extremity injuries, poor proprioception, weakness of muscles for potential transfer, and the need for multiple operations. The most important aspect of a rehabilitation program is the patient's acceptance of the responsibility and initiative for his own recovery.[8]

LOW MEDIAN-ULNAR NERVE PALSY

This is the most common combined nerve palsy, and the complete loss of volar sensation and intrinsic motor muscles produces an almost useless claw-hand (Fig. 40-1). Reconstruction of the thumb is extremely important,[45] and special effort must be made to prevent adduction contractures. There is a flat transverse palmar arch (metacarpal arch), with hyperextension at the MP joints and hyperflexion at the PIP joints. An abducted little finger may be associated with the flat transverse metacarpal arch.[16] The patient uses flexion of the wrist as a functional tenodesis to obtain greater finger exten-

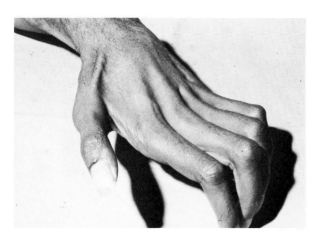

Fig. 40-1. A combined median-ulnar palsy, with intrinsic motor atrophy and atrophy of volar pulps of the fingers. The thumb has developed an adduction contracture.

sion, but with prolonged use, this results in a fixed flexion contracture of the wrist[52] (Ahern GS: Personal communication, 1969). Following individualized transfers, the residual loss of sensibility should be a greater functional problem than patterns for grasp and pinch (Table 40-1).

Table 40-1. Combined Low (Distal) Median and Ulnar Palsy

Needed Function	Preferred Transfer	Alternate Transfer
Thumb adduction—key pinch	Brachioradialis with free graft between third and fourth metacarpals, to abductor tubercle of thumb[3]	Flexor digitorum superficialis (long) to abductor tubercle of thumb with palmar fascia and flexor tendons as pulleys[30,53]
Thumb abduction[27] (opposition)	Extensor indicis proprius to insertion of abductor pollicis brevis[17] and extensor pollicis longus tendons[49]	Palmaris longus tendon transfer[10] or Extensor carpi ulnaris with free graft[26,28]
Thumb–index tip pinch	Abductor pollicis longus slip to first dorsal interosseous tendon[34] and arthrodesis of thumb MP joint[43]	Extensor pollicis brevis to first dorsal interosseous tendon[14] (if thumb MP joint is fused)
Metacarpal (palmar) transverse arch, and adduction for little finger	Extensor digiti minimi to deep transverse metacarpal ligament[1] (extensor digitorum communis to little finger must be active)	Flexor digitorum superficialis of little finger to deep transverse metacarpal ligament between fourth and fifth metacarpals (Ahern, 1969) or Combined as single transfer with thumb adduction transfer[41,43]
Power flexion—proximal phalanx and integration of MP and interphalangeal motion (clawed fingers)	Extensor carpi radialis longus to all four fingers using four-tailed free graft and flexor sheath insertion (A2 pulley)[4,5,7,11,18,60]	Flexor carpi radialis (if wrist flexion contracture) with four-tailed graft and flexor sheath insertion or dorsal apparatus[49-51]
Volar sensibility	Free neurovascular cutaneous island flap[21]	Cross-finger index–to–thumb neurocutaneous flap[23,42] (Radial nerve)

HIGH MEDIAN-ULNAR NERVE PALSY

The hand will rarely be used for precision activities following this severe injury, even if minimal muscle balance is restored. Atrophy of the finger pulps will discourage both power and precise grip. If the other hand is normal, it is best to direct surgical endeavors toward a key pinch and simple grasp (Table 40-2).

Sensibility can be transferred to the radiovolar aspect of the hand.[37,41,43] Careful testing of the superficial radial nerve will demonstrate the distal level of sensibility on the dorsum of the index finger. The skeleton of the index finger is removed distal to the proximal third of the second metacarpal. The index ray is excised through a racquet incision at the distal end of good dorsal index sensibility and a longitudinal palmar incision between the second and third metacarpals (see Chapter 3).

The insensitive distal index skin is discarded. The filleted index finger flap is then fitted into an additional volar defect created for it in the insensitive palmar skin (Fig. 40-2). This broad-based finger flap is innervated by the superficial radial nerve and will provide protective sensibility within the web space, which seems to be of benefit in such activities as holding a steering wheel.

Elbow flexion may be weaker due to involvement of the pronator-flexor forearm muscle mass. These muscles initiate flexion against gravity, and are critical if there is weakness of muscles innervated by the musculocutaneous nerve. The extensor carpi radialis brevis has the best mechanical advantage for wrist extension and should be retained in this capacity, but all other extrinsic wrist muscles on the extensor aspect can be redirected for alternate functions. There is no wrist extensor muscle with adequate amplitude for full flexion of the digits unless the motion is reinforced by active wrist extension (Fig. 40-3). Abduction of the thumb for opposition does not require great strength, and the thumb extensor muscles can be

Table 40-2. Combined High (Proximal) Median and Ulnar Palsy

Needed Function	Preferred Transfer	Alternate Transfer
Thumb adduction—key pinch	Brachioradialis with free graft between third and fourth metacarpals[3] to abductor tubercle of thumb	Extensor indicis proprius between third and fourth metacarpals[13]
Thumb flexion (IP joint)	Extensor indicis proprius through carpal tunnel to flexor pollicis longus	Tenodesis of flexor pollicis longus distal to MP joint
Thumb abduction (opposition)	Extensor pollicis brevis around tendon of flexor carpi radialis[56,58] (if thumb MP joint is fused)	Extensor pollicis longus rerouted around pisiform[48] (if thumb MP joint is fused and no active flexion at thumb IP joint)
Thumb-long (index) pinch (tip pinch)	Arthrodesis of thumb MP joint (and) abductor pollicis longus slip to first dorsal interosseous tendon[34,41]	Extensor digitorum communis of index to second dorsal interosseous tendon (if index fillet flap is used)
Finger flexion	Extensor carpi radialis longus to tendons of flexor digitorum profundus[36] with tenodesis of DIP joint of three ulnar fingers[7,36]	Biceps brachii extended with flexor carpi radialis tendon to tendons of flexor digitorum profundus[24]
Power flexion—proximal phalanx and integration of MP and interphalangeal motion (clawed fingers)	Tenodesis of all digits with free tendon graft from dorsal apparatus to deep transverse metacarpal ligament[47]	Capsulodesis of MP volar capsule[60] or Arthrodesis of PIP joints[24]
Metacarpal (palmar) arch and adduction for little finger	Extensor digiti minimi to deep transverse metacarpal ligament[1] (extensor digitorum communis of little finger must be active)	
Wrist flexion	Extensor carpi ulnaris to insertion of flexor capri ulnaris	
Radiovolar sensibility	Superficial radial innervated index fillet flap to palm[37,41,43,45]	Free vascularized nerve graft[55]

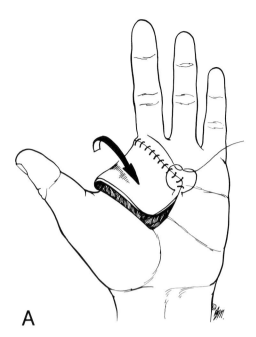

A

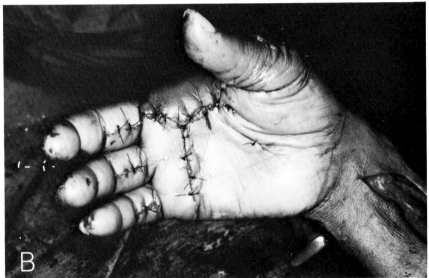

B

Fig. 40-2. **(A)** A radial-innervated dorsal skin flap for combined high median-ulnar palsy. The insensitive palmar skin is excised to create space for the fillet flap, which brings radial-innervated skin into the radial side of the palm. **(B)** Intraoperative photograph.

rerouted to clear the thumb from the palm.[48,56,58] Although there is active thumb extension, the interphalangeal joint may assume a flexed position. This deformity is improved by using Riordan's insertion for opponensplasty (see Chapter 38), where the transferred tendon is first sutured to the abductor pollicis brevis tendon and is then carried on to be inserted into the long extensor tendon just proximal to the interphalangeal joint.[31,49–51]

The loss of simultaneous MP flexion with either interphalangeal extension or flexion disrupts the rhythm necessary to grasp large and small objects. There are no available motors to provide dynamic integration of these motions, so that static techniques must be used. Parkes[47] placed a free tendon graft between the radial lateral band of the dorsal apparatus of the finger and the deep transverse metacarpal ligament. Zancolli[58] opens the proximal

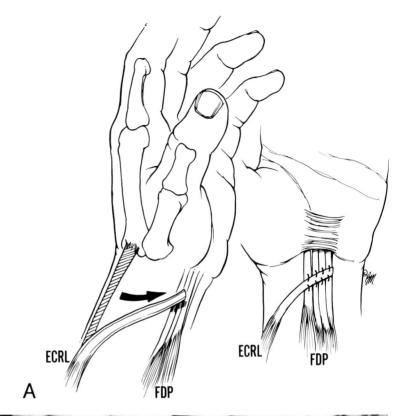

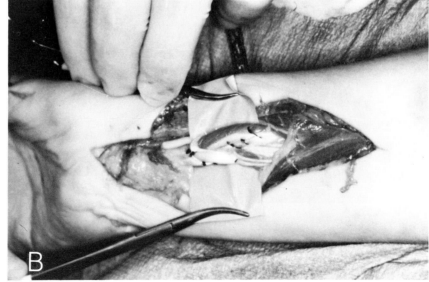

Fig. 40-3. (A) Transfer of the extensor carpi radialis longus *(ECRL)* around the radial aspect of the forearm to the tendons of the flexor digitorum profundus for finger flexion. The tendon juncture should be proximal to the carpal tunnel. The range of finger motion is less than normal because of the limited excursion of the ECRL. (B) Intraoperative photograph. The transfer has been secured well proximal to the transverse carpal ligament.

(A1) pulley of the flexor sheath and a flap is removed from the volar plate (see Chapter 39). Long-term results of the capsulodesis procedure of Zancolli have demonstrated indifferent results in isolated ulnar nerve palsy,[13] but it has been effective in combined palsies.

HIGH ULNAR-RADIAL NERVE PALSY

These patients retain radiovolar sensibility, and reconstruction is a useful surgical investment to improve function (Table 40-3). Although more than 30 different procedures are described for isolated radial nerve palsy,[2,32] the combination of ulnar and radial palsy leaves few expendable muscle-tendon units for transfer.

Transfer of the pronator teres to the extensor carpi radialis brevis for wrist extension in a high ulnar-radial nerve palsy may result in radial deviation of the hand, and a balanced yoke insertion into both the extensor carpi ulnaris and the extensor carpi radialis longus is preferable[6] (Fig. 40-4). The extensor carpi ulnaris tendon is cut at the muscle-tendon junction, and the proximal (high) end of the tendon is sutured to the extensor carpi radialis longus tendon to provide balanced extension. A low ulnar-radial nerve palsy retains wrist flexion,

Table 40-3. Combined High (Proximal) Ulnar and Radial Palsy

Needed Function	Preferred Transfer	Alternate Transfer
Wrist extension	Pronator teres (yoke insertion) to extensor carpi radialis longus and extensor carpi ulnaris[6]	
Thumb adduction—key pinch	One-half flexor digitorum superficialis (long) as split transfer, to abductor tubercle of the thumb[38,41,43]	Palmaris longus extended with free graft around palmar fascia pulley
Clawed fingers { Metacarpal (palmar transverse arch) (and) Power flexion —proximal phalanx (and) Integration of MP and interphalageal motion	One-half flexor digitorum superficialis (long) in two slips to A2 pulley as flexor sheath insertion to ring and little fingers[11,38,41,43,60] (and, later) Arthrodesis of PIP joints, ring and little fingers if unable to fully extend[36,41]	Tenodesis with free tendon graft from radial lateral band of dorsal apparatus to deep transverse metacarpal ligament[47] or Capsulodesis of MP volar capsule[43,60]
Wrist flexion (ulnar aspect)		Palmaris longus to insertion of flexor carpi ulnaris
Proximal thumb abduction stability and wrist flexion (radial aspect)	Flexor carpi radialis (yoke insertion) to abductor pollicis longus and extensor pollicis brevis[41,43]	Tenodesis of abductor pollicis longus to radius[6]
Thumb–index tip pinch	Arthrodesis of thumb MP joint[36,43]	
Finger and thumb extension	Flexor digitorum superficialis (index and ring) through interosseous membrane to extensor digitorum communis and extensor pollicis longus[2]	Palmaris longus to extensor digitorum communis and extensor pollicis longus[51]
Finger flexion (ring and little)	Tenodesis of flexor digitorum profundus index and long fingers (active motors) to ring and little flexor digitorum profundus[7,57] (and) Tenodesis of DIP joint of ring and little fingers, using flexor digitorum profundus[36]	
Volar sensibility—ring and little fingers	Free vascularized nerve grafts[55]	Free neurovascular cutaneous island flap on pedicles[21]

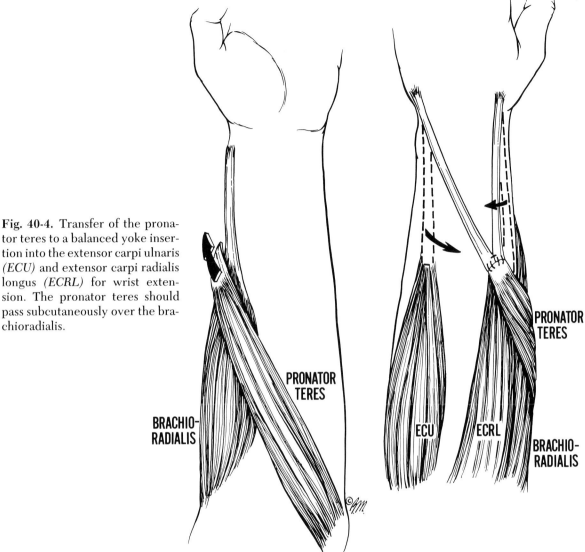

Fig. 40-4. Transfer of the pronator teres to a balanced yoke insertion into the extensor carpi ulnaris *(ECU)* and extensor carpi radialis longus *(ECRL)* for wrist extension. The pronator teres should pass subcutaneously over the brachioradialis.

PRONATOR TERES

BRACHIO-RADIALIS

PRONATOR TERES

BRACHIO-RADIALIS

ECU

ECRL

and the yoke insertion should not be done. Instead, the pronator teres should insert into the tendon of the extensor carpi radialis brevis.

The ring superficialis tendon may be used in low ulnar palsy to improve the integration of MP and interphalangeal joint flexion, key pinch for the thumb, and the flattened metacarpal arch (see Chapter 39), but in a high ulnar palsy, the long superficialis tendon is preferred (Table 40-3) (Fig. 40-5). The superficialis tendon of the little finger is often congenitally absent, or not functionally independent, and should therefore not be used for tendon transfers. The loss of balanced power across the PIP joints caused by removing the superficialis may result ultimately in either a flexion contracture or a swan-neck deformity of these joints. Since one cannot accurately predict which of these deformities may result in an individual patient, I believe that it is preferable to await the onset of the deformity before treating it. The most predictable corrective procedure may be arthrodesis of the PIP joint.

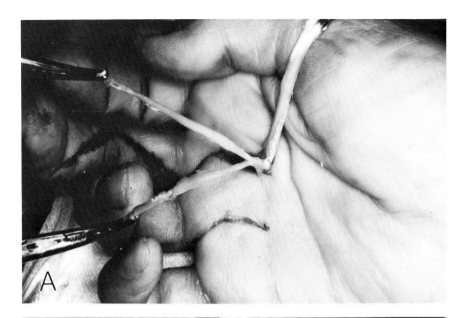

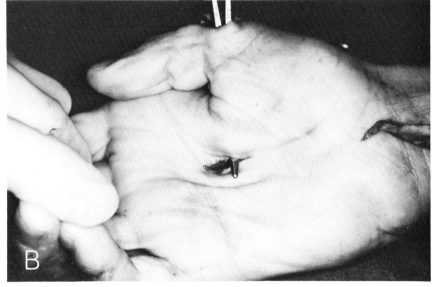

Fig. 40-5. The long finger flexor digitorum superficialis as a split transfer. One half of the tendon is separated into two slips, which will be inserted into the flexor sheaths at the level of the A2 pulleys in the ring and little fingers. (B) The other half of the tendon is passed dorsal to the index flexor sheath, on the surface of the adductor pollicis muscle, to be inserted into the tendon of the abductor pollicis brevis.

HIGH MEDIAN-RADIAL NERVE PALSY

Tendon transfers in this combined nerve lesion will result in a hand that functions only slightly more effectively than a prosthesis[12] (Table 40-4). All wrist motors are lost except the flexor carpi ulnaris, and radiocarpal (wrist) arthrodesis is indicated. The flexor profundus tendons are sutured side-to-side for ulnar-innervated mass action (Fig. 40-6). The profundus tendons to the index and long fingers must be under greater tension at the suture line in order to obtain appropriate flexion.

Transfer of the abductor digiti quinti for thumb abduction should not be attempted until the wrist is stabilized and there is normal adduction power.[15,31] The neurovascular pedicle to the abductor digiti quinti is proximally situated, and the muscle should be freed distally to proximally, then turned like a page in a book, to its new position

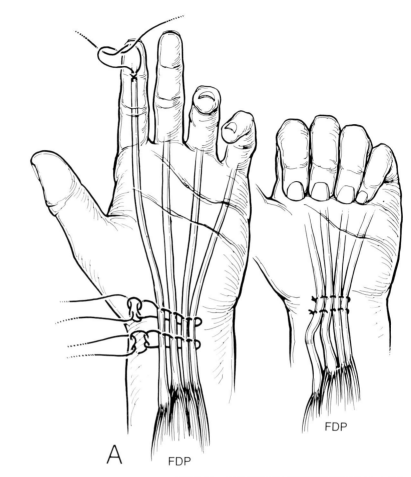

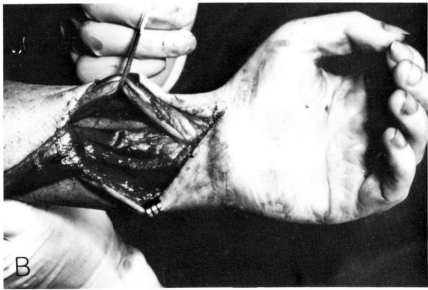

Fig. 40-6. (A) Tenodesis of the denervated index and long finger tendons to the innervated ring and little finger tendons of the flexor digitorum profundus *(FDP)* to provide flexion of all fingers. A double line of sutures is important to prevent "whip sawing" of the tendons with power grip. The index profundus has been tenodesed across the DIP joint to eliminate one joint in the arc of motion. **(B)** Intraoperative photograph. The finger pulps are in a "straight," rather than oblique, line; i.e., with more tension in the index and long fingers (see text).

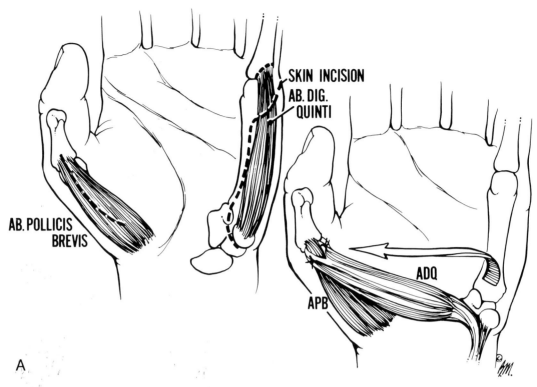

A

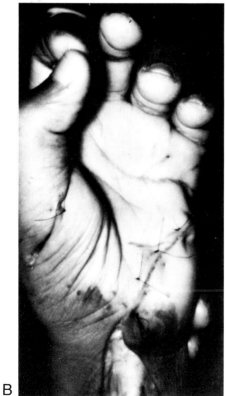

B

Fig. 40-7. (A) Transfer of the abductor digiti quinti *(ADQ)* from its hypothenar position to the thenar area for abduction. Two incisions are made, to minimize damage to the superficial nerves and grasping surface of the palm. The muscle is folded over 170 degrees and passed subcutaneously, to be inserted into the tendon of the abductor pollicis brevis *(APB)*. (B) Intraoperative photograph.

Table 40-4. Combined High (Proximal) Median and Radial Palsy

Needed Function	Preferred Transfer	Alternate Transfer
Forearm pronation	Biceps brachii tendon rerouting around the radius[46,59]	
Wrist extension and flexion	Radiocarpal arthrodesis[25,54]	
Finger flexion	Tenodesis of flexor digitorum profundus ring and little fingers (active motors) to index and long flexor digitorum profundus[7,57]	
Finger and thumb extension	Flexor carpi ulnaris to tendon of extensor digitorum communis and extensor pollicis longus[36,51]	
Proximal thumb abduction stability	Arthrodesis of thumb MP joint[36,43] and Tenodesis abductor pollicis longus to radius[6]	
Thumb abduction (opposition)	Abductor digiti quinti to the insertion of abductor pollicis brevis[31]	Adductor pollicis tendon from adductor tubercle to abductor tubercle[7,20]
Thumb flexion	Tenodesis of flexor pollicis longus across thumb interphalangeal joint[43]	Biceps brachii extended with flexor carpi radialis tendon to tendon of flexor pollicis longus[24]
Radiovolar sensibility	Cross-finger index–to–thumb neurocutaneous flap[23,42]	Free neurovascular cutaneous island pedicle flap on long nerve pedicles or Neurovascular cutaneous island pedicle from ring finger[37,42]

(Fig. 40-7). This muscle has inadequate excursion, but will provide functional thumb opposition. Nonetheless, it is questionable that total hand function is improved, since the little finger, with sensation intact, has now lost its ability for opposition.

new ones. The key to success for the surgical techniques is simplicity, since complexity invites failure. The specific details of these operative procedures are described in Chapters 37, 38, and 39. Tables 40-1 to 40-4 summarize how these operations might best be used in these difficult reconstructive problems.

SUMMARY

Surgeons concerned with reconstruction of the upper extremity after combined nerve palsies have occurred should be experienced enough to select appropriate procedures based on the individual case. Procedures to restore motor function should be done prior to procedures to improve sensibility, such as neurovascular island transfer. The anticipated result should be a balanced simplification of functional performance, because surgery will redistribute a few remaining assets rather than create

REFERENCES

1. Blacker GJ, Lister GD, Kleinert HE: The abducted little finger in low ulnar nerve palsy. J Hand Surg 1:190–196, 1976
2. Boyes JH: Tendon transfers for radial palsy. Bull Hosp Joint Dis 21:97–105, 1959
3. Boyes JH: Bunnell's Surgery of the Hand. 4th Ed. JB Lippincott, Philadelphia, 1964
4. Brand PW: Paralytic claw hand. J Bone Joint Surg 40B:618–632, 1958

5. Brand PW: Tendon grafting. Illustrated by a new operation for intrinsic paralysis of the fingers. J Bone Joint Surg 43B:444–453, 1961

6. Brand PW: Tendon transfers in the forearm. pp. 331–342. In Flynn JE (ed): Hand Surgery. Williams & Wilkins, Baltimore, 1966

7. Brand PW: Tendon transfers for median and ulnar nerve paralysis. Orthop Clin North Am 1:447–454, 1970

8. Brand PW: Timing and objectives of tendon transfers after nerve injury. In Fredericks S, Brody GS (eds): Symposium on the Neurologic Aspects of Plastic Surgery. Educ Found Am Soc Plast Reconstr Surg 17:67–69. CV Mosby, St Louis, 1978

9. Brand PW, Beach RB, Thompson DE: Relative tension and potential excursion of muscles in the forearm and hand. J Hand Surg 6:209–219, 1981

10. Braun RM: Palmaris longus tendon transfer for augmentation of the thenar musculature in low median palsy. J Hand Surg 3:488–491, 1978

11. Brooks AL, Jones DS: A new intrinsic transfer for the paralytic hand. J Bone Joint Surg 57A:730, 1975

12. Brown PW: The time factor in surgery of upper extremity peripheral nerve injury. Clin Orthop 68:14–21, 1970

13. Brown PW: Reconstruction for pinch in ulnar intrinsic palsy. Orthop Clin North Am 5:323–342, 1974

14. Bruner JM: Tendon transfer to restore abduction of the index finger using the extensor pollicis brevis. Plast Reconstr Surg 3:197–201, 1948

15. Bunnell S: Opposition of the thumb. J Bone Joint Surg 20:269–284, 1938

16. Burge P: Abducted little finger in low ulnar nerve palsy. J Hand Surg 11B:234–236, 1986

17. Burkhalter WE, Christensen RC, Brown PW: Extensor indicis proprius opponensplasty. J Bone Joint Surg 55A:725–732, 1973

18. Burkhalter WE, Strait JL: Metacarpophalangeal flexor replacement for intrinsic paralysis. J Bone Joint Surg 55A:1667–1676, 1973

19. Burkhalter WE: Early tendon transfer in upper extremity peripheral nerve injury. Clin Orthop 104:68–79, 1974

20. Curtis RM: Opposition of the thumb. Orthop Clin North Am 5:305–321, 1974

21. Daniel RK, Terzis J, Midgley RD: Restoration of sensation to an anesthetic hand by a free neurovascular flap from the foot. Plast Reconstr Surg 57:275–280, 1976

22. Fleeter TB, Adams JP, Brenner B, Podolsky RJ: A laser diffraction method for measuring muscle sarcomere length in vivo for application to tendon transfers. J Hand Surg 10A:542–546, 1985

23. Gaul JS Jr: Radial-innervated cross finger flap from index to provide sensory pulp to injured thumb. J Bone Joint Surg 51A:1257–1263, 1969

24. Goldner JL: Tendon transfers for irreparable peripheral nerve injuries. Orthop Clin North Am 5:343–375, 1974

25. Haddad RJ, Riordan DC: Arthrodesis of the wrist. A surgical technique. J Bone Joint Surg 49A:950–954, 1967

26. Henderson ED: Transfer of wrist extensors and brachioradialis to restore opposition of the thumb. J Bone Joint Surg 44A:513–522, 1962

27. Hill NA: Restoration of opposition for the paralyzed thumb. Clin Orthop 61:234–240, 1968

28. Kessler I: Transfer of extensor carpi ulnaris to tendon of extensor pollicis brevis for opponensplasty. J Bone Joint Surg 51A:1303–1309, 1969

29. Labosky DA, Waggy CA: Apparent weakness of median and ulnar motors in radial nerve palsy. J Hand Surg 11A:528–533, 1986

30. Littler JW: Tendon transfers and arthrodesis in combined median and ulnar nerve paralysis. J Bone Joint Surg 31A:225–234, 1949

31. Littler JW, Cooley SGE: Opposition of the thumb and its restoration by abductor digiti quinti transfer. J Bone Joint Surg 45A:1389–1396, 1963

32. Moberg E, Nachemson A: Tendon transfers for defective long extensors of the wrist and fingers. Acta Chir Scand 133:31–34, 1967

33. Moneim MS, Omer GE Jr: Latissimus dorsi muscle transfer for restoration of elbow flexion after brachial plexus disruption. J Hand Surg 11A:135–139, 1986

34. Neviaser RJ, Wilson JN, Gardner MM: Abductor pollicis longus transfer for replacement of first dorsal interosseous. J Hand Surg 5:53–57, 1980

35. Omer GE Jr, Vogel JA: Determination of physiological length of a reconstructed muscle-tendon unit through muscle stimulation. J Bone Joint Surg 47A:304–310, 1965

36. Omer GE Jr: Evaluation and reconstruction of the forearm and hand after acute traumatic peripheral nerve injuries. J Bone Joint Surg 50A:1454–1478, 1968

37. Omer GE Jr, Day DJ, Ratcliff H, Lambert P: Neurovascular cutaneous island pedicles for deficient median nerve sensibility. J Bone Joint Surg 52A:1181–1192, 1970

38. Omer GE Jr: Restoring power grip in ulnar palsy. In Proceedings of the American Society for Surgery of the Hand. J Bone Joint Surg 53A:814, 1971

39. Omer GE Jr: Injuries to nerves of the upper extremity. J Bone Joint Surg 56A:1615–1624, 1974

40. Omer GE Jr: The technique and timing of tendon transfers. Orthop Clin North Am 5:243–252, 1974

41. Omer GE Jr: Tendon transfers in combined nerve lesions. Orthop Clin North Am 5:377–387, 1974

42. Omer GE Jr: Neurovascular sensory island transplants. In Fredericks S, Brody GS: Neurologic Aspects of Plastic Surgery. Educ Found Amer Soc Plast Reconstr Surg 17:52–60. CV Mosby, St Louis, 1978

43. Omer GE Jr: Tendon transfers for reconstruction of the forearm and hand following peripheral nerve injuries. pp. 817–846. In Omer GE, Spinner M (eds): Management of Peripheral Nerve Problems. WB Saunders, Philadelphia 1980

44. Omer GE: Early tendon transfers in the rehabilitation of median, radial, and ulnar palsies. Ann Chir Main 1:187–190, 1982

45. Omer GE Jr: Reconstruction of a balanced thumb through tendon transfers. Clin Orthop 195:104–116, 1985

46. Owings R, Wickstrom J, Perry J, Nickel VL: Biceps brachii rerouting in treatment of paralytic supination contracture of the forearm. J Bone Joint Surg 53A:137–142, 1971

47. Parkes A: Paralytic claw fingers—A graft tenodesis operation. Hand 5:192–199, 1973

48. Riley WB, Mann RJ, Burkhalter WE: Extensor pollicis longus opponensplasty. J Hand Surg 5:217–220, 1980

49. Riordan DC: Tendon transplantation in median-nerve and ulnar-nerve paralysis. J Bone Joint Surg 35A:312–320, 1953

50. Riordan DC: Surgery of the paralytic hand. pp. 79–90. AAOS Instructional Course Lectures, Vol. 16. CV Mosby, St Louis, 1959

51. Riordan DC: Tendon transfers for nerve paralysis of the hand and wrist. Curr Pract Orthop Surg 2:17–40, 1964

52. Riordan DC: Tendon transfers in hand surgery. J Hand Surg 8:748–753, 1983

53. Srinivasan H: Correction of the paralytic claw-thumb by two-tailed transfer of the superficialis tendon through a window in the flexor retinaculum. Plast Reconstr Surg 69:90–95, 1982

54. Stein I: Gill turnabout radial graft for wrist arthrodesis. Surg Gynecol Obstet 106:231–232, 1958

55. Taylor GI: Nerve grafting with simultaneous microvascular reconstruction. Clin Orthop 133:56–70, 1978

56. Tubiana R: Anatomic and physiologic basis for the surgical treatment of paralysis of the hand. J Bone Joint Surg 51A:643–660, 1969

57. White WL: Restoration of function and balance of the wrist and hand by tendon transfers. Surg Clin North Am 40:427–459, 1960

58. Zancolli E: Tendon transfers after ischemic contracture of the forearm. Am J Surg 109:356–360, 1965

59. Zancolli EA: Paralytic supination contracture of the forearm. J Bone Joint Surg 49A:1275–1284, 1967

60. Zancolli EA: Structural and Dynamic Bases of Hand Surgery. 2nd Ed. p. 174. JB Lippincott, Philadelphia, 1979

Brachial Plexus

41

Robert D. Leffert

The treatment of injuries to the brachial plexus is a demanding and difficult area of surgery of the upper extremity. Not only is the anatomy complex and variable, but the skills required to render comprehensive care cross specialty barriers and require both extensive training and innovative application. Furthermore, the field is by no means static; it continues to evolve as controversies are generated and resolved with the hope of providing better care for these often disastrously impaired patients.

The first report of successful surgery on a traction injury of the brachial plexus appeared in 1900, when William Thornburn of Manchester, England, described improved function in a 16-year-old girl whose plexus had been injured and whose lesion was treated by secondary suture.[80] By 1920, Taylor[79] had accumulated a series of 70 cases of birth palsy treated surgically, and other surgeons had reported their experiences.[61,71] However, the initial enthusiasm for operative treatment, both in obstetric palsy and adult injury, was often engendered by anecdotal reporting and poor documentation, so that by the third decade of this century the tide had turned against direct surgical

attack on the plexus.[39] As recently as 1963, Sir Herbert Seddon stated: "Repair of the brachial plexus has proved so disappointing that it should not be done except for the upper trunk."

In practice, surgery on these nerves was largely limited to exploration for prognosis so that peripheral orthopedic reconstruction or amputation could be performed without delay. By 1973, however, technical improvements in optics, instruments, and suture material revitalized the field with the emergence of microsurgery. Millesi, Meissl, and Katzer[55] in Vienna, Narakas[57] in Lausanne, and Lusskin, Campbell, and Thompson[51] in New York, as well as Alnot, Augereau, and Frot,[4] Allieu,[3] Sedel,[68] Gilbert,[28] and Benassy and colleagues[6] in France reported their experience in surgery of the brachial plexus. A new era of investigation and encouragement had arrived. The reader is referred to the above-mentioned works, since a detailed presentation of these authors' results is not possible in this brief chapter. In addition, several general discussions of the subject are available for review.[23,45,46,47,48,81] Nevertheless, it should be remembered that each patient must be evaluated individually in terms of the specific techniques that should be employed to restore as much function as possible; these are herein described.

THE SCOPE OF THE PROBLEM

Although injuries of the brachial plexus can occur under a wide variety of circumstances, they may be considered under the headings listed below.

    I. Open injuries of the brachial plexus
    II. Closed (traction) injuries of the brachial plexus
       A. Supraclavicular injuries
          1. Supraganglionic
          2. Infraganglionic
       B. Infraclavicular injuries
       C. Postanesthetic palsy
    III. Radiation injury to the brachial plexus
    IV. Obstetric palsy

Open Injuries

These injuries may by caused by a variety of instruments and missiles. They may or may not be accompanied by life- or limb-threatening vascular injury[59] that, if present, mandates immediate operative exploration. Where there is no vascular injury, direct operative intervention should be determined by the nature of the wound. If caused by a sharp instrument, such as a knife or glass, the assumption may be made that whatever nerve deficit exists may be attributed to a division of nerve rather than a contusion or stretch, as might result from a bullet. Operative repair in stab wounds can be done as soon as the patient's condition permits, unless there is a strong likelihood of sepsis. Precisely when such surgery should be done depends on several factors. Since operative exposure, technical requirements, and potential complications require a full and efficient team with potential backups, it is prudent not to start surgery in the middle of the night with a fatigued "skeleton"

crew. Assuming there is minimal contamination of the wound, there would be little objection to applying a dressing and proceeding with surgery within 24 hours on an elective basis. Otherwise, I see no objection to closing the wound and waiting for primary healing before doing the exploration and repair.

The question of which sharp injuries merit exploration in the absence of vascular injury depends on several factors. The first is whether there is a significant neural deficit that could be expected to benefit from surgical repair, and second is which portions of the plexus have been injured. For example, a patient in whom a very minimal deficit exists might well be expeditiously treated by means of tendon transfer rather than direct attack on the nerves if the deficit is localized and sensory function not severely compromised. Furthermore, experience has shown that the upper and intermediate trunks affected by sharp lacerations have a much better prognosis than the lower trunk and its outflow following surgical repair. In the case of children with sharp lacerations, everything that can be repaired should be, since their ability to regenerate and regain function is far superior to that of adults.

A subdivision of open lacerations that presents very severe problems is the chainsaw injury. Unfortunately, these have increased as the number of unskilled "do-it-yourselfers" have included the chainsaw among their tools. The kick-back from the chainsaw may result in a fatal injury when a ragged laceration of the supraclavicular fossa occurs. In patients who are lucky enough to survive, there is usually extensive damage that involves not only laceration of the nerves, but, in cases that I have observed, sufficient traction to produce root avulsion from the spinal cord. If these patients are seen at the time of injury, the nerves should be identified and tagged for later repair unless it is quite clear that avulsion is not a possibility. In the event that it is, myelography should precede secondary exploration. Open wounds of the lower trunk of the brachial plexus are far more likely to be accompanied by vascular injury than those of the upper or intermediate trunks. In addition to their obvious life-threatening nature, they are also liable to further injury of the neural elements during frantic attempts to arrest hemorrhage.

Gunshot wounds differ from sharp lacerations in terms of the wounding mechanism and its effect on nerves. They are rarely initially complete and if so, usually become partial fairly quickly. The reason this occurs is because of the concussive effect of a bullet, which may deform the nerves nearby, thus temporarily interrupting their function.

Assuming there is no significant pulmonary or vascular injury accompanying a bullet wound of the brachial plexus, conservative therapy with local wound care is indicated. If no recovery is seen within 3 months, or there is a major area of neurologic deficit, I believe that they should be explored secondarily.

For patients who develop pain and neurologic dysfunction following the placement of subclavian lines or as a consequence of arteriography,[10,20] the brachial plexus should be explored as soon as there is evidence of increasing local or referred pain or neurologic deficit.

Operative injuries to the brachial plexus not due to position on the operating table or traction on the limb may occur in operations about the shoulder girdle. If they are realized as resulting from sharp injury, they should be immediately repaired. Unfortunately, their effect is often not appreciated until the patient has awakened from general anesthesia, at which time there may be difficulty in differentiating them from traction lesions due to operative positioning on the operating table. Since the latter usually recovers substantially within 6 weeks, it may well be prudent to wait that long to observe what happens before advocating second-

ary exploration. For patients who sustain injury to the lower trunk of the brachial plexus during performance of transaxillary first rib resection, the prognosis for recovery of major deficits is extremely poor. These patients usually require reconstruction of their hands by means of tendon transfer.

Closed (Traction) Injuries

SUPRACLAVICULAR INJURIES

Most supraclavicular injuries result from falls from motorcycles or in motor vehicle accidents in which the head and shoulder are forcibly separated, causing a variable degree and distribution of stretch on the elements of the plexus.[5,8] All combinations of injury are possible, which results in a variety of clinical pictures of paralysis, paresis, and sensory loss. In adults these results may be generally classified as outlined in Table 41-1, with some allowance for variation in innervation.

Clinical evaluation must be directed toward determination not only of which root levels of the plexus have been damaged, but whether root avulsion (supraganglionic) or distal rupture (infraganglionic) has occurred. Table 41-2 summarizes the clinical assessment of this aspect of the problem, which is absolutely essential information, since preganglionic or supraganglionic lesions are irreparable, while those more distally may be reparable. It should be categorically stated that all of

Table 41-1. Neurologic and Functional Consequences of Brachial Plexus Injury

Roots Involved	Muscles Affected	Functional Loss	Sensory Loss
C5–6	Deltoid, supraspinatus and infraspinatus, biceps, brachialis, coracobrachialis, brachioradialis, (±) radial wrist extensors, clavicular pectoralis major	Shoulder lateral rotation, abduction and forward flexion, elbow flexion, (±) wrist extension	Thumb and index finger
C5–6–7	As above, plus triceps, ECRL and ECRB, FCR, EDC, EPL, EPB, APL	As above, plus elbow, wrist, finger and thumb extensors	As above, plus middle finger
C(7)–8, 1	(EDC, EPL) FDS, FDP, FPL, lumbricals and interossei, thenars and hypothenars	(Finger extension) Finger and thumb flexion, median and ulnar intrinsics	(Middle finger) Little and ring fingers
C5–T1	All of above	All of above	Anesthesia except for medial brachium

(±) = may or may not be present.

Table 41-2. Differentiation of Supra- and Infraganglionic Lesions of the Brachial Plexus

Evaluation Technique	Supraganglionic Lesion	Infraganglionic Lesion
Inspection	Flail arm, winged scapula, Horner's syndrome	Flail arm
Manual muscle testing	Paralysis of serratus anterior, rhomboids, (±) diaphragm and limb musculature	Paralysis of limb musculature
Sensation	Absent in involved dermatome	Absent in involved dermatome
Tinel's sign	Absent	Present (unless supraganglionic lesions are present at the same level)
Myelography	Traumatic pseudomeningoceles, obliteration of root detail	Normal
EMG	Paravertebral muscle and limb muscle denervation	Limb muscle denervation
Nerve conduction	Motor conduction absent, (±) sensory conduction	Motor and sensory conduction absent
Axon response	Normal. Absent if infraganglionic lesion is present at the same level	Absent

(±)=may or may not be present.

these evaluation methods are indirect in nature and none of them is totally reliable. Myelography and electromyography should be delayed for 1 month to provide more accurate information in a patient with a totally flail, anesthetic limb. Patients who have Horner's syndrome, severe pain, fractures of the clavicle, or winged scapulae generally have poorer prognosis for recovery than those in whom these signs and symptoms are absent. The fractured clavicle usually allows for greater traction-elongation of the nerves than would have been possible with an intact shoulder girdle, which decreases the incidence of root avulsion. The finding of Horner's syndrome is presumptive evidence of avulsion of the first thoracic nerve root. Although myelography cannot be regarded as absolutely reliable in the demonstration of the avulsion,[34,38] I believe that it still should be done in cases where that possibility exists. The use of water-soluble contrast material with computed tomographic imaging is an improvement over the older techniques.

Electromyography[14] should include needle examination of the posterior cervical musculature to help define root avulsions from distal ruptures of the nerve, since the former have no potential for either spontaneous recovery or surgical manipulation. Sensory nerve action potentials and somatosensory-evoked potentials should be obtained in addition to motor nerve conduction velocity determinations.[9,40] I no longer use intradermal histamine[7] to test axon responses for differentiation of root avulsion versus distal rupture, since interpretation of the technique may be extremely difficult and the potential of histamine allergic response exists.

INFRACLAVICULAR INJURIES

Infraclavicular injuries to the brachial plexus may result from closed skeletal injury in the shoulder girdle, which injures the nerves by local compression or traction. Since the potential excursion of a dislocated humeral head or fragments of a fractured humerus is considerably limited by soft tissue attachments, the extent of damage is usually less than that found in supraclavicular injuries. Unless there is actual tearing apart of the neural elements by sharp bone fragments or serious vascular injury, these injuries may usually be managed conservatively with a good prognosis.[49] If, however, there is evidence of supraclavicular injury in addition to that below the clavicle, management will be determined by the former, more serious injury. In other words, extensive supraclavicular injuries may extend below the clavicle. In these cases, if surgery is done on the nerves, the infraclavicular plexus and its terminal branches will have to be thoroughly explored. Direct blunt injury to the infraclavicular portions of the plexus may occur in the absence of supraclavicular injury and may produce extensive localized scarring. A recent patient of mine incurred his injury when he ran into a moose on the highway while riding a motorcycle. He had a neurologic deficit localized to the infraclavicular plexus, but had not dislocated his shoulder or sustained any local fractures. Complete exploration of the plexus failed to demonstrate any lesion above the level of the clavicle. At this writing, he has begun to experience considerable recovery following extensive neurolysis of the scarred infraclavicular plexus. It should be emphasized that fresh fractures of the clavicle usually cause extensive supraclavicular traction injuries to the plexus because they allow even greater excursion than normal between the head and shoulder. Malunion and nonunion of clavicular fractures and those fractures that heal with excessive callus in the retroclavicular space can cause signs and symptoms either of brachial plexus compression or thoracic outlet syndrome, and may require either clavicular correction, excision, or resection of the first rib (Fig. 41-1).

POSTOPERATIVE BRACHIAL PLEXUS PALSY

Postanesthetic palsy results from injury to the brachial plexus with the patient undergoing either general or regional anesthesia for the performance of a surgical procedure that is unrelated to the plexus. In the former case, its cause is the patient's position on the operating table and is not directly caused by the surgical manipulation. It is usually due to traction on the plexus of an unconscious and therefore unguarded patient and usually represents a first degree injury or neurapraxia. As such, the prognosis for recovery is excellent and it is usually substantially improved by 6 weeks from the time of injury. This injury may be prevented in most cases by careful attention to the position of the patient on the operating table. There are no indications for surgical exploration in these cases.

Radiation Neuropathy of the Brachial Plexus

Radiotherapy for breast cancer has been used with increasing frequency as a modality of treatment because of comparable survival rates with radical surgery in many cases. Although for many years it was considered that nerve tissue was radioresistant,[22] further study revealed that these assumptions were unwarranted.[32] An early axonal effect of radiation on peripheral nerves is an actual increase in conduction velocity, which then declines with time.[76] Later effects, which are angiomesenchymal, result in changes in the vasonervorum, and ultimately obliterate the blood vessels and produce progressive scarring, with ultimate disappearance of the neural elements. This is clinically expressed in patients who have had radiation as pain and paresthesias, with ultimate progressive loss of neurologic function. Unfortunately, for patients who have had a near-by malignancy such as breast cancer, the clinician may be hard-pressed to define whether the deficit is due to the effects of radiation or recurrent tumor. Although pain may be found in both groups of patients, it tends to be more severe in the case of patients with malignant plexopathy. Since the natural history of both radiation neuropathy and neoplastic brachial plexopathy is a progressive loss of neurologic function in most cases, in addition to the question of establishment of the diagnosis, there is the question of therapy. The use of CT scanning often may be of value in defining those patients who have tumor, but this is not invariably so, and some of these patients will have to undergo complete exploration of the plexus in order to settle the issue. It should be emphasized that limited explorations are not only inadequate for complete diagnosis, but may be very dangerous because of the possibility of increased risk of hemorrhage from vessels that have been damaged by radiation.

The treatment of patients presumed to have radiation neuropathy and who are experiencing progression of their symptoms and signs is one that has not been resolved. Unfortunately, there are significant hazards for such operative procedures, as documented by Match.[52] Reports by Brunelli[13] from Brescia, Italy and Ulschmid and Clodius[83] have described the results of neurolysis accompanied by transplantation of omentum in an attempt to revascularize the plexus damaged by radiation fibrosis. The reported results are favorable with reference to pain and in some cases, neurologic function, as well. Because of the hazardous nature of operative procedures in these patients, indications for neurolysis must be very carefully considered. My personal experience has been limited to a few cases of neurolysis without free omental grafts, and in these patients, pain relief was temporary and the neurologic deficit was not improved.

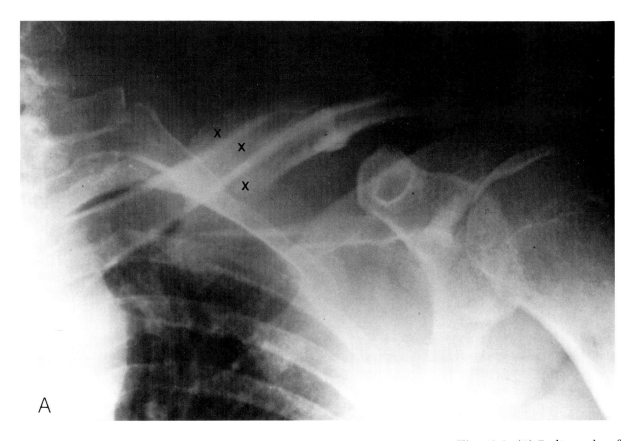

A

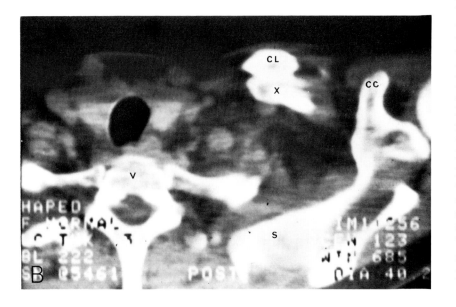

B

Fig. 41-1. (A) Radiographs of the left clavicle of a 42-year-old man 4 months after he sustained a closed midshaft fracture of the clavicle, which was treated with a figure-of-eight harness. He returned to work as a dentist within 2 weeks of his fracture and was asymptomatic until 4 months later when, within a 4-day period, he developed an upper trunk palsy. Note the large amount of callus at the fracture site (indicated by the Xs above, below, and behind the clavicle). **(B)** CT scan of same area. (*V*, vertebral body; *S*, scapula; *CC*, coracoid; *CL*, clavicle; *X*, callus impinging on the brachial plexus.) *(Figure continues.)*

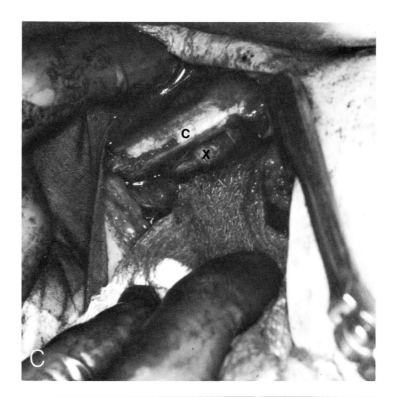

Fig. 41-1 *(Continued)*. (**C**) Operative photograph showing clavicle (*C*) and excess callus (*X*).(**D**) The subclavian vein has been dissected off the callus, the brachial plexus has been identified and retracted, and the excess bone has been carefully excised from the clavicle (*C*). Neurologic function returned to normal within 3 weeks of surgery.

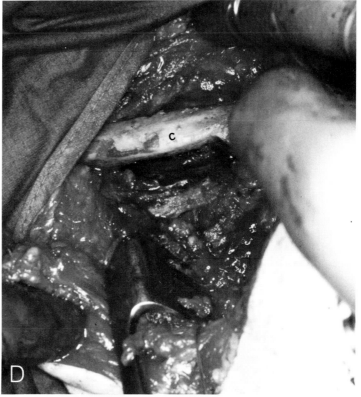

TECHNIQUE OF OPERATIVE TREATMENT OF THE BRACHIAL PLEXUS

General Considerations and Equipment

Surgeons who treat injuries of the brachial plexus must be prepared to confront the pathologic complexities of the area with a full knowledge of the relevant anatomy. Although numerous treatises on the subject are available for review,[35,36,41,70] it is also mandatory that experience be gained in the anatomy laboratory prior to an actual surgical approach in a patient.

The patient's general condition must be adequate to tolerate up to 8 to 10 hours of general anesthesia in the supine, semi-sitting position. Prepping and draping must allow extensile exposure from the neck into the shoulder girdle and arm, as well as access to both legs, should nerve grafts be required. An anesthetic technique without total motor paralysis that will allow the use of a nerve stimulator intraoperatively should be employed. The techniques of somatosensory-evoked potentials and the physiologic monitoring that they permit are an indispensable aid in the intraoperative evaluation of lesions of the brachial plexus. As has been previously stated, although myelography and electrodiagnostic studies done preoperatively are helpful, they are not infallible, nor is the ability of the surgeon, either by gross inspection or with the use of the operative microscope, to define whether a proximal stump of the nerve is capable of regeneration and whether it retains its central connections. The use of this electrophysiologic equipment requires trained personnel who can cooperate with the surgeon during the course of the procedure. The study of the nerve action potentials in the more distal parts of the plexus can also be extremely valuable.[43]

Several units of blood must be available for use in the event of inadvertent injury to large vessels in the field. Personnel adequate in number and training should be present, depending on local custom and practice. It does not matter what surgical specialties, or combination thereof, are represented in the operating team, as long as the surgeons are knowledgeable about the anatomic and technical problems that will have to be faced, and can assist or relieve each other to avoid fatigue. The use of either an operating microscope or loupes with magnification of 6× is suggested. Exactly which optical aids are elected depends on the experience and preference of the operator. Because of the variable topography and size of the operative field, I use 3.5× and 6× loupes and a fiberoptic headlight, and I have found this combination quite satisfactory. In some cases, the operating microscope is preferable.

Surgical Approach

The incision used in most cases is shown in Figure 41-2A. It begins at the midpoint of the posterior border of the sternomastoid muscle and drops to the clavicle. If a strictly vertical incision is used, there is greater danger of producing a hypertrophic scar. This can be minimized by making the incision more obliquely than vertically oriented and carrying it more medially before curving horizontally beneath the level of the clavicle. It then continues laterally one fingerbreadth below the clavicle to enter the deltopectoral groove. From here it can be continued down into the arm as necessary (Fig. 41-2B). The platysma muscle is divided in line with the skin incision and preserved for layered closure at the end of the procedure. The external jugular vein will be encountered at this stage of the procedure, running vertically from its termination in the subclavian vein just posterior to the sternomastoid muscle. It is a good landmark for the location of the brachial plexus, which lies between the scalenes directly under it. It is wise to ligate and excise the vein to prevent annoying bleeding during the course of the procedure. The spinal accessory nerve lies relatively superficially on the fascial carpet in the apex of the wound, and it must be protected from harm. The transverse cervical artery and vein cross the plexus in the posterior triangle and must be ligated. The suprascapular vessels are located more inferiorly in the region of the clavicle and they, too, must be found and divided. The plexus lies between the anterior and middle scalene muscles deep to the fascia, and although it is readily apparent in the dissecting room

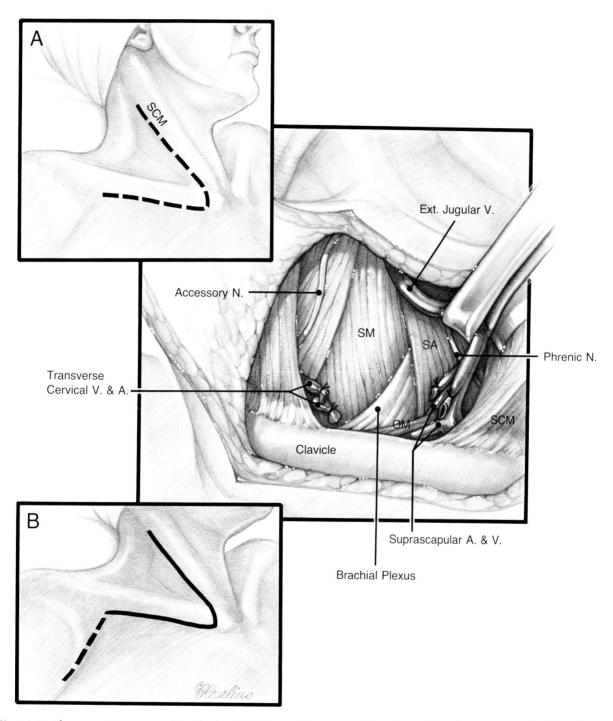

Fig. 41-2. The operative approach to the brachial plexus. The external jugular vein has been retracted rather than excised to show its relationships. Figure **B** shows the extension of the skin incision into the deltopectoral groove.

specimen, in the living patient with a traction injury, there may be a solid wall of scarred muscle that makes the precise identification of individual nerves difficult. Fortunately, the phrenic nerve can usually be located by means of a stimulator probe. Contraction of the diaphragm on stimulation will allow the operator to trace the phrenic nerve upward and ultimately identify C5 and the upper trunk at the level of the intervertebral foramen. Electrical stimulation, in addition to evoked potentials, is useful in demonstrating those elements of the plexus that are intact or potentially capable of spontaneous recovery. Therefore, the limb musculature must be palpable within the operative field or through the drapes. In situations where precise anatomic localization is difficult, it may be extremely helpful to temporarily suspend operation in the supraclavicular fossa and go directly to the infraclavicular portion of the plexus. This is readily identifiable by detachment of the pectoralis minor and as much of the pectoralis major from the clavicle as is necessary for exposure. The omohyoid muscle should be divided at midpoint for exposure but saved for later reattachment.

The question of division of the clavicle is to be considered in terms of whether it is possible to gain exposure without osteotomy and the subsequent risk of nonunion. Because the necessary soft tissue dissection virtually skeletonizes the clavicle and its medullary blood supply is meager, the risk of nonunion is very real. Usually, by placing a bolster pillow beneath the scapula posteriorly, the clavicle may be sufficiently raised off the vessels and nerves so that it is possible to work beneath it. Retraction on the clavicle and positioning the arm may further facilitate exposure (Fig. 41-3). However, the lower trunk and vessels are dealt with more easily if the clavicle is divided. In those cases where it is necessary, an osteotomy should be done and repair at the end of the procedure should be completed by means of a suitable compression plate.

Options and Specific Techniques in Neurologic Reconstruction of the Brachial Plexus

Once the elements of the injured plexus have been identified as completely as possible, the surgeon must formulate a plan that can be integrated with what has already been learned by preoperative assessment. Consideration should be given to what can also be provided ultimately by other means of restoration or peripheral reconstruction using arthrodesis and tendon transfers. For the patient with a totally flail, anesthetic arm, anything that is recovered will usually come from rejoining the nerves. Therefore, in this case, nerve repair or grafting is indispensable, particularly for sensibility.

The timing of operative intervention requires emphasis, since most authors believe that delay of more than 6 months after injury will diminish the chances of functional recovery. It is therefore of advantage to explore these patients prior to that

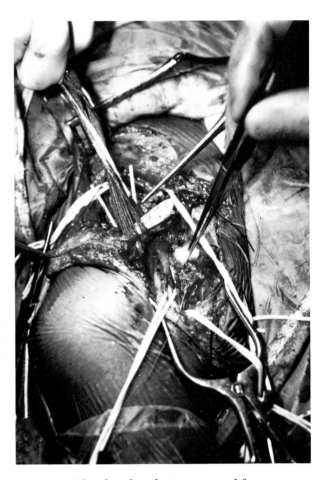

Fig. 41-3. The clavicle is being retracted for exposure. The patient's head is toward the top of the figure, and the neural elements are retracted with small silicone tubes.

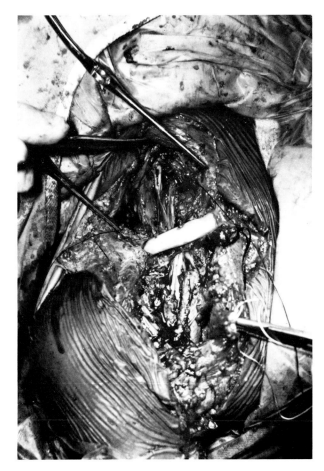

Fig. 41-4. Sural nerve grafts extend from the upper trunk, beneath the clavicle to the lateral cord. In this case, the intervening, scarred plexus was by-passed, not resected.

time, which also would minimize scarring. Again, it is the patient with a completely flail and anesthetic arm for whom neurologic reconstruction will make the most difference. In adults, it is the outflow of C5, C6, and C7, the upper and intermediate trunks, that can be used as a source of axons for those patients in whom neurotmesis has been demonstrated. For those who are found to have scarring encompassing the neural elements, with neuroma-in-continuity, neurolysis is indicated. For patients with partial lesions of this type, there is a very definite risk of increasing the deficit, especially with internal neurolysis. Allieu and co-workers[3] emphasized the danger of attempting neurolysis of the upper trunk in a patient who has regained elbow

flexion without shoulder abduction, since there is a possibility of losing what has already been recovered. In their series of 14 neurolyses, there were only two cases in which recovery absolutely attributed to the neurolysis could be documented. Neurolysis can, in most cases, be external and done with the aid of high magnification, as well as electrical monitoring.

Because of the nature of traction injuries, direct suture generally is impossible, and gaps must be overcome by means of intercalated grafts of autogenous nerve (Figs. 41-4 and 41-5). The choice of donor nerves depends on the individual require-

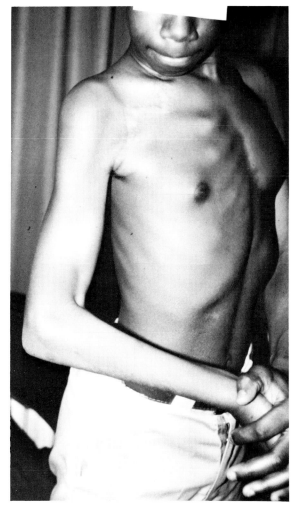

Fig. 41-5. The biceps is able to contract against strong resistance 18 months later.

ments and what can be sacrificed. In the average adult, the sural nerves may yield as much as 35 cm from each leg, although the medial cutaneous nerve of the forearm may be taken in the arm. In cases where there has been documented avulsion of C8 and T1, the main trunk ulnar nerve may be harvested and used as a graft, although it is usually wise to diminish the diameter of the nerve by stripping out the dorsal sensory branch. In addition to the usual problems of dealing with scarred nerve, which require resection of all neuroma prior to grafting, there is a further difficulty found in proximal lesions of the brachial plexus that must be considered. With lesions at the level of the intervertebral foramina or within the scalene muscles, the retrograde effect on parent neurons may be so devastating that the cells may die and the axons disappear from the proximal stumps, making successful repair of any type impossible. This has been well documented by Narakas[56] in his consideration of muscle recovery as a function of where in the plexus the suture was done. When grafting is considered feasible and resection of scar from both ends of the neuroma has been accomplished, the lengths of the graft should be increased by 15 percent to allow for shrinkage. Usually 9–0 nylon suture is used, although for main trunk grafts, 8–0 may be sufficient. Some authors have used plasma clot and find that it is helpful.[77] Plasma clot may also be substituted for suture. For the present time, I continue to use as few sutures as possible to obtain coaptation of the nerves.

As much reconstruction as possible is done if there is adequate root stock, although the lower trunk is rarely successfully grafted in adults and function usually does not return. The results of plexus surgery in several large series have been documented by Millesi,[54] Narakas,[58] and Sedel.[68] In my experience, the results of neurologic reconstruction for restoration of elbow flexion have been that approximately 75 percent of patients regain flexion against gravity and moderate resistance; this is better than anything that can be produced by means of tendon transfer. Unless the outflow of the suprascapular nerve can be reconstituted, useful shoulder function is unlikely even if the deltoid can be recovered, because the lack of control of lateral rotation deprives the shoulder of good control and power equivalent to what might be experienced

with a complete traumatic rupture of the rotator cuff.

The prognosis for recovery of significant hand function is generally the least favorable of the area under consideration as documented by several series.[51,54,56,57,68]

Whether the use of vascularized nerve grafts has a place in the treatment of brachial plexus injuries remains to be seen.

For patients who have partial function and in whom motor control of the hand is intact, but with no good alternatives available from peripheral reconstruction because of paucity of motors, consideration should be given to neurologic reconstruction, using the outflow of C5 and C6 distal to the takeoff of the branches supplying the rhomboids and serratus anterior. This, of course, presupposes that there is distal rupture rather than avulsion. The restoration of elbow flexion is favorable in these cases. However, one must weigh those potential gains against the loss of sensibility in the thumb and index finger, if it is intact prior to surgery. Such lesions do exist in partial injury to the upper trunk, and one must be careful not to disconnect the nerves if such is the case.

The question of neurotization is one that has appeal for the patient with a totally flail, anesthetic limb as a result of complete avulsion of the brachial plexus. Historically, although nerve crossing operations have been reported as far back as 1903,[31] they have not been very popular. In 1961 Yeoman and Seddon[85] successfully grafted intercostals three and four to the musculocutaneous nerve, using the ulnar nerve as a free graft from a forearm amputation specimen. The experience of the Japanese[44,82] as well as Millesi,[54] Narakas,[58] and others, has proved that the procedure can be done successfully. It should be remembered that when Yeoman and Seddon performed the operation, they transected the intercostal nerves as close to the intervertebral foramina as possible, using a costotransvasectomy approach. Subsequent surgeons have not found this to be necessary and, in fact, if the entire intercostal nerve is dissected out to the midline, an intercalated graft would not be necessary. However, much of the motor supply will then have been dissipated. A reasonable compromise is to transect the intercostal nerve at the anterior axillary line and then cable graft to the musculocutaneous nerve. Usually three intercostals provide enough axons to achieve functional elbow flexion. Patients initially find that elbow flexion is synchronous with inspiration and may occur involuntarily with coughing or sneezing. However, it is possible to achieve independent action for voluntary elbow flexion.

The other nerves that have been used for provision of axons for neurotization of a totally avulsed brachial plexus are the cervical plexus and the spinal accessory nerve. The latter has a significant disadvantage in that if the function is lost to the trapezius, it cannot be replaced by any other means, and the possibility of abduction of a shoulder fusion would be impossible if that were an option.

RECONSTRUCTION OF THE UPPER EXTREMITY IN PATIENTS WITH IRREPARABLE INJURIES

Timing

The timing of peripheral reconstruction if it is employed depends on determining that spontaneous neurologic recovery is unlikely or impossible, based on either time elapsed since injury or direct knowledge of the status of the nerves. In general, patients more than $1\frac{1}{2}$ years postinjury have reached the chronic state where no further recovery is anticipated unless nerve repair has been previously done. In such cases, it may take as long as 18 months postoperatively for recovery of active elbow flexion. For the shoulder, under any circumstances, failure to achieve significant voluntary control at 1 year usually indicates the permanence of the lesion.

Shoulder Reconstruction

The mobility of the shoulder should be preserved if there is any possibility of providing muscular control by means of multiple tendon transfers.[64] In patients who have either suffered partial lesions or experienced partial recovery, it

may be possible to use multiple adjacent muscles to augment shoulder control. The procedure must be very carefully and individually planned and executed, as shown by Ober[60] and Harmon.[30] If it is working, the posterior deltoid may be rotated anteriorly, and the long heads of the biceps and triceps may be advanced to the acromion with benefit. The L'Episcopo procedure,[50] in which the insertions of the latissimus dorsi and teres major are transposed posterolaterally to achieve active lateral rotation, can be employed alone when indicated or in combination with other transfers. The results are extremely useful.

For the patient with total loss of shoulder control or in whom transfers are not possible, arthrodesis of the glenohumeral joint is the salvage procedure. In order to have maximal control of the shoulder-arm complex, the patient must have preserved at least the function of the serratus anterior and the trapezius.

ARTHRODESIS OF THE SHOULDER

At the present time I employ two methods of fixation for shoulder fusion, with the same approach used in both. The patient is placed on the operating table in the lateral decubitus position. The surgical approach is posterior, with the incision extending parallel to and one fingerbreadth beneath the spine of the scapula. The incision continues anterolaterally across the humeral head to the midlateral line, from which it goes distally along the shaft of the humerus for about 5 cm. Electrocautery is used to traverse the posterior musculature. This method provides an excellent view of the glenohumeral joint and head, as well as the proximal lateral shaft of the humerus. During the entire procedure, the affected arm is supported by a padded, sterile Mayo stand, which holds it in the intended position for fusion. The shaft of the humerus and the scapula and its vertebral border are palpable within the field and serve as reference landmarks. The position I strive for is approximately 20 to 30 degrees of glenohumeral abduction, 30 degrees forward flexion, and 30 to 40 degrees of internal rotation, using the medial border of the scapula and the humerus as landmarks. This combination appears to provide the most useful and comfortable function for the fused shoulder.

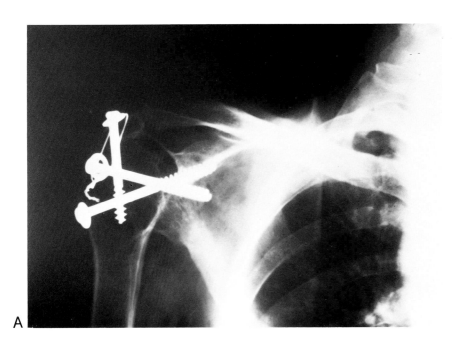

A

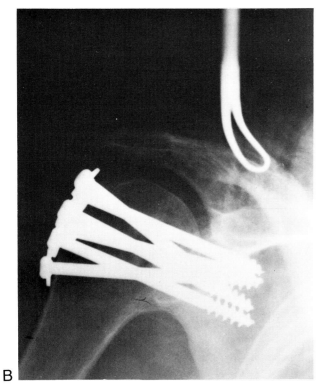

B

Fig. 41-6. **(A)** Radiograph of a shoulder fusion incorporating the acromion. Usually more than two screws traverse the glenohumeral joint. **(B)** Note the compression produced by having the threads extend beyond the fusion site to securely anchor in the scapula.

The glenoid and then the humeral head are decorticated and shaped for a smooth fit without gaps, usually with broad osteotomes for a planar surface, and internal fixation is used in all cases. Three, four, or five 75- to 85-mm half-threaded cancellous screws with washers are drilled through the head. They should penetrate into the relatively more dense subchondral bone of the neck of the glenoid. The acromion may be denuded of soft tissue, partially osteotomized, hinged down, and fixed to the humeral head with an additional screw or wire to serve as an extraarticular site for fusion (Fig. 41-6). For this technique, I employ a spica cast, which is applied a few days postoperatively when the patient can stand comfortably to have it applied. In the interval, a commercially available and adjustable metal abduction brace or simple pillow splint can be used to safeguard the fusion.

In very reliable patients, or in those in whom a spica is either contraindicated or undesirable, this method can be avoided by using the second method, that of fixation with compression plates.[62] The identical technique is used as that described above, except that instead of compression screws and a spica, I use two plates. One 10-hole plate is carefully contoured to a gentle 90-degree torsional bend and is secured to the spine of the scapula and then down over the humeral head and shaft. A sec-

ond buttress or DCP plate is secured posteriorly to the glenoid and neck of the scapula (Figs. 41-7 and 41-8). The fixation of the plate to the spine of the scapula may be difficult to achieve, particularly where the contour of the bone will not allow intramedullary placement of screws, or the spinous process is thin or porotic. In these situations, nuts may be used on cortical screws to enhance fixation. For patients with very thin subcutaneous tissue, the position of the plate may present a problem with skin closure or subsequent skin breakdown. Therefore, the plates may be contraindicated in very thin individuals. However, with this method, the postoperative period may be considerably more pleasant for the patient, since a light brace or simple sling may be used. With either method, the time for solid fusion has averaged 12 weeks, at which time all immobilization can be discontinued. In general, if shoulder fusion is to be one of several staged reconstructive procedures, it should be done as the last operation, except when a pectoralis major transfer is planned to restore elbow flexion.

Restoration of Elbow Flexion

Although surgical reconstruction of the plexus can restore excellent elbow flexion, the predictability of peripheral reconstruction by means of

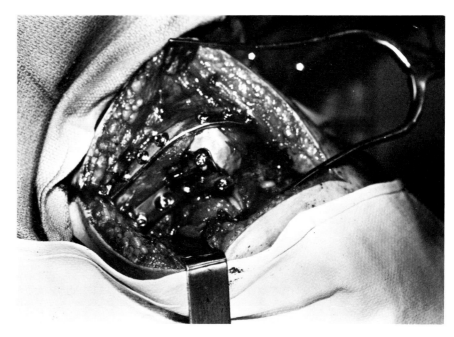

Fig. 41-7. Posterior approach for shoulder fusion showing a contoured 10-hole plate fixed to the spine of the scapula, humeral head, and proximal shaft. The buttress plate is applied posteriorly to the humeral head and neck of the scapula.

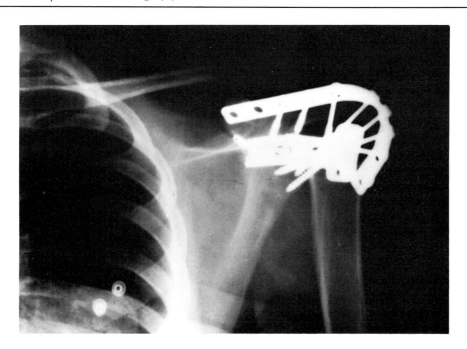

Fig. 41-8. Radiograph of the arthrodesis in Figure 41-7. Because of the amount of metal obscuring the bone detail on plane radiographs, tomography is usually required to assess the adequacy of fusion.

tendon transfer without sacrifice of sensibility in the hand, if it is present, has maintained my preference for it in patients who have partial lesions. Although active control of extension is important, if there is a relative paucity of available motors, flexion is the more important function to regain. A number of useful alternatives are available, but a prerequisite to all methods is a functional arc of passive motion in the elbow.

STEINDLER FLEXORPLASTY

The procedure that has been used most successfully in more paralytic elbows from any cause is the flexorplasty devised by Arthur Steindler in 1918.[73,74] The flexor-pronator muscles arising from the medial epicondyle are transposed to a more proximal point on the humerus so that their moment for elbow flexion is increased enough to permit active control. Although most patients can flex through a useful range against gravity, it is rare for them to be able to lift more than 5 pounds following such a transfer.[42] Nevertheless, it is a useful approach. As with all potential candidates for tendon transfer, the preoperative evaluation of the strength of the proposed motors is critical to the success of Steindler flexorplasty or any of its variations. Since the muscles originating from the me-

dial epicondyle of the humerus—the pronator teres, flexor carpi radialis, palmaris longus, flexor carpi ulnaris, and flexor digitorum superficialis— will now serve to flex the elbow in addition to their usual functions, they must have normal or near-normal power to achieve a meaningful result. Patients who already have weak elbow flexion or who can achieve flexion by the so-called Steindler effect preoperatively are most likely to have satisfactory results from surgery. The Steindler effect makes use of contraction of those muscles in a supplementary movement as follows: the patient may achieve elbow flexion by flexing wrist and fingers and pronating the forearm, usually while the arm is forward flexed to the horizontal to eliminate the effect of gravity. Since this is precisely the muscular activity that is enhanced by moving the origins more proximally, it may be used to identify those patients whose muscles are adequate for transfer. Although one may proceed in the absence of a demonstrable Steindler effect, the postoperative result is likely to be barely functional.

The modified technique that I prefer was described by Mayer and Green.[53] The incision (Fig. 41-9A) begins posterior to the medial epicondyle of the humerus and is then directed proximally and anteriorly for 7.5 cm over the distal brachium. The incision curves distally over the anterior forearm

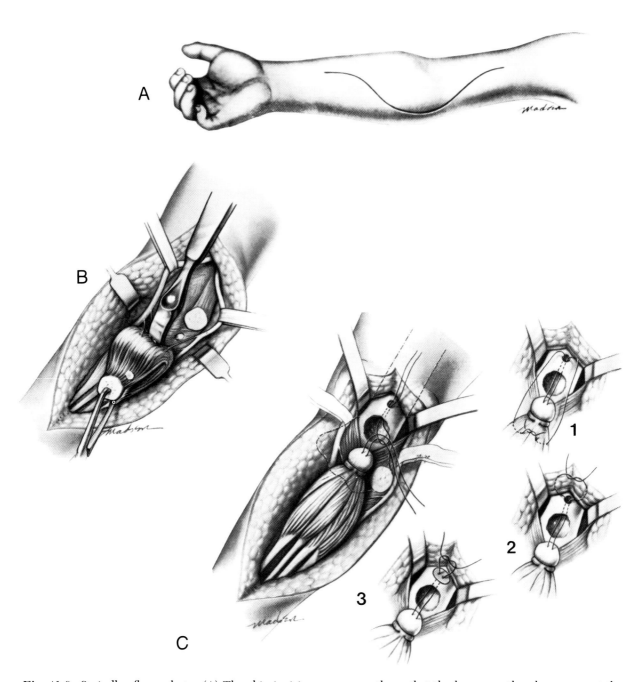

Fig. 41-9. Steindler flexorplasty. (**A**) The skin incision curves gently so that the humerus, the ulnar nerve at the elbow, and the muscles arising from the medial epicondyle are exposed. (**B**) The muscles are stripped from the anterior portion of the elbow joint capsule and ulna. Note the small capsular rent created by the stripping; it should be closed by fine nylon sutures. (**C**) Alternative methods of fixation. That shown in 3, without the additional button, has proved most satisfactory. (Mayer L, Green W: Experiences with the Steindler flexorplasty at the elbow. J Bone Joint Surg 36A:775-789, 1954.)

for 10 cm following the outline of the pronator teres muscle. The skin flap thus formed is retracted gently with the full thickness of subcutaneous tissue, and the incision is then undermined posteriorly to identify the ulnar nerve, which is mobilized from behind the elbow. The articular branch must be sacrificed, but the branches to the flexor carpi ulnaris are preserved and protected as the nerve is mobilized for about 5 cm distal to the elbow. The median nerve is then identified after the fascia over the pronator teres has been incised. The branch of the median nerve to the pronator is usually found on the medial side of the median nerve, 2.5 to 5 cm proximal to the elbow, and it too must be preserved as the nerve is mobilized. The common origin of the pronator and wrist flexor muscles is dissected from above downward and then detached with a fragment of bone from the medial epicondyle using an osteotome. Usually 0.5 to 0.75 cm of bone is sufficient, and the muscles are gently retracted while their nerve supply is protected from injury (Fig. 41-9B). Distal stripping of the muscles is continued until, with the elbow acutely flexed to 130 degrees,

the bone fragment and muscle origin have been advanced 5 to 7 cm proximally. Although in the original Steindler technique the transfer was attached to the medial intermuscular septum and fascia, Mayer used bony fixation to the anterior aspect of the humerus.

The reason for this type of attachment is twofold: (1) the attachment to bone is stronger than to fascia, and (2) the more lateral the insertion, the less the pronatory effect of the muscles. The original technique had a significant drawback, since with the increased tension on the pronator teres, flexion was usually accompanied by marked pronation of the forearm, a functionally compromised attitude for hand function.

The methods of attachment of the bone and muscle pedicle are shown in Figure 41-9C. The median nerve and brachial artery are retracted gently, and the brachialis is incised so that the humerus can be prepared for receipt of the transfer. I usually use two 0 synthetic sutures to ensure retention against the humeral shaft during healing. The distal portion of the wound is closed before the pedicle is

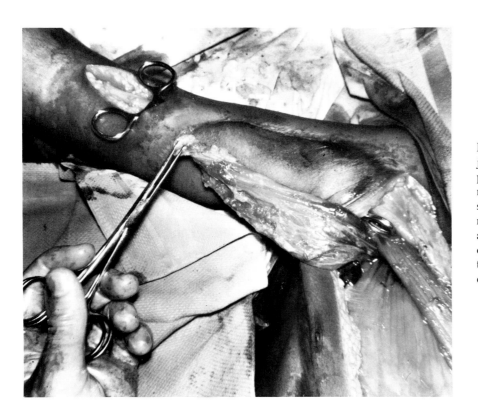

Fig. 41-10. Pectoralis major transfer. The pedicle of pectoralis major, with the nerve and vessels preserved, has been allowed to retract. At resting length, and including the rectus fascia, it just reaches the biceps tendon with the arm adducted.

secured in its new site and after the tourniquet has been removed and hemostasis has been achieved. The suture of the pedicle to the humerus and soft tissue is then accomplished with the elbow flexed 130 degrees and the forearm supinated. The proximal portion of the wound is then closed and the dressing applied. A posterior plaster splint maintains this position for 4 weeks. The postoperative rehabilitation and muscle re-education take several months, and no attempt should be made to overcome the last 30 degrees of elbow flexion contracture, since the mechanical advantage in initiation of flexion from a partially flexed position would be lost. For further discussion of this procedure, I would recommend the articles by Segal, Seddon, and Brooks[69] and Kettlekamp and Larson.[42]

PECTORALIS MAJOR TRANSFER

In 1945, Clark[21] devised an ingenious transfer of the sternocostal portion of the pectoralis major muscle for restoration of elbow flexion. The procedure has not been as popular as it should be because of failure to appreciate several technical points.

The shoulder must either be strong or fused, since with a flail shoulder the power and excursion of the transfer will dissipate in shrugging, adduction, and medial rotation of the humerus rather than in elbow flexion. The muscle pedicle must be carefully elevated from the chest wall with its nerve and major vessels intact and then routed subcutaneously down the arm to be inserted into the biceps tendon at the elbow. In order to reach the antecubital fossa, the muscle should preserve the fascia from the rectus sheath attached to it so that this tissue, rather than the muscle, is used for the suture (Fig. 41-10). As in the Steindler flexorplasty, the elbow is immobilized in acute flexion by means of a posterior plaster splint with a sling added for 4 weeks. Furthermore, the postoperative power of flexion is enhanced if there is some preoperative function and if the arm can be flexed forward to eliminate gravity. In my experience, the functional results of Clark's transfer (Fig. 41-11) have been so superior to those of the Steindler operation that I reserve the latter procedure for those patients in whom a pectoral transfer is less desirable or impossible. Although the vast majority of my patients with brachial plexus palsy are men, an occasional woman presents with this problem. Thus far, because of the large pectoral incision, I have not done the procedure in a woman. Schottstaedt, Larsen, and Bost,[65] D'Aubigne, Benassy, and Ramadieu[24] and recently Carroll and Kleinman[19] have proposed modifications of the basic technique aimed at improving the line of pull of the transfer. The Brooks-Seddon pectoral transfer,[12] in which a surgically devascularized biceps brachii is used as the tendon, has not achieved popularity.

As an alternative to the above procedures, the latissimus dorsi, when it is available, may be trans-

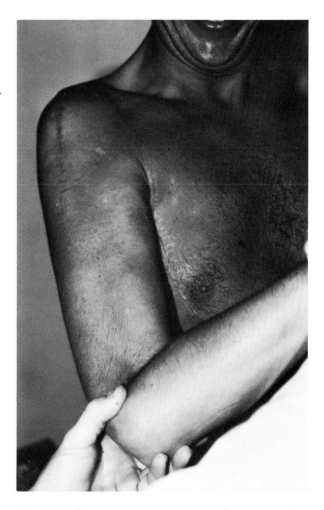

Fig. 41-11. Postoperative appearance of a patient with a Clark's pectoral transfer. Note the bulk of the muscle, which has the ability to support 4.5 kg with comfort.

ferred to the arm as either a replacement for elbow flexion or, less commonly, extension. First proposed by Schottstaedt, Larsen, and Bost in 1955,[65] it has also been described in clinical cases by Hovnanian[37] and Zancolli and Mitre.[86] These authors have reported excellent results.

TRICEPS TRANSFER

The triceps transfer, first described by Bunnell[15] and then modified by Carroll and Hill,[18] has been the subject of much controversy and often heated debate. In a patient who has an intact triceps but lacks active elbow flexion, the triceps may be brought forward and attached to the biceps tendon to regain flexion. The entire muscle must be mobilized and detached distally, and, as Carroll has shown, if a tongue of ulnar periosteum is elevated along with muscle, the need for an intercalated fascial graft to the biceps tendon is obviated (Fig. 41-12). There has been little difficulty in achieving postoperative phase conversion, and the power and excursion of the transfer are satisfactory. What makes this transfer non grata to many surgeons contemplating reconstruction for elbow flexion is the loss of what they consider the "all-important"

triceps. Several of the objections hark back to the polio patients for whom the operation was originally done. Many of these patients had bilateral disease and many walked with crutches. Loss of triceps power in these patients could seriously impair their getting out of chair or crutch walking. However, the usual patient with a brachial plexus injury has neither of these significant problems. The serious negative factors that remain are as follows: (1) the lack of triceps precludes working with the arm in front of the body or at the horizontal or using the arm as a stabilizer; and (2) although elbow extension can obviously be achieved by the effect of gravity, the smooth action of elbow flexion is materially aided by the presence of an active antagonist, which will, in addition, offset the annoying tendency to otherwise develop a contracture of the unopposed transfer.

STERNOCLEIDOMASTOID TRANSFER

The use of the sternocleidomastoid for elbow flexion was first described by Bunnell.[15] Although it can produce excellent elbow flexion, it has the disadvantage of causing an unsightly web in the neck, and occasionally, rather grotesque manipula-

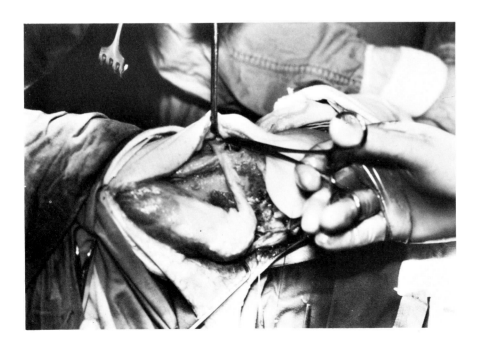

Fig. 41-12. Triceps transfer. The triceps has been elevated from the distal half of the humeral shaft, and the periosteal tongue is being directed subcutaneously and anteriorly to be sutured to the biceps tendon.

tions of the face and neck to activate the transfer. These cosmetic reasons have been sufficient for many surgeons to avoid doing this transfer. I have had the opportunity to observe several cases done by Carroll, and their strength was quite good. Most reconstructive surgeons today regard the procedure as mainly of historic interest.

AUTHOR'S PREFERRED METHOD

In my experience, the pectoral transfer provides the strongest transfer, assuming that the ipsilateral shoulder is near-normal or is fused so that the power of the muscle is not dissipated in unwanted movements. The Steindler flexorplasty, and modifications thereof, give active control that tends to be weaker. The triceps transfer is reserved for those situations where no better alternative exists and the patient has unilateral paralysis.

The Wrist

In reconstruction of an upper extremity weakened by nerve injury, it is desirable to maintain the mobility of the wrist whenever possible, since the functional excursion of all tendons and transfers that cross it are thereby improved. If two tendons of adequate power will not be available for wrist flexion and extension, or preservation of this motion will make it impossible to adequately reconstruct a functional hand, it is necessary and permissible to arthrodese the wrist. Numerous dependable techniques for achieving solid fusion are available[23] (see Chapter 6). For the paralytic wrist where a subsequent tendon transfer for finger extension is planned, or has already been done, the tendons must be able to glide unimpeded across the joint. In patients who have had wrist fusions done from the dorsal approach, a danger of scarring that will compromise excursion of the finger extensors exists. Both Smith-Peterson[72] and Seddon[66] described fusion using the distal ulna as a bone graft placed across the radiocarpal joint. This requires sacrifice of a normal distal radioulnar joint, and the stability thereby conveyed. It is for this reason that the technique described by Haddad and Riordan[29] is so attractive. Their radial approach uses an iliac graft slotted between the radius and the bases of

the second and third metacarpals. It produces an excellent fusion with minimal disturbance to the surrounding structures, and spares the extensor surface the risks of scarring (Fig. 41-13). The Haddad-Riordan fusion remains my preferred technique despite the fact that of 32 such fusions over the past 15 years, I have had three patients who sustained subsequent fractures. All of them were the result of significant trauma that would probably have caused fractures in normal wrists, and two of the three united following closed treatment. The third required a bone graft, which resulted in union.

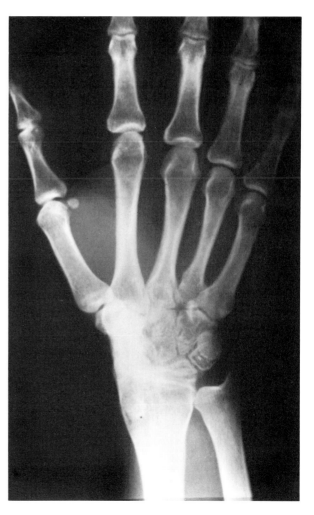

Fig. 41-13. A wrist fused by the Haddad-Riordan technique.

The Hand

The techniques for restoration of active control and stability in the weakened hand of a patient with a brachial plexus injury do not differ from those employed in cases of multiple peripheral nerve injuries. These techniques are discussed in detail in other chapters in this book. However, their application to the hand must be properly timed with reference to reconstruction of the remainder of the limb and modified accordingly if, for example, the same potential motor must be used actively at both ends of the forearm. Unless there is significant reason for doing otherwise, the hand should be reconstructed before the remainder of the limb.

The Dilemma of the Flail, Anesthetic Arm

The flail, anesthetic arm that results from neurotmesis of the brachial plexus poses a grave problem, not only for the patient, but for the surgeon as well. Before the resurgence of neurologic reconstruction, there were three general approaches — no active treatment, surgical reconstruction, and amputation. For patients whose deficit, although complete, results from a mixture of root avulsions and distal ruptures, there is usually the possibility of attempting some restoration of function by means of neurologic reconstruction. Therefore, while formerly I would suggest the option of simply placing the insensate upper limb in a sling, I am now much more confident in recommending surgical exploration to attempt to repair what can be repaired. Furthermore, some of these patients can benefit from functional bracing, which allows use of the limb as an assistive one, without using the hand in contact with objects that are grasped. This is made possible by various adaptive devices or cable-activated hooks. In order for the brace to be effective, however, the shoulder must be fused and there must be some way to achieve elbow flexion. Nevertheless, it does provide some function, for which patients are grateful.

Surgical reconstruction of the flail, anesthetic arm and hand would conceivably consist of arthrodesis of the shoulder, posterior bone block at the elbow and various combinations of arthrodeses

and tenodeses for the hand and wrist. This approach was advocated by Hendry in 1949[33] and is, in my opinion, most undesirable. It represents the surgical expression of a "very long run for a short slide," in that function is minimal and the insensate limb is vulnerable to fractures and skin breakdown.

The final solution, that of amputation of the limb, is performed far less frequently today than it was in the past, but must still be considered as a potential rehabilitative procedure for appropriate patients. Fortunately, recent advances in surgical reconstruction of the plexus have diminished the need for consideration of amputation. Nevertheless, patients whose limbs become the site of chronic infection or multiple fractures or nonunions with no

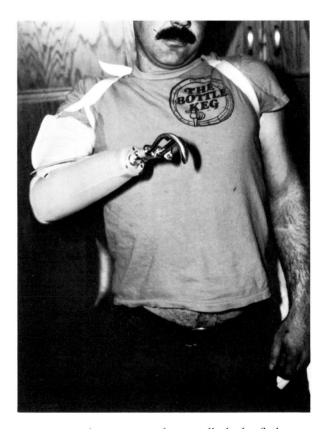

Fig. 41-14. This patient, who initially had a flail-anesthetic arm, regained active elbow flexion by means of a nerve graft from the upper trunk to the lateral cord. A shoulder fusion provided proximal control. Because no recovery was expected or occurred in the hand, the patient elected to undergo forearm amputation and prosthetic fitting. He uses the prosthesis on a regular basis.

hope of functional healing should be advised to have an amputation. If a functional prosthetic fitting is desired, an arthrodesis of the shoulder will be required in those patients who have no shoulder control (Fig. 41-14). As is well-known, the incidence of acceptance of upper extremity prostheses and their habitual use after major amputations is quite low, and in brachial plexus injury patients, it is even more prejudiced because of sensory loss and the shoulder deficit. For patients who have a contralateral normal limb, the tendency is to use it rather than the prosthesis, and for those with severe phantom pain for more than 2 years postinjury, the possibility of successful prosthetic fitting is unlikely. Since retention of the elbow, if it has position sense, is an important prognostic factor in prosthetic use, all efforts should be expended to amputate below the elbow in these cases, even if the skin sensibility is absent over the potential stump. If elbow proprioception is absent on gross testing, there is no advantage in retaining the joint. The management of the flail, anesthetic arm has been discussed by Yeoman and Seddon on the basis of their extensive experience.[85]

OBSTETRICAL BRACHIAL PLEXUS INJURY (BIRTH PALSY)

Brachial plexus injury sustained by the neonate during difficult delivery has become considerably less common because of modern obstetric management.[1] Nevertheless, such patients are still sporadically seen by pediatricians and orthopaedic surgeons who must manage them through childhood. Growth is a significant factor that can alter form and function in a manner not found in the mature individual who sustains a brachial plexus injury. Specifically, in the growing child, asymmetric muscle forces due to paralysis will be expressed as contractures and bony deformity. These must be anticipated and prevented or treated to diminish their deleterious effects.

The etiology of the nerve injury in obstetrical palsy is traction, usually due to fetal malposition, cephalopelvic disproportion, or the use of forceps. The distribution of the lesion is as follows: (1) C5 – 6 (Erb's palsy); (2) entire plexus or diffuse partial involvement; and (3) C8, T1 (Klumpke's palsy). This last group is rarely seen in its pure form.

Early diagnosis is aided by a high index of suspicion in those neonates who exhibit asymmetric active upper extremity motion in the presence of a good passive range. Skeletal injuries, such as a fractured clavicle, may result in similar disinclination to move the limb, but they may also accompany brachial plexus injury. Although a clavicle fracture is usually recognizable on x-ray examination, it may be difficult to define other bony injuries that involve the proximal humerus and its epiphysis.

As already stated, during the first two decades of this century, there was considerable enthusiasm for surgical exploration of these traction injuries.[69] However, the following 40 years saw a parallel to the management of adult traction lesions: traction injuries were not to be explored. There recently has been renewed interest in the surgical approach. The experience of Gilbert of Paris[28] has been very carefully documented and was originally presented in Tassin's thesis at the University of Paris in 1983.[78] In Tassin's paper, a series of 44 patients were observed for a 5-year period (1977 through 1982) to provide further data on the natural history of spontaneous recovery of obstetrical palsy, and these were compared with the results of the 100 neonates operated upon by Gilbert. Most of these patients were seen almost immediately following birth and were very carefully clinically evaluated. At 3 months, the final evaluation for those infants with residual paralysis consisted of a new manual muscle test, an electromyogram, and a myelogram. A paralyzed biceps at 3 months was considered an indication for surgery. Surgery was performed under general anesthesia with monitoring equipment to allow for the measurement of somatosensory-evoked potentials intraoperatively. This was found helpful in defining pathology in the presence of traumatic pseudomeningocele. Tassin's analysis of Gilbert's first 100 cases of surgical reconstruction of the plexus revealed that the timing and quality of recovery were variable and very good for the biceps, with 75 percent of the muscles able to contract to full range against gravity at 2 years, but less good for the deltoid and external rotators. The results were said to be especially good if paralysis was less extensive in the plexus. Tassin concluded that the type of surgical intervention demonstrated by Gilbert improves the prognosis of obstetrical paralysis by increasing the number of good shoulders and diminishing the number of very bad ones.

The question of neurologic reconstruction of the brachial plexus in birth palsy continues to be evaluated. Although I have no personal experience in the neurologic reconstruction of these lesions in newborns, I believe that those patients who show no evidence of recovery by 3 months should be systematically evaluated with a view toward surgical exploration.

For children with partial lesions, conservative treatment in the form of range of motion exercises in an attempt to maintain the bimanual character of the child's activities is of greatest importance, since many of the deformities that develop in the growing child can be ameliorated or prevented.

The shoulder will tend to assume an internally rotated and adducted attitude that will require constant vigilance and gentle stretching by those caring for the child. The deficit in those patients who do not respond to treatment or who are neglected will be functionally obvious. Posterior subluxation or dislocation of the glenohumeral joint may be missed, which complicates management greatly. Fixed contractures must be overcome by release of tight anterior structures, using the procedures described by Fairbank[27] and Sever,[70] and active lateral rotation, reinforced by means of tendon transfer if possible.[84] If there is significant incongruity of the glenohumeral joint, osteotomy of the proximal humerus or open reduction of the joint may be required.[63] Rarely, anterior dislocation may be encountered, and this may be dealt with accordingly, assuming the correct diagnosis has been made.

The elbow may develop abnormally in a high percentage of children with significant residual weakness of the upper extremity. Aitken's work[2] is particularly valuable when planning management and should be consulted. Aitken studied 107 cases of obstetrical paralysis and found 33 cases of bony deformity of the elbow region, an incidence of 30.8 percent of the series. From his observations, he was able to define the radiographic features of poste-

rior subluxation of the radial head. One can initially observe clubbing of the upper radial metaphysis followed by notching of its anterior aspect and increased ulnar curvature, with posterior displacement of the upper end of the radius. With growth, these changes progress so that by 5 to 8 years of age, the head becomes completely dislocated. Aitken made the point that if the radiographic changes could be identified early, complete dislocation could be prevented by splinting and range of motion exercises. For cases in which the dislocation was established, Aitken had formerly advised operative removal of the radial head. After completion of the investigation described in his article, the operation advised was osteotomy through the proximal third of the ulna, which allowed reposition of the radial axis. Results in two cases were encouraging.

The forearm and hand of a child with obstetrical palsy will often not be used in daily activities. If this is so, or if the patient is embarrassed by the abnormal limb and tends to hide it from view, even the most exquisitely planned and executed surgical reconstruction will be little more than a futile technical exercise. Sometimes the correction of an obvious deformity will have significant psychological benefit for the child, even if the functional benefit is not great. Hence, surgical procedures to be applied to the child or adolescent must be very carefully considered. Finally, growth centers must not be damaged in these paretic limbs that are invariably smaller than their normal counterparts.

REFERENCES

1. Adler JB, Patterson RL: Erb's palsy. Long time results of treatment in eighty-eight cases. J Bone Joint Surg 49A:1052–1064, 1967
2. Aitken J: Deformity of the elbow joint as a sequel to Erb's obstetrical palsy. J Bone Joint Surg 34B:352–365, 1952
3. Allieu Y: Exploration et traitement direct des lesions nerveuses dans les paralysies traumatiques par elongation du plexus brachial chez l'adulte. Rev Chir Orthop 63:107–122, 1977

4. Alnot JY, Augereau B, Frot B: Traitement direct des lesions nerveuses dans les paralysies traumatiques par elongation du plexus brachial chez l'adulte. Chirurgie 103:935–947, 1977

5. Barnes R: Traction injuries of the brachial plexus in adults. J Bone Joint Surg 31B:10–16, 1949

6. Benassy J, Held JP, Bernardeau D, Monteard J: Traumatismes fermes due plexus brachial. Chirurgie 100:374–381, 1973

7. Bonney G: The value of axon responses in determining the site of lesion in traction injuries to the brachial plexus. Brain 77:588, 1954

8. Bonney G: Prognosis in traction lesions of the brachial plexus. J Bone Joint Surg 41B:4–35, 1959

9. Bonney G, Gilliat RW: Sensory nerve conduction after traction lesions of the brachial plexus. Proc R Soc Med 51:365, 1958

10. Braun RM, Newman J, Thacher B: Injury to the brachial plexus as a result of diagnostic arteriography. J Hand Surg 3:90–97, 1978

11. Brooks DM: Open wounds of the brachial plexus. J Bone Joint Surg 31B:17–33, 1949

12. Brooks DM, Seddon HJ: Pectoral transplantation for paralysis of the flexors of the elbow. A new technique. J Bone Joint Surg 41B:36–50, 1959

13. Brunelli G: Neurolysis and free microvascular omentum transfer in the treatment of postactinic palsies of the brachial plexus. Int Surg 65:6, 1980

14. Bufalini C, Pescatori G: Posterior cervical electromyography in the diagnosis and prognosis of brachial plexus injuries. J Bone Joint Surg 51B:627–631, 1969

15. Bunnell S: Restoring flexion to the paralytic elbow. J Bone Joint Surg 33A:566–571, 1951

16. Carroll RE: Restoration of flexor power to the flail elbow by transplantation of the triceps tendon. Surg Gynecol Obstet 95:685, 1952

17. Carroll RE, Gartland JJ: Flexorplasty of the elbow. An evaluation of a method. J Bone Joint Surg 35A:706–710, 1953

18. Carroll RE, Hill NA: Triceps transfer to restore elbow flexion: A study of fifteen patients with paralytic lesions and arthrogryposis. J Bone Joint Surg 52A:239–244, 1970

19. Carroll RE, Kleinman WB: Pectoralis major transplantation to restore elbow flexion to the paralytic limb. J Hand Surg 4:501–507, 1979

20. Carroll SE, Wilkins WW: Two cases of brachial plexus injury following percutaneous arteriograms. Can Med Assoc J 102:862, 1970

21. Clark JMP: Reconstruction of biceps brachii by pectoral muscle transplantation. Br J Surg 34:180, 1946

22. Clemedson CJ, Nelson A: In Errera M, Fossberg A

(eds): Mechanisms in Radiobiology. Vol. 2. Academic Press, New York, 1960

23. Crenshaw AH: Campbell's Operative Orthopaedics, 5th Ed. Ch. 14, CV Mosby, St Louis, 1971

24. D'Aubigne M, Benassy J, Ramadieu JO: Chirurgie Orthopedique des Paralysies. pp. 122-139. Masson, Paris, 1956

25. Davis DH, Onofrio BH, MacCarthy CS: Brachial plexus injuries. Proc Mayo Clin 53:799–807, 1978

26. Delbet P, Cauchoix A: Les paralysies dans les luxations de l'epaule. Rev Chir Orthop 41:327, 1910

27. Fairbank HAT: Birth palsy: subluxation of shoulder-joint in infants and young children. Lancet 1:1217, 1913

28. Gilbert A, Tassin JL: Surgical repair of the brachial plexus in obstetric paralysis. Chirurgie 110(1):70–75, 1984

29. Haddad RJ, Riordan DC: Arthrodesis of the wrist. A surgical technique. J Bone Joint Surg 49A:950–954, 1967

30. Harmon PH: Surgical reconstruction of the paralytic shoulder by multiple muscle transplantation. J Bone Joint Surg 32A:583–595, 1950

31. Harris W, Low VW: The importance of accurate muscle analysis in lesions of the brachial plexus. Brit Med J 2:1035–1038, 1903

32. Haymaker W, Lindgren M: Nerve disturbances following exposure to ionizing radiation. In Vinker DJ, Bruyn GW (eds): Handbook of Clinical Neurology, Vol. VII. Diseases of Nerves, Part II. North-Holland Publishing, Amsterdam, 1970

33. Hendry AM: The treatment of residual paralysis after brachial plexus injury. J Bone Joint Surg 31B:42–49, 1949

34. Heon M: Myelogram: A questionable aid in diagnosis and prognosis in avulsion of brachial plexus components by traction injuries. Conn Med 29:260, 1965

35. Hollinshead WH: Anatomy for Surgeons: The Back and Limbs. Vol. 3, Ch. 4. Harper and Row, New York, 1969

36. Hovelacque A: Anatomie des Nerfs Craniens et Rachidiens et du Systeme. Grande Sympathhique. pp. 385-513. Gaston, Doin et Cie, Paris, 1927

37. Hovnanian AP: Latissimus dorsi transplantation for loss of flexion or extension at the elbow. A preliminary report of technique. Ann Surg 143:493, 1956

38. Jelasic F, Piepgras U: Functional restitution after cervical avulsion injury with "typical" myelographic findings. Europ Neurol 11:158, 1974

39. Jepson PN: Obstetrical paralysis. Ann Surg 91:724–730, 1930

40. Jones SJ, Wynn-Parry CB, Landi A: Diagnosis of

brachial plexus traction lesions by sensory nerve action potentials and somatosensory evoked potentials. Injury 12:376, 1981

41. Kerr AT: The brachial plexus of nerves in man. The variations in its formation and branches. Am J Anat 23:285, 1918

42. Kettlekamp DB, Larson CB: Evaluation of the Steindler flexorplasty. J Bone Joint Surg 45A:513–518, 1963

43. Kline DG: Evaluation of the neuroma-in-continuity. In Omer GE Jr, Spinner M (eds): Management of Peripheral Nerve Problems. WB Saunders, Philadelphia, 1980

44. Kotani T, Toshima Y, Matsuda H, Suzuki T: Postoperative results of nerve transposition and brachial plexus injury. Orthop Surg Tokyo 22:963, 1971

45. Leffert RD: Brachial plexus injuries. Orthop Clin North Am 1:399–417, 1970

46. Leffert RD: Brachial plexus injuries. N Engl J Med 291:1059–1067, 1974

47. Leffert RD: Lesions of the brachial plexus, including thoracic outlet syndrome. AAOS Instructional Course Lectures. Vol. 26. CV Mosby, St Louis, 1977

48. Leffert RD: Brachial Plexus Injuries. Churchill Livingstone, New York, 1985

49. Leffert RD, Seddon H: Infraclavicular brachial plexus injuries. J Bone Joint Surg 47B:9–22, 1965

50. L'Episcopo JB: Restoration of muscle balance in the treatment of obstetrical paralysis. NY State J Med 39:357–363, 1939

51. Lusskin R, Campbell JB, Thompson WAL: Posttraumatic lesions of the brachial plexus: Treatment by transclavicular exploration and neurolysis or autograft reconstruction. J Bone Joint Surg 55A:1159–1176, 1973

52. Match RM: Radiation induced brachial plexus paralysis. Arch Surg 110:384, 1975

53. Mayer L, Green W: Experiences with the Steindler flexorplasty at the elbow. J Bone Joint Surg 36A:775–789, 1954

54. Millesi H: Surgical management of brachial plexus injuries. J Hand Surg 2:367–379, 1977

55. Millesi H, Meissl G, Katzer H: Zur Behandlung der Verletzungen des Plexus Brachialis. Vorchlag einer inegrierten Therapie. Bruns Beitr Klin Chir 220:429, 1973

56. Narakas A: Indications et resultats du traitement chirurgical direct dans les lesions par elongation du plexus brachial. Rev Chir Orthop 63:88–107, 1977

57. Narakas A: The surgical management of brachial plexus injuries. p. 443. In Daniel RK, Terzis JK (eds): Reconstructive Microsurgery. Vol. 1, Ch. 9. Little, Brown, Boston, 1977

58. Narakas A: Brachial plexus surgery in symposium on peripheral nerve injuries. Orthop Clin North Am 12:303–323, 1981

59. Nelson KG, Jolly PC, Thomas PA: Brachial plexus injuries associated with missile wounds of the chest. A report of nine cases from Viet Nam. J Trauma 8:268–275, 1968

60. Ober FR: Transplantation to improve the function of the shoulder joint and extensor function of the elbow joint. AAOS Instructional Course Lectures on Reconstructive Surgery. JW Edwards, Ann Arbor, 1944

61. Platt H: Opening remarks on birth paralysis. J Orthop Surg 2:272, 1920

62. Riggins R: Shoulder fusion without external fixation. A preliminary report. J Bone Joint Surg 58A:1007–1008, 1976

63. Rogers MH: An operation for the correction of the deformity due to "obstetrical paralysis." Boston Med Surg J 174:163, 1916

64. Saha AK: Surgery of the paralyzed and flail shoulder. Acta Orthop Scan suppl. 97, 1967

65. Schottstaedt ER, Larsen LJ, Bost FC: Complete muscle transposition. J Bone Joint Surg 37A:897–919, 1955

66. Seddon HJ: Reconstructive Surgery of the Upper Extremity. Poliomyelitis. Second International Poliomyelitis Congress. JB Lippincott, Philadelphia, 1952

67. Seddon HJ: Nerve grafting. J Bone Joint Surg 45B:447–461, 1963

68. Sedel L: Results of surgical repair in brachial plexus injuries. J Bone Joint Surg 64B:54–66, 1982

69. Segal A, Seddon HJ, Brooks DM: Treatment of paralysis of the flexors of the elbow. J Bone Joint Surg 41B:44–50, 1959

70. Sever JW: Obstetrical paralysis: Report of eleven hundred cases. JAMA 85:1862, 1925

71. Sharpe W: The operative treatment of brachial plexus paralysis. JAMA 66:876, 1916

72. Smith-Petersen, MN: A new approach to the wrist joint. J Bone Joint Surg 22:122, 1940

73. Steindler A: Reconstruction work on hand and forearm. NY State Med J 108:117–119, 1918

74. Steindler A: Muscle and tendon transplantation at the elbow. In Thompson JEM (ed): Instructional Course Lectures on Reconstructive Surgery. Vol. 2. AAOS, Chicago, 1944

75. Stevens JH: Brachial plexus paralysis. In Codman EA (ed): The Shoulder. G Miller, Brooklyn, 1934

76. Sunderland S: Nerves and Nerve Injuries. 2nd Ed. Churchill Livingstone, Edinburgh, 1978

77. Tarlov IM: Autologous plasma clot suture of nerves. Its use in clinical surgery. JAMA 126:741, 1944

78. Tassin JL: Paralysies obstetricales du plexus brachial

evolution spontance, resultats des interventions reparatrices precoces. Thesis, University of Paris, VII, 1983

79. Taylor AS: Brachial birth palsy and injuries of similar types in adults. Surg Gynecol Obstet 30:495–502, 1920

80. Thornburn W: A clinical lecture on secondary suture of the brachial plexus. Br Med J 1:1073–1075, 1900

81. Tracy JF, Brannon EW: Management of brachial plexus injuries (traction type). J Bone Joint Surg 40A:1031–1042, 1958

82. Tsuyama N, Hara T: Intercostal nerve transfer in the treatment of brachial plexus injury of root avulsion type. p. 351. Proc 12th Cong International Soc Orthop Surg Traumatol, Tel Aviv. Exerpta Medica Amsterdam, 1972

83. Uhlschmid G, Clodius L: A new use for the freely transplanted omentum. Management of a late radiation injury of the brachial plexus using freely transplanted omentum and neurolysis. Chirugie 49(11):714, 1978

84. Wickstrom J: Birth injuries of the brachial plexus: Treatment of defects in the shoulder. Clin Orthop 23:187–196, 1962

85. Yeoman PM, Seddon HJ: Brachial plexus injuries— Treatment of the flail arm. J Bone Joint Surg 43B:493–500, 1961

86. Zancolli E, Mitre H: Latissimus dorsi transfer to restore elbow flexion. An appraisal of eight cases. J Bone Joint Surg 55A:1265–1275, 1973

Tetraplegia

42

Charles L. McDowell

PATIENT SELECTION AND CLASSIFICATION

For the surgeon considering operative treatment in a tetraplegic patient, patient selection is the most difficult task to confront. The difficulty lies in the complexity of the physical examination, in which conditions change, especially during the first 12 months after injury, and where spasticity often exists. In addition, there are subjective factors that have a different emphasis in tetraplegic patients than in patients with other conditions. The dramatic change in the patient's life requires a long and arduous psychological adjustment, and some patients fail to adjust sufficiently to handle surgical reconstruction. Other factors to consider include the patient's age, occupation, interests, level of education, learning capacity, economic support, family and agency support, personality type, and understanding of what can and cannot be expected from surgical treatment. Patient selection is not simply a matter of obtaining the objective information and applying a set method of treatment.

Classically, tetraplegic patients have been classified by the cervical spine segment injured by fracture or dislocation, and there has been an assumption that the level of paralysis and sensory loss coincided exactly with the bony injury, producing a precise transverse spinal cord lesion (Fig. 42-1). Careful examination of patients rendered tetraplegic has shown that (1) there is frequently little relationship between the level of the skeletal lesion and the spinal cord lesion; (2) lesions may be asymmetrical; and (3) there may be unusual patterns of sparing of sensory or motor function. Thus a more useful classification had to be developed that used spared functions as its basis. The classification (Table 42-1) used in this chapter was approved by an international group of surgeons working with tetraplegics[25] and modified in 1984 at Giens, France.[26]

Sensory Classification

The sensory classification has two categories: O for ocular or visual afferent input and Cu for cutaneous afferent input. The two-point discrimination test described by Moberg is used to determine cutaneous sensibility. A patient must demonstrate discrimination of 10 mm or less (using the blunt points of a paper clip) to be classified in Group Cu, as it is assumed that the minimum cutaneous sensibility to control grip is 10 mm two-point discrimination. The O (ocular) group depends on vision for afferent information and grip control.

1597

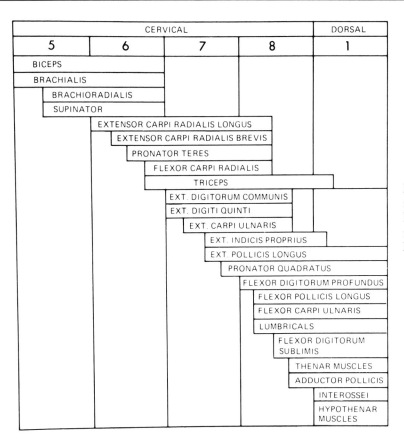

Fig. 42-1. Segmental innervation of muscles of the elbow, forearm, and hand. (Zancolli EA: Structural and Dynamic Bases of Hand Surgery. 2nd Ed. p. 231. JB Lippincott, Philadelphia, 1979.)

Motor Classification

Muscles are included in the classification of a patient only if they are of at least Grade 4 MRC (Medical Research Council)[27] (Table 42-2). Surgeons disagree as to whether it is possible to distinguish between function of the extensor carpi radialis longus and extensor carpi radialis brevis. Some believe that they can test and grade each muscle separately; others do not. Fortunately, both groups agree that the extensor carpi radialis brevis can be assessed best by exposing the tendon at the wrist level under local anesthesia and testing it with weights attached to a sterile pin through the tendon.[4] The patient should be able to lift 3 to 5 pounds of weight for the muscle to be considered classifiable.

Most patients rendered tetraplegic by an injury will fall under the first half of the classification. Moberg points out that significantly more high-level cases with more severe paralysis were seen in Scandinavia and the United States than in Argentina. He suggests that the difference might be due to the lower mortality rate in Scandinavia and the United States.[32] If this is true, it means that surgeons in areas with a high survival rate of spinal cord–injured patients will encounter more difficult cases.

Timing of Operative Treatment

Additional guidelines for patient selection, apart from the subjective factors or the patient's classification, are based on information acquired from experience in treating tetraplegic patients. The conference surgeons agreed that serial sensory and muscle testing should be done at about 3-month intervals for at least 1 year after injury before considering operative procedures. Surgical recon-

Table 42-1. International Classification for Surgery of the Hand in Tetraplegia
Edinburgh 1978 (Modified—Giens 1984)

Sensibility	Motor[a]		Description
O or Cu	Group	Characteristics	Function
	0	No muscle below elbow suitable for transfer	Flexion and supination of the elbow
	1	BR	
	2	ECRL	Extension of the wrist (weak or strong)
	3°	ECRB	Extension of the wrist
	4	PT	Extension and pronation of the wrist
	5	FCR	Flexion of the wrist
	6	Finger extensors	Extrinsic extension of the fingers (partial or complete)
	7	Thumb extensor	Extrinsic extension of the thumb
	8	Partial digital flexors	Extrinsic flexion of the fingers (weak)
	9	Lacks only intrinsics	Extrinsic flexion of the fingers
	X	Exceptions	

[a] BR, Brachioradialis; ECRL, Extensor carpi radialis longus; ECRB, Extensor carpi radialis brevis; PT, Pronator teres; FCR, Flexor carpi radialis.
° Caution: It is not possible to determine the strength of the ECRB without surgical exposure.

1. This classification does not include the shoulder. It is a guide to the forearm and hand only. Determination of patient suitability for posterior deltoid to triceps transfer or biceps to triceps transfer is considered separately.
2. The need for triceps reconstruction is stated separately. It may be required in order to make brachioradialis transfers function properly (see text).
3. There is a sensory component to the classification. Afferent input is recorded using the method described by Moberg and precedes the motor classification. Both ocular and cutaneous input should be documented. When vision is the only afferent available the designation is "Occulo" (abbreviated O). Assuming there is 10 mm or less two-point discrimination in the thumb and index finger, the correct classification would be Cu, indicating that the patient has adequate cutaneous sensibility. If two-point discrimination is greater than 10 mm (meaning inadequate cutaneous sensibility), the designation O would precede the motor group (example O 2).
4. Motor grouping assumes that all listed muscles are grade 4 (MRC) or better and a new muscle is added for each group; for example, a Group 3 patient will have BR, ECRL, and ECRB rated at least grade 4 (MRC).
(Modified from McDowell CL, Moberg EA, House JH: The Second International Conference on Surgical Rehabilitation of the Upper Limb in Tetraplegia (Quadriplegia). J Hand Surg 11A:604–608, 1986.)

Table 42-2. Currently Accepted Muscle Grading System First Devised by the British Medical Research Council[27]

0	No contraction
1	Flicker or trace of contraction
2	Active movement with gravity eliminated
3	Active movement against gravity
4	Active movement against gravity and resistance
5	Normal

struction should rarely be considered prior to 1 year following spinal cord injury to allow the patient sufficient time to make major psychological adjustments, especially to understand that there is no hope for further recovery. Further delay of reconstruction is indicated if there is evidence of any neurologic recovery; operative treatment is considered only after the motor and sensory improvement has stopped.[16]

Role of Spasticity

Spasticity is a serious consideration in reconstructive surgery for the tetraplegic patient. The degree of spasticity is difficult to evaluate, and its presence may severely compromise results. The conference surgeons agreed that muscles exhibiting uncontrolled spasticity, even though of adequate strength, should not be transferred.[25] Lesser degrees of spasticity constitute a relative contraindication to transfer operations. There are a few situations in which a spastic muscle can be rendered flaccid by neurectomy or tendon release, thus making tenodesis or arthrodesis procedures reasonable possibilities.

Goals of Operative Treatment

Preoperative observation of patients who have enough muscle strength to actively dorsiflex the wrist reveals a tendency to utilize the natural "tenodesis" effect for function; that is, with wrist dorsiflexion, the digital extensor tendons are slack and the digital flexor muscle-tendon units are placed under sufficient tension to cause the thumb to adduct against the side of the index finger and the fingers to flex. This effect should be enhanced whenever possible. Arthrodeses, especially wrist fusion, should be avoided because fusion interferes with the pattern of function that the patient has learned to use.

A formerly popular method used to try to obtain grasp in patients with wrist extension only (Groups 2, 3, and 4) had as its goal a three-point "chuck"-type pinch. The operations employed to achieve this included combinations of tendon transfers, tenodesing procedures, and joint fusions.[1,34] The results of such procedures have been judged unacceptable by most surgeons and patients because the thumb and fingers are rendered rigid. Key pinch (i.e., thumb to the radial side of the index finger) is easier to accomplish with surgery and is more useful and acceptable to the patient.[31,44] The conference surgeons recommended side pinch (key grip) as a better goal of surgical reconstruction.[25]

DEVELOPMENT OF THE SURGICAL TREATMENT PLAN

Planning of surgical procedures should take into account other needs that may have priority over upper extremity reconstruction. Pressure sores must be cared for, and all scars should be well healed. The patient should be mobilized in a wheelchair so that upper extremity use and training can be optimized. Treatment of other systems, such as urogenital and cardiopulmonary, may also take priority. Appropriate expert consultation for these other systems must be sought.

General anesthesia and axillary regional block have been successful in this type of surgery. Few complications have been reported with either method, probably due to the high quality of anesthesia available to the reporting surgeons.[10,33] My preferred method is the axillary regional block. I do not recommend supraclavicular block because of the risk of pneumothorax and/or paralysis of the diaphragm.

Precise muscle and sensory testing should be recorded so that the patient can be properly classified. Both upper extremities should be classified separately, as they may not be the same.

If reconstructive surgery to restore active elbow extension by deltoid-to-triceps transfer is indicated, the transfer should precede other operations. Moberg reasoned that a patient who obtained grasp capability by surgery on the forearm would be frustrated by a deltoid-to-triceps transfer performed later since he would not be able to grasp objects during the prolonged period of elbow immobilization. In addition, an active elbow extensor improves the function of a brachioradialis transfer because it acts as an antagonist.[31]

Only one operation should be performed at a time. This does not mean that small joint fusions or other synergistic procedures should not be combined, but rather that complex operations should be carefully staged. My own experiences indicate that the best outcomes have resulted from the least complex operations. In addition, operations that impair the use of both upper extremities at the same time must be avoided (Zuelzer W: personal communication).

Whether stated or implied by the way they managed their cases, Moberg[32] and House, Gwathmey, and Lundsgaard[17] believe that reconstruction should begin on the dominant extremity if both are classified at the same level. If sparing of function is not symmetrical, reconstruction should begin on the side with better function. I use this approach because some patients, particularly those with significant loss, may be content with reconstruction of only one side. Obviously, if there is inadequate cutaneous sensibility, surgery should be done only on the side with the better sensibility.

At this stage of planning, the surgeon must consider, according to his own experience and judgment, the best functional goals that can be obtained for this patient. Moberg has departed from the priorities established by earlier authors. Prior to his articles, surgeons designed reconstructive procedures that would restore as many lost motor functions as possible. Moberg has emphasized the fact that the hand's function is not simply motor function, but also sensation. He believes that people are very interested in human contact and that hands that are made more rigid by multiple tendon transfers and/or small joint arthrodeses are not well accepted by patients. His concept of the patient's priorities justifies his more conservative approach to surgical reconstruction in cases with few spared muscles.[31]

Contraindications to Operative Treatment

In my experience two factors have had a uniformly adverse effect on results of surgical treatment: spasticity and psychoneurosis. Spasticity that cannot be controlled by the patient is a strong contraindication to surgery. Freehafer, Vonhaam, and Allen[11] and Moberg have stated that some spasticity might be helpful, but judging the degree of spasticity compatible with good results is difficult. In fact, Moberg noted such an error in his poor result group.[30]

Psychoneurosis should be controlled prior to surgery. When the condition was not detected and left untreated, the results of surgery were unsatisfactory from the patient's point of view. Also, psychological problems can interfere significantly with postoperative training.

ELBOW EXTENSION

Elbow extension should be provided in patients whose spinal cord lesion spares the function of the deltoid. This operation has proved useful in pa-

tients who are not candidates for any other reconstructive surgery because elbow extension helps the patient stabilize himself in the wheelchair and improves control of self-help devices. It is required where transfer of the brachioradialis is being considered in Group 0 to Group 5 or 6 when the triceps is not innervated. Moberg has shown that active elbow extension improved the function of the transferred brachioradialis. As the brachioradialis is not only a supinator but also an elbow flexor, the deltoid-to-triceps transfer provides an antagonist. Most surgeons agree that the deltoid-to-triceps transfer should be the first operation performed.[25]

DELTOID-TO-TRICEPS TRANSFER (MOBERG)

A curved incision is made along the posterior border of the deltoid muscle, and the muscle is exposed to its insertion on the humerus. The posterior third (spinous portion) of the deltoid origin is separated from the middle or acromial portion distal to the axillary nerve by blunt dissection. The anterior border is dissected free, preserving the fibrous band to the brachialis, if present, which is useful in attaching the graft to the deltoid. The axillary nerve, whose course is about 4 to 5 cm distal to the acromion, must be protected. The posterior portion of the muscle belly is isolated (Fig. 42-2A), and the posterior portion of the insertion is carefully stripped away from the humerus to preserve as much tough tendinous tissue and periosteum as possible. Moberg recommends proximal dissection of the belly to increase the excursion of the muscle to 30 mm. To avoid damage to the axillary nerve, only the superficial aponeurosis is divided at the upper end of the muscle. The tendon of insertion of the triceps into the olecranon is then exposed through a separate curved incision. Tendon grafts to connect the deltoid to the triceps insertion can be obtained from many locations. Moberg prefers the toe extensors to the second, third, and fourth toes, which he obtains through multiple incisions on the dorsum of the foot and anterior surface of the ankle. The additional length required is obtained by adding more small incisions about the ankle or by using a tendon stripper. There should be adequate tendon graft material to make at least three loops at the attachment site.

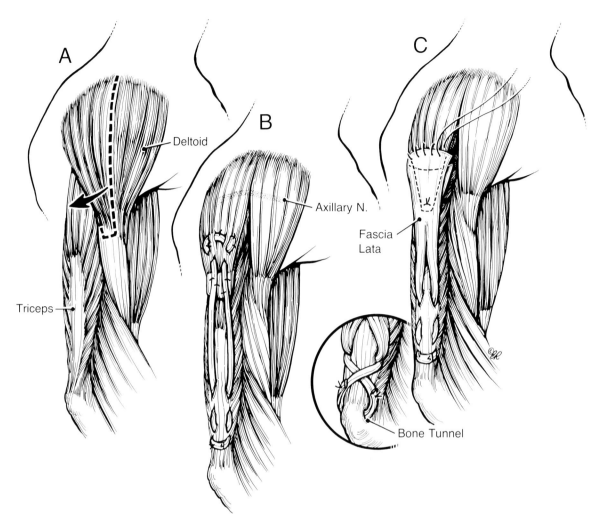

Fig. 42-2. Deltoid-to-triceps transfer (Moberg). **(A)** The posterior border of the muscle belly is isolated, preserving as much of the tendinous insertion as possible. **(B)** Tendon grafts are laced into the distal end of the deltoid muscle belly and triceps aponeurosis. **(C)** Use of fascia lata rather than tendon grafts. Direct insertion into the olecranon through a bone tunnel can also be done with either type of graft.

Next, a tunnel is made between the two incisions on the arm in the plane between subcutaneous fat and the triceps muscle. The tendon grafts are laced into the distal end of the deltoid muscle belly and into the triceps aponeurosis (Fig. 42-2B). The laced tendon grafts are sutured into place with moderate tension while the elbow is held in full extension and the humerus abducted 30 to 40 degrees.

I prefer Hentz's method[16] of using fascia lata as the interposition graft because of the large contact surface into the triceps tendon insertion and into the muscle belly of the posterior deltoid (Fig. 42-2C). Also, enough length can be obtained to attach the graft to the most distal end of the triceps and even directly to the olecranon if the surgeon wishes. There is not enough experience with any alternative tendon graft method to suggest that these other techniques shorten the time of immobilization and staged rehabilitation described by Moberg. There is enough experience to recommend that the transfer be set relatively tight. Moberg has advanced the triceps insertion distalward in some cases where the transfers were too loose (Moberg E: personal communication).

Postoperative Management. A well-padded long arm plaster cylinder is applied to hold the elbow in 10 degrees flexion. The plaster stops just proximal to the wrist. Moberg recommends strapping the cast to the patient's waist until he is able to protect himself to prevent inadvertent stretching of the transfer. Also, he uses a local anesthetic in the deltoid muscle to prevent any inadvertent contraction of the muscle sufficient to rupture or stretch the suture lines during recovery from anesthesia. He administers 20 ml of 1 percent Xylocaine or Carbocaine with 1 : 200,000 epinephrine. The elbow is immobilized in 10 degrees flexion in the cast for 6 weeks. Gentle active exercises are then done to slowly gain flexion for the next 3 months (at a rate of 5 to 10 degrees of flexion per week). For the first 2 months in this phase of rehabilitation, the patient should use a padded night splint designed to hold the elbow in 0 to 10 degrees flexion. The patient may be eager to gain elbow flexion too rapidly, and the surgeon may have to consider the use of a re-movable splint during part of the day also. Resistive exercises should be delayed until 4 months after surgery.

My patients prefer an elbow brace with a dial-lock hinge that can be used during the stage of progressive elbow flexion beginning at 6 weeks after surgery. It is lighter, cooler, and can be used many times.[16]

FOREARM PRONATION

Pronation is important to patients who have active wrist extension only (Group 2 and 3). These patients use the automatic or "tenodesis" effect for grasp, but if the hand cannot be pronated, gravity cannot be used to produce palmar flexion and digital extension for release of grasp. Also, those patients using a "tenodesis" brace need pronation for the same reason. Zancolli produces pronation by converting the biceps into a forearm pronator. He reroutes the tendon around the radius in the opposite direction[44] (Fig. 42-3).

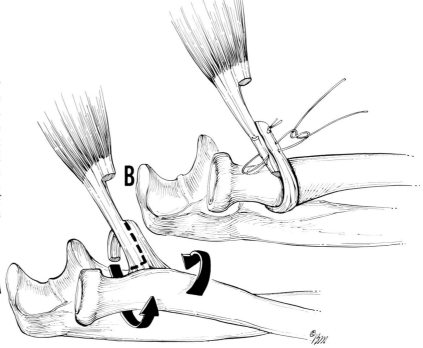

Fig. 42-3. Zancolli's method for rerouting the insertion of the biceps tendon to provide pronation of the forearm. Half of the tendon is passed behind the neck of the radius (**A**), and then sutured into the remaining biceps tendon (**B**). (Redrawn from Zancolli EA: Structural and Dynamic Bases of Hand Surgery. 2nd Ed. p. 236. JB Lippincott, Philadelphia, 1979.)

PROCEDURES ACCORDING TO CLASSIFICATION

Group 0

Patients whose spinal cord injury level is high enough to be classified under Group 0 may nonetheless be candidates for deltoid-to-triceps transfer for elbow extension. These patients should be considered for orthoses powered by an external source, such as the "CO_2 muscle" or an electric motor. Almost all of these patients can use some assistive devices attached to one hand.

A few patients in Group 0 may have a weak brachioradialis and a weak extensor carpi radialis longus. Tendon transfer may be considered if the surgeon thinks that the brachioradialis is strong enough to transfer to the weak radial wrist extensors and thus achieve sufficient strength to dorsiflex the wrist against resistance. If this is accomplished, the patient may be able to use a wrist-driven flexor hinge splint (Fig. 42-4) or a flexor pollicis longus tenodesis.

Few patients in this group will qualify for transfer. Assessing the strength of the brachioradialis muscle is difficult and requires an experienced examiner. It is best performed by having the patient flex his elbow against resistance, while the examiner evaluates muscle tension by trying to deflect the muscle belly. It is important to remember that the patient will need elbow extension to make good use of a brachioradialis transfer.

It is not likely that a patient in this group will have enough dorsiflexion strength to consider constructing a Moberg-type of simple grip.

BRACHIORADIALIS TO RADIAL WRIST EXTENSOR TRANSFER

Freehafer and Mast have described a useful method of transfer of the brachioradialis to the radial wrist extensors[10] (Fig. 42-5). They make an S-shaped or slightly curved incision on the radial side of the forearm near the junction of the proximal and middle thirds. At this site the brachioradialis is on the radial aspect of the forearm, the extensor carpi radialis longus is dorsal and parallel to it, and the extensor carpi radialis brevis is on the

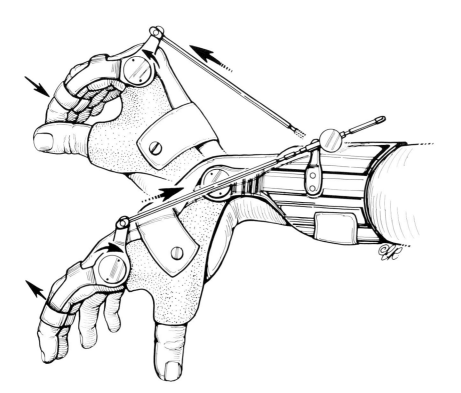

Fig. 42-4. The wrist-driven flexor hinge splint uses the principle of synergistic action. As the wrist is dorsiflexed, the fingers are flexed to bring them into contact with the thumb, which is fixed. As the wrist is volar flexed, the fingers are extended. In patients in Group 0, the splint may be powered by an external source, such as the "CO_2 muscle" or an electric motor.

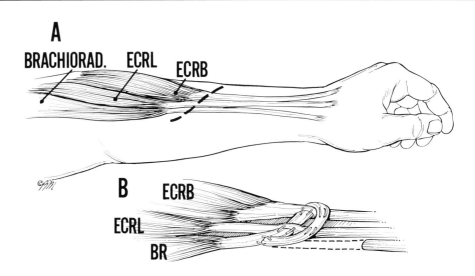

Fig. 42-5. A brachioradialis transfer to extensor carpi radialis longus and extensor carpi radialis brevis. An important technical detail is that the brachioradialis muscle belly must be mobilized completely to the elbow, taking care to protect its nerve supply from the radial nerve.

ulnar side of the longus. The tendons are exposed by opening their sheaths. The brachioradialis tendon is divided, preserving sufficient length of the proximal stump so that it can be threaded through the tendons of the extensor carpi radialis longus and brevis for a strong anastomosis. Special care is required to protect the branches of the superficial radial nerve beneath the brachioradialis muscle and tendon. Another critical technical detail is adequate proximal dissection of the brachioradialis muscle belly. It must be mobilized toward the elbow sufficiently to increase its excursion to 3 cm or more. The brachioradialis tendon is passed through a small slit in the two radial wrist extensors, looped back, and sutured to itself. The brachioradialis tendon is also sutured to each of the radial wrist extensors. The tension should be sufficient to hold the wrist in 0 degrees, but not so tight that the wrist cannot be fully flexed passively.

Postoperative Management. A long arm cast is applied at operation to hold the elbow in 90 degrees flexion and the wrist in 45 degrees dorsiflexion. The cast is removed at 4 weeks, and the patient is started on active strengthening exercises. A removable splint is worn to support the wrist when the patient is not exercising for an additional 3 weeks.

Group 1

Patients in Group 1 have a strong brachioradialis. Transfer of the brachioradialis to weak or nonfunctioning radial wrist extensors should provide suffi-

cient strength to allow the patient to dorsiflex his wrist against at least 5 pounds of resistance. This is sufficient strength to operate a wrist-driven flexor hinge splint satisfactorily, or to consider a Moberg-type of simple hand grip reconstruction to be performed at the same time as the brachioradialis–to–radial wrist extensor transfer is done. As Moberg and others have suggested, the brachioradialis transfer will function better if it has an antagonist. Thus, a deltoid-to-triceps transfer should be done before the brachioradialis is transferred.[25]

The simple hand grip procedure was designed to produce a key grip of thumb–to–radial side of index finger. Moberg[31] believes that the key grip is more useful to the tetraplegic patient. His procedure does not interfere with the interlacing grip used by patients who have no finger motors. The interlacing grip is accomplished by passively weaving a utensil through the fingers. The simple hand grip does not produce a stiff hand, which Moberg believes is unacceptable to the tetraplegic patient because it makes contact with other people less pleasant.[6,32]

The alternative operation is the wrist-driven flexor hinge hand described by Nickel, Perry, and Garrett.[34] Their operation includes making a post of the thumb in an abducted position by arthrodesis of the interphalangeal and MP joints and by insertion of a bone block between the first and second metacarpals. In addition, the interphalangeal joints of the index and long fingers are fused. The profundus tendons of the index and long fingers are tenodesed to the distal radius so that, upon wrist dorsiflexion, the tips of those two fingers are brought into contact with the thumb in a three-point palmar pinch. Their operation has been further modified by Beasley.[1]

In my experience, patient acceptance and functional improvement have been better with a simple hand grip rather than the wrist-driven flexor hinge hand.

MOBERG'S SIMPLE HAND GRIP (KEY PINCH) PROCEDURE

Moberg described the simple hand grip reconstruction in six steps (Fig. 42-6).

1. Strong wrist dorsiflexion is a prerequisite, and brachioradialis transfer, if needed, can be done at the same operation. Gravity provides wrist palmar flexion.
2. The annular ligaments of the thumb are released to permit bowstringing of the flexor pollicis longus. This is done through an oblique incision over the flexor surface of the proximal phalanx. The digital nerves and arteries are carefully retracted and the annular ligaments divided. The results of this phase should be checked by lifting the flexor pollicis longus tendon out of the wound.
3. Release of the annular ligaments will improve the mechanical advantage of the flexor pollicis longus tenodesis to the volar surface of the distal radius. A curved 6- to 7-cm incision is made from the proximal wrist flexion crease along the radial volar side of the forearm. The palmar cutaneous branch of the median nerve should be preserved. The flexor tendons and the median nerve are retracted to expose the flexor pollicis longus tendon. The distal muscle fibers are removed from the tendon, and the tendon is divided 6 to 7 cm proximal to the wrist. An incision is made in the pronator quadratus along its radial border, and the muscle is elevated as a flap toward the ulna. Two holes are made into the metaphysis of the radius and connected, leaving a bridge of cortex between them. The distal stump of the flexor pollicis longus tendon is pulled into the bone through the ulnar hole and out through the radial hole with a wire loop.

This wound is then closed temporarily with a single stitch.

4. The surgeon then proceeds to the dorsal tenodesis of the extensor hood mechanism to the metacarpal of the thumb for prevention of hyperflexion of the MP joint. This part of the operation is strongly recommended. A dorsal midline incision is made, the extensor mechanism is displaced, about 3 cm of the periosteum on the dorsum of the metacarpal is scraped, and three or four pairs of holes are made in the cortex. Nonabsorbable sutures are used to compress the extensor mechanism against the scraped periosteum. An arthrodesis of this joint can be used to salvage a failed tenodesis.
5. The thumb interphalangeal joint is fixed with a large threaded K-wire at about 0 degrees. The wire should be buried beneath the cortex of the distal phalanx. This can be accomplished by measuring and cutting the pin preoperatively. A slot is made in the blunt end of the pin, which will receive a small screwdriver. At operation the short pin is inserted as far as possible with a drill and driven farther with a screwdriver.
6. Resection or division of the retinaculum over the extensor carpi radialis longus and brevis is done to allow bowstringing and thus improve the mechanical advantage. However, this procedure decreases the amplitude of wrist motion. In a patient with a supination deformity, the tendons may displace to the radial side of the wrist and act as wrist flexors. Finally, the surgeon returns to the forearm where the tenodesis of the flexor pollicis longus is completed. It is attached to itself with a few sutures to make a loop and to test the tension. The thumb should contact the radial side of the index finger with the wrist in neutral.

Since Moberg first reported his simple "key grip" procedure, considerable experience with it has accumulated. Hentz, Brown, and Keoshian reviewed their experience in 1983.[16] They agreed that key grip was an achievable functional goal that was well accepted by their patients, but they described a number of complications, which included stretching out of the flexor pollicis longus tenodesis, excessive flexion of the MP joint secondary to stretching of the extensor pollicis longus tenodesis,

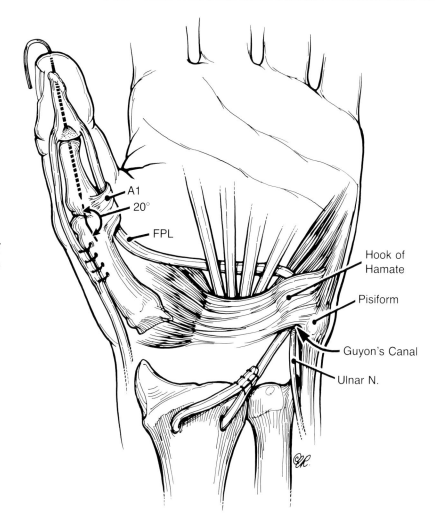

Fig. 42-6. A modification of Moberg's operation to create a "simple hand grip" (see text).

and frequent breakage of the pin used to fix the thumb interphalangeal joint. My own experience parallels that of Hentz, Brown, and Keoshian. I have accepted their suggestions for modifying the original description by increasing the immobilization time to 4 weeks to try to prevent flexor pollicis longus tenodesis stretching, making a slot in the shaft of the metacarpal for tenodesis of the extensor pollicis longus to try to prevent stretching of that tenodesis, and fusing the thumb interphalangeal joint to try to avoid complications with pin breakage.

In addition, a more significant modification of the tenodesis has been suggested by Brand,[2] who modified Moberg's flexor pollicis longus tenodesis by changing the course of the flexor pollicis longus.

After dividing the flexor pollicis longus near the musculotendinous junction and withdrawing it into the palm, he passes the tendon obliquely across the palm behind the flexor tendons and passes it through Guyon's canal back to the tenodesis site on the radius (Fig. 42-6). Further, he believes that releasing the pulleys of the flexor pollicis longus tendon sheath produces bowstringing and a tendency to hyperflexion of the thumb at the MP joint and does not increase the strength of pinch.

He has added a third interesting option that calls for tenodesis of the extensor pollicis longus to the radius radial to Lister's tubercle, which will make it function much like the abductor pollicis longus to open the thumb-index web space upon flexion of the wrist. He stresses the need for careful tension adjustment at surgery so that the tension on the extensor pollicis longus is not so great that it prevents the thumb from reaching the index finger upon wrist dorsiflexion. Brand also agrees that fusion of the thumb interphalangeal joint is a better choice than pin stabilization.

My experience with the modifications suggested by Hentz and his co-workers[16] and by Brand[2] has resulted in a better quality of result.

Postoperative Management. A thumb spica cast is applied with the wrist in slight dorsiflexion to reduce the tension on the brachioradialis transfer, and the thumb is adducted under the fingers to prevent tension at the tenodesis site. Casting is continued for 4 weeks before an active exercise program is started. The program of education in the use of the grip is graduated so that maximum stress on the hand is delayed until 2 months after surgery.

Group 2

This group has active wrist extension because the extensor carpi radialis longus is functioning at MRC Grade 4 or better. In this group the extensor carpi radialis brevis is not functioning or is too weak to change the patient's classification.

Patients in this group can operate a tenodesis splint and are candidates for the simple hand grip reconstruction or any of the other procedures that depend on active wrist extension for some form of automatic grip discussed in Group 1.

The brachioradialis is available for transfer and has been used in a variety of ways. Street and Stambaugh[42] recognized the value of side pinch or "key grip" in 1959 and, in an attempt to increase the strength of pinch, transferred the brachioradialis to the flexor pollicis longus. Moberg reported four patients with brachioradialis transfer to flexor pollicis longus, and, upon comparison he found the flexor pollicis longus tenodesis to be stronger than the transfer. Also, Moberg used the brachioradialis to open the thumb-index web space to improve the release phase of the grasp-release sequence. He tested the extensor pollicis longus, extensor pollicis brevis, and abductor pollicis longus at surgery to determine which gave the best abduction and then transferred the brachioradialis to that one. He

did this operation as a second-stage procedure, following construction of a simple hand grip. He reported that the additional abduction was not as useful to the patient as he had anticipated.[32]

I do not transfer the brachioradialis in Group 2 patients.

Group 3

As the level of spinal cord injury moves distally, the next muscle innervated is the extensor carpi radialis brevis. Proof of strength of both radial wrist extensors depends on testing by the method of Curtis[4] as described on page 1598. When both radial wrist extensors are stong, one is available for transfer. Most surgeons recommend leaving the extensor carpi radialis brevis in place because its insertion is more central and is a better wrist extensor.[17,22,44]

Patients in Group 3 have strong wrist dorsiflexion and might be content with a flexor hinge splint, but surgical reconstruction should be considered. The surgeon can keep reconstruction simple by performing a simple hand grip procedure or some other tenodesis operation. If a more complex method is selected, the brachioradialis and extensor carpi radialis longus are available for transfer. Zancolli prefers tendon transfers in this group. His procedure is divided into two stages because different positions of immobilization are required for proper healing after each stage.[44]

ZANCOLLI'S TWO-STAGE RECONSTRUCTION

Stage I

At the first stage, Zancolli's goals are to construct finger and thumb extension tenodeses, prevent or reduce claw deformity with intrinsic tenodeses and stabilize the thumb by interphalangeal joint fusion. (Capsulodesis of the MP joint is done at the second stage if the joint hyperextends too much for good contact.)

Zancolli makes an 8- to 10-cm longitudinal incision on the radial side of the forearm and exposes the dorsum of the radius proximal to the extensor retinaculum. A window, large enough to accept the distal stumps of the common extensor tendons (which have been divided just distal to the musculotendinous junction), is made on the dorsum of the radius. Tendon balance is preserved by suturing the distal stumps together. The ends of the sutures are brought through two drill holes made proximal to the window, drawing the tendon stumps snugly into the bone window. The sutures are tied to each other for fixation. Zancolli sets the tension so that the finger MP joints will be extended to 0 degrees with the wrist in slight palmar flexion. (In patients in Group 5 who have a functional flexor carpi radialis, he sets the tension in the MP joints with the wrist at 0 degrees.)

Zancolli's original description of the procedure utilized a modified Fowler-type intrinsic tenodesis, but he has subsequently described a simpler and more useful method of reducing claw deformity that is called the lasso operation (Fig. 42-7).[44] The operation uses the superficialis to flex the MP joints. In patients with no voluntary flexion of the superficialis, the muscle tone alone can assist. Chevron-shaped incisions are made across the MP joint flexion creases, and the A1 and A2 pulleys are exposed. An incision is made in the A2 pulley distal to the MP joint. The superficialis tendon is divided through the hole in the A2 pulley. The proximal

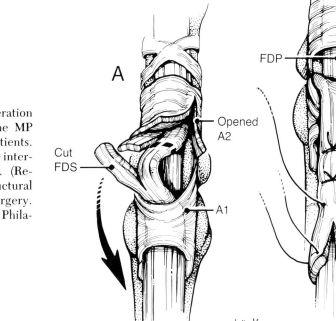

Fig. 42-7. Zancolli's lasso operation can be used to produce some MP joint flexion in Groups 3–9 patients. This facilitates extension of the interphalangeal joints (see text). (Redrawn from Zancolli EA: Structural and Dynamic Bases of Hand Surgery. 2nd Ed. p. 117. JB Lippincott, Philadelphia, 1979.)

stump is pulled through the incision in the A2 pulley and it is attached to itself in the form of a loop or "lasso" with side-to-side sutures. Enough tension is applied to produce mild MP joint flexion so that the interphalangeal joints can be extended by the extensor tenodesis when it is activated by wrist palmar flexion.

A strip of the abductor pollicis longus tendon is freed up through the original radial longitudinal incision and is kept small enough to pass it proximally through the tunnel of the extensor pollicis longus around Lister's tubercle and into the window on the dorsum of the radius, where it and the tendon of the extensor pollicis longus are sutured to the bone with wire, as described for the common extensor tendons. This tenodesis will produce thumb extension.

Arthrodesis of the thumb interphalangeal joint is done to prevent hyperflexion of the joint and to facilitate side pinch. I prefer Carroll's technique of small joint fusion (see Chapter 4).

Postoperative Management. Zancolli recommends immobilization for 5 weeks in a cast, with the wrist, thumb, and fingers in extension. He also suggests an additional week of immobilization when the patient has a strong flexor carpi radialis (Group 5). Active extension exercises are then begun; gentle passive exercises are necessary when there is no active flexor carpi radialis. Pins used for fixation of the thumb interphalangeal joint arthrodesis are left in until the fusion is solid at about 8 to 12 weeks.

Stage II

When scar resolution is complete and the preoperative range of motion is restored, the second-stage operation is done. The objective of this operation is to establish some digital flexion.

The same radial lateral incision used in Stage I is reopened to expose the extensor carpi radialis longus and the flexor digitorum profundus tendons. The extensor carpi radialis longus is detached at its insertion and transferred to the flexor digitorum profundus tendons with a side-to-side connection. Tension is set so that the fingers and thumb come together in a lateral pinch with the wrist in about 20 degrees dorsiflexion. The tension is set loosely enough to allow easy release of the fingers during wrist flexion.

The brachioradialis is detached from its insertion (leaving a short stump) and dissected well proximally so that maximum excursion can be obtained. The brachioradialis is sutured to the flexor pollicis longus, with tension set to achieve lateral pinch with the wrist in about 20 degrees dorsiflexion (the same as in the extensor carpi radialis longus transfer).

If the thumb MP joint is hyperextended, a capsulodesis should be done. The volar capsule should be fixed to bone. The flexor tendon sheath is exposed through a transverse incision just proximal to the thumb MP joint flexion crease. The sheath is opened and the flexor pollicis longus retracted away from the volar plate. Care should be taken to protect the digital nerves. A longitudinal incision is made in the volar plate to expose the neck of the metacarpal. Two holes are drilled in the bone to receive a nonabsorbable suture. The volar plate is pulled proximally and sutured against the bone. Tension is set with the MP joint in 10 degrees flexion.

Zancolli also constructs a volar tenodesis of the extensor pollicis brevis tendon if the thumb is in excessive extension and lateral pinch is impaired. Through the radial incision, the extensor pollicis brevis tendon is divided as far proximally as possible. The tendon is passed through the flexor carpi radialis tunnel and sutured into the short distal stump of the brachioradialis, which was left in place when it was divided for transfer previously. Tension is set to hold the thumb in complete abduction with the wrist in moderate flexion.

Postoperative Management. Immobilization in a cast for 5 weeks precedes gentle active range of motion exercises.

Group 4

In patients in Group 4 the pronator teres is intact and is available for transfer, but has been used only by Zancolli. The pronator teres is useful in its role as an antagonist to the biceps. By providing active pronation, it enhances the effect of gravity on the wrist-activated tenodeses. Zancolli has transferred the pronator teres to the flexor carpi radialis to strengthen wrist flexion and further enhance the usefulness of the wrist-activated tenodesis operations.

In patients in this group, I prefer not to transfer the pronator teres to reduce the complexity of the operation. Patients like their ability to control pronation and supination and I believe that preserving this function improves results after tenodesing operations.

In Groups 2, 3, and 4 where the patient has strong wrist extension, Moberg prefers the simpler key grip operation and I agree with his plan with the modifications described.

I reserve the more complex operations for patients in Group 5 and lower where there is also strong wrist flexion and the quality of sensibility is better.

Group 5

The flexor carpi radialis is intact in this group, and the patients have active control of wrist flexion as well as extension. The brachioradialis, extensor carpi radialis longus, and pronator teres muscles are available for transfer. In 1958 Lipscomb, Elkins, and Henderson[22] and in 1971 Lamb and Landry[21] reported transfer of the flexor carpi radialis in this group. The current approach favors leaving the flexor carpi radialis in place to preserve maximum wrist control.

The operative plan described by House, Gwathmey, and Lundsgaard[17] conforms to this proposition. These authors leave the extensor carpi radialis brevis and the flexor carpi radialis in place for wrist control and combine extensor tenodeses and tendon transfers to activate the digits in a two-stage operation. House and colleagues call the two stages the *extensor phase* (the wrist is palmar flexed and the digits extend) and the *flexor phase* (the wrist is dorsiflexed to supplement the action of the tendon transfer to the digital flexors). House has been comparing the results of two methods of reconstruction in group 5 patients. The first two-stage method was described in 1976[17] and the second in 1985.[18] His second method uses Zancolli's techniques for thumb stabilization and control of claw deformity of the fingers.[44,45] House concludes in his comparative study that both methods are satisfactory and have slightly different indications.

I prefer his second method because thumb positioning and stabilization is assured if the fusion is successful and there are less chances for error when balancing transfers to activate the thumb for key pinch. I favor Zancolli's lasso method (Fig. 42-7) of controlling clawing of the fingers because it leaves the hand in a more flexible condition. In addition, it does not prevent extension of the finger MP joints, allowing the patient to open his grasp wide enough to accept larger objects.

HOUSE'S TWO-STAGE RECONSTRUCTION

Extensor Phase

The extensor phase requires either a tenodesis of the common extensor and the extensor pollicis longus to the distal radius or a transfer of the brachioradialis to the common extensors and the extensor pollicis longus for digital extension. The thumb is stabilized by carpometacarpal joint arthrodesis (my preference) or tenodesis of the abductor pollicis longus.

To accomplish either tenodesis or tendon transfer, a gently curved dorsal incision is begun just proximal to Lister's tubercle and is extended in a line convex to the radial side of the forearm for approximately 6 to 8 cm. The branches of the radial nerve must be protected. The skin flap should be dissected far enough to the radial side to expose the insertion of the brachioradialis into the radius if one has chosen the tendon transfer. If the transfer is the method chosen, then the brachioradialis is detached from its insertion into the radius and carefully dissected proximally to detach it from the forearm fascia, which limits its excursion. The brachioradialis is then attached to the extensor pollicis longus and the common extensors to the fingers by passing the distal stump of the brachioradialis through each individual tendon. Tension should be set so that the thumb is in full extension and the MP joints of the fingers are at 0 degrees with the wrist in 35 to 40 degrees of flexion.

If the choice is to do a tenodesing operation, the extensor pollicis longus and the common extensors are set at the same tension as described for brachioradialis transfer but they are attached to a window made in the distal and dorsal portion of the radius (Fig. 42-8).

Carpometacarpal joint arthrodesis to stabilize the base of the thumb is performed through a transverse incision or an oblique incision at the base of

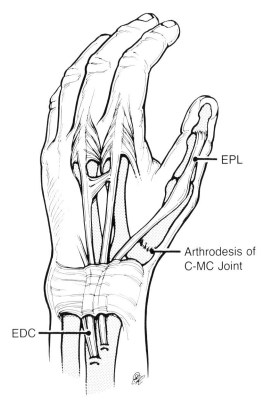

Fig. 42-8. Stage I (extensor phase) of House's two-stage reconstruction for patients in Group 5 (modified—see text). (Redrawn from House JH, Gwathmey FW, Lundsgaard DK: Restoration of strong grasp and lateral pinch in tetraplegia due to cervical spinal cord injury. J Hand Surg 1:152, 1976.)

the thumb metacarpal. Care must be taken to identify and protect the multiple branches of the superficial radial nerve and the radial artery as it passes dorsal to the capsule of the thumb carpometacarpal joint. The base of the thumb metacarpal and the distal articular surface of the trapezium are removed by osteotomy so that the metacarpal is placed in a position of approximately 40 to 45 degrees of palmar abduction, 20 to 25 degrees extension, and 10 to 15 degrees pronation. Either internal or percutaneous fixation is important to increase the chances for union. After carpometacarpal joint fusion some patients may develop a collapse deformity of the thumb, with MP joint hyperextension and IP joint hyperflexion. If that occurs, it can be corrected by arthrodesis of the IP joint or capsulodesis of the MP joint.[18]

Postoperative Management. Postoperative immobilization should hold the wrist in 40 to 45 degrees extension and the cast should include the thumb in the position described above. Immobilization is maintained with a cast or plaster splints for 4 weeks. At this stage, the cast is removed but the thumb carpometacarpal joint arthrodesis should be protected with an orthosis that will still allow wrist flexion and extension and finger flexion and extension for gentle active and passive mobilization. The arthrodesis site at the base of the thumb is to be protected until there is evidence of solid union.

When the patient has a solid union and passive range of motion is restored so that the tenodesis of the extensor pollicis longus and common extensors is functioning, the second phase can be performed.

Flexor Phase

In the flexor phase, (Fig. 42-9) the available extensor carpi radialis longus and pronator teres are employed for active digital flexion and pinch. All of the transfers are done during one operation. A gently curved incision is made on the flexor surface of the forearm. It should begin distally at the proximal wrist flexion crease and extend proximally about 8 to 10 cm, with the skin flap being convex to the ulnar side. Through this incision, the flexor digitorum profundus and flexor pollicis longus tendons are exposed at and distal to their musculotendinous junctions. Next, the extensor carpi radialis longus is exposed through a small incision over its insertion into the base of the second metacarpal, where it is divided. A portion of the proximal end of the previous (extensor phase) dorsal incision can be used to expose the extensor carpi radialis longus proximal to the bellies of the extensor pollicis brevis and abductor pollicis longus. The tendon is withdrawn into this incision, and the belly is dissected away from its investing fascia to improve its excursion and to create a straight line to its new insertion. It is passed from the proximal dorsal wound through a subcutaneous tunnel around the radial side of the forearm into the volar wound.

The pronator teres is then detached from the radius. A strip of periosteum should be raised distal to its insertion to make the tendon long enough for strong connection to the flexor pollicis longus. A weaving type of juncture is created between the

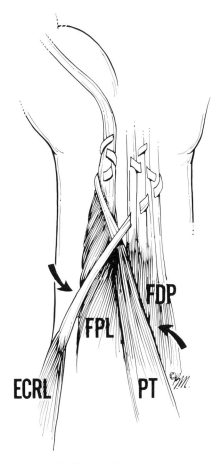

Fig. 42-9. Stage II (flexor phase) of House's two-stage reconstruction for patients in Group 5 (modified — see text). (Redrawn from House JH, Gwathmey FW, Lundsgaard DK: Restoration of strong grasp and lateral pinch in tetraplegia due to cervical spinal cord injury. J Hand Surg 1:152, 1976.)

pronator teres and the flexor pollicis longus and between the extensor carpi radialis longus and the profundus tendons to the index, long, ring, and little fingers. Tension is adjusted so that with the wrist in about 30 degrees of extension the thumb will touch the radial side of the index finger. To be certain that the tension is not too tight, the wrist should be flexed to check for adequate passive thumb and finger extension by the tenodesis or brachioradialis transfer. In setting the tension at the junction between the extensor carpi radialis longus and the flexor digitorum profundus, one should err on the side of looseness, as it is better too

loose than too tight, since when it is too tight, the patient cannot get enough extension to grasp larger objects.

The final step in the flexor phase is to perform the "lasso" intrinsic transfer (see Fig. 42-7). This part of the procedure can be performed through a single transverse incision across the palm just proximal to the MP joint flexion creases of the fingers. Through this incision, the flexor tendons proximal to the A1 pulley, the A1 pulley, and the proximal portion of the A2 pulley are exposed. The distal portion of the A1 pulley or the proximal portion of the A2 pulley is grasped with a skin hook or other instrument and pulled upon to be certain that it causes flexion of the MP joint. At this site, an L-shaped incision is made in the pulley as depicted in the illustration. Then the superficialis tendon is pulled as far proximal as possible with the PIP joint in flexion, and both tails of the tendon are divided. The two tails are then withdrawn through the L-shaped incision, folded over the intact A1 pulley and sutured to the superficialis proximal to the A1 pulley, thus creating a loop of superficialis tendon around the A1 pulley. Tension is set against the viscoelastic force of the superficialis, as it is paralyzed and will not function actively. Enough tension is applied so that the MP joints extend to 0 degrees when the wrist is flexed to 35 to 40 degrees. If more extension is allowed at the MP joint with the wrist in flexion, the claw deformity will not be ameliorated.

Postoperative Management. The hand is immobilized using plaster splints with the wrist dorsiflexed about 25 degrees and the fingers flexed at the MP joints and gently extended at the interphalangeal joints for about 3 weeks. This should be followed by 4 weeks of graduated active and passive range of motion exercises and muscle re-education. The patient should not be allowed to push a wheelchair, transfer, or engage in any other activity that causes full wrist dorsiflexion for at least 10 weeks.

Group 6

At this level, the finger extensors are strong but extensor pollicis longus function is either absent or too weak to extend the thumb adequately. For patients in this group the extensor phase of reconstruction as described for Group 5 is modified. Tenodesis of the common extensors to the radius is not required. The extensor pollicis longus can be sutured to the common extensors so that active extension of the fingers will produce extension of the thumb.

A gently curved incision is made over the distal forearm, beginning proximal to the dorsal retinaculum. The common extensor tendons and the extensor pollicis longus tendon are identified. Peritenon is scraped away from the extensor pollicis longus tendon and the common extensor tendon to the index finger on the adjacent surfaces for about 2 to 3 cm. They are firmly sutured together with 3 or 4 horizontal mattress sutures of a nonabsorbable material. If the common extensor tendon to the index finger is small, additional common extensor tendons can be included to produce a strong union. Tension is set with all extensors in the relaxed posture.

Postoperative Management. A short arm cast is applied at operation with the thumb, fingers, and wrist in slight dorsiflexion. The cast is removed in 4 weeks, and the patient begins gentle active extension exercises. Resistance exercises for the thumb and fingers are not allowed until 6 weeks after the operation.

After rehabilitation from this phase is completed, the flexor phase operation is performed as described for Group 5.

Group 7

Patients in this group have a strong extensor pollicis longus, so extensor phase reconstruction is not required. Results following surgery in patients in Groups 6 and 7 are much better than in higher groups because normal extensor function gives the patient more precise control.

Group 8

This group includes all patients who have weak activity of the long flexors. Usually, the long flexors to the ulnar digits (ring and small fingers) are strong and those to the thumb, index, and long fingers are weak.

Flexion of the index and long fingers can be improved or strengthened by connecting all four profundus tendons together. An active motor should be transferred to give independent function of the flexor pollicis longus. Finally, an intrinsic replacement using the "lasso" procedure will ameliorate the tendency toward clawing of the fingers. The thumb can be positioned either by carpometacarpal joint arthrodesis as described with Group 5 or an opponens transfer. I prefer the two-staged reconstruction as described by Zancolli.[45]

Stage I

At the first stage, the profundus tendons are united and a transfer of the brachioradialis to the flexor pollicis longus is done. Both procedures can be done through a gently curved volar incision that should begin near the palmaris longus at the distal wrist flexion crease, making the curve convex to the radial side, and extending to the proximal one-third of the forearm. The palmar cutaneous branch of the median nerve should be protected. The skin should be undermined on the radial side of the forearm sufficiently to expose the brachioradialis for detachment from its insertion and adequate proximal dissection. The median and radial nerves must be protected. The four profundus tendons are exposed by opening the forearm fascia and retracting ulnarward the median nerve with its palmar cutaneous branch and the four superficial tendons. A site in the distal forearm is selected for side-to-side suture of the four profundus tendons. The peritenon is scraped away from the tendons for a distance of 3 cm, and the tendons are sutured together with horizontal mattress sutures using nonabsorbable material. The fingers should be evenly balanced during the connection. Next, the brachioradialis is transferred directly to the flexor pollicis longus and connected by braiding the tendon of the brachioradialis into the tendon of the flexor pollicis longus with the wrist in neutral and the thumb just touching the side of the index finger, with mild tension on the brachioradialis.

Postoperative Management. A thumb spica cast is applied to the fingertips for 4 weeks, with each joint held in about 20 to 30 degrees flexion, the thumb straight at the MP and interphalangeal joints, and the wrist at 30 degrees flexion. Gentle active and passive range of motion and muscle re-education can begin immediately and should be carried on until a full range of motion is restored.

Stage II

At the second stage, an opponens transfer is used to abduct the thumb, and Zancolli's "lasso" procedure is used to control claw deformity of the fingers. Zancolli recommends transfer of the extensor carpi radialis longus to the flexor digitorum superficialis tendons, to produce active control of the "lasso" intrinsic replacement. The opponens transfer can be motored by the flexor carpi ulnaris, and the palmaris longus can be used as a free tendon graft (if it is not present, a toe extensor or the plantaris tendon may be used) to extend the tendon of the flexor carpi ulnaris to its insertion into the ulnar side of the base of the proximal phalanx of the thumb. The flexor carpi ulnaris is exposed through an L-shaped incision over its insertion, which is split in half for a distance of 3 to 4 cm proximal to its insertion. One-half of the tendon is left attached to the pisiform, and this segment is divided 3 to 4 cm proximal to the insertion. The proximal end of this segment is sutured to the insertion to create a loop. The other half is detached from the pisiform and attached to the proximal end of the free tendon graft using a braiding technique. A subcutaneous tunnel is created from the loop to the MP joint of the thumb. The tendon graft is passed around the loop at the pisiform and through the subcutaneous tunnel to be attached to the tendon of the abductor pollicis brevis at the base of the proximal phalanx. Tension is adjusted so that with the wrist at neutral the thumb pulp will just touch the radial side of the index finger.

The intrinsic replacement procedure is modified as described by Zancolli by transferring the extensor carpi radialis longus tendon to the superficialis tendons in the forearm. Tension on the transfer is set only after the distal portion of the lasso procedure is done at the base of the fingers (see page 1609). Once that portion of the procedure is completed, the union is completed in the forearm. Tension is set so that with the wrist at neutral the MP joints of the fingers are at 0 degrees.

Postoperative Management. A thumb spica cast is applied, extending across the MP joints of the fingers so the wrist is fixed at about 30 degrees flexion, the MP joints of the fingers in about 30 degrees flexion, and the thumb in wide abduction and opposition. The cast is removed after 4 weeks, and gentle active motion and muscle re-education are started. Progression to full active and passive motion should be started 6 weeks after surgery.

This group also includes patients who have Grade 4 MRC strength in all the profundus tendons and the flexor pollicis longus. Because they lack superficialis and intrinsic muscle function only, the reconstruction can be accomplished in a one-stage procedure. That includes an opponens transfer and the lasso operation with an active motor to improve thumb control and reduce the claw deformity.

Group 9

Patients in Group 9 have functioning superficialis muscles as well as all the other extrinsic flexors and extensors, but do not have intrinsic muscle innervation. In this situation, an opponens transfer is performed as in the second stage for Group 8. The lasso operation can be further modified by doing the loop around the A1 pulley as described earlier, and expecting the superficialis muscles, which are under voluntary control, to ameliorate the claw deformity. The postoperative management is the same as that described for Group 8.

Group X

This group was created so that those few patients who cannot be classified with the above scheme can still be included. A careful description of the motor and sensory function should be made and reconstructive procedures will have to be tailored even more carefully for these patients.

REFERENCES

1. Beasly RW: Surgical treatment of hands for C5-C6 tetraplegia. Orthop Clin North Am 14:893–904, 1983

2. Brand PW: Clinical Mechanics of the Hand. CV Mosby, St Louis, 1985

3. Bryan RS: The Moberg deltoid-triceps replacement and key-pinch operations in quadriplegia: Preliminary experiences. Hand 9:207–214, 1977

4. Curtis RM: Tendon transfers in the patient with spinal cord injury. Orthop Clin North Am 5:415–423, April 1974

5. DeBenedetti M: Restoration of elbow extension power in the tetraplegic patient using the Moberg technique. J Hand Surg 4:86–89, 1979

6. Dolphin JA: Surgery to the quadriplegic hand: A new operative approach to achieve thumb-finger pinch. In Proceedings of the American Society for Surgery of the Hand. J Bone Joint Surg 52A:1060, 1970

7. Flatt AE: An indication for shortening of the thumb. J Bone Joint Surg 46A:1534–1539, 1964

8. Freehafer AA: Flexion and supination deformities of the elbow in tetraplegics. Paraplegia 15:221–225, 1977

9. Freehafer AA, Kelly CM, Peckham HP: Tendon transfer for the restoration of upper limb function after a cervical spinal cord injury. J Hand Surg 9A:887–893, 1984

10. Freehafer AA, Mast WA: Transfer of brachioradialis to improve wrist extension in high spinal-cord injury. J Bone Joint Surg 49A:648–652, 1967

11. Freehafer AA, Vonhaam E, Allen V: Tendon transfer to improve grasp after injuries of the cervical spinal cord. J Bone Joint Surg 56A:951–959, 1974

12. Friedenberg ZB: Transposition of the biceps brachii for triceps weakness. J Bone Joint Surg 36A:656–658, 1954

13. Grigg P, Finerman GA, Riley LH: Joint-position sense after total hip replacement. J Bone Joint Surg 55a:1016–1025, 1973

14. Hanson RW, Franklin MR: Sexual loss in relation to other functional losses for spinal cord injured males. Arch Phys Med Rehabil 57:291–293, 1976

15. Henderson ED, Lipscomb PR, Elkins EC, Auerback AM, Magness JL: Review of the results of surgical treatment of patients with tetraplegia. J Bone Joint Surg 52A:1059, 1970

16. Hentz VR, Brown M, Keoshian LA: Upper limb reconstruction in quadriplegia: Functional assessment and proposed treatment modifications. J Hand Surg 8:119–131, 1983

17. House JH, Gwathmey FW, Lundsgaard DK: Restoration of strong grasp and lateral pinch in tetraplegia due to cervical spinal cord injury. J Hand Surg 1:152–159, 1976

18. House JH: Reconstruction of the thumb in tetraplegia following spinal cord injury. Clin Orthop 195:117–128, 1985

19. Kiwerski J: Recovery of simple hand function in tetraplegia patients following transfer of the musculocutaneous nerve into the median nerve. Paraplegia 20:242–247, 1982

20. Lamb DW, Chan KM: Surgical reconstruction of the upper limb in traumatic tetraplegia: A review of 41 patients. JBJS 65B:291–298, 1983

21. Lamb DW, Landry R: The hand in quadriplegia. Hand 3:31–37, 1971

22. Lipscomb PR, Elkins EC, Henderson ED: Tendon transfers to restore function of hands in tetraplegia, especially after fracture-dislocation of the sixth cervical vertebra on the seventh. J Bone Joint Surg 40A:1071–1080, 1958

23. Maury M, Guillaumat M, Francois N: Our experience of upper-limb transfers in cases of tetraplegia. Paraplegia 11:245–251, 1973

24. McDowell CL: Tendon transfer to augment wrist extension in the tetraplegic patient. Proc Eighteenth Veterans Administration Spinal Cord Injury Conf. 18:78, 1971

25. McDowell CL, Moberg EA, Graham-Smith A: International conference on surgical rehabilitation of the upper limb in tetraplegia. J Hand Surg 4:387–390, 1979

26. McDowell CL, Moberg EA, House JH: The Second International Conference on Surgical Rehabilitation of the Upper Limb in Tetraplegia (Quadriplegia). J Hand Surg 11A:604–608, 1986

27. Medical Research Council: Aids to the investigation of peripheral nerve injuries. War Memorandum No. 7, 2nd Ed. (revised) PL London, His Majesty's Stationary Office, 1943

28. Moberg E: Criticism and study of methods for examining sensibility in the hand. Neurology 12:8–19, 1962

29. Moberg E: Fingers were made before forks. Hand 4:201–206, 1972

30. Moberg E: Surgical treatment for absent single-hand grip and elbow extension in quadriplegia. J Bone Joint Surg 57A:196–206, 1975

31. Moberg E: Reconstruction hand surgery in tetraplegia, stroke and cerebral palsy: Some basic concepts in physiology and neurology. J Hand Surg 1:29–34, 1976

32. Moberg E: The Upper Limb in Tetraplegia. George Thieme, Stuttgart, 1978

33. Newman JH: The use of the key grip procedure for improving hand function in quadriplegia. Hand 9:215–220, 1977

34. Nickel VL, Perry J, Garrett AL: Development of

useful function in the severely paralyzed hand. J Bone Joint Surg 45A:933–952, 1963

35. Norris-Baker C, Stephens M, Rintala D, Willems E: Patient behavior as a predictor of outcomes in spinal cord injury. Arch Phys Med Rehabil 62:602–608, 1981

36. Ober FR, Barr JS: Brachioradialis muscle transposition for triceps weakness. Surg Gynecol Obstet 67:105–107, 1938

37. Omer GE Jr: Evaluation and reconstruction of the forearm and hand after acute traumatic peripheral nerve injuries. J Bone Joint Surg 50A:1454–1478, 1968

38. Peckham PH, Marsolais EB, Mortimer JT: Restoration of key grip and release in the C6 tetraplegic patient through functional electrical stimulation. J Hand Surg 5:462–469, 1980

39. Racxzka R, Braun R, Waters RL: Posterior deltoid-to-triceps transfer in quadriplegia. Clin Orthop 187:163–167, 1984

40. Riordan DC: Surgery of the paralytic hand. pp. 79–90. AAOS Instructional Course Lectures. Vol. 16. CV Mosby, St Louis, 1959

41. Smith, AG: Early complications of key grip hand surgery for tetraplegia. Paraplegia. 19:123–126, 1981

42. Street DM, Stambaugh HD: Finger flexor tenodesis. Clin Orthop 13:155–163, 1959

43. Wilson JN: Providing automatic grasp by flexor tenodesis. J Bone Joint Surg 38A:1019–1024, 1956

44. Zancolli EA: Structural and Dynamic Bases of Hand Surgery. 2nd Ed. pp. 229–262. JB Lippincott, Philadelphia, 1979

45. Zancolli E: Surgery for the quadriplegic hand with active strong wrist extension preserved. A study of 97 cases. Clin Orthop 112:101–113, 1975

Open Injuries of the Hand 43

Paul W. Brown

PRINCIPLES AND PRIORITIES

The Patient

Most severe injuries of the hand are open injuries and how intriguing they are! The surgeon is fascinated by the appearance of a laid-open distorted hand and feels challenged to restore it, or at least, to improve it. So he should be—but he should proceed cautiously lest the fascination lead to surgical myopia with such concentration on the surgical problem that the patient is neglected, leaving him under the care of a surgical technician and badly in want of a physician. A broader view must be taken from the beginning. The patient with an open wound of the hand presents a triple challenge: the overall welfare of the patient, the general nature of the wound, and the specific structures injured in the hand.

The first priority is the the patient, both as an injured person and as an injured body. When associated injuries threaten life itself, their immediate management, of course, assumes precedence, but when resuscitation is successful and the patient's strength returns, the surgeon must remember this dual consideration of mind and body.

With regard to the person, suffice it to say that the wounded hand belongs to a human being who has many fears and questions, and for whom this injury has posed many problems. The hand surgeon is as responsible for assuaging the patient's fears as he is for easing his pain. The surgeon must give as much attention to his patient's reaction to injury as he does to the specific tissues that are injured. Comunication is at least as valuable as penicillin, and technical proficiency, though indispensable, is no substitute for compassion.[16,26,29,30,50,61,83,84,107,110,123,150]

Multiple Injury

The problem of multiple injury is always complex. Bodily injury requires a triage, a sorting out and assessment of priorities, followed by a plan of treatment. The patient requires a physician—one doctor, not a committee of specialists—and this physician must assume primary responsiblity for orchestrating treatment. Such direction is generally best given by the general surgeon, although any surgical specialist may take command if his particular specialty requires priority. In cases of multiple injury, this is seldom the hand surgeon. When vital organ systems are in jeopardy, the injured hand may be given a low priority for treatment,

1619

which may lead to problems of proper surgical timing for the hand, and later, to problems of rehabilitation. This should not be seen as a fight for turf, but as an attempt to understand the patient's needs. Thus, it is essential that open communication among the patient's attending physicians is established.

When other injuries or medical conditions preempt the hand surgeon's priorities, he must be flexible enough to buy time for the injured hand. He must be able to surrender the ideal treatment and find alternative methods that will minimally compromise the end result. If, for instance, skin coverage cannot be done at the best time (i.e., best, only for the hand itself), a way must be found to keep the hand supple and well maintained until the next best time is available. Thoracic, abdominal, or cranial problems may interfere with or prevent proper timing for debridement or staged surgery of the hand. This, in turn, may lead to other problems and complications. Adaptability to the less than ideal situation is essential, and unfortunately, there will be occasions when unavoidable compromise in the treatment of the hand will result in a hand less good than it might have been were it the only injury.[55]

Assessment of Injury

HISTORY

The essentials of the history of injury are "when," "where," and "how." The amount of time elapsed may be the determinate of how the wound is to be managed. The longer contaminants are present, the more entrenched they become. After 6 hours, closure becomes progressively more dangerous.[24]

The "where" of an injury, that is the environment in which the injury occurred, may tell something about the type of contamination. Wounds occuring in a relatively clean area, such as in the kitchen, may require less attention to debridement and may be closed more safely than those occurring on the battlefield. This parameter of "where" is only one of many and not a very important one, as even a "clean" area may be laden with all sorts of potential pathogens, such as clostridial spores.

Nevertheless, the relative import of "where" must be weighed in assessing any wound.

How an injury was incurred will reveal something about the forces expended within the hand and may be a measure of the degree of tissue damage, such as in the distinction between a high and low-velocity missile. It is particularly important to know if there have been crushing forces or if materials have been injected under high pressure. Such information may dictate more meticulous exploration and debridement and decompression of spaces. It is useful to know what objects caused puncture wounds. Pieces of glass are often hard to find and may not be shown on radiographs, whereas metallic and organic foreign bodies are usually more apparent.

The significance of the injury may also dictate the type of treatment. An on-the-job injury for which all medical expenses will be paid by a third party may allow the patient to opt for more involved salvage procedures than one incurred at home or one incurred by a self-employed individual. The circumstances of the injury may affect the patient's reaction to injury and may determine how well he will cooperate with the surgeon and participate in treatment and rehabilitation. Personality, age, dependency and vocation must also be considered. Attempts to salvage a severed flexor tendon may not be practical for a clerk, but might be mandatory for a musician. A mangled digit with only a 10 percent chance for survival might be better amputated in a self-employed farmer, whereas a young woman might wish every effect made to save the finger regardless of cost and time.

PHYSICAL EXAMINATION

Examination of the hand should be done when the patient is conscious, before any anesthesia is given and without tourniquet. If done in an orderly fashion, with the patient supine and with good lighting, an accurate appraisal of the extent of injury can be obtained in a few minutes. First in importance is circulation. A white hand or digit implies arterial impairment. In dark-skinned patients, the color of the palm and nail beds must be closely observed. A blue, purplish, or dusky color suggests mounting edema and lack of venous drainage. Skin edges and flaps must be scrutinized carefully to

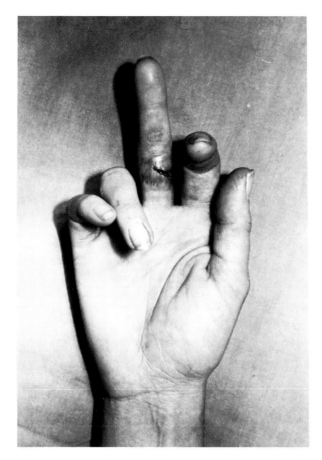

Severed extensor tendons should be suspected with dorsal wounds even if finger extension is possible. Flexor tendon damage is usually apparent when the patient attempts to actively flex his fingers. If he cannot or will not flex a finger, the resting position of the digits may suggest the damage. The position of "hang-out" is especially valuable in demonstrating flexor tendon damage in children, or in unconscious patients (Figs. 43-1 and 43-2).[24,91]

Nerve injury is frequently missed in emergency room examinations, but always becomes apparent later on, when the best opportunity for repair has

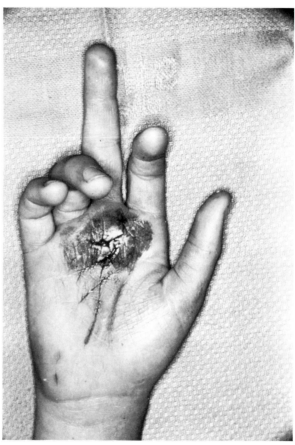

Fig. 43-1. Laceration with a kitchen knife. Flexor digitorum profundus, both slips of flexor digitorum superficialis, and the radial digital nerve were transected 1 hour ago. The position of the middle finger indicates that both tendons are severed. The patient denied sensory loss until his visual field was blocked and sensory examination was repeated.

assess vascularity. Grease and dirt may be ground into the skin, making the condition appear worse than it is: aesthetics should not be confused with blood supply.

Bone and joint damage may or may not be apparent on visual and manual examination and radiographs should be obtained if in doubt. In cases of crush injury, or where great forces have been expended within the hand, radiographic examination should always be done. In carpal injures, particularly in children, comparative views of the opposite hand are helpful.

Fig. 43-2. Window pane laceration. Both flexor tendons of the middle finger were severed, as well as the common digital nerve to the third cleft. (Brown PW: Lacerations of the flexor tendons of the hand. Surg Clin North Am 49:1259, 1969. Reprinted with permission of WB Saunders, Philadelphia.)

been lost. Testing for sensibility must be done before any anesthetic is given. The simplest method is to have the patient discriminate between sharp and dull sensation using alternately the head and the point of a pin. This test should be done with the patient's visual view of the hand blocked: if the patient sees the examination he may report feeling where there is none. Injured patients are frightened, feel vulnerable, and often wish to please the examiner; or they may simply confuse visual with sensory input. If in doubt, a more accurate assessment can be done by using the two ends of a paper clip fashioned to form a horseshoe to test two-point discrimination. Holding the two points approximately 1 cm apart and touching the tactile pads at random with one or two points is a more objective and accurate test of sensibility. Motor nerves are tested by asking the patient to abduct the thumb, small, and index fingers or simply by palpating the thenar eminence and first dorsal interosseous muscle while the patient pinces thumb and index finger together forcibly.[92,113]

Part of the examination is consideration of the patient's complaints of pain. Pain is subjective and dependent on many factors. Seldom can it be accurately evaluated during the initial examination, but extremes, either very severe pain, or the complete lack of it, are significant. Lack of pain may signify nerve damage or psychic problems, whereas agonizing pain, particularly if progressive, may indicate a pressure phenomenon, such as a compartment syndrome.[81]

BLOOD FLOW

Tissue will die without sufficient blood supply; contamination will become infection and infection will proceed unchecked. The fate of the hand and the outcome of all surgery depend on vascularity. Blood supply has the highest priority (the patient excepted) in the treatment plan, for without it, all else fails.[68,115,129,130]

Inadequate blood flow may be primary, that is, impaired ingress due to severed or occluded arteries, or secondary, due to restricted egress resulting from occluded veins, which then results in compartment pressures and edema, which in turn restrict arterial inflow. Severed arteries must be repaired quickly, since ischemic meat starts to spoil

after 4 hours. Venous repair is seldom required, but decompression of tight spaces—fingers, carpal tunnel, and anterior forearm compartment may be necessary. Compartment syndromes and progressive edema must be looked for attentively, lest all other problems of the hand become academic.[149,152]

THE WOUND ITSELF

With the patient out of danger and adequate blood flow present, the wound itself must be considered, not simply the specific tissues and structures that have been damaged, but the overall concept of the wound. The term *open wound* is significant in that the mucocutaneous barrier has been violated: not only is the skin and its contents damaged, but bacterial contaminants have been introduced. "Open" implies the threat of infection and the interruption of the healing process. It should also imply that certain urgencies and disciplines are now required that might not be necessary were the skin intact.[26,62,63,101,102,132–134]

Contaminants, as long as they remain simply that, are not harmful. When they begin to proliferate, they then assume ascendancy over the body's defenses, and when this happens the harmless condition of contamination phases over to infection— a pathologic condition. Either the quality or quantity of bacteria, or a reciprocal combination of the two, may contribute to this. Some bacteria are more virulent than others, but any, in sufficient quantity, may interfere with healing. If bacteria exist in quantities of 100,000 or more per gram of tissue, the tissue is infected and will show some or all of the classic signs of infection (i.e., heat, erythema, induration, pain, and usually purulence).[12,36,65,69,74,89,100,117,118,126,128,137,138,142,147]

To prevent contamination from becoming infection, the surgeon must launch a three-pronged attack: he must remove as many bacteria as possible; he must prepare the tissue of the wound to resist the multiplication of bacteria; and he must attempt to poison the bacteria without damaging the host —in essence, debridement for the first two and antibiotics for the last. It is impossible to sterilize a wound, but cleaning a wound properly will decrease the quantity of contaminating bacteria to below the level of 100,000/gram, after which the natural defense mechanisms of the body will take care of the rest, provided the next step is properly performed.[20]

This next, important step is to prepare the contaminated tissues so that they may effectively mobilize the body's defenses. This requires enhancing good blood supply by removing all tissue without supportive blood supply and then stimulating blood flow by allowing free drainage, proper dressings, splinting, active motion, and all of the other proper means of supporting an injured hand in the early postinjury stages. The condition of the contaminated tissue — the environment of the contaminating bacteria — is as influential on subsequent events as the bacteria themselves. Healthy tissue with a good blood supply will actively resist the development of infection.[3,39,100,121]

Debridement

Debridement is the first and most important overt surgical act in treating the open wound. Its purpose is to decrease contamination and to prepare the damaged tissues for healing. If debridement is not done well, infection may develop, tissues will not heal, and all else done surgically will fail.[26,73,76,114,167,171]

Debridement is performed in two ways: by cleansing and by excision. Cleansing is best done with sterile saline, which is delivered to the wound in a jet stream that flushes out contaminants, tissue debris, and foreign material. A simple, but effective arrangement is to use a medicine dropper tip attached by tubing to an overhead reservoir. The gravity feed of the saline through the nozzle gives a gentle fluid jet that can be used to explore the entire wound. The pressure head can be varied by lowering or elevating the reservoir. Working the jet through all nooks and crannies will open up closed planes and spaces and float out debris and a significant number of bacteria. For large, mangling wounds of the hand, 2 or more liters of fluid should be used. There is no sufficiently convincing evidence that the addition of antibiotics to the lavage solution significantly decreases the chance of infection. Until this point is better proven, their topical use is not warranted.[123]

Intermittent or pulsating jet lavage from a me-chanical pump increases the efficiency of cleansing even further. The force of the jet should be kept low; if too strong it may distend spaces with fluid and force debris and bacteria into uncontaminated tissue.[19,24,67,142]

Debridement lavage is seldom popular among emergency and operating room personnel as it is messy, time-consuming, and boring. Support personnel must understand that it is the best available deterrent to the development of infection.

Surgical debridement, defined by some as wound excision, is as much an art as it is a science. The objective is to remove everything detrimental to wound healing and, at the same time, preserve all possible that is useful to hand function or necessary to future reconstruction. There is little that is expendable in the hand: aside from some fat and muscle, everything is necessary to normal function. Conversely, any contaminated or devascularized tissue that is left in the hand may increase the chance of wound breakdown and thereby jeopardize all tissue. A compromise must sometimes be made, and later replacement of the structure may be preferable to its retention. Accurate assessment of vascularity is the key to thorough debridement, and seldom will a tourniquet be necessary or useful.[20]

It has been traditional to excise skin edges of the wound but this is not necessary unless they are crushed or of questionable viability. It is often impossible to be certain of their condition, as in the tangential distally based flap. It may be preferable to retain the questionable tissue and be prepared to remove it later in redebridement if one has guessed wrong. Bone fragments completely free of soft tissue attachment are better removed and replaced later by bone graft if necessary. Meanwhile, the skeletal framework and the normal length of fingers can be maintained by K-wires. The initial appearance of battered tendons and nerves can be quite deceptive; they may look damaged beyond repair, but if there is some semblance of continuity their true state of vascularity may not be apparent for several days and often they can be preserved if carefully cleansed and properly dressed.

Extensive hand injuries, particularly the crushed hand, may develop extreme edema, which, in turn, may cause increasing pressure and ischemia within restrained spaces. During debridement, poten-

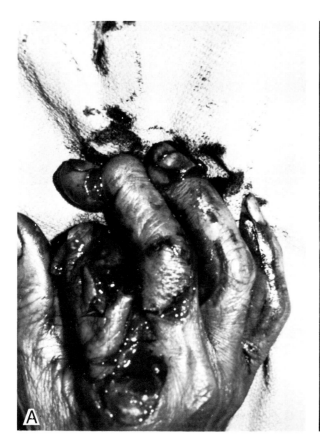

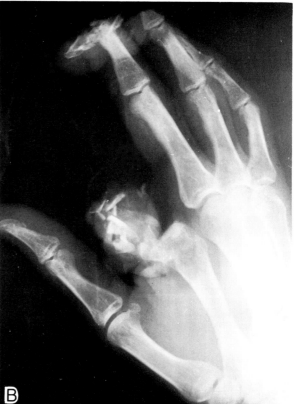

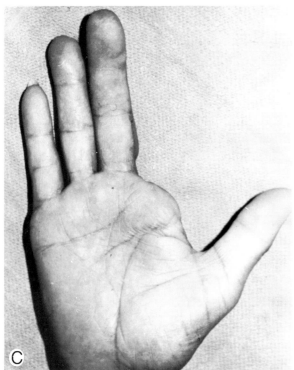

Fig. 43-3. (A,B) A manual laborer's hand mangled by a snow blower. Multiple fractures of the index finger phalanges, and multiple injuries of the extensor and flexor tendons and digital nerves and arteries are noted. The index finger is clearly unsalvageable. There is partial amputation of the tips of the middle and ring fingers. (C) MP disarticulation allowed prompt healing and early rehabilitation.

tially tight compartments such as the carpal tunnel should be opened and left open. The surgeon may be reluctant to open spaces not yet contaminated, but decompression is better when done early and can be safely done if lavage is thorough.

The Second Look Concept

A second look and redebridement 3 or 4 days later gives the surgeon the opportunity to remove those pieces of tissue that were questionable earlier but now clearly show their nonsalvageable state. At this time delayed primary repair of tendons and nerves and further skeletal realignment and fixation may be accomplished. On occasion, a third or fourth look may be required. Open wounds require a wide spectrum of surgical timing, ranging from those that can be safely closed immediately to those that should never be closed. Most severe wounds lie somewhere between these two extremes. The doctrines of "delayed emergency" of Iselin[80] and "staged wound reconstruction" of Burkhalter and colleagues[32] conceive of time as an ally of the surgeon, allowing him to choose the safest and most appropriate time to repair tissue in contrast to the compulsion to close or cover, wherein time is viewed as an opponent. Properly used, time ensures that the disasters of wound breakdowns due to premature closure will be avoided.[17,26,80,16]

Indications for Amputation

The severely mangled hand, or parts of it, may clearly be beyond repair (Fig. 43-3). One must be prepared to amputate those parts that would endanger other parts if they were retained. A hand or digit that will have no useful function or that will be grotesque or painful may not serve the patient as well as an amputation would. It is often impossible to predict the outcome, but as long as there is any reasonable hope for useful salvage, the part should be preserved. There are no easy answers for mangled hands in which survival seems marginal; the surgeon must temper realism with optimism. When in doubt, the part should be retained, since it can be removed later if the need becomes obvious, and at that time the patient may accept the loss with better grace than if it were done primarily.

Skeletal Stability

There are many paradoxes in body kinetics, and none are more dramatic than in the hand where a happy marriage of reciprocal opposites — motion versus stability — results in the essentials of useful function. While truly sophisticated function requires the addition of sensibility to this duo, these two basic elements of movement and stability are fundamental to usefulness. They, in turn, dependent as they are on girders, cross members, levers, fulcrums, moments of force, pivots, and motors, must have a sound architectural framework. When trauma has distorted or disrupted this framework, it must be realigned before the parts can function again.

With the patient stable and tissues perfused and cleansed, a golden opportunity awaits the surgeon. In the first few days — or even better, within the first few hours, at the time of debridement — reduction of fractures and correction of distortion are relatively easy (Fig. 43-4). With each passing day, bony displacement becomes progressively more difficult to correct as edema phases over to fibrosis and contracture. Poor reduction, or poor retention of reduction, rapidly becomes malunion, and unreduced joints ankylose as ligaments and capsules congeal and shorten.

Even the most disrupted and mangled hand will usually have bits and pieces of bony scaffolding that can be reassembled. Although gaps and defects may be present here and there, the basic framework must be reassembled if the hand is to function again. Reconstruction is not the term used here, but rather, *reconstitution* (Fig. 43-5). The skin can wait, and so can nerves and tendons: they are only the roof and furnishings of the house, whereas the foundation is basic and one must start with that.[59,122,153]

The 0.045-inch K-wire has almost universal applicability for the internal stabilization of fractures. It may be used for intramedullary or oblique transcortical fixation of fractures, or as an internal splint to maintain reduction of joints or to temporarily prevent joint motion. It may be used as a springy double bayonet (Fig. 43-6) to maintain bone length until a segmental defect can be filled in with bone graft, or it may be used to transfix two or more metacarpals to maintain normal length of the unsta-

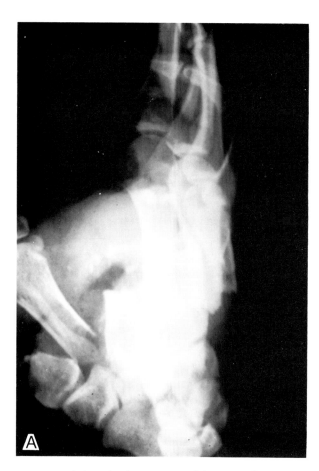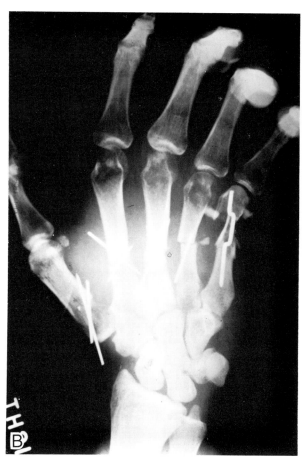

Fig. 43-4. (A) Multiple metacarpal fractures from a high-velocity missile. (B) Extensive debridement and skeletal fixation. The wounds were closed 2 weeks later, and tendon and nerve reconstruction were carried out 2 months later. (Brown PW: The management of phalangeal and metacarpal fractures. Surg Clin North Am 53:1408, 1973. Reprinted with permission of WB Saunders, Philadelphia.)

ble or deficient metacarpal. The K-wire is best inserted with a power drill that can be controlled by one hand, leaving the other hand free to stabilize the parts being wired.[21,81,122]

Traction devices to maintain length or position of damaged digits, though successfully used by some, are hazardous, unwieldy, and difficult to maintain, and usually create more problems than they solve.

Static splinting for skeletal instability is far less satisfactory than is internal or percutaneous K-wire fixation. The latter allows some active motion in all or most of the hand, whereas the splint impedes early motion and is clumsy and difficult to maintain. Although the splint is useful for short periods of time for soft tissue problems, as in some types of

skin and tendon repairs, it is second best to the K-wire for skeletal problems. The same is true for internal fixation of fractures with percutaneous wires and braces.

Bone plates, screws, encircling wire loops, and other orthopaedic gadgetry, intriguing as they may be, are generally inferior to the K-wire. Their application often requires excessive tissue manipulation; their complexities are proportionate to their complications, the right size always seems to be out of stock, and their removal requires another operation.[109]

Despite these very real disadvantages there is growing acceptance for the primary application of these devices for the open fracture in the hand —

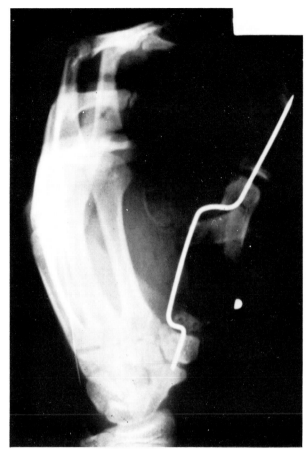 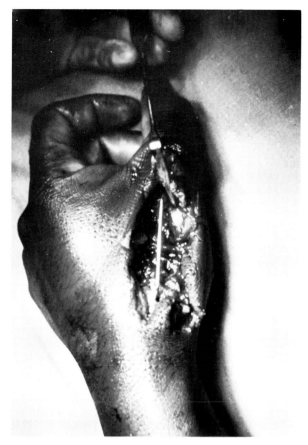

Fig. 43-5. Shotgun muzzle blast injury with avulsion of skin, flexor and extensor tendons, and most of the first metacarpal. After debridement, collapse of the thumb was prevented by a K-wire double bayonet spacer. The wound and K-wire were covered with a dorsal rotation flap 2 weeks later. Bone graft and tendon replacement were done 6 weeks after injury when all wounds were healed.

often followed by primary closure or coverage. The techniques are demanding and unforgiving; those who use them must be well schooled both in their application and in their hazards.[5,41,64,146]

External fixation devices have come into widespread use in the past decade and have proven adaptable and useful for the manaagement of some long bone and pelvic fractures. They, too, are dangerous, but properly applied they can assist in the reduction of very unstable and complex fractures, and can maintain the reduction very well. They also have the advantage of allowing easy access to wounds overlying the fracture, although this may be a disadvantage if it leads to unnecessary poking and prying at the wound.[13,]

There is little that the external fixators can ac-complish for fractures in the hand that the K-wire cannot, although when expertly used the device can be quite useful in maintaining length of shattered metacarpals. More useful is their application to extremely unstable forearm fractures; the stability they impart may enable the patient to more quickly mobilize his hand than if he were in a plaster cast.[145,146]

Deeper Structures

Last priority goes to tendons, nerves, ligaments, and tissues other than vessels and bone. Open wounds often expose these structures to the outside world. Contrary to the belief of many sur-

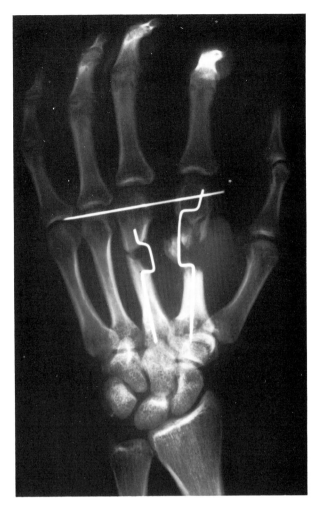

Fig. 43-6. Two months after gunshot wounds with comminution and partial loss of the second and third metacarpals and extensor tendon loss. K-wire spacers and a transverse wire maintain length, preventing shortening until the wound was healed, after which segmental bone grafts were added. (Jabaley ME, Peterson HD: Early treatment of war wounds of the hand and forearm in Vietnam. Ann Surg 177:163–173, 1973.)

on the higher priorities and leave coverage to a more opportune time, he has then bought time in which to more effectively stage surgical repair and reconstruction. More importantly, by deferring reconstructive work in badly contaminated cases or in hands that may need further debridement, the surgeon greatly decreases the chances of infection. There are no exact criteria for timing. Some tissues and wounds can be safely repaired or covered primarily, whereas repair or coverage in others should be delayed. Each hand, each wound, and each damaged structure must be individually assessed. There is one rule, however, that can be applied to most open injuries: *when in doubt, leave open!*[23,57,105,166]

Skin and Closure

There is no surplus skin in the hand; or at least there is very little to spare. Dorsal skin can be replaced with reasonably good results but there is no really satisfactory substitute for palmar skin. If skin is damaged beyond repair or is devoid of good blood supply, it must be removed—but every tag, flap, or island that is potentially viable is worthy of strenuous salvage efforts. Where viability is in question, removal can be deferred for a few days. Digits so badly mangled that they must be removed may contribute viable skin flaps that can be used to replace missing skin in contiguous parts of the hand. Free skin grafts from damaged parts are seldom very successful: only skin still attached to a good blood supply and venous drainage should be used.

Following debridement, a decision regarding closure or coverage must be made. Certainly it is most desirable to obtain healing by primary intention but there are some wounds that can not be safely closed primarily: those in which the "golden period" is far exceeded, those in which the degree of contamination is very great, or those in which the adequacy of debridement or of circulation is questionable; healing cannot be imposed on such wounds. To try it is to invite wound breakdown and worse. Many open wounds of the hand may be safely closed and will proceed to orderly healing by primary intention. Some should have closure deferred for a few days; if they show no sign of infec-

geons, exposure in itself is not harmful; rather it is the drying out of these structures that may cause irreversible changes. If kept moist by proper dressings and if adequately supplied with blood, any of these structures will tolerate exposure without a harmful effect for varying degrees of time—often many days. If the surgeon is relieved of the compulsion to cover or close exposed tissue prematurely, and if he can with equanimity concentrate

tion they may then be safely closed: this is called *delayed primary closure.* If closure is effected before granulations have formed, that is, within the first week, the wound will still heal by primary intention. More contaminated wounds, or wounds with tissues of marginal circulation should be closed secondarily, and a few, such as human bite wounds, should never be closed, but instead allowed to heal by secondary intention. It's worth noting that healing by secondary intention is the *natural* method of wound healing and evolved long before there were surgeons.[52,95,97,170]

The relative advantages and disadvantages of closure must be weighed and many factors carefully assessed. The degree and nature of contamination is important: a wound incurred in the home is less likely to contain as many virulent bacteria as a wound incurred in the barnyard. Time, too, is important; antibiotics have not appreciably changed the concept of the "golden period," but have only extended it a bit. Wounds should not be closed later than about 8 hours postinjury. The state of the contaminated tissues is just as important as the contaminating bacteria. Marginally vascular tissues are at higher risk if the skin is closed and the same is true of puncture wounds where contaminants have been introduced deep into spaces and tissues of the hand. If there is a probability of bleeding or fluid accumulation in the wound, closure will inhibit its free drainage, thereby increasing the risk of infection.[112,141]

When the degree of contamination or the extent of vascular imparment is in doubt the wound should be left open. If, by the fourth or fifth day, there is no sign of infection, edema, erythema, or pus, the wound can then be closed with a much higher chance of undelayed healing. Although many hand wounds can be closed primarily, more are closed than should be. Those wounds that do not accept closure but go on to infection and breakdown ultimately result in more damage to the hand than the original injury.[161]

Rank and Wakefield's[127] concept of *tidy* and *untidy* wounds is useful in roughly classifying the amount of tissue damage and the degree of contamination. The laceration caused by a knife has relatively little tissue damage, even though important structures may be transected, and usually there are relatively few bacteria in such a wound. Such wounds lend themselves well to primary repair, provided all other factors are safely accounted for. The mangled hand from a farm machinery accident or from an explosion may well require a second look and redebridement. Closure of such a wound may well jeopardize uneventful healing. Appearance may be deceptive: a hand through which a high-velocity bullet has passed may look quite benign for the first few hours but may have large amounts of devitalized tissue within it, and may later become terribly edematous.[6,26,127]

When in doubt as to whether to close a wound, a useful middle course is to effect a loose closure with adhesive tape strips. The strips can be laid on without tension to loosely approximate wound edges and to control distortion of flaps of skin. If there is subsequent edema, the strips will allow the wound to gape, whereas sutures would tend to progressively strangle the skin as tension increased.

Charles F. Gregory once said in a lecture: "Primary closure should be based on judgement — plus willingness to take a chance." There is great pressure on the surgeon to close wounds, both pressures from without, and pressures from within. The lay public expects wounds to be closed. If emergency room personnel do not understand the principles of wound management, they too may add to the pressure. Pressures from within the surgeon are generated by misconceptions, lack of experience, an erroneous belief that exposed tissue will "get infected," and a compulsion to suture.[6,11,159–161]

Experience in past wars has convincingly demonstrated not only that wounds of the hand may be safely left open, but that many will do better if they are left open. This knowledge has been acquired at great cost, but as the memories of the last war fades, so too do its lessons, and the old compulsion to suture revives and the lessons must be learned all over again. It's been said that if we do not learn from history we are doomed to repeat our mistakes.[32,33,50,51,94,155,162,163,167–169,170,171]

Worse than ill-advised primary closure is the compulsion to cover the avulsed wound with primary skin flaps (Fig. 43-7). When skin transfer — either split- or full-thickness, free or pedicle — is required, the transfer can be done more efficiently and safely by deferring it until one is reasonably certain that infection will not occur and that the

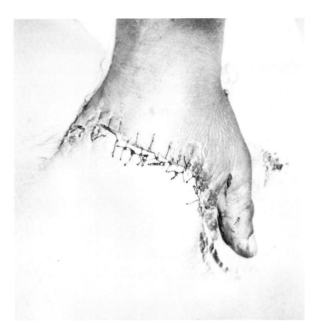

Fig. 43-7. The compulsion to suture. This farmer avulsed four digits in a machine. His surgeon buried the hand in the abdominal wall. When it began to smell bad, some days later, the patient was transferred to another hospital.

tissues appear receptive to coverage. Though widely applied— usually for the convenience of the surgeon and operating room schedules—it is potentially unsafe and is usually quite unnecessary. Consistently better results will be obtained by delayed skin transfer, when the tissues are receptive to the transfer and when proper attention can be given to planning, operating room availability, and other details (Fig. 43-8).

The development of microsurgical techniques has given us the ability to transfer full-thickness skin and subcutaneous tissue coverage to wounds and to revascularize them in their new site (see Chapter 27). This exciting addition to our skills offers great promise for dealing with the devastating hand wound where there has been avulsion of large amounts of skin leaving bone, joints, tendons, nerves and vessels exposed. Such skin transfers are called "microvascular free flaps"—a misleading term, as they are neither free nor are they flaps. Some very impressive results have been demonstrated with this technique; where the transfer has been successful it has facilitated staged reconstruc-

tion and rehabiliation of the hand. The costs and complications of such transfer may be considerable. Success depends on a highly skilled team working in a hospital that will consistently give that team all necessary personnel and logistical support, which few community hospitals can afford. Unless done well, such surgery will fail and further jeopardize an already badly damaged hand. Where the highest standards for microvascular surgery — and its postoperative sequelae — cannot be maintained, it is far safer to defer closure or coverage until the nature of the wound allows it to be done safely and when proper attention can be given to planning, operating room availability, and other details.[9,64,87]

Dressings

The postdebridement dressing (Fig. 43-9) has several functions: to keep wounds and exposed tissues moist, to prevent further contaminaton, and most of all, to enhance circulation by the prevention of edema. The wound is covered with fine mesh gauze, lightly impregnated with petrolatum. The fingers are separated by lightly tucking a folded surgical gauze sponge in each finger cleft. A bulky dressing of multiple fluffed-up gauze sponges is then applied from elbow to fingertips while holding the hand and wrist in the position of function with the wrist slightly extended, MP and interphalangeal joints slightly flexed, and thumb abducted and slightly flexed. Dead spaces should be left open; if it seems likely that they will be occluded by tissue flaps, they should be drained with a short length of 8- or 10-gauge tubing. Packing wounds open is not only unnecessary but may be harmful, as the packing may block free drainage. The entire dressing is then wrapped with a nonelastic conforming roller gauze bandage. An elastic bandage may be used but is potentially dangerous, as it is deceptively easy to apply it too tightly or to create constricting bands of uneven tension. The entire dressing should apply mild and uniform pressure throughout the hand, wrist, and forearm.

This type of dressing is applicable to most injured hands. It is safe and comfortable and has enough "give" to allow a slight amount of active finger motion, and yet it provides enough stability

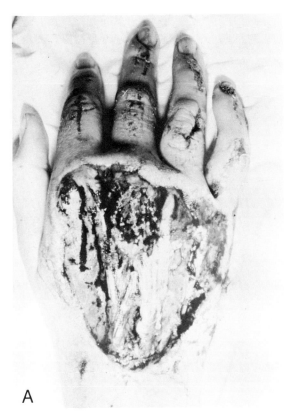
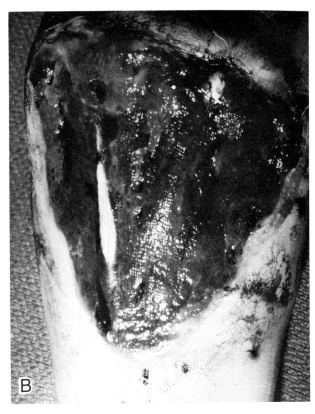

Fig. 43-8. (A) An automobile overturned on the hand of this 16-year-old girl, avulsing skin, extensor tendons and joint capsules of the knuckles. A lot of dirt and debris was ground into the wound. Extensive debridement was done, and the wound was covered with fine mesh gauze and compression dressing. Active assisted exercises were started a few days later. (B) Thirteen days later. Healthy granulations cover the wound. There is no erythema, induration, edema, pus, or pain. The wound is now an ideal recipient for properly planned skin coverage — in this case, a cross-arm pedicle flap. *(Figure continues.)*

to make rigid splints unnecessary. If special positions are required, a plaster splint may be molded to either the dorsal or volar side of the dressing. An intrinsic-plus position of acutely flexed MP joints and fully extended interphalangeal joints is desirable where there has been loss of dorsal skin of the hand or fingers, as in the case of burns, or where there has been extensive damage to these joints. Immediately following application of the dressing, the extremity should be suspended with the hand held higher than the heart, and this elevation should be maintained until it is certain that edema has either been avoided or controlled. More satisfactory for this elevation than actually suspending the arm from a bedframe is to use one of the light plastic foam elevating blocks made especially for

this purpose.[40] They enhance mobility of both the extemity and the patient and are better accepted by the patient than suspension.

Antibiotics and Tetanus Prophylaxis

Antibiotics are useful adjuncts, but not substitutes, to proper wound care. Overdependence on them to the neglect of meticulous debridement and good tissue management will result in many unnecessary infections. Most open wounds of the hand (or elsewhere) do not require antibiotics. Their use should be reserved for wounds where the risk of infection is high. Such wounds would include bites;

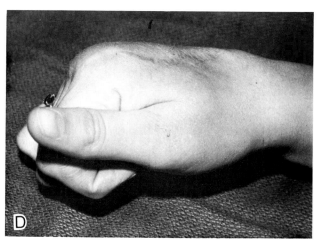

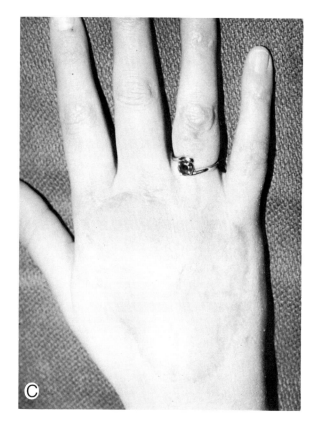

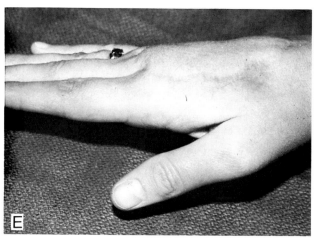

Fig. 43-8 *(Continued).* **(C,D)** The hand 9 months after injury. Three months after detachment of the pedicle flap, four extensor tendon grafts were inserted. Appearance and function compare favorably with results from primary coverage. The delayed transfer of skin decreased the probability of complications and the amount of cicatrix. **(E)** Extensor tendon excursion was excellent beneath the flap on the dorsum of the hand.

deep, penetrating wounds; and mangling or crushing wounds in which the degree of contamination is great or in which debridement has been delayed for more than a few hours. Such wounds should be cultured aerobically and anaerobically at the time of debridement. The appropriate antibiotic can then be selected on the basis of the culture and sensitivity studies. Most hand infections are caused by gram-positive staphylococci and streptococci, although the incidence of infection caused by various gram-negative bacteria seems to be steadily increasing as overzealous users of antibiotics create resistant strains. While waiting for the bacteriology

laboratory results hospital patients with severe wounds can be given intravenous methicillin or oxacillin. If gram-negative organisms are present in significant numbers a cephalosporin should also be used. Outpatients with high-risk wounds can be started on an oral cephalosporin such as cephradine pending the laboratory reports. Other than in the burn wound, topical antibiotics, or, for that matter, any type of locally applied medication, solution, or ointment, have nothing to offer in the treatment of open wounds.[85]

Tetanus prophylaxis is required for all but the most minor open wounds of the hands. The guide-

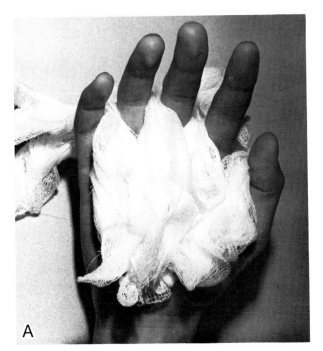

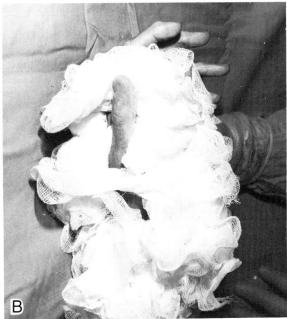

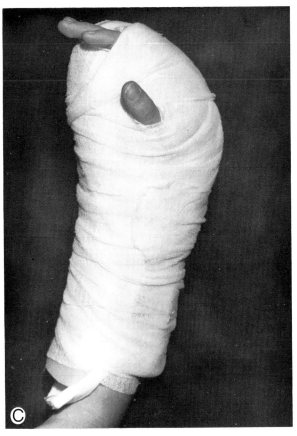

Fig. 43-9. The hand compression dressing. (A) The fingers are lightly separated. (B) Many fluffed-up surgical sponges. (C) Firm, but not tight, uniform compression with the hand in the "position of function." The extremity should now be elevated. (Brown PW: The hand. pp. 643-686. In Hill GJ III (ed): Outpatient Surgery. 2nd Ed. WB Saunders, Philadelphia, 1980.)

A guide to prophylaxis against tetanus in wound management

1979 revision

**Prepared by
The Committee on Trauma
of the American College of Surgeons**

General principles

I. The attending physician must determine for each patient with a wound, individually, what is required for adequate prophylaxis against tetanus.

II. Regardless of the active immunization status of the patient, meticulous surgical care, including removal of all devitalized tissue and foreign bodies, should be provided immediately for all wounds. Such care is essential as part of the prophylaxis against tetanus.

III. Passive immunization with Tetanus Immune Globulin—Human (called human T.A.T.) must be considered individually for each patient. The characteristics of the wound, conditions under which it was incurred, its treatment, its age, and the previous active immunization status of the patient must be considered. It is not indicated, however, if the patient has ever received two or more injections of toxoid.[4]

IV. To every wounded patient, give a written record of the immunization provided, instructing him to carry the record at all times, and if indicated, to complete active immunization. For precise tetanus prophylaxis, an accurate and immediately available history regarding previous active immunization against tetanus is required.

V. Immunization in *adults* requires at least three injections of toxoid. A routine booster of adsorbed toxoid is indicated every ten years thereafter.[1] In *children* under seven, immunization requires four injections of diphtheria and tetanus toxoids combined with pertussis vaccine. A fifth dose may be administered at four to six years of age. Thereafter, a routine booster of tetanus and diphtheria toxoid is indicated at ten-year intervals.[2]

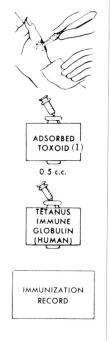

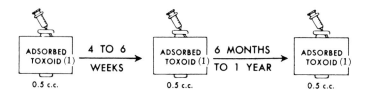

Fig. 43-10. Reprinted from American College of Surgeons: Bulletin, July 1979.

1634

Specific measures for patients with wounds

I. Previously immunized individuals

A. When the attending physician has determined that the patient has been previously fully immunized and the last dose of toxoid was given *within ten years:*

1. For nontetanus-prone wounds, no booster dose of toxoid is indicated;

2. For tetanus-prone wounds and if more than five years has elapsed since the last dose, give 0.5 cc adsorbed toxoid. If excessive prior toxoid injections have been given, this booster may be omitted.

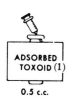

B. When the patient has had two or more prior injections of toxoid and received the last dose *more than ten years previously,* give 0.5 cc adsorbed toxoid for both tetanus-prone and nontetanus-prone wounds. Passive immunization is not considered necessary.

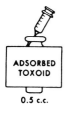

II. Individuals NOT adequately immunized

A. When the patient has received only one or no prior injection of toxoid, or the immunization history is unknown:

1. For nontetanus-prone wounds:
   a. Give 0.5 cc adsorbed toxoid,[1]

2. For tetanus-prone wounds:
   a. Give 0.5 cc adsorbed toxoid,[1]
   b. Give 250 units (or more) of human T.A.T.,[3]
   c. Consider providing antibiotics, although the effectiveness of antibiotics for prophylaxis of tetanus remains unproved.

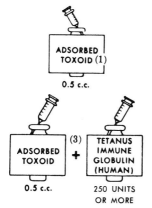

Footnotes

(1) The Public Health Service Advisory Committee on Immunization Practices in 1977 recommended DTP (diphtheria and tetanus toxoids combined with pertussis vaccine) for basic immunization in infants and children from two months through the sixth year of age, and Td (combined tetanus and diphtheria toxoids: adult type) for basic immunization of those over six years of age. For the latter group, Td toxoid was recommended for routine or wound boosters; but if there is any reason to suspect hypersensitivity to the diphtheria component, tetanus toxoid (T) should be substituted for Td.
(Morbidity and Mortality Weekly Report, Vol. 26, No. 49, p 402, Dec 9, 1977, Center for Disease Control.)

(2) Report of the Committee on Infectious Diseases, ed 18. Evanston, IL. American Academy of Pediatrics, 1977, p 2-11, 278-285.

(3) Use different syringes, needles, and sites of injection.

(4) Equine Tetanus Antitoxin: *Do not* administer equine T.A.T. except when human T.A.T. is not available, and only if the possibility of tetanus outweighs the danger of reaction to horse serum.

This guide from the Committee on Trauma of the American College of Surgeons is the work of an ad hoc subcommittee on prophylaxis against tetanus: Roger T. Sherman, MD, FACS, Tampa, Florida, Chairman; Wesley Furste, MD, FACS, Columbus, Ohio; and Richard Faust, MD, FACS, New Orleans, Louisiana.

Posters and reprints may be obtained from the Committee on Trauma, American College of Surgeons, 55 East Erie Street, Chicago, Illinois 60611.

Fig. 43-10 *(Continued).*

lines, published by the Committee for Trauma of the American College of Surgeons, should be followed (Fig. 43-10). Particular attention must be given to those patients not previously immunized, those who have not had a booster injection within the past 5 years, and all those with very severe or neglected wounds.[4]

SPECIFIC INJURIES

Abrasions

An abrasion is a split-thickness skin loss in which enough of the deeper layers remain to fully regenerate the lost tissue. If stratum germinativum has been lost, the wound is considered an avulsion.

The tissue loss from abrasions is not serious. If they are well cleansed, abrasions usually heal quickly, either exposed to air, or under fine mesh gauze and a dry dressing, and without benefit of topical or systemic antibiotics. During the exudative and proliferative phases of wound healing, they become crusted over with a scab, which is an amalgam of precipitated and clotted blood proteins, dead white cells, and bacteria. The scab and its underlying bed develop a high bacterial count that then rapidly declines as healing progresses and the scab begins to separate, a process usually lasting 2 or 3 weeks.

The clinical significance of abrasions lies in their association with injury to deeper tissues. During the healing period, the high bacterial count poses a threat to the deeper tissues if they were exposed at the time of injury or during subsequent reparative surgery. Where possible, one should defer surgery until the abrasion is completely reepithelialized. If this is not possible, the abrasion should be thoroughly scrubbed with a povidone-iodine solution before surgery and the operative wound left open. A delayed primary closure can be done 3 to 7 days later if the wound appears benign.

Lacerations

The primary concern with lacerations is what lies beneath them. Have nerves or tendons been damaged, or have joints been exposed? One of the most common emergency room mistakes is for the physician to concentrate on suturing the skin and fail to

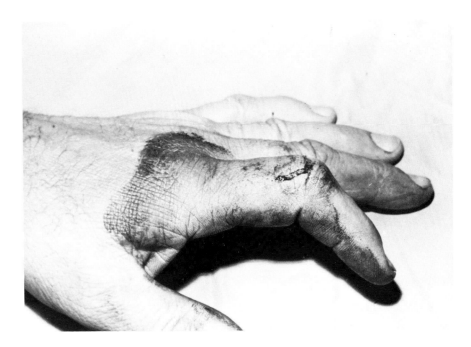

Fig. 43-11. Knife wound. The central slip of the extensor tendon is severed. Repair is needed before the lateral bands migrate volarward, causing boutonnère deformity.

detect the severed or damaged structures underlying it. Failure to detect severed flexor tendons or digital nerves under small transverse lacerations through the proximal flexion creases of the fingers, and especially of the thumb, is the most common error.

Particularly deceptive is the laceration over the dorsum of the PIP joint of a finger with a severed central extensor slip underneath (Fig. 43-11). The patient initially lacks only about 30 degrees of full active extension of the middle phalanx, but if this is missed, so is the one good opportunity to prevent the insidious development of a boutonnière deformity. Another common, but less serious, oversight is to miss the severed extensor digitorum communis in a laceration over the MP joint, wherein the patient initially has lost only the last 30 or 40 degrees of extension.

The laceration—often quite small and not very painful—of a child's midpalm caused by a fall on a broken bottle may look rather innocuous, but deep to it may be found transection of all of the common digital nerves where they spread out from the main trunk of the median nerve (Fig. 43-12).

Lacerations on the volar side of the wrist are often accompanied by severed flexor tendons, nerves and vessels in many different combinations. Such injuries often lend themselves well to primary repair of the deep structures. They require careful debridement and thorough examination under ideal circumstances; that is, in the operating room with adequate anesthesia. Seldom is the emergency room an adequate locale for this. Dorsal wrist lacerations may overlie severed extensor tendons, and careless examination may fail to reveal severed extensor tendons of the thumb or fingers.

Lacerations tend to heal themselves very well by secondary intention, and they should be allowed to do so if they are badly contaminated or have been untreated for more than 7 or 8 hours. They do particularly well without benefit of suture if they lie in or parallel to flexion creases or on the dorsum or lateral aspect of the finger. Most lacerations, of course, are sutured primarily, but too often the emphasis is on closure, to the neglect of what lies below.[142]

Crush and Burst

Great pressures applied to the hand shear, compress, and twist tissues, creating havoc in the vascular bed and in the cellular structures of the tissues, causing hemorrhage and the escape of intra- and extracellular fluids into potential spaces and tissue planes. The net result is the formation of hematoma and a progressive edema that, in turn, leads to the precipitation of proteins, fibrosis, and stiffness. Although crush affects all tissues adversely and its sequelae may be irreversible, prompt surgical measures may, nevertheless, salvage much that at first looks hopeless. The fundamental principles of early debridement, decompression, effective dressing, and postoperative elevation are the basics

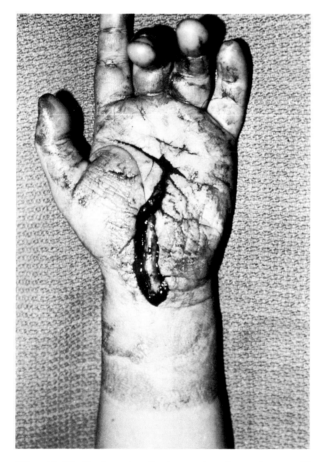

Fig. 43-12. Broken bottle laceration in a 4-year-old child. All branches of the median nerve and both flexor tendons of the index finger are severed. Note "hangout" of the index finger.

of treatment. Primary reconstructive measures, other than skeletal realignment and stabilization, are seldom applicable, as a weeping tissue base, or one laced with microhemorrhage, offers a poor substrate for satisfactory healing.[60,104]

With such a picture of widespread tissue destruction and its subsequent impairment of blood supply, the crushed hand is particularly vulnerable to the proliferation of contaminating bacteria. It follows then, just as with most severe injuries, that measures that improve arterial input and venous and lymphatic drainage are the key to healing without infection. Accurate assessment of irreversible ischemia of the intrinsic musculature, fascia, and other connective tissue may be impossible in the initial debridement. A second or third look and redebridement are often necessary. Wound culture and careful selection of antibiotics are important as well, but only as an adjunct to the surgical support of tissue vascularity. It follows that primary closure of an open wound in which crush has been a significant wounding factor will seriously jeopardize healing, but, perhaps fortunately, closure is often impossible. Postdebridement edema must be expected; any sutures, no matter how loosely placed, may become tight and will then strangle the tissue in which they are placed. Crush

injuries frequently split the skin with shear and torque forces, or the skin may burst from pressure generated from within, just as a grape will burst if compressed (Fig. 43-13). The burst finger or palm may result from industrial presses, pistons, and gears, or the dropping of heavy objects on the hand. The burst finger often has a longitudinal rent the length of the flexor surface. The underlying tendons, nerves and vessels may be quite salvageable if the finger is properly managed by avoiding closure under tension. The burst palm may have masses of muscle extruding from the lateral margins of the hand, or from the thumb web space. Often these muscle masses are viable and should not be removed unless obviously avascular or hopelessly contaminated.[40,79,157]

Avulsion and Degloving

Parts of the hand that are torn or ground off, either partially or completely, may or may not be suitable for salvage. There are great pressures on the surgeon, from the public and from within himself, to preserve everything and to reattach all that is detached. The specifics of the how and when of amputation management, as well as the principles

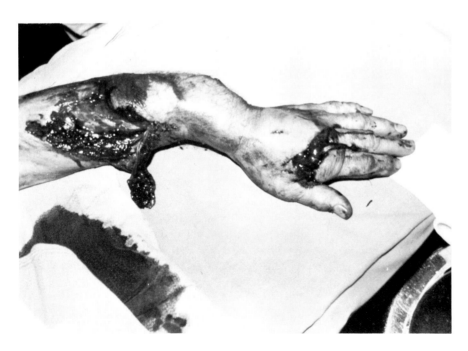

Fig. 43-13. Roller press crush injury with multiple hand and forearm fractures, avulsion of muscles and tendons, and burst injuries of the forearm and hand. Extensive debridement of devascularized tissue and forearm were done. The wounds were left open to be covered with skin grafts 2 weeks later.

of skin transfer, are covered elsewhere in this text. Other than amputation, most avulsion injuries involve mainly the loss of skin or the creation of distally based flaps of skin. Completely avulsed skin is seldom retrievable, but the distal flap may be.

Full-thickness skin loss from the dorsum of the hand may leave the underlying extensor tendons relatively unscathed with paratenon intact, or the tendons may be avulsed with the skin, or damaged beyond repair. In the former, split-thickness skin replacement will generally allow satisfactory gliding of the minimally damaged tendon. The time to apply the graft will vary with the degree of contamination, how soon and how well the debridement is done, and all the other factors bearing on good wound management. Primary skin replacement, immediately following debridement, is not necessary and has all the potential risks (considerable) and gains (minimal) of other forms of primary closure.

If the tendons are avulsed or mangled, their replacement with segmental tendon grafts, or occasionally by transfer, must be preceded by full-thickness skin replacement, as subdermal fat will be required to prevent tendon adherence. Staged reconstruction in such cases requires careful planning and timing. Wound breakdown and infection, or persistent edema will result in a stiff hand and poor function. Again, primary attention must be paid to the fundamentals of debridement and preparation of the tissue base for uneventful healing. Premature coverage may create more problems than it will solve. The skin flap can be transferred any time in the first 2 or 3 weeks after injury. The ideal time is about the ninth or tenth day, early in the proliferative phase of wound healing, when granulation tissue has just started to appear. In the interim it is important to prevent edema and stiffness with proper dressings, elevation, and a combination of active and passive exercises of the digits. The exercise program is particularly important if the avulsion has included the extensor mechanism and capsules of the MP joints.

Full-thickness avulsion of the volar skin of the proximal palm, the "heel of the hand," is often caused by falls from motorcycles or bicycles. Skin in this area has an impressive regenerative capacity, and most of these wounds can be allowed to heal by secondary intention (Fig. 43-14). During the healing process the patient should be encour-

aged to use his hand actively; dressings need not be bulky or complex. This seems to be an unorthodox, even risky, method to the advocates of immediate skin replacement, but I have found that the nature and amount of cicatrix formed compare most favorably with that of successful skin grafts. The healing time is about the same, but with the open method the patient is able to use his hand sooner and is spared additional operations.[37,48]

The vascularity and potential viability of the distally based flap are often difficult to assess (Fig. 43-15). Unless the flap is obviously without hope of survival, the best course is to debride carefully and to replace the flap without benefit (?) of sutures, using adhesive strips instead. Examination of the flap on the third or fourth day will usually reveal whether or not it must be removed or trimmed.

Degloving of digits, most commonly the ring finger, frequently leaves underlying tendons and joints intact. The problem is generally one of devascularized skin. If the avulsion is complete, with skin completely detached and the finger denuded, skin replacement with either the avulsed skin or by skin graft will not produce a result as satisfactory to the rest of the hand as amputation. Replacement may sometimes succeed where the skin is still attached, or where revascularization is possible, but very careful assessment of the degree of avulsion, the state of the tissues, and the patient's individual requirements and wishes must be made before the salvage attempt is made. Microsurgical reanastomosis of both arteries and veins offers promise of salvage in some degloving injuries that have hitherto been hopeless, but the functional results have seldom been very good, though the cosmetic results are sometimes more acceptable to the patient than amputation. (see Chapter 25).[38,58,93,107,136,164]

Amputation

In a sense, an amputation is the ultimate open wound. Amputations in the hand are covered in detail in Chapter 3, but it is appropriate to give some consideration to the amputation simply as a wound of the hand. The simplest way to treat one is by applicaton of the basic wound care principles already described: debridement, appropriate closure or cover, and early rehabilitation. *For most*

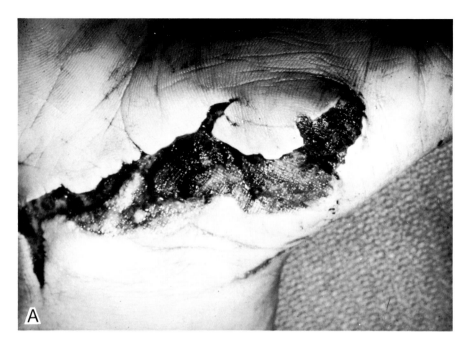

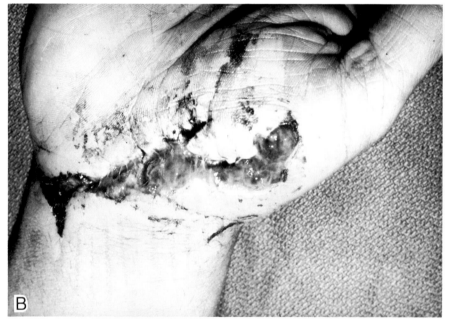

Fig. 43-14. (A) Crush, burst, and avulsion of the base of the palm from industrial machinery. The wound was debrided and left open, with compression dressing for several days. Active motion was started at the end of the third day. **(B)** Five days after injury. There is no erythema, induration, pus, or pain. Granulations have appeared earlier than usual. *(Figure continues.)*

amputations, for most individuals, in most of the world's medical installations, this simplest course is the best course. For some type of amputations, in some individuals, in some places, and in some circumstances, reattachment of the severed part may be feasible and may be preferable, but this depends on many factors: the nature of the wound itself, the requirements, wishes and condition of the patient, and the uncompromised availability of competent, reattachment teams in institutions prepared to give them all the logistical support necessary for this highly specialized surgery. Compromise with these principles will yield compromised results.[25,27,90,143]

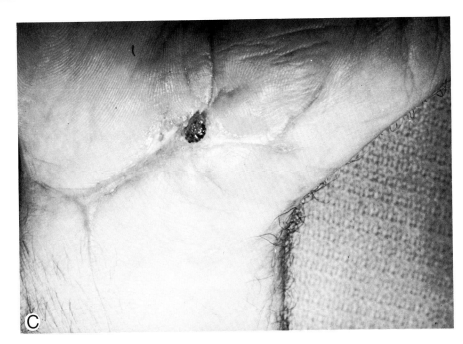

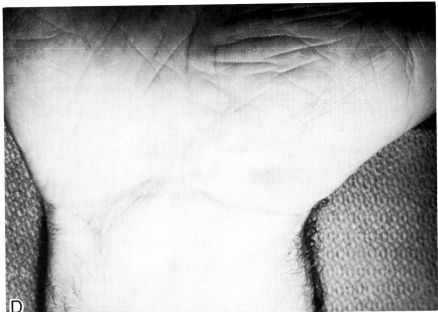

Fig. 43-14 *(Continued).* (**C**) At 6 weeks, the wound has almost completely healed by secondary intention. The patient returned to manual work at 4 weeks. (**D**) Seven weeks after injury, there is normal function and minimal cicatrix.

Machine Mangling

Power machines of industry, farm, and home can cause hand injuries of many types and combinations. Power saws, the whirling blades of automotive radiator fans, lawn mowers and snow blowers, the meshing gears and pulleys of machinery, punch and molding presses, corn pickers and harvesters, meat grinders and shredders, pulverizers, mills, and conveyor belts all make their regular contribution to the emergency room. These moving parts coupled with inattentiveness or human foolishness do great damage: hand parts are avulsed, sliced off, crushed, ground, twisted and lacerated. The inju-

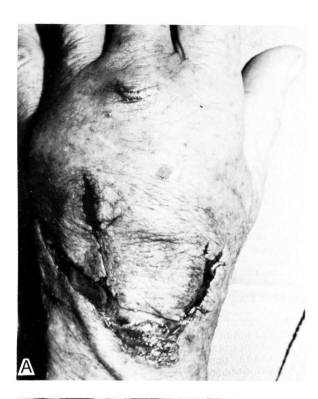

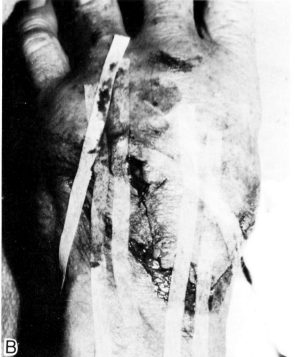

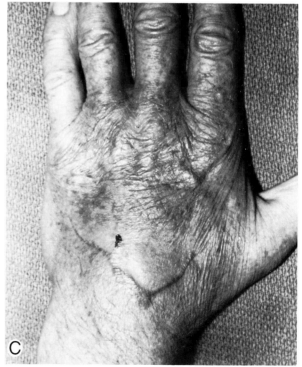

Fig. 43-15. (**A**) Deceleration on concrete caused this combination of avulsion, abrasion, and a distally based flap. (**B**) Wound debrided. The flap is held lightly in place with paper strip tapes. (**C**) Two months later.

ries are complex, with combined elements of contamination, structural disruption, crush, and often thermal and chemical injury as well.[28,110,143]

The basic fundamentals of treatment apply for these injuries: all repairs must be built on a foundation of the history of the injury, a careful appraisal of the damage, and good overall care of the patient followed by painstaking debridement. Many of these wounds are highly contaminated, and often the history of the injury will tell more of the degree and hazard of contamination than will the appearance of the wound. Industrial accident wounds often appear very dirty due to grease and other lubricants, but grease and grime are far less dangerous than those contaminants that are difficult or impossible to see, such as meat particles, pieces of vegetation, or the myriad of bacteria found in the soil of a lawn or farmland.[18,34,105,108,135]

There are often multiple fractures and widespread skeletal disruption and distortion in the mangled hand. The architectural framework of the hand must be reconstituted. Skeletal realignment and stabilization must be accomplished early and the best opportunity for this is during the initial operation. Reduction of dislocations and fractures — re-establishment of the surgical scaffolding — are much easier to accomplish in the newly injured hand. Satisfactory reduction may be impossible to attain even a few days after the injury.

Premature closure of these complex, heavily contaminated wounds is dangerous; delayed closure, or, in some cases, nonclosure, is a safer course. The timing of closure must be predicated on a careful and accurate appraisal of the vascular state of the tissue, the degree of contamination, and the effectiveness of the debridement (Fig. 43-16).

Some of these hands are beyond repair. After careful examination and meticulous debridement, it may still be impossible to determine what will survive and what will be useful. The hand surgeon must walk an uncertain line between realism and optimism. He is obligated to discard all parts that may be detrimental to ultimate hand function, and yet, sometimes seemingly hopelessly damaged tissue will survive the insult of injury. The surgeon must consider the alternatives with every decision he makes; the basic alternative is amputation and he must consider its advantage as measured against its cost to the patient. Realism may dictate amputa-

tion: optimism may counsel retention. Sometimes the outcome is uncertain enough to dictate retention, subject to a second or third look – and consultation with the patient.[22]

Penetration, Injecton, and Bites

Sharp instrument penetration, or stab wounds, cause little tissue disruption even though important structures may be damaged. The wound is often small and undramatic and frequently causes little discomfort. Careful examination of the hand for tendon, nerve, and artery damage is necessary. Although the wound itself may be of little import, primary repair of these deeper, more important, structures is frequently feasible and advisable. Arterial transection or puncture may cause aneurysm or fistula formation that will not be apparent until several days or even months later. It is helpful to know what caused the injury. Wounds from knives or other sharp metal objects seldom need much in the way of exploration or debridement provided a careful examination of hand function has been done. Thorough lavage is usually all that is required. If the wounding instrument was glass or an organic material, such as a tree branch or pencil, the wound should be explored if there seems a probability that a piece of the material has been left in the depths of the hand.[49]

Penetration of the hand by fluids under pressure, such as paints, lubricants, abrasives or hydraulic solutions, or organic solvents, requires wide surgical opening of the hand, careful lavage and mechanical debridement. For the first hour or two after injury, these injuries seem deceptively benign, but rapidly increasing pain and edema then indicate the severity and magnitude of the damage. The management of this type of injury is discussed in Chapter 16.

Carnivore bites are mostly penetrating wounds, although all have an element of crush proportionate to the size and ferocity of the animal. The animal's teeth carry many types of bacteria deep beneath the skin and deposit them in tissue whose vascularity may have been compromised by crush. Most of these wounds respond well to lavage and nonclosure. Human bites cause more crush and shear, and the extent of tissue damage is greater

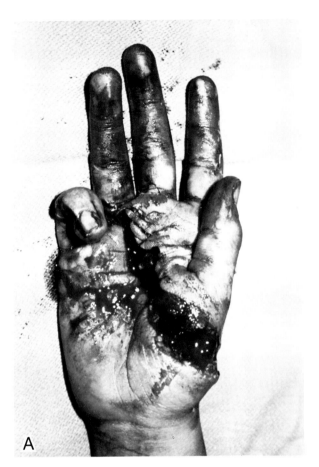

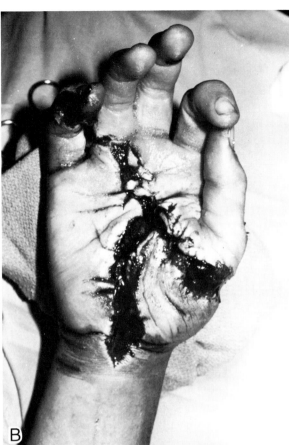

Fig. 43-16. (A) The hand of a teenage boy mangled by a power saw. There are comminuted fractures of the first metacarpal; severed extensor and flexor tendons and intrinsic muscles and digital nerves of the thumb; severed flexor tendons and digital nerves of the index, middle and ring fingers; and avulsion of the ulnar border of the small finger. Exploration and debridement were done, the wounds were left open, and no sutures were used. **(B)** On the fourth day, the wound appears benign and ready for delayed primary closure. *(Figure continues.)*

than from a dog or cat bite. Furthermore, the microbial flora of human saliva appears to be more varied and virulent than that of the "lower" animals. Careful debridement, copious lavage, nonclosure, and prophylactic antibiotics are all important to their care and will generally allow orderly healing by secondary intention. If the wounds are surgically closed, not only will they often break down, but the resultant infection will often be particularly malignant (often a mixed aerobe-anaerobe type) and may cause widespread tissue destruction and permanent hand impairment.

The clenched fist injury incurred by the sharp encounter of a metacarpal head with a human inci-

sor will often open and innoculate an MP joint (Fig 43-17). If debridement is skimped, or it the wound is closed, pyarthrosis commonly results, followed by articular cartilage degradation, degenerative arthritis, and a stiff, painful, or deformed joint.[44,98]

Gunshot Wounds

In the evaluation of gunshot wounds, it helps to know the type of weapon and how far it was from the patient. Projectiles shot through the hand may be fast or slow, single or multiple, large or small. The surgeon mainly wishes to know how much en-

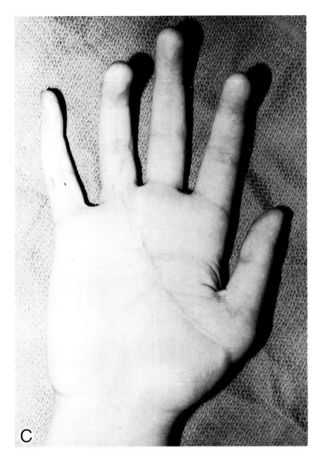

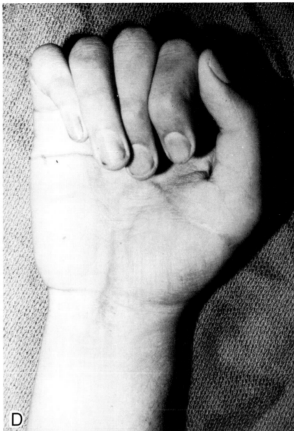

Fig. 43-16 *(Continued).* **(C,D)** Three months after injury and 6 weeks after tendon and nerve grafts. The hand is supple. At 1 year, there was good tendon function and fair sensibility with two-point discrimination to 8 mm.

ergy was expended within the hand. Since energy equals mass times velocity squared ($E=MV^2$), the size (M) of the missile is of some importance and its velocity (V) is very important. Velocity depends on the type of weapon, the explosive charge, and the distance the projectile has traveled.[72]

High-velocity missiles, (those moving faster than 2000 ft/sec) are shot from sporting and military rifles and from machine guns. Most remain in a high-velocity category for a range of several hundred yards. Fragments from artillery shells, bombs, and grenades may sometimes attain high velocities, but their speed (and hence, their destructive energy) usually drops off rapidly within a hundred yards.

Low-velocity missiles come from most .22 caliber weapons and almost all pistols. Shotguns throw a mass of pellets in a spreading pattern for a short distance. Individual shot pellets of buckshot size may retain lethal energy for over 100 yards, but smaller pellets of birdshot size lose most of their energy in less than half that distance. Shotgun injuries of the hand are seldom of much consequence beyond a distance of a few yards. Most shotgun injuries are incurred at close range, frequently with the hand held over the muzzle, and these may be terribly destructive as the compressed wad of shot acts as a single large projectile with considerable energy. This shot wad does not begin to disperse until several yards from the muzzle of the gun.[54,158]

The low-velocity missile, generally from a .22 caliber weapon, or from a .32 or .38 caliber pistol, may fracture a bone or disrupt a joint, but often

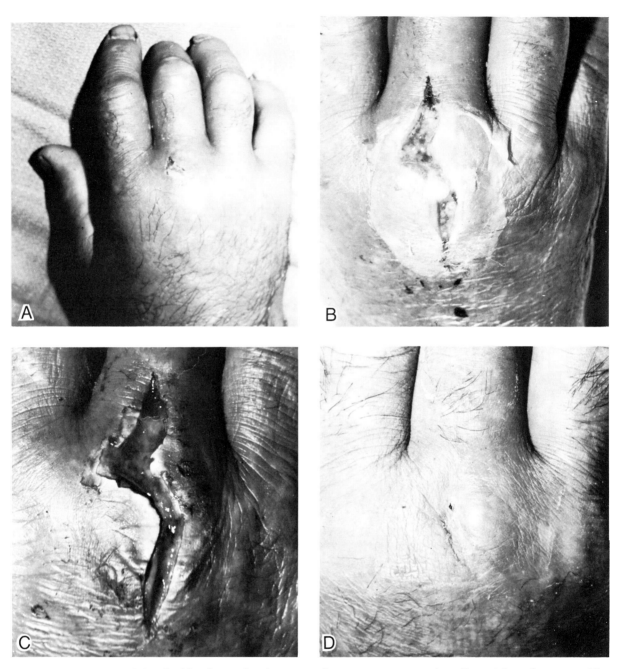

Fig. 43-17. (**A**) A typical clenched fist (human bite) injury with progressive pain and swelling, 4 days after injury. The patient now has active pyarthrosis of the MP joint of the middle finger. In the operating room, the joint was opened widely, debrided of thick pus and torn capsule, and lavaged copiously. No attempt was made to close the joint or wound. Compression dressing, elevation, antibiotics, and early motion were part of the treatment plan. (**B**) Seven days after injury. Pain, erythema, induration, and fever have subsided. Pus is still extruding from the wound as the patient moves the finger. The wound (and the joint) will close spontaneously as the pyarthrosis subsides, and should be allowed to do so. (**C**) Ten days after injury. The joint has closed and the wound is in the proliferative phase of healing. (**D**) Six weeks after injury. The wound is healed, with the joint functional and comfortable.

does surprisingly little damage to a hand. Occasionally a tendon or a nerve may be damaged or a vessel disrupted, but more often the relatively slow-moving bullet tends to deflect these mobile structures rather than transect them. There is usually not much tissue damage, and extensive debridement or decompression is seldom necessary. The entrance wound is small and the exit wound only a bit larger. If examination reveals no tendon or nerve damage, and if the hand was not gloved, opening the wound further or exploring its depths is usually not necessary. Through-and-through lavage, fixation of fractures, nonclosure, a bulky dressing and elevation will suffice. Tetanus prophylaxis is imperative, and a short course of antibiotics is advisable. Active motion should be started early.[1,14,54,70–72,78,154]

High-velocity missile wounds, as well as shotgun blasts at close range, are far more serious. Large amounts of tissue are damaged and the requirements for exploration, debridement, and decompression are much greater. The assessment of tissue viability is more difficult, and no wounds in this category should be closed primarily. If the missle has struck bone, and sometimes if it has not, the degree of comminution, distortion, dispersion of bone fragments, and bone loss may be great and skeletal realignment becomes much more of a challenge. These factors make it even more imperative to concentrate on the re-establishment of the skeletal architecture of the hand at this primary surgical session; with each succeeding day the task will become more difficult, and after a few days, may well be impossible. Segmental defects of bone will require cross-K-wire fixation of fragments to adjacent intact bones or K-wire spacers (K-wires bent into a bayonet configuration) to prevent collapse. External fixation devices are enjoying a revival in orthopaedics and are occasionally useful in the hand, but only by those skilled in their application and maintenance. For most surgeons, the K-wire is more adaptable, more useful, more forgiving, and more safe.

The shotgun charge wad, which may be plastic, felt, or cardboard, should always be looked for in close-range shotgun wounds. The entrance wound of the high-velocity missile is small unless the bullet was tumbling or ricocheting, but the exit wound is very large and may avulse great amounts of tissue from the hand or amputate a digit. In debriding the high-velocity missile wound, it is advisable for the surgeon to visualize the course of the missile through the hand and to reflect that the missile has probably expended tremendous energy within the hand, causing momentary, but extreme distortion and insult to all tissues in the hand. The high-velocity missile imparts an explosive force to the hand, frequently damaging tissue quite remote from the track of the bullet.[11,34,53,66,78,96,119,120]

There is an erroneous tendency to dissociate military from civilian wounds, particularly in the treatment of gunshot wounds of the hand. It is true that there are some differences between the two: military weapons, in general, are more destructive and the wounding environment and degree of contamination are usually worse in military combat than in the civilian millieu, but the degree of destruction, the physiology of wound healing, and the fundamentals of wound care are basically not different. The real difference lies in the surgeon's experience, his prejudices, and his relationship to the patient, and in the pressures to which he is subjected. These pressures are considerable. The civilian patient, even though he is usually less seriously injured, makes far greater emotional, economic, and vocational demands on the surgeon, and usually his expectations for a good hand are far greater than those of the combat-injured soldier. The latter is happy to get out of combat alive, whereas the civilian's injury is often just the beginning of his trouble.[2,31,45–47,70,81]

Explosion and Blast

Bombs, firecrackers, and other explosive devices may injure hands in many ways. Military high explosive weapons, homemade pipe bombs, dynamite, and blasting caps may tear off a hand or several fingers or blast a hand wide open. There are several elements to the injury: blast effect from the explosion, missile injury from flying debris and container fragments, and thermal injury from burning gunpowder, cordite, or other explosive agents. These may cause a complex injury, resulting from any combination of avulsion, laceration, blast, crush, and burns. Contamination with multiple foreign bodies, often driven deep into the tissues of the hand, contributes to the complexities of the injury. Tissue may be torn apart, shredded and impregnated with debris. Tattooing of the skin also commonly occurs.[156]

The effects of explosives and the direction in which their energy is expended are capricious and unpredictable. A mortar shell is capable of killing large numbers of people within a radius of many yards, yet in some freak accidents the same shell may be detonated in a soldier's hands with only minor injury resulting. A small, seemingly benign, firecracker, if compressed within the fist, may mangle the hand terribly, The small blasting cap of fulminate of mercury has a very destructive force if contained within the hand, and the same is true of cartridge primers, which are made of a similar material. Fireworks, flares, and other pyrotechnical devices also have explosive force when contained and will add chemical and thermal damage to the injury.

The spectrum of injury from explosive devices is so varied that no specifics for treatment can be given here. The hand surgeon must apply the principles that have been delineated and reiterated throughout this chapter. The plan and course of treatment are based on decision making; decisions are made by considering the alternatives, and alternatives are classified according to the priorities given to surgical principles and the individual patient's needs.[86]

RECAPITULATION OF THE ORDER OF PRIORITY FOR OPEN WOUND MANAGEMENT[42,43]

1. The patient as person and body
2. Other injuries; resuscitation
3. History
4. Physical examination
5. Blood supply
6. Debridement
7. Skeletal stability
8. Repair of damaged structures (sometimes)
9. Appropriate timing of closure or coverage
10. Proper dressings and elevation
11. Tetanus prophylaxis and antibiotics
12. Secondary reconstruction
13. Rehabilitation — should be started as early as possible, preferably while the hand is still in the primary dressing

REFERENCES

1. Adams RW: Small caliber missile blast wounds of the hand. Mechanism and early management. Am J Surg 82:219–226, 1951
2. Allen HA: Hand Injuries in the Mediterranean (North African) Theater of Operations. pp. 79–153. In Bunnell S (ed): Surgery in World War II - Hand Surgery. Office of the Surgeon General, Dept. of the Army, Washington DC, 1955
3. Altemeier WA: The significance of infection in trauma. Bull Am Coll Surg 57:7–16, February 1972
4. American College of Surgeons, Committee on Trauma: Early Care of the Injured Patient. 2nd Ed. WB Saunders, Philadelphia, 1976
5. Anderson JT, Gustilo RB: Immediate internal fixation in open fractures. Orthop Clin North Am 11:569–578, 1980
6. Ariyan S, Krizek TJ: In defense of the open wound. Arch Surg 111:293–296, 1976
7. Arons MS, Fernando L, Polayes IM: Pasteurella multicida -The major cause of hand infections following domestic animal bites. J Hand Surg 7:47–52, 1982
8. Bailey BN: Skin cover in hand injuries. Injury 2:294–304, 1970
9. Beasley RW: Principles of soft tissue replacement for the hand. J Hand Surg 8:781–784, 1983
10. Bell MJ: The management of shotgun wounds. J Trauma 11:522–527, 1971
11. Bennett JE: Skin and soft tissue injuries of the hand in children. Pediatr Clin North Am 22:443–449, 1975
12. Billmire DA, Neale HW, Stern PJ: Acute management of severe hand injuries. Surg Clin North Am 64:683–697, 1984
13. Bornside GH, Bornside BB: Comparison between moist swab and tissue biopsy methods for quantitation of bacteria in experimental incisional wounds. J Trauma 19:103–105, 1979
14. Bowers WH, Preston ET: Low velocity bullet wounds. Contemp Surg 1:57–59, 1973

15. Boyes JH: A philosophy of care of the injured hand. Bull Am Coll Surg 50:341–348, 1965

16. Boyes JH (ed): Bunnell's Surgery of the Hand. 5th Ed. JB Lippincott, Philadelphia, 1970

17. Bragdon RW: Delayed excision in the severely injured hand. Orthop Trans 3(1): 70, 1979

18. Brown HC, Williams HB, Woolhouse FM: Principles of salvage in mutilating hand injuries. J Trauma 8:319–332, 1968

19. Brown LL, Shelton HT, Bornside GH, and Cohn J Jr: Evaluation of wound irrigation by pulsatile jet and conventional methods. Ann Surg 187:170–173, 1978

20. Brown PW: The prevention of infection in open wounds. Clin Orthop 96:42–50, 1973

21. Brown PW: The management of phalangeal and metacarpal fractures. Surg Clin North Am 53:1393–1437, 1973

22. Brown PW: Sacrifice of the unsatisfactory hand. J Hand Surg 4:417–425, 1979

23. Brown PW: The fate of exposed bone. Am J Surg 137:464–469, 1979

24. Brown PW: The hand. In Hill GJ III (ed): Outpatient Surgery. 2nd Ed. WB Saunders, Philadelphia, 1980

25. Brown PW: The rational selection of treatment for upper extremity amputations. Orthop Clin North Am 12:843–849, 1981

26. Brown PW: Complications following wound care. pp. 314–324. In Boswick JA Jr (ed): Complications in Hand Surgery. WB Saunders, Philadelphia, 1986

27. Brown PW: Complications following amputation of parts of the hand. pp. 197–204. In Boswick JA Jr (ed): Complications in Hand Surgery, WB Saunders, Philadelphia, 1986

28. Bruner JM: Cornpicker injuries of the hand. Plast Reconstr Surg 21:306–313, 1958

29. Bunnell S: Suggestions to improve the early treatment of hand injuries. Bull US Army Med Dept 3:78–82, 1945

30. Bunnell S: The early treatment of hand injuries. J Bone Joint Surg 33A:807, 1951

31. Bunnell S (ed): Hand Surgery in World War II. Office of the Surgeon General, Dept of the Army, Washington DC, 1955

32. Burkhalter WE, Butler B, Metz W, Omer GE Jr: Experience with delayed primary closure of war wounds of the hand in Vietnam. J Bone Joint Surg 50A:945, 1968

33. Burkhalter WE: Care of war injuries of the hand and upper extremity. Report of the War Injury Committee. J Hand Surg 8:810–813, 1983

34. Burkhalter WE: Complex injuries of the hand In Sandzen SC Jr (ed): The Hand and Wrist: Current Management of Complications in Orthopaedics. Williams & Wilkins, Baltimore, 1985

35. Butler B Jr: Initial management of hand wounds. Milit Med 134:1–7, 1969

36. Cabot H: The doctrine of the prepared soil: A neglected factor in surgical infections. Can Med Assoc J 11:610–614, 1921

37. Carrell A: Cicatrization of wounds. XII. Factors initiating regeneration. J Exp Med 34:425–434, 1921

38. Carrol RE: Ring injuries in the hand. Clin Orth 104:175–182, 1974

39. Carrico TJ, Mehrhof AI, Cohen IK: Biology of wound healing. Surg Clin North Am 64:721–733, 1984

40. Carter PR: Crush injury of the upper limb: Early and late management. Orthop Clin North Am 14:719–747, 1983

41. Chapman MW: The use of immediate internal fixation in open fractures. Orthop Clin North Am 11:579–591, 1980

42. Chase RA: Surgery of the hand. N Engl J Med 287:1227–1234, 1972

43. Chase RA, Laub DR: The hand: Therapeutic strategy for acute problems. Curr Probl Surg, June 1966

44. Chuinard RG, D'Ambrosia RD: Treatment of human bite infections. Orthop Trans 1(2):158, 1977

45. Churchill ED: The surgical management of the wounded in the Mediterranean Theater at the time of the Fall of Rome. Ann Surg 120:268–283, 1944

46. Cleveland M: Hand injuries in the European Theater of Operations. pp. 155–184. In Bunnell S (ed): Surgery in World War II - Hand Surgery. Office of the Surgeon General, Dept. of the Army, Washington DC 1955

47. Cleveland M, Manning JG, Stewart WJ: Care of battle casualties and injuries involving bones and joints. J Bone Joint Surg 33A:517, 1951

48. Conolly WB: Spontaneous healing and wound contraction of soft tissue wounds of the hand. Hand 6:26–32, 1974

49. Cutler CW Jr.: Injuries of hand by puncture wounds and foreign bodies. Surg Clin North Am 21:485, 1941

50. Cutler CW Jr: The Hand: Its Disabilities and Diseases. WB Saunders, Philadelphia, 1942

51. Cutler CW Jr: Early management of wounds of the hand. Bull US Army Med Dept 85:92–98, 1945

52. deHoll D, Rodeheaver GT, Edgerton MT, Edlich RF: Potentiation of infection by suture closure of dead space. Am J Surg 127:716–720, 1974

53. DeMuth WE Jr, Smith JM: High velocity bullet wounds of muscle and bone: The basis of rational early treatment. J Trauma 6:744–755, 1966
54. Duncan J, Kettelkamp DB: Low Velocity gunshot wounds of the hand. Arch Surg 109:395–397, 1974
55. Dunphy JE, VanWinkle W Jr: Repair and regeneration: The Scientific Basis for Surgical Practice. p. 353. McGraw-Hill, New York, 1968
56. Dziemian AJ, Mendelson JA, Lindsey D: Comparison of the wounding characteristics of some commonly encountered bullets, J Trauma 1:341–353, 1961
57. Edgerton MT: Immediate reconstruction of the injured hand. Surgery 36:329–343, 1954
58. Elliott RA, Hoehn JG, Stayman JW: Management of the viable soft tissue cover in degloving injuries. Hand 11:69–71, 1979
59. Elton RC, Bouzard WC: Management of gunshot and fragment wounds of the metacarpus (Abstract). J Bone Joint Surg 55A:887, 1973
60. Entin MA: Crushing and avulsing injuries of the hand. Surg Clin North Am 44:1009–1018, 1964
61. Flatt AE: The Care of Minor Hand Injuries. 3rd Ed. CV Mosby, St Louis, 1972
62. Flynn JE: Compound wounds of the hand. Ann Surg 135:500–507, 1952
63. Flynn JE: Acute trauma in the hand. Surg Clin North Am 46:797–812, 1966
64. Freeland AE, Jabaley ME, Burkhalter WE, Chaves MV: Delayed primary bone grafting in the hand and wrist after traumatic bone loss J Hand Surg 9A:22–28, 1984
65. Friedrich PL: Die aeseptische Versorgung frischer Wunden. Arch Klin Chir 57:288–310, 1898
66. Granberry WM: Gunshot wounds of the hand. Hand 5:220–228, 1973
67. Gross A, Cutright DE, Bhaskar SN: Effectiveness of pulsating water jet lavage in treatment of contaminated crushed wounds. Am J Surg 124:373–377, 1972
68. Gryska PF, Darling RC Jr, Linton RR: Management of acute vascular injuries of the extremities. pp. 84–101. In Adams JP (ed): Current Practices Orthopedic Surgery, CV Mosby, St Louis, 1964
69. Hamer ML, Robson MC, Krizek TJ, Southwick WO: Quantitative bacterial analysis of comparative wound irrigations. Ann Surg 181:819–828, 1975
70. Hampton OP Jr: Wounds of the Extremities in Military Surgery. CV Mosby, St Louis, 1951
71. Hampton OP Jr: The indications for debridement of gunshot (bullet) wounds of the extremities in civilian practice. J Trauma 1:368–372, 1961
72. Harvey EN, McMillen JH, Butler EG, Puckett WO: Mechanism of wounding. In Coates JB (ed): Wound Ballistics. pp. 143–235, Medical Department, US Army, 1962
73. Haury B, Rodeheaver G, Vensko J, Edgerton MT, Edlich RF: Debridement: An essential component of traumatic wound care. Am J Surg 135:238–242, 1978
74. Heggers JP, Robson MC, Ristroph JD: A rapid method of performing quantitative wound cultures. Milit Med 134:666–667, 1969
75. Hennessy MJ, Banks HH, Leach RD, Quigley TB: Extremity gunshot wound and gunshot fracture in civilian practice. Clin Orthop 114:296–303, 1976
76. Hoover NW, Ivins JC: Wound debridement. Arch Surg 79:701–710, 1959
77. Hopkinson DAW, Marshall TK: Firearm injuries. Br J Surg 54:344–353, 1967
78. Howland SW, Ritchey SJ: Gunshot wounds in civilian practice. J Bone Joint Surg 53A:47–55, 1971
79. Hueston JT: The mechanism and management of the burst finger. Plast Reconstr Surg 39:432, 1967
80. Iselin M: Emergency with delayed operation for wounds of the limbs. J Int Coll Surg 36:374–376, 1961
81. Jabaley ME, Peterson HD: Early treatment of war wounds of the hand and forearm in Vietnam. Ann Surg 177:167–173, 1973
82. James JIP: The assessment and management of the injured hand. Hand 2:97–105, 1970
83. Kaplan I: The management of injuries to the hand. Surg Ann 6:283–308, 1974
84. Kilgore ES Jr, Graham WP III: The Hand: Surgical and Non-Surgical Management. Lea & Febiger, Philadelphia, 1977
85. Kilgore ES Jr: Hand infections. J Hand Surg 8:723–726, 1983
86. Kleinert HE, Williams DJ: Blast injuries of the hand. J Trauma 2:10–35, 1962
87. Kleinman WB, Dustman JA: Preservation of function following complete degloving injuries to the hand: Use of simultaneous groin flap, random abdominal flap, and partial-thickness skin graft. J Hand Surg 6:82–89, 1981
88. Koch SL: Treatment of hand injuries. N Engl J Med 225:105–109, 1941
89. Krizek TJ, Robson MC: Evolution of quantitative bacteriology inwound management. Am J Surg 130:579–584, 1975
90. Lamon RP, Cicero JJ, Frascone RJ, Hass WF: Open treatment of fingertip amputations. Ann Emerg Med 12:358–360, 1983
91. Lindsay WK: Hand injuries in children. Clin Plast Surg 3:65–75, 1976

92. Lister G: The Hand: Diagnosis and Indications. Churchill Livingstone, Edinburgh, 1977

93. London PS, Clarke R: Severe accidental flaying. A plea for initial conservatism. J Bone Joint Surg 41B:658–670, 1959

94. Louis DS, Palmer AK, Burney RE: Open treatment of digital tip injuries. Orthop Trans 3:332, 1979

95. Lowry KF, Curtis GM: Delayed suture in the management of wounds. Analysis of 721 traumatic wounds illustrating the influence of time interval in wound repair. Am J Surg 80:280–287, 1950

96. Luce EA, Griffen WO: Shotgun injuries of the upper extremity. J Trauma 18:487–492, 1978

97. Madden JW: Wound healing: The biological basis of hand surgery. Clin Plast Surg 3:3–11, 1976

98. Mann RJ, Hoffeld TA, Farmer CB: Human bites of the hand: Twenty years of experience. J Hand Surg 2:97–104, 1977

99. Margles SW: Principles of management of acute hand injuries. Surg Clin North Am 60:665–686, 1980

100. Marshall KA, Edgerton MT, Rodeheaver GT, Magee CM, Edlich RF: Quantitative microbiology: Its application to hand injuries. Am J Surg 131:730–733, 1976

101. Mason ML: Principles of management of open wounds of the hand. Am J Surg 80:767–771, 1950

102. Mason ML: Treament of open wounds. Bull Am Coll Surg 42:33–38, 1957

103. Mason ML, Bell JL: The crushed hand. Clin Orthop 13:84–96, 1959

104. Maxim ES, Webster FS, Willender DA: The cornpicker hand. J Bone Joint Surg 36A:21–29, 1954

105. McCormack RM: Reconstructive surgery in the immediate care of the severely injured hand. Clin Orthop 13:75–82, 1959

106. McCormack RM: Acute injuries of the hand. pp. 1574–1575. In Converse JM (ed): Reconstructive Plastic Surgery. WB Saunders, Philadelphia, 1974

107. McGregor IA: Degloving injuries. Hand 2:130–133, 1970

108. Melvin PM: Cornpicker injuries of the hand. Arch Surg 104:26–29, 1972

109. Meyer VE, Chiu DT, Beasley RW: The place of internal fixation in surgery of the hand. Clin Plast Surg 1:51–64, 1981

110. Midgley RD, Entin M: Management of mutilating injuries of the hand. Clin Plast Surg 3:99–109, 1976

111. Milford LW: The Hand. In Crenshaw AH (ed): Campbell's Operative Orthopaedics. 4th Ed. CV Mosby, St Louis, 1963

112. Millard DR Jr, Cooley SGE: A solution to coverage in severe compound dorsal hand injuries. Case Report. Plast Reconstr Surg 49;215–219, 1972

113. Moberg E: Emergency Surgery of the Hand. E & S Livingstone, Edinburgh, 1968

114. Morgan MM, Spencer AD, Hershey FB: Debridement of civilian gunshot wounds of soft tissue. J Trauma 1:354–360, 1961

115. Morton JH, Southgate WA, DeWeese JA: Arterial injuries of the extremities. Surg Gynecol Obstet 123:611–627, 1966

116. Newmeyer WL: Primary Care of Hand Injuries. Lea & Febiger, Philadelphia, 1979

117. Newmeyer WL: Problems in primary emergency care of hand injuries. pp. 39–57. In Sandzen SC Jr (ed): The Hand and Wrist: Current Management of Complications in Orthopaedics. Williams & Wilkins, Baltimore, 1985

118. Nicols HM: Manual of Hand Injuries. 2nd Ed. pp. 276–290. Yearbook Medical Publishers, Chicago 1957

119. Omer GE Jr: The early management of gunshot wounds of the extremities. South Da J Med 9:340, 1956

120. Paradies LH, Gregory CF: The early treatment of close range gunshot wounds to the extremities. J Bone Joint Surg 48A:425–435, 1966

121. Peacock EE Jr, VanWinkle W Jr: Surgery and Biology of Wound Repair. WB Saunders, Philadelphia, 1970

122. Peimer CA, Smith RJ, Leffert RD: Distraction-fixation in the primary treatment of metacarpal bone loss. J Hand Surg 6:111–124, 1981

123. Petty W: Evaluation of the efficacy of topical antimicrobial solutions in reducing bacterial contamination in an experimental wound. Orthop Trans 3(2):132, 1979

124. Pulvertaft RG: Operative surgery series, Vol II. In Rob C, Smith R (eds): The Hand. JB Lippincott, Philadelphia, 1970

125. Pulvertaft RG: Twenty five years of hand surgery. Personal reflections. J Bone Joint Surg 55B:32–55, 1973

126. Raahave D: New technique for quantitative bacteriological sampling of wounds by velvet pads: Clinical sampling trial. J Clin Microbiol 2:277–280, 1975

127. Rank BK, Wakefield AR: Surgery of Repair as Applied to Hand Injuries. 2nd Ed. E & S Livingstone, Edinburgh, 1970

128. Remington JS: The compromised host. Hosp Pract 7:59–70, 1972

129. Rich NM: Vascular trauma in Vietnam. J Cardiovasc Surg 11:368–377, 1970

130. Rich NM, Baugh JH, Hughes CW: Acute arterial

injuries in Vietnam: 1000 cases. J Trauma 10:359, 1970

131. Riggs SA, Cooney WP: External fixation of complex hand and wrist fractures. J Trauma, 23:332–336, 1983

132. Riordan DC: The primary treatment of acute hand injuries. New Orleans Med Surg J 103:365–371, 1951

133. Riordan DC: Primary treatment of soft tissue injuries of the hand. J La State Med Soc 106:300–304, 1954

134. Riordan DC: Emergency treatment of compound injury of the hand. Am J Orthop 1:30–32, 1958

135. Robinson DC, Hardin CA: Cornpicker injuries. Am J Surg 89:780–783, 1955

136. Robinson DW, Masters FW: Severe avulsion injuries of the extremities including the degloving type. Surg Clin North Am 47:379–388, 1967

137. Robson MC, Duke WF, Krizek TJ: Rapid bacterial screening in the treatment of civilian wounds. J Surg Res 14:426–430, 1973

138. Robson MC, Heggers JP: Bacterial quantification. Milit Med 134:19–24, 1969

139. Robson MC, Heggers JP: Delayed wound closures based on bacterial counts. J Surg Oncol 2:379–383, 1970

140. Robson MC, Krizek TJ, Heggers JP: Biology of surgical infection. Curr Probl Surg, March 1973

141. Robson MC, Lea CE, Dalton JB, Heggers JP: Quantitative bacteriology and delayed wound closures. Surg Forum 19:501–502, 1968

142. Rodeheaver GT, Pettry D, Thacker JG, Edgerton MT, Edlich RF: Wound cleansing by high pressure irrigation. Surg Gynecol Obstet, 141:357–362, 1975

143. Rosenthal EA: Treatment of fingertip and nailbed injuries. Orthop Clin North Am 14:675–697, 1983

144. Sandzen SC Jr: Treating acute hand and finger injuries. Am Fam Physician 9:74–97, 100–117, 1974

145. Sandzen SC Jr: Complications of external, percutaneous and internal fixation. pp. 192–205. In Sandzen SC Jr (ed): The Hand and Wrist: Current Management of Complications in Orthopaedics. Williams & Wilkins, Baltimore, 1985

146. Sanzen SC Jr: Complications of the skeletal system of the hand. pp. 107–158. In Sandzen SC Jr (ed): The Hand and Wrist: Current Management of Complications in Orthopaedics. Williams & Wilkins, Baltimore, 1985

147. Saymen DG, Nathan P, Holder IA, Hill EO, MacMillan BG: Infected surface wound: An experimental model and a method for the quantitation of bacteria in infected tissues. Appl Microbiol 23:509–514, 1972

148. Schneewind JH: Surgical emergencies of the hand. Surg Clin North Am 52:203–218, 1972

149. Scherr DD, Lichti EL, Lambert KL: Tissue-viability assessment with Doppler ultrasonic flow meter in acute injuries of extremities. J Bone Joint Surg 55A:157–161, 1973

150. Scott FA: Complications following replantation and revascularization. pp. 205–214. In Boswick JA Jr (ed): Complications in Hand Surgery. WB Saunders, Philadelphia, 1986

151. Smith RJ, Leffert RD: Open wounds. In Flynn JE (ed): Hand Surgery. 2nd Ed. Williams & Wilkins, Baltimore, 1975

152. Spencer FC, Grewe RV: The management of arterial injuries in battle casualties. Ann Surg 141:304–313, 1955

153. Stark HH: Troublesome fractures and dislocations of the hand. p. 130 AAOS Instructional Course Lectures. Vol. 29, CV Mosby, St Louis, 1970

154. Stromberg BV: Management of low velocity gunshot wounds of the hand. South Med J 71:1087–1088, 1978

155. Swanson AB: The treatment of war wounds of the hand. Clin Plast Surg 2:615–626, 1975

156. Symonds FC, Garnes NL: Tear gas gun injury of hand. Plast Reconstr Surg 39:175–177, 1967

157. Tajima T: Treatment of open crushing type of industrial injuries of the hand and forearm: Degloving open circumferential, heat press and nail bed injuries. J Trauma 14:995–1011, 1974

158. Thoresby FP, Darlow HM: The mechanism of primary infection of bullet wounds. Br J Surg 54:359–361, 1967

159. Tobin GR: Closure of contaminated wounds: Biologic and technical considerations. Surg Clin North Am 64:639–652, 1984

160. Tobin GR: An improved method of delayed primary closure: An aggressive management approach to unfavorable wounds. Surg Clin North Am 64:659–661, 1984

161. Tophoj K, Madsen E: Delayed primary operation for open injuries of the extremities, especially the hand (two-stage treatment). Injury 2:51–54, 1970

162. Trueta J: Treatment of War Wounds and Fractures. Paul B Hoeber, New York, 1940

163. Trueta J: The Principles and Practice of War Surgery: With Reference to the Biological Method of the Treatment of War Wounds and Fractures. CV Mosby, St Louis, 1943

164. Urbaniak JR, Bright DS, Evans JP: Microvascular

managment of ring avulsion injuries. Orthop Trans 3:306, 1979

165. Wagensteen OH, Wagensteen SD: Carl Ryher (1846-1890), great Russian military surgeon: His demonstration of the role of debridement in gunshot wounds and fractures. Surgery 74:641–649, 1973

166. Walker DH: The fate of exposed bone. Reconstr Surg Traumatol 13:141–158, 1972

167. Whelan TJ: Emergency War Surgery. First U.S. Revison of the Emergency War Surgery NATO Handbook, US Dept of Defense, Washington, DC, 1975

168. Whelan TJ: Surgical lessons learned and relearned in Vietnam. Surg Ann. 7:1–23, 1975

169. Whelan TJ, Burkhalter WE, Gomez A: Management of war wounds. In Welch CE (ed): Advances in Surgery. Vol 3. Yearbook Medical Publishers, Chicago, 1968

170. Wilson H: Secondary suture of war wounds. A clinical study of 305 secondary closures. Ann Surg 121:152–156, 1945

171. Ziperman HH: The management of soft tissue missile wounds in war and peace. J Trauma 1:361–367, 1961

Index

Note that page numbers followed by "f" designate figures and those followed by "t" designate tables. Abbreviations: DIP = distal interphalangeal; IP = interphalangeal; MP = metacarpophalangeal; PIP = proximal interphalangeal.